The
MOLECULAR
BASIS
of
CANCER

JOHN MENDELSOHN, M.D.

Chairman, Department of Medicine
Memorial Sloan-Kettering Cancer Center;
Professor of Medicine and Pharmacology
Cornell University Medical College
New York, New York

PETER M. HOWLEY, M.D.

Professor and Chairman, Department of Pathology
Harvard Medical School
Boston, Massachusetts

MARK A. ISRAEL, M.D.

Director, Preuss Laboratory of Molecular Neuro-oncology
   Brain Tumor Research Center;
Professor of Neurological Surgery and Pediatrics
University of California San Francisco
San Francisco, California

LANCE A. LIOTTA, M.D., Ph.D.

Chief, Laboratory of Pathology
National Cancer Institute
National Institutes of Health
Bethesda, Maryland

The
MOLECULAR
BASIS
of
CANCER

W. B. SAUNDERS COMPANY
A Division of Harcourt Brace & Company
PHILADELPHIA, LONDON, TORONTO, MONTREAL, SYDNEY, TOKYO

W. B. SAUNDERS COMPANY
A Division of Harcourt Brace & Company

The Curtis Center
Independence Square West
Philadelphia, PA 19106

Library of Congress Cataloging-in-Publication Data

The molecular basis of cancer / John Mendelsohn . . . [et al.].
    p. cm.
   ISBN 0-7216-6483-0
   1. Cancer—Molecular aspects.   2. Carcinogenesis.   I. Mendelsohn,
John
   [DNLM: 1. Neoplasms—metabolism. 2. Cell Transformation,
Neoplastic—genetics. 3. Neoplasm Metastasis—genetics.
4. Neoplasms—therapy.   QZ 202 M7176 1995]
RC268.5.M632   1995
616.99′4071—dc20
DNLM/DLC   94-36487

The Molecular Basis of Cancer   ISBN   0-7216-6483-0

Printed in the United States of America.

Last digit is the print number: 9   8   7   6   5   4   3   2   1

This book is dedicated to our wives

Anne C. Mendelsohn
Ann Howley
Susan Jean Israel
Linda Liotta

CONTRIBUTORS

STUART A. AARONSON, M.D.
Director, Ruttenberg Cancer Center, Mount Sinai Medical Center, New York, New York
Growth Factors and Signal Transduction

W. FRENCH ANDERSON, M.D.
Director, Gene Therapy Laboratories, University of Southern California School of Medicine; Professor of Biochemistry and Pediatrics, University of Southern California School of Medicine, Los Angeles, California
Gene Therapy

JOSEPH R. BERTINO, M.D.
Professor of Medicine and Pharmacology, Cornell University Medical College; Attending Physician, Department of Medicine, Memorial Hospital; Member and Program Chairman, Molecular Pharmacology and Therapeutics, Memorial Sloan-Kettering Cancer Center, New York, New York
Chemotherapy Susceptibility and Resistance

CLAYTON A. BUCK, Ph.D.
Director, The Wistar Institute, The University of Pennsylvania Medical School; Wistar Professor of Medicine in Pediatrics, Children's Hospital of Philadelphia and Hospital of the University of Pennsylvania, Philadelphia, Pennsylvania
Adhesion Mechanisms Controlling Cell-Cell and Cell-Matrix Interactions During the Metastatic Process

MICHAEL J. CAMPBELL, Ph.D.
Assistant Professor, Stanford University School of Medicine, Department of Surgery, Stanford, California
Monoclonal Antibody Therapy

ADELAIDE M. CAROTHERS, Ph.D.
Assistant Professor, School of Public Health/Division of Environmental Sciences, Columbia University, College of Physicians and Surgeons, New York, New York
Molecular Mechanisms of Mutagenesis and Multistage Carcinogenesis

DAVID CLAXTON, M.D.
Assistant Professor, M.D. Anderson Cancer Center, The University of Texas, Houston, Texas
Molecular Diagnosis and Therapy of Hematopoietic Neoplasms

CARLO M. CROCE, M.D.
Director, Jefferson Cancer Institute, Jefferson Cancer Center, Thomas Jefferson University, Philadelphia, Pennsylvania
Molecular Genetics and Cytogenetics of Hematopoietic Malignancies

RICCARDO DALLA-FAVERA, M.D.
Uris Professor of Pathology, Genetics and Development, Columbia University College of Physicians and Surgeons, New York, New York
Molecular Biology of Lymphoid Neoplasms

ALBERT B. DEISSEROTH, M.D., Ph.D.
Professor of Medicine, Chairman, Department of Hematology, The University of Texas, M.D. Anderson Cancer Center, Houston, Texas
Molecular Diagnosis and Therapy of Hematopoietic Neoplasms

ROBERT B. DICKSON, Ph.D.
Professor, Department of Cell Biology, Department of Pharmacology, Georgetown University; Associate Director for Basic Science, Lombardi Cancer Research Center, Georgetown University, Washington, D.C.
Molecular Basis of Breast Cancer

ERIC R. FEARON, M.D., Ph.D.
Assistant Professor of Pathology and Biology, Yale University School of Medicine, New Haven, Connecticut
Molecular Abnormalities in Colon and Rectal Cancer

JUDAH FOLKMAN, M.D.
Andrus Professor of Pediatric Surgery, Professor of Cell Biology, Harvard Medical School; Director, Surgical Research, Children's Hospital, Boston, Massachusetts
Tumor Angiogenesis

ZVI FUKS, M.D.

Professor of Medicine, Cornell University Medical College; Attending Physician, Department of Medicine, New York Hospital; Attending Physician and Chairman, Department of Radiation Oncology, Memorial Sloan-Kettering Cancer Center, New York, New York
Radiation Therapy

JANICE GABRILOVE, M.D.

Associate Professor of Medicine, Cornell University Medical College; Associate Member, Memorial Sloan-Kettering Cancer Center, New York, New York
Growth Factors in Malignancy

GIANLUCA GAIDANO, M.D., Ph.D.

Associate Research Scientist, Columbia University College of Physicians and Surgeons, New York, New York
Molecular Biology of Lymphoid Neoplasms

CHARLOTTE E. GAUWERKY, M.D.

Assistant Professor, Department of Microbiology and Immunology, Jefferson Cancer Institute, Thomas Jefferson University, Philadelphia, Pennsylvania
Molecular Genetics and Cytogenetics of Hematopoietic Malignancies

TERESA GILEWSKI, M.D.

Instructor, Cornell University Medical College; Clinical Assistant, Memorial Sloan-Kettering Cancer Center, New York, New York
Cytokinetics of Neoplasia

RONALD B. HERBERMAN, M.D.

Professor of Medicine and Pathology, Hillman Professor of Oncology, University of Pittsburgh School of Medicine; Attending Physician, Montefiore University Hospital and Presbyterian University Hospital, Pittsburgh, Pennsylvania
Cellular Immunity

PETER M. HOWLEY, M.D.

Professor and Chairman, Department of Pathology, Harvard Medical School, Boston, Massachusetts
Viral Carcinogenesis

MARK A. ISRAEL, M.D.

Professor, Departments of Neurological Surgery and Pediatrics; Director, The Preuss Laboratory for Molecular Neuro-oncology, Brain Tumor Research Center, University of California, San Francisco, San Francisco, California
Molecular Biology of Childhood Neoplasms

BRUCE E. JOHNSON, M.D.

Chief, Lung Cancer Biology Section, NCI-Navy Medical Oncology Branch, National Naval Medical Center, Bethesda, Maryland
Molecular Biology of Lung Cancer

HAGOP KANTARJIAN, M.D.

Professor of Medicine and Internist, M.D. Anderson Cancer Center, University of Texas, Houston, Texas
Molecular Diagnosis and Therapy of Hematopoietic Neoplasms

ISSA KHOURI, M.D.

Instructor, Assistant Internist, M.D. Anderson Cancer Center, University of Texas, Houston, Texas
Molecular Diagnosis and Therapy of Hematopoietic Neoplasms

STEVEN KORNBLAU, M.D.

Assistant Professor, The University of Texas, M.D. Anderson Cancer Center, Houston, Texas
Molecular Diagnosis and Therapy of Hematopoietic Neoplasms

ARNOLD J. LEVINE, Ph.D.

The Harry C. Weiss Professor in Life Sciences, Department of Molecular Biology Princeton University, Princeton, New Jersey
Tumor Suppressor Genes

RONALD LEVY, M.D.

Robert K. Summy and Helen K. Summy Professor, Stanford University School of Medicine; American Cancer Society Clinical Research Professor; Chief, Division of Oncology, Stanford University School of Medicine, Stanford, California
Monoclonal Antibody Therapy

LANCE A. LIOTTA, M.D., Ph.D.

Chief, Laboratory of Pathology, National Cancer Institute, National Institute of Health, Bethesda, Maryland
Molecular Mechanisms of Tumor Cell Metastasis

MARC E. LIPPMAN, M.D.

Professor, Department of Medicine, Department of Pharmacology, Georgetown University; Director, Lombardi Cancer Research Center, Georgetown University, Washington, D.C.
Molecular Basis of Breast Cancer

DAVID G. MALONEY, M.D., Ph.D.

Clinical Associate Physician, Division of Oncology, Department of Medicine, Stanford University School of Medicine, Stanford, California
Monoclonal Antibody Therapy

JOHN MENDELSOHN, M.D.

Chairman, Department of Medicine, Memorial Sloan-Kettering Cancer Center, New York, New York, and incumbent of the Winthrop Rockefeller Chair in Medical Oncology; Professor of Medicine and Pharmacology, Cornell University Medical College, New York, New York
Growth Factors in Malignancy

MONICA S. MURAKAMI, Ph.D.

ABL-Basic Research Program, NCI-FCRDC, Frederick, Maryland

Cell Cycle Regulation, Oncogenes, and Antineoplastic Drugs

LARRY NORTON, M.D.

Professor of Medicine, Cornell University Medical College; Chief, Breast and Gynecologic Cancer Medicine Service, Memorial Sloan-Kettering Cancer Center, New York, New York

Cytokinetics of Neoplasia

FREDERICA P. PERERA, Dr. P.H.

Associate Professor, Columbia University School of Public Health, New York, New York

Molecular Mechanisms of Mutagenesis and Multistage Carcinogenesis

NEAL ROSEN, M.D., Ph.D.

Associate Member, Memorial Sloan-Kettering Cancer Center; Associate Attending, Memorial Hospital, New York; Associate Professor of Medicine, Cornell University Medical College, New York, New York

Oncogenes

REGINA M. SANTELLA, Ph.D.

Associate Professor of Public Health, Columbia University College of Physicians and Surgeons, New York, New York

Molecular Mechanisms of Mutagenesis and Multistage Carcinogenesis

KATHLEEN W. SCOTTO, Ph.D.

Assistant Professor, Pharmacology, Cornell Graduate School of Medical Sciences; Assistant Member, Molecular Pharmacology and Therapeutics Program, Sloan-Kettering Institute, Memorial Sloan-Kettering Cancer Center, New York, New York

Chemotherapy Susceptibility and Resistance

MARY L. STRACKE, M.D.

Senior Staff Fellow, Laboratory of Pathology, National Cancer Institute, National Institute of Health, Bethesda, Maryland

Molecular Mechanisms of Tumor Cell Metastasis

MARJORIE C. STROBEL, Ph.D.

ABL-Basic Research Program, NCI-FCRDC, Frederick, Maryland

Cell Cycle Regulation, Oncogenes, and Antineoplastic Drugs

MOSHE TALPAZ, M.D.

Professor of Medicine, M.D. Anderson Cancer Center, The University of Texas, Houston, Texas

Molecular Diagnosis and Therapy of Hematopoietic Neoplasms

PAUL TOLSTOSHEV, Ph.D.

Vice President and Director of Research, Genetic Therapy, Inc., Gaithersburg, Maryland

Gene Therapy

STEVEN R. TRONICK, Ph.D.

Laboratory of Cellular and Molecular Biology, National Cancer Institute, Bethesda, Maryland

Growth Factors and Signal Transduction

GEORGE F. VANDE WOUDE, Ph.D.

ABL-Basic Research Program, NCI-FCRDC, Frederick, Maryland

Cell Cycle Regulation, Oncogenes, and Antineoplastic Drugs

RALPH R. WEICHSELBAUM, M.D.

Harold H. Hines Professor and Chairman of Department of Radiation and Cellular Oncology, University of Chicago, Chicago, Illinois

Radiation Therapy

I. BERNARD WEINSTEIN, M.D.

Director, Columbia Presbyterian Cancer Center; Attending Physician, Presbyterian Hospital, New York, New York

Molecular Mechanisms of Mutagenesis and Multistage Carcinogenesis

PREFACE

Molecular biology has revolutionized our understanding of malignant transformation and the pathogenesis of cancer. Conversely the study of malignancy has "transformed" our understanding of the molecular and genetic processes that govern the growth and proliferation of normal cells.

Our knowledge has expanded to the point where a textbook describing *the molecular basis of cancer* will be useful to students, investigators, physicians, and providers of clinical care in a variety of disciplines. The aim is to explain, rather than to merely recount, the discoveries and observations that form the basis for understanding a disease which until recently was thought about in purely descriptive terms.

Four editors, selected for their expertise and for their reputations as educators, met to design a sequence of chapters that will lead the reader from the basic mechanisms of malignant transformation of cells, to the molecular and biological features of tumor growth and metastasis in the body, then to a description of the molecular abnormalities found in the common types of cancer, and finally to the molecular basis for new approaches to therapy.

In this textbook, we do not provide a detailed description of the clinical manifestations of cancer, or its diagnosis and management with specific treatments. We do pursue the scientific underpinnings that will enable clinicians and other professionals who manage cancer patients to better understand the disease and its therapy. We perceive that this information base is of equal interest to laboratory and clinical investigators in biomedical research, as well as advanced students and trainees, who need to understand the molecular mechanisms that govern the function of malignant cells.

While the chapters follow a sequence that moves from pathogenesis to therapy, each chapter stands alone in its treatment of the subject matter. Certain important topics are presented in more than one context. For example, growth factors and their receptors are discussed in different chapters as oncogene products, regulators of signal transduction, activators of malignant cell proliferation, mediators of angiogenesis and metastasis, and therapeutic agents. The p53 suppressor gene is described as a regulator of cell cycle traversal, a site of mutation, a key step in transformation, a target for viral oncogenesis, and a hereditary or acquired genetic factor in the pathogenesis of many of the common human cancers.

We now know that cancer arises as result of accumulated genetic alterations that either enhance or diminish the activity of pathways mediating normal cellular events. A remarkable lesson of cancer research is that the strategies utilized by widely divergent cell lineages to regulate growth and differentiation share common molecular pathways. The sequential mutation of genes critical for these pathways is a recurrent theme observed in many different tumor types. Tumors of specific tissues appear to select certain of these genetic abnormalities that may be most advantageous for escape of these cell lineages from normal regulatory mechanisms in particular microenvironments within the body. These selected molecular aberrations may, in turn, identify specific therapeutic approaches to eliminating the malignant cells.

Cancer is not merely a disorder of individual cells. Transformed cells grow into tumor masses, and they invade and metastasize through surrounding tissues. Knowledge of the kinetics and the molecular basis for these complex processes is important for understanding the natural history of malignant disease. The molecular mechanisms that enable tumors to grow and spread also point to novel therapeutic approaches, which are already entering the clinic.

What is most impressive and exciting today is the active dialogue between clinicians and laboratory scientists who share an interest in applying the new knowledge of molecular biology to the diagnosis, treatment and prevention of disease. It is clear that during this decade we will be experimenting with many new biological and chemical agents which will be targeted towards the specific molecular irregularities that characterize malignant cells. The research literature is filled with publications exploring these approaches in cultured cells and model animal systems, and early clinical trials have begun with a number of such agents. In this textbook we provide a number of examples of clinical interventions which utilize new drugs, biological agents, engineered antibody molecules and gene therapies. We hope that the information in this book will supply a basis upon which new approaches to therapy can be evaluated by those interested in understanding and critically assessing the products of the biotechnology revolution that is occurring in academic centers and the pharmaceutical industry.

The editors are delighted that we were able to recruit outstanding investigators who are excited about the challenge of presenting their areas of expertise in a textbook format. In many cases this has required more time and effort than they initially anticipated, and we are grateful for their dedication. We hope that we have come at least part way in achieving what we set out to undertake. We have been assisted and encouraged by Mr. Richard Zorab and the staff of the W. B. Saunders Company, as well as the patient and ever-essential help of the secretaries in our offices.

The Editors

CONTENTS

SECTION II
GROWTH AND SPREAD OF CANCER

SECTION III
MOLECULAR ABNORMALITIES IN SPECIFIC MALIGNANCIES

SECTION IV
MOLECULAR BASIS OF CANCER THERAPY

SECTION

I

MALIGNANT TRANSFORMATION

CELL CYCLE REGULATION, ONCOGENES, AND ANTINEOPLASTIC DRUGS

MOLECULAR GENETICS AND CYTOGENETICS OF HEMATOPOIETIC MALIGNANCIES

VIRAL CARCINOGENESIS

MOLECULAR MECHANISMS OF MUTAGENESIS AND MULTISTAGE CARCINOGENESIS

TUMOR SUPPRESSOR GENES

ONCOGENES

GROWTH FACTORS AND SIGNAL TRANSDUCTION

1

CELL CYCLE REGULATION, ONCOGENES, AND ANTINEOPLASTIC DRUGS

MONICA S. MURAKAMI
MARJORIE C. STROBEL
GEORGE F. VANDE WOUDE

Our understanding of the events governing cell cycle progression has increased at an astonishing rate over the past several years. Much of this progress has been fueled by the need to understand how oncogenes and tumor suppressor genes deregulate cell growth. Genetic, biochemical, and cell biological studies carried out in diverse eukaryotic systems have generated a general picture of the components that regulate cell cycle progression. This regulation ensures the faithful duplication and partitioning of genetic information. Although cell type–specific nuances have been and are continuing to be discovered, the remarkable feature of cell cycle control is the functional conservation of the basic regulatory mechanisms and components across vast evolutionary distances, from yeast to mammalian cells. This fundamental conservation was illustrated by the demonstration that a human gene product could substitute for a defective cell cycle gene in yeast.[1] Such conservation of components has led to the convergence of information from many separate areas of research, such as yeast cell cycle genetics, DNA tumor virus transformation, oocyte maturation biochemistry, and cancer biology. The identification of proto-oncogene and tumor suppressor gene products as participants in normal cell cycle control provides valuable insights into the means by which oncogenic activation or loss of tumor suppressor function can lead to deregulated growth and the abnormal genetic constitution of transformed cells.

We begin with a general description of the cell cycle, followed by discussion of the various molecular components that control the cell cycle. We conclude with discussions of the role of oncogenes and tumor suppressor genes in cell cycle progression and checkpoint control. We also discuss how compromise of checkpoint function can lead to an understanding of antineoplastic drug therapy at the molecular level.

THE CELL CYCLE

The interval between each cell division is defined as a cell cycle. Each cell cycle consists of four ordered, strictly regulated phases referred to as G_1 (gap 1), S (DNA synthesis), G_2 (gap 2), and M (mitosis/meiosis) (Fig. 1–1A). DNA replication occurs during S phase; chromosome separation (karyokinesis) and cell division (cytokinesis) occur during M phase; and G_1 and G_2 are gap or growth phases. Quiescent mammalian cells that are not actively growing reside in G_0, a resting state. In mammalian cells, cell growth control is exerted primarily in the G_1 phase. The factors modulating exit from G_0 and progression through G_1 are critical for determining overall growth rate.

The cell cycle regulates the faithful duplication of genetic information and accurate partitioning of duplicated chromosomes to daughter cells. Checkpoints are pauses in the cell cycle during which the fidelity of DNA duplication and the accuracy of chromosome segregation are monitored. Checkpoint pauses permit editing and repair of genetic information so that each daughter cell receives a full compliment of genetic information identical to that of the parent cell (Fig. 1–1B).

The restriction point or ''competence'' in somatic cells was identified in early studies as the point in the cell cycle at which a cell becomes committed to completing the cy-

3

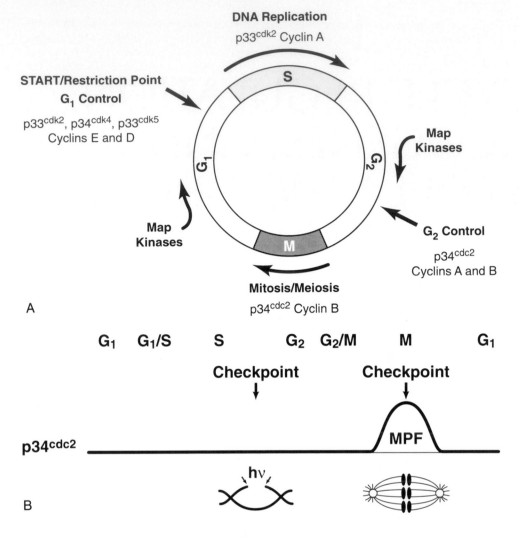

Figure 1–1. Schematic representation of cell cycle and checkpoints. *A,* Schematic representation of the eukaryotic cell cycle. The major regulatory kinases are indicated at their approximate points of action in the cell cycle. *B,* Schematic illustration of the two major checkpoints in the cell cycle: arrest after DNA damage at the G_2/M border and arrest at metaphase of mitosis/meiosis.

cle. In the budding yeast *Saccharomyces cerevisiae,* cells arrest at START, a point analogous to the mammalian restriction point. Before a non-transformed cell passes the restriction point, it requires specific growth factors and nutrients; after passage through the cell cycle restriction point, progression is factor and nutrient independent. The restriction point divides G_1 into two stages: pre–restriction point, a growth factor–dependent stage; and post–restriction point, a growth factor–independent stage. The specific growth factors required for G_1 progression are cell type specific; for example, murine NIH 3T3 cells require platelet-derived growth factor (PDGF), epidermal growth factor (EGF), insulin, and insulin-like growth factor I (IGF-I). Because the cell is responsive to and dependent on many extracellular stimuli during G_1, this phase is considered a primary point of growth regulation. Many oncogenes promote progression through G_1 because they are inappropriately expressed growth factors (v-*sis*/PDGF), constitutively activated growth factor receptors (v-*erbB*/EGF-R, v-*fms*/CSF-1-R, *trk*/NGF-R, *met*/HGF-R), or activated forms of the downstream components in signal transduction pathways (*ras* and *raf*). These alterations mimic a mitogenic signal, resulting in uncontrolled cell proliferation. After the restriction point (competence or START), extracellular factors are usually unnecessary. The cell pro-

ceeds through the cell cycle and a complex intracellular program guides the cell through S, G_2, and M (for review, see refs. 2,3).

Mammalian cells normally arrest in G_0, a quiescent state, however progression through the cell cycle can also be arrested at the G_1/S boundary (restriction point or START), or at the G_2/M boundary. For example, in fission yeast, growth arrest occurs during G_2. In this organism, START occurs at the G_2/M border, not G_1/S. Similarly, vertebrate oocytes show phenomenal growth during G_2, and arrest either in the pachytene stage or at the G_2/M border prior to meiotic maturation. After oocyte maturation, the unfertilized egg arrests at metaphase II of meiosis. The examination of these systems has revealed that the mechanisms regulating progression from G_1 to S phase and from G_2 to M phase are quite similar.

MOLECULAR COMPONENTS CONTROLLING THE CELL CYCLE

Universal Cell Cycle Regulator (p34^{cdc2})

Genetic studies in both fission and budding yeast have identified a critical gene, *cdc2*, that controls cell cycle progression. *cdc2* was first identified as a temperature-sensitive mutation (*S. cerevisiae, cdc28; Schizosaccharomyces pombe, cdc2*) that resulted in cell cycle arrest.[4,5] In fission yeast, cdc2 cells incubated at the nonpermissive temperature arrest at the G_2/M border. However, in budding yeast, the *cdc2* mutation causes arrest at the G_1/S border (START). Thus, the *cdc2* gene product regulates the transition into both S phase and M phase.[6–8] Sequence analyses showed that the *cdc2* gene encodes a 34-kDa serine-threonine protein kinase, $p34^{cdc2}$.[9,10] Functional complementation of a *cdc2*-deficient fission yeast cell with a human cDNA library identified a functional human equivalent that shared 64 per cent amino acid sequence identity with the yeast *cdc2* gene.[1] This was an extraordinary discovery because it demonstrated that a billion years of evolution had not significantly changed the structure and function of the cdc2 kinase. There are now many homologues of cdc2; they are referred to as cyclin-dependent kinases (cdks).[11,12] The function and activities of the various cdks are now being investigated.[13] A working hypothesis has been that the cdks are potentially promiscuous kinases that are activated by and directed to substrates by specialized regulators known as cyclins.

Concurrent with the studies of cell cycle mutations in yeast, biochemical analysis of oocyte maturation in invertebrates and vertebrates was focused on an activity called maturation promoting factor, or M-phase promoting factor (MPF). In *Xenopus laevis* ovaries, fully grown immature oocytes are arrested in meiotic prophase I. Completion of meiosis or maturation, typified by germinal vesicle (nuclear) membrane breakdown (GVBD) and chromosome condensation, is induced naturally by the hormone progesterone. MPF initially was recognized as a cytoplasmic component present in progesterone-treated maturing oocytes. When extracts from these oocytes are injected into immature *Xenopus* oocytes arrested in meiotic prophase I, the injected oocytes mature into unfertilized eggs.[14,15] This process of maturation involves the exit from meiosis I prophase arrest, completion of meiosis I, initiation of meiosis II, and finally arrest at meiotic metaphase II. At this point the unfertilized egg or mature oocyte awaits fertilization. Purified MPF activity[16] consists of two proteins of 45 and 32 kDa. Subsequent experiments identified the cdc2 kinase as the 32-kDa component of MPF.[17–20] Henceforth, MPF can be considered to be the form of cdc2 ($p34^{cdc2}$) that is associated with cyclin B (see below and, for review, ref. 21).

Cyclins

Biochemical studies showed that the cdc2 protein was present at a constant level throughout the cell cycle even though cdc2 activity oscillated (as measured by histone H1 phosphorylation). These observations implied that exogenous factors were regulating the cdc2 kinase activity. Recent work has revealed that the cdc2 kinase is regulated by two classic posttranslational mechanisms: association with a second, activating subunit and covalent modification by phosphorylation. The first of these activating proteins, cyclins, were identified by and initially named for their cyclic appearance during the cell cycle.[22] In invertebrate oocytes, it was observed that cyclins were synthesized during interphase and abruptly destroyed at the end of mitosis. Initially, two cyclins, A and B, distinguished by slight differences in molecular weight, were identified. Subsequently, six families of mammalian cyclin genes have been identified; they are classified by the extent of sequence homology and by the point in the cell cycle at which they function. Cyclins are divided into two functional classes: those that act at the G_2/M boundary (cyclins B1 and B2) and those that act at the G_1/S boundary (cyclins C, D, and E). Cyclin A is the exception; it is present and presumably functioning from S through M phase.[23,24]

p21/p16: Cyclin/cdk Kinase Inhibitors

Recent reports have uncovered a new family of tumor suppressor genes that directly implicate aberrant cell cycle regulation in tumorigenesis. The general function of these new products is that they prevent cell cycle progression by directly interfering with cyclin/cdk kinase activation. The first protein, a 21 kDa protein cdk kinase inhibitor, p21, was discovered in three independent studies: 1) as a protein which inhibits cyclin/cdk activation (Cip1)[116b,116c]; 2) as a gene product induced by p53 (WAF1)[116d]; and 3) as a gene product highly expressed in senescent cells (SDI1).[116a] A cdk kinase inhibitor that shares homology with p21, p27 (or Kip1) was isolated from mink cells that had been growth arrested with the negative growth regulator TGFβ.[116e] A third protein, a 16 kDa product, p16, also an inhibitor of cyclin/cdk kinase activity[116f] was recently discovered to be deleted from a large number of human tumor cell lines (MTS1), and possibly tumors as well.[116g] Collectively, these gene products mediate growth arrest in the absence of growth factors, by negative regulators of growth such as TGFβ or by DNA damaging agents which induce p53 expression. In each case, cells respond by producing these cyclin/cdk inhibitor proteins.

The role of p53 in cell cycle arrest and checkpoint control has been discussed earlier. The induction of p21 (WAF1) by p53 may partially explain how host DNA synthesis is shut down after DNA damage has occurred. p53 activates the transcription of WAF1 which in turn inhibits cyclin/cdk complexes arresting the cell in G_1. These studies provide a direct link between activation of p53 and cell cycle arrest. The loss of these small cyclin/cdk inhibitors or the inability to activate their expression (i.e., in p53 deficient cells) would be expected to enhance tumor cell progression. These discoveries make a dramatic contribution to our understanding of cell cycle progression and checkpoint control.

Mitotic G_2/M Cyclins

In 1986, Swenson et al.[25] demonstrated that injection of cyclin mRNA could induce oocyte maturation, indicating that the cyclins were an essential component of MPF. The B cyclins are synthesized during the G_2 phase and levels peak at mitosis. The B cyclins are necessary and sufficient for entry into mitosis and the degradation of cyclin is necessary for exit out of mitosis.[26] B cyclins are degraded abruptly at the metaphase-anaphase transition by a ubiquitin-dependent pathway.[27] Normal degradation can be inhibited by using a truncated cyclin that is resistant to degradation. These mutated cyclins have MPF activity, but they result in metaphase arrest because they are not degraded.[28] Additional experiments have demonstrated that cyclins physically associate with and activate the cdc2 protein kinase.[29-31]

Cyclins may have other properties in addition to cdc2 kinase activation. One possible function of the cyclins may be to direct cell cycle–dependent subcellular location. The cyclin B-cdc2 complex is localized in the cytoplasm during interphase and is transported to the nucleus at mitosis, whereas the cyclin A-cdc2 complex is always nuclear.[32,33] Cyclin B also may regulate the tyrosine phosphorylation of cdc2. In vivo and in vitro, the wee 1 kinase, a negative regulator of M phase, will only phosphorylate cdc2 complexed to cyclin B (see later in this chapter).[34,35] In addition, cyclin B also may regulate the activity of cdc25 tyrosine phosphatase.[36,37] Both the wee 1 kinase and cdc25 phosphatase are direct regulators of cyclin B-cdc2 (see later in this chapter).

Cyclin A

Because both cyclins A and B could induce oocyte maturation, they were thought to be functionally identical. Subsequently, clear distinctions were revealed in their expression patterns and substrate preferences during the cell cycle. Cyclin B is synthesized during G_2 and M phase; cyclin A is synthesized during S phase and is degraded during metaphase, slightly before cyclin B destruction. Moreover, during Drosophila embryogenesis,[38,39] mutations in cyclin A prevent passage through mitosis 14, even in the presence of wild-type cyclin B. Injection of antisense cDNA or antibodies to cyclin A into somatic fibroblastic cells prevents their progression into both S phase and mitosis,[40,41] suggesting that cyclin A may play a role in the G_1/S transition. Furthermore, cyclin A, but not cyclin B, associates with several cell growth regulatory proteins, such as the retinoblastoma (Rb) tumor suppressor gene product,[42] the p 107 Rb-related protein, the transcription factor E2F,[43] and the adenovirus E1A oncoprotein.[44-46] These interactions provide clues to the unique role of cyclin A in the cell cycle. To date, no cyclin A homologues have been isolated from yeast, suggesting that cyclin A may integrate complex signals that are critical for cell cycle control in higher eukaryotes.

G₁ Cyclins

Cyclins A and B first were characterized by their ability to promote the G_2/M transition in clam S. pombe and Xenopus oocytes. However, in S. cerevisiae and mammalian cells, cell cycle arrest occurs at the G_1/S border (START or restriction point). In yeast, cdc2 kinase activity regulates entry into both S phase and M phase. Cyclins activate the cdc2 kinase at G_2/M; therefore, it was assumed that cyclin-like proteins would be essential for progression through the G_1/S boundary.

S. cerevisiae cells can be arrested at the G_1/S border (START) by starvation or mating pheromone treatment; however, S. cerevisiae mutations have been isolated that allow cells to progress through START under conditions that should cause cells to arrest. Some of these mutations identified cyclin-like proteins or CLNs that have limited homology to the G_2/M cyclins.[47,48] Three functionally redundant CLN proteins have been identified in S. cerevisiae, and all three CLN genes must be inactivated simultaneously to invoke G_1/S arrest.[49] Through functional complementation of a triple CLN-deficient mutant, Lew et al.[50] and Xiong et al.[51] were able to clone human G_1/S cyclin homologues. Interestingly, Matsushime et al.[52] also isolated G_1 cyclins while screening for genes expressed in response to colony-stimulating factor 1 (CSF-1) treatment. By sequence homology, the three types of mammalian G_1/S cyclins are classified as C, D, and E.[23,24]

The C, D, and E cyclins are expressed specifically during the G_1 and S phases of the mammalian cell cycle. The mammalian G_1/S cyclins associate with cdks, not cdc2 kinase; for instance, the E-type cyclins are associated primarily with cdk2.[53-55] The cyclin E-cdk2 complex also associates with other cellular regulatory proteins, including the Rb-related p107 protein and the E2F transcription factor.[56] The D-type cyclins associate with cdks 2,4, and 5 [57,58] (for review, see refs. 23, 24). The cyclin D-cdk4 complex is reported to specifically phosphorylate the Rb gene product.[57] In addition, cyclin D1- and D3-cdk2 complexes associate with, but do not phosphorylate, proliferating cell nuclear antigen (PCNA), a well-characterized protein essential for replication of the SV40 DNA tumor virus.[58]

Regulation of cdc2 by Covalent Modification

In Xenopus oocytes, cyclin B was shown to be associated with cdc2 in a kinase-inactive complex,[59] implying that cdc2 kinase activity is not regulated solely by cyclin B association. The cdc2 kinase is subject to cell cycle–dependent phosphorylation and dephosphorylation.[60,61] Three functional phosphorylation sites have been identified on the cdc2 protein: threonine 14, tyrosine 15, and threonine 161. Biochemical analysis has demonstrated that threonine 161 phosphorylation activates cdc2 kinase, whereas threonine 14 and tyrosine 15 phosphorylation inhibits the kinase activity.[62] Threonine 161 is phosphorylated by CAK (cdc2-activating kinase).[63] CAK recently has been shown to be MO-15, a cdc2-like kinase initially isolated by its sequence homology to cdc2.[64-66]

The proteins that phosphorylate and dephosphorylate the negative regulatory sites of cdc2 have been well characterized. The genes encoding these kinases were identified as S. pombe mutations that resulted in altered cell size.[67] The wee 1 mutation caused cells to enter mitosis prematurely, resulting in very small cells. Conversely, mutations in the cdc25 gene delayed entry into mitosis, generating very large cells.[68] Genetically, these mutations can complement each other: A wee 1/cdc25 double mutant cell is normal in size.

The wee 1 protein, purified by expression of the cloned

gene, was shown to be a bifunctional serine-threonine tyrosine kinase, with sequence homology to the activating kinase for mitogen-activated protein kinase (MAPK) from higher eukaryotes.[69] Parker and Piwnica-Worms[35,70] determined that the human wee 1 kinase specifically phosphorylates cdc2 on tyrosine 15 only when cdc2 kinase is complexed with cyclin A or B.

The wee 1–mediated, inactivating phosphorylation of cdc2 tyrosine 15 is overcome by dephosphorylation of this residue by the cdc25 protein, a tyrosine-threonine phosphatase.[71-74] The *S. pombe cdc25* gene was first recognized as a mutation that caused cell cycle arrest at G_2. Subsequently, multiple *cdc25* homologues have been isolated from *Xenopus*, mouse, and humans by complementation of the yeast *cdc25* defect. Study of these homologues indicates that the *cdc25* gene can be regulated at several levels. The human cdc25A and cdc25B proteins appear to be activated by cyclin B, but not by cyclins A or D,[36,37] whereas the *Xenopus* and human cdc25C protein is regulated by phosphorylation.[75,76] A homologous *Drosophila* gene, *string*, is regulated at the transcriptional level.[77] Furthermore, there is evidence that the different cdc25 variants may function at specific points in the cell cycle or in development.[78] For example, the *Drosophila string* gene was identified by an embryonic lethal mutation, whereas the *Drosophila twine* gene, a *string/cdc25* homologue, is expressed solely in the *Drosophila* germ line.[79]

In summary, MPF employs at least three modes of regulation—cyclin B association, as well as both inhibitory and activating phosphorylations. Perhaps cyclin B association is the first step toward the assembly of pre-MPF. After the addition of the inhibitory and activating phosphates, pre-MPF awaits a signal that will result in its rapid, complete conversion to MPF.[80]

Substrates of the cdc2 Protein Kinase

Although the multiplicity and conservation of cdk homologues and their regulatory molecules emphasize the requirement for the activity of these kinases in regulation of the G_1/S and G_2/M progression, the targets of this regulation remain elusive. Considerable effort is being directed toward the elucidation of bona fide cdc2 and cdk2 substrates.

S-PHASE SUBSTRATES

Depletion of the cdk2 kinase from *Xenopus* oocyte extracts prevents initiation of DNA replication,[81,82] suggesting an essential role for this kinase in regulating DNA replication. DNA replication of the SV40 tumor virus can be reconstituted in vitro, and many of the cellular components required for replication have been identified. SV40 DNA replication is executed primarily by cellular proteins and requires only one viral protein, the large T antigen (TAg). D'Urso et al. demonstrated that the essential cellular replication factor C (RFC), contains cdc2 or cdk2 kinase.[83-85] TAg binds the SV40 origin of replica-

tions and possesses ATP-dependent helicase activity. Active TAg requires phosphorylation, and this phosphorylation can be mediated by cdc2 in vitro.[86] However, the TAg isolated from the SV40 DNA replication extracts is already phosphorylated; therefore, the in vivo substrate for the RFC-cdc2/cdk2 kinase activity may be another cellular replication protein.

Whereas initiation of SV40 DNA replication requires TAg helicase activity and cellular topoisomerase I, elongation of the SV40 DNA strands needs other cellular factors: replication protein A (RPA), DNA polymerases α and δ, PCNA, and RFC. RPA is a multisubunit complex consisting of 11-, 34-, and 70-kDa proteins. The 70-kDa subunit possesses single-strand DNA binding activity. Although the function of the other subunits is unclear, antibodies directed against the 34-kDa subunit inhibit DNA replication. The 34-kDa subunit is phosphorylated specifically during the S and G_2 phases of the cell cycle, and the kinetics of RPA activation suggest this phosphorylation is mediated by cyclin A-cdk2[84,85] (for review, see ref. 87). Although a cyclin A-cdk2 complex appears to stimulate the initiation of replication, DNA elongation may depend on cyclin D-cdk2. An association between cyclin D-cdk2 and PCNA has been reported. PCNA is an accessory factor for DNA polymerase δ, which is essential for leading and lagging strand synthesis.[13,58,88]

M-PHASE SUBSTRATES

Chromosome partitioning at mitosis requires a dramatic rearrangement of cellular components; this includes breakdown of the nuclear envelope, formation of the mitotic spindle apparatus, and reorganization of the cytoskeleton. One component of the nuclear envelope, nuclear lamin C, is phosphorylated in a cell cycle–dependent manner. In vitro nuclear lamin C is phosphorylated by cdc2 on sites that are found to be phosphorylated in vivo.[89,90] This phosphorylation promotes the disassembly of lamin polymers.[91,92] cdc2 also can phosphorylate and promote depolymerization of another intermediate filament protein, vimentin.[13,93,94]

Cyclins, the cdc2 Family, and Oncogenesis

The analysis of cyclins and their association with cdc2, homologous kinases, and other cellular growth-control proteins provides a link between signal transduction, cell cycle regulation in normal cells, and the perturbations of cell growth control associated with tumor formation. Perhaps the simplest way to achieve uncontrolled cellular proliferation is to inappropriately or constitutively express components of the cell cycle machinery. Alternatively, functional ablation of growth-inhibiting tumor suppressor genes, such as *Rb*, can result in deregulated, neoplastic growth. Because a cell at the G_0/G_1 transition is responsive to and dependent on many extracellular stimuli, G_1 is considered a primary point of growth regulation. Not surprisingly, numerous oncogenes have been found to promote entry into progression through G_1. Inappropriately expressed growth factors (TGF-α, PDGF) and constitutively activated growth factor receptors (v-*erbB*/EGF receptor, V-*fms*/CSF-1 receptor) can mimic progression through G_1, causing uncontrolled cell proliferation (for review, see ref. 95).

CYCLINS

Matsushime et al.[52] found that levels of G_1 cyclins are increased after treatment with CSF-1. If mouse macrophages are deprived of CSF-1, they arrest in early G_1 and the G_1 cyclins are rapidly degraded. However, within 1 hour after stimulation with CSF-1, high levels of G_1 cyclin mRNAs are observed. These findings suggest a mechanism by which *fms*, an oncogene that encodes a truncated CSF-1 receptor, affects transformation. *fms*-transformed macrophages may constitutively express G_1 cyclins, leading to accelerated progression to S phase. It has also been suggested that PDGF and other growth factors may stimulate G_1 cyclin synthesis.[23,24]

Aberrant G_1 cyclin expression has been associated directly with several types of human tumors, underscoring the importance of these cell cycle regulatory proteins in the etiology of human cancer.[96] Genomic rearrangements in some parathyroid adenomas result in increased expression of the *PRAD1* oncogene (Table 1–1). Molecular cloning revealed that *PRAD1* encodes cyclin D. Also, overabundant levels of cyclin D transcripts are observed in some breast cancer cell lines, and the cyclin D locus is amplified in several human esophageal tumors.[97] Similarly, the cyclin A gene is the site of hepatitis B virus integration in some hepatocellular carcinomas [98] (Table 1–1) (see refs. 23, 95 for reviews).

RETINOBLASTOMA

Wild-type tumor suppressor genes, or antioncogenes, inhibit cell growth, but mutation or deletion of these genes can result in neoplastic transformation and genetic instability. The retinoblastoma susceptibility gene (*Rb*) was the first tumor suppressor gene identified (reviewed in ref. 99). Loss or mutation of *Rb* is associated with several human cancers. The *Rb* gene product was found to be present in most normal proliferating cells, a surprising observation for a putative growth/tumor suppressor.[100] The activity of *Rb* was found to be cell cycle dependent and regulated by phosphorylation.[101,102] *Rb* is underphosphorylated until late G_1, at which time it becomes phosphorylated. This phosphorylation inactivates the growth-inhibiting properties of the *Rb* gene product. In vitro, *Rb*

phosphorylation can be mediated by cdc2 kinase on the same sites that are phosphorylated in vivo.[103] However, the phosphorylation profile of *Rb* during the cell cycle reflects the activity of G_1 cyclin-cdk complexes (for review, see refs. 100, 104). What is the function of this cell cycle–dependent phosphorylation? The answer may lie in the affinity of the *Rb* gene product for various DNA tumor virus proteins. The underphosphorylated form of *Rb* associates with a variety of viral tumor antigens, such as the SV40 T antigen, [105,106] adenovirus E1A,[107] and the human papillomavirus E7 protein.[108] These observations suggest that the association with tumor virus proteins inactivates the *Rb* tumor suppressor protein, resulting in accelerated growth. Thus, in wild-type cells, the growth-suppressing activities of *Rb* can be ablated by two mechanisms: binding to tumor antigens and phosphorylation by cyclin-cdks.

Another key observation that may illuminate the growth regulatory function of *Rb* is the affinity of *Rb* for the transcription factor E2F.[42,109] E2F was identified initially as a cellular protein required for the transcription of adenovirus early genes; however, the E2F binding site is found in a variety of cellular genes, including c-*myc*, N-*myc*, c-*myb*, cdc2, DNA polymerase α, and dihydrofolate reductase. Studies have shown that *Rb* inhibits transcriptional activation by E2F; therefore, the growth-suppressive properties of *Rb* could be mediated through inactivation of E2F. *Rb* phosphorylation or the binding of the E1A tumor antigen disassociates the *Rb*-E2F complex. Free E2F proceeds to activate transcription and promote progression to S phase. In addition, it has been proposed that the E2F-*Rb* complex may actively repress transcription of other cellular genes, including proto-oncogenes, that have an E2F binding site.[110,111]

E2F is a component of two other cell cycle–regulated complexes. Both cyclins A and E associate with E2F, cdk2 and the *Rb*-related p107 protein.[42,43,56,113,114] The cdk2-cyclin A-p107-E2F complex appears to be S-phase specific,[114,115] whereas the cdk2-cyclin E-p107-E2F complex is found primarily during G_1.[56] Because these complexes have both histone H1 kinase and DNA binding activities,[116] complex formation may serve to target the kinase to specific genomic sequences of substrates.

p16/p21

An exciting series of recent reports has identified a new family of tumor suppressors. The importance of these genes was immediately recognized, they are potent inhib-

TABLE 1–1. CYCLIN GENES ASSOCIATED WITH HUMAN TUMORS

GENE	TUMOR	REFERENCE
Cyclin A	Hepatocellular carcinoma (HBV insertion)	98
Cyclin D*		
D11S287E	Benign parathyroid adenoma (11q13)	95
or *PRAD 1*	B-cell malignancies (11q13)	96
or *bcl1*?	B-cell and breast cancer (amplified)	97

*Characterized as G_1 cyclins in refs. 57,58.
Abbreviation: HBV, hepatitis B virus.

itors of cdks, and they are induced by p53. Incredibly, a large percentage of melanoma cell lines have deletions of this gene.[116a]

Checkpoints

The successful completion of a cell cycle demands a highly ordered, strictly regulated series of events. To ensure that the daughter cells possess a full complement of genetic information, control mechanisms must exist to sense the readiness of the cell. These control mechanisms regulate, positively or negatively, progression through the cycle. Specifically, DNA replication must be completed before mitosis begins; chromosome partitioning and cell division must be concluded before the next round of DNA synthesis commences.

In wild-type cells, agents that damage DNA or inhibit DNA synthesis prevent entry into mitosis, and agents that interfere with microtubule assembly and spindle formation restrict exit from mitosis (Figure 1–1B). From their characterization of an extensive battery of *S. cerevisiae* mutants, Weinert and Hartwell[117] identified mutations that allow cell cycle progression in the presence of such deleterious agents. They found that a subset of these genes encode the "checkpoint control functions"—receptors, transducers, and effectors that constitute a surveillance system in which the initiation of late events is coupled to and restricted by the completion of earlier events.

CHECKPOINTS FOR INITIATION OF MITOSIS

When yeast cells are exposed to DNA-damaging agents, wild-type cells arrest in G_2, presumably to repair their DNA prior to chromosome segregation. Mutation of the checkpoint genes allows a cell to enter mitosis after x-ray irradiation. These cells enter mitosis prematurely, resulting in an increased sensitivity to DNA-damaging agents. Although this increased sensitivity to x-ray irradiation could result simply from defective DNA repair processes, several *S. cerevisiae* loci, notably the *rad9* gene, are sensitive to agents that inhibit DNA synthesis as well as DNA-damaging agents. Therefore, *rad9* is defined as a G_2/M checkpoint gene because it responds to two different types of signals.[118,119]

RCC1

The temperature-sensitive baby hamster kidney cell line, tsBN2, ceases DNA synthesis and undergoes premature chromosome condensation at the nonpermissive temperature. This phenotype was associated with mutation of the *RCC1* (repressor of chromosome condensation) gene that encodes a 45-kDa DNA-binding protein. On shifting to the nonpermissive temperature, the level of RCC1 protein declines, leading to premature mitosis. However, the microinjection of wild-type RCC1 protein rescues this defect. Further analysis demonstrated that the loss of active RCC1 protein coincided with the activation of cdc2 kinase activity, and this activation requires additional protein synthesis. These observations suggest that the wild-type *RCC1* gene product regulates entry into mitosis by acting on the cdc2 kinase[120] (see ref. 121 for review).

Matsumoto and Beach[122] isolated a fission yeast homologue of *RCC1* called *pim-1* (premature initiation of mitosis). The *pim-1* gene shares significant sequence identity with *RCC1* and, phenotypically, *pim* mutant yeast cells are very similar to *RCC1*-deficient mammalian cells. Loss of *pim-1* function induces premature mitosis in yeast cells at any point in the cell cycle except G_1. The *spi-1* gene was identified as a suppressor of *pim-1* and possesses significant homology to *TC4*, a gene isolated from a teratocarcinoma cell cDNA library by its homology to the *ras* proto-oncogene. Bischoff and Ponstingi[123] have demonstrated that the *TC4* gene product, a G protein called RAN (*ras*-related nuclear protein), co-purified with RCC1 in HeLa cells. Furthermore, they showed that RCC1 can catalyze the exchange of GDP for GTP on RAN. Therefore, the apparent G_2/M checkpoint control mediated by *RCC1* occurs through another classical signal transduction mechanism. Unreplicated DNA signals the maintenance of high levels of the RCC1 protein; this protein may prevent activation of cdc2 kinase by inhibiting the presumed GTPase activity of the RAN protein. Conversely, loss of RCC1 protein, by mutation or degradation on completion of DNA synthesis, permits elevated cdc2 kinase activity and entry into mitosis (for review, see ref. 121).

CHECKPOINTS FOR INITIATING S PHASE

p53

In wild-type mammalian cells, γ irradiation leads to cell cycle arrest at the G_1/S border. The study of several factors that modulate this arrest has led to a model of G_1 checkpoint control. Kastan et al.[124] observed that levels of the *p53* tumor suppressor gene product increased after γ irradiation, whereas cells that carry two mutant *p53* alleles do not undergo G_1 arrest after radiation treatment.[125] These observations suggest that *p53*, recently shown to be a transcriptional activator,[126–128] may be critical for G_1 checkpoint control.

Ataxia-telangiectasia (AT) is a recessive genetic disorder that predisposes patients to a high incidence of cancer and hypersensitivity to ionizing radiation. In AT cells, Kastan et al.[129] demonstrated that p53 levels do not increase in response to γ irradiation and G_1 arrest does not occur. Similarly, the *GADD45* gene, induced in wild-type Chinese hamster ovary and human cells upon growth arrest and DNA damage,[130] does not respond to γ irradiation in AT cells. A p53 binding site is present in the third intron of both the human and hamster genomic *GADD45* genes. This sequence can bind recombinant p53 in vitro and is sufficient to confer p53 dependence on the transcription of a heterologous reporter gene. These observations suggest the AT gene encodes a protein(s) that initiates a checkpoint cascade in response to γ irradiation. Increased p53 levels result in activation of *GADD45* (and other genes), which, in turn, promotes G_1 growth arrest in response to damaged DNA. Interestingly, mutation of either the AT or *p53* genes in vivo does not interfere with embryonic development, but rather promotes high-frequency gene amplification and increases the overall genetic instability of adult cells[125] (see ref. 131 for review).

ONCOGENES, CELL CYCLE, AND ANTINEOPLASTIC DRUGS

With the wealth of new information describing the molecular phenotype of cancer, we can begin to explain how oncogenes and tumor suppressor genes contribute to neoplastic transformation. Functionally diverse groups of oncoproteins that include growth factors, their tyrosine kinase receptors, the *ras* family of GTPases, cytoplasmic serine-threonine kinases, and transcription factors define a signal transduction cascade that ultimately regulates cell cycle progression. The inappropriate activation or inactivation of any component in the signaling pathway can result in a transformed cell phenotype. It is likely that the transforming activity of the oncogene product is related to its normal activity; therefore, it is critical to understand the normal function of such oncogene products. For example, the *mos* proto-oncogene regulates the meiotic cell cycle in vertebrates. This observation has led us to propose that the phenotype of *mos*-transformed somatic cells results from the inappropriate expression of meiotic M-phase activities during all stages of the cell cycle (Fig. 1–

2). This model of transformation may provide an explanation for many phenotypes of transformed cells.[132]

Mos is Required for M Phase of Meiosis

The *mos* proto-oncogene is expressed at high levels in the germ cells of testes and ovaries. The 39-kDa *mos* product (pp39^{mos}) is expressed during the maturation of both mouse and *Xenopus* oocytes.[132–135] In amphibians, progesterone induces fully grown oocytes to reinitiate meiotic maturation. Biochemically, maturation involves the activation of MPF from preexisting stores of inactive pre-MPF.[136–138] MPF activity cycles through meiosis I, but is stabilized at metaphase of meiosis II. The mature unfertilized egg is maintained in metaphase II arrest until fertilization triggers completion of meiosis II.[14,15] Sagata et al.[139] first demonstrated that Mos is both expressed during and required for progesterone-induced oocyte maturation. Meiosis does not occur in the absence of endogenous pp39Mos.[139–143] Mos also is required after GVBD, either in late meiosis I or during meiosis ll.[144,145] Although Mos-depleted oocytes can be induced to undergo GVBD by injecting MPF, the MPF activity required for meiosis II does not reappear.[144] Likewise, when *mos* RNA is depleted after meiosis I, MPF activity disappears and fails to reappear.[145] These results indicate that de novo synthesis of Mos is required after meiosis I for the reappearance of MPF during meiosis II, emphasizing the critical link

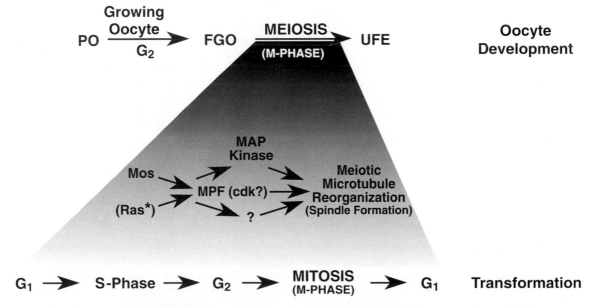

Figure 1–2. Mos in oocyte development and transformation. The Mos product is a regulator of meiotic maturation. The association of Mos with tubulin[153–155] and MPF (p34^{cdc2} [and other cdk family members]),[152] as well as with MAP kinase activation,[165–167] suggests that Mos may contribute to the reorganization of microtubules that leads to spindle formation and the partitioning of chromosomes that occurs during meiosis I and II. The participation of Mos in other meiotic activities, such as nuclear envelope breakdown and chromosome condensation, is not excluded (as indicated by the question mark). The Ras oncoprotein (Ras*) can mimic the activity of Mos during oocyte maturation and in embryonic cleavage-arrest assay.[150,151] It is suggested that the M-phase activity of Mos or Ras, inappropriately expressed during interphase of the somatic cell cycle, is responsible for the phenotype of transformed cells. Abbreviations: PO, primordial oocyte; FGO, fully grown oocyte; UFE, unfertilized egg.

between *mos* proto-oncogene function and MPF. Mos synthesis is induced within 1 hour of hormone treatment of fully grown oocytes, before the appearance of MPF. Using a recombinant Mos fusion protein produced in *Escherichia coli*, it was shown that the addition of Mos protein is necessary and sufficient to initiate meiosis during the early cycloheximide-sensitive period.[146]

Cytostatic factor (CSF) is an activity found in metaphase II–arrested unfertilized eggs. CSF is believed to stabilize MPF, thus causing arrest of meiosis at metaphase II. Sagata et al.[147] noted the similarities between Mos protein and CSF. CSF-containing extracts, assayed by injection into two-cell embryos, arrest blastomere cleavage at metaphase. CSF activity can be depleted from these extracts with anti-Mos antibodies. Moreover, *mos*RNA[142,147] or the soluble Mos protein made in *E. coli*[146] mimics CSF activity when injected into one blastomere of a two-cell embryo. These experiments demonstrate that Mos is an integral component of CSF; however, the complete biochemical composition of CSF and its mechanism of action are still unknown.

Soluble Mos fusion protein will induce meiosis I in the presence of cycloheximide; however, the reappearance of MPF, indicative of oocytes entering meiosis II, does not occur.[146] This suggests that the protein(s) essential for MPF reactivation at Meiosis II are synthesized during or after meiosis I. This protein(s) also could interact directly or indirectly with Mos to induce metaphase II arrest/CSF activity. Similar component(s) also must be present in cleaving embryos, because injection of Mos alone into one blastomere results in metaphase arrest.[142,147] Recently, the Maller laboratory has implicated cdk2 and MAPK as components of CSF.[148,149] The interaction of these three proteins is currently under investigation.

We have previously shown that the Ras oncoprotein mimics CSF and induces cleavage arrest in the absence of Mos.[150,151] These results suggest that Mos and Ras function along parallel pathways to activate a common downstream target. Recent studies suggest that activation of MAPK via a Ras/Raf or Mos pathway is this common target (Fig. 1–2).

Candidate Mos Substrates

The mitotic spindle apparatus is thought to play a role at the mitotic checkpoint.[119,138] The spindle apparatus may function to stabilize MPF, and our studies suggest that Mos may stabilize the spindle by interacting with tubulin. Mos co-elutes in a high-molecular-weight complex with tubulin in extracts prepared from either *mos* transformed NIH 3T3 cells or unfertilized *Xenopus* eggs.[152] Moreover, in these extracts β-tubulin and Mos are found in stoichiometric amounts. Mos specifically phosphorylates tubulin when an in vitro kinase reaction is performed on these Mos-immune complexes.[152–155] In vivo, microtubule-mediated mitochondria and organelle transport does not occur when endogenous Mos is depleted from mouse oocytes undergoing meiotic maturation.[133,156] Strikingly, this same phenotype is observed when maturation is blocked by the antineoplastic, microtubule-stabilizing drug taxol.

In contrast, microtubule destabilizing drugs do not have this effect.[157,158]

How does Mos and its interaction with tubulin result in CSF arrest? Disruption of microtubules with nocodazole or other microtubule depolymerizing drugs prevents cyclin degradation[159–161] and stabilizes MPF activity,[162,163] arresting the cells in a pseudo-metaphase state. This observation suggests that there is a surveillance system that couples microtubules to MPF regulation.[119,138] Presumably, this system ensures the integrity of the mitotic spindle and the proper segregation of chromosomes. In oocytes, Mos co-localizes with the meiotic spindle and the spindle pole. We have shown that Mos also associates with these structures in *mos*-transformed somatic cells.[153] Therefore, it is possible that Mos directs the microtubule reorganization that leads to the formation of the spindle and the spindle pole,[153,154,164] as well as the process of chromosome partitioning during M phase. If Mos acts on tubulin in a manner that produces a stabilized meiotic spindle, the checkpoint system would sense this stabilized spindle and maintain high levels of MPF. In addition, an interaction may exist between Mos and MPF at the biochemical level because p34^{cdc2} and B cyclins also have been localized to the spindle.[136,163] In any case, the process of reductive division is likely to employ additional proteins and checkpoints.

Activation of MAPK during Meiosis

Recently, MAPK has been shown to be rapidly activated after fully grown oocytes are injected with either the Mos fusion protein[165] or the Ras oncoprotein,[166,167] suggesting that MAPK is a common downstream target (Fig. 1–2). The role of MAPK in meiotic maturation is obviously different than its role in mitogenic signaling. MAPK recently has been shown to facilitate the interphase-metaphase transition of microtubule arrays in vitro and has been shown to localize to the spindle pole.[168–170] Thus, the CSF arrest induced by Mos and Ras[150,151] could be mediated by MAPK-induced spindle formation.

Mos Expression and the Transformed Phenotype

The *mos, src,* and *ras* oncogenes are considered the paradigm for transforming genes, and each has M-phase activity.[133] Mos is a critical regulator of meiotic M phase; it is required for the initiation of meiosis and the activation of MPF during meiosis I and II, and is a component of CSF, stabilizing MPF during metaphase II. We have proposed that neoplastic transformation is due to the imposition of the Mos M-phase program on all stages of the somatic cell cycle. Similar proposals have been made for *src*[171] and the Ras oncoprotein.[150,151]

In the model of multistep carcinogenesis, cancer results from at least two damaging events. The previously described rat embryo fibroblast cooperating oncogene assay (Table 1–2)[172] is believed to mimic tumor progression. A careful examination of the activities of cooperating on-

TABLE 1–2. ONCOGENE COMPLEMENTATION GROUPS IN RAT EMBRYO FIBROBLAST TRANSFORMATION ASSAY

GROUP I RESCUE FROM SENESCENCE (S PHASE)	GROUP II MORPHOLOGIC TRANSFORMATION (M PHASE)
E1A	E1B
SV40 large T	Polyoma middle T
Polyoma large T	H-*ras*
c-*myc*	K-*ras*
N-*myc*	N-*ras*
Mutant *p53*	

From Hunter T: Cooperation between oncogenes. Cell 64:249, 1991. Copyright held by Cell Press, with permission.

cogenes reveals that one class of oncogenes rescues cells from senescence, and the second class are responsible for morphologic transformation. Oncogenes that rescue cells from senescence promote entry into S phase; for instance, G_1 cyclins clearly fit into this class. The second class of oncogenes, those responsible for morphologic transformation, may act by promoting expression of M-phase events during interphase.[133] Constitutive MAPK activation may be the event common to both classes of oncogenes. It is possible that the many oncogenes and tumor suppressor genes may elicit one of two critical effects on the cell cycle: entry into S phase or inappropriate expression of M-phase activities during all stages of the cell cycle. Cellular transformation may result from the combination of these events within a single cell. Tumor invasion and metastasis are likely to require additional changes that affect other biologic processes[173] (Table 1–3).

Tumor progression is due to genetic instability (Table 1–3), a property central to the cancer process. We have proposed that the genetic instability of transformed cells is due to the compromise of checkpoint functions by oncogene activation.[133] Presumably, checkpoints work by acting, directly or indirectly, on the ability of a cell to proceed through the cell cycle (Fig. 1–1B); therefore, oncogenes with downstream M-phase activity could compromise or override checkpoint functions when expressed during interphase. In addition, some proto-oncogenes and tumor suppressor genes may normally serve as checkpoint genes. Therefore, there may be two possible mechanisms to interfere with normal checkpoint function: to fool the cell into thinking it is in M phase or to directly inactivate the checkpoint genes.

If oncogenes and tumor suppressor genes act by compromising checkpoints, then a tumor cell should be more vulnerable to antineoplastic drugs than a normal cell. When a normal cell is treated with a DNA-damaging agent, its checkpoint system will be activated, allowing the cell to repair the DNA before resuming the cell cycle. However, transformed cells with a defective checkpoint system will tolerate the damaged DNA and proceed through the cell cycle, accumulating errors. This proposal can explain how the same tumor lineage can harbor different genomic alterations, such as translocations, deletions, and point mutations. Thus, compromise of checkpoint function can explain the genetic instability of tumor cells and tumor progression, as well as the sensitivity of tumor cells to antineoplastic agents.

At present, antineoplastic drugs are discovered through empirical testing. By understanding the mechanisms by which oncogene activation or loss of tumor suppressor gene function renders tumor cells more sensitive to these drugs, it may be possible to improve the use of existing antineoplastic drugs. It is rather striking that many antineoplastic drugs act either on S-phase or M-phase targets (Table 1–4)[132]: These drugs either damage DNA or affect chromosome partitioning during M phase. If, as suggested, oncogenes promote unchecked cell cycle progression, a transformed cell will tolerate the damage caused by these agents. Therefore, drugs acting at different stages of the cell cycle would be expected to act in synergy. This

TABLE 1–3. ALTERED PROPERTIES OF TUMOR CELLS

	G^1S	G^2M
Cellular morphology		+
Nuclear structure		+
Cytoskeleton		+
Growth characteristics and cell metabolism	+	+
Anchorage independence and loss of contact inhibition		+
Changes in extracellular matrix		+
Growth factor independence		+
Genetic instability	+	

Adapted from Vande Woude GF, Schulz N, Zhou R, et al: Cell cycle regulation, oncogenes and antineoplastic drugs. *In* Fortner JG, Rhoads JE (eds): 1990 Views of Cancer Research. Philadelphia, JB Lippincott Company/General Motors Cancer Research Foundation, 1991, pp 128–143, with permission.

TABLE 1–4. SELECTED ANTINEOPLASTIC AGENTS

G₁ + S PHASE (UPSTREAM)	M PHASE (DOWNSTREAM)
Tamoxifen (antiestrogen)	Vincristine (tubulin binding)
Prednisone (corticosteroid)	Vinblastine (tubulin binding)
Dacarbazine (DNA alkylation)	Taxol (tubulin binding)
Mechlorethamine (DNA alkylation)	Doxorubicin (topoisomerase II inhibitor)
Cisplatin (DNA cross-linking)	Daunorubicin (topoisomerase II inhibitor)
Methotrexate (DNA synthesis)	Etoposide (topoisomerase II inhibitor)
5'-fluorouracil (DNA synthesis)	Bleomycin (DNA cross-linking)
Cytosine arabinoside (DNA synthesis)	

From Vande Woude GF, Schulz N, Zhou R, et al: Cell cycle regulation, oncogenes and antineoplastic drugs. *In* Fortner JG, Rhoads JE (eds): 1990 Views of Cancer Research. Philadelphia, JB Lippincott Company/General Motors Cancer Research Foundation, 1991, pp 128–143, with permission.

suggestion may explain why tumor cells are more vulnerable to combinations of drugs that target both S phase (DNA alkylating agents) and M phase (the tubulin-binding vinca alkaloids or taxol and topoisomerase II inhibitors). In essence, the tumor cells continue through the cell cycle, passing through checkpoints and accumulating errors, whereas the normal cell stops at the appropriate checkpoints and makes the necessary repairs or undergoes apoptosis. Certain empirically established protocols are combinations of S-phase and M-phase drugs (Table 1–5); clinical regimens for treating acute lymphocytic leukemia, acute nonlymphocytic leukemia, testicular cancer, and Hodgkin's lymphoma employ a combination of drugs that act at S phase and M phase. The balance of S-phase and M-phase agents in the MOPP versus ABVD regimens for Hodgkin's lymphoma might explain the efficacy of one as a salvage chemotherapy after the other. One rather somber scenario, however, is that drug treatment protocols may select tumor cells that have increased genetic instability (e.g., cells harboring *p53* mutations). These cells may fail to undergo apoptosis—for instance, by expressing *bcl-2*,[174] resulting in cells that may be less responsive to subsequent treatment.

With the discoveries of the genes that regulate the cell cycle and checkpoint function, we can develop new approaches to identify and design antineoplastic drugs that will specifically target the biochemical activities of oncoproteins (e.g., the use of drugs that inhibit farnesylation to inhibit Ras function)[175,176] and altered tumor suppressor gene products. Knowledge of how oncogenes function in the cell cycle may, in the very near future, serve to elucidate the mechanisms of antineoplastic drug action. In addition, we may improve the usefulness of existing drugs by identifying more drugs that act synergistically. The knowledge that a particular oncogene compromises a specific checkpoint would lead to the selection of very specific drugs, resulting in a more effective way to target tumor cells. Another potential benefit would be the reduction of drug dosage: Lower doses of a combination of drugs that target multiple checkpoints would enhance the accumulation of cytotoxic errors, whereas a drug protocol that targets a single checkpoint may require greater amounts to have the same effect. We are actively involved in examining the cell cycle in greater detail; ultimately, such knowledge will enable us to develop novel strategies to treat cancer.

ACKNOWLEDGMENTS: Research sponsored by the National Cancer Institute, DHHS, under contract No. NO1-CO-74101

TABLE 1–5. SELECTED CHEMOTHERAPEUTIC REGIMENS

MALIGNANCY	G₁ OR S PHASE (UPSTREAM)	M PHASE (DOWNSTREAM)
Acute lymphocytic leukemia	Prednisone L-Asparaginase Cytosine arabinoside	Vincristine Daunorubicin Etoposide
Acute nonlymphocytic leukemia	Cytosine arabinoside	Daunorubicin
Testicular cancer	Cis-plantinum Mechlorethamine	Bleomycin Vinblastine or etoposide
Hodgkin's lymphoma	Procarbazine Prednisone Dacarbazine	Vincristine Doxorubicin Vincristone Bleomycin

From Vande Woude GF, Schulz N, Zhou R, et al: Cell cycle regulation, oncogenes and antineoplastic drugs. *In* Fortner JG, Rhoads JE (eds): 1990 Views of Cancer Research. Philadelphia, JB Lippincott Company/General Motors Cancer Research Foundation, 1991, pp 128–143, with permission.

74101 with ABL. The contents of this publication do not necessarily reflect the views or policies of the Department of Health and Human Services, nor does mention of trade names, commercial products, or organizations imply endorsement by the U.S. Government. We thank Michelle Reed and Lori Summers for expert secretarial assistance, Nelson Yew for his valuable input, and past and present members of the Vande Woude laboratory for discussion and comments.

REFERENCES

1. Lee MG, Nurse P: Complementation used to clone a human homologue of the fission yeast cell cycle control gene cdc2. Nature 327:31, 1987
2. Pardee AB: Molecules involved in proliferation of normal and cancer cells: Presidential address. Cancer Res 47:1488, 1987
3. Pardee AB: G1 events and regulation of cell proliferation. Science 246:603, 1989
4. Hartwell LH, Culotti J, Pringle JR, et al: Genetic control of the cell division cycle in yeast. Science 183:46, 1974
5. Nurse P, Thuriaux P, Nasmyth K: Genetic control of the cell division cycle in the fission yeast Schizosaccharomyces pombe. Mol Gen Genet 146:167, 1976
6. Piggot JR, Rai R, Carter BLA: A bifunctional gene product involved in two phases of the yeast cell cycle. Nature 298:391, 1982
7. Nurse P, Bissett Y: Gene required in G1 for commitment to cell cycle and in G2 for control of mitosis in fission yeast. Nature 292:558, 1981
8. Reed SI, Wittenberg C: A mitotic role for the Cdc28 protein kinase of S. cerevisiae. Proc Natl Acad Sci USA 87:5697, 1990
9. Lorincz AT, Reed SI: Primary structure homology between the product of yeast cell division control gene cdc28 and vertebrate oncogenes. Nature 308:183, 1987
10. Simanis V, Nurse P: The cell cycle control gene cdc2+ of fission yeast encodes a protein kinase potentially regulated by phosphorylation. Cell 45:261, 1986
11. Paris J, Le Guellec R, Couturier A, et al: Cloning by differential screening of a Xenopus cDNA coding for a protein highly homologous to cdc2. Proc Natl Acad Sci USA 88:1039, 1991
12. Myerson M, Enders GH, Wu C-L, et al: A family of human cdc2 related protein kinases. EMBO J 11:2909, 1992
13. Nigg EA: Targets of cyclin dependent protein kinases. Curr Opin Cell Biol 5:187, 1993
14. Masui Y, Markert CL: Cytoplasmic control of nuclear behavior during meiotic maturation in frog oocytes. J Exp Zool 177:129, 1971
15. Smith LD, Ecker RE: The interaction of steroids with Rana pipens oocytes in the induction of maturation. Dev Biol 25:233, 1971
16. Lohka MJ, Hayes MK, Maller JL: Purification of maturation-promoting factor, an intracellular regulator of early mitotic events. Proc Natl Acad Sci USA 85:3009, 1988
17. Arion D, Meijer L, Briquela L, Beach D: cdc2 is a component of M phase-specific histone H1 kinase: Evidence for identity with MPF. Cell 55:371, 1988
18. Dunphy WG, Brizuela L, Beach D: The Xenopus cdc2 protein is a component of MPF, a cytoplasmic regulator of mitosis. Cell 54:423, 1988
19. Gautier J, Norbury C, Lohka M, et al: Purified maturation-promoting factor contains the product of a Xenopus homolog of the fission yeast cell cycle control gene cdc2+. Cell 54:433, 1988
20. Labbé JC, Lee MG, Nurse P, et al: Activation at M-phase of a protein kinase encoded by a starfish homolog of the cell cycle control gene cdc2+. Nature 335:251, 1988
21. Nurse P: Universal control mechanism regulating onset of M-phase. Nature 344:503, 1991
22. Evans T, Rosenthal ET, Youngblom J, et al: Cyclin: A protein specified by maternal mRNA in sea urchin eggs that is destroyed at each cleavage division. Cell 33:389, 1983
23. Sherr C: Mammalian G₁ cyclins. Cell 73:1059, 1993
24. Pines J: Cell proliferation and control. Curr Opin Cell Biol 4:144, 1992
25. Swenson KI, Farrell KM, Ruderman JV: The clam embryo protein cyclin A induces entry into M phase and the resumption of meiosis in Xenopus oocytes. Cell 47:861, 1986
26. Murray AW, Kirschner MW: Cyclin synthesis drives the early embryonic cell cycle. Nature 339:275, 1989
27. Glotzer M, Murray AW, Kirschner MW: Cyclin is degraded by the ubiquitin pathway. Nature 349:132, 1991
28. Murray AW, Solomon MJ, Kirschner WM: The role of cyclin synthesis and degradation in the control of maturation promoting factor activity. Nature 339:280, 1989
29. Meijer L, Arion D, Golsteyn R, et al: Cyclin is a component of the sea urchin egg M-phase specific histone H1 kinase. EMBO J 8:2275, 1989
30. Gautier J, Minshull J, Lohka M, et al: Cyclin is a component of maturation-promoting factor from Xenopus. Cell 60:487, 1990
31. Solomon MJ, Glotzer M, Lee TH, et al: Cyclin activation of p34cdc2. Cell 63:1013, 1990
32. Pines J, Hunter T: Human cyclins A and B1 are differentially located in the cell and undergo cell cycle-dependent nuclear transport. J Cell Biol 115:1, 1991
33. Gallant P, Nigg EA: Cyclin B2 undergoes cell cycle dependent nuclear translocation and when expressed as a non-destructible mutant causes mitotic arrest in HeLa cells. J Cell Biol 117:213, 1992
34. Parker LL, Atherton-Fessler S, Lee MS, et al: Cyclin promotes the tyrosine phosphorylation of p34cdc2 in a wee 1 dependent manner. EMBO J 10:1255, 1991
35. Parker LL, Piwnica-Worms H: Inactivation of the p34cdc2 cyclin B complex by the human WEE 1 tyrosine kinase. Science 257:1955, 1992
36. Jessus C, Beach D: Oscillation of MPF is accompanied by periodic association between cdc25 and cdc2 cyclin B. Cell 68:323, 1992
37. Galaktionov K, Beach D: Specific activation of cdc25 tyrosine phosphatases by B-type cyclins: Evidence for multiple roles of mitotic cyclins. Cell 67:1181, 1991
38. Lehner CF, O'Farrell PH: Expression and function of Drosophila cyclin A during embryonic cell cycle progression. Cell 56:957, 1989
39. Lehner CF, O'Farrell P: The roles of Drosophila cyclins A and B mitotic control. Cell 61:535, 1990
40. Girard F. Strausfeld U, Fernandez A, et al: Cyclin A is required for the onset of DNA replication in mammalian fibroblasts. Cell 67:1169, 1991
41. Pagano M, Pepperkok R, Verde F, et al: Cyclin A is required at two points in the human cell cycle. EMBO J 11:961, 1992
42. Bandara LR, Adamczewski JP, Hunt T, et al: Cyclin A and the retinoblastoma gene product complex with a common transcription factor. Nature 352:249, 1991
43. Mudryi M, Devoto SH, Hiebert SW, et al: Cell cycle regulation of the E2F transcription factor involves an interaction with cyclin A. Cell 65:1243, 1991
44. Pines J, Hunter T: Human cyclin A is adenovirus E1A associated protein p60 and behaves differently from cyclin B. Nature 346:760, 1990
45. Tsai LH, Harlow E, Myerson M: Isolation of the human cdk2 gene that encodes the cyclin A an adenovirus E1A associated p33 kinase. Nature 353:174, 1991
46. Giordano A, Whyte P, Harlow E, et al: A 60 kd cdc2 associated polypeptide complexes with the E1A proteins in adenovirus-infected cells. Cell 58:961, 1989
47. Hadwiger JA, Wittenberg C, Richardson HE, et al: A family of cyclin homologs that control the G1 phase in yeast. Proc Natl Acad Sci USA 86:6255, 1989
48. Wittenberg C, Sugimoto K, Reed SI: G1 specific cyclins of S. cerevisiae: Cell cycle periodicity, regulation by mating pheromone and association with the p34 cdc28 protein kinase. Cell 62:225, 1990

49. Richardson HE, Wittenberg C, Cross F, et al: An essential G1 function for cyclin-like proteins in yeast. Cell 59:1127, 1989

50. Lew DJ, Dulic V, Reed SI: Isolation of three novel human cyclins by rescue of G1 cyclin(Cln) function in yeast. Cell 66:1197, 1991

51. Xiong X, Connolly T, Futcher B, et al: Human D-type cyclin. Cell 65:691, 1991

52. Matsushime H. Roussel MF, Ashmun RA, et al: Colony-stimulating factor 1 regulates novel cyclin during the G1 phase of the cell cycle. Cell 65:701, 1991

53. Dulic V, Lees E, Reed SI: Association of human cyclin E with a periodic G1-S phase protein kinase. Science 257:1958, 1992

54. Koff A, Cross F, Fisher A, et al: Human cyclin E, a new cyclin that interacts with two members of the CDC2 gene family. Cell 66:1217, 1991

55. Koff A, Giordano A, Desai D, et al: Formation and activation of a cyclin E-cdk2 complex during the G1 phase of the human cell cycle. Science 257:1689, 1992

56. Lees E. Faha B, Dulic V, et al: Cyclin E/cdk2 and cyclin A/cdk2 kinases associate with p107 and E2F in a temporally distinct manner. Genes Dev 6:1874, 1992

57. Matsushime H, Ewen ME, Strom DK, et al: Identification and properties of an atypical catalytic subunit (p34 pskj-3/cdk4) for mammalian D type G1 cyclins. Cell 71:323, 1992

58. Xiong Y, Zhang H, Beach D: D type cyclin associate with multiple protein kinases and the DNA replication and repair factor PCNA. Cell 71:505, 1992

59. Gautier J, Maller JL: Cyclin B in Xenopus oocytes: Implications for the mechanism of pre-MPF activation. EMBO J 10:177, 1991

60. Gould KL, Nurse P: Tyrosine phosphorylation of the fission yeast cdc2+ protein kinase regulates entry into mitosis. Nature 342:39, 1989

61. Moria AO, Draetta G, Beach D, et al: Reversible tyrosine phosphorylation of cdc2: Dephosphorylation accompanies activation during entry into mitosis. Cell 58:193, 1989

62. Norbury C, Blow J, Nurse P: Regulatory phosphorylation of the p34 cdc2 protein kinase in vertebrates. EMBO J 10:3321, 1991

63. Solomon MJ, Lee TH, Kirschner MW: Role of phosphorylation in p34^{cdc2} activation: Identification of an activating kinase. Mol Biol Cell 3:13, 1992

64. Poon RYC, Yamashita K, Adamczewski JP, et al: The cdc2-related protein P40^{MO15} is the catalytic subunit of a protein kinase that can activate p33^{cd2} and p34^{cdc2}. EMBO J 12:3123, 1993

65. Fesquet D, Labbe J-C, Derancourt J, et al: The MO15 gene encodes the catalytic subunit of a protein kinase that activates cdc2 and other cyclin-dependent kinase (CDKs) through phosphorylation of Thr161 and its homologues. EMBO J 12:3111, 1993

66. Solomon MJ, Harper JW, Shuttleworth J: CAK, the p34^{cdc2} activating kinase, contains a protein identical or closely related to p40^{MO15}. EMBO J 12:3133, 1993

67. Lundgren K, Walworth N, Booher R, et al: mik1 and wee1 cooperate in the inhibitory tyrosine phosphorylation of cdc2. Cell 64:1111, 1991

68. Russell P, Nurse P: cdc25+ functions as an inducer in the mitotic control of fission yeast. Cell 45:145, 1986

69. Featherstone C, Russell P: Fission yeast p107 wee1 mitotic inhibitor is a tyrosine serine kinase. Nature 349:808, 1991

70. Parker LL, Atherton-Fessler S, Piwnica-Worms H: p107 wee1 is a dual specificity kinase that phosphorylates p34cdc2 on tyrosine 15. Proc Natl Acad Sci USA 89:2917, 1992

71. Dunphy WG, Kumagai A: The cdc25 protein contains an intrinsic phosphatase activity. Cell 67:189, 1991

72. Gautier J, Solomon MJ, Booher RN, et al: cdc25 is a specific tyrosine phosphatase that directly activates p34cdc2. Cell 67:197, 1991

73. Millar JBA, McGowan CH, Lenaers G, et al: p80cdc25 mitotic inducer is the tyrosine phosphatase that activates p34cdc2 kinase in fission yeast. EMBO J 10:4301, 1991

74. Strausfeld U, Labbé JC, Fesquet K, et al: Dephosphorylation and activation of a p34cdc3/cyclin B complex in vitro by human cdc25 protein. Nature 351:242, 1991

75. Kumagai A, Dunphy WG: Regulation of the cdc25 protein phosphatase during the cell cycle in Xenopus extracts. Cell 70:139, 1992

76. Hoffmann E, Clarke PR, Marcote MJ, et al: Phosphorylation and activation of human cdc25-C by self amplification of MPF at mitosis. EMBO J 12:53, 1993

77. Edgar BA, O'Farrell PH: The three postblastoderm cell cycles of Drosophila embryogenesis are regulated in G2 by string. Cell 62:469, 1990

78. Kakizuka A, Sebastian B, Borgmeyer U, et al: A mouse cdc25 homolog is differentially and developmentally expressed. Genes Dev 6:578, 1992

79. Alphy L, Jimenez J, White-Cooper H, et al: Twine, a cdc25 homolog that functions in the male and female germline of Drosophila. Cell 69:977, 1992

80. Draetta G: Cell cycle control in eukaryotes: Molecular mechanisms of cdc2 activation. Trends Biochem Sci 15:378, 1990

81. Blow JJ, Nurse P: A cdc2-like protein is involved in the initiation of DNA replication in Xenopus egg extracts. Cell 62:855, 1990

82. Fang F, Newport JW: Evidence that the G1/s and G2-M transitions are controlled by different cdc2 proteins in higher eukaryotes. Cell 66:731, 1991

83. D'Urso G, Marraccino RL, Marshak DR, et al: Cell cycle control of DNA replication by a homologue from human cells of the p34 cdc2 protein kinase. Science 250:786, 1990

84. Dutta A, Stillman B: cdc2 family kinases phosphorylate a human cell DNA replication factor, RPA, and activate DNA replication. EMBO J 11:2189, 1992

85. Fotedar R, Roberts JM: Cell cycle regulated phosphorylation of RPA-32 occurs within the replication initiation complex. EMBO J 11:2177, 1992

86. McVey D, Brizuela L, Mohr I, et al: Phosphorylation of large tumor antigen by cdc2 stimulates SV40 DNA replication. Nature 341:503, 1989

87. Borowiec JA, Dean FB, Bullock, PA, et al: Binding and unwinding—how T antigen engages the SV40 origin of DNA replication. Cell 60:181, 1990

88. Roberts JM: Turning DNA replication on and off. Curr Opin Cell Biol 5:201, 1993

89. Ward GE, Kirschner MW: Identification of cell cycle-regulated phosphorylation sites on nuclear lamin C. Cell 61:561, 1990

90. Heald R, McKeon F: Mutations of phosphorylation sites in lamin A that prevent nuclear lamina disassembly in mitosis. Cell 61:579, 1990

91. Peter M, Heitlinger E, Häner M, et al: Disassembly of in vitro formed lamin head-to-tail polymers by cdc2 kinase. EMBO J 10:1535, 1991

92. Lüscher B, Brizuela L, Beach D, et al: A role for the p34cdc2 kinase and phosphatases in the regulation of phosphorylation and disassembly of lamin B2 during the cell cycle. EMBO J 10:865, 1991

93. Chou Y-H, Bischoff JR, Beach D, et al: Intermediate filament reorganization during mitosis is mediated by P34cdc3 phosphorylation of vimentin. Cell 62:1063, 1992

94. Nigg EA: Assembly-disassembly of the nuclear lamina. Curr Opin Cell Biol 4:105, 1992

95. Hunter T, Pines J: Cyclins and cancer. Cell 66:1071, 1991

96. Motokura T, Kim HG, Jüppner H, et al: A novel cyclin encoded by a bcl1-linked candidate oncogene. Nature 350:512, 1991

97. Jiang W, Kahn SM, Tomita N, et al: Amplification and expression of the human cyclin D gene in esophageal cancer. Cancer Res 52:2980, 1992

98. Wang J, Chenivesse X, Henglein B, et al: Hepatitis B virus integration in a cyclin A gene in a hepatocellular carcinoma. Nature 343:555, 1990

99. Cobrinik D, Dowdy SF, Hinds PW, et al: The retinoblastoma protein and the regulation of cell cycling. Trends Biochem Sci 17:312, 1992

100. Hollingsworth RE, Hensey CE, Lee W-H: Retinoblastoma protein and the cell cycle. Curr Opin Genet Dev 3:55, 1993

101. Chen P-H, Shew J-Y, Wang JY, et al: Phosphorylation of the

retinoblastoma gene product is modulated during the cell cycle and cellular differentiation. Cell 58:1193, 1989

102. Buchkovich K, Duffy LA, Harlow E: The retinoblastoma protein is phosphorylated during specific phases of the cell cycle. Cell 58:1097, 1989

103. Lin BT-Y, Gruenwald S, Moria AO, et al: Retinoblastoma cancer suppressor gene product is a substrate of the cell cycle regulator cdc2 kinase. EMBO J 10:857, 1991

104. Hamel PA, Gallie BL, Phillips RA: The retinoblastoma protein and cell cycle regulation. Trends Genet 8:180, 1992

105. DeCaprio JA, Ludlow JW, Figg J, et al: SV40 large tumor antigen forms a specific complex with the product of the retinoblastoma susceptibility gene. Cell 54:275, 1988

106. Ludlow JW, DeCaprio JA, Huang CM, et al: SV40 large T antigen binds preferentially to an underphosphorylated member of the retinoblastoma susceptibility gene product family. Cell 56:57, 1989

107. Whyte P, Buchkovich KJ, Horowitz JM, et al: Association between an oncogene and an anti-oncogene: The adenovirus E1A proteins binds to the retinoblastoma gene product. Nature 334:124, 1988

108. Dyson N, Howley PM, Munger K, et al: The human papilloma virus-16 E7 oncoprotein is able to bind to the retinoblastoma gene product. Science 243:934, 1989

109. Chellappan S, Kraus VB, Kroger B, et al: Adenovirus E1A, simian virus 40 tumor antigen, and human papillomavirus E7 protein share the capacity to disrupt the interaction between transcription factor E2F and the retinoblastoma gene product. Proc Natl Acad Sci USA 89:4549, 1992

110. Nevins JR, Chellappan SP, Mudryj M, et al: E2F transcription factor is a target for the Rb protein and the cyclin A protein. Cold Spring Harb Symp Quant Biol LVI:157, 1991

111. Nevins JR: E2F: A link between the Rb tumor suppressor protein and viral oncoproteins. Science 258:424, 1992

112. Ewen ME, Faha B, Harlow E, et al: Interaction of p107 with cyclin A independent of complex formation with viral oncoproteins. Science 255:85, 1992

113. Faha B, Ewin ME, Tsai L-H, et al: Interaction between human cyclin A and adenovirus E1A-associated p107 protein. Science 255:87, 1992

114. Pagano M, Draetta G, Jansen-Durr P: Association of cdk2 kinase with the transcription factor E2F during S phase. Science 255:1144, 1992

115. Shirodkar S, Ewen M, DeCaprio JA, et al: The transcription factor E2F interacts with the retinoblastoma product and a p107-cyclin A complex in a cell cycle-regulated manner. Cell 68:157, 1992

116. Devoto SH, Mudryj M, Pines J, et al: A cyclin A-protein kinase complex possesses sequence-specific DNA binding activity: p33cdk2 is a component of the E2F cyclin A complex. Cell 68:167, 1992

116a. Hunter T: Braking the cycle. Cell 75:839, 1993

116b. Harper JW, Adam GR, Wei N, et al: The p21 Cdk-interacting protein Cip1 is a potent inhibitor of G1 cyclin-dependent kinases. Cell 75:805, 1993

116c. Xiong Y, Hannon GJ, Zhang H, et al: p21 is a universal inhibitor of cyclin kinases. Nature 366:701, 1993

116d. El-Deiry WS, Tokino T, Velculescu VE, et al: WAF1, a potential mediator of p53 tumor suppression. Cell 75:817, 1993

116e. Polyak K, Kato JY, Solomon MJ, et al: p27Kip1, a cyclin-cdk inhibitor, links transforming growth factor-beta and contact inhibition to cell cycle arrest. Genes Dev 8:9, 1994

116f. Serrano M, Hannon GJ, Beach D: A new regulatory motif in cell-cycle control causing specific inhibition of cyclin D/CDK4. Nature 366:704, 1993

116g. Kamb A, Gruis NA, Weaver-Feldhaus J, et al: A cell cycle regulator potentially involved in genesis of many tumor types. Science 264:436, 1994

117. Weinert TA, Hartwell LA: The RAD9 gene controls the cell cycle response to DNA damage in Saccharomyces cerevisiae. Science 241:317, 1988

118. Hartwell LH, Weinert TA: Checkpoints: Controls that ensure the order of cell cycle events. Science 246:629, 1989

119. Murray AW: Creative blocks: Cell-cycle checkpoints and feedback controls. Nature 359:599, 1992

120. Nishitani H, Ohtsubo M, Yamashita K, et al: Loss of RCC1, a nuclear DNA-binding protein uncouples the completion of DNA replication from the activation of cdc2 protein kinase and mitosis. EMBO J 10:1555, 1991

121. Dasso M: RCC1 in the cell cycle: The regulator of chromosome condensation takes on new roles. Trends Biochem Sci 18:96, 1993

122. Matsumoto T, Beach D: Premature initiation of mitosis in yeast lacking RCC1 or an interacting GTPase. Cell 66:347, 1991

123. Bischoff FR, Ponstingi H: Catalysis of guanine nucleotide exchange on Ran by the mitotic regulator RCC1. Nature 354:80, 1991

124. Kastan MB, Onyekwere O, Sidransky D, et al: Participation of p53 protein in the cellular response to DNA damage. Cancer Res 51:6304, 1991

125. Livingstone LR, White A, Sprouse J, et al: Altered cell cycle arrest and gene amplification potential accompany loss of wild-type p53. Cell 70:923, 1992

126. Bargonetti J, Reynisdottir I, Friedman PN, et al: Site-specific binding of wild type p53 to cellular DNA is inhibited by SV40 T antigen and mutant p53. Genes Dev 6:1886, 1992

127. Zambetti GP, Bargonetti J, Walker K, et al: Wild type p53 mediates positive regulation of gene expression through a specific DNA sequence element. Genes Dev 6:1143, 1992

128. Prives C: Doing the right thing: Feedback control and p53. Curr Opin Cell Biol 5:214, 1993

129. Kastan MB, Zhan Q, El-Deiry WS, et al: A mammalian cell cycle checkpoint pathway utilizing p53 and GADD45 is defective in ataxia-telangiectasia. Cell 71:587, 1992

130. Papathanasiou MA, Kerr NC, Robbins NC, et al: Induction by ionizing radiation of the GADD45 gene in cultured human cells: Lack of mediation by protein kinase C. Mol Cell Biol 11:1009, 1991

131. Hartwell L: Defects in a cell cycle checkpoint may be responsible for the genomic instability of cancer cells. Cell 71:543, 1992

132. Vande Woude GF, Schulz N, Zhou R, et al: Cell cycle regulation, oncogenes and antineoplastic drugs. In Fortner JG, Rhoads JE (eds): 1990 Views of Cancer Research, Philadelphia, JB Lippincott Company/General Motors Cancer Research Foundation, 1991, pp 128–143

133. Vande Woude GF, Zhou R, Paules RS, et al: mos proto-oncogene product and cell cycle control. In Brugge J, Curran T, Harlow E, McCormick F (eds): Origins of Human Cancer: A Comprehensive Review, Cold Spring Harbor, NY, CSHL Press, 1991, pp 65–75

134. Freeman RS, Donoghue DJ: Protein kinase and protooncogenes: Biochemical regulators of the eukaryotic cell cycle. Biochemistry 30:2293, 1991

135. Yew N, Strobel M, Vande Woude GF: Mos and the cell cycle: The molecular basis of the transformed phenotype. Curr Opin Genet Dev 3:19, 1993

136. Cyert MS, Kirschner MW: Regulation of MPF activity in vitro. Cell 53:185, 1988

137. Kobayashi H, Minshull J, Ford C, et al: On the synthesis and destruction of A- and B-type cyclins during oogenesis and meiotic maturation in Xenopus laevis. J Cell Biol 4:755, 1991

138. Murray AW, Kirschner MW: Dominoes and clocks: The union of two views of the cell cycle. Science 246:614, 1989

139. Sagata N, Oskarsson M, Copeland T, et al: Function of c-mos proto-oncogene product in meiotic maturation in Xenopus oocytes. Nature 335:519, 1988

140. Sagata N, Daar I, Oskarsson M, et al: The product of the mos protooncogene as a candidate "initiator" for oocyte maturation. Science 245:643, 1989

141. Freeman RS, Pickham KM, Kanki JP, et al: Xenopus homolog of the mos protooncogene transforms mammalian fibroblasts and induces maturation of Xenopus oocytes. Proc Natl Acad Sci USA 86:5805, 1989

142. Freeman RS, Kanki JP, Ballantyne SM, et al: Effects of the v-mos oncogene on Xenopus development: Meiotic induction in oocytes and mitotic arrest in cleaving embryos. J Cell Biol 111:533, 1990

143. Barrett CB, Schroetke RM, Van der Hoorn FA, et al: Ha-

ras^{val12thr59} activates S6 kinase and p34^{cdc2} kinase in Xenopus oocytes: Evidence for c-mos^{xe} dependent and independent pathways. Mol Cell Biol 10:310, 1990

144. Daar I, Paules RS, Vande Woude GF: A characterization of cytostatic factor activity from *Xenopus* eggs and c-*mos*-transformed cells. J Cell Biol *114*:329, 1991

145. Kanki JP, Donoghue DJ: Progression from meiosis I to meiosis II in *Xenopus* oocytes required *de novo* translation of the *mos*□e proto-oncogene. Proc Natl Acad Sci USA 88:5794, 1991

146. Yew N, Mellini ML, Vande Woude G: Meiotic initiation by the Mos protein in *Xenopus*. Nature 355:649, 1992

147. Sagata N, Watanabe N, Vande Woude GF, et al: The c-*mos* proto-oncogene product is a cytostatic factor responsible for meiotic arrest in vertebrate eggs. Nature 342:512, 1989

148. Gabrielli BG, Roy LM, Maller JL: Requirement for cdk2 in cytostatic factor-mediated metaphase II arrest. Science 259:1766, 1993

149. Haccard O, Sarcevic B, Lewellyn A: Induction of metaphase arrest in cleaving *Xenopus* embryos by MAP kinase. Science 262:1262, 1993

150. Daar I, Nebreda AR, Yew N, et al: The *ras* oncoprotein and M-phase activity. Science 253:74, 1991

151. Daar I, Zhou R, Shen R-L, et al: *Mos* and *Ras*: Two oncoproteins that display M-phase activity. Cold Spring Harb Symp Quant Biol 56:477, 1991

152. Zhou R, Daar IO, Ferris D, et al: pp39^{mos} is associated with p34^{cdc2} kinase in c-*mos*^{xe}-transformed NIH/3T3 cells. Mol Cell Biol *12*:3583, 1992

153. Zhou R, Oskarsson M, Paules RS, et al: Ability of the c-*mos* product to associate with and phosphorylate tubulin. Science 251:671, 1991

154. Zhou R, Schen R, Pinto da Silva P, et al: *In vitro* and *in vivo* characterization of pp39Mos association with tubulin. Cell Growth Differ 2:257, 1991

155. Bai W, Singh B, Yang Y, et al: The physical interactions between p37$^{env-mos}$ and tubulin structures. Oncogene 7:493, 1992

156. Paules RS, Buccione R, Moschel RC, et al: The mouse c-*mos* proto-oncogene product is present and functions during oogenesis. Proc Natl Acad Sci USA 86:5395, 1989

157. Albertini DF: Cytoplasmic reorganization during the resumption of meiosis in cultured preovulatory rat oocytes. Dev Biol *120*:121, 1987

158. Van Blerkom J: Microtubule mediation of cytoplasmic and nuclear maturation during the early stages of resumed meiosis in cultured mouse oocytes. Proc Natl Acad Sci USA 88:5031, 1991

159. Alfa CE, Ducommun B, Beach D, et al: Distinct nuclear and spindle pole body population of cyclin-cdc2 in fission yeast. Nature 347:680, 1990

160. Hoyt MA, Totis L, Roberts BT: *S. cerevisiae* genes required for cell cycle arrest in response to loss of microtubule function. Cell 60:507, 1991

161. Li R, Murray AW: Feedback control of mitosis in budding yeast. Cell 66:519, 1991

162. Sunkara PS, Wright DA, Rao PN: Mitotic factors from mammalian cells induce germinal vesicle breakdown and chromosome condensation in amphibian oocytes. Proc Natl Acad Sci USA 76:2799, 1979

163. Pines J: Cyclin: Wheels within wheels. Cell Growth Differ 6:305, 1991

164. Zhao X, Singh B, Batten BE: The role of the c-*mos* proto-oncogene in mammalian meiotic maturation. Oncogene 6:43, 1991

165. Posada J, Yew N, Vande Woude GF, et al: Mos activates the MAP kinase signalling pathway in *Xenopus* oocytes. Mol Cell Biol *13*:2546, 1993

166. Nebreda AR, Porras A, Santos E: p21^{ras}-induced meiotic maturation of *Xenopus* oocytes in the absence of protein synthesis: MPF activation is preceded by activation of MAP and S6 kinases. Oncogene 2:467, 1993

167. Shibuya EK, Polverino AJ, Change E, et al: Oncogenic Ras triggers the activation of 42-kDa mitogen-activated protein kinase in extracts of quiescent Xenopus oocytes. Proc Natl Acad Sci USA 89:9831, 1992

168. Gotoh Y, Nishida E, Matsuda S, et al: In vitro effects on microtubule dynamics of purified *Xenopus* M phase activated MAP kinase. Nature 349:251, 1991

169. Nishida E, Gotoh Y: Mitogen-activated protein kinase and cytoskeleton in mitogenic signal transduction. Int Rev Cytol 138:211, 1992

170. Verlhac MH, Pennart HD, Maro B, et al: MAP kinase becomes stably activated at metaphase and is associated with microtubule organizing centers during meiotic maturation of mouse oocytes. Dev Biol 158:330, 1993

171. Chackalaparampil I, Shalloway D: Altered phosphorylation and activation of pp60^{c-src} during fibroblast mitosis. Cell 52:801, 1988

172. Hunter T: Cooperation between oncogenes. Cell 64:249, 1991

173. Rong S, Segal S, Anver M, et al: Invasiveness and metastasis of NIH/3T3 cells induced by Met-HGF/SF autocrine stimulation. Proc Natl Acad Sci USA, 1994 (in press)

174. Korsmeyer ST: Bcl-2 initiates a new category of oncogenes: Regulators of cell death. Blood 80:879, 1992

175. James GL, Goldstein JL, Brown MS, et al: Benzodiazepine peptidomimetics: Potent inhibitors of Ras farnesylation in animal cells. Science 260:1937, 1993

176. Kohl NE, Mosser SD, deSolms SJ, et al: Selective inhibition of *ras*-dependent transformation by a farnesyltransferase inhibitor. Science 260:1934, 1993

2

MOLECULAR GENETICS AND CYTOGENETICS OF HEMATOPOIETIC MALIGNANCIES

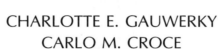

CHARLOTTE E. GAUWERKY
CARLO M. CROCE

Advances in cytogenetics, molecular biology, and biochemistry have contributed to our understanding of the role of chromosomal abnormalities in human cancer. Especially for a variety of hematologic malignancies, consistently occurring chromosomal abnormalities have been identified; such abnormalities underlie the process of oncogenesis in these tumors.

The initial cytogenetic finding was made in 1960, when Nowell and Hungerford discovered the Philadelphia chromosome (Ph′) as the chromosomal abnormality consistently associated with chronic myelogenous leukemia (CML).[1] The Philadelphia chromosome is a small marker chromosome 22, which results from a reciprocal translocation between chromosome 9 and chromosome 22 [t(9;22)(q32;q11)],[2] and which is now one of the best understood chromosomal abnormalities in molecular terms. Most human hematologic malignances exhibit nonrandom chromosomal translocations of the sort found in CML.

A second striking observation was made in 1972 by Manolov and Manolova, who described a chromosome 14q⁺, associated with 80 per cent of cases of Burkitt's lymphoma[3]; Zech et al. subsequently showed that this 14q⁺ chromosome is caused by a t(8;14)(q24;q32) translocation.[4]

Interestingly, some of these somatic genetic changes in chromosomal translocations occur near or at a protooncogene locus. For example, in Burkitt's lymphoma the c-*myc* oncogene—the human homologue of the v-*myc* on-cogene of the avian myelocytomatosis virus located at chromosome 8q24—translocates into the immunoglobulin heavy chain locus on chromosome 14q32,[5] and in CML the c-*abl* gene—which is the human homologue of the v-*abl* oncogene of the Abelson leukemia virus—is translocated from its normal position at chromosome 9q34 to chromosome 22q11 in the t(9;22) translocation.[6] For these two intensively studied neoplasms, a clear association exists between a chromosomal alteration and the location of a cellular proto-oncogene. Thus, one might conclude that malignancy in these hematopoietic tumors results from a malfunctioning oncogene and oncogene product that is overexpressed or structurally altered in tumor-specific chromosomal abnormalities.

These initial observations have provided more precise information on the molecular genetics of oncogene activation in chromosomal abnormalities for several leukemias and lymphomas. In the example of Burkitt's lymphoma, c-*myc* is juxtaposed to the immunoglobulin heavy chain locus by the t(8;14) translocation, and it becomes deregulated by its proximity to *cis*-acting elements within the immunoglobulin heavy chain (IgH) complex. Similar mechanisms of oncogene activation are found for other malignancies, such as follicular lymphomas or T-cell leukemias and lymphomas.

A different mechanism of oncogene activation is suggested for CML cases carrying a Philadelphia chromosome. In this translocation the c-*abl* oncogene is fused with the *bcr* gene, resulting in a hybrid gene that gives rise to an abnormal *bcr/abl* protein product. This abnormal fusion protein exhibits an elevated tyrosine kinase activity that is thought to play a key role in the development of this leukemia. In this example, a chromosomal translocation results in an abnormal protein product that is essential for the development of the malignant phenotype.

In this chapter, we summarize our current understanding of some of the translocations that occur in hematopoietic tumors. We discuss the molecular findings, mechanisms by which these translocations arise, and the role of oncogene activation, and we include aspects of the biochemistry of abnormal oncogene products relevant for the process of malignancy in these tumors.

LYMPHOID MALIGNANCIES

Among lymphoid malignancies, which include non-Hodgkin's lymphoma (NHL) of high-, intermediate-, and low-grade malignancy and the acute and chronic lymphoblastic and lymphocytic leukemias, the majority of cases have B-cell characteristics. Among those with B-cell features, 60 per cent carry chromosomal abnormalities that involve on one site chromosome 14q32, the locus of the immunoglobulin heavy chain.[7-9] This situation has been investigated specifically with regard to Burkitt's lymphoma,[4] chronic lymphocytic leukemia,[10] and follicular lymphoma.[11,12] However, these disorders also exhibit variant translocations with alternative chromosomal aberrations, which involve the loci for the immunoglobulin light-chain genes κ and λ at chromosome 2q11 and chromosome 22p11, respectively.[13-15] The consistent involvement of the immunoglobulin loci in these disorders is remarkable, and, in particular, the participation of the immunoglobulin heavy-chain gene in the cytogenetic abnormalities found in most of these tumors underscores the key role played by these genes in B-cell oncogenesis.

THE BURKITT'S LYMPHOMA TRANSLOCATIONS AND c-*myc*

Burkitt's lymphoma is a very aggressive neoplastic condition involving B cells that strikes children and young adults.[16] Burkitt's lymphoma—originally described by Burkitt as "a sarcoma involving the jaw of African children"—has a characteristic clinical presentation pattern that is different for African children and for North American children.[17,18] This lymphoma also continues to represent both a chemotherapeutic success story and a continuing challenge, because it currently represents a subset of NHL accounting for treatment failures.

Several differences are apparent between African children and North American children (Table 2–1). Epstein-Barr virus DNA is nearly always noted in tumor cells of African children,[19] but not in American children. The majority of the African tumors express surface IgM, and some IgG; and only a small portion are surface immunoglobulin negative.[20,21] Because of the prevalence of this tumor in central Africa, it is also called endemic Burkitt's lymphoma. In contrast, this malignancy is less common in North America and in Europe, and is termed sporadic Burkitt's lymphomas in those regions. Cell lines derived from the sporadically occurring tumors possess more surface immunoglobulin and secrete more immunoglobulin than those derived from endemic cases, suggesting that there might be differences in the genetics giving rise to these two types of Burkitt's lymphomas.[21-23] Differences in the molecular genetics in these tumors correlate with apparent differences in the clinical presentation, with African children having a very high proportion of primary jaw lesions and American children presenting nearly always with abdominal disease.[16]

Burkitt's lymphoma is one of the better understood malignancies in molecular terms. In 80 per cent of Burkitt's cases, the distal end of the long arm of chromosome 8 (q24-qter) translocates to the long arm of chromosome 14 at band q32,[5,7,8] thus displaying a t(8;14)(q24;q32) translocation. The remaining cases display variant translocations: The t(8;22)(q24;q11) or the t(2;8)(p11;q24) translocations occur in 15 per cent and 5 per cent of cases, respectively[24] (Fig. 2–1).

By using somatic cell hybridization techniques, several important genes have been shown to map precisely to the chromosomal bands involved in these translocations. The cellular proto-oncogene c-*myc* was localized to chromosome 8 band q24—the chromosomal region consistently involved in all Burkitt's lymphoma translocations.[5] This assignment of c-*myc* was confirmed by in situ hybridization studies.[25] Then, in collaboration with Riccardo Dalla-

TABLE 2–1. FEATURES OF SPORADIC AND ENDEMIC BURKITT'S LYMPHOMAS

	SPORADIC	ENDEMIC
Geographic location	Europe and North America	Central Africa
Age affected	Young adults, children	Children
Organ involvement	Abdomen, bone marrow	Jaw
Epstein-Barr virus	−	+
IgM secretor	+	−
c-*myc* rearranged	+	−
c-*myc* sequence	Decapitation	Point mutations
Recombinase-mediated translocation	−	+
Isotype switch-mediated translocation	+	−

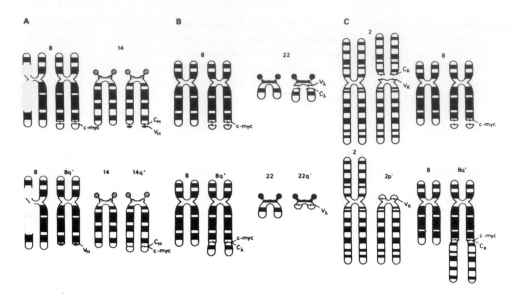

Figure 2–1. In Burkitt's lymphoma with the t(8;14) translocation, c-*myc* from chromosome 8 translocates to the heavy-chain locus (*A*), and a portion of the immunoglobulin locus (VH) is translocated to chromosome 8. In Burkitt's lymphomas with the less frequent t(8;22) (*B*) and t(2;8) (*C*) translocations, the c-*myc* oncogene remains on the involved chromosome 8, but the genes for the immunoglobulin light-chain constant regions (Cκ and Cλ) translocate to a region 3′ (distal) to the c-*myc* oncogene on the involved chromosome 8 (8q⁺). Again, with these translocations, the immunoglobulin loci are split so that sequences that encode for the variable portion of the immunoglobulin (Vκ or Vλ) remain on chromosome 2 or 22, respectively.

Favera, we found that c-*myc*—the human homologue of v-*myc*—translocates from chromosome 8q24 to chromosome 14 band q32 in Burkitt's lymphomas with the t(8;14) translocations.[8] Like all avian myelocytomatosis viruses, the avian myelocytomatosis virus oncogene v-*myc* can transform normal B cells into lymphoma cells by integrating in proximity to the normal c-*myc* homologue,[26] a phenomenon that argued for the importance of c-*myc* in the pathogenesis of human B-cell malignancy. In some cases the translocated c-*myc* gene remains intact, whereas in others it is disrupted, with only a portion of the c-*myc* gene translocated or rearranged with head-to-head orientation to one of the immunoglobulin heavy-chain region genes on chromosome 14, or is decapitated, with a loss of a portion of its 5′ end.[8,25] In the variant translocations t(8;22) and t(2;8), the c-*myc* gene does not translocate but remains intact on the involved chromosome 8q.[24]

Somatic cell hybridization techniques have been used to demonstrate that the immunoglobulin heavy-chain locus is located at chromosome 14q32—the other site involved in the majority of the Burkitt's lymphoma t(8;14) translocations.[9] In addition, the variant translocations were shown to involve the immunoglobulin light-chain loci: The λ locus was mapped to chromosome 22q11[13] and the κ locus to chromosome 2p11;[14,15] thus, the constant-region genes of the Igλ or the Igκ locus were found to translocate 3′ into the vicinity of c-*myc* to form a chromosome 8q⁺ in the t(2;8) and t(8;22) translocations[27,28] (Fig. 2–1).

Precise understanding of the organization of the trans-located chromosomes has been obtained by analyzing many Burkitt's lymphomas by cloning and sequencing the chromosomal breakpoint regions (Fig. 2–2). In this way, it was possible to localize the breakpoints of the t(8;14) translocation on chromosome 14 and on chromosome 8 precisely. Breakpoints in the IgH locus at chromosome 14q32 occur in the DH segments,[29] within the JH segments,[30,31] upstream of the Sμ region,[32–34] and within the Sμ,[35–37] Sγ,[38,39] Sα,[40] and Cγ[41] regions. For the variant translocations, the breaks may occur within the VK[28] or JK[42] segments on chromosome 2, or 5′ to Cλ on chromosome 22.[27] Thus, the chromosomal breaks, especially those on chromosome 14 but also those on chromosome 2 and on chromosome 22, are situated at sites where normal physiologic rearrangement occurs.[43]

The translocation breakpoints on chromosome 8 are also dispersed (Fig. 2–2). In Burkitt's lymphoma with the t(8;14) chromosome translocation, the breaks always leave the c-*myc* coding sequence intact. Thus, they occur far 5′ (up to 200 to 300 kb) to c-*myc*,[29,31] immediately or within the first intron of c-*myc*, when a reciprocal translocation takes place with chromosome 14.[32–34,36,37,40] However, in both types of variant translocations, the breakpoint regions are at variable distances (up to 300 kb) 3′ to the c-*myc* coding regions.[27,28,42,44]

We have mentioned the differences in endemic and sporadic Burkitt's lymphoma. Although both forms carry a t(8;14)(q24;q32) translocation, cloning and sequencing studies revealed differences at the molecular level. In en-

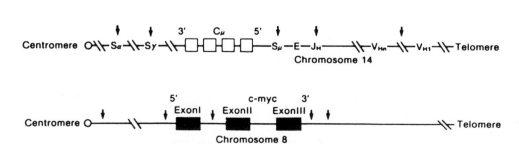

Figure 2–2. Heterogeneity of translocation breakpoints in Burkitt's lymphomas. On chromosome 14 (top), chromosome breakage has been demonstrated in the Cα, Cγ, Cμ, JH, and DH regions, as indicated by arrows. On chromosome 8 (bottom), breakpoints are 5′ to c-*myc* or within the first intron in cases carrying t(8;14) translocations. The variant translocations resulted in breakage 3′ to an intact c-*myc*.

demic Burkitt's, sequences far upstream of c-*myc* (approximately 300 kb 5' to exon 1) are involved in the translocation and join into the JH or DH region on chromosome 14, apparently leaving the entire c-*myc* locus "intact."[22,29,31] However, sequencing data of the c-*myc* exons and introns showed that around 60 per cent of those cases have characteristic point mutations in the 5' flanking region, in the first exon, and in the first intron of c-*myc*. It was soon noted that the Pvull site of exon 1 is especially subject to these somatic mutations.[23,41] These alterations may alter c-*myc* expression by blocking transcription termination or by changing promoter or coding sequences.[23,45,46] Thus, in these cases the c-*myc* gene cannot be considered as "intact," and detailed molecular studies are necessary to elucidate these sequence alterations. In contrast, in sporadic Burkitt's sequences within the 1. intron, the 1. exon and the 5' flanking region of c-*myc* participate in the translocation to chromosome 14, and join into the switch or constant region of the immunoglobulin heavy-chain locus.[40,41]

Molecular and cellular biology aspects of the c-*myc* gene have been reviewed elsewhere,[47–49] and only the most important features of c-*myc* as they influence the process of malignancy in leukemias and lymphomas should be mentioned. The normal human c-*myc* gene is formed by three exons, which are separated by two short introns (Fig. 2–3). The first exon cannot be translated, because it contains termination condons in all three reading frames and it represents an untranslated leader sequence.[50,51] At the beginning of the second exon, there is the first ATG (methionine) signal for protein synthesis. There is a single open reading frame involving the second and the third exon, which encodes for a protein of 439 amino acids and a molecular mass of 48,312 Da.[51] The c-*myc* protein becomes phosphorylated and is localized to the cell nucleus,[48] and has been shown to be functionally involved in DNA synthesis.[52]

Under normal physiologic conditions, c-*myc* transcription occurs from two promoters, designated P1 and P2, that initiate transcription of distinct mRNAs estimated as 2200 (P2) or 2400 (P1) nt in length.[53] Recognition sites for negative and positive control elements are clustered at the 5' end of c-*myc*, in the first exon, and in the first intron.[54–56] Another level of control occurs at the posttranscriptional levels. c-*myc* mRNA transcripts are unstable, with a half-life of around 10 minutes.[57] Because the c-*myc* mRNA rates are high in resting fibroblasts, and because there is no significant change after growth factor stimulation, it is thought that alterations of the mRNA level are modulated at the posttranscriptional level.[58]

Studies on the function of c-*myc* have included investigations of c-*myc* expression in normal tissue and in leukemias, lymphomas, and solid tumors.[59–61] It was soon noticed that c-*myc* expression can be modulated by various growth stimuli in normal cells. That is, within hours the expression of c-*myc* can be induced in lymphocytes by polysaccharide or concanavalin A, and in fibroblasts by platelet-derived growth factor (PDGF);[60–62] in the latter system, the requirement for PDGF to obtain competence for cell division can be abrogated by the introduction of c-*myc* expressing DNA constructs.[62] Thus, cells stimulated to divide show a transient increase in c-*myc* expression that correlates with transition from the G_0 to G_1 phase of the cell cycle.[48]

Elevated levels of c-*myc* expression and increased proliferation rates are characteristic findings in tumor cells.[61] Although we do not know the mechanisms of c-*myc* activation for many of them, for those acute lymphoblastic leukemias and lymphomas with translocations involving c-*myc* and the immunoglobulin loci, these rearrangements cause elevated transcription of c-*myc*.

When c-*myc* at chromosome 8 band q24 becomes involved in a chromosomal translocation either in the first intron or in the first exon, new cryptic promoters become activated within the first intron. Because the coding region of c-*myc* stays intact in almost all Burkitt's lymphomas, the c-*myc* protein is unaffected in those chromosomal translocations. However, as a result of the translocation, c-*myc* is transcribed constitutively at high levels, similar to what is seen in proliferating normal cells.[28,30,32,39,63–67] Several hypotheses have been proposed to explain this phenomenon, such as the loss of c-*myc*'s natural promoter and positive and negative regulatory region in the 5' segment of the coding sequence, the loss of transacting control on c-*myc* expression, nucleotide changes in the coding and noncoding regions,[68] and increased stability of mRNA from translocated genes.[68,69] However, none of these hypotheses has been able to explain satisfactorily the deregulated c-*myc* expression resulting from the Burkitt's lymphoma translocation.

It is most likely that the alterations in c-*myc* regulation are due to activation of c-*myc* transcription by *cis*-acting enhancers within the immunoglobulin loci.[27,28,32] This has been confirmed by transfection experiments using constructs that contain c-*myc* plus the IgH enhancer of the Cμ segment, which in some cases of Burkitt's lymphoma is juxtaposed to c-*myc*.[32,70] Transfection with c-*myc* plus the Cμ enhancer resulted in high levels of c-*myc* transcription, whereas transfection with constructs of only the c-*myc* coding region without the 5' exon or a viral or an

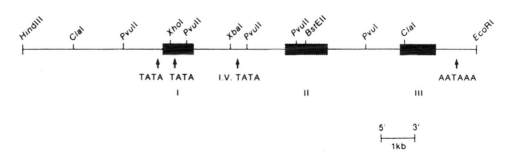

Figure 2–3. Schematic representation of the c-*myc* locus as determined by us by sequencing and S1 nuclease analysis, including approximate location of the authentic TATA boxes found by us and others. TATA box–like sequences (I.V. TATA) found within the first intron are indicated. Location of the recognition signal sequence (AATAAA) for polyadenylation also is indicated.

immunoglobulin enhancer did not result in c-*myc* transcription, suggesting that decapitation of c-*myc* per se is not sufficient to explain deregulation of c-*myc* expression. It also appears that transcription deregulation of the translocated allele requires a certain B-cell environment: Transfection of Burkitt's constructs into fibroblasts resulted in the identical level of expression for the translocated and for the normal c-*myc* alleles.

A second line of evidence is derived from somatic cell hybrid studies showing that, in all cases of Burkitt's lymphoma, the translocated allele is constitutively expressed, whereas the nontranslocated c-*myc* allele is transcriptionally silent.[63] However, it seems that expression of the translocated allele is specific to the differentiated state of the Burkitt's lymphoma cell. The translocated allele is expressed in hybrids between Burkitt's lymphoma cells and mouse myeloma cells,[71,72] in which the normal untranslocated c-*myc* gene is transcriptionally silent. The translocated c-*myc* gene of endemic Burkitt's lymphoma is deregulated in hybrids with lymphoblastoid cells, but the translocated c-*myc* gene of sporadic Burkitt's is not, suggesting that different *cis*-acting enhancer elements are involved in endemic and in sporadic Burkitt's lymphomas.[73] Thus, *cis*-acting elements within the immunoglobulin locus influence the transcription of c-*myc* in these translocations, and it is the juxtaposition of c-*myc* to such enhancers that leads to c-*myc* deregulation.

A third aspect supporting this *cis*-acting transcriptional control model of c-*myc* deregulation comes from studies using transgenic mice into which activated c-*myc* genes were introduced.[74,75] c-*myc* genes under the influence of enhancer sequences from the μ or the κ locus caused aggressive B-cell tumors in these animals,[74] whereas c-*myc* alone or in a truncated form was ineffective. In these young animals, polyclonal B-cell hyperplasia was observed prior to B-cell tumor development, suggesting that tissue-specific activation of c-*myc* in Burkitt's lymphoma also occurs through some sort of *cis*-regulated mechanism of transcriptional control.

Criticism of this hypothesis has arisen, because for many cases of Burkitt's lymphoma the immunoglobulin enhancer located in proximity to JH is placed far away from c-*myc*. The endogenous immunoglobulin heavy-chain enhancer, however, can activate tandem VH promoters separated by a large distance.[76]

MOLECULAR BIOLOGY OF AIDS-ASSOCIATED LYMPHADENOPATHY

Malignant lymphomas of the non-Hodgkin's type represent a major clinical manifestation in patients with acquired immunodeficiency syndrome (AIDS). Large series of malignant lymphomas that occur in homosexual men and that are observed during human immunodeficiency virus (HIV) infection have been reported. In a major study of 90 cases of malignant lymphoma in homosexual men, histopathology readings indicated that 70 per cent of the cases were high-grade lymphomas, mostly of the small noncleaved cell variety or showing a large-

cell immunoblastic-plasmacytoid histology, and 30 per cent were of intermediate grade, with a diffuse large-cell histology.[77] Interestingly, acute B-cell leukemias[78] and terminal deoxynucleotidyltransferase-positive pre–B-cell leukemias in patients with AIDS also have been described.[79] These AIDS-associated lymphoid malignancies share several features with Burkitt's lymphoma. Many of them occur in conjunction with the presence of Epstein-Barr virus (EBV);[80,81] they develop in a situation of severe immunosuppression, which is considered an important cofactor for the development of endemic Burkitt's lymphoma; and they often are preceded by the expansion of an oligoclonal B-cell population.[82]

AIDS-associated malignant lymphomas have been found to carry chromosomal translocation characteristics for Burkitt's lymphoma:[78,83–85] Many of them have a t(8;14)(q24;q32) translocation, but variant translocations t(2;8) or t(8;22) also have been found for some of the cases. In addition, EBV sequences could be identified for many of the cases, and also rearrangement of c-*myc*.[84,86]

We have studied the molecular genetics in AIDS-associated Burkitt's lymphoma, and we have analyzed cases with the Burkitt's-specific t(8;14) translocation and proven HIV infection. We found a molecular pattern as in endemic Burkitt's: There was rearrangement of the immunoglobulin heavy-chain locus and c-*myc* was in germline configuration, indicating that the break on chromosome 8 had occurred far 5' to c-*myc*, as in endemic Burkitt's, and then had directly involved the IgH locus on chromosome 14 in the t(8;14) translocation. Cloning of the breakpoint region of these t(8;14) translocations could show that the break had occurred nearly at the identical JH site previously described for the endemic Burkitt's lymphoma cell line P3HRI in the very 5' region of c-*myc* by the same mechanisms as in endemic Burkitt's lymphoma.[87,88]

Interestingly, other authors had investigated many cases of AIDS-associated lymphoma, and found rearrangement patterns suggesting sporadic Burkitt's with a rearranged c-*myc* gene in 11 out of 16 cases in which the c-*myc* gene had joined into the switch region of the heavy-chain locus of chromosome 14.[46,84]

In summary, AIDS-associated lymphoma might develop under conditions similar to those for Burkitt's lymphoma in conjunction with immunosuppression, in the presence of EBV and/or HIV infection. A distinctive follicular hyperplasia with polyclonal B-cell proliferation is characteristic of the prelymphomatous state, and the molecular pattern identical to that in Burkitt's translocation indicates that similar molecular mechanisms are involved.

MOLECULAR GENETICS OF FOLLICULAR LYMPHOMA: *bcl-2* AND THE t(14;18) TRANSLOCATION BREAKPOINT

The t(14;18)(q32;q21) translocation is the chromosomal abnormality consistently occurring in follicular lymphoma.[89] In about 85 per cent of cases of follicular lymphoma, the malignant cells carry the t(14;18)(q32q21) translocation—the chromosomal marker and the hallmark of the disease.

Because this translocation involves the immunoglobulin heavy-chain locus at band q32 of chromosome 14, probes from the JH region were used in molecular analysis of the DNA region joining chromosomes 14 and 18.[90-92] By screening a genomic library made from DNA of the pre-B-cell leukemia cell line 380, which contains the t(18;14) and t(14;18) translocations, two sets of clones were obtained that correspond to the translocation breakpoints from both 14q⁺ chromosomes.[90,91] One of them had joined into a locus at chromosome 18 band q21, which was designated as bcl-2 (B-cell leukemia/lymphoma 2).[90-94] DNA probes from this region were able to detect a transcriptional unit near the breakpoint at chromosome 18q21, and they were found to recognize DNA rearrangements in more than 60 per cent of cases of follicular lymphoma.

Nowadays, the bcl-2 gene is very well characterized.[95] bcl-2 is a very large gene; its final length is not known yet, but data from pulse-field electrophoresis and chromosome walking studies indicate that it might have a length of over 200 kb (Fig. 2–4). Gene structure data from Seto et al. indicate three exons for the bcl-2 gene, and they further showed that exon 1 as described by Tsujimoto is actually two exons that are separated by intron 1, which consists of only 220 nucleotides.[96] Interestingly, the murine bcl-2 genomic sequence published by Negrini et al. suggests such a conserved 220-bp intron 75 per cent homologous with the human sequence.[97]

bcl-2 has two distinct promoter regions with a TATA box plus a CAAT box for exon 2 and a GC-rich region with seven SP1 binding motifs for exon 1.[96] Also, a decanucleotide motif could be identified that has sequence homology to the immunoglobulin variable region enhancer and that most likely serves as a tissue-specific enhancer for this B cell–specific gene.[11,95,96] The bcl-2 gene is transcribed into three messages of 3.5, 5.5, and 8.5 kb[90,95] generated by differential splicing and polyadenylation. Two proteins are encoded by these transcripts: bcl-2α comprises 239 amino acids and bcl-2β has 205 amino acids; the proteins differ only at their carboxyl termini. The molecular masses are 26 kDa and 22 kDa, respectively.[95,98,99]

Investigations in our own laboratory have indicated that bcl-2 might be located on the cell membrane, and might have an associated GTP binding activity.[100] Thus, the bcl-2 protein product might function in signal transduction. As shown by subcellular fractionation studies, the bcl-2 protein is located to where it co-migrates with fractions possessing succinate dehydrogenase activity.[101,102]

We now know that bcl-2 is expressed in a variety of lymphomas with and without rearrangement of the bcl-2 locus, in B cells and in T cells, and bcl-2 expression also is modulated in response to mitogenic stimuli,[103] but a high expression is detected in follicular lymphoma cells carrying a t(14;18) translocation and a deregulated bcl-2 gene.[104] Deregulation takes place as a consequence of enhanced bcl-2 transcription.[90] It is likely that this occurs because of the abnormal proximity of the bcl-2 gene to enhancer elements within the IgH locus. Because the chromosome breakpoints all fall into the 5' end of JH segments, the IgH enhancer, which lies immediately 3' to the JH segment, is positioned close to the chromosome junction.[91,92,94,105,106] We believe that, in parallel to our investigation in Burkitt's lymphoma, the consistent transcriptional deregulation of bcl-2 in the setting of follicular lymphoma strongly argues for the oncogenic potential of bcl-2 in B cells.

Molecular probes for the bcl-2 locus have been used to study the involvement of bcl-2 in follicular lymphoma and related disorders.[94,107] In this way it was possible to identify a major breakpoint cluster region (MBCR), which is a stretch of approximately 200 nucleotides in the 3' untranslated region of exon 3, where the breaks occur for 60 per cent of patients from the United States.[94] Then, a region 13 to 20 kb 3' to the major breakpoint cluster region was identified, where breaks were found in up to 35 per cent of cases with follicular lymphoma; it was called a minor breakpoint cluster region (mbcr).[94,108] Later, a single case of follicular lymphoma was described in which the translocation breakpoint was detected close to the 5' region of exon 1 of bcl-2[105] (Fig. 2–4). Although the 5' region of bcl-2 appears to be involved in a very small number of cases of follicular lymphoma, approximately 10 per cent of the cases of chronic lymphocytic leukemia recently have been found to exhibit a ''variant'' translocation of bcl-2 involving the 5' region of exon 1 of bcl-2 and one of the immunoglobulin light-chain loci—Igλ or Igκ on chromosome 22 or on chromosome 2, respectively.[89-91] Thus, it appears that the bcl-2 gene is especially involved in low-grade B-cell malignancies, with a translocation at one of the breakpoint cluster regions of bcl-2 on one side and at an immunoglobulin locus either of the heavy-chain or light-chain type at chromosome 14q32, chromosome 2p11, or chromosome 22q11.

The molecular characterization of the breakpoint region of the t(14;18) translocation indicated that the breaks cluster within a 2000-bp stretch of bcl-2 in the 3' untranslated region of exon 3. In most cases, the J4, J5, and J6 segments of the immunoglobulin heavy-chain joining region

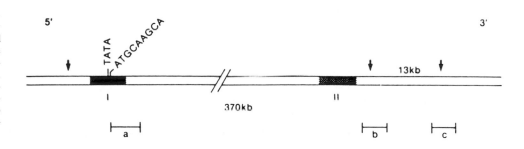

Figure 2–4. Schematic representation of the bcl-2 locus as described by us and others. Exon I/II is separated by a large intron of 370 kb from the exon I/II complex. There are two promoters in exon I/II, SPI binding sites, and a deconucleotide motif with similarity to those found in immunoglobulin variable regions. Probes used to identify the major and minor breakpoint cluster regions are indicated.

were involved close to the 5' end of each JH region, at the position, where D (diversity) segments recombine with JH DNA segments to generate a productively rearranged heavy-chain gene.[43] The consistency of this nucleotide sequence involved in this translocation therefore made it possible to design polymerase chain reaction technology for the MBCR and for the mbcr, taking advantage of the consensus sequence for the JH regions on chromosome 14.[41,109,110] This technology is of special importance in terms of identifying minimal numbers of circulating tumor cells and also of diagnosing clinically silent disease, which is characteristic of the early stages of this indolent lymphoma.[111]

Initial data of Tsujimoto and Croce[94] indicated the involvement of the MBCR in 60 per cent of a National Cancer Institute (NCI) patient group, and Lee et al.[107] reported rearrangement in 69 per cent of follicular lymphomas, 60 per cent of transformed follicular lymphomas, 40 per cent of diffuse large cell lymphomas, and 29 per cent of small noncleaved cell lymphomas. During the last several years, observations from the NCI suggest involvement of bcl-2 in around 70 per cent of follicular lymphomas. However, of some interest are ethnic-associated differences in frequency of bcl-2 gene involvement in lymphomas. Studies from Asia revealed the involvement of bcl-2 in a small number of follicular lymphomas; in China only 5 per cent of all malignant lymphomas display a follicular subtype, and only very few of those have rearrangement for bcl-2. Similar findings were reported in Japanese and Russian lymphoma patients,[112] but involvement of bcl-2 in the European population is similar to that in the United States.[113]

The physiologic role of bcl-2 is under investigation, but gene transfer experiments have shown that overproduction of the bcl-2 protein induces a growth advantage in EBV-immortalized B cells,[114] prevents apoptotic cell death in pre–B cells,[102] and increases the clonogenicity of LCL cells.[115,116]

In transgenic mice carrying a bcl-2 transgene that is controlled by the IgH enhancer, B-cell hyperplasia develops, with an accumulation of small noncycling B cells that survive well in vitro but do not show spontaneous tumor growth.[117] In c-myc mice, bcl-2 cooperates with c-myc to promote proliferation of B-cell precursors, some of which become tumorigenic. Thus, it appears that bcl-2 has an important function in B cell survival, and it increases the likelihood of B-cell tumor development.[118,119]

bcl-1 AND THE t(11;14) TRANSLOCATION IN CHRONIC LYMPHOCYTIC LEUKEMIA AND IN LYMPHOMAS OF INTERMEDIATE DIFFERENTIATION

B-cell chronic lymphocytic leukemia (CLL) is characterized by different clonal chromosomal abnormalities; one of these is the t(11;14)(q13;q32) translocation, which is found in 10 to 15 per cent of cases of CLL in this country. Other chromosomal abnormalities include a trisomy 12,[120,121] which may be found in around 17 per cent of cases and is considered a poor prognostic sign; a 14q+ chromosome found in 10 per cent of cases[10]; structural abnormalities at 11q13 or interstitial deletions involving chromosome 13q14,[122] the site of the retinoblastoma antioncogene;[123] and translocations with one breakpoint at chromosome 13q14. We also know now that there are further chromosomal translocations that are characteristic for CLL and are cytogenetically masked, but they are detectable using molecular biology techniques.[124,125] The t(11;14) translocation also has been demonstrated in multiple myeloma,[126] in plasmacytoma, in some cases of diffuse B-cell lymphoma,[127] and recently in prolymphocytic leukemia.[128] The t(11;14)(q13;q32) translocation in CLL has been intensively studied by us. It was shown to involve the IgH locus directly, and molecular cloning of the breakpoint region indicated that the 5' region of the IgH segment is involved in most of the cases.[129] We suggested that an oncogene named bcl-1 (B-cell leukemia/lymphoma 1) must be localized to the involved chromosome 11.[127] On chromosome 11q13, the translocation breakpoints appear to be clustered for most of the cases, but translocation breakpoints also have been reported to occur 27 kb,[130] 36 kb, or 67 kb telomeric from the cluster region.[131]

Recently, a gene involved in parathyroid adenomatosis (PRAD1) has been cloned. This gene maps at 11q13 and is involved in an inversion with the parathyroid hormone gene at 11p15.[132] It shows sequence homology with cyclin genes that are involved in control of the cell cycle.[133] The PRAD1 gene was found to be located close to the t(11;14) translocation breakpoint in some cases of CLL and is consistently highly expressed in B-cell malignancies carrying the t(11;14) chromosome translocation. The PRAD1 gene seems to be the bcl-1 that we have hypothesized. This gene codes for a G_1 cyclin, a protein involved in the control of cell cycle progression.

MOLECULAR GENETICS OF T-CELL LEUKEMIAS

The molecular organization of T-cell receptor genes bears remarkable similarity to that of the immunoglobulin genes. During early T-cell development, variable (V), diversity (D), and joining (J) segments rearrange to form a full variable exon, and then transcription of the variable and constant exons follows. The T-cell receptor α locus (TCR-α) is located at chromosome 14 band q11 and is most frequently involved in inversions and translocations found in T-cell leukemias and lymphomas.[134,135] Less frequent are the translocations involving chromosome 7 band q35, the location of the TCR-β locus,[136] and chromosome 7 band p13, the location of the TCR-γ locus.[137] In T-cell and B-cell leukemias, the TCR loci, like the immunoglobulin loci, are subject to abnormal recombination; and in chromosomal abnormalities they promote tissue-specific expression of genes translocated nearby[138] (Fig. 2–5).

The t(8;14)(q24;q11) translocation is one of the best understood T-cell–specific translocations. In this translocation, the c-*myc* gene joins with the TCR-α/δ locus on chromosome 14.[139–143] Somatic cell hybridization studies indicated that the translocation interrupts the TCR-α locus in the Jα region on one side, and involves the 3' sequences of the c-*myc* locus on the other side of the translocation.[140,143] These data were confirmed by other investigators by molecularly cloning breakpoint regions from different leukemia cell lines.[139,141,142] In all cases, the analyzed chromosomal break occurs 3' to the intact c-*myc* gene, and nucleotide sequence analysis indicated that the region 3' to c-*myc* had joined to a TCR Jα segment.[139] Interestingly, hybrids carrying the translocated c-*myc* gene expressed it inappropriately in a manner previously shown for Burkitt's lymphoma. These studies strengthen the analogy between chromosome translocations in T cells and in B cells by demonstrating that the TCR loci may function to translocate and activate oncogenes.

Another important T-cell–specific chromosomal aberration involves chromosome 14q32, the location of the IgH gene. Such T-cell neoplasms carry either the inv[14] (q11;q32) inversion or a t(14;14)(q11;q32) chromosomal translocation. In these inversions, the TCR-α gene joins into the IgH locus, resulting in a chimeric gene.[144–146] Interestingly, in these tumors IgH loci recombine with TCR loci, and it is not surprising that a small fraction of T and B cells rearrange both their immunoglobulin and TCR genes, and express those genes on the cell surface at some stage early in T-cell or B-cell differentiation by using the same enzymes, which are involved in both processes of recombination.[146–149] This locus at chromosome 14q32 also is involved in the t(7;14) translocation found in ataxia-telangiectasia, and involves the TCR-γ/β locus at chromosome 7q35 or the TCR-δ locus at 7p13.[150–155] Our investigations suggest that these inversions involving either the TCR-α, TCR-β, or TCR-γ locus activate a region, termed *tcl-1*, at chromosome 14q32, which is proximal to the IgH locus[152] (Fig. 2–5).

Chromosome 10 band q24 harbors the *tcl-3* locus, renamed *hox*11, which involved in the t(10;14)(q24;q11) translocation found in 5 to 10 per cent of all T-cell leukemias and high-grade T-cell lymphomas[156,157] (Fig. 2–5). On chromosome 14, this translocation splits the TCR-δ locus, which is located within the TCR-α locus between the cα and vα segments;[158–160] on chromosome 10, the break occurs distal to the terminal deoxynucleotidyltransferase gene.[158] Because breaks were found to cluster within a 0.5-kb chromosomal region, a polymerase chain

reaction could be designed as a valuable diagnostic tool for patients with this T-cell malignancy.[161] Then, DNA probes from the breakpoint region on chromosome 10 were able to identify a gene—*hox*11—that encodes 330 amino acids of a new homeobox protein, and has been demonstrated to be a candidate for the *tcl-3* gene. *hox*11 possesses similarity to the murine *hox* gene and is remarkable glycine rich. *hox*11 is expressed in the liver, but not in the thymus or T cells; however, it is deregulated in the t(10;14) translocation in acute T-cell leukemias, where it may act as an oncogene.[162]

In association with the TCR-δ locus from chromosome 14q11, a gene—the rhombotin gene or *tgl*—was found at the site of a rare translocation in T-cell acute lymphoblastic leukemia (T-ALL), the t(11;14)(p15;q11) translocation.[163] The rhombotin gene encodes a protein that is highly conserved among the human, mouse, and fly, and possesses a cystein-rich domain—the LIM domain—present in some transcription regulators. Two genes with homology to rhombotin have been characterized. One of them is located at chromosome 11p13 at the site of the break of the more frequent t(11;14)(p13;q11) translocation found in 10 to 15 per cent of cases of T-ALL.[164] On chromosome 14 breaks occur within the TCR-δ locus, and on chromosome 11p13 they cluster within a 25-kb region.[165,166] The LIM domain gene involved in this translocation was called *rhom 2* and possesses 50 per cent homology to rhombotin. It is located 26 kb telomeric to the breakpoint cluster region and starts at an HTF region, which is about 8 kb from the nearest translocation breakpoint. *rhom 2* is expressed in a number of tissues, including the brain in the adult mouse, but interestingly not in the thymus.[163] Apparently, *rhom 2* represents a putative oncogene at 11p13, for which we previously had proposed the name *tcl-2*, involved in T-cell leukemias (Fig. 2–5).

Chromosome 1 band p32 abnormalities are described to occur in acute T-cell leukemias,[157] in human cutaneous malignant melanoma,[167] and in human neuroblastoma.[168] The *tcl-5/SCL/TAL* gene (T-cell leukemia/lymphomas/stem cell leukemia/T-cell acute leukemia) located at chromosome 1p32 was recently cloned and analyzed by us and others from the t(1;14)(p32;q11) translocation found in certain cases of T-cell leukemias and also T-cell leukemia cell lines,[170] and in several melanoma cell lines[167] (Fig. 2–5).

We and Begley et al. have used the T-cell leukemia cell line DU528 to clone the t(1;14) translocation break-

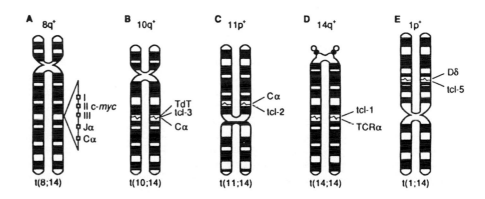

Figure 2–5. Translocations commonly observed in various T-cell leukemias and lymphomas. *A*, The t(8;14)(q24;q11) translocation; we have cloned the breakpoint from this tumor and demonstrated the juxtaposition of sequences 3' to c-*myc* and the TCR Jα segment. The locations of putative T-cell oncogenes are illustrated.

point.[168,169] Sequence analysis of the breakpoint regions shows involvement of the TCR-δ locus (Dδ2) at chromosome 14q11, and DNA fragments from the joining region at chromosome 1p32 were able to identify a transcript of 5 kb.[168] All translocation breakpoints at chromosome 1 that have been cloned so far were found to accumulate within a 10-kb distance, thus suggesting a breakpoint cluster region at 1p32 for the tcl-5 locus.

The cDNA of the tcl-5 gene sequence suggests a protein with a helix-loop-helix binding motif that has 80 per cent homology to those found for other genes, such as lyl-1.[169–172] tcl-5, like lyl-1, is expressed at the early stages of hematopoietic cell differentiation.[170,171] It encodes for two distinct proteins with molecular masses of 37 and 41 kDa that could be precipitated by antibodies to tcl-5–derived specific peptides.[172]

MECHANISMS OF CHROMOSOMAL TRANSLOCATIONS IN B- AND T-CELL NEOPLASIA

For B- and T-cell malignancies, similar mechanisms exist that lead to oncogene deregulation. Within the immunoglobulin and TCR loci, the sites of physiologic rearrangement become subject to abnormal chromosomal breakage, resulting in malignancy. Thus, during early B- or T-cell development, the normal process of genetic recombination takes place and confers a genetic predisposition for translocations in these lymphocytes.[22]

Breaks within switch regions of the immunoglobulin locus at chromosome 14 were described for sporadic Burkitt's lymphoma[35–37] and for mouse plasmacytoma.[173,174] Immunoglobulin switch regions are characterized by switch-like repeat units,[43] which represent motifs of oligonucleotides with a typical base pair pattern. Because similar oligonucleotide units are found for the involved portion of c-myc, it seems possible that these translocations have occurred because of mistakes in the function of enzymes that normally catalyze immunoglobulin isotype switching.

For endemic Burkitt's lymphoma with the t(8;14) translocation, the breakpoints occur far from c-myc, and the breakpoint region displays a DNA sequence pattern as we described for the t(14;18) translocation in follicular lymphoma[106] or the t(11;14) translocation in CLL.[129] In endemic Burkitt's, the translocations involve the DH regions,[29] the JH segments,[31] and, in the variant translocations, the VK[28] and JK[42] segments. The other B-cell tumors (follicular lymphoma and CLL) exhibit clustering at the 5' ends of JH segments at the position where D (diversity) segments recombine with JH DNA segments to generate a productively rearranged heavy-chain gene.[43]

Cloning and sequencing data of the breakpoint region have implicated the involvement of the V-D-J recombinase system in these translocations. The breakpoints exhibit V regions, which are short stretches of nucleotides associated with the operation of terminal transferase, the presence of heptamer-nonamer motifs near DH, or the 5' region of J segments—all of these are hallmarks for en-

zymes involved in recombination and functioning during V-D-J to V-J joining. Thus, the translocations of endemic Burkitt's lymphoma, follicular lymphoma, and CLL result from mistakes in V-D-J or V-J joining (Fig. 2–6).

T cells use the same enzyme system involved in V-D-J joining in order to rearrange their TCR genes.[147] Studies of the t(8;14)(q24;q11), the t(10;14),[159] the t(11;14),[175] and the t(1;14)[168] translocations revealed features of breakpoint sequence that are identical to those described for the B-cell recombinase-mediated translocation.[175] Thus, the mechanisms giving rise to T-lymphocyte chromosomal abnormalities are functionally identical to those in B cells.

MOLECULAR BIOLOGY AND BIOCHEMICAL CONSEQUENCES OF THE PHILADELPHIA CHROMOSOME: THE t(9;22) TRANSLOCATION

The Philadelphia chromosome is the cytogenetic marker of chronic myelogenous leukemia (CML), a chronic myeloproliferative disorder that is characterized by an excessive proliferation of abnormal bone marrow stem cells. The initial or chronic phase of the disease is represented by an overproduction of neoplastic myeloid elements. Then, after several months to several years, the disease progresses into the accelerated phase, which finally develops into the terminal phase of the disease, the blastic crisis, with an accumulation of cells from a single lineage—usually of an immature myeloid or a pre–B lymphoid cell type.[16] The Ph' chromosome was the first chromosomal abnormality understood to be associated with a specific malignant disease.[1] It is a small marker chromosome 22 that is the result of a reciprocal t(9;22)(q34;q11) translocation.[2] This cytogenetic abnormality is detected in 95 per cent of patients with CML, in around 10 per cent of the patients with ALL, and in 5 per cent of the cases with acute myelogenous leukemia (AML).[176,177]

The first indication that the t(9;22) translocation might involve a cellular proto-oncogene came from mapping the c-abl gene to chromosone 9, and further studies showed that the c-abl gene translocates to form the Ph' chromosome 22.[6,178] The c-abl gene is the cellular homologue of the Abelson murine leukemia transforming gene v-abl. The Abelson murine leukemia virus (MULV) is a retrovirus that infects granulocytes or lymphocytes in vitro[179] and causes leukemias and lymphosarcomas in the mouse.[180] Like several other viral oncogenes, it is formed by fusion of the viral gag sequences into the 5' end of mouse c-abl sequences.[181,182] Addition of the gag sequences at the 5' end of c-abl stabilizes the 160-kDa protein, and they have been shown to explain the promiscous tyrosine kinase activity.[182–184] These polypeptide sequences added to the 5' end of the c-abl tyrosine kinase domain confer the ability to transform hematopoietic cells by activation of the kinase activity. Thus, the transforming potential of v-abl correlates with aberrations in the amino-terminal end of the protein.[185] This situation parallels the molecular changes of the c-abl organization in the chromosomal alteration in CML and Ph+ ALL (Fig. 2–7).

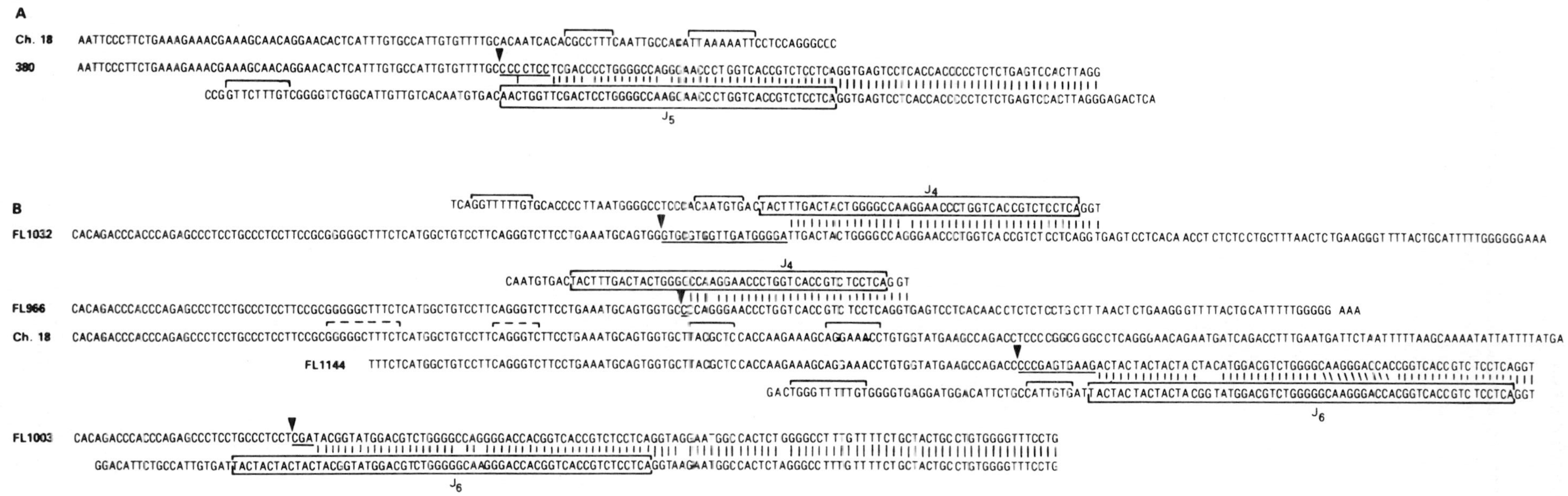

Figure 2–6. Sequences of breakpoints derived from samples carrying t(14;18) translocations. For each case, the position of the breakpoint is indicated by the arrow. Heavy chain JH segments are bracketed. Heptamer-nonamers motifs are also bracketed, and N-regions are underlined.

27

The genomic organization of the human c-*abl* locus has been studied extensively. The c-*abl* locus spans at least 230 kb, and it contains at least 11 exons (exon 1a and exon 1b). Exon 1a is 19 kb proximal to exon 2, and exon 1b is 200 kb or more proximal to exon 2.[186,187] The c-*abl* gene is transcribed into two messages of either 6 or 7 kb. The 6-kb message is derived from exons 1a through 11; the 7-kb message is derived from exon 1b through exon 11 by excluding exon 1a. An analogous situation exists for the mice that have four types of c-*abl* message with distinct first exons.[188] The c-*abl* messages share a set of 3′ exons starting from exon 2. The acceptor splice site associated with exon 2 is unusual: It can accept multiple exon donor sites, it can omit near exons in favor of those far away, and it can jump long distances. These features are important for the tumorigenicity of the gene, because they allow c-*abl* to be fused to non-*abl* sequences, as in chromosomal translocations.

In the t(9;22) translocation, the breakpoints on chromosome 9 occur 5′ to c-*abl*, and on chromosome 22 the breakpoints are clustered within a 5.8-kb region—designated as the breakpoint cluster region (*bcr*)[189] (Fig. 2–7). This DNA segment belongs to the breakpoint cluster region that has a size of at least 90 kb[190] and that is involved in the t(9;22) translocation in CML. *bcr* is one member of a family of four closely related genes distributed along chromosome 22. The *bcr* gene is transcribed as messages of 4.5 or 6.7 kb, and it is expressed ubiquitously.[186] The translational product is a 160-kDa protein, but its function is unknown.[191]

In Ph+ chromosome–positive CML with the t(9;22) translocation, the breakpoint on chromosome 22 is between exons 2 and 3 or between exons 3 and 4 of the *bcr* gene and, as a result of the reciprocal exchange, the 3′ *bcr* gene exons distal to the breakpoint within *bcr* are relocated to chromosome 9. Proximal 5′ *bcr* exons remain on chromosome 22. At the same time, c-*abl* is transferred from chromosome 9q34 to chromosome 22q11. Although only a small DNA segment is involved in rearrangement on chromosome 22, the chromosome 9 breakpoints can span over an extended region of 200 kb or more at the 5′ end of the c-*abl* gene.[192] Exons 2 through 11 are always included in the translocation, but exons 1a and 1b can be

included as well,[186] thus forming a chimeric *bcr-abl* gene on chromosome 22 (Fig. 2–7).

Then, when transcription occurs, the splice acceptor site associated with c-*abl* exon 2 can skip splice donor sites in c-*abl* exon 1a and 1b and can fuse with donor splice sites of the *bcr* gene.[187] The *bcr-abl* fusion gene gives rise to an abnormal 8.5-kb fusion transcript that is translated into a chimeric protein of 210 kDa.[193,194] Molecular variants of the *bcr-abl* p210 protein can occur as a consequence of the variability of the exact localization of the *bcr* breakpoints.[190] The p210 *bcr-abl* protein has a very high tyrosine kinase activity. The activation of the tyrosine kinase activity by the added aminoterminal sequences in p210 is directly analogous to its activation by fusion of c-*abl* to gag-encoded sequences in *abl*-MULV.

It is thought that the aminoterminal sequences of p210 encoded on chromosome 22 activate tyrosine kinase of the c-*abl*–encoded segment, and it could be that those sequences are involved in the effect of p210, especially that on hematopoietic cells. Thus, it seems likely that the tyrosine kinase activity of p210 is a major factor in the pathogenesis of CML, based on its analogy to v-abl and other activated tyrosine kinases, although there is no formal proof for this hypothesis.

The molecular basis for the Ph′ chromosome is different in Ph+ ALL.[195] These ALLs carry the same reciprocal t(9;22) translocation as in CML, but there are differences at the molecular level. Some cases of Ph+ ALL carry *bcr* rearrangements and others exhibit germline *bcr* configuration,[196,197] suggesting that different mechanisms may be involved in *abl* activation in these cells. It has been shown that the breakpoint in Ph+ ALL is located in the first intron of the *bcr* gene, and thus closer to the centromere. As a consequence, a different *bcr-abl* fusion gene is formed that results in a 7.0-kb *bcr-abl* transcript that encodes a p185 fusion protein with elevated tyrosine kinase activity.[197,198] Because these acute leukemias can be confused with CML that has progressed to the blast crisis stage with lymphoid predominance, the association of the more acute disease with the smaller *bcr-abl* protein and message should be useful diagnostically.

The similarities of these altered forms of *abl* in CML and ALL to the gag-*abl* fusion product has suggested that

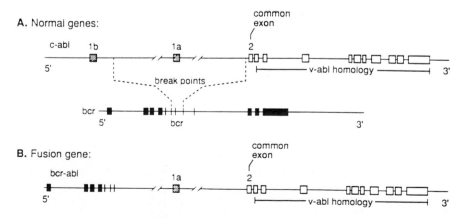

Figure 2–7. Molecular rearrangement of the Philadelphia chromosome. *A,* The germline organization of the c-*abl* and *bcr* genes. In the 3′ region of c-*abl*, there are several exons homologous to v-*abl* coding sequences. Use of one or more promoters and differential splicing of 5′ exons results in several different c-*abl* transcripts. The molecular breakpoint within c-*abl* in different Ph′ chromosomes is highly variable and occurs within the segment between the vertical dashed lines. The *bcr* locus is only partially characterized. The *bcr* (5.8-kb) region where breaks occur in all Philadelphia chromosomes is indicated. *B,* One example of a rearrangement between the *bcr* and c-*abl* genes. The fusion transcript is spliced from the small exon in the *bcr* region across the sequences transcribed from the 5′ c-*abl* exons to form a junction with the 5′ end of the common exon.

the bcr-abl fusion gene is a functional oncogene. To test this hypothesis, transfection experiments recently were carried out using bcr-abl constructs that copy for the p210 and the p185 proteins. Data indicate that the bcr-abl gene acts as a growth stimulus for murine B-hematopoietic cells; and, interestingly, the kinetics were faster for the p185 gene product than for the p210 gene product. Growth factor independence for the DA 3.15 GM-CSF dependent cell line could be generated by introducing either p185 or p210, but a fully transformed phenotype could not be obtained, suggesting that additional factors might be necessary. However, the subsequent introduction of v-myc into p210-expressing RAT-1 cells converted the cells into a fully malignant phenotype, thus indicating that the c-myc gene cooperates with bcr-abl to create fully immortalized and transformed cells, which are able to form aggressive tumors in nude mice.[199-202]

In a certain way these findings parallel the situation we have mentioned for the bcl-2 gene and its interaction with c-myc when used for experiments in transgenic mice. bcl-2, like the bcr-abl gene, is able to create some growth advantage in vitro and to cause a chronic hematologic disorder in humans, but the cooperation with other factors or with an oncogene such as c-myc is necessary to generate a fully immortalized and transformed cell type in vitro that results in the formation of an aggressive hematolymphoid malignancy when inoculated into animals.

SOMATIC MUTATIONS OF A TRANSCRIPTION FACTOR: THE t(1:19) TRANSLOCATION IN PRE–B-CELL LEUKEMIAS

The t(1;19)(q23;p13) chromosome translocation found in 30 per cent of pediatric pre–B-cell ALL cases was first described in 1978.[163,203,204] Recently, the gene E2A, which codes for a protein with the property of an immunoglobulin enhancer binding factor, was mapped to the chromosomal region 19p13.2–p13.3, the site of the nonrandom t(1;19) translocations in ALL.[205] This translocation event splits the E2A gene on chromosome 19,[205-207] and thus produces a molecular marker for this chromosomal translocation. Further molecular characterization of this translocation revealed that the E2A gene joins into the PRL gene—a homeobox gene located at chromosome 1q23—by the formation of a fusion gene.[206,207] This fusion gene has characteristics of a chimeric transcription factor, in which the DNA binding domain of E2A has been replaced by the putative DNA binding domain of the PRL gene. Using the polymerase chain reaction, identical fusion transcripts have been detected for several t(1;19)-carrying cell lines, and they appear to be a consistent phenomenon also in patients with a pre–B-ALL and a t(1;19) translocation.[206,208] Two forms of this fusion protein exist that have molecular masses of 80 and 85 kDa and that result from alternative splicing.[206,207]

The E2A gene codes for two proteins, E12 and E47, that bind the Igκ gene E box motif.[209] The E2A protein product seems to function in Igκ chain expression through a helix-loop-helix DNA binding and dimerization motif, but there are also reports indicating that it is expressed in many nonlymphoid tissues.[210-212] Probably essential is that the E2A-encoded proteins are ubiquitous components of an enhancer binding regulatory system whose specificity is determined by heterodimerization with tissue-specific proteins, resulting in sequence-specific transcription factors.

The PRL gene has features suggesting a role in regulation of gene expression. It contains a homeodomain of the sort that was first described for Drosophilia homeotic proteins[213] and that regulates the expression of developmentally important genes.[214] Thus, the PRL gene appears to be a new member of the family of homeotic genes, and apparently it functions as do sequence-specific DNA binding proteins, with a probable role in development.

In the t(1;19) translocation, the E2A effector domain joins into the PRL DNA binding site, resulting in a chimeric transcription factor. The t(1;19) translocation appears to result in transcriptional deregulation of the PRL gene: Using Northern blot analysis, expression of the nontranslocated PRL gene is not observed in a number of lymphoid cell lines[206]; also, PRL is not expressed in pre-B cells that do not carry the t(1;19) translocation. E2A, in contrast, appears to be constitutively expressed, and in the t(1;19) translocation the entire fusion gene is expressed at levels known for E2A.

Activation of PRL by E2A puts an important function onto the E2A proteins. The E2A gene contains a helix-loop-helix motif, which is consistently deleted in the t(1;19) translocation.[206,207] However, it is possible that a region with leucine residues, which could represent a leucine zipper element, or a prolin-rich region in the E2A effector domain, which is closely located to the breakpoint region in this translocation, is of more importance. Both elements could have important and new functions in transcription activation in this translocation that is deleting the helix-loop-helix motif. The t(1;19) translocation therefore can be considered as an important somatic mutation of a transcriptional activator that contributes to oncogenesis in this neoplasia.

ALL-1 AND TRANSLOCATIONS INVOLVING CHROMOSOME 11q23

The frequent involvement of the region of chromosome 11 band q23 in rearrangements seen in human ALL and AML has made this locus attractive for molecular characterization. Reciprocal translocations t(14;11)(q21;q23), t(11;19)(q23;p13), and t(1;11)(p32;q23) are found in up to 10 to 15 per cent of ALL cases. Translocations between 11q23 and chromosomal regions at 9p23, 6q27, 1p21, 2p21, 10p11, 17q23, and 19p13 are found in 5 to 6 per cent of AML cases, and interstitial deletions at 11q23 have been detected in both ALL and AML. Translocations involving 11q23 occur frequently in childhood acute leukemia and account for two thirds of the chromosome abnormalities in acute leukemia of children under 1 year of age. These leukemias, in particular those with t(4;11), are characterized by a heavy tumor load and poor prognosis, and often exhibit both lymphoblastic and myeloid/monocytoid surface markers.[215]

Because the *CD3* gene was found to map to the chromosomal band of chromosomal translocations in patients' samples and in cell lines carrying an 11q23 abnormality, a clone containing the *CD3* gene was obtained from a human YAC library. From the same YAC clone a probe was developed that by Southern blot analysis was able to detect rearrangements in leukemic cells with 11q23 abnormalities, and that could show that the breaks of cases with t(4;11) translocation cluster within a region of 8 kb. Molecular sequence analysis of the breakpoint region identified heptamer and monamer sequences, suggesting that the same mechanisms of V-D-J joining that are functional in T-cell and B-cell leukemia translocations also are involved in the mechanisms of the t(4;11) translocations.[216]

Adjacent to the breakpoint, we identified a gene with a transcript of approximately 15 kb that we termed *ALL-1*. The *ALL-1* gene is composed of at least 21 exons spanning over 100 kb of genomic DNA. It encodes 3962 amino acids, giving rise to a protein exceeding a mass of 400 kDa. Interestingly, three regions with homology to the trithorax gene of *Drosophila* could be identified containing zinc finger motifs. Therefore, it is thought that the *ALL-1* gene is a transcription factor and that it is involved in regulation of genes controlling human development and/or differention.[215]

MOLECULAR EVENTS IN TUMOR PROGRESSION

The clinical term "tumor progression" is derived from the observation that many tumors acquire over time more aggressive characteristics and more malignant behavior. Foulds pointed out that this phenomenon develops in a stepwise fashion through qualitatively different stages.[217] Nowell integrated cytogenetic aspects indicating that the stepwise events in tumor progression are accompanied by the sequential appearance of specific somatic genetic and also cytogenetic changes.[218] Thus, characteristic phenomena of tumor progression (e.g., metastasis, change in growth rate, acquisition of drug resistance) are due to changes in the genes that regulate these functions.

In terms of cytogenetic studies, evidence for sequential genetic changes during tumor evolution comes from studies of CML. As already discussed, the early and chronic phase of CML is characterized by a malignant myeloid cell population carrying a single cytogenetic alteration— the t(9;22) translocation that produces the Philadelphia chromosome. In this translocation, the c-*abl* proto-oncogene is fused with the *bcr* gene, resulting in a hybrid gene that codes for a markedly elevated tyrosine kinase activity that plays a key role in the tumorigenesis of this neoplasia. When CML progresses into the accelerated or blastic phase, additional karyotypic changes develop: a second Ph' chromosome, a trisomy 8, and an isochromosome for the long arm of chromosome 17q.[219] Abnormalities on the short arm of chromosome 17 also may include alterations

of the *p53* gene, indicating that the gene may be important in tumor progression in CML.[220] Also, the *bcr/abl* fusion product is altered de novo in Ph+ ALL. Cytogenetically, the t(9;22) translocation is indistinguishable from that in CML, but at the molecular level the breakpoint in the *bcr* gene is closer to the centromere. Thus, an altered *bcr/abl* fusion product results that has a different function than in the chronic disorders with regard to growth rate, rapid expansion of the malignant cell clone, and clinical presentations of acute leukemia.

In B-cell lymphomas, we and others were able to show that clinical progression has been associated with sequential cytogenetic changes involving genes we recently have characterized. The t(14;18) translocation involving the *bcl-2* gene occurs in the majority of the low-grade and indolent follicular lymphomas. It has been shown in several cases that, when such a lymphoma progresses to a more aggressive stage, this is associated with overgrowth by a subclone containing additional karyotypic changes (Fig. 2–8). In some cases, the additional alteration is a t(8;14) translocation we know from Burkitt's lymphoma and is responsible for the very aggressive type of the disease.[221,222] Also, circumstances may occur in which other chromosomes and genes may become associated with progression from a low-grade B-cell lymphoma carrying a t(14;18) translocation. We recently have analyzed the cytogenetic and molecular patterns in a case with very aggressive B-cell leukemia that appeared to have evolved from an earlier indolent lymphoma with a t(14;18) translocation. Molecular studies confirmed the presence of an additional translocation involving c-*myc*, and karyotype analysis showed an additional chromosomal abnormality, chromosome 17q+. In this case, c-*myc* from chromosome 8 had joined into the promoter region of a new locus *bcl-3* at chromosome 17q22. This association resulted in a high expression of c-*myc* that presumably contributed to the aggressive nature of the patient's B-cell disorder. We also found *bcl-3* highly expressed in a variety of hematopoietic lineages, but not in other cell types, suggesting that it may play an important role in the regulation of hematopoietic cells.[223]

SOLID TUMORS

Chromosomal abnormalities may be involved not only in hematopoietic malignancies but also in solid tumors. Some chromosomal rearrangements observed in solid tumors may be DNA amplification and interstitial deletions. For example, amplification of the *bcl-1* gene we have studied in CLL is also a characteristic finding in 20 per cent of breast cancer cases, as well as in squamous cell tumors of head and neck. c-*myc* amplification has been detected in a variety of solid tumors.[224–226] Deletion of genomic material usually is suggestive of a gene (tumor suppressor gene) whose loss of function is important in the pathogenesis of malignancy. Most solid malignancies carry aberrations that implicate the loss of chromosomal material. The regions that are deleted in these solid tumors harbor tumor suppressor genes. The nature of these genes is recessive, and both copies must be inactivated to initiate tumor formation. Although many tumor-specific deletions are noted, only very few have been cloned and characterized, such as the del(13)(q14q14) deletion observed in retinoblastoma, or the 11p13 deletion, which is restricted to Wilms' tumor, or the deletions at 17p and 18q in colonic cancer.

There are also certain chromosomal aberrations common to tumors of different cellular origin. For example, deletions at the 3p13–23 region have been observed in small-cell carcinoma and in adenocarcinoma of the lung, melanoma, renal cell carcinoma, and ovarian adenocarcinoma. Although no tumor suppressor gene has yet been identified in this region, a potential candidate gene *PTPG*, encoding a receptor protein with tyrosine phosphatase activity, was mapped to the region of 3q21. It is possible that *PTPG* may be a tumor suppressor gene whose functional loss is involved in the pathogenesis of solid malignancies.[227]

CONCLUSIONS THAT CAN BE DRAWN FROM CYTOGENETIC INVESTIGATIONS

Most human neoplasms carry specific chromosomal abnormalities that are specifically linked to the pathogenesis of malignancy. In B-cell malignancies, the scenarios of malignant transformation are well understood. In these cases, the neoplastic phenotype is the consequence of a reciprocal translocation involving loci of an activator gene such as the human immunoglobulin heavy-chain enhancer or *bcl-3* and, on the other side, a well-characterized proto-oncogene or a putative proto-oncogene. The

juxtaposition of an oncogene to such an activator results in their transcriptional deregulation because of their proximity to genetic elements capable of gene activation in *cis* over considerable distances. Sequence analysis of the translocation breakpoints has provided insights with regard to the molecular mechanisms involved in these translocations in B cells. It appears that the reciprocal translocations in B-cell malignancies are catalyzed by the same enzymes that are involved in physiologic immunoglobulin gene rearrangements.

Similar scenarios most likely are responsible for the neoplastic transformation in T-cell malignancies, in which the TCR-α/δ locus is directly involved in those translocations in T-cell neoplasms and is juxtaposed to proto-oncogenes or putative proto-oncogenes, leading to their transcriptional deregulation. Again, the enzyme system involved in the causation of these rearrangements is related to those of B-cell malignancies. Thus, it appears that the molecular basis of T-cell and B-cell malignancies is quite similar.

The other common mechanism of oncogene activation in leukemias and lymphomas and in sarcomas is gene fusion. Such a mechanism results in the formation of transforming chimeric genes. In addition to CMLs and Ph+ ALLs, this mechanism has been shown to be involved in pre–B-cell leukemias with the t(1;19) translocation, in promyelocytic leukemias with the t(15;17) translocation, in AMLs with the t(8;21) translocation, in acute leukemias with translocations involving 11q23, and, more recently, in a variety of sarcomas, including Ewing sarcoma, rhabdomyosarcoma, and liposarcoma. Consistent chromosomal alterations, predominantly deletions, also are involved in loss of function of tumor suppressor genes. Such alterations are quite common in carcinomas.

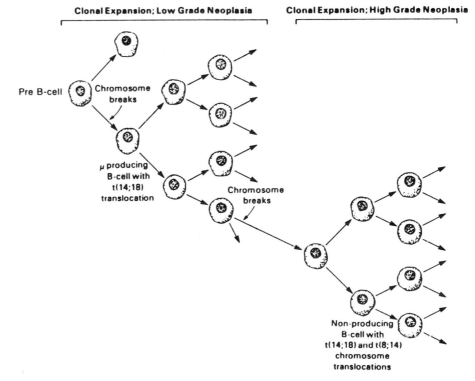

Figure 2–8. Model of tumor progression in B-cell neoplasms carrying two reciprocal translocations involving human chromosomes 14 and 18 and 8.

Thus, cytogenetic studies combined with molecular techniques have proved useful to unravel intracellular phenomena that contribute to the process of malignancy. They have shown the tremendous complexity and how much more needs to be learned in the future. We have to know the cytogenetics, and we need to identify the specific genes and the protein products that underline the process of oncogenesis. We also have to understand the mechanism of genetic instability that converts normal cells into tumor cells, or that leads to sequential genetic changes and to tumor evolution. In the future, further development of technology in molecular genetics, biochemistry, and cell biology is needed to clarify more details for the understanding of cancer, leading to an application in clinical diagnostics and a rationally designed therapy based on a molecular understanding.

REFERENCES

1. Nowell PC, Hungerford DA: A minute chromosome in human chronic granulocytic leukemia. Science 132:1497, 1960
2. Rowley GD: A new consistent chromosomal abnormality in chronic myelogenous leukemia identified by quinacrine fluorescence and giemsa staining. Nature 243:290, 1973
3. Manolov G, Manolova Y: Marker band in one chromosome 14 from Burkitt's lymphomas. Nature 237:33, 1972
4. Zech L, Haglund U, Nilsson K, Klein G: Characteristic chromosomal abnormalities in biopsies and lymphoid cell lines from patients with Burkitt's and non-Burkitt's lymphomas. Int J Cancer 17:47, 1976
5. Dalla-Favera R, Bregni M, Erikson J, et al: Human c-myc oncogene is located on the region of chromosome 8 that is translocated in Burkitt's lymphoma cells. Proc Natl Acad Sci USA 79:7824, 1982
6. Heisterkamp N, Stephenson JR, Groffen J, et al: Localization of the c-abl oncogene adjacent to a translocation breakpoint in chronic myelocytic leukemias. Nature 306:239, 1983
7. Haluska FG, Tsujimoto Y, Croce CM: Oncogene activation by chromosomal translocation in human malignancy. Annu Rev Genet 21:321, 1987
8. Croce CM, Nowell PC: Molecular basis of human B-cell neoplasia. Blood 65:1, 1985
9. Croce CM, Shander M, Martinis J, et al: Chromosomal location of the genes for human immunoglobulin heavy chains. Proc Natl Acad Sci USA 76:3416, 1979
10. Juliusson G, Oscur DG, Fitdiett M, et al: Prognostic subgroups in B-cell chronic lymphocytic leukemia defined by specific chromosomal abnormalities. N Engl J Med 323:720, 1990
11. Yunis JJ: The chromosomal basis of human neoplasia. Science 221:227, 1983
12. Yunis JJ, Frizzera G, Oken MM, et al: Multiple recurrent genomic defects in follicular lymphoma. N Engl J Med 316:79, 1987
13. Erikson J, Martinis J, Croce CM: Assignment of the genes for human λ immunoglobulin chains to chromosome 22. Nature 294:173, 1981
14. McBride OW, Hieter DA, Hollis GF, et al: Chromosomal location of human kappa and lambda immunoglobulin light chain constant region genes. J Exp Med 155:1480, 1982
15. Malcolm S, Barton P, Murphy C, et al: Localization of human immunoglobulin κ light chain variable region genes to the short arm of chromosome 2 by in situ hybridization. Proc Natl Acad Sci USA 74:4957, 1982
16. DeVita VT, Hellman S, Rosenberg SA: Cancer, Principles and Practice of Oncology. Philadelphia, JB Lippincott Company, 1983
17. Burkitt DP: The trail to a virus. In Biggs PM, DeTheg F, Payne LN (eds), Oncogenesis and Herpes Viruses. Lyon, France, International Agency for Research in Cancer, 1972, pp 345–348
18. Burkitt DP: A sarcoma involving the jaws of African children. Br J Surg 46:218, 1958
19. Klein G, Klein E: Evolution of tumors and the impact of molecular oncology. Nature 315:190, 1985
20. Gunven P, Klein G, Klein E, et al: Surface immunoglobulins on Burkitt's lymphoma biopsy cell from 91 patients. Int J Cancer 25:711, 1984
21. Benjamin D, Magrath IT, Maguire R, et al: Immunoglobulin secretion by cell lines derived from African and American undifferentiated lymphomas of Burkitt's and non-Burkitt's type. J Immunol 129:1336, 1982
22. Haluska FG, Tsujimoto Y, Croce CM: Mechanisms of chromosome translocation in B- and T-cell neoplasia. Trends Genet 3:11, 1987
23. Pelicci P, Knowles DM, Magrath I, Dalla-Favera R: Chromosomal breakpoints and structural alterations of the c-myc locus differ in endemic and sporadic forms of Burkitt's lymphoma. Proc Natl Acad Sci USA 83:2984, 1987
24. Croce CM, Nowell PC: Molecular genetics of human B-cell neoplasia. Adv Immunol 38:245, 1986
25. Taub R, Kirsch J, Morton C, et al: Translocation of the c-myc gene into the immunoglobulin heavy chain locus in human Burkitt's lymphoma and murine plasmacytoma cells. Proc Natl Acad Sci USA 79:7837, 1982
26. Hayward WS, Neel BG, Astrin SM: Activation of a cellular onc gene by promoter insertion in ALV-induced lymphoid leukosis. Nature 290:475, 1981
27. Croce CM, Thierfelder W, Erikson J, et al: Transcriptional activation of an unrearranged untranslocated c-myc oncogene by translocation of a cλ locus in Burkitt's lymphoma. Proc Natl Acad Sci USA 80:6922, 1983
28. Erikson J, Nishikura K, ar-Rushdi A, et al: Translocation of an immunoglobulin κ locus to a region 3' of an unrearranged c-myc oncogene enhances c-myc transcription. Proc Natl Acad Sci USA 80:7581, 1983
29. Haluska FG, Tsujimoto Y, Croce CM: The t(8;14) translocation of the Daudi endemic Burkitt's lymphoma occurred during immunoglobulin gene rearrangement and involved the DH region. Proc Natl Acad Sci USA 84:6835, 1987
30. Erikson J, ar-Rushdi A, Orwinga H, et al: Transcriptional activation of the translocated c-myc oncogene in Burkitt's lymphoma. Proc Natl Acad Sci USA 80:820, 1983
31. Haluska FG, Finver S, Tsujimoto Y, Croce CM: The t(8;14) chromosomal translocation occurring in B-cell malignancies results from mistakes in V-D-J joining. Nature 324:158, 1986
32. Hayday AC, Gillies SD, Saito H, et al: Activation of a translocated human c-myc gene by an enhancer in the immunoglobulin heavy-chain locus. Nature 307:334, 1984
33. Saito H, Hayday AC, Wiman K, et al: Activation of the c-myc gene by translocation: A model for translational control. Proc Natl Acad Sci USA 80:7476, 1983
34. Wiman KG, Clarkson B, Hayday AC, et al: Activation of a translocated c-myc gene: Role of structural alterations in the upstream region. Proc Natl Acad Sci USA 81:6798, 1984
35. Battey J, Maulding C, Taub R, et al: The human c-myc oncogene: Structural consequences of translocation into the IgH locus in Burkitt's lymphoma. Cell 34:779, 1983
36. Gelman EP, Psallidopoulos MC, Papas T, Dalla-Favera R: Identification of reciprocal translocation sites within the c-myc oncogene and immunoglobulin μ locus in a Burkitt's lymphoma cell line. Nature 306:799, 1983
37. Murphy W, Sarid J, Taub R, et al: A translocated human c-myc oncogene is altered in a conserved coding sequence. Proc Natl Acad Sci USA 83:2939, 1986
38. Hamlyn PH, Rabbitts TH: Translocation joins c-myc and immunoglobulin γ1 genes in a Burkitt's lymphoma revealing a third exon in the c-myc oncogene. Nature 304:135, 1983
39. Rabbitts TH, Forster A, Baer R, Hamlyn PH: Transcriptional enhancer identified where the human cμ immunoglobulin heavy chain gene is unavailable to the translocated c-myc gene in a Burkitt's lymphoma. Nature 306:806, 1983
40. Showe LC, Ballantine M, Nishikura K, et al: Cloning and sequencing of a c-myc oncogene in a Burkitt's lymphoma cell line that is translocated to a germ line alpha switch region. Mol Cell Biol 5:501, 1985

41. Gauwerky CE, Haluska FG, Tsujimoto Y, et al: Evolution of B-cell malignancy: Pre B-cell leukemia resulting from MYC activation in a B-cell neoplasm with a rearranged bcl-2 gene. Proc Natl Acad Sci USA 85:8548, 1988

42. Lipp M, Hartl P: Possible role of immunoglobulin recombination sequences in the genesis of variant t(2;8) translocations of Burkitt's lymphoma. Curr Top Microbiol Immunol 132:162, 1986

43. Tonegawa S: Somatic generation of antibody diversity. Nature 302:575, 1983

44. Sun LK, Showe LC, Croce CM: Analysis of the 3' flanking region of the human c-myc gene in lymphomas with the t(8;22) and t(2;8) chromosomal translocation. Nucleic Acids Res 14:4037, 1986

45. Bentley DL, Groudine M: Novel promoter upstream of the human c-myc gene and regulation of c-myc expression in B-cell lymphomas. Mol Cell Biol 6:3481, 1986

46. Neri A, Barriga F, Knowles DM, Different regions of the immunoglobulin heavy chain locus are involved in chromosomal translocations in distinct pathogenetic forms of Burkitt's lymphoma. Proc Natl Acad Sci USA 85:2748, 1988

47. Alt FW, DePinho R, Zimmerman K, et al: The human myc gene family. Cold Spring Harb Symp Quant Biol 51:931, 1986

48. Cole MD: The myc oncogene: Its role in transformation and differentiation. Annu Rev Genet 20:361, 1986

49. Piechaczyk M, Blanchard JM, Jeanteur P: c-myc gene regulation still holds its secret. Trends Genet 3:47, 1987

50. Watt R, Stanton LW, Morank B, et al: Nucleotide sequence of cloned cDNA of the human c-myc gene. Nature 303:725, 1983

51. Watt R, Nishikura K, Sorrentino J, et al: The structure and nucleotide sequence of the 5' end of the human c-myc gene. Proc Natl Acad Sci USA 80:6307, 1983

52. Studzinski GP, Brelvi ZS, Feldman SC, Watt RA: Participation of c myc protein in DNA synthesis of human cells. Science 234:467, 1986

53. Stewart TA, Bellve AR, Leder P: Transcription and promoter usage of the c-myc gene in normal somatic and spermatogenic cells. Science 226:707, 1984

54. Siebenlist TU, Hennighausen L, Battey J, Leder PP: Chromatin structure and protein binding in the putative regulatory region of the c-myc gene in Burkitt's lymphoma. Cell 37:381, 1984

55. Chung J, Sinn E, Reed RR, Leder P: Trans-acting elements modulate expression of the human c-myc gene in Burkitt's lymphoma cells. Proc Natl Acad Sci USA 83:7918, 1986

56. Remmers EF, Young J-Q, Marcu KB: A negative transcriptional control element located upstream of the murine c-myc gene. EMBO J 5:899, 1986

57. Dani C, Blanchard JM, Piechaczyk M, et al: Extreme instability of myc mRNA in normal and transformed human cells. Proc Natl Acad Sci USA 81:7046, 1984

58. Blanchard JM, Piechaczyk M, Dani C, et al: c-myc gene is transcribed at high rate in G0-arrested fibroblasts and is post-transcriptionally regulated in response to growth factors. Nature 317:443, 1985

59. Slamon D, de Kernion JB, Verma JM, Cline MJ: Expression of cellular oncogenes in human malignancies. Science 224:256, 1984

60. Greenberg ME, Ziff EB: Stimulation of 3T3 cells induces transcription of the c-fos proto-oncogene. Nature 311:433, 1984

61. Kelly K, Cochran B, Stiles CD, Leder P: Cell-specific regulation of the c-myc gene by lymphocyte mitogens and platelet-derived growth factor. Cell 35:603, 1983

62. Armelin HA, Armelin MCS, Kelly K, et al: Functional role for c-myc in mitogenic response to platelet-derived growth factor. Nature 310:655, 1984

63. ar-Rushdi A, Nishikura K, Erikson J, et al: Differential expression of the translocated and the untranslocated c-myc oncogene in Burkitt's lymphoma. Science 222:390, 1983

64. Bernard O, Cory S, Gerondakis S, et al: Sequence of the murine and human cellular myc oncogenes and two modes of myc transcription resulting from chromosome translocations in B-lymphoid tumors. EMBO J 2:2395, 1983

65. Leder P, Battey J, Lenoir G, et al: Translocations among antibody genes in human cancer. Science 222:7650, 1983

66. Campisi J, Gray HE, Pardee AB, et al: Cell-cycle control of c-myc but not c-ras expression is lost following chemical transformation. Cell 36:241, 1984

67. Keath EJ, Kelekar A, Cole MD: Transcriptional activation of the translocated c-myc oncogene in mouse plasmacytomas: Similar RNA levels in tumor and proliferating normal cells. Cell 37:521, 1984

68. Rabbits TH, Forster A, Hamlyn P, Baer R: Effect of somatic mutation within translocated c-myc genes in Burkitt's lymphoma. Nature 309:592, 1984

69. Rabbitts PH, Forster A, Stinson MA, Rabbits TH: Truncation of exon 1 from the c-myc gene results in prolonged c-myc mRNA stability. EMBO J 4:3727, 1985

70. Feo S, Harvey RC, Moore RCA, et al: Regulation of translocated c-myc genes transfected into plasmacytoma cells. Proc Natl Acad Sci USA 83:706, 1986

71. Richman A, Hayday A: Normal expression of a rearranged and mutated c-myc oncogene after stable transfection into fibroblasts. Science 246:494, 1989

72. Croce CM, Erikson J, ar-Rushdi A, et al: Translocated c-myc oncogene of Burkitt's lymphoma is transcribed in plasma cells and repressed in lymphoblastoid cells. Proc Natl Acad Sci USA 81:3170, 1984

73. Nishikura K, Erikson J, ar-Rushdi A, et al: The translocated c-myc oncogene of Raji Burkitt's lymphoma cells is not expressed in human lymphoblastoid cells. Proc Natl Acad Sci USA 82:2900, 1985

74. Adams JM, Harris AW, Pinkert CA, et al: The c-myc oncogene driven by immunoglobulin enhancers induces lymphoid malignancy in transgenic mice. Nature 318:533, 1985

75. Schmidt EV, Pattengale PK, Weir L, Leder P: Transgenic mice bearing the human c-myc activated by an immunoglobulin enhancer: A pre B-cell lymphoma model. Proc Natl Acad Sci USA 85:6047, 1988

76. Yancopoulos GD, Alt FW: Developmentally controlled and tissue specific expression of unrearranged VH gene segments. Cell 40:271, 1985

77. Ziegler JL, Beckstead JA, Volberding PA, et al: Non-Hodgkin's lymphoma in 90 homosexual men: Relation to generalized lymphodenapathy and the acquired immunodeficiency syndrome (AIDS). N Engl J Med 311:565, 1984

78. Richardi G, Ben-Bassat I, Berkowicz M, et al: Molecular analysis of Burkitt's leukemia in two hemophilic brothers with AIDS. Blood 70:1713, 1987

79. Ciobanu N, Andreef M, Safai B, et al: Lymphoblastic neoplasia in a homosexual patient with Kaposi's sarcoma. Ann Intern Med 78:151, 1983

80. Ziegler JL, Miner RC, Rosenbaum E, et al: Outbreak of Burkitt's-like lymphoma in homosexual men. Lancet 2:631, 1982

81. Klein G, Klein E: Evolution of tumors and the impact of molecular oncology. Nature 315:190, 1985

82. Meyer PR, Yanagihara E, Taylor CR, et al: Abnormal hyper-B cell proliferation in AIDS and related disorders with evolution of B-cell lymphoma: An immunomorphologic study of lymph node biopsies in 29 cases. Hematol Oncol 7:219, 1989

83. Chaganti RSK, Suresh C, Jhanwar SC: Specific translocations characterize Burkitt's like lymphoma of homosexual men with the acquired immunodeficiency syndrome. Blood 61:1265, 1983

84. Pelicci PG, Knowles DM, Arlin ZA, et al: Multiple monoclonal B-cell expansions and c-myc oncogene rearrangements in acquired immune deficiency syndrome related lymphoproliferative disorders. J Exp Med 164:2049, 1986

85. Petersen JM, Tubbs RR, Savage RA, et al: Small noncleaved B-cell Burkitt's-like lymphoma with chromosome t(8;14) translocation and Epstein-Barr virus nuclear-associated antigen in a homosexual man with acquired immune deficiency syndrome. Am J Med 78:141, 1985

86. Subar M, Neri A, Inghirami G, et al: Frequent c-myc oncogene activation and infrequent presence of Epstein-Barr virus genome in AIDS-associated lymphoma. Blood 72:667, 1988

87. Haluska FG, Russo G, Andreeff M, Croce CM: Molecular analysis of an AIDS-associated Burkitt's lymphoma: Near-identity with endemic cases. Curr Top Microbiol Immunol 141:76, 1988

88. Haluska FG, Russo G, Kant J, et al: Molecular resemblance of an AIDS-associated lymphoma and endemic Burkitt's lymphomas: Implications for their pathogenesis. Proc Natl Acad Sci USA 86:8907, 1989

89. Rowley JD: Identification of the constant chromosomal regions involved in human hematologic malignant disease. Science 216:749, 1983

90. Tsujimoto Y, Cossman J, Jaffe E, Croce CM: Involvement of the bcl-2 gene in follicular lymphoma. Science 228:1440, 1985

91. Tsujimoto Y, Finger LR, Yunis J, et al: Cloning of the chromosomal breakpoint of neoplastic B-cells with t(14;18) chromosome translocation. Science 226:1390, 1985

92. Cleary MC, Sklar G: Nucleotide sequence of a t(14;18) chromosomal breakpoint in follicular lymphoma and demonstration of a breakpoint cluster region near a transcriptionally active locus on chromosome 18. Proc Natl Acad Sci USA 82: 7439, 1985

93. Bakhshi A, Jensen JP, Goldman P, et al: Cloning the chromosomal breakpoint of t(14;18) human lymphomas: Clustering around JH on chromosome 14 and near a transcriptional unit on chromosome 18. Cell 41:899, 1985

94. Pegoraro L, Palumbo A, Erikson, J, et al: A t(14;18) and a t(8;14) chromosomal translocation in a cell line derived from an acute B-cell leukemia. Proc Natl Acad Sci USA 81:7166, 1984

95. Tsujimoto Y, Croce CM: Analysis of structure, transcripts and protein products of bcl-2, the gene involved in follicular lymphoma. Proc Natl Acad Sci USA 83:5214, 1986

96. Seto M, Jeager U, Hockett RD, et al: Alternative promoters and exons, somatic mutation and deregulation of the bcl-2 Ig fusion gene in lymphoma. EMBO J 7:123, 1988

97. Negrini M, Silini E, Kozak C, et al: Molecular analysis of mbcl-2: Structure and expression of the murine gene homologous to the human gene involved in follicular lymphoma. Cell 49: 455, 1987

98. Tsujimoto Y, Ikegaki N, Croce CM: Characterization of the protein product of bcl-2, the gene involved in follicular lymphoma. Oncogene 2:3, 1987

99. Chen-Levy Z, Nourse J, Cleary M: The bcl-2 candidate protooncogene product in a 24 Kb integral membrane protein highly expressed in lymphoid cell lines and lymphomas carrying the t(14;18) translocation. Mol Cell Biol 9:701, 1989

100. Haldar S, Beatty C, Tsujimoto Y, Croce CM: The bcl-2 gene encodes a novel G protein. Nature 342:195, 1989

101. Monica K, Chen-Levy Z, Cleary M: Small G proteins are expressed ubiquitously in lymphoid cells and do not correspond to bcl-2. Nature 346:184, 1990

102. Hockenberry D, Nuñez G, Milliman C, et al: Bcl-2 is an inner mitochondrial membrane protein that blocks programmed cell death. Nature 348:334, 1990

103. Reed JC, Tsujimoto Y, Alpers JD, et al: Regulation of bcl-2 proto-oncogene expression during normal human lymphocyte proliferation. Science 236:1295, 1987

104. Pezella F, Tse A, Cordell JL, et al: Expression of the bcl-2 oncogene protein is not specific for the (14;18) chromosomal translocation. Am J Pathol 137:225, 1990

105. Tsujimoto Y, Bashir M, Givol I, et al: The DNA rearrangements in human follicular lymphoma can involve the 5′ or the 3′ region of the bcl-2 gene. Proc Natl Acad Sci USA 84:1329, 1987

106. Tsujimoto Y, Gorham J, Cossman J, et al: The t(14;18) chromosome translocation involved in B-cell neoplasms result from mistakes in V-D-J joining. Science 229:1390, 1985

107. Lee MS, Blick MB, Pathak S, et al: The gene located at chromosome 18 band q21 is rearranged in uncultured diffuse lymphomas as well as follicular lymphoma. Blood 70:90, 1987

108. Cleary ML, Galleli N, Sklar, J: Detection of second t(14;18) breakpoint cluster region in human follicular lymphoma. J Exp Med 164:315, 1986

109. Crescenci M, Seto M, Herzig G, et al: Thermostable DNA polymerase chain amplification of t(14;18) chromosome breakpoints and detection of minimal residual disease. Proc Natl Acad Sci USA 85:4869, 1988

110. Lee MS, Chong KS, Cabanillas F, et al: Detection of minimal residual cell carrying the t(14;18) by DNA sequence amplification. Science 237:175, 1987

111. Smith Br, Weinberg DS, Robert NJ, et al: Circulating monoclonal B lymphocytes in non-Hodgkin's lymphoma. N Engl J Med 311:1476, 1984

112. Fleischman EW, Prigogina EC, Dynskaya GW, et al: Chromosomal characteristics of malignant lymphoma. Hum Genet 82: 343, 1989

113. Gauwerky CE, Pierotti M, Croce CM, Bcl-2 in malignant non-Hodgkin lymphoma in Italy: Involvement of major and minor breakpoint cluster regions. (submitted)

114. Tsujimoto Y: Overexpression of the human bcl-2 gene product results in growth enhancement of Epstein Barr virus immortalized B-cells. Proc Natl Acad Sci USA 86:1958, 1989

115. Nuñez G, Seto M, Seremetis S, et al: Growth- and tumor-promoting effect of deregulated bcl-2 in human lymphoblastoid cell. Proc Natl Acad Sci USA 86):4589, 1989

116. Reed J, Cuddy M, Slabiak T, et al: Oncogenic potential of bcl2 demonstrated by gene transfer. Nature 336:259, 1988

117. McDonnell JT, Deane N, Platt IM, et al: Bcl-2-immunoglobulin transgenic mice demonstrate extended B-cell survival and follicular lymphoproliferation. Cell 57:79, 1989

118. Vaux DL, Long S, Adams JM: Bcl-2 gene promotes hematopoietic cell survival and co-operates with c-myc to immortalize pre B-cell Nature 335:440, 1988

119. Strasso A, Harris AW, Bath ML, Cory S: Novel primitive lymphoid tumors induced in transgenic mice by cooperation between myc and bcl-2. Nature 348:331, 1990

120. Julisson G, Gahrton G: Chromosomal aberrations in B-cell chronic lymphocytic leukemia: Pathogenetic and clinical implications. Cancer Genet Cytogenet 45:143, 1990

121. Gahrton G, Robert KH, Friberg K: Cytogenetic mapping of the duplicated segment of chromosome 12 in lymphoproliferative disorders. Nature 297:513, 1982

122. Fitchett M, Griffiths MJ, Oscier DG, et al: Chromosome abnormalities involving band 13q14 in hematologic malignancies. Cancer Genet Cytogenet 24:143, 1987

123. Yunis JJ, Ramsey N: Retinoblastoma and subband deletion of chromosome 13. Am J Dis Child 132:161, 1978

124. Adachi M, Cossman J, Longo D, et al: Variant translocation of the bcl-2 gene in chronic lymphocytic leukemia. Proc Natl Acad Sci USA 86:2771, 1989

125. Adachi M, Tefferi A, Gripp PR, et al: Preferential linkage of bcl2 to immunoglobulin light chain gene in chronic lymphocytic leukemia. J Exp Med 171:559, 1990

126. Van den Berghe H, Vermaelen K, Lanwagie A, et al: High incidence of chromosome abnormalities in Ig63 myeloma. Cancer Genet Cytogenet 11:381, 1984

127. Erikson J, Finan J, Tsujimoto Y, et al: The chromosome 14 breakpoint in neoplastic B cells with the t(11;14) translocation involves the immunoglobulin heavy chain locus. Proc Natl Acad Sci USA 81:4144, 1984

128. Melo JV, Brito-Babapulle V, Foroni F, et al: Two new cell lines from B-prolymphocytic leukemia: Characterization by morphology, immunological markers, karyotype and Ig gene rearrangement. Int J Cancer 38:531, 1986

129. Tsujimoto Y, Jaffe E, Cossman J, et al: Clustering of breakpoints on chromosome 11 in human B-cell neoplasms with the t(11;14) chromosome translocation. Nature 315:340, 1985

130. Louie E, Tsujimoto Y, Huebner K, Croce CM: Molecular cloning of the chromosomal breakpoint isolated from a B-prolymphocytic leukemia patient carrying a t(11;14)(q13;q32) Am Hum Genet 41(suppl):31, 1987

131. Rabbits P, Douglas J, Fischer P, et al: Chromosome abnormalities at 11q13 in B-cell tumors. Oncogene 3:99, 1988

132. Arnold A, Kim HG, Gar RD, et al: Molecular cloning and chromosomal mapping of DNA rearranged with the parathyroid hormone gene in parathyroid adenoma. J Clin Invest 83:2034, 1989

133. Withers DA, Harvey RC, Faust JB, et al: Characterization of a candidate bcl-1 gene. Mol Cell Biol 11:4846, 1991

134. Croce CM, Isobe M, Palumbo A, et al: Gene for α-chain of human T-cell receptor: Location on chromosome 14 region involved in T-cell neoplasms. Science 227:1044, 1985

135. Collins MKL, Goodfellow PN, Spurr NK, et al: The human Tcell receptor α-chain gene maps to chromosome 14. Nature 314: 273, 1985

136. Isobe M, Erikson J, Emanuel BS, et al: Location of gene for β subunit of human T-cell receptor at band 7q35, a region prone to rearrangements in T-cells. Science 228:580, 1985

137. Murre C, Waldmann RA, Morton CC, et al: Human γ-chain genes are rearranged in leukemic T-cells and map to the short arm of chromosome 7. Nature 316:549, 1985

138. Minden MD, Mak TW: The structure of the T-cell antigen receptor genes in normal and malignant T-cells. Blood 68:327, 1986

139. Finger LR, Harvey RC, Moore RCA, et al: A common mechanism of chromosomal translocation in T- and B-cell neoplasia. Science 234:982, 1986

140. Erikson J, Finger L, Sun L, et al: Deregulation of c-myc by translocation of the T-cell receptor in T-cell leukemias. Science 232:884, 1986

141. Mathieu-Mabul D, Canbet JF, Bernheim A, et al: Molecular cloning of a DNA fragment from human chromosome 14(14q11) involved in T-cell malignancies. EMBO J 4:3427, 1985

142. McKeithan T, Shima EA, LeBeau MM, et al: Molecular cloning of the breakpoint junction of a human chromosomal 8;14 translocation involving the T-cell receptor α-chain gene and sequences on the 3' side of myc. Proc Natl Acad Sci USA 83:6636, 1986

143. Shima EA, LeBeau MM, McKeithan TW, et al: Gene encoding the α chain of the T-cell receptor is moved immediately downstream of c-myc in a chromosomal 8;14 translocation in a cell line from a human T-cell leukemia. Proc Natl Acad Sci USA 83:3439, 1986

144. Baer R, Chen KC, Smith SD, Rabbitts TH: Fusion of an immunoglobulin variable gene and a T-cell receptor constant gene in the chromosome 14 inversion with T-cell fusions. Cell 43:705, 1985

145. Denny CT, Yoshikai Y, Mak TW, et al: A chromosome 14 inversion in a T-cell lymphoma is caused by site specific recombination between immunoglobulin and T-cell receptor loci. Nature 320:549, 1986

146. Towa A, Hozumi N, Minden, et al: Rearrangement of the T-cell receptor β chain gene in non T-cell non-B-cell acute lymphoblastic leukemia of childhood. N Engl J Med 312:1393, 1985

147. Yancopoulos GD, Blackwell TU, Suh H, et al: Induced T-cell receptor variable region gene segments recombine in pre-B cells: Evidence that B- and T-cells use a common recombinase. Cell 44:251, 1986

148. Steon MH, Lipkowitz S, Aurias A, et al: Inversion of chromosome 7 in ataxia telangiectasia is generated by a rearrangement between T-cell receptor β and T-cell receptor γ genes. Blood 74:2076, 1989

149. Tycko B, Palmer JD, Sklar J: T-cell receptor gene trans-rearrangements: Chimeric γ/δ genes in normal lymphoid tissues. Science 245:1242, 1987

150. Mengle-Gaw L, Albertson DG, Sherrington PD, Rabbitts TH: Analysis of a T-cell tumor specific breakpoint cluster at human chromosome 14q32. Proc Natl Acad Sci USA 85:9171, 1988

151. Russo G, Isobe M, Gatti R, et al: Molecular analysis of a t(14;14) translocation in leukemic T-cells of an ataxia telangiectasia patient. Proc Natl Acad Sci USA 86:602, 1989

152. Russo G, Isobe M, Pegoraro L, et al: Molecular analysis of a t(7;14)(q35;q32) chromosome translocation in a T-cell leukemia of a patient with ataxia telangiectasia. Cell 53:137, 1988

153. Mengle-Gaw L, Willard HF, Smith CIE, et al: Human T-cell tumors containing chromosome 14 inversions or translocation with breakpoints proximal to immunoglobulin joining region at 14q32. EMBO J 6:2273, 1987

154. Baer R, Heppel A, Taylor AMR, et al: The breakpoint of an inversion chromosome 14 is a T-cell leukemia: Sequences downstream of the immunoglobulin heavy chain locus are implicated in tumorigenesis. Proc Natl Acad Sci USA 84:9069, 1987

155. Bertness VL, Felix CA, McBride OW, et al: Characterization of the breakpoint of a t(14;14)(q11.2;q32) from the leukemic cells of a patient with T-cell acute lymphoblastic leukemia. Cancer Genet Cytogenet 44:47, 1990

156. Hecht F, Morgan R, Hecht BKM, Smith SD: Common region on

157. Raimondi S, Behm FG, Roberson PK, et al: Cytogenetics of childhood T-cell leukemia. Blood 72:1560, 1988

158. Kagan J, Finan J, Letofsky J, et al: α-chain locus of the T-cell antigen receptor is involved in the t(10;14) chromosome translocation of T-cell acute lymphocytic leukemia. Proc Natl Acad Sci USA 84:4543, 1987

159. Kagan J, Finger LR, Letofsky J, et al: Clustering of breakpoints on chromosome 10 in acute T-cell leukemias with the t(10;14) chromosome translocations. Proc Natl Acad Sci USA 86:4161, 1989

160. Zutter M, Hockett RD, Roberts CWM, et al: The t(10;14)(q24;q11) of T-cell acute lymphoblastic leukemia juxtaposes the δ T-cell receptor with tcl-3, a conserved and activated locus at 10q24. Proc Natl Acad Sci USA 87:3161, 1990

161. Kagan J, Finger LR, Besa E, Croce CM: Detection of minimal residual disease in leukemic patients with the t(10;14)(q24;q11) chromosome translocation. Cancer Res 50:5240, 1990

162. Hatano M, Roberts CWM, Minden M, et al: Deregulation of a homeobox gene, HOXII, bu the t(10;14) in T cell leukemia. Science 253:79, 1991

163. Boehm T, Foroni L, Kaneko Y, et al: The rhombotin family of cysteine rich LIM domain oncogenes: Distinct members are involved in T-cell translocations to human chromosomes 11p15 and 11p13. Proc Natl Acad Sci USA 88:4367, 1991

164. Williams DL, Look AT, Melvin SL, et al: New chromosomal translocations correlate with specific immunophenotypes of childhood acute lymphoblastic leukemia. Cell 36:101, 1984

165. Boehm T, Buluwela L, Williams SD, et al: A cluster of chromosome 11p13 translocations found via distinct D-D and D-DJ rearrangements of the human T-cell receptor δ chain gene. EMBO J 7:2011, 1988

166. Foroni L, Boehm T, Lampert F, et al: Multiple methylation-free islands flank small breakpoint cluster region on 11p13 in the t(11;14)(p13q11) translocation. Genes Chromosom Cancer 1:301, 1990

167. Balaban GB, Herlyn M, Clark WM, Nowell PC: Karyotypic evolution in human malignant melanoma. Cancer Genet Cytogenet 19:113, 1986

168. Finger LR, Kagan J, Christopher G, et al: Involvement of the TCL-5 gene on human chromosome 1 in T-cell leukemia and melanoma. Proc Natl Acad Sci USA 86:5039, 1989

169. Begley CG, Aplan PD, Davey MP, et al: Chromosomal translocation in human leukemic stem-cell line disrupts the T-cell antigen receptor δ-chain diversity region and results in previously unreported fusion transcripts. Proc Natl Acad Sci USA 86:2031, 1989

170. Chen Q, Cheng JT, Tsai LH, et al: The tal gene undergoes chromosome translocation in T-cell leukemia and potentially encodes a helix-loop-helix protein. EMBO J 9:415, 1990

171. Begley CG, Aplan PD, Danning SM, et al: The gene SCL is expressed during early hematopoiesis and encodes a differentiation-related DNA binding motif. Proc Natl Acad Sci USA 86:10128, 1989

172. Mellentin SD, Smith SD, Cleary ML: lyl-1, a novel gene altered by chromosomal translocation in T-cell leukemia, codes for a protein with a helix-loop-helix DNA binding motif. Cell 58:77, 1989

173. Dunwick W, Shell B, Dery C: DNA sequences near the site of reciprocal recombination between a c-myc oncogene and an immunoglobulin switch region. Proc Natl Acad Sci USA 80:7269, 1983

174. Gerondakis S, Cory S, Adams JM: Translocation of the myc cellular oncogene to the immunoglobulin heavy chain locus in murine plasmacytomas is an imprecise reciprocal exchange. Cell 36:973, 1984

175. Boehm T, Baer R, Lavenir I, et al: The mechanism of chromosomal translocation t(11;14) involving the T-cell receptor cδ locus on human chromosome 14q11 and a transcribed region of chromosome 11p15. EMBO J 7:385, 1988

176. Rowley JD: Chromosome abnormalities in human leukemia. Annu Rev Genet 14:17, 1980

177. Look AT: The emerging genetics of acute lymphoblastic leuke-

mia: Clinical and biologic implications. Semin Oncol *12*:92, 1985

178. Bartram GR, de Klein A, Hageneijer A, et al: Translocation of c-abl oncogene correlates with the presence of a Philadelphia chromosome in chronic myelocytic leukemia. Nature *306*:277, 1983

179. Rosenberg N, Baltimore, D, Schen CD: In vitro transformation of lymphoid cells by Abelson murine leukemia virus. Proc Natl Acad Sci USA *72*:1932, 1975

180. Oliff A, Agranovsky O, McKinney MD, et al: Friend murine leukemia virus-immortalized myeloid cells are converted into tumorigenic cell lines by Abelson leukemia virus. Proc Natl Acad Sci USA *82*:3306, 1985

181. Ponticelli AS, Whitlock CA, Rosenberg N, Witte ON: In vivo tyrosine phosphorylations of the Abelson virus transforming protein are absent in its normal cellular homolog. Cell *29*:953, 1982

182. Wang J, Baltimore D: Cellular RNA homologues to the Abelson murine leukemia virus transforming gene expression and relationship to the viral sequences. Mol Cell Biol *3*:773, 1983

183. Witte ON, Rosenberg N, Paskind M, et al: Identification of an Abelson murine leukemia virus-encoded protein present in transformed fibroblast and lymphoid cell. Proc Natl Acad Sci USA *75*:2488, 1978

184. Drywes R, Hoag J, Rosenberg N, Baltimore D: Protein stabilization explains the gag requirement for transformation of lymphoid cell by Abelson murine leukemia virus. J Virol *53*:123, 1985

185. Mathy-Prevat B, Baltimore D: Specific transforming potential of oncogenes encoding protein-tyrosine kinases. EMBO J *4*:1769, 1985

186. Shtivelman E, Lipshitz B, Gale RP, Canaani E: Fused transcript of abl and bcr genes in chronic myelogenous leukemia. Nature *315*:550, 1985

187. Shtivelman E, Lipshitz B, Gale RP, et al: Alternative splicing of RNAs transcribed from human abl gene and from the bcr-abl fused gene. Cell *47*:277, 1986

188. Ben-Neriah Y, Bernardes A, Baltimore D: Alternative 5' exons in c-abl in RNA. Cell *44*:577, 1986

189. Groffen J, Stephenson JR, Heisterkamp N, et al: Philadelphia chromosome breakpoints are clustered within a limited region, bcr, on chromosome 22. Cell *36*:93, 1984

190. Heisterkamp N, Stam K, Groffen J, et al: Structural organization of the bcr gene and its role in the Ph' translocation. Nature *315*:758, 1985

191. Stam K, Heisterkamp N, Reynolds FH, Groffen J: Evidence that the Ph' gene encodes a 160,000 dalton phosphoprotein with associated kinase activity. Mol Cell Biol *7*:1955, 1987

192. Bernards A, Rubin CM, Westbrook CH, et al: The first intron in the human c-abl gene is at least 200 Kb long and is a target for translocations in chronic myelogenous leukemia. Mol Cell Biol *7*:3231, 1987

193. Kloetzer W, Kurzock R, Smith L, et al: The human cellular abl gene product in the chronic myelogenous leukemia cell line K562 has an associated tyrosine protein kinase activity. Virology *140*:230, 1985

194. Konopka JB, Watanabe SM, Witte ON: An alteration of the human c-abl protein in K562 leukemia cells unmasks associated tyrosine kinase activity. Cell *37*:1035, 1984

195. Catovsky D: Ph'-positive acute leukemia and chronic granulocytic leukemia: One or two diseases? Br J Haematol *42*:493, 1979

196. Rodenhuis S, Smets LA, Slater RM, et al: Distinguishing the Philadelphia chromosome of acute lymphoblastic leukemia from its counterpart in chronic myelogenous leukemia. N Engl J Med *313*:51, 1985

197. Kurzock R, Shtalrid M, Romero P, et al: A novel c-abl protein product in Philadelphia-positive acute lymphoblastic leukemia. Nature *325*:631, 1987

198. Walker X: Novel chimeric protein expressed in Philadelphia positive acute lymphoblastic leukemia. Nature *329*:851, 1987

199. McLaughlin J, Chianese E, Witte ON: In vitro transformation of immature hematopoietic cells by the P210 BCR/ABL oncogene product of the Philadelphia chromosome. Proc Natl Acad Sci USA *84*:6558, 1987

200. Young J, Witte ON: Selective transformation of positive lymphoid cells by the BCR/ABL oncogene expressed in long-term lymphoid and myeloid cultures. Mol Cell Biol *8*:4079, 1988

201. Lugo TG, Witte ON: The BCR/ABL oncogene transforms Rat-1 cells and co-operates with v-myc. Mol Cell Biol *9*:1263, 1989

202. McLaughlin J, Chianese E, Witte ON: Alternative forms of the BCR-ABL oncogene have quantitatively different potencies for stimulation of immature lymphoid cells. Mol Cell Biol *9*: 1866, 1989

203. Vogler LB, Crist WM, Bockman DE, et al: Pre B-cell leukemia: A new phenotype of childhood lymphoblastic leukemia. N Engl J Med *298*:872, 1978

204. Carroll AJ, Crist WM, Parunley RT, et al: Pre B-cell leukemia associated with chromosome translocation 1;19. Blood *63*:721, 1984

205. Mellentin J, Murre C, Darlon TA, et al: The gene for enhancer binding proteins E12/E47 lies at the t(1;19) breakpoint in acute leukemias. Science *246*:379, 1989

206. Nourse J, Mellentin J, Galili N, et al: Chromosomal translocation t(1;19) results in synthesis of a homeobox fusion mRNA that codes for a potential chimeric transcription factor. Cell *60*:535, 1990

207. Kamps MP, Murre C, Sun S-H, Baltimore D: A new homeobox gene contributes the DNA binding domain of the t(1;19) translocation protein in pre B-ALL. Cell *60*:547, 1990

208. Hunger S, Galili N, Carroll AJ, et al: The t(1;19)(q23p13) results in consistent fusion of E2A and PBX1 coding sequences in acute lymphoblastic leukemias. Blood *77*:687, 1991

209. Murre C, McCaw PS, Vaessin H, et al: Interactions between heterologous helix-loop-helix proteins generate complexes that bind specifically to a common DNA sequence. Cell *58*:537, 1989

210. Church GM, Ephrussi A, Gilbert W, Tonegawa S: Cell type specific contacts to immunoglobulin enhancers in nuclei. Nature *313*:798, 1985

211. Ephrussi A, Church GM, Tonegawa S, Gilbert W: B-lineage specific interactions of an immunoglobulin enhancer with cellular factors in vivo. Science *227*:134, 1985

212. Moss LG, Moss GB, Rutter WJ: Systematic binding analysis of the insulin gene transcription control region: Insulin and immunoglobulin enhancers utilize similar transactivators. Mol Cell Biol *8*:2670, 1988

213. Scott MP, Tamkun JW, Hartzell GW: The structure and function of the homeodomain. Annu Rev Biol *3*:345, 1987

214. Gehring WJ: Homeo boxes in the study of development. Science *236*:1245, 1987

215. Gu Y, Nakamura T, Alder H, et al: The t(4:11) chromosome translocation of human acute leukemias fuses the ALL-1 gene, related Drosophila trithorax, to the AF-4 gene. Cell *71*:701, 1992

216. Gu Y, Cimino G, Alder H, et al: The t(4:11) (q21;q23) chromosome translocations in acute leukemia involve the VDJ recombinase. Proc Natl Acad Sci USA *89*:10464, 1992

217. Foulds L: Tumor progression. Cancer Res *17*:355, 1957

218. Nowell PC: The clonal evolution of tumor cell populations. Science *194*:23, 1976

219. Rowley JD: Ph-positive leukemia, including chronic myelogenous leukemia. Clin Haematol *9*:55, 1980

220. Bar-Eli M, Advani SH, et al: Alterations in the p53 gene during clonal evolution of the blast crisis of chronic myelocytic leukemia. Proc Natl Acad Sci USA *86*:6783, 1989

221. Gauwerky CE, Hoxie J, Nowell PC, et al: Pre B-cell leukemia with a t(14;18) and a t(8;14) translocation is preceded by follicular lymphoma. Oncogene *2*:431, 1988

222. de Jong D, Voetdijk KBMH, Beverstock GL, et al: Activation of the c-myc oncogene in a precursor B-cell blast crisis of follicular lymphoma, presenting as composite lymphoma. N Engl J Med *318*:1378, 1988

223. Gauwerky CE, Huebner K, Isobe M, et al: Activation of c-myc in a masked t(8;17) translocation results in an aggressive Bcell leukemia. Proc Natl Acad Sci USA *85*:8867, 1989

224. Möröy T, Mardino A, Etiemble T, et al: Rearrangement and en-

hanced expression of c-myc in hepatocellular carcinoma of hepatitis virus infected woodchucks. Nature *324*:276, 1986

225. Lammie GA, Fantl V, Schwiring E, et al: DIIS287, a putative oncogene on chromosome 11q13, is amplified and expressed in squamous cell and mammary carcinomas and linked to Bcl-1. Oncogene *6*:439, 1991

226. Rosenberg CL, Kim HG, Shows TB, et al: Rearrangement and overexpression of DIIS287E, a candidate oncogene on chromosome 11q13 in benign parathyroid tumors. Oncogene *6*: 449, 1991

227. LaForgia S, Morse B, Levy J, et al: Receptor protein-tyrosine phosphatase γ is a candidate tumor suppressor gene at human chromosome region 3p21. Proc Natl Acad Sci USA *88*:5036, 1991

3

VIRAL CARCINOGENESIS

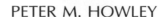

PETER M. HOWLEY

Viral carcinogenesis dates back to observations made during the early part of this century, when the transmissibility of avian leukemia was first described by Ellermann in Denmark in 1908 and the transmissibility of an avian sarcoma in chickens was described by Rous in 1911.[1,2] The importance of these findings was not appreciated at the time, and the full impact on virology and medicine was not recognized until the 1950s. Indeed, the work of Peyton Rous[2] from the first part of this century showing that cell-free extracts containing a filterable agent from a sarcoma in chickens could induce tumors in injected chickens within a few weeks finally was recognized by a Nobel prize in 1968. Rous' original work pointed out that a filterable agent (the working definition of a virus at that time) not only was capable of inducing tumors, but also was responsible for determining the phenotypic characteristics of the tumor. Because these studies were carried out in birds and not in mammals, however, this early work was consigned to the rank of avian curiosities by some.

In the 1930s, Richard Shope published a series of papers demonstrating cell-free transmission of tumors in rabbits. The first studies involved fibromatous tumors found in the footpads of wild cottontail rabbits that could be transmitted by injecting cell-free extracts in either wild or domestic rabbits.[3] Subsequent studies have shown that this virus, now referred to as the Shope fibroma virus, is a pox virus. Additional studies carried out by Shope demonstrated that cutaneous papillomatosis in wild cottontail rabbits also could be transmitted by cell-free extracts. In a number of cases, these benign papillomas would progress spontaneously into squamous cell carcinomas in infected domestic rabbits or in the infected cottontail rabbits.[4,5] In general, however, the field of viral oncology lay dormant until the early 1950s, when it was revitalized with the discovery of the murine leukemia viruses by Ludwig Gross[6] and of the mouse polyoma virus by Gross, Stewart, and Eddy.[7,8] These findings of tumor viruses in mice led many cancer researchers and virologists to the field of viral oncology. These researchers had the hope that these initial observations in mammals could be extended to humans and that some human tumors also might be found to have a viral etiology. The Special Viral Cancer Program at the National Cancer Institute grew from this intense interest in viral oncology and the hope that human tumor viruses would be identified.

Many of the most important developments in modern molecular biology derive from studies in viral oncology from the 1960s and 1970s. The discovery of reverse transcriptase, the development of recombinant DNA technology, the discovery of messenger RNA splicing, and the discovery of oncogenes and, more recently, tumor suppressor genes all derive directly from studies in viral oncology. Oncogenes first were recognized as cellular genes that had been acquired by retroviruses through recombinational processes to convert them into acute transforming RNA tumor viruses. It is now recognized that oncogenes participate in many different types of tumors and can be involved at different stages of tumorigenesis and viral oncology. This has contributed significantly to our concepts of nonviral carcinogenesis. It is likely that the direct-transforming, oncogene-transducing retroviruses do not play a major causative role in naturally occurring cancers in animals or in humans, but rather represent laboratory-generated recombinants. A list of human viruses with oncogenic properties is presented in Table 3–1. This list includes viruses such as the transforming adenoviruses, which are capable of transforming normal cells into malignant cells in the laboratory but which have not been associated with any known human tumors. The list also includes viruses such as the papillomaviruses, which have been etiologically associated with specific human cancers and which have been shown to encode transforming viral oncogenes. Finally, it includes viruses, such as the hepatitis B virus, that have been linked closely with a specific human tumor, hepatocellular carcinoma, for which the evidence of a bona fide viral oncogene is still unclear. This chapter focuses on those viruses that have been associated with specific human cancers and discusses the biology and pertinent molecular biology of these viruses. The evidence pertaining to the association of each of these viruses with specific types of human neoplasia is presented and the mechanisms by which these viruses may contribute to malignant transformation are discussed. Much of the information presented here has been updated from a previous chapter.[8a]

Also listed in Table 3–1 are co-factors that are believed to be important in the carcinogenic processes associated with each of these viruses. It is clear that none of these viruses by themselves is sufficient for the induction of the specific neoplasias with which they have been associated. Each of the viruses associated with these human cancers is thought to be involved at an early step in carcinogenesis. Additional cellular genetic events are thought to be important at the subsequent steps involved in the multistep process of malignant progression.

HUMAN RETROVIRUSES

The first tumor viruses described at the turn of the century were retroviruses: the avian leukemia virus described by Ellermann and Bang[1] and the avian sarcoma virus described by Peyton Rous.[2] Historically, the retroviruses have held a prominent place among investigators studying tumor viruses, and have provided many significant advances whose impact extends well beyond viral oncology. The retroviruses have provided us with reverse transcriptase and oncogenes, and over the past decade have been engineered into vectors that are being used in clinical trials for gene therapy. Interest in viruses as infectious tumor agents was spurred by the finding that retroviruses were associated with leukemias in mammals. The initial studies of Ludwig Gross in the 1950s established that retroviruses could cause tumors in mice.[6,7] Soon thereafter, William Jarrett discovered the feline leukemia virus (FeLV), which was capable of inducing leukemia as well as aplasia in cats.[9] This discovery was particularly important because the leukemia associated with FeLV could be communicated in the natural setting and was not limited to the laboratory. These early studies with the animal retroviruses provided a major impetus to look for human retroviruses as possible causative agents of cancer and leukemia in humans. The initial studies relied heavily on the electron microscope, looking for morphologic evidence of viral particles in blood cells from patients with blood disorders. This is because there is extensive viral replication, and retrovirus particles often were visualized easily in the retrovirus-associated leukemias in chickens, mice, and cats.[10] However, these early studies did not yield a human cancer virus.

A second strategy that was used was to look for the reverse transcriptase enzymatic activity associated with retroviruses in cells and tissues suspected of harboring a retrovirus. The Nobel Prize–winning experiments of David Baltimore and the late Howard Temin showed that retroviruses contain enzymes called reverse transcriptases that are involved in transcribing the single-stranded RNA copy of the input viral genomic RNA into DNA.[11,12] This enzymatic activity is associated with retrovirus particles and can be assayed readily from infected cells. Thus, assays for reverse transcriptase activity, which is unique to retroviruses, provided an alternative and sensitive assay for these viruses. This approach also failed to find evidence of a retrovirus associated with the common or usual human cancers or leukemias; however, almost 70 years after Peyton Rous's initial description of the avian sarcoma virus, unequivocal evidence of the first human retrovirus emerged.

TABLE 3–1. HUMAN TUMOR VIRUSES

VIRUS FAMILY	TYPE	HUMAN TUMOR	CO-FACTORS
Adenovirus	Types 2, 5, 12	None	—
Hepadnavirus	Hepatitis B	Hepatocellular carcinoma	Aflatoxin, alcohol, smoking
Herpesvirus	Epstein-Barr	Burkitt's lymphoma	Malaria
		Immunoblastic lymphoma	Immunodeficiency
		Nasopharyngeal carcinoma	Nitrosamines, HLA genotype
		? Hodgkin's disease	
Flavivirus	Hepatitis C virus	Hepatocellular carcinoma	?
Papillomaviruses	HPV-16, -18, -33, -39	Anogenital cancers and some upper airway cancers	Smoking, oral contraceptives, ? other factors
	HPV-5, -8, -17	Skin cancer	Genetic disorder, sunlight
Polyomavirus	BK, JC	?Neural tumors, ?insulinomas	—
Retroviruses	HTLV-1	Adult T-cell leukemia/ lymphoma	Uncertain
	HTLV-2	Hairy-cell leukemia	Unknown

HLA, human lymphocyte antigen; HPV, human papillomavirus; HTLV, human T-cell leukemia virus.

Human T-Cell Leukemia Virus Type I

Although there were prior claims, the first credible reports of a human retrovirus were published in 1980 and 1981 by Robert Gallo and his colleagues[13,14] and soon after by Yoshida and his colleagues in Japan.[15] These isolates were from human T-cell leukemia cell lines. The human T-cell leukemia virus type I (HTLV-1) is recognized as the etiologic agent of adult T-cell leukemia (ATL). A causal relationship between HTLV-1 and ATL initially was suggested by epidemiologic studies showing geographic clustering of ATL, a pattern that was consistent with an infectious agent.

ATL first was described by Takatsuki and his colleagues in 1977[16] before the virus was discovered; it is a malignancy of mature CD4-positive lymphocytes.[17] It is endemic in parts of Japan,[18] as well as in the Caribbean and in parts of Africa.[19,20] Clinically the tumor resembles mycosis fungoides and Sezary syndrome but is more aggressive than these other two syndromes, with a median survival from the time of diagnosis of only 3 to 4 months. In addition to the skin involvement, it affects visceral organs and there is often an associated hypercalcemia. An important contributing factor to the isolation of HTLV-1 from a leukemia cell line from the patient in the Gallo laboratory[14] was the basic research that had been carried out in that laboratory identifying the T-cell growth factor (now known as interleukin 2, or IL-2),[21] which allowed Gallo and his colleagues to maintain the human leukemic cell line in culture in the laboratory.

Serologic assays specific for HTLV-1 viral antigens revealed that virus infection is more widespread in the endemic areas than is ATL.[18] It is estimated that an HTLV-1–infected individual has about a 3 per cent lifetime risk of developing ATL. HTLV-1 infection is most marked in the southernmost islands of Japan and the Caribbean. After Japan and the Caribbean, parts of Africa appear to have the next largest reservoirs of infection. The prevalence in the United States and in Europe is low in the general population, although it is quite high among intravenous drug abusers. A preleukemic disease in the form of a chronic lymphocytosis often precedes the development of acute leukemia or lymphoma.[22] ATL usually occurs in early adulthood, and this is believed to be approximately 20 to 30 years after the initial infection in the subset of individuals who develop it.

HTLV-1 infection has been associated with a second clinical entity: HTLV-1–associated myelopathy/tropical spastic paraparesis (HAM/TSP), a chronic degenerative neurologic syndrome that primarily affects the spinal cord.[23–25] Specific risk factors that may be important in determining the development of ATL or HAM/TSP in the HTLV-1–infected individual currently are not known. Transmission, when it occurs in childhood, is usually from the mother through breast milk, and can result in ATL in the small percentage of patients seen as adults several decades later. The factors that contribute to disease progression in the few percent of HTLV-1–infected individuals who will develop ATL are not known. HAM/TSP, in contrast, usually occurs in individuals through parenteral transmission by blood transfusion or intravenous drug use, or through sexual transmission. It generally is believed that HAM/TSP primarily is the result of an autoimmune process against the central nervous system somehow initiated by the viral infection.

Human T-Cell Leukemia Virus Type II

Another human retrovirus, referred to as human T-cell leukemia virus type II (HTLV-2) initially was isolated in 1982 from a cell line established from a patient with an unusual form of hairy-cell leukemia.[26] Morphologically, the cells resemble those of a hairy-cell leukemia; however, they contain markers of a T-cell lineage, whereas most hairy-cell leukemias contain B-cell markers. HTLV-2 has not yet been found to be endemic in any specific population of humans. Its association with specific malignancies or pathologic disorders is not yet established. Although there is some serologic cross reactivity and considerable nucleic acid homology shared between HTLV-1 and HTLV-2, these two viruses are distinct.[27,28]

Human Immunodeficiency Virus

The human immunodeficiency viruses (HIV-1 and HIV-2) are retroviruses that initially were referred to as HTLVs but now are recognized to be members of a distinct subclass of retroviruses called lentiviruses.[29] Similar to HTLV-1 and HTLV-2, the HIVs also infect T4-positive cells; however, beyond that, the viruses are not closely related and do not share serologic cross reactivity. HIV-1 and HIV-2 are associated with the acquired immunodeficiency syndrome (AIDS); however, these viruses themselves do not appear to play a major direct etiologic role in any specific human tumors. Patients with AIDS do have a high incidence of specific tumors, including Kaposi's sarcoma (KS) and cancers that often are caused by specific viruses.[30] Indeed, one of the earliest diagnostic features of AIDS in homosexual males can be KS, a tumor that was regarded as extremely rare prior to the current AIDS epidemic. The etiology of KS is unclear, however, and the tumor may be due to the uncontrolled proliferation of an activated microvascular endothelial cell, which is believed to be the cell of origin in KS. KS appears to be not clonal in origin but, rather, polyclonal. The cells proliferate in response to specific cytokines such as basic fibroblast growth factor and other diffusible factors that have not yet been identified, some of which may be released by HIV-infected cells.[31] There have been attempts to identify a specific virus in KS, but to date there are no convincing candidates. The role of HIV in KS appears to be indirect, through the stimulation of endothelial cell proliferation through cytokine pathways.[32]

Other tumors often seen in AIDS patients include non-Hodgkin's lymphomas and papillomavirus-associated cancers, including perianal squamous cell carcinomas and cervical cancer. Because of the immunodeficiency in AIDS patients, viral infections are common and some of the tumors seen in these patients likely have a viral etiology. For instance, a high percentage of AIDS patients develop lymphomas, including central nervous system lymphomas. Some of these lymphomas may be accounted for in part by the emergence of B lymphocytes transformed by the Epstein-Barr virus progressing to malignancy; this is discussed later in this chapter. It is also possible that HTLV-1 may account for some lymphomas in patients with AIDS. AIDS patients often are infected by papillomaviruses and hepatitis B virus. The genital warts, anal and perianal squamous cell carcinomas, and cervical cancers seen in these patients are due to specific human papillomavirus types that also are discussed below.

Cellular Transformation HTLV-1

Epidemiologic studies have shown that about 2 to 5 per cent of individuals seropositive for HTLV-1 will develop ATL. The virus is not casually transmitted. It can be transmitted from mother to infant through the mother's milk, and in adults is transmitted through sexual contact and through contaminated blood.[33,34] The latency period between the time of infection and the development of ATL can vary from a few to as long as 40 years. The specific mechanisms through which HTLV-1 is involved in leukemogenesis are not yet known. There is some evidence to suggest that the virus's role may be direct. First, infants born in an endemic area who have been infected have the same likelihood of developing ATL if they remain in the endemic area or if they move to some other part of the world. Thus, it appears that the virus alone is sufficient to initiate a series of events that may lead to leukemia independent of subsequent environmental factors.

Second, molecular studies suggest a possible role of HTLV-1 as an etiologic agent in ATL. In the life cycle of a retrovirus, the provirus (i.e., the double-stranded DNA copy of the viral RNA genome) becomes integrated into the cellular genome at random positions. Thus, within an HTLV-1–infected cell, the provirus is integrated randomly into the host chromosome and the integration site varies from cell to cell.[35] In the leukemic cells of an ATL patient, however, the viral sequences are found integrated in the same place in each cell, although the site of integration varies from leukemia to leukemia.[36,37] This indicates that ATL is clonal and all of the leukemic cells necessarily must derive from a single cell. Furthermore, the viral infection must precede the origin of the tumor.

HTLV-1 is also a transforming virus capable of transforming normal human umbilical cord blood lymphocytes (T cells) in vitro from normal cells into immortalized precancerous cells. The mechanism by which HTLV-1 induces leukemogenesis is different from that of the other chronic leukemia retroviruses studied in animals, such as the avian leukosis virus or the murine leukemia virus (MuLV). The combination of the clonality of the tumor cells and the random nature of the integration sites of the provirus from tumor to tumor are not characteristics of the animal leukemia viruses and indicate that HTLV-1 transforms by a different mechanism. Prior to the studies of HTLV-1 transformation, two mechanisms were known by which a retrovirus could induce malignancy. The first mechanism involved the transduction of an oncogene directly by the retrovirus. Indeed, the avian sarcoma virus studied by Peyton Rous is capable of inducing tumors in chickens because it has acquired extra nucleic acids from the cellular oncogene called *src*. Retroviruses such as the avian sarcoma virus, which contain an oncogene, are themselves defective for viral replication and are considered acute transforming viruses because they give rise to a rapidly developing cancer following infection of the appropriate cell. The tumors that result from infection with an acute transforming retrovirus are not necessarily monoclonal. It should be noted that the genetic events leading to the recombination between the cellular and viral nucleic acids are rare, and that, although acute transforming retroviruses are of importance to the molecular virologist in the laboratory, they are of little or no consequence to the etiology of naturally occurring cancers either in humans or in animals.

The second mechanism by which retroviruses can cause malignancies is used by the slow-acting leukemogenic retroviruses such as FeLV and MuLV. These viruses do not contain oncogenes and induce leukemia in only a minority of the animals infected by the virus. As with the HTLV-1 leukemias, there is also a long latency between the time of viral infection and the time of tumor formation, and the tumors are clonal. The mechanism of leukemogenesis by these slow-acting animal retroviruses differs from that of HTLV-1, however. Although the provirus integrates randomly into the cellular chromosomes in infected cells, for the slow-acting leukemogenic animal retroviruses, integration occurs preferentially in the vicinity of cellular proto-oncogenes in the tumors that develop. The provirus for these viruses must integrate into a region of the cellular genome in a manner that allows the regulatory sequences of the provirus to activate a nearby oncogene to stimulate cellular proliferation. This mechanism is called promoter insertion if the proviral long terminal repeat (LTR) acts as a promoter to initiate transcription of the proto-oncogene, or enhancer insertion if the LTR acts as an enhancer to activate the expression of proto-oncogene. For the avian leukosis virus, the integration of the retrovirus occurs in the vicinity of the c-myc oncogene, resulting in the deregulation of its expression and cellular proliferation.[38]

The HTLV-1 provirus is integrated in a clonal manner in the leukemias with which it is associated; however, the integration site varies from leukemia to leukemia, suggesting that the provirus can function at a distance. Therefore, this mechanism is different from those described above for the well-studied animal retroviruses. Furthermore, the pattern of different integration sites suggests that the HTLV-1 genome encodes a factor that is critical in the early stages of leukemogenesis. The specific integration site is not critical to leukemogenesis, but the expression of a viral gene product is important. HTLV-1 and its relative HTLV-2 belong to a distinct group of retroviruses that have been referred to as *trans*-regulating retroviruses, which include the bovine leukemia virus, the biology of which is actually quite similar to that of HTLV-1 and HTLV-2.[39] This group of retroviruses differs from the chronic leukemia viruses and the acute leukemia viruses, as depicted in Figure 3–1, by the fact that they contain additional genes at the 3' end of the genome. This region originally was called the X region by Yoshida when he first described it.[40] The X region encodes *trans*-regulatory factors involved in transcriptional activation, translational control, and mRNA transport from the nucleus.[41-44] Two unique regulatory genes, *tax* and *rex,* encoded by this region have been studied particularly well.[45] The *tax* gene serves as a master key for activating transcription from the viral LTR and the *rex* gene is involved in the transport of specific viral messenger RNA species from the nucleus to the cytoplasm. The *tax* gene product acts to increase the transcriptional activity of the viral promoter in the LTR through *tax*-responsive elements (TREs).[43,46,47] These TREs turn out to be binding sites for cellular transcription factors such as CREB and NF-κB, which are activated as a consequence of their interaction with *tax.*[48-50]

In addition, the *tax* gene product has been shown to activate transcription of specific cellular genes, including the IL-2 gene and the IL-2 receptor gene.[51] It is believed that HTLV-1 may initiate the leukemogenic process through activation of specific cellular genes by *tax.* One mechanism by which HTLV-1 could induce cellular proliferation and immortalization could involve an autocrine loop through the *tax*-mediated stimulation of both IL-2 and its receptor. *Tax*-mediated activation of cellular genes also may involve paracrine mechanisms. Among the cellular genes that *tax* has been shown to activate is the granulocyte-macrophage colony-stimulating factor (GM-CSF).[52] *Tax*-stimulated GM-CSF secreted by T cells could affect T-cell growth by activating or increasing the number of macrophages that could then activate T cells through the release of additional cytokines such as IL-1. It is also possible that HTLV-1 could contribute to leukemogenesis through a direct stimulation of T cells by the virus itself or some viral structural component through

interaction with cellular receptors in a mechanism independent of the *tax* gene product.

HEPATITIS B VIRUS

Hepatitis B virus (HBV) is the cause of hepatitis B, which is a major worldwide public health problem. It is one of several human viruses associated with acute hepatitis, and also is associated with chronic hepatitis, cirrhosis, and hepatocellular carcinoma (HCC). In areas of the world such as Far East Asia and tropical Africa, where infection by HBV is endemic, approximately 10 per cent of the population are chronic carriers of HBV, and, in these areas, chronic active hepatitis and liver cirrhosis associated with HBV infection are the major causes of death. HBV has been shown by epidemiologic studies to be of major importance in the etiology of HCC.[53] In China alone, there are between 500,000 and 1 million cases of HCC per year.

HBV is a member of a group of animal viruses referred to as the hepadnaviruses (for hepatotropic DNA viruses). HBV is the only human member of this group of viruses.[54] Other members of this group include the woodchuck hepatitis virus (WHV), the Beechey ground squirrel hepatitis virus (GSHV), the Pekin duck hepatitis B virus (DHBV), and the grey heron hepatitis virus.[55-57] Other hepadnaviruses likely exist. These viruses share a similar structure and each is hepatotropic, leading to persistent viral infections of the liver. The animal hepatitis viruses have been very important contributors to our understanding of the molecular biology of these viruses. Of the hepadnaviruses, only HBV and WHV have been associated with chronic active hepatitis and HCC. A culture system for this group

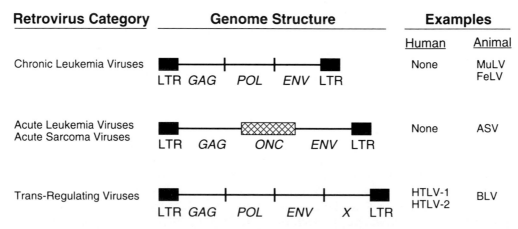

Figure 3–1. The genomic organization of different types of retroviruses. The prototype retrovirus is represented in the figure by the chronic leukemia viruses. It contains regulatory sequences at each end derived from the long terminal repeat (LTR) elements of the virus as well as the coding sequences for the viral proteins *gag, pol,* and *env.* The acute transforming retroviruses are defective viruses. Acquired *onc* sequences from the cellular genome replace critical viral gene segments. These defective viruses therefore can replicate only in the presence of a replication competent helper virus. The *trans*-regulatory retroviruses contain sequences, 3' to the *env* gene, that encode regulatory factors. This region has been referred to as the X region and encodes the *tax* and *rex* genes. ASV, avian sarcoma virus; BLV, bovine leukemia virus. (Modified from Howley PM: Principles of carcinogenesis: Viral. *In* DeVita VT, Hellman S, Rosenberg SA (eds): Cancer: Principles and Practice of Oncology, ed. 4. Philadelphia, JB Lippincott Company, 1993, pp. 182–199, with permission.)

of viruses was not available until 1986, when Summers and his colleagues found that hepatocytes from ducklings could be infected by DHBV in culture, yielding infectious virus.[58]

The hepatitis B surface antigen (HBsAg) was discovered in 1963 by Baruch Blumberg, who at the time was studying human serum protein polymorphisms.[59,60] Subsequent studies demonstrated that this antigen was associated with acute hepatitis B infection, ultimately leading to its current name.[61,62] This antigen is the surface or envelope protein of the hepatitis B virus particle, and its presence in the serum of infected patients serves as a useful marker of an active HBV infection.[63]

During an HBV infection, virus particles are present at high titer in the serum, with up to 10^5 to 10^9 virions/mL, visible by electron microscopy.[64] In addition to the complete virion particles, the serum also contains empty viral envelopes consisting of spherical or filamentous particles 22 nm in diameter.[65] The virion is 42 nm in diameter and consists of an envelope surrounding a nucleocapsid that contains the double-stranded circular DNA molecule and the DNA polymerase. This virion particle, which first was described by Dane, sometimes is referred to as the "Dane" particle.[63] It is the outer envelope that contains the HBsAg, consisting of protein, carbohydrate, and lipid. The capsid carries the hepatitis B core antigen (HBcAg). The concentrations of the incomplete viral forms in the serum can exceed the concentrations of the complete virions greatly. This spectrum of virus forms described for HBV also is found in the serum of animals infected with respective hepadnaviruses.[55–57]

Hepatitis B viral particles contain small, circular DNA molecules that are only partially double stranded.[66,67] The DNA consists of a long strand with a constant length of 3220 bases and a shorter strand that varies in length from 1700 to 2800 bases in different molecules. A map of the HBV DNA genome is shown in Figure 3–2.[67] The virion particles contain a DNA polymerase activity that is capable of repairing the single-stranded DNA region to make two fully double-stranded molecules, each approximately 3220 bases in length.[68] For this reaction, DNA synthesis initiates at the 3' end of the short strand, which, as noted above, is heterogeneous among different DNA molecules. DNA synthesis terminates at the uniquely located 5' end of the short strand when it is reached. The long strand is not a closed molecule but contains a nick at a unique site approximately 300 bp from the 5' end of the short strand.

The HBV genome has four open reading frames (ORFs) and encodes four genes. These ORFs are designated as S and pre-S, C, P, and X.[67,69] S and pre-S represent two contiguous reading frames and code for the viral surface glycoproteins. C contains the coding sequences for the core structural protein of the nucleocapsid. The P gene encodes the viral polymerase, which contains reverse transcriptase activity. The X open reading frame encodes a basic polypeptide that has transcriptional transactivation properties that can up-regulate the activity of hepadnavirus promoters.[70,71] The overall structure of the genomes of all of the animal hepadnaviruses is quite similar.[69] The WHV and GSHV genomes are approximately 3300 bp in

size and that of the DHBV is approximately 3000 bp in size. The genomic organization of the different hepadnaviruses is similar and there is extensive nucleotide homology between them. The mammalian hepadnaviruses differ from the avian hepadnaviruses in that only the mammalian hepadnaviruses contain an X gene.[69]

HBV Replication

HBV DNA can be either free or integrated in the host chromosome of the hepatocyte.[72,73] Free HBV DNA represents intermediate forms of replication for the viral genome and can be detected during acute infections and some chronic stages of HPV infection. Integrated sequences usually are found during chronic virus infection and in HCC. The replication mechanism for the hepadnaviruses, first discovered by Summers and Mason for DHBV[74] and later confirmed for HBV, is different from that of other DNA viruses.[75] The replication cycle involves a reverse transcription step resembling that of the retroviruses in that it goes through an RNA copy of the genome as an intermediate in replication. The hepadnaviruses differ from the retroviruses, however, in that, whereas retrovirus virions contain RNA and the intermediate form of replication is integrated DNA, the virions of the hepadnaviruses contain DNA and the intermediate replication form is RNA. Also, integration of the hepadnavirus genome as a provirus is not a necessary intermediate step for viral genome replication, as it is for a

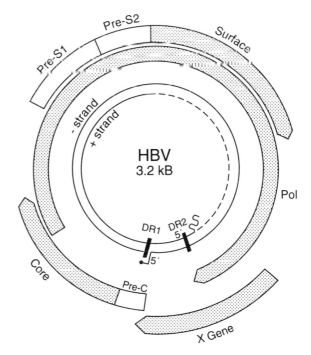

Figure 3–2. Map of the HBV genome. The arrows surrounding the genome represent the four large open reading frames of the L(−) strand with the genes they encode indicated. The broken line is the S(+) DNA strand. The positions of the 5' ends of the DNA strands are indicated. The location of the direct repeats (DR1 and DR2) involved in the initiation of DNA replication also are indicated.[69,75] (Modified from Howley PM: Principles of carcinogenesis: Viral. In DeVita VT, Hellman S, Rosenberg SA (eds): Cancer: Principles and Practice of Oncology, ed. 4. Philadelphia, JB Lippincott Company, 1993, pp. 182–199, with permission.)

retrovirus. The similarity between the retroviruses and the hepadnaviruses extends to the overall genomic organization, in which all of the genes are encoded on only one strand. The order of the genes within the retroviruses (*gag, pol,* and *env*) is similar to that of their counterparts for the hepadnaviruses (core, polymerase, and surface antigen). Other subtle differences exist in the transcriptional programs utilized to generate the messenger RNAs for these different viruses. A further similarity between these viruses is that some members of each group of these viruses encode transcriptional regulatory factors. For HTLV-1, described earlier in this chapter, the X region encodes the transcriptional activator *tax* as well as the *rex* gene product involved in messenger RNA transport to the cytoplasm. The X genes encoded by the mammalian hepadnaviruses similarly encode proteins with transcriptional activator properties, although the X gene product and its properties still are not very well understood.

Hepatocellular Carcinoma

There is compelling epidemiologic evidence supporting the etiologic role of HBV in human HCC. There is a striking correlation between the worldwide geographic incidence of HCC and the prevalence of HBsAg chronic carriers.[76] Important evidence for the role of HBV in HCC was provided by the prospective epidemiologic studies of Palmer Beasley in Taiwan.[53] A relative risk of 217 for the development of HCC was found for HBsAg-positive males as compared to noncarriers. Furthermore, 51 per cent of the deaths from these carriers were caused by cirrhosis of the liver or HCC, compared with only 2 per cent among the control population. Among the noncarriers, 90 per cent had evidence of a prior HBV infection even though they did not have evidence of the HBsAg chronic carrier state. Therefore, the high incidence of HCC clearly was related to the carrier state and not to a prior HBV infection, per se. The age distribution of HBV infections, which occurs at early ages in this population of Taiwanese, indicated that the tumors appear after a mean duration of 35 years of HBV infection. Between 60 and 90 per cent of the HCC patients also had cirrhosis.

These strong epidemiologic data do not preclude a role for additional factors in HCC. On the contrary, other factors such as aflatoxin have been recognized as having a role in some cases of liver cancer. Also, chronic hepatitis resulting from infection with hepatitis C virus (HCV), an RNA virus with similarities to flaviviruses, also has been implicated strongly in some cases of HBV-negative HCC. Even in those cases of HCC where HBV plays a causative role, other factors may be contributing to carcinogenesis.

The mechanistic role of HBV in HCC has not yet been determined. Usually in HBV-positive liver cancers, the viral DNA sequences are found integrated into the host cellular DNA. Different tumors display different patterns of integration, indicating that the insertion of the viral DNA into the host chromosome is not site specific. In a given tumor, however, all cells have the same pattern of HBV DNA integration, indicating that the integration event preceded the clonal expansion of the tumor. This clonal pattern of HBV DNA integration supports the etiologic role of HBV in HCC. The HBV-integrated genomes often are highly rearranged within tumors, displaying a variety of deletions, inversions, and point mutations. Although occasional integrated genomes do retain one or more viral genes intact, there does not appear to be a consistent pattern in which one gene regularly is preserved intact. This indicates that the continued expression of a specific viral gene is not required for the maintenance of the malignant phenotype in an HBV-positive liver cancer.

So the main question is, how does HBV cause HCC? There is no compelling evidence that HBV encodes a transforming protein. The viral X protein has been shown to have transcriptional activation properties, and it is possible that it could directly or indirectly contribute to growth deregulation as a transcription factor. Indeed, there has been a report that under some conditions transgenic mice, which overexpress the HBV X protein, can develop liver tumors.[77] The role of the HBV X gene product in tumorigenesis in these mice may be indirect, however, as appears to be the case in HBV transgenic mice that overexpress the large surface antigen of HBV.[78] In the latter case, the role of HBV is indirect, through provoking an immune-mediated liver injury and triggering hepatocellular regeneration. Such regeneration expands the pool of cells at risk for additional genetic lesions. Those cells with the appropriate genetic mutations then could undergo clonal expansion and ultimately progression to HCC.

Mechanisms by which HBV DNA integration could contribute directly to tumorigenesis could be either (1) proto-oncogene activation as a result of the insertion of the viral DNA or (2) the inactivation of tumor suppressor alleles by such integration. Indeed, there is compelling evidence that insertional activation in WHV-induced hepatomas is important in hepatocellular carcinogenesis in the woodchuck model. Approximately 20 per cent of the tumors show WHV DNA inserted into the N-*myc* locus. However, an extensive search for comparable events in HBV-associated human HCC has turned up only rare examples.[79,80] It seems likely that many different mechanisms may contribute to the role of HBV in HCC. Insertional mutagenesis or specific oncogene activation may be important in some cases of HCC. It is difficult to conclude at this time that a specific viral gene product is functioning as an oncogene; however, such a role cannot be ruled out completely. It does seem likely, however, that the induction of cellular injury by HBV, with the resulting immune response and hepatic regeneration, may be a very important common event, perhaps initiating the multistep process that results in HCC.

HUMAN PAPILLOMAVIRUSES

The human papillomaviruses (HPVs) cause warts and papillomas, and now have been associated with some human cancers. The viral nature of human warts was demonstrated at the turn of the century by transmission using a cell-free filtrate.[81] However, detailed studies on this group of viruses did not begin until recombinant DNA techniques could be applied to their analysis, because none of the papillomaviruses has ever been propagated successfully in the laboratory in tissue culture in a way that allowed standard virologic studies on this group of viruses to be carried out. There has been a significant advance in our knowledge of the papillomaviruses during the past decade, principally as a result of advances in basic research.

The papillomaviruses are found in many higher vertebrate species, ranging from birds to humans. Although originally classified as papovaviruses because of their icosohedral shape and circular, double-stranded DNA genome, the papillomaviruses now are recognized to be separate from the other papovaviruses, such as polyomavirus and simian virus 40 (SV40), based on different biologic and genetic characteristics. The papillomaviruses contain a double-stranded circular DNA genome of 8000 bp, which is larger than the polyomaviruses (5000 bp), and the virion particles have a correspondingly larger capsid diameter (55 versus 40 nm). The papillomaviruses have not yet been propagated in tissue culture under standard conditions. The development of a permissive cell culture system for papillomavirus replication would be a major advance to the study of the biology of this virus.

There are over 65 different types of HPVs.[82] Unlike some human viruses, such as adenoviruses, it has not been possible to type the papillomaviruses by serologic methods because antisera that can distinguish between the different HPV types currently are not available. As a consequence, the viruses have been "typed" by DNA hybridization under controlled conditions of stringency. Viruses differing by more than 50 per cent DNA homology when assayed under stringent conditions are considered as different types.[82] Over 65 types of HPV now have been categorized, and new types still are being recognized on a regular basis. Some of these viruses, as well as the clinical syndromes with which they are associated, are presented in Table 3–2.

The functions of the papillomaviruses necessary for production of infectious virions, which include vegetative viral DNA replication and the synthesis of the capsid proteins, occur only in the fully differentiated squamous epithelial cells of a papilloma. Viral DNA replication for progeny virion production can be detected by in situ hybridization only in the more differentiated squamous epithelial cells of the stratum spinosum and of the granular layer of the epidermis, but not in the basal layer or in the underlying dermal fibroblasts. Viral capsid protein synthesis and virion assembly occur only in the upper stratum spinosum and in the granular layer, in which the epithelial cells are terminally differentiated. The viral genome is present in the epithelial cells of the basal layer. It generally is believed that the expression of specific viral genes in the basal layer and in the lower layers of the epidermis stimulates cellular proliferation and alters the keratinocyte differentiation profile, characteristics of a wart. As the cells of the epidermis migrate upward through the stratum spinosum into the granular layer, they undergo a program of differentiation. The control of papillomavirus late gene expression is linked tightly to the differentiation state of the squamous epithelial cells.[83] The basis of this control

TABLE 3–2. ASSOCIATION OF HPVs AND CLINICAL LESIONS

CLINICAL ASSOCIATION	HPV TYPES
Cutaneous Lesions and HPVs	
Plantar wart	1
Common wart	2, 4
Mosaic wart	2
Multiple flat warts	3, 10, 28, 41
Macular plaques in epidermodysplasia verruciformis	5, 8, 9, 12, 14, 15, 17, 19, 20, 21, 22, 23, 24, 25, 36, 47, 50
Butcher's warts	7
Genital Tract and Other Mucosal HPVs	
Condyloma acuminata (exophytic)	6, 11
Giant condyloma (Bushke-Lowenstein tumor)	6, 11
Subclinical infection	All genital tract types
Squamous intraepithelial lesions	16, 18, 31, 33, others
Bowenoid papulosis	16
Cervical cancer	
Strong association ("high risk")	16, 18, 31, 45
Moderate association	33, 35, 39, 51, 52, 56, 58, 59, 68
Weak or no association ("low risk")	6, 11, 26, 42, 43, 44, 51, 53, 54, 55, 66
Respiratory papillomas	6, 11
Conjunctival papillomas	6, 11
Focal epithelial hyperplasia (oral cavity)	13, 32

is not fully understood but involves the activation of a "late" promoter and altered patterns of viral messenger RNA processing.

Papillomaviruses have a specific tropism for keratinocytes, and the different HPV types have specificity for different anatomic sites. For instance, HPV-1, which is associated with plantar warts, has been observed to replicate only in heavily keratinized epithelium such as the palm or the sole, whereas HPV-16 has a preference for mucosal squamous epithelium characteristic of the genital tract. HPV-1 does not replicate in cervical epithelium and HPV-16 generally is not observed in the skin of the hand or foot. Specialized keratinocytes from different anatomic sites may be likely to have distinct differentiation patterns, as is evident from the distinct types of keratin proteins that they synthesize and from the pattern of synthesis of other epithelial-specific proteins, such as involucrin. The ability of HPVs to proliferate at a particular anatomic site therefore may reflect a specific interaction between viral and cellular gene regulatory factors involved in transcription. The tropism of the HPVs for squamous epithelial cells appears to be due in part to epithelial-specific enhancer elements in the viral transcriptional control region.[84]

HPV Genomic Organization

All of the papillomaviruses share a similar genomic organization. The DNA genomes of many of the HPVs as well as some of the animal papillomaviruses have been sequenced. The viral genomes consist of approximately 8000 bp. All of the ORFs that could serve to encode proteins for these viruses are located on only one of the two viral DNA strands, and only one strand is transcribed.[85]

The HPV genome can be divided into three distinct regions: (1) an "early" region that encodes the viral proteins involved in viral DNA replication, transcriptional regulation, and cellular transformation; (2) a "late" region that encodes the viral capsid proteins; and (3) a region called the long control region (LCR), or sometimes the upstream regulatory region (URR), that does not contain any genes but does contain the origin of DNA replication and important transcription regulatory elements. A diagram of the organization of the HPV-16 genome, which is typical of all the HPVs, is shown in Figure 3–3. The genes located in the early region of the genome are designated as E1, E2, and so forth, and the genes located in the late region are designated as L1 and L2. From studies with the HPVs, it is likely that E4 encodes a "late" gene that is expressed only in productively infected keratinocytes.[86] Thus, although this ORF is located with the early ORFs, its function may be important only in virion production, by causing the disruption of keratin intermediate filaments.[87]

In productively infected tissue (i.e., tissues in which viral particles are made, such as a wart), messenger RNA is transcribed from the early *and* late regions of the genome.[83] The nonproductive phase of the infectious cycle of the cells in the lower epithelium is accompanied by mRNA being transcribed only from the early region of the genome. The restriction of expression of the genome to only the early region involves regulation of transcription at the levels of the initiation of RNA synthesis, RNA stability, and transcriptional termination.[83]

The functional analysis of the molecular biology of papillomaviruses has been studied most extensively for the bovine papillomavirus type 1 (BPV-1), which is capable of transforming a variety of rodent fibroblast cell lines in tissue culture.[88] In these transformed cells, the DNA remains as a stable extrachromosomal plasmid, and this system has served as an excellent model for studying the latent nonproductive phase of the papillomavirus infectious cycle. In many ways, BPV has served as the prototype for unraveling aspects of the biology of the papillomaviruses. Three independent transforming genes have been mapped in BPV-1: E5, E6, and E7 (reviewed in ref. 88). BPV also encodes regulatory genes that have roles in viral DNA replication and in controlling viral transcription. The E2 gene of BPV-1 has a critical role regulating viral transcription but also has a direct role in viral DNA replication.[89] The full-length BPV E2 protein known as E2TA is a DNA-binding protein that can either activate or repress transcription depending on the context of the E2-binding sites within the promoter sequences. BPV encodes two additional E2 proteins that are shorter truncated forms of E2 and can inhibit the transactivation functions of the full-length E2 protein.[89] The E2 genes of other papillomaviruses, including the HPVs, also have been shown to encode transcriptional regulatory functions but in general have been less well studied.[90,91] The E1 gene encodes a protein that is the major viral DNA replication factor that is necessary for the initiation of viral DNA synthesis. E1 is a DNA-specific binding protein[92] that has properties necessary for its replication functions, including helicase and ATPase activities. E1 and E2 complex together and as a complex are necessary for origin-dependent DNA replication.[93] No function has yet been found for the BPV E3 ORF or the E8 ORF. The L1 ORF of the papillomaviruses encodes the major capsid protein and the L2 ORF encodes a minor capsid protein.[94,95] The L1 and L2 ORFs are expressed only in the terminally differentiated keratinocytes.[83]

The initial cellular transformation studies with the papillomaviruses focused on BPV-1 because it was so effective at transforming rodent cells in tissue culture. The major transforming gene for BPV-1 is E5, which has been shown to transform cells by affecting the turnover and activity of cellular growth factor receptors, specifically the platelet-derived growth factor (PDGF) receptor.[96,97] E5 also has been shown to associate with the 16-kDa component of the vacuolar ATPase enzyme complex, but the functional significance of this association is unclear at this time.[98] As noted above, the E6 and E7 genes also have been shown to have transforming properties, but there have not yet been studies that have examined mechanistically the oncogenic nature of the proteins encoded by these two genes.

Recent transformation studies have focused on HPV-16

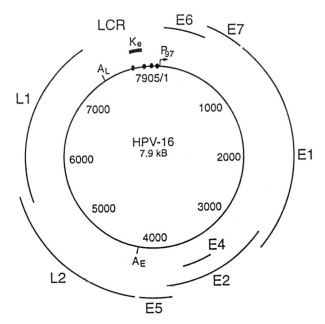

Figure 3–3. Map of the HPV-16 genome. The nucleotide numbers are noted within the circular maps, transcription proceeds clockwise, and the major open reading frames (E1 to E7, L1, and L2) are indicated. The transcriptional promoter that directs the expression of E6 and E7 is designated (P_{97}). A_E and A_L represent the polyadenylation signals for the early and late transcripts, respectively. The viral long control region (LCR) contains the viral transcriptional and replication regulatory elements. The solid circles on the genome represent the four E2-binding sites that have been noted in the LCR. A keratinocyte-dependent enhancer in the LCR is indicated by the bold bar and is designated K_e.[84] (Modified from Howley PM: Principles of carcinogenesis: Viral. *In* DeVita VT, Hellman. S, Rosenberg SA (eds): Cancer: Principles and Practice of Oncology, ed. 4. Philadelphia, JB Lippincott Company, 1993, pp. 182–199, with permission.)

and HPV-18, which are associated with human cervical cancer. Although the genomic organization of the HPVs is quite similar to that of BPV-1, there appear to be important differences in the mechanisms by which they transform cells. The principal transforming genes for the cancer-associated HPVs have been mapped to E6 and E7, as is discussed in the next section. E7 is by itself sufficient for the transformation of established rodent cells, such as NIH 3T3 cells.[99–101] E7 also is capable of cooperating with an activated *ras* oncogene to transform primary rodent cells.[100] Expression of E6 and E7 together is sufficient for the efficient immortalization of primary human cells, most notably primary human keratinocytes, which are the normal host cell for the HPVs.[102,103] There have been a number of papers demonstrating that the HPV E5 genes also have transforming activities in a variety of assays. The HPV viral oncoproteins and their roles in carcinogenic progression are discussed in more detail in the next section.

Papillomaviruses and Cancer

Only a subgroup of the papillomaviruses are associated with lesions that may progress to cancer. These viruses and their associated malignancies are listed in Table 3–3. The Shope papillomavirus (CRPV), which infects cottontail rabbits in nature, first was identified by Richard Shope as the etiologic agent of cutaneous papillomatosis in rabbits.[4] CRPV has been studied extensively as a model for papillomavirus-induced carcinogenesis.[5,104] One of the principle features of the carcinogenic progression associated with the papillomaviruses is the synergy observed between the virus and carcinogenic external factors (Table 3–3). In the case of CRPV, carcinomas develop at an increased frequency in papillomas that are painted with coal tar or methylcholanthrene.[105,106] These CRPV-associated carcinomas contain copies of the viral DNA that are transcriptionally active, and the carcinogenic properties are believed to map to specific viral genes.[107,108]

In cattle, BPV-4 causes esophageal papillomatosis and also is associated with squamous cell carcinomas of the upper alimentary tract.[109,110] Interestingly, however, only those cattle from the highlands of Scotland that feed on bracken fern (known to contain a radiomimetic substance) and also are infected by BPV-4 have a high incidence of squamous cell carcinomas of the esophagus and of the foregut.[109] In contrast to the CRPV-associated carcinomas, in which the viral DNA invariably can be found, extensive analysis of the squamous cell carcinomas of the upper alimentary tract in these cattle infected with BPV-4 have failed to reveal a consistent pattern of viral DNA sequences within the malignant tumors.[111] In the case of these alimentary tract tumors, it is possible that the continued presence of BPV-4 DNA sequences is not required for the maintenance of the cancer.

EPIDERMODYSPLASIA VERRUCIFORMIS

Epidermodysplasia verruciformis (EV) is a very rare genetic disease in humans that usually begins in infancy or childhood. Patients with this disease display disseminated polymorphic cutaneous lesions that resemble flat warts, and reddish macules sometimes referred to as "pityriasis-like" lesions.[112] Approximately one third of the patients with EV develop multiple skin cancers, usually during the third of fourth decade of their lives. Papillomavirus particles can be detected within the benign lesions but not in the carcinomas. It is thought that EV is linked to a rare, recessive, abnormal allele of an X-linked gene. Patients with EV often have impaired cell-mediated immunity, which is believed to be important with regard to the manner in which they respond to infections by this subset of cutaneous HPVs. The EV carcinomas usually arise in sun-exposed areas, suggesting that ultraviolet radiation may play a co-carcinogenic role with the specific HPVs in the etiology of these cancers. Despite the fact that EV is a very rare disease, it has received intense study by dermatologists and virologists, and over 15 different HPV types now have been isolated from individual lesions in the small number of patients studied (see Table 3–2).

The spectrum of skin cancers that have been described in patients with EV include bowenoid carcinomas, in situ carcinomas, and invasive squamous cell carcinomas. Of the many HPV types that have been found in patients with EV, only a subset of them appear to be associated with the cancers, most notably HPV-5 and HPV-8. Extensive studies have been carried out by Gerard Orth from the Pasteur Institute in Paris and Stephania Jablonska in Warsaw in analyzing the HPVs in skin cancers from patients with EV; these workers have documented the presence of HPV DNA in the vast majority of EV cancers examined. Most of them contained either HPV-5 or HPV-8 DNA, and one contained HPV-14 DNA.[113] HPV-5 also has been found in metastatic squamous cell carcinoma lesions in some patients with EV.[114,115] Additional HPVs have been

TABLE 3–3. MALIGNANCIES ASSOCIATED WITH PAPILLOMAVIRUSES

PAPILLOMAVIRUSES	CANCERS	OTHER FACTORS
CRPV	Skin cancer	Methylcholanthrene
BPV-4	Tongue, esophageal, foregut cancers	Bracken fern
BPV (not typed)	Ocular cancers	Ultraviolet light
Ovine papillomavirus	Skin cancer	Ultraviolet light
HPV-5, -8, others	Skin cancer in patients with EV	Ultraviolet light
HPV-16, -18, -31, other high-risk types	Anogenital cancers, some oral and upper airway cancers	Smoking?, herpes virus?, other factors?

CRPV, cottontail rabbit papillomavirus; EV, epidermodysplasia verruciformis.

found in carcinomas in EV patients, including HPV-3 in an in situ vulvar carcinoma[116] and HPV-17 in a cutaneous EV carcinoma.[117] Thus, the association of a specific HPV in cancers in patients with EV is not strictly limited to HPV-5 and HPV-8. Although metastasis is uncommon in the cancers in these patients, the presence of HPV-5 in the two metastatic lymph node lesions examined strengthens the agreement on an etiologic role for HPV in these carcinomas.[113,114] Further studies have established that the viral genomes are transcriptionally active within these carcinomas[118] and that HPV-5 and HPV-8.[119]

GENITAL TRACT CARCINOMAS

The epidemiology of genital warts indicates that it is a venereal transmitted disease and that there is a high prevalence in populations of men and women with multiple sexual partners.[120,121] There are two types of genital wart virus infections that generally can be differentiated by their clinical appearance: condyloma acuminata and flat genital warts. Condyloma acuminata (also known as venereal warts) can be localized to the penis, the vulva, the perineum, the anus, and rarely the uterine cervix, and are caused by papillomaviruses. Papillomaviruses have been demonstrated in such lesions by the electron microscope,[122,123] and papillomavirus-specific capsid antigens have been detected using antisera that can cross react among all papillomavirus types.[124] HPV-6 and the closely related HPV-11 DNAs are present in over 90 per cent of the condyloma acuminata lesions.[125,126] Less frequently, other HPV types can be found in condyloma acuminata. Malignant conversion of condyloma acuminata into squamous cell carcinoma occurs but is quite uncommon. Buschke and Lowenstein described a lesion, which was designated as a giant condyloma, that has characteristics similar to those of a locally invasive squamous cell carcinoma.[127] These tumors are associated with HPV-6 and HPV-11.[128,129] The majority of cervical carcinomas and other genital tract carcinomas, however, are negative when examined for HPV-6 and HPV-11.

Compelling evidence linking an HPV infection with cervical carcinoma followed the observation that some of the morphologic changes characteristic of cervical dysplasia seen previously on Pap smears were due to a papillomavirus infection.[130–132] With its characteristic perinuclear clearing and abnormally shaped nucleus, the cell that is diagnostic for a cervical papillomavirus infection is the koilocyte.[133] Papillomavirus particles have been demonstrated in the koilocytotic cells supporting the papillomavirus etiology.[134,135] Furthermore, papillomavirus-specific capsid antigens and HPV DNA can be demonstrated readily within cervical dysplastic lesions, providing confirmation of the viral etiology of cervical dysplasia.

Epidemiologic studies that implicate an infectious agent in the etiology of human cervical carcinoma date back to the 1960s.[136,137] Venereal transmission of a carcinogenic factor with a long latency has been suggested by such studies. Sexual promiscuity, an early age of onset of sexual activity, and poor sexual hygienic conditions are revealed by these studies as risk factors for cervical carcinoma in women. The counterpart to cervical cancer in the male appears to be penile cancer, because there is a correlation between the incidence rates of these two cancers in different geographic areas. The incidence rates for penile carcinoma, however, are on the order of 20-fold lower compared to those of cervical carcinoma. A similar ratio of incidence between cervical carcinoma and penile carcinoma is maintained in areas of high, medium, or low prevalence, however, suggesting that the etiologic factors for penile and cervical carcinoma may be the same.

The possible involvement of an infectious agent in the etiology of cervical carcinoma has prompted many studies evaluating genital pathogens as potential causative agents over the years. There is no evidence linking infections by *Trichomonas, Chlamydia,* and bacteria such as those causing syphilis and gonorrhea with cervical carcinoma. In the late 1960s and early 1970s, genital infection by herpes simplex virus (HSV) type 2 was considered as a possible etiologic candidate.[138,139] A principle role for HSV in cervical cancer was not supported by molecular studies. Attempts to demonstrate HSV RNA or DNA in cervical cancer tissues were unsuccessful and therefore did not provide convincing evidence for a role for HSV in cervical cancer.[140] Furthermore, a large prospective epidemiologic study carried out by Vonka, published in 1984, also did not support the involvement of HSV-1 or HSV-2 infections in cervical cancer.[141,142]

The association of a HPV with the preneoplastic lesions of the cervix (also referred to as cervical intraepithelial neoplasia, or CIN) prompted the search for HPV sequences in cervical cancers. The natural history of the disease progression in women linking CIN to carcinoma in situ and to invasive squamous cell carcinoma of the cervix was well established and indeed is the basis of the Pap screening program. Women with cervical dysplasia are at an increased risk for the development of cervical cancer.[143–145] Using radioactively labeled HPV-11 DNA under low-stringency annealing conditions, zur Hausen and his colleagues examined human cervical carcinomas for related HPV DNAs. They were able to identify two new papillomavirus DNAs, HPV-16 and HPV-18.[146,147] Using the HPV-16 and HPV-18 cloned DNAs as probes, approximately 70 per cent of cervical carcinomas could be shown to harbor these two HPV DNAs.[148] Subsequent studies have led to the identification of approximately 25 different HPVs that are associated with genital tract lesions. Of these, HPV-31, HPV-33, HPV-39, HPV-42, and several others each are associated with a small percentage of cervical carcinomas.[149,150] Specific HPVs can be found in approximately 85 to 90 per cent of human cervical carcinomas. In addition, these same DNAs can be found in other human genital carcinomas, including penile carcinomas, some vulvar carcinomas, and some perianal carcinomas. The availability of HPV DNA probes has permitted the extensive analysis of specific clinical lesions, and it is now recognized, for instance, that bowenoid papulosis of the penis[151,152] is associated with HPV-16, and therefore is the male counterpart of CIN in the female.

The genital tract–associated HPVs generally can be classified further as either ''high risk'' or ''low risk'' based on whether or not the lesions with which they are associated are at significant risk for malignant progression. The low-risk viruses, such as HPV-6 and HPV-11, are associated with venereal warts, lesions that only rarely progress to cancer. The high-risk viruses, such as HPV-16 and HPV-18, are associated with CIN and cervical cancer. The other high-risk viruses include HPV-31, HPV-33, HPV-35, HPV-39, HPV-45, HPV-51, HPV-52, and HPV-56. As noted earlier, approximately 80 to 90 per cent of cervical carcinomas contain a high-risk DNA. HPV-positive cervical cancers and cell lines derived from HPV-positive cervical cancer tissues often contain integrated viral DNA, although there are some cases in which DNA is apparently also extrachromosomal. In those cancers in which the viral DNA is integrated, the pattern of integration is clonal, indicating that the integration event preceded the clonal outgrowth of the tumor. Integration of the viral DNA does not occur at specific sites in the host chromosome, although integration can occur in some cases in the vicinity of known oncogenes. For instance, in the HeLa cell line (which is an HPV-18–positive cervical carcinoma cell line), the integration of the viral genome is within approximately 50 kb of the c-myc locus on human chromosome 8.[153] It is not known whether such an integration event provides a selective growth advantage to the cell and therefore might contribute to neoplastic progression. However, it seems quite plausible that, in some cancers, the integration of the viral DNA could result in genetic changes that could contribute to carcinogenic progression.

In the HPV-positive cancers, there is a selection for the integrity of the E6-E7 coding region and the URR. Furthermore, the E6 and E7 genes are expressed regularly in HPV-positive cervical cancers.[153–155] Integration of the HPV genome into the host chromosome in the cancers often results in the disruption of the viral E1 or E2 genes.[153,154] As in BPV, the HPV E2 gene encodes transcriptional regulatory factors[90,91]; however, in HPV-16 and HPV-18, it appears that E2 negatively regulates expression of the E6 and E7 genes. Thus integration of the viral genome disrupting the E2 gene could result in the depres-

sion of the promoter upstream of E6 and E7, leading to deregulated expression of the viral E6 and E7 genes. A recent study has confirmed that disruption of either the E1 or the E2 regulatory gene of HPV-16 increases the immortalization capacity of the viral genome.[156]

Support for a role for the E6 and E7 genes in cervical carcinogenesis comes from the studies that have established that transforming properties of these two proteins mirror their clinical associations. The cloned DNAs of the high-risk HPVs are efficient at being able to extend the life span and contribute to the immortalization of squamous epithelial cells.[157,158] This immortalization property is not shared by the DNAs of the low-risk HPVs. A genetic dissection of the viral genome revealed that the high-risk HPV E6 and E7 genes together were necessary and sufficient for the efficient immortalization of primary squamous epithelial cells.[102,103] In contrast to the immortalization properties of the HPV-16 and HPV-18 E6 and E7 proteins, E6 and E7 encoded by the low-risk viruses are either inactive or only weakly transforming in the same assays.

An emerging theme among DNA tumor viruses (including the HPVs) is that the immortalization and transformation properties of the proteins encoded by these viruses may, in part, be due to their interactions with critical cellular regulatory proteins (Fig. 3–4). As noted above, the E7 proteins encoded by the high-risk HPVs share sequence similarity to adenovirus E1A. This sequence similarity also can be extended to SV40 large T antigen and in all three proteins involves regions that are critical for the transformation properties of these oncoproteins. The regions of amino acid sequence similarity between E7 and adenovirus E1A that are shared with SV40 large T antigen are regions that have been shown to participate in the binding of a number of important cellular regulatory proteins, including the product of the retinoblastoma tumor suppressor gene, pRb.[159–162]

The immortalization/transformation properties of the E6 protein first were revealed by studies using primary human cells, including the normal host cell for HPV-16,

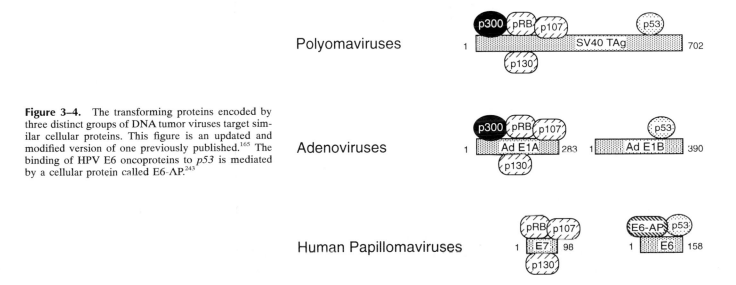

Figure 3–4. The transforming proteins encoded by three distinct groups of DNA tumor viruses target similar cellular proteins. This figure is an updated and modified version of one previously published.[165] The binding of HPV E6 oncoproteins to p53 is mediated by a cellular protein called E6-AP.[243]

the human genital squamous epithelial cell.[102,103] Efficient immortalization of primary human cells by HPV-16 or HPV-18 requires both the E6 and E7 genes.[102,103,163] The ability of the E6 and E7 proteins to cooperate and efficiently immortalize primary human keratinocytes is a characteristic of the high-risk HPVs but not of the low-risk HPVs.[157,164] Like SV40 large T antigen and the 55-kDa protein encoded by adenovirus E1B, the E6 proteins of the high-risk HPVs can enter into a complex with p53.[165] E6 is capable of inactivating the function of p53[166] and apparently does so by promoting the degradation of p53 as revealed by in vitro studies.[167] Consequently, the half-life and level of p53 are low in E6-immortalized cell lines and in HPV-positive cancers.[168,169]

The functional inactivation of p53 and pRb through their interactions with E6 and E7, respectively, appears to be an important event in cervical carcinogenesis. Analysis of human cervical carcinoma cell lines has revealed that the *p53* and *pRb* genes are intact and expressed in those cervical carcinoma cell lines that are HPV positive. In contrast, mutations were identified in both the *p53* and *pRb* genes in two HPV-negative cervical carcinoma cell lines.[169,170] These results support the hypothesis that the inactivation of the normal functions of the tumor suppressor proteins, pRb and p53, can be important steps in human cervical carcinogenesis, either by mutation (as in the case of HPV-negative cancers) or from complex formation with the HPV oncoproteins in HPV-positive cell lines.[171] Several groups have extended the analysis of *p53* mutations to cervical cancer specimens and have confirmed that, indeed, *p53* mutations are rare in cervical cancers but have shown that these few mutations can be seen in HPV-positive as well as HPV-negative cancers.[172,173]

It is clear that HPV infections by themselves are not sufficient for carcinogenic progression. Only a small fraction of HPV-infected individuals eventually develop cervical carcinoma. Expression of the E6 and E7 oncogenes per se is therefore not sufficient for malignant progression. Other factors are involved in the progression to cancer. Epidemiologic studies have suggested that smoking is a risk factor for developing cervical carcinoma.[174–176] The recognition that other factors are involved in the progression to cervical carcinomas suggest that papillomavirus infections may work synergistically with these other factors. It has been suggested that tobacco condensate in women who smoke could accumulate in the vaginal fluids, bathing the cervix and acting as a co-factor with the papillomavirus infection,[177] and it has been postulated that herpesvirus infection might act synergistically with specific papillomaviruses to induce human cervical carcinoma.[178]

OTHER HUMAN CANCERS ASSOCIATED WITH PAPILLOMAVIRUSES

Specific HPV DNA probes have been used by many investigators to carry out extensive screening of a variety of different human cancers for HPV sequences. Based on the animal models, any squamous carcinomas or any cancers involving an epithelium that has the potential to undergo squamous metaplasia would be reasonable candidates to investigate for an association with HPV. Studies examining oral carcinomas and upper airway carcinomas have revealed some HPV-positive carcinomas.[179–181] HPV has been associated with some benign oral papillomas,[182–185] and a papillomavirus etiology involving HPV types 13 and 32 has been firmly established for oral focal epithelial hyperplasia.[186,187] In addition, papillomavirus DNA sequences have been reported in a low percentage of cases of oral leukoplakia.[183,188] HPV-16 sequences have been described in a verrucous carcinoma of the larynx. HPV-11 has been found in a squamous cell carcinoma of the lung arising in a young adult with a history of laryngeotracheobronchial papillomatosis.[189] In this case, HPV-11 DNA also was found within metastatic lesions in the liver and lymph nodes. The viral genome was transcriptionally active, suggesting that expression of the virus may have played an active role in the carcinogenic progression.

Esophageal carcinomas in humans also have been reported to have some association with HPVs; however, the data as yet are not as convincing as they are with the anogenital cancers and with some of the oral and upper airway cancers. The esophagus is lined by a squamous epithelium, and squamous cell papillomas of the esophagus have been described in humans.[190,191] Additional studies would seem warranted to investigate a possible role of HPV in human esophageal cancers. There also have been sporadic reports in the literature associating occasional human tumors, including colon cancer, ovarian cancer, prostate cancer, and even melanomas, with the presence of HPV DNA. In general, it seems prudent to be skeptical of such reports until systematic and well-carried-out studies are confirmed in more than one laboratory.

EPSTEIN-BARR VIRUS

The Epstein-Barr virus (EBV) was discovered from studies of a lymphoma described in young children in certain parts of East Africa. Although this childhood lymphoma had been recognized previously, it first was defined clearly as a unique entity with characteristic clinical, pathologic, and epidemiologic features by Dennis Burkitt in 1958.[192,193] In these early descriptive studies, it was speculated that the lymphoma could be due to a virus because its geographic distribution in a belt across equatorial Africa was similar to that of yellow fever. In 1964, Epstein and Barr described virus particles of the herpesvirus family in lymphoblastoid cells from patients with Burkitt's lymphoma (BL).[194,195] The finding of such virus particles in lymphoid lines, however, was not restricted to tissues from BL patients, because these particles also could be observed in cell lines established from patients with other malignancies, from patients with infectious mononucleosis, and even occasionally from normal individuals. Nonetheless, EBV was the first virus to be recognized as a human tumor virus.

EBV is a double-stranded DNA virus and is a member of the herpesvirus family. Other members of the human herpesvirus family include HSV-1 and HSV-2, varicella zoster virus, cytomegalovirus, and the more recently described human herpesvirus types 6 and 7. The mature EBV particle is essentially indistinguishable from those of the other herpesviruses. Herpesviruses are large viruses, measure 150 to 180 nm in diameter, and contain a large double-stranded DNA genome of about 170,000 bp of genetic information. In addition to this central core of genetic material, the virus particle consists of a capsid layer made up of capsomeres in an icosahedral shape and an outer lipoprotein envelope. EBV is considered a member of the γ herpesviruses because of its tropism for lymphoid cells, both in vivo and in vitro. The γ herpesviruses are specific for either B or T lymphocytes; other members include Marek's disease virus of chickens and two viruses that infect New World monkeys: herpes ateles and herpes saimiri.

EBV Genome

As noted, the genome is a double-stranded DNA molecule of approximately 170,000 bp.[196] The organization of the EBV genome is complex, with regions of repeated DNA sequences and a variable number of tandem copies (6 to 12) of a 500-bp terminal repeat unit located at the ends of the linear genome. When the virus is in the latent state, the genome is found in a circular form in the cell nucleus. It is thought that the ability of the viral genome to circularize may involve homologous recombination through these terminal-repeated DNA sequences. The DNA sequence of the EBV genome has been determined in its entirety,[197] which has led to the identification of the specific ORFs and genes and has permitted an extensive genetic and molecular dissection of the virus over the past decade.

EBV Proteins

A variety of antigens have been identified and described in the literature in EBV-infected and transformed cells using immunologic means. The viral capsid antigens (VCAs) are detected in cells producing EBV particles,[198] as are the membrane antigens (MAs). These are late antigens, because their expression occurs after the onset of vegetative viral DNA synthesis in the life cycle of the virus. The MAs are responsible for eliciting virus-neutralizing antibody.[199]

In a productive infection, the first genes to be expressed are the ''immediate early'' genes, which in turn trigger the expression of the next set of genes, or ''early genes.'' One of the EBV immediate early genes that has been studied extensively is the *BZLF-1* gene, which is a transcriptional activator that can disrupt latency by initiating the expression of the viral genes necessary for viral replication.[200] There are also antigens referred to as the EBV-induced early antigens (EAs), which are synthesized early, before the onset of DNA replication in the virus replication cycle. The EAs can be subdivided into diffuse (D) and restricted (R) components based on the distribution of the antigens and the sensitivity of the patterns to fixation.[201]

All cells that harbor and express the EBV genome in a latent state express a viral antigen complex in the nucleus, which is referred to as the EBV-induced nuclear antigen (EBNA).[202] This antigen complex can serve as an immunologic marker for the presence of the viral DNA because it is expressed in virtually every cell containing the viral genome. EBNA now is known to consist of a group of at least six different EBV-encoded proteins that individually are referred to as EBNAs. The individual EBNA gene products and the genes that encode them now have been identified and antisera have been developed to specific proteins encoded by specific genes. Two of these proteins, EBNA 2 and one of the latent membrane proteins (LMPs) called LMP1, are important with regard to viral latency and the immortalization of human lymphocytes by EBV. EBNA 1 is a DNA-binding protein that binds to a specific portion of the EBV genome called oriP and is involved in replication of the viral DNA in the latent state.[203] EBNA 2 is an acidic protein that can serve as a transcriptional activator of both viral and cellular genes. Viral proteins whose expression can be increased by EBNA 2 include LMP[204,205] and another membrane protein that is expressed in latently infected cells called terminal protein.[206] Cellular proteins that can be activated by EBNA 2 include the B-cell activation antigens, CD21, CD23, and the proto-oncogene c-*fgr*.[207–209]

Other EBV proteins expressed in latently infected cells include the EBNA 3A, EBNA 3B, and EBNA 3C proteins. These proteins are found in the nuclear matrix, chromatin, and nuclear plasmic fractions, but their functions still are unknown. EBNA-LP is encoded in a leader segment for each of the EBNA mRNAs and is translated from some of these mRNAs, and therefore is referred to as the leader protein. The function of this protein is not known. Several LMPs are encoded by the virus. The expression of one of these, LMP1, is itself activated by EBNA 2. As noted above, LMP1 along with EBNA 2 is required for immortalization of B lymphocytes. LMP1 has been shown to alter the effect of the growth properties of rodent cells, epithelial cells, and B lymphocytes. LMP1 is a membrane protein that is predicted based on its amino acid structure to span the plasma membrane six times, with both the amino terminus and carboxyl terminus located in the cytoplasm. The function of LMP1 is not yet known; however, based on its amino acid sequence, it has been noted to resemble certain transport properties such as the product of the multiple drug resistance (*mdr*) gene. A full discussion of all of the EBV-encoded proteins and their functions is well beyond the scope of this chapter. Readers interested in further information on these proteins as well as a more thorough review of the virus are referred to the excellent recent review by Liebowitz and Kieff.[210]

The role of specific EBV genes in EBV-associated malignancies is not yet clear. Immortalization genes have now been mapped to EBNA 2 and LMP1 as noted above. It is presumed that these two genes may play a direct role in inducing cellular immortalization in B lymphocytes as an early event in leukemogenesis. The role of other genes in this process, however, cannot be ruled out because genetic studies on the immortalizing and transforming functions of EBV have been limited.

Burkitt's Lymphoma

Burkitt's lymphoma in Africa occurs several years after the primary infection with EBV. BL is a monoclonal lymphoma,[211] as opposed to infectious mononucleosis, which is a polyclonal disease caused by EBV. African BL is characterized clinically by rapid growth of the tumor at nonlymphoid sites such as the jaw or the retroperitoneum. The tumor is of B-cell origin and is morphologically similar to the small noncleaved cells of normal lymphoid follicles.[212] The biopsy specimens from African BL invariably contain the EBV genome and are positive for EBNA.[213] This is in contrast to the non-African BL, in which only 15 to 20 per cent of the tumors contain the EBV genome. EBV is a common virus with a worldwide distribution. More than 90 per cent of individuals worldwide have been infected by the time they reach adulthood. The clustering of BL in the equatorial belt of East Africa, therefore, cannot be explained solely on the basis of EBV infection. Potential effects on the immune system, possibly resulting from hyperstimulation by endemic malaria, have been postulated to play an important role in the outcome of an EBV infection in this region of Africa.[214,215] Individuals from this region do have impairment of virus-specific cytotoxic T-cell activity, and it is the T-cell response to EBV infection that limits B-cell proliferation resulting from EBV stimulation.[216] The failure of the T-cell immune response to control this proliferation might be an early step providing the enhanced opportunity for further mutation, oncogenic transformation, and lymphomagenesis. BLs regularly contain chromosomal abnormalities, often in regions that contain the immunoglobulin genes, most notably chromosomes 2, 14, and 22. In greater than 90 per cent of BL, a translocation of the long arm of chromosome 14 (containing the heavy-chain immunoglobulin genes) to chromosome 8 (containing the c-*myc* oncogene) is observed.[217] Less frequent translocations involve chromosome 2 (κ light chain) and chromosome 22 (λ light chain).[218] These translocations to chromosomes 2 and 22 generally involve reciprocal translocations to the distal arm of chromosome 8, containing c-*myc*.[219] BLs are believed to deregulated expression of the c-*myc* oncogene following this translocation, and it is thought that abnormal expression may be due to the proximity of the c-*myc* oncogene to the transcriptional control elements of the immunoglobulin genes.[219,220]

The chromosomal abnormalities noted above are not detected in the peripheral blood lymphocytes of BL patients, nor are they found in nonmalignant lymphoblastoid cell lines that can be derived from such patients. Thus, the translocation appears to be specific for BL and appears to occur at a step following the immortalization by EBV. George Klein has suggested a possible scenario to explain a role for EBV in the etiology of African BL.[221] The first step involves the EBV-induced immortalization of B lymphocytes in a primary infection. The second step involves the stimulated proliferation of EBV-positive B cells, a step that is facilitated in the geographic areas where BL is endemic (presumably because of the presence of malaria), through B-cell triggering and the suppression of T cells that are involved in the control of the proliferation of EBV-infected cells. This pool of EBV-immortalized cells would become increased in size and serve as a target cell population for random chromosomal rearrangements. The third and final step is the reciprocal translocation involving a chromosomal locus involving an immunoglobulin gene and the c-*myc* gene on chromosome 8. This leads to the deregulation of the c-*myc* gene, to the development of the malignant clone, and finally to the appearance of a tumor mass.[222] The order of these individual steps probably can be rearranged, with the B-cell activation by malaria preceding the chromosomal translocation and followed by the EBV infection, as has been proposed alternatively.[223] Regardless, the components of these two scenarios each account for the geographic distribution of BL, the critical involvement of EBV in lymphomagenesis, and the eventual selection and clonal outgrowth of a population of cells with the critical translocation involving the deregulation of the *myc* gene on chromosome 8.

What is the role of specific EBV genes in the maintenance of BL? As noted above, EBNA 2 and LMP1 appear to be the mediators of EBV-induced growth effects in B lymphocytes. However, these are not expressed in BL and therefore are not required for BL growth. It is possible that altered *myc* expression may replace the need for EBV oncogenic functions. Furthermore, the down-modulation of the EBV EBNA and LMP functions actually may be advantageous to tumor development, allowing the cell to escape from T-cell–mediated immune surveillance. It has been shown that the EBNAs and LMPs can serve as targets of immune cytotoxic T cells, and that LMP1 induction of cell adhesion molecules can enhance the human lymphocyte antigen (HLA)–restricted killing of EBV-infected T cells.[224,225]

Nasopharyngeal Carcinoma

Nasopharyngeal carcinoma (NPC) also is linked to EBV (reviewed in ref. 226). NPC occurs in adults from ages 20 to 50, although in certain parts of Africa the age distribution extends to children as well. In general, males outnumber females 2 to 1, and, although worldwide the annual incidence rates are low, there are areas in China (especially the southern providence) in which there is a high rate of approximately 10 cases per 100,000 population per year. Because the incidence among individuals of Chinese descent remains high, irrespective of where they live, a genetic susceptibility has been proposed. For the Cantonese in Singapore, the annual rates of 29/100,000 are higher than for other racial groups living in the same locale. A correlation of certain HLA haplotypes has been noted among the Chinese. Environmental factors have been implicated as risk factors for NPC, including fumes, chemicals, smoke, and ingestion of salt-cured fish.

EBV genomes are found in nearly all biopsies of undifferentiated NPC specimens from all over the world.[227,228] The genome has been demonstrated to exist in the epithelial cells of the tumors.[229] The EBV genome is transcriptionally active within these tumors, and the regions that are transcribed in the NPC biopsies are the same as those expressed in latently infected lymphocytes.[230] These molecular observations are consistent with an active role for EBV in the neoplastic processes involved in NPC. Patients with NPC have elevated levels of immunoglobulin (Ig) G antibodies to EBV capsid and early antigens. Indeed, the association of EBV with NPC first was suggested based on serologic evidence of higher antibody levels to EBV proteins.[231] NPC patients have serum IgA antibodies to capsid and early antigen, likely reflecting the local production of such antibodies in the nasopharynx. Cytogenetic studies on NPC xenografts have identified abnormal markers on a number of different chromosomes. Loss of heterozygosity has been noted by studies using restriction fragment length polymorphism on two different regions of chromosome 3, mapping to 3p25 and 3q14 in a very high percentage of NPC specimens.[232]

The presence of immunoglobulin markers for EBV (IgA/VCA and IgA/EA) has provided the opportunity for early serologic identification of patients with NPC. The frequency of IgA antibody to the EBV capsid antigen of 150,000 Chinese studied was found to be 1 per cent. About 20 per cent of the patients with elevated IgA antibodies to VCA had NPC, however, when biopsied. Thus, early detection using serologic tests can be applied in areas where NPC is prevalent, possibly leading to early therapeutic intervention.[233,234]

Lymphoma in Immunodeficient Individuals

EBV is also associated with lymphomas in patients with acquired or congenital immunodeficiencies. These lymphomas differ from the classical BLs in that the tumors are often polyclonal and do not demonstrate the characteristic chromosomal abnormalities of BL described earlier in this chapter. The pathogenesis of these lymphomas involves a deficiency in the mechanisms needed to control EBV-transformed cells. The prototypic model for this disease has been the X-linked lymphoproliferative syndrome (XLP).[235] Patients with XLP who develop acute infectious mononucleosis exhibit the usual atypical lymphocytosis and polyclonal elevation of serum immunoglobulins as well as increases in specific antibody to VCA and to EA. However, patients with XLP do not mount or sustain an anti-EBNA response following acute infection. The susceptibility of males with XLP to EBV infection appears to be due to an inherited immune regulatory defect resulting in a failure to govern the cytotoxic T cells and natural killer cells required to handle an EBV infection.

Patients with iatrogenic immunodeficiencies, such as organ transplant recipients, are also at an increased risk for lymphomas, which can contain EBV DNA and EBNA. As noted earlier in the chapter, some of the lymphomas observed in AIDS patients may be due in part to the malignant progression of B lymphocytes transformed by EBV.

Hodgkin's Disease

Serologic and epidemiologic studies have suggested a possible link between Hodgkin's disease and EBV; how-ever, the high EBV infection rate in humans has made interpretation of these data difficult. Recent molecular studies have demonstrated EBV DNA, RNA, and proteins in Hodgkin's disease pathologic specimens.[236-242] These analyses have shown that, whereas the mixed cellularity (MC) and nodular sclerosing (NS) subtypes are often EBV positive, the lymphocyte-depleted (LD) or lymphocyte-predominant subtypes usually are negative. Interestingly, in a positive specimen, it is usually the large binucleate Reed-Sternberg cells and the mononuclear variant Hodgkin's cells that are EBV positive. The nonmalignant cells in the tissues generally do not contain demonstrable levels of EBV DNA, RNA, or protein. Studies have shown expression of LMP1 in the Reed-Sternberg and Hodgkin's cells in a large percentage of the EBV-positive cases of MC and NS subtypes, although EBNA 2 expression could not be detected.[240,241]

REFERENCES

1. Ellermann V, Bang O: Experimentelle leukamie bei huhnern. Zentralbl Bakteriol Abt I 46:595, 1908
2. Rous P: A sarcoma of the fowl transmissible by an agent separable from the tumor cells. J Exp Med 13:397, 1911
3. Shope RE: A filtrable virus causing a tumor-like condition in rabbits and its relationship to virus myxomatosum. J Exp Med 56:803, 1932
4. Shope RE: Infectious papillomatosis of rabbits. J Exp Med 58:607, 1933
5. Rous P, Beard JW: The progression to carcinoma of virus-induced rabbit papillomas (Shope). Exp Med 62:523, 1935
6. Gross L: Pathogenic properties and "vertical" transmission of the mouse leukemia agent. Proc Soc Exp Biol Med 62:523, 1951
7. Gross L: A filtrable agent, recovered from Akr leukemia extracts, causing salivary gland carcinomas in C3H mice. Proc Soc Exp Biol Med 83:414, 1953
8. Steward SE: Leukemia in mice produced by a filterable agent present in AKR leukemic tissues with notes on a sarcoma produced by the same agent. Anat Rev 117:532, 1953
8a. Howley PM: Principles of carcinogenesis: Viral. In DeVita VT, Hellman S, Rosenberg SA (eds): Cancer: Principles and Practice of Oncology, ed. 4. Philadelphia, JB Lippincott Company, 1993, pp 182–199
9. Jarrett W, Martin WB, Crighton GW, et al: Transmission experiments with leukemia (lymphosarcoma). Nature 202:566, 1964
10. Bernard W: The detection and study of tumor viruses with electron microscopy. Cancer Res 20:71, 1960
11. Temin HM, Mizutani S: RNA-dependent DNA polymerase in virions of Rous sarcoma virus. Nature 226:1211, 1970
12. Baltimore D: RNA-dependent DNA polymerase in virions of RNA tumor viruses. Nature 276:1209, 1970
13. Poiesz BJ, Ruscetti FW, Gazdar AF, et al: Detection and isolation of type C retrovirus particles from fresh and cultured lymphocytes of a patient with cutaneous T-cell lymphoma. Proc Natl Acad Sci USA 77:7415, 1980
14. Poiesz BJ, Ruscetti FW, Reitz MS, et al: Isolation of a new type C retrovirus (HTLV) in primary uncultured cells of a patient with Sezary T-cell leukemia. Nature 294:268, 1981
15. Yoshida M, Miyoshi I, Hinuma Y: Isolation and characterization of retrovirus from cell lines of human adult T-cell leukemia and its implication in disease. Proc Natl Acad Sci USA 79:2031, 1982
16. Uchiyama T, Yodoi J, Sagawa K, et al: Adult T-cell leukemia—clinical and hematological features of 16 cases. Blood 50:481, 1977
17. Hattori T, Uchiyama T, Tibana K, et al: Surface phenotype of

Japanese adult T-cell leukemia cell characterized by monoclonal antibodies. Blood 58:645, 1981

18. Hinuma T, Nagata K, Misoka M, et al: Adult T cell leukemia: Antigen in an ATL cell line and detection of antibodies of the antigen in human sera. Proc Natl Acad Sci USA 78:6476, 1981

19. Blattner WA, Kalyanararaman VS, Robert GM, et al: The human type C retrovirus, in HTLV, in blacks from the Caribbean region, and relationship to adult T cell leukemia/lymphoma. Int J Cancer 30:257, 1982

20. Hunsman G, Schneider J, Schmitt J, et al: Detection of serum antibodies to adult T-cell leukemia virus in non-human primates and in people from Africa. Int J Cancer 32:329, 1983

21. Morgan DA, Ruscetti FW, Gallo RC: Selective in vitro growth of T-lymphocytes from normal human bone marrows. Science 193:1007, 1981

22. Yamaguchi K, Nishimura H, Kawano K, et al: A proposal for smoldering adult T-cell leukemia; diversity in clinical pictures of adult T-cell leukemia. Jpn J Clin Oncol 13:189, 1983

23. Gessain A, Barin F, Vernant JC, et al: Antibodies to human lymphotropic virus type-I in patients with tropical spastic paraparesis. Lancet 2:407, 1985

24. Bartholomew C, Cleghorn F, Charles W, et al: HTLV-1 and tropical spastic paraparesis. Lancet 2:99, 1986

25. Osame M, Usuku K, Izumo S, et al: HTLV-I associated myelopathy: A new clinical entity. Lancet 1:1031, 1986

26. Kalyanaraman VS, Sarngadharan MG, Robert-Guroff M, et al: A new su type of human T-cell leukaemia virus (HTLV-11) associated with a T-cell variant of hairy cell leukemia. Science 218:571, 1982

27. Gelmann EP, Franchini G, Manzari V, et al: Molecular cloning of a unique human T-cell leukemia virus (HTLV-II). Proc Natl Acad Sci USA 81:993, 1984

28. Shaw GM, Gonda MA, Flickinger GH, et al: Genomes of evolutionary divergent members of human T-cell leukemia virus family (HTLV-I and HTLV-II) are highly conserved, especially in pX. Proc Natl Acad Sci USA 81:4544, 1984

29. McClure MO, Weiss RA: Human immunodeficiency virus and related viruses. Curr Top AIDS 1:95, 1987

30. Pinching A, Weiss RA: AIDS and the spectrum of HTLV-III/LAV infection. Int Rev Exp Pathol 28:1, 1986

31. Ensoli B, Nakamura S, Salahuddin SZ, et al: AIDS–Kaposi's sarcoma derived cells express cytokines with autocrine and paracrine growth effects. Science 243:223, 1989

32. Barillari G, Buonaguro L, Fiorelli V, et al: Effects of cytokines from activated immune cells on vascular cell growth and HIV-1 gene expression: Implications for AIDS-Kaposi's sarcoma pathogenesis. J Immunol 149:3727, 1992

33. Tajima K, Tominaga S, Suchi T, et al: Epidemiological analysis of the distribution of antibody to adult T-cell leukemia virus. Gann 73:893, 1982

34. Okochi K, Sato H, Hinuma Y: A retrospective study on transmission of adult T-cell leukemia virus by blood transfusion: Sero-conversion in recipients. Vox Sang 46:245, 1983

35. Seika M, Eddy R, Shows TR, et al: Non-specific integration of the HTLV provirus genome into adult T-cell leukemia cells. Nature 309:640, 1984

36. Yoshida M, Sciki M, Yamaguchi K, et al: Monoclonal integration of human T-cell leukemia provirus in all primary tumors of adult T-cell leukemia suggest causative role of human T-cell leukemia virus in the disease. Proc Natl Acad Sci USA 81:2534, 1984

37. Wong-Staal F, Hahn B, Manzari V, et al: A survey of human leukemias for sequences of a human retrovirus, HTLV. Nature 302:626, 1983

38. Hayward WS, Neel BG, Astrin SM: Activation of a cellular onc gene by promoter insertion in ALV-induced lymphoid leukosis. Nature 290:475, 1981

39. Burny A, Buck C, Chantrenne H, et al: Bovine leukemia virus: Molecular biology and epidemiology. In Klein G (ed): Viral Oncology. New York, Raven Press, 1980, p 231

40. Seiki M, Hattori S, Hirayama Y, et al: Human adult T-cell leukemia virus: Complete nucleotide sequence of provirus genome integrated in leukemia cell DNA. Proc Natl Acad Sci USA 80:3618, 1983

41. Sodroski JG, Rosen CA, Haseltine WA: Trans-acting transcriptional activation of the long terminal repeat of human T lymphotropic viruses in infected cells. Science 225:381, 1984

42. Fujisawa J, Seiki M, Kiyokawa T, et al: Functional activation of long terminal repeat of human T cell leukemia virus type 1 by transacting factor. Proc Natl Acad Sci USA 82:2277, 1985

43. Febler BK, Paskalis H, Klienman EC, et al: The pX protein of HTLV-I is a transcriptional activator of its long terminal repeats. Science 229:675, 1985

44. Chen I, Slamon DJ, Rosenblatt JD, et al: The x gene is essential for HTLV replication. Science 229:54, 1985

45. Kiyokawa T, Seiki M, Iwashita S, et al: p27x-III and p21x-III proteins encoded by the pX sequence of human T-cell leukemia virus type I. Proc Natl Acad Sci USA 82:8359, 1985

46. Fujisawa J, Seika M, Sato M, et al: A transcriptional enhancer sequence of HTLV-1 is responsible for trans-activation mediated by p40 or HTLV-1. EMBO J 5:713, 1986

47. Rosen CA, Sodroski JG, Haseltine WA: Location of cis-acting regulatory sequences in the human T-cell leukemia virus type 1 long terminal repeat. Proc Natl Acad Sci USA 82:6502, 1985

48. Suzuki T, Fujisawa J-I, Toita M, et al: The trans-activator Tax of human T-cell leukemia virus type 1 (HTLV-1) interacts with cAMP-responsive element (CRE) binding and CRE modulator proteins that bind to the 21-base-pair enhancer of HTLV-1. Proc Natl Acad Sci USA 90:610, 1993

49. Zhao LJ, Giam CZ: Human T-cell lymphotropic virus type 1 (HTLV-1) transcriptional activator, Tax, enhances CREB binding to HTLV-1 21-base-pair repeats by protein-protein interaction. Proc Natl Acad Sci USA 89:7070, 1992

50. Hirai H, Fujisawa J, Suzuki T, et al: Transcriptional activator Tax of HTLV-1 binds to the NF-kappaB precursor p105. Oncogene 7:1737, 1992

51. Greene WC, Leonard WJ, Wano Y, et al: Trans-activator gene of HTLV-11 induces IL-2 cellular gene expression. Science 232:877, 1986

52. Wano Y, Feinberg M, Hosking JB, et al: Stable expression of the tax gene of type I human T-cell leukemia virus in human T cells activates specific cellular genes involved in growth. Proc Natl Acad Sci USA 85:9733, 1988

53. Beasley RP, Lin CC, Hwang L, et al: Hepatocellular carcinoma and hepatitis B virus: A prospective study of 22,707 men in Taiwan. Lancet 2:1129, 1981

54. Robinson WS, Marion PL, Feitelson M, et al: The hepadnavirus group: Hepatitis B and related viruses. In Szmuness W, Alter HJ, Maynard JW (eds): Viral Hepatitis—1981 International Symposium. Philadelphia, Franklin Institute Press, 1982, p 57

55. Summers J, Smolec JM, Snyder R: A virus similar to human hepatitis B virus associated with hepatitis and hepatoma in woodchucks. Proc Natl Acad Sci USA 74:4533, 1978

56. Marion PL, Oshiro L, Regnery DC, et al: A virus in Beechey ground squirrels that is related to hepatitis B virus of man. Proc Natl Acad Sci USA 77:2941, 1980

57. Mason WS, Seal G, Summers J: Virus of Peking ducks with structural and biological relatedness to human hepatitis B virus. J Virol 36:829, 1980

58. Tuttleman JS, Pugh JC, Summers JW: In vitro experimental infection of primary duck hepatocyte cultures with DHBV. J Virol 58:17, 1986

59. Blumberg BS, Alter HJ, Visnich S: A "new" antigen in leukemia sera. JAMA 191:541, 1965

60. Alter HJ, Blumberg BS: Further studies on a "new" human isoprecipitin system (Australia antigen). Blood 27:297, 1966

61. Blumberg BS, Gerstley BJS, Hungerford DA, et al: A serum antigen (Australia antigen) in Down's syndrome leukemia and hepatitis. Ann Intern Med 66:924, 1967

62. Prince AM: An antigen detected in the blood during the incubation period of serum hepatitis. Proc Natl Acad Sci USA 60:814, 1968

63. Dane DS, Cameron CH, Briggs M: Virus-like particles in serum of patients with Australia antigen associated hepatitis. Lancet 2:695, 1970

64. Almeida JD: Individual morphological variation seen in Australia antigen positive sera. Am J Dis Child 123:303, 1972

65. Kim CY, Tilles JG: Purification and biophysical characterization of hepatitis B antigen. J Clin Invest 52:1176, 1970

66. Summers JA, O'Connell A, Millman I: Genome of hepatitis B virus: Restriction enzyme cleavage and structure of DNA extracted from Dane particles. Proc Natl Acad Sci USA 72:4597, 1975

67. Tiollais P, Pourcel C, Dejean A: The hepatitis B virus. Nature 317:489, 1985

68. Landers TA, Greenberg HB, Robinson WS: Structure of hepatitis B Dane particle DNA and nature of the endogenous DNA polymerase reaction. J Virol 23:368, 1977

69. Ganem D, Varmus HE: The molecular biology of hepatitis B virus. Annu Rev Biochem 56:651, 1987

70. Spandau D, Lee C: Trans-activation of viral enhancers by the hepatitis B virus X protein. J Virol 62:427, 1988

71. Colgrove R, Simon G, Ganem D: Transcriptional activation of homologous and heterologous genes by the hepatitis B virus X gene product in cells permissive for viral replication. J Virol 63:4019, 1989

72. Shafritz DA, Shouval D, Sherman H, et al: Integration of hepatitis B virus DNA into the genome of liver cells in chronic liver disease and hepatocellular carcinoma. N Engl J Med 305:1067, 1981

73. Brechot C, Pourcel C, Hadchouel M, et al: State of hepatitis B virus DNA in liver diseases. Hematology 2:27, 1982

74. Summers J, Mason WS: Replication of the genome of a hepatitis B-like virus by reverse transcription of an RNA intermediate. Cell 29:403, 1982

75. Seeger C, Ganem D, Varmus HE: Biochemical and genetic evidence for the hepatitis B virus replication strategy. Science 232:477, 1986

76. Szmuness W: Hepatocellular carcinoma and the hepatitis B virus: Evidence for a causal association. Prog Med Virol 24:40, 1978

77. Kim C-Y, Koike K, Saito I, et al: HBx gene of hepatitis B virus induces liver cancer in transgenic mice. Nature 351:317, 1991

78. Chisari FV, Klopchin K, Moriyama T, et al: Molecular pathogenesis of hepatocellular carcinoma in hepatitis B virus transgenic mice. Cell 59:1145, 1989

79. Dejean A, Bougueleret K, Grzeschik K, et al: Hepatitis B virus DNA integration in a sequence homologous to v-erbA and steroid receptor genes in a hepatocellular carcinoma. Nature 322:70, 1986

80. Wang J, Chenivesse X, Henglein B, et al: Hepatitis B virus integration in a cyclin A gene in a hepatocellular carcinoma. Nature 343:555, 1990

81. Ciuffo G: Imnfesto positivo con filtrato di verruca volgare. Giorn Ital Mal Venereol 48:12, 1907

82. DeVilliers EM: Heterogeneity of the human papillomavirus group. J Virol 63:4898, 1989

83. Baker CC, Howley PM: Differential promoter utilization by the bovine infected wart tissues. EMBO J 6:1027, 1987

84. Cripe TP, Haugen TH, Turk JP, et al: Transcriptional regulation of the human papillomavirus E6-E7 promoter by a keratinocyte-dependent enhancer, and by viral E2 trans-activator and repressor gene products: Implications for cervical carcinogenesis. EMBO J 6:3745, 1987

85. Howley PM: Papillomavirinae and their replication. In Fields BN, Knipe DM (eds): Fundamental Virology. New York, Raven Press, 1991, p 743

86. Doorbar J, Campbell D, Grand RJA, et al: Identification of the human papilloma virus-1a E4 gene products. EMBO J 5:355, 1986

87. Doorbar J, Ely S, Sterling J, et al: Specific interaction between HPV-16 E1-E4 and cytokeratins results in the collapse of the epithelial cell intermediate filament network. Nature 352:824, 1991

88. Spalholz BA, Howley PM: Papillomavirus-host cell interactions. In Klein G (ed): Advances in Viral Oncology. New York, Raven Press, 1989, p 27

89. McBride AA, Romanczuk H, Howley PM: The papillomavirus E2 regulatory proteins. J Biol Chem 266:18411, 1991

90. Phelps WC, Howley PM: Transcriptional trans-activation by the human papillomavirus type 16 E2 gene product. J Virol 61:1630, 1987

91. Hirochika H, Broker TR, Chow LT: Enhancers and transacting E2 trancriptional factors of papillomaviruses. J Virol 61:2599, 1987

92. Wilson VG, Ludes-Meyers J: A bovine papillomavirus E1-related protein binds specifically to bovine papillomavirus DNA. J Virol 65:5314, 1991

93. Mohr IJ, Clark R, Sun S, et al: Targeting the E1 replication protein to the papillomavirus origin of replication by complex formation with the E2 transactivator. Science 250:1694, 1990

94. Pilacinski WP, Glassman DL, Krzyzek RA, et al: Cloning and expression in Escherichia coli of the bovine papillomavirus L1 and L2 open reading frames. Biotechnology 1:356, 1984

95. Komly CA, Breitburd F, Croissant O, et al: The L2 open reading frame of human papillomavirus type 1a encodes a minor structural protein carrying type-specific antigens. J Virol 60:813, 1986

96. Martin P, Vass WC, Schiller JT, et al: The bovine papillomavirus E5 transforming protein can stimulate the transforming activity of EGF and CSF-1 receptors. Cell 59:21, 1989

97. Petti L, Nilson L, DiMaio D: Activation of the platelet-derived growth factor receptor by the bovine papillomavirus E5 transforming protein. EMBO J 10:845, 1991

98. Goldstein DJ, Schlegel R: The E5 oncoprotein of bovine papillomavirus binds to a 16kD cellular protein. EMBO J 9:137, 1990

99. Bedell MA, Jones KH, Laimins LA: The E6-E7 region of human papillomavirus type 18 is sufficient for transformation of NIH 3T3 and rat-1 cells. J Virol 61:3635, 1987

100. Phelps WC, Yee CL, Munger K, et al: The human papillomavirus type 16 E7 gene encodes transactivation and transformation functions similar to those of adenovirus E1A. Cell 53:539, 1988

101. Matlashewski G, Schneider J, Banks L, et al: Human papillomavirus type 16 DNA cooperates with activated ras in transforming primary cells. EMBO J 6:1741, 1987

102. Munger K, Phelps WC, Bubb V, et al: The E6 and E7 genes of the human papillomavirus type 16 together are necessary and sufficient for transformation of primary human keratinocytes. J Virol 63:4417, 1989

103. Hawley-Nelson P, Vousden KH, Hubbert NL, et al: HPV16 E6 and E7 proteins cooperate to immortalize human foreskin keratinocytes. EMBO J 8:3905, 1989

104. Rous P, Kidd JG, Smith WE: Experiments on the cause of the rabbit carcinomas derived from virus-induced papillomas. J Exp Med 96:159, 1953

105. Rous P, Kidd JG: The carcinogenic effect of a virus upon tarred skin. Science 83:468, 1936

106. Kidd JG, Rous P: Effect of the papillomavirus (Shope) upon tar warts of rabbits. Proc Soc Exp Biol Med 37:518, 1937

107. Wettstein FO, Stevens JG: Variable-sized free episomes of Shope papilloma virus DNA are present in all non-virus-producing neoplasms and integrated episomes are detected in some. Proc Natl Acad Sci USA 79:790, 1982

108. Nasseri M, Wettstein FO: Differences exist between viral transcripts in cottontail rabbit papillomavirus-induced benign and malignant tumors as well as non-virus-producing and virus-producing tumors. J Virol 51:706, 1984

109. Jarrett WFH, McNeil PE, Grimshaw WIR, et al: High incidence area of cattle cancer with a possible interaction between an environmental carcinogen and a papillomavirus. Nature 274:215, 1978

110. Jarrett WFH, Murphy J, O'Neill BW, et al: Virus-induced papillomas of the alimentary tract of cattle. Int J Cancer 22:323, 1978

111. Campo MS, Moar MH, Sartirana ML, et al: The presence of bovine papillomavirus type 4 DNA is not required for the progression to, or the maintenance of, the malignant state in cancers of the alimentary canal in cattle. EMBO J 4:1819, 1985

112. Lutzner M: An autosomal recessive disease characterized by viral warts and skin cancer: A model for viral oncogenesis. Bull Cancer 65:169, 1978

113. Orth G: Epidermodysplasia verruciformis: A model for understanding the oncogenicity of human papillomaviruses. Ciba Found Symp 120:157, 1986

114. Ostrow RS, Bender M, Niimura M, et al: Human papillomavirus DNA in cutaneous primary and metastasized squamous cell carcinomas from patients with epidermodysplasia verruciformis. Proc Natl Acad Sci USA 79:1634, 1982

115. Pfister H, Gassenmaier A, Nurnberger F, et al: Human papilloma virus 5-DNA in a carcinoma of an epidermodysplasia verruciformis patient infected with various human papillomavirus types. Cancer Res 43:1436, 1983

116. Green M, Brackmann KH, Sanders PR, et al: Isolation of a human papillomavirus from a patient with epidermodysplasia verruciformis: Presence of related viral DNA genomes in human urogenital tumors. Proc Natl Acad Sci USA 79:4437, 1982

117. Yutsudo M, Shimakage T, Hakura A: Human papillomavirus type 17 DNA in skin carcinoma tissue of a patient with epidermodysplasia verruciformis. Virology 144:295, 1985

118. Yutsudo M, Hakura A: Human papillomavirus type 17 transcripts expressed in skin carcinoma tissue of a patient with epidermodysplasia verruciformis. Int J Cancer 39:586, 1987

119. Iftner T, Bierfelder S, Csapo Z, et al: Involvement of human papillomavirus type 8 genes E6 and E7 in transformation and replication. J Virol 62:3655, 1988

120. Underwood PB, Hester L: Diagnosis and treatment of premalignant lesions of the vulva. Am J Obstet Gynecol 110:849, 1971

121. Waugh M: Condylomata acuminata. BMJ 2:527, 1972

122. Dunn AE, Ogilvie MM: Intranuclear virus particles in human genital wart tissue: Observation on the ultrastructure of epidermal layer. J Ultrastruct Res 22:282, 1968

123. Oriel JD, Almeida JD: Demonstration of virus particles in human genital warts. Br J Vener Dis 46:37, 1970

124. Woodruff JD, Braun L, Cavalieri R, et al: Immunologic identification of papillomavirus antigen in condyloma tissues from the female genital tract. Obstet Gynecol 56:727, 1980

125. Gissmann L, Diehl V, Schultz CH, et al: Molecular cloning and characterization of human papillomavirus DNA derived from a laryngeal papilloma. J Virol 44:393, 1982

126. Gissmann L, Wolnik L, Ikenberg H, et al: Human papillomavirus types 6 and 11 DNA sequences in genital and laryngeal papillomas and in some cervical cancers. Proc Natl Acad Sci USA 80:560, 1983

127. Buschke A, Lowenstein L: Uber carcinomahnliche condylomata acumina des penis. Arch Dermatol Syph 163:30, 1931

128. Gissmann L, de Villiers EM, zur Hausen H: Analysis of human genital warts (condylomata acuminata) and other genital tumors for human papillomavirus type 6 DNA. Int J Cancer 29:143, 1982

129. Boshart M, zur Hausen H: Human papillomaviruses in Buschke-Lowenstein tumors: Physical state of the DNA and identification of a tandem duplication in the noncoding region of a human papillomavirus 6 subtype. J Virol 58:963, 1986

130. Meisels A, Fortin R: Condylomatous lesions of the cervix and vagina. I. Cytologic patterns. Acta Cytol 20:505, 1976

131. Purola E, Savia E: Cytology of gynecologic condyloma acuminatum. Acta Cytol 21:26, 1977

132. Laverty CR, Russell P, Hills E, et al: The significance of noncondylomatous wart virus infection of the cervical transformation zone. Acta Cytol 22:195, 1978

133. Koss LG, Durfee GR: Unusual patterns of squamous epithelium of the uterine cervix: Cytologic and pathologic study of loilocytotic atypia. Ann N Y Acad Sci 63:1245, 1956

134. Della Torre G, Pilotti S, De Palo G, et al: Viral particles in cervical condylomatous lesions. Tumori 64:549, 1978

135. Hills E, Laverty CR: Electron microscopic detection of papilloma virus particles in selected koilocytotic cells in a routine cervical smear. Acta Cytol 23:53, 1979

136. Kessler IL: Human cervical cancer as a venereal disease. Cancer Res 36:783, 1976

137. zur Hausen H: Human papillomaviruses and their possible role in squamous cell carcinomas. Curr Top Microbiol Immunol 78:1, 1977

138. Rawls WE, Tompkins WAF, Figueroa ME, et al: Herpes simplex virus type 2: Association with carcinoma of the cervix. Science 161:1255, 1968

139. Nahmias AJ, Josey WE, Naib ZM, et al: Antibodies to herpes virus hominus types 1 and 2 in humans. II. Women with cervical cancer. Am J Epidemiol 91:547, 1970

140. zur Hausen H: Herpes simplex virus in human genital cancer. Int Rev Exp Pathol 25:307, 1983

141. Vonka V, Kanda J, Hirsch I, et al: Prospective study on the relationship between cervical neoplasia and herpes simplex type-2 virus. II. Herpes simplex type-2 antibody presence in sera taken at enrollment. Int J Cancer 33:61, 1984

142. Vonka V, Kanda J, Jelinek J, et al: Prospective study on the relationship between cervical neoplasia and herpes simplex type-2 virus. I. Epidemiological characteristics. Int J Cancer 33:49, 1984

143. Peterson O: Spontaneous course of cervical precancerous conditions. Am J Obstet Gynecol 72:1063, 1956

144. Kinlen LJ, Spriggs AI: Women with positive cervical smears but without surgical intervention: A follow up study. Lancet 2:463, 1978

145. Richart RM, Barrow BA: A follow-up study of patients with cervical dysplasia. Am J Obstet Gynecol 105:386, 1969

146. Durst M, Gissmann L, Idenburg H, et al: A papillomavirus DNA from a cervical carcinoma and its prevalence in cancer biopsy samples from different geographic regions. Proc Natl Acad Sci USA 80:3812, 1983

147. Boshart M, Gissmann L, Idenberg H, et al: A new type of papillomavirus DNA, its presence in genital cancer biopsies and in cell lines derived from cervical cancer. EMBO J 3:1151, 1984

148. Gissmann L, Schwarz E: Persistence and expression of human papillomavirus DNA in genital cancer. In Evered D, Clark S (eds): Papillomaviruses. Chichester, England, John Wiley & Sons, 1986, p 190

149. Beaudenon S, Kremsdorf D, Croissant O, et al: A novel type of human papillomavirus associated with genital neoplasias. Nature 321:246, 1986

150. Beaudenon S, Kremsdorf D, Obalek S, et al: Plurality of genital human papillomaviruses: Characterization of two new types with distinct biological properties. Virology 161:374, 1987

151. Ikenberg H, Gissmann L, Gross G, et al: Human papillomavirus-16-related DNA in genital Bowen's disease and in Bowenoid papulosis. Int J Cancer 32:563, 1983

152. Gross G, Hagedorn M, Ikenberg H, et al: Presence of human papillomavirus (HPV) structural antigens and of HPV-16 related DNA sequences. Arch Dermatol 121:858, 1985

153. Durst M, Croce C, Gissmann L, et al: Papillomavirus sequences integrate near cellular oncogenes in some cervical carcinomas. Proc Natl Acad Sci USA 84:1070, 1987

154. Schwarz E, Freese UK, Gissmann L, et al: Structure and transcription of human papillomavirus sequences in cervical carcinoma cells. Nature 314:111, 1985

155. Yee CL, Krishnan-Hewlett I, Baker CC, et al: Presence and expression of human papillomavirus sequences in human cervical carcinoma cell lines. Am J Pathol 119:361, 1985

156. Romanczuk H, Howley PM: Disruption of either the E1 or the E2 regulatory gene of human papillomavirus type 16 increases viral immortalization capacity. Proc Natl Acad Sci USA 89:3159, 1992

157. Schlegel R, Phelps WC, Zhang YL, et al: Quantitative keratinocyte assay detects two biological activities of human papillomavirus DNA and identifies viral types associated with cervical carcinoma. EMBO J 7:3181, 1988

158. Durst M, Dzarlieva PR, Boukamp P, et al: Molecular and cytogenetic analysis of immortalized human primary keratinocytes obtained after transfection with human papillomavirus type 16 DNA. Oncogene 1:251, 1987

159. DeCaprio JA, Ludlow JW, Figge J, et al: SV40 large tumor antigen forms a specific complex with the product of the retinoblastoma susceptibility gene. Cell 54:275, 1988

160. Whyte P, Williamson NM, Harlow E: Cellular targets for transformation by the adenovirus E1A proteins. Cell 56:67, 1989

161. Ewen MB, Ludlow JW, Marsilio E, et al: An N-terminal transformation-governing sequence of SV40 large T antigen contributes to the binding of both p110RB and a second cellular protein, p120. Cell 58:257, 1989

162. Munger K, Werness BA, Dyson N, et al: Complex formation of human papillomavirus E7 proteins with the retinoblastoma tumor suppressor gene product. EMBO J 8:4099, 1989

163. Hudson JB, Bedell MA, McCance DJ, et al: Immortalization and altered differentiation of human keratinocytes in vitro by the E6 and E7 open reading frames of human papillomavirus type 18. J Virol 64:519, 1990

164. Barbosa MS, Vass WC, Lowy DR, et al: In vitro biological activities of the E6 and E7 genes vary among HPVs of different oncogenic potential. J Virol 65:292, 1991

165. Werness BA, Levine AJ, Howley PM: Association of human papillomavirus types 16 and 18 E6 proteins with p53. Science 248:76, 1990

166. Mietz JA, Unger T, Huibregtse JM, et al: The transcriptional transactivation function of wild-type p53 is inhibited by SV40 large T-antigen and by HPV-16 E6 oncoprotein. EMBO J 11:5013, 1992

167. Scheffner M, Werness BA, Huibregtse JM, et al: The E6 oncoprotein encoded by human papillomavirus types 16 and 18 promotes the degradation of p53. Cell 63:1129, 1990

168. Hubbert NL, Sedman SA, Schiller JT: Human papillomavirus type 16 E6 increases the degradation rate of p53 in human keratinocytes. J Virol 66:6237, 1992

169. Scheffner M, Munger K, Byrne JC, et al: The state of the p53 and retinoblastoma genes in human cervical carcinoma cell lines. Proc Natl Acad Sci USA 88:5523, 1991

170. Crook T, Wrede D, Vousden KH: p53 point mutation in HPV negative cell lines. Oncogene 6:873, 1991

171. Munger K, Yee CL, Phelps WC, et al: Biochemical and biological differences between E7 oncoproteins of the high- and low-risk human papillomavirus types are determined by amino-terminal sequences. J Virol 65:3943, 1991

172. Paquette RL, Lee YY, Wilczynski SP, et al: Mutations in p53 and human papillomavirus infection in cervical carcinoma. Cancer 72:1272, 1993

173. Crook T, Vousden KH: Properties of p53 mutations detected in primary and secondary cervical cancers suggest mechanisms of metastasis and involvement of environmental carcinogens. EMBO J 11:3935, 1992

174. Clarke EA, Morgan RW, Newman AM: Smoking as a risk factor in cancer of the cervix: Additional evidence from a case control study. Am J Epidemiol 115:59, 1982

175. Wigle DT: Smoking and cancer of the cervix: Hypothesis. Am J Epidemiol 111:125, 1980

176. Winkelstein WJ: Smoking and cancer of the uterine cervix. Am J Epidemiol 106:257, 1977

177. Hoffmann D, Hecht SS, Haley NJ, et al: Tumorigenic agents in tobacco products and their uptake by chewers, smokers and nonsmokers. J Cell Biochem 9C:33, 1985

178. zur Hausen H: Human genital cancer: Synergism between two virus infections or synergism between a virus infection and initiating events. Lancet 2:1370, 1982

179. Kahn T, Schwarz E, zur Hausen H: Molecular cloning and characterization of the DNA of a new human papillomavirus from a laryngeal carcinoma. Int J Cancer 37:61, 1986

180. Loning T, Ikenberg H, Becker J, et al: Analysis of oral papillomas, leukoplakias, and invasive carcinomas for human papillomavirus type related DNA. J Invest Dermatol 84:417, 1985

181. Brandsma JL, Steinberg BM, Abromson AL, et al: Presence of human papillomavirus type 16 related sequences in verrucous carcinoma of the larynx. Cancer Res 46:2185, 1986

182. Jenson AB, Lancaster WD, Hartmann DP, et al: Frequency and distribution of papillomavirus structural antigens in verrucae, multiple papillomas, and condylomata of the oral cavity. Am J Pathol 107:212, 1982

183. Lind P, Syrjanen K, Koppang HS, et al: Immunoreactivity and human papillomavirus (HPV) on oral precancer and cancer lesions. Scand J Dent Res 94:419, 1986

184. DeVilliers EM, Neumann R, Le JY, et al: Infection of the oral mucosa with defined types of human papillomaviruses. Med Microbiol Immunol (Berl) 174:287, 1986

185. Naghashfar Z, Sawada E, Kutcher MK, et al: Identification of genital tract papillomaviruses HPV-6 and HPV-16 in warts of the oral cavity. J Med Virol 17:313, 1989

186. Pfister H, Hettich I, Runne U, et al: Characterization of human papillomavirus type 13 from focal epithelial hyperplasia Heck lesions. J Virol 47:363, 1983

187. Beaudenon S, Praetorius F, Kremsdorf D, et al: A new type of human papillomavirus associated with oral focal epithelial hyperplasia. J Invest Dermatol 88:130, 1987

188. Syrjanen S, Syrjanen K, Lambert MA: Detection of human papillomavirus DNA in oral mucosal lesions using in situ DNA hybridization applied on paraffin sections. Oral Surg Oral Med Oral Pathol 62:660, 1986

189. Byrne JC, Tsao MS, Fraser RS, et al: Human papillomavirus-11 DNA in a patient with chronic laryngotracheobronchial papillomatosis and metastatic squamous-cell carcinoma of the lung. N Engl J Med 317:873, 1987

190. Syrjanen K, Pyrhonen S, Aukee S, et al: A tumor probably caused by human papillomavirus (HPV). Diagn Histopathol 5:291, 1982

191. Winkler B, Capo V, Reumann W, et al: Human papillomavirus infection of the esophagus. Cancer 55:149, 1985

192. Burkitt D: A sarcoma involving the jaws in African children. Br J Surg 46:218, 1958

193. Burkitt D: Determining the climatic limitations of a children's cancer common in Africa. BMJ 2:1019, 1962

194. Epstein MA, Barr YM: Cultivation in vitro of human lymphoblasts from Burkitt's malignant lymphoma. Lancet 1:252, 1964

195. Epstein MA, Achong BG, Barr YM: Virus particles in cultured lymphoblasts from Burkitt's lymphoma. Lancet 1:702, 1964

196. Kieff E, Dambaugh T, Heller M, et al: The biology and chemistry of Epstein-Barr virus. J Infect Dis 146:506, 1982

197. Baer R, Bankier AT, Biggin MD, et al: DNA sequence and expression of B95-8 Epstein Barr virus genome. Proc Natl Acad Sci USA 310:207, 1984

198. Hummel M, Kieff E: Mapping of polypeptides encoded by the Epstein-Barr virus genome in productive infection. Proc Natl Acad Sci USA 79:5678, 1982

199. de Schryver A, Klein G, Henle W, et al: Comparison of EBV neutralization tests based on abortive infection or transformation of lymphoid cells and their relation to membrane reactive antibodies (anti-MA). Int J Cancer 13:353, 1974

200. Grogan E, Jenson H, Countryman J, et al: Transfection of a rearranged viral DNA fragment, WZhet, stably converts latent Epstein-Barr viral infection to productive infection in lymphoid cells. Proc Natl Acad Sci USA 84:1332, 1987

201. Henle G, Henle W, Klein G: Demonstration of two distinct components in the early antigen complex of Epstein-Barr virus-infected cells. Int J Cancer 8:272, 1971

202. Reedman BM, Klein G: Cellular localization of an Epstein-Barr virus (EBV) associated complement-fixing antigen in producer and non-producer lymphoblastoid cell lines. Int J Cancer 11:499, 1973

203. Yates J, Warren N, Reisman D, et al: A cis-acting element from the Epstein-Barr viral genome that permits stable replication of recombinant plasmids in latently infected cells. Proc Natl Acad Sci USA 81:3806, 1984

204. Abbot SD, Rowe M, Cadwallader K, et al: Epstein-Barr virus nuclear antigen 2 induces expression of the virus-encoded latent membrane protein. J Virol 64:2126, 1990

205. Wang F, Tsang S, Kurilla MG, et al: Epstein-Barr virus nuclear antigen 2 transactivates latent membrane protein LMP 1. J Virol 64:3407, 1990

206. Zimber-Strobl U, Suentzenich KO, Laux G, et al: Epstein-Barr virus nuclear antigen-2 activates transcription of the terminal protein gene. J Virol 65:415, 1991

207. Cordier M, Calender A, Billaud M, et al: Stable transfection of Epstein-Barr virus nuclear antigen 2 in lymphoma cells containing the EBV P3HR1 genome induces expression of B-cell activation molecules CD21 and CD23. J Virol 64:1002, 1990

208. Wang F, Gregory C, Sample C, et al: Epstein-Barr virus latent membrane protein (LMP 1) and nuclear proteins 2 and 3C are effectors of phenotypic changes in B-lymphocytes: EBNA 2 and LMP 1 cooperatively induce CD23. J Virol 64:2309, 1990

209. Knutson JC: The level of c-fgr RNA is increased by EBNA-2, Epstein-Barr virus gene required for B-cell immortalization. J Virol 64:2530, 1990

210. Liebowitz D, Kieff E: Epstein-Barr virus. In Roizman B, Whitley RJ, Lopez C (eds): The Human Herpesviruses. New York, Raven Press, 1993, p 107

211. Fialkow PJ, Klein E, Klein G, et al: Immunoglobulin and glucose-6-phosphate dehydrogenase as markers of cellular origin in Burkitt lymphoma. J Exp Med 138:89, 1973

212. Mann RB, Bernard CW: Burkitts tumor: Lessons from mice, monkeys, and man. Lancet 2:84, 1979

213. Magrath I: Clinical and pathobiological features of Burkitt's lymphoma and their resistance to treatment. In Levine PH, et al (eds): Epstein-Barr Virus and Associated Diseases. Boston, Martinus Nijhoff, 1986, p 631

214. Kafuko GW, Burkitt DP: Burkitt's lymphoma and malaria. Int J Cancer 6:1, 1970

215. Morrow RHJ: Epidemiological evidence for the role of falciparum malaria in the pathogenesis of Burkitt's lymphoma. In Lenior GM, O'Connor G, Olweny CLM (eds): A Human Cancer Model. Lyon, IARC Scientific Publications, 1985, p 177

216. Moss DJ, Burrows SR, Catelino DJ, et al: A comparison of Epstein-Barr virus-specific T-cell immunity in malaria-endemic and nonendemic regions of Papua New Guinea. Int J Cancer 31:727, 1983

217. Manolov G, Manolova Y: Marker band in one chromosome 14 from Burkitt lymphomas. Nature 237:33, 1972

218. Lenoir GM, Taub R: Chromosomal translocations and oncogenes in Burkitt's lymphoma. In Goldman JM (ed): Leukaemia and Lymphoma Research: Genetic Rearrangements in Leukaemia and Lymphoma. London, DG Harnden, 1986, p 152

219. Leder P, Battey J, Lenoir G, et al: Translocations among antibody genes in human cancer. Science 222:765, 1983

220. Erikson J, Finan J, Nowell PC, et al: Translocation of immunoglobulin V H genes in Burkitt's lymphoma. Proc Natl Acad Sci USA 79:5611, 1982

221. Klein G: Lymphoma development in mice and human: Diversity of initiation is followed by convergent cytogenetic evolution. Proc Natl Acad Sci USA 76:2442, 1979

222. Klein G, Klein E: Evolution of tumors and the impact of molecular oncology. Nature 315:190, 1985

223. Lenoir GM, Bornkamm GW: Burkitt's lymphoma, a human cancer model for the study of multistep development of cancer: Proposal for a new scenario. Adv Viral Oncol 7:173, 1987

224. Murray R, Wang D, Young L, et al: Epstein-Barr virus-specific cytotoxic T-cell recognition of transfectants expressing the virus-coded latent membrane protein LMP. J Virol 62:3747, 1988

225. Gregory CD, Murray RJ, Edwards CF, et al: Down regulation of cell adhesion molecules LFA-3 and ICAM-1 in Epstein-Barr virus-positive Burkitt's lymphoma underlies tumor cell escape from virus-specific T cell surveillance. J Exp Med 167:1811, 1988

226. Henle W, Henle G: Epstein-Barr virus and human malignancies. Adv Viral Oncol 5:201, 1985

227. zur Hausen H, Schulte-Holthausen H, Klein G, et al: EBV DNA in biopsies of Burkitt tumors and anaplastic carcinomas of the nasopharynx. Nature 228:1056, 1970

228. Andersson-Anvret M, Forsby N, Klein G, et al: Relationship between the Epstein-Barr virus and undifferentiated nasopharyngeal carcinoma: Correlated nucleic acid hybridization and histopathological examination. Int J Cancer 20:486, 1977

229. Raab-Traub N, Flynn K, Pearson G, et al: The differentiated form of nasopharyngeal carcinoma contains Epstein-Barr virus DNA. Int J Cancer 39:25, 1987

230. Pagano JS: Epstein-Barr virus transcription in nasopharyngeal carcinoma. J Virol 48:580, 1983

231. Old LJ, Boyse AE, Oettgen HF, et al: Precipitation antibody in human serum to an antigen present in cultured Burkitt's lymphoma cells. Proc Natl Acad Sci USA 56:1699, 1966

232. Huang DP, Lo KW, Choi PH, et al: Loss of heterozygosity on the short arm of chromosome 3 in nasopharyngeal carcinoma. Cancer Genet Cytogenet 54:91, 1991

233. De The G, Zeng Y: Population screening for EBV markers: Toward improvement of nasopharyngeal carcinoma control. In Epstein MA, Achog BS (eds): The Epstein-Barr Virus. New York, John Wiley & Sons, 1986, p 237

234. Zhu XX, Zheng Y, Wolf H: Detection of IgG and IgA antibodies to Epstein-Barr virus membrane in sera from patients with nasopharyngeal carcinoma and from normal individuals. Int J Cancer 37:689, 1986

235. Purtilo DT, Sakamoto K, Barnabai V, et al: Epstein-Barr virus-induced diseases in boys with the X-linked lymphoproliferative syndrome (XLP): Updates on studies of the registry. Am J Med 73:49, 1982

236. Weiss LM, Movahed LA, Warnke RA, et al: Detection of Epstein-Barr viral genomes in Reed-Sternberg cells of Hodgkin's disease. N Engl J Med 320:502, 1989

237. Weiss LM, Strickler JG, Warnke RA, et al: Epstein-Barr viral DNA in tissues of Hodgkin's disease. Am J Pathol 129:86, 1987

238. Wu TC, Mann RB, Charache P, et al: Detection of EBV gene expression in Reed-Sternberg cell of Hodgkin's disease. Int J Cancer 46:801, 1990

239. Staal SP, Ambinder R, Beschorner WE, et al: A survey of Epstein-Barr virus DNA in lymphoid tissue: Frequent detection in Hodgkin's disease. Am J Clin Pathol 91:1, 1989

240. Pallesen G, Hamilton-Dutoit SJ, Rowe M, et al: Expression of Epstein-Barr virus latent gene products in tumour cells of Hodgkin's disease. Lancet 337:320, 1991

241. Herbst H, Dallenbach F, Hummel M, et al: Epstein-Barr virus latent membrane protein expression in Hodgkin and Reed-Sternberg cells. Proc Natl Acad Sci USA 88:4766, 1991

242. Herbst H, Niedobitek G, Kneba M, et al: High incidence of Epstein-Barr virus genomes in Hodgkin's disease. Am J Pathol 137:13, 1990

243. Huibregtse JM, Scheffner M, Howley PM: A cellular protein mediates association of p53 with the E6 oncoprotein of human papillomavirus types 16 or 18. EMBO J 10:4129, 1991

4

MOLECULAR MECHANISMS OF MUTAGENESIS AND MULTISTAGE CARCINOGENESIS

I. BERNARD WEINSTEIN
ADELAIDE M. CAROTHERS
REGINA M. SANTELLA
FREDERICA P. PERERA

HISTORICAL BACKGROUND

As we approach the 21st century, it is instructive to look back at the remarkable progress that has been made in our understanding of cancer causation during the past three centuries and the exciting crescendo of knowledge obtained at the cellular and molecular levels during the latter half of this century. The first insights into human cancer causation occurred in the 18th century with the astute clinical observations by John Hill of the association of the use of snuff with nasal polyps, by Percival Pott of the association of soot with scrotal cancer in chimney sweeps, and by Bernadino Ramazzini of the association of reproductive factors with breast cancer. The 19th century provided a foundation for the pathophysiology of cancer, through classic descriptions of the pathology of specific tumors. It also focused attention on the cancer cell, rather than the host, as the major site of the pathology. In the last decade of the 19th century, L. Rehn reported an association between occupational exposure to aromatic amines and bladder cancer, thus setting the stage for the identification during the 20th century of other specific carcinogens in the workplace and the environment. Early evidence for the multistage and multifactor nature of the carcinogenic process was revealed by the experimental studies of Yamagiwa and Ichikawa at the beginning of this century. This evidence was extended by Peyton Rous, Isaac Berenblum, Leslie Foulds, and others in the middle decades of this century. Now, in the final decade of this century, studies on the molecular biology of cancer have revealed that these multiple steps appear to reflect, at least in part, the progressive accumulation of mutations in cellular oncogenes and growth suppressor genes. The 20th century also witnessed the emergence of modern genetics, first with studies at the level of whole organisms (mainly inbred strains of mice and *Drosophila*) and of chromosomes. These advances in genetics provided important new concepts and tools for studying cancer causation. For comprehensive reviews of this history of cancer research, the reader is referred to refs.1–3.

Within the past few decades, the focus in cancer research has shifted to studies at the macromolecular level, yielding profound insights into the biochemistry and molecular biology of cancer cells. Within the past 10 to 15 years, this approach has led to the discovery of cellular oncogenes, growth suppressor genes, and derangements in regulatory circuits that control gene expression, the cell cycle, and cell proliferation and differentiation.[4-9] Thus, as we look toward the 21st century, we have entered the era of "molecular oncology." Indeed, molecular oncology should provide a bridge between basic research, cancer prevention, and cancer treatment, thus joining together laboratory and clinical investigators. The current central dogma of molecular oncology actually was formulated about 80 years ago by Theodor Boveri,[10] who recognized that the fundamental defects in cancer reside in the genetic material of the cell, which at that time was conceptualized at the level of chromosomes rather than DNA. His insights were even more profound because he hypothesized that cancers might arise from defects in chromosomes that have either growth-promoting or growth-inhibitory effects. Thus, he anticipated the genetic elements that we now call oncogenes and tumor suppressor genes.

The exciting advances during this century in the genetics and molecular biology of cancer have been paralleled by major advances in chemical carcinogenesis and other areas of cancer research. During the middle decades of this century, a good deal of cancer research was concentrated on the biochemistry of cancer, particularly intermediary metabolism thus providing important insights into derangements in energy metabolism and biosynthetic and catabolic pathways in cancer cells. This knowledge provided a rationale for developing several very useful chemotherapy agents, especially antimetabolites and various cytotoxic compounds. Parallel biochemical studies in the field of chemical carcinogenesis revealed insights into carcinogen metabolism, activation, macromolecular binding, and detoxification.[3,11,12] Current biochemical studies, fortified by the powerful tools of molecular genetics, are focused on pathways of signal transduction and the control of gene expression.[6,13] This exploration holds even greater promise in cancer research because it deals with the intelligence system of the cell, rather than its building blocks and energy sources. Research in this field also has merged with studies on carcinogenesis, especially the action of tumor promoters and the field of hormonal carcinogenesis.[13] Indeed, recent results from several disciplines suggest that the multistage carcinogenic process is best understood as a "progressive disorder in signal transduction and gene expression.[13]

With this history as background, the purpose of this chapter is to review recent findings on molecular mechanisms of chemical mutagenesis and multistage carcinogenesis, to discuss the possible relevance of these findings to cancer prevention and therapy, and to suggest future directions of research in this area. For other recent reviews on this and related subjects, the reader is referred to refs. 3,4,12,14–18.

ROLES OF EXOGENOUS AGENTS IN HUMAN CANCER CAUSATION

Fortunately, several types of evidence indicate that a major fraction (50 to 80 per cent) of human cancer is potentially preventable, because its causation (i.e., the factors that determine incidence) is largely exogenous.[14,16]

This evidence comes mainly from epidemiologic studies, including: (1) time trends in cancer incidence and mortality; (2) geographic variations and the effects of migration; (3) the identification of specific causative factors (cigarette smoking, occupational and environmental chemicals, radiation, dietary factors, socioeconomic factors, and specific viruses); and (4) the fact that the majority of human cancers do not show simple patterns of inheritance. We should, of course, emphasize that genetic factors are also extremely important in terms of influencing individual susceptibility, and that, in certain less common (but highly instructive) forms of human cancer, hereditary factors play a more decisive role. For the majority of human cancers, however, modification of the external factors, and/or the response of the host to these factors, is the most promising approach to cancer prevention. This is an optimistic message because it means that the development of several forms of cancer is not an inherent consequence of the aging process per se and that the human species is not inevitably destined to suffer a high incidence of cancer.[14] In principle, the majority of cancers are therefore preventable if the external causative factors can be identified. This constitutes a major challenge because, for several prevalent forms of human cancer (i.e., cancers of the breast, prostate, colon, and several other organ sites), the precise causes are not known with certainty. Therefore, basic research on cancer causation is an essential component of a comprehensive approach to cancer prevention and control. Furthermore, advances in secondary prevention are also highly dependent on basic research on the carcinogenic process, because there are major gaps in our current armamentarium of methods for the early detection of several types of cancer, and also in rational approaches to intervention.

Known causes of human cancer include specific chemicals or mixtures of chemicals present in various sources (cigarette smoke, various therapeutic agents, diet, the workplace, and the general environment); radiation (both ultraviolet and ionizing radiation); and specific viruses (hepatitis B, Epstein-Barr, papilloma, and certain retroviruses) (for review, see refs. 15,16). In addition, oxidative damage to DNA as a result of endogenous metabolic reactions that generate highly reactive forms of oxygen,[19-21] and certain bacterial or parasitic infections,[16] also have been implicated, but the roles of these factors are less well understood. This review concentrates on the chemical carcinogens because of their abundance and the fact that they illustrate several general principles in cancer causation.

BIOCHEMICAL AND MOLECULAR MECHANISMS OF MULTISTAGE CARCINOGENESIS

Diversity of Structures and Sources of Chemical Carcinogens

The known human chemical carcinogens consist of a broad diversity of compounds, in terms of both their chemical structures and their sources (for review, see refs. 3,15,16). They include numerous man-made or industrial compounds, as well as naturally occurring chemicals. Their chemical structures include polycyclic aromatic hydrocarbons, aromatic amines, nitrosamines and nitrosoureas, alkylating agents, alkyl and aryl halides, steroid hormones, mycotoxins, metals, and asbestos fibers. Aflatoxin B_1, the product of a mold that frequently contaminates peanuts, cereals, and grains as a result of improper storage and processing techniques, is an important example of a naturally occurring, highly potent carcinogen. It is thought to contribute (probably in combination with hepatitis B virus infection) to the high incidence of liver cancer in certain regions of Africa and Asia.[22] In addition to plant and fungal products, certain cooking and food preparation practices may generate carcinogenic substances. Highly potent mutagens that are carcinogenic in rodents have been identified recently as products of certain amino acids that are formed during the broiling of fish or meat.[17,23] These heterocyclic amines[17,23] and a number of other constituents of the human diet[14,16,24,25] cause cancer in laboratory animals, but the extent to which they contribute to human cancer is not known with certainty. The important roles of dietary factors such as fat, fiber, vitamins, and minerals in human cancer causation is discussed in greater detail later in this chapter.

The most important known source of chemical carcinogens for humans is, of course, cigarette smoke, because smoking causes about one third of all the cancer deaths in the United States. Most of these deaths are due to lung cancer, but smoking also increases the risk of cancers of the bladder, esophagus, and pancreas.[15,16] Although there has been an encouraging decline in smoking in white American males, this is not the case in black American males, and there has been a shocking increase in smoking and lung cancer deaths in American women.[15] Cigarette smoke is a complex chemical mixture that includes several known genotoxic carcinogens and tumor promoters. The precise chemicals in cigarette smoke that are responsible for human cancers are not known. Polycyclic aromatic hydrocarbons and N-nitrosonornicotine have been implicated in lung cancer, and aromatic amines in bladder cancer.[16,26] Thus, cigarette smoking provides strong and direct evidence that, as in other species, specific classes of chemicals can be potent carcinogens in humans. At least 50 other types of chemicals or mixtures of chemicals have been implicated in human cancer causation.[16] The production of various species of activated oxygen (including superoxide anion, perhydroxy radical, H_2O_2, the OH radical, alkoxy- and peroxy- radicals, organic hydroperoxides, and singlet oxygen) can enhance carcinogenesis in experimental systems by producing oxidative damage to DNA or cellular membranes and proteins, thereby causing mutations and/or altered gene expression and enhanced cell proliferation.[19–21,24] As mentioned earlier in this chapter, the extent to which oxidative stress contributes to human cancer is not known at the present time.

Metabolic Activation and Detoxification of Carcinogens

A basic principle in the biochemistry of carcinogenesis is that several chemical carcinogens are not active in their native forms. They undergo metabolic activation by various tissues and thereby are converted to highly reactive electrophilic species. These then can react with nucleophilic residues in cellular proteins and nucleic acids to form covalent adducts.[11,12,18] The polycyclic aromatic hydrocarbon benzo[a]pyrene (BP), for example, is not highly reactive chemically. The cellular endoplasmic reticulum, however, which is present in cells of a variety of tissues and species, contains a group of enzymes, the cytochrome P-450 system (also called the microsomal mono-oxygenase system), that can convert BP and related polycyclic aromatic hydrocarbons (PAHs) to a variety of derivatives. The normal role of this system is to convert lipid-soluble foreign substances to more water-soluble substances that can be excreted. However, some of the intermediates in this oxidative process are epoxides, which can form covalent bonds with bases in DNA. In the case of BP, the critical intermediate is a specific diol epoxide that forms a covalent adduct with the 2-amino group of guanine residues in DNA.[12] Biochemical and DNA cloning studies indicate that the mammalian genome encodes a large number of P-450 enzymes that differ in terms of their specificity for oxidizing different drugs and potential carcinogens.[27,28] There also exists a series of enzymes (so-called phase II enzymes) that are involved in the further metabolism and detoxication of activated carcinogens and other xenobiotics, thus preventing their binding to DNA. These include epoxide hydrolase, glutathione-S-transferase, sulfotransferase, UDP-glucuronyl transferase, and NADPH quinone reductase.[27,28] As discussed later in this chapter, inter-individual variation in carcinogen activation or detoxification probably plays an important role in susceptibility to certain forms of cancer.

Structures of Carcinogen-DNA Adducts

The metabolic activation and interactions with nucleic acids of several types of carcinogens have been elucidated in considerable detail.[3,12,18] The simple alkylating agents can methylate or ethylate any of the nitrogens or oxygens in all four bases in DNA, as well as the sugar residues and phosphates of the DNA backbone. Although the N^7 position of guanine is generally the most extensive site of modification, current evidence indicates that the O^6 position of guanine is often the most important site of attachment with respect to mutagenesis and carcinogenesis by these alkylating agents. Because the O^6 position of guanine is involved in Watson-Crick base pairing, alkylation of O^6 interferes with hydrogen bonding, and thus produces base pairing errors during nucleic acid replication. The interaction of bulky carcinogens is more complex, as illustrated by the aromatic amine carcinogen N-2-acetylaminofluorene (AAF), which, like BP, undergoes metabolic activation. Activation of AAF occurs on the amino group, and the major nucleic acid adduct results from linkage to the C^8 position of guanine residues. This presents steric (or space filling) problems in terms of accommodating the bulky AAF residue within the nucleic acid helix. Therefore, AAF modification of DNA can result in a distortion in the conformation of the DNA helix known as base displacement, in which the AAF residue is inserted into the DNA helix, displacing the modified guanine residue.[12,18] Recent studies using two-dimensional nuclear magnetic resonance (NMR) analysis of the structures of carcinogen-modified oligonucleotides have provided detailed information on the conformational changes produced by activated forms of AAF and BP.[29,30] In the case of the diol epoxide of BP (BPDE), opening of the epoxide ring to form a covalent DNA adduct creates four spacially different stereoisomers. Hence, the precise conformation of the complex with DNA depends on the chirality of the BPDE. Thus in one case the BP residue lies in the minor groove of the DNA helix, whereas in another case it is inserted into the helix.[30] As discussed later in this chapter, this detailed structural information has provided insights into the molecular mechanisms of mutagenesis. Different carcinogens can attack different sites on the DNA molecule and produce different distortions in the structure of DNA, and even a single carcinogen can form multiple types of adducts. This complicates attempts to formulate a unified or simple theory relating specific types of DNA damage to the mechanism of carcinogenesis. However, the major carcinogen-DNA adducts are often the same in diverse species and tissues. This evidence provides some unity to the comparative chemistry of carcinogen-DNA adducts.[12,18] Representative structures of carcinogen-nucleoside adducts are shown in Figure 4–1.

Mutational Spectra in Mammalian Cells

Within the past few years, exciting progress has been made in elucidating the types of mutations produced by different lesions in DNA and the roles of DNA repair and other host responses in this process. These topics will therefore be reviewed in this section and the following two sections. During the process of DNA replication, carcinogen-DNA adducts are either miscoding or noninstructional; hence these lesions can cause a variety of mutations. Carcinogen-induced mutational spectra have been examined extensively in bacteria; for this purpose, the *Escherichia coli lacI* gene has been very useful. For reasons discussed below, mammalian cell culture and whole animal mutation systems are more relevant to the process of carcinogenesis. In the last decade, mutational mechanisms in mammalian cells have been studied using various types of model systems (Table 4–1). In the first category are *shuttle vectors*, which are plasmids consisting of sequences that direct episomal replication, a selectable marker, and a target sequence for mutations. An advantage

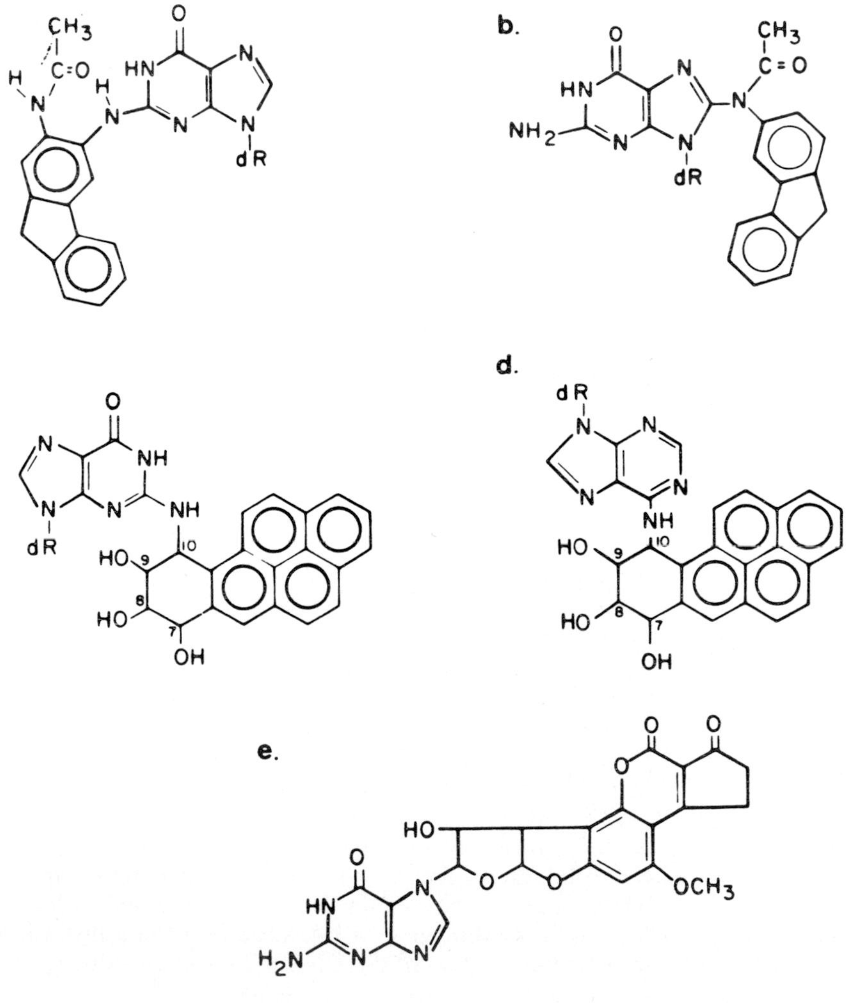

Figure 4–1. The structures of several carcinogen–nucleoside adducts. *a*, 2-acetamido-3-(2'-deoxy-N^2-guanosyl)fluorene. *b*, 3-[N-(2'-deoxy-8-iguanosyl)acetamido]fluorene. *c*, 2'-deoxy-N^2-(7,8,9,10-tetrahydro-7β,8α,9α-trihydroxybenzo[a]pyrene-10-yl) guanosine. *d*, 2'-deoxy-N^6(7,8,9,10-tetrahydro-7β,8α,9α-trihydroxybenzo[a]pyrene-10-yl) adenosine. *e*, 7-guanyldihydrohydroxyaflatoxin B$_1$. For additional details, see text and related references in the section on ''Structures of Carcinogen DNA Adducts.''

of this approach is that the construct DNA is first modified by the carcinogen of interest in vitro, and damage levels can be accurately quantitated. Mammalian cells receive the modified vectors by transfection, and are spared the toxic and lethal effects of the physical or chemical treatment. Thus, the mutations observed may more directly reflect the specificity of the lesion. The most widely used shuttle vector employs the bacterial tyrosine amber suppressor tRNA gene, *supF*, designated pZ189.[31] The advantage of this shuttle vector is that the mutational target sequence is only about 200 bp in size and almost every single base substitution creates a selectable mutant phenotype.

The second approach listed in Table 4–1 is *targeted mutagenesis*. This method demonstrates the biologic effects of DNA-damaging agents through the use of single,

TABLE 4–1. ASSAYS TO DETERMINE MUTATIONAL SPECIFICITIES OF CARCINOGENIC AGENTS AT THE DNA LEVEL IN MAMMALIAN CELLS

SYSTEMS*	EXAMPLES OF AGENTS STUDIED†
1. Shuttle vectors	UV, 1NOP, H_2O_2, AFB$_1$, AF, AAF, BPDE, BcPHDE, EMS, MNU, *cis*-Pt, melphalan, spontaneous
2. Targeted mutagenesis	AAF & AF, O^6-methyl-dG, O^4-ethyl-T, *cis*-Pt, BPDE, 8-OH-dG
3. Null mutants selected at autosomal, heterozygous markers	UV, EMS, BrdUrd, IR, spontaneous
4. Forward/reverse mutants in transfectants with single-copy mutant constructs	UV, EMS, AAF, IR, spontaneous
5. Forward mutations in endogenous hemizygous genes	UV, *cis*-Pt, carbo-Pt, EMS, BPDE, AAF, N-OH-AF, BcPHDE, 1NOP, N-OH-PhIP, BCNU, IR, spontaneous

*For additional details, see text and references cited in "Mutation Spectra in Mammalian Cells."
†Abbreviations for carcinogens and physical damaging agents: UV, ultraviolet light; 1NOP, 1-nitrosopyrene; H_2O_2, hydrogen peroxide; AFB$_1$, aflatoxin B$_1$; AF, 2-aminofluorene; AAF, 2-acetylaminofluorene; BPDE, (±)-7α, 8α-dihydroxy-9α, 10α-epoxy-7,8,9,10-tetrahydrobenzo [α]pyrene; BcPHDE; (±)-3α,4β-dihydroxy-1α, 2α-epoxy-1,2,3,4-tetrahydrobenzo[c]phenanthrene; EMS, ethyl methanesulfonate; MNU, *N*-methyl-*N*-nitrosourea; *cis*-DDP, *cis*-diamminedichloroplatinum^{11}; melphalan, 4-([bis(2-chloroethyl)-amino]-L-phenylalanine; O^6-methyl-dG, O^6-methyldeoxyguanosine, O^4-ethyl-T, O^4-ethylthymine, 8-OH-dG, 7,8-dihydro-8-oxodeoxyguanosine; BrdUrd, 5-bromo-2′-deoxyuridine; IR, ionizing radiation; carbo-PT, *cis*-diammine-1, 1-cyclobutane dicarbylate; *N*-OH-AF, *N*-hydroxyamino-fluorene; PhIP, 1-amino-1-methyl-6-phenylimidazo[4,5-β]pyridine; BCNU, 1-3-bis(2- chloroethyl)1-nitrosourea.

structurally defined adducts. As indicated earlier in this chapter, genotoxic agents typically create a heterogeneous mixture of electrophilic species when they are metabolized to reactive intermediates by cellular enzymes. Hence, several structurally distinct adducts often form upon treatment of cells in vivo with a single chemical agent. Recent advances in molecular biology and nucleic acid chemistry have made it possible to examine the biologic effects of individual adducts. For targeted mutagenesis studies, oligonucleotides are synthesized in vitro that contain a modified base centrally positioned at a specific site in a given sequence.[32] This molecule then is annealed into a gapped duplex vector, ligated, and introduced into cells to generate mutants, or annealed with a complementary primer for in vitro translesion synthesis. After transfection into cells and replication, mutants are selected and analyzed at the modification site by DNA sequencing. These modified oligonucleotides also can be used as templates in subcellular replication assays, and the effects of different variables in the reaction on mutational specificity can be evaluated by sequencing gels. For example, the relative fidelities of different DNA polymerases can be compared for a given lesion. This approach is especially informative when carried out in parallel with proton NMR structural analysis of the modified oligonucleotide. Moreover, because the sequence context in which the adduct is placed is predetermined, this method can be used to reveal the basis for mutational hot spots. However, because the sequence context is often arbitrary, the results obtained may not necessarily reflect the in vivo situation.

Another mutagenesis approach is to induce a *null phenotype* using a mammalian cell line that is heterozygous for the target gene. Employing this approach, studies of spontaneous or induced thymidine kinase deficient (*TK*$^-$) human cells indicated that allele loss is a more common type of mutation than either intragenic rearrangement or point mutation.[33] Allelic loss may be underrepresented in other assay systems as a result of constraints on deletion. For example, elimination of the targeted locus also may remove an adjacent critical sequence. Indeed, this problem arises in the case of the adenosine phosphoribosyltransferase gene (*APRT*), because in Chinese hamster ovary (CHO) cells deletion of the *APRT* 3′ flanking sequence is apparently lethal.[34] A model for evaluating the induction of very large chromosomal deletions and/or rearrangements is the A$_L$ hybrid rodent cell line that stably maintains a dispensible human chromosome 11.[35]

Mutagenesis studies have been performed using *transfected mammalian cells* carrying a single copy of a selectable target gene on a construct that subsequently can be rescued in bacteria[36] (Table 4–1, item 4). The selectable marker used for much of this work was the *E. coli* gene encoding xanthine (guanine) phosphoribosyltransferase (*gpt*), introduced into hypoxanthine guanine phosphoribosyltransferase–deficient (*HPRT*$^-$) rodent cell lines. Cells expressing the bacterial gene are rendered resistant to 6-thioguanine (TG^r). In addition to determining the nature of induced point mutations, transfected markers have been used to study the ability of chemical and physical agents to induce homologous recombination. Thus, an interrupted *TK*$^-$ construct introduced in mouse *LTK*$^-$

cells was induced to recombine to yield a TK^+ phenotype using the chemicals, N-methyl-N'-nitro-N-nitrosoguanidine (MNNG), mitomycin C, or BPDE, as well as ultraviolet and ionizing radiation.[37] In another type of assay, a transfected mutant target gene can be tested for reversion instead of forward mutation. Treatment of cells carrying an integrated mutant gpt^- marker with specific chemicals was followed by selection of clones that display a positive TG^r phenotype.[38] Because reversion assays are restricted with respect to the types of mutations that will satisfy the phenotypic requirement, they are limited in their utility. A novel reversion assay was used, however, to show that point mutations induced by a PAH in the dihydrofolate reductase (*DHFR*) gene preferentially arose on the DNA coding strand.[39]

The use of transfected or retrovirally introduced sequences for mutational studies may bias the results for several reasons. The transfection process itself is mutagenic and can introduce chromosome rearrangements, other types of mutations, and epigenetic changes in recipient cells.[40] The marker DNA used for transfection is also subject to numerous kinds of spontaneous alterations. Integration sites for transfected DNA in the recipient genome often are situated in repetitive elements that may be intrinsically unstable. Introduction of a target gene by transduction with a retroviral vector can lead to nonrandom integration (reviewed in ref. 41), including preferential integration at methylated runs of CpG dinucleotides.[42] Spontaneous mutation rates for a target gene carried on a retroviral vector can vary depending on the site of chromosomal integration, and can be more than ten-fold higher than that of an endogenous target.[43] Because the chromosomal location of a marker may influence the types of mutations produced, this approach also can bias the results obtained in mutation assays.

The last approach listed in Table 4–1 is the use of *endogenous genes* in rodent and human cells in culture.[44] Markers of this type that have been used for the analysis of induced forward mutations include *APRT*, *DHFR*, and *HPRT*. Unambiguous analysis of induced mutations requires the use of actual or functional hemizygous cells (i.e., cells that carry a single functional copy of the selectable locus). As noted earlier in this chapter, this requirement may be a disadvantage in terms of detecting all possible types of induced mutations. Nonetheless, there are several advantages. The spontaneous mutation rate for endogenous mammalian genes is, in general, low (10^{-7} to 10^{-8}), and induction by chemicals or radiation typically causes mutations to occur at frequencies greater than tenfold over background. *Cis*-acting regulatory elements in DNA exert effects on transcription through interactions with specific *trans*-acting protein factors. Examples of such elements are enhancers, pre-mRNA splice sites, attenuators, and 3' untranslated sequences that affect mRNA stability. These elements are also targets for mutations in addition to coding sequences. Thus, mutational studies of an endogenous gene can reveal the presence of these sequences,[45] and the fact that they can be preferential targets for certain carcinogens.[46] In addition, because these model genes reside in their normal chromosomal locations and in their natural chromatin environment, cellular repair and replicative processes can be inferred to be normal. Finally, mutations in endogenous genes can reveal hot spots and target sites that are specific for a given carcinogen, as well as for spontaneous mutations. Deducing the mechanisms for these events then provides a better understanding of the in vivo situation.

The foregoing discussion emphasizes the need for comparative data because each of the approaches listed in Table 4–1 has advantages and disadvantages. The types of mutations obtained in the assays listed in Table 4–1 are too extensive to describe in detail here; therefore, in Table 4–2, we have provided only examples of some of the major results obtained. Alkylation of DNA bases by small residues (methyl or ethyl) generally induces transition mutations, with O^6-alkylguanine causing guanine-to-adenine (G → A) substitutions and O^4-alkylthymine causing thymine-to-cytosine (T → C) substitutions.[18] Exposure to ultraviolet light induces pyrimidine dimers and the (4-6) pyrimidine-pyrimidone photoproduct[47]; both DNA lesions are mutagenic. The latter, unlike the pyrimidine dimer, is not known to be corrected by photoreactivation in mammalian cells. Dimer and photoproduct modifications cause single or tandem double transitions at dipyrimidines, with the 3' base most commonly mutated.[47] Transitions are also preferred changes induced by oxygen radicals produced by transition metal ions (ref. 48 and references therein). The most prevalent damage induced by oxidative processes is 7,8-dihydro-8-oxodeoxyguanosine (8-OH-dG).[49] This adduct, and purine adducts formed by bulky carcinogens, tend to induce transversion substitutions. The modified purine is mutated to thymine. This effect has been explained by the A-rule,[50] the hypothesis that DNA polymerase preferentially incorporates deoxyadenosine opposite a noninstructional base. This suggestion fits well for carcinogen adducts that interfere with base pairing (e.g.,

TABLE 4–2. SUMMARY OF MAJOR TYPES OF MUTATIONS FOUND WITH DIFFERENT CLASSES OF CARCINOGENIC AGENTS IN VARIOUS MAMMALIAN SYSTEMS*

AGENT[†]	MUTATION TYPE
Polycyclic aromatic hydrocarbons: BPDE, BcPHDE, DMBA, etc.	purine→T
Heterocyclic and aromatic amines: PhIP, AAAF, 1NPO	G→T
Alkylating agents: MNU, EMS, vinyl chloride	G→A
Oxidative damage: 8-OH-dG	G→T
oxygen radicals from Fe^{2+}, Cu^{1+}, or Cu^{2+} and H_2O_2	CC→TT
UV light: cyclobutane pyrimidine dimer and/or (6-4) pyrimidine-pyrimidone photoproduct	CC→TT CC→CT

*It should be emphasized that this table indicates only the most frequent types of mutation produced by these agents. Each of these agents can produce other types of mutations (e.g., other base substitutions, frameshifts, deletions, etc.) depending on the system or DNA sequence examined.

[†]For abbreviations, see Table 4–1.

BPDE, which binds at the N^2 position of guanine). As indicated earlier in this chapter, adducts such as AAF or the deacetylated form (AF) modify the C-8 position of guanine, a position not involved in base pairing. Proton NMR analysis revealed that the deoxyguanosine-AF (dG-AF) adduct may allow pairing of adenine opposite the modified base because of hydrophobic interactions between the carcinogen situated in the minor groove and an opposing adenine.[51] In the case of 8-OH-dG, moreover, Hoogsteen base pairing can occur when the modified base is opposite dA [8-OH-dG (*syn*) · dA (*anti*)] in DNA.[51a] Hence, adduct-directed mispairing in certain circumstances may provide an alternative explanation for mutational specificity. Thus, in some cases structurally different types of DNA damage can have similar mutational specificity. However, the probability of mutagenesis by lesion is also influenced by the sequence context at the modification site. Finally, host systems (discussed in "DNA Repair," later in this chapter) that are specific for different types of DNA lesions are also important modulators of the extent and type of mutagenesis observed in vivo.

Not mentioned in Table 4–1 are approaches to evaluate mutagenesis in the intact rodent or in humans, using either the endogenous *HPRT* locus[52] or transgenic mice.[53] This newer field has focused mainly on spontaneous mutation rates for target sequences. The origin(s) and nature of spontaneous mutations in vivo are of particular interest in view of the possible destabilization of the genome during the carcinogenic process (as discussed in "Genomic Instability and Inducible Responses to DNA Damage," later in this chapter). Studies in transgenic mice should indicate the effects of the chromosomal location of the integrated transgene and tissue-specific effects. Studies in humans will provide insights into inter-individual susceptibility Furthermore, low doses of agents can be used in transgenic animals over prolonged periods of time, which will better approximate human exposures. The examination of in vivo mutations in humans is discussed in greater detail later in this chapter under the topic "Molecular Epidemiology."

Mutations Seen in Oncogenes and Tumor Suppressor Genes

Induced tumors in whole animals provide a means of identifying oncogenes as potential targets for the mutagenic action of chemical carcinogens and for establishing that these mutated genes play a causative role in specific types of cancer. These have been studied extensively with respect to the H-*ras* oncogene. Two examples illustrate this point. Female rats were exposed at puberty to the alkylating chemical methylnitrosourea (MNU).[54,55] This treatment induces mammary tumors, and the incidence of $G_{35} \rightarrow A$ transitions detected in the H-*ras* oncogene of these tumors was 86 per cent. The PAH 7,12-dimethylbenz[*a*]anthracene (DMBA) is a potent initiator of papillomas and carcinomas in mouse skin.[56] The metabolized diol epoxide of DMBA primarily binds to adenine residues in DNA.[57] When H-*ras* mutations were analyzed in skin tumors of DMBA-treated mice, the mutations were $A_{181} \rightarrow T$ transversions with an incidence of 45/50.[58] Thus, in these examples, the nature of the oncogene mutations detected in treated animals reflected the chemical specificity of the carcinogen. These findings are summarized in Table 4–3.[59–63] Although various other chemicals have been used in similar studies examining H-*ras* mutations, the results obtained are difficult to interpret because precise knowledge of the adducts formed by the chemicals is not available.

Recently, there has been considerable interest in evaluating mutations in the human *p53* tumor suppressor gene because changes in this gene in tumors are so prevalent in several types of human cancer. The product of this gene is a transcriptional activator that appears to play a role in checkpoint control and other cellular functions (as discussed in "Genomic Instability and Inducible Responses to DNA Damage," later in this chapter, and in Chapter 5). Exons 4 through 9 are conserved evolutionarily, and most of the mutations seen in cancers occur in these regions. In its role as an activator of transcription, the *p53* protein binds to DNA in a sequence-specific manner, and it appears that the point mutations detected in this gene in tumors alter this property. The diversity of sequence changes in *p53* that occur in human tumors is of interest from the point of view of mutagenesis. Unlike the *ras* gene, in which only a small subset of base substitutions yield the activated phenotype, in the *p53* gene a wide variety of mutations have been detected.[64] Thus, the mutations seen in this gene may provide a useful fingerprint of the causative agents.

The *p53* mutational spectra observed in different human cancers is summarized in Table 4–4.[65–83a] Three major types of mutations have been found, and it is of interest that these relate to specific types of cancers. In colon and brain tumors, the mutations are usually transitions from guanine to adenine or from cytosine to thymine. These changes tend to be concentrated at CpG dinucleotide sequences. Because in the latter sequences the cytosine res-

TABLE 4–3. MUTATIONS IN THE H-*ras* ONCOGENE PUTATIVELY INDUCED BY CHEMICAL CARCINOGENS WITH DEFINED DNA ADDUCTS

CHEMICAL	PROBABLE ADDUCT	CODON AFFECTED	MUTATION
7,12-Dimethylbenz[a]anthracene[58–62]	N^6-dA-DMBA	61	A:T→T:A
N-methyl-N'-nitro-N-nitrosoguanidine[58]	O^6-methyl-dG	12	G:C→A:T
Methylnitrosourea[58]	O^6-methyl-dG	12	G:C→A:T
β-Propriolactone[63]	1-carboxyethyl-dA	61	A:T→T:A

idue is often actually 5-methylcytosine, it is thought that the C → T mutations arise by deamination of this residue, to yield thymidine.[84] This can occur spontaneously or be enhanced by certain chemicals, because it is known that chemicals such as 5-azacytosine can have this effect. The presence of 8-OH-dG in DNA at CpG dinucleotide sequences in an in vitro system containing methylase and S-adenosyl lead to significant changes in methylation suggesting that oxidative damage may have epigenetic consequences.[84a] Additionally, O^6-methyl-dG was shown to stimulate methyltransferase activity in vitro, therefore induction of this lesion by alkylating agents may cause de novo changes in the methylation of CpG dinucleotides.[84b] Transition mutations accounted for 25/27 point mutations detected in *p53* in ovarian cancers, and 16 (60 per cent) of these changes were G → A substitutions that did not arise in a CpG context.[7] It is not known whether the G → A mutations occur spontaneously (e.g., as a result of depurination) or reflect the action of other factors. Mutations in the *p53* gene occur relatively late in the evolution of both colon and brain tumors, but the cause of these mutations is not known.

In contrast to the situation in colon and brain tumors, mutations in the *p53* gene in human tumors of the lung, liver, and breast are frequently G → T transversions. This is of interest because, in experimental systems, this type of mutation often is induced by external agents that covalently modify the guanine residue in DNA (e.g., BPDE).[85] In the case of lung cancer, G → T transversions account for half of all the point mutations detected in the *p53* gene, and this change could reflect the formation of deoxyguanosine adducts by carcinogens in cigarette smoke. In 90 per cent of these cases, the mutated purine is on the nontranscribed strand, presumably because of transcription-coupled repair of adducts from the transcribed strand (as discussed in "DNA Repair," later in this chapter). In the case of certain liver cancers, the G → T transversion mutations could reflect the action of aflatoxin B$_1$, which is known to modify deoxyguanosine residues. It is of interest that, in certain regions of Africa and China where aflatoxin has been implicated as a risk factor, the G → T mutations appear to be concentrated specifically at codon 249. The factor that causes G → T

transversion mutations in breast cancer is not known. It could reflect oxidative damage leading to the formation of 8-OH-dG adducts in cellular DNA. Oxidized bases have been detected in breast tissue and the concentration of total modified bases was increased 9-fold in tumor samples compared with normal control values.[85a] As previously noted, 8-OH-dG lesions primarily induce G→T transversions,[49,86] the type of base substitution observed in the *p53* gene from breast tumor DNA. Dietary factors may play a mutagenic role, as well. For example, certain heterocyclic amines that are formed when cooking meat and fish at high temperature have been shown to induce mammary tumors in rodents[17,23] and to induce this type of base change in a forward mutation assay.[86a]

A third category of mutations in the *p53* gene is seen in skin cancers, which display transitions characteristic of photoproduct lesions (see Table 4–2). This finding is consistent with the fact that the ultraviolet radiation present in sunlight, particularly UVB (wavelength 280 to 320 nm), induces the formation of pyrimidine dimers and (4-6) pyrimidine-pyrimidone photoproducts in DNA. Moreover, it is well known that the risk of squamous cell carcinoma is increased in individuals who have increased exposure to sunlight. Interestingly, in the *p53* gene of irradiated human fibroblasts, slow DNA repair of pyrimidine dimers at the sequence level was demonstrated to be coincident with the hotspots for mutations detected in skin cancers (e.g., those positions noted in Table 4–4).[86b] However, two alternative explanations for the mutations putatively induced by radiation in the ultraviolet range are worthy of mention. Firstly, 8-OH-dG in DNA induced by reactive oxygen species in conjunction with endogenous sensitizers such as riboflavin may induce mutations at the 5′ site of 5′-GG-3′ sequences.[87] Secondly, the codon 248 mutational hotspot in *p53* may undergo transitions at the CpG sequence because this site is consistently observed to be methylated and hence may undergo spontaneous deamination.[87b] Another physical damaging agent that acts as a cancer initiator is ionizing radiation. This type of damage mainly induces large deletions, inversions, and chromosomal rearrangements in model systems.[88] In particular, radon gas is believed to contribute to lung cancer incidence in the United States.[89] Radon is an odorless gas

TABLE 4–4.   HUMAN *p53* SUPPRESSOR GENE MUTATIONAL SPECTRA

BASE SUBSTITUTION	PREVALENT TARGET SITE(S)	PUTATIVE INDUCER*	CANCER TYPE
G→A	175, 248, 273	Unknown	Colon[64–69]
C→T	CpG dinucleotides	Deamination of 5-MeC*	Ovary[70] Brain[69,71]
G→T	157, 273, 249	Tobacco smoke, e.g., PAHs; Reactive oxygen species, e.g., 8-OH-dG; Diet, e.g., aflatoxin for liver; unknown for breast	Lung[69,72–74] Liver[75,76] Breast[77–79]
TC→TT CC→TT	196, 248, 278	Ultraviolet light	Skin[80–82]

*Abbreviations: 5-MeC, 5-methylcytosine; PAHs, polycyclic aromatic hydrocarbons; 8-OH-dG, 7,8-dihydro-8-oxodeoxyguanosine.

composed of α-particle–emitting decay products from [214]Po and [218]Po that are naturally present in soil. Individuals at highest risk for radon-induced lung cancer are uranium miners and those living in private dwellings that are situated where radon emissions are especially high. Cigarette smokers who are also exposed to radon have an additional tenfold higher risk for lung cancer. Presumably, deposition of these particles on the epithelium of the respiratory tract leads to the induction of DNA lesions, eventually resulting in mutations, oncogenic transformation, or cell death. Interestingly, radon-associated *p53* mutations in lung tumors of uranium miners were mainly transversions and deletion mutations in 7/19 samples studied.[90]

Thus, the types of mutations seen in certain genes in a given type of human cancer may provide clues to the general category of causative agents that was involved in the induction of those cancers. This approach must be used with caution because different types of exogenous agents may produce similar mutations, a single agent can produce multiple types of DNA adducts and mutations, and endogenous mutagenic agents can mimic the effects of exogenous mutagens. Nevertheless, when combined with other molecular epidemiology methods (discussed later in this chapter), these mutation spectra may provide important insights into the causation of specific human cancers.

DNA Repair

As mentioned earlier in this chapter, the frequency and specificity of spontaneous or induced mutations is also a function of DNA repair systems in the host cell. Much of the current knowledge of repair mechanisms is derived from the genetic and biochemical analyses of repair-deficient *E. coli* mutants. In bacteria, DNA damage by ultraviolet light or chemicals triggers the SOS response and induces expression of a regulon consisting of about 20 genes.[91] Genes in this regulon encode proteins that mediate DNA repair, mutagenesis, and recombination. Repair via this pathway is error prone. Error-free pathways exist for the repair of alkylation damage and mismatch correction. In general, the proteins involved in all of these processes are conserved across the phylogenetic spectrum. Inducible gene expression upon DNA damage also occurs in eukaryotes. In yeast, there appear to be up to 80 DNA damage–inducible genes; the estimate in mammalian cells is 100 to 200.[92,93]

Five major repair pathways can be briefly summarized:

1. *Base excision*—Glycosylases recognize and remove specific altered bases, such as alkylation products of adenine and guanine. They excise the affected base, leaving an apurinic site that is further processed by endonucleases. The types of damage recognized by these enzymes are, for example, adducts produced by the mutagens ethyl methanesulfonate (EMS) and MNU. A formamidopyrimidine (FAPY) glycosylase repairs the prevalent 8-OH-dG adduct resulting from oxidative processes.[94]

2. *Direct damage reversal*—Examples of enzymes that carry out this type of repair are alkyltransferases, per-

oxide scavengering enzymes, and photolyase. An example of the former enzyme class is methyltransferase; it is specific for O^6-alkylguanine-DNA and catalyzes the transfer of small alkyl adducts (e.g., methyl or ethyl) from the O^6 position of the base to an internal cysteine, yielding *S*-alkyl cysteine and guanine.[95] The latter photolyase binds in a light-independent manner to ultraviolet-induce pyrimidine dimers, absorbs a photon, and reverses the dimer. Recently, a photoreactivating activity from *Drosophila melanogaster* was identified for the (6-4) photoproduct.[96]

3. *Recombination repair*—The mechanism of this type of repair involves strand exchange between homologous DNA duplexes. It occurs after replication and mediates repair of double-strand breaks induced by ionizing radiation, as well as cross-link damage created by mitomycin C and the therapeutic drugs *cis*-platinum, psoralen, and melphalan.

4. *Mismatch repair*—This pathway corrects errors that occur during DNA synthesis or after recombination, or that arise spontaneously as a result of the deamination of 5-methylcytosine. Since this repair pathway is methyl-directed, incision which is specifically targeted to the unmethylated strand results in enhanced replication fidelity. For a review on cancer susceptibility due to defects in mismatch repair see reference.[96a]

5. *Nucleotide excision repair*—This mechanism involves placement of two single-strand nicks on the damaged strand on either side of the modified base. In human cells, these nicks on the damaged strand are located about 21 and 5 nucleotides 5′ and 3′ to the lesion, respectively.[97] The types of damage recognized by excision endonucleases are ultraviolet photoproducts and bulky carcinogen adducts, as well as cross-linking drugs (e.g., those noted in pathway 3). Excision is completed by release of the damaged segment in a reaction that is carried out by helicase(s) to unwind the duplex DNA and single-strand binding protein(s).[98] The resulting gap then is filled in by DNA polymerase δ and/or ε. For this step, proliferating cell nuclear antigen (PCNA) also is required.[99] Finally, DNA ligase seals the remaining two nicks. A detailed review of DNA repair mechanisms can be found in ref. 100.

The five categories of repair summarized above apply to the overall genome. In addition, there is preferential repair of transcriptionally active genomic regions.[101] Generally, overall genome repair is slow in comparison to this rapid preferential repair. There are exceptions, however, for certain types of adducts. For example, deoxyguanosine-C^8 adducts (dG-AF) appear to be more rapidly repaired from the overall genome of mammalian cells than deoxyguanosine-N^2 adducts (e.g., dG-BP). The overall genome repair rate differences for these two adducts possibly reflect the difference in conformational distortion each creates in DNA structure. The relatively slow overall genome repair may reflect hindered accessibility of DNA adducts that are embedded in chromatin. In vivo, the chromatin structure of constitutively expressed domains is different from that of inducible regions. The structure of expressing genomic regions is regulated by the nucleosome core particles.[102] Evidence that chromatin structure regulates gene expression and cell cycle progression is indicated by the requirements of transient histone acetylation for transcriptional activation,[103] and the observation that transcriptionally active chromatin domains have a specific nuclear localization.[104] Thus, factors dictating the changing nature of chromatin structure also can modulate DNA repair indirectly.

In addition to the preferential repair provided by an open chromatin structure, repair is coupled with gene transcription. This phenomenon was first observed by Hanawalt and coworkers,[105] and has been detected in human, rodent, yeast, and bacterial cells. RNA polymerase is required for the recruitment of repair enzymes to the damaged site, and repair is specific for the transcribed strand of a gene. In eukaryotic cells, it appears that only RNA polymerase II mediates this recruitment response.[39,106] Presumably a stalled transcriptional complex leads to the recruitment of repair factors because a modified base on the template strand is either noncoding or causes a conformational change in DNA structure that arrests elongation. Indeed, a variety of lesions located on the transcribed strand of a gene can block transcription in vitro. These blocking lesions include ultraviolet-induced pyrimidine dimers,[107] deoxyguanosine-AAF,[108] 8-OH-dG, 3-hydroxy-2-hydroxymethyltetrahydrofuran,[109] and alkylguanines induced by nitrogen mustard.[110] Transcription elongation is unaffected by damaged bases on the nontranscribed strand.

Transcription-coupled DNA repair in bacteria requires at least one coupling factor to facilitate removal of the elongation complex from the site of damage. In a concerted manner, this factor also may recruit the repair enzymes. An *E. coli* mutant that is deficient in the function of this coupling factor (*mfd⁻*; "mutation frequency decline") originally was isolated by Witkin.[111] Recently, this factor was purified and shown to complement in vitro transcription-coupled repair using extracts from *mfd⁻* bacteria.[112] The *mfd* gene encodes a 130-kDa protein containing helicase (DNA-unwinding) and leucine zipper (DNA-binding) motifs. It acts to displace the stalled elongation complex from the damaged site on the template DNA strand via a reaction that requires ATP hydrolysis. The factor then facilitates binding by the excision enzyme complex UvrABC, and stimulates the rate of repair.[113]

Exciting progress is being made in the identification and characterization of the genes involved in DNA repair in humans (for recent reviews, see ref. 114 and 96a), and these studies ultimately will provide insights into how DNA repair influences genomic stability and carcinogenesis. In humans, the inheritance of defects in DNA repair is associated with cancer predisposition. Examples of autosomal recessive diseases linked to early cancers resulting from defects in repair include xeroderma pigmentosum (XP), ataxia-telangiectasia (AT), Fanconi's anemia (FA), and Bloom syndrome. The major types of cancers associated with these diseases are skin cancer (XP), lymphoma (AT), and leukemia (FA). In the case of Bloom syndrome, various types of neoplasias are noted. Like XP, two other heritable diseases are associated with hypersensitivity to ultraviolet light: Cockayne syndrome and the brittle hair disease trichothiodystrophy. Common clinical

consequences of these latter diseases are growth and mental retardation.

Repair-deficient strains of the yeast *Saccharomyces cerevisiae* and of cultured rodent cells have been isolated and characterized. Furthermore, seven complementation groups for XP (designated A through G) have been identified. In addition, there are at least four distinct groups for FA, two groups for Cockayne syndrome (A and B), and four groups for AT (A through D). Several human repair genes have been cloned after finding that they were able to correct defects in repair-deficient rodent cell lines. Many of these genes, in turn, share homology with yeast repair genes. Table 4–5[115–130d] lists several of the human repair genes that have been cloned thus far and indicates their chromosomal locations. Cells from AT-affected individuals show enhanced killing by ionizing radiation,[131] and those from FA patients show a similar sensitivity to cross-linking agents.[132] In the case of cells derived from Bloom syndrome, there also is an increased sensitivity to these drugs, but their most striking abnormality is a high spontaneous frequency of sister chromatid exchanges (SCEs).[133] The gene defective in a variant of Bloom syndrome was found to be DNA ligase 1 (Table 4–5). A cDNA for the gene that is defective in FA group C recently was cloned, and it encodes a 1677–amino acid protein that is ubiquitously expressed but whose function is not known.[134] The genes involved in three AT groups (A, C, and D) all are localized in the vicinity of chromosome 11q23 (Table 4–5).[123–125] Consistent with the observation that defects in DNA repair may confer a mutator phenotype to affected cells, it is noteworthy that AT fibroblast cell lines display spontaneous intrachromosomal recombination rates 30–200 times higher than in normal cells.[134a] That AT genes are involved in a pathway for response to DNA damage is a topic for further discussion in "Genomic Instability and Inducible Responses to DNA Damage," later in this chapter.

In many cases, the cloned genes that correct DNA re-

TABLE 4–5. CLONED HUMAN DNA REPAIR GENES

GENE	LOCATION	REFERENCE
LIG	19q13.2-13.3	115
ERCC1	19q13.2	116
ERCC2	19q13.2	117
ERCC3 (XPBC)	2q21	118
ERCC4	16p13.13-13.2	119
ERCC5	13q32-33	120
ERCC6	10q11-q21	121
XPAC	9q34	122
AT-A	11q22-23	123
AT-C	11q22-23	124
AT-D	11q22-23	125
XPC	3p25	126
XRCC1	19q13	130
XRCC5	2q35	130a
FACC	9q22	129
APE (REF-1,HAP1)	14q11.2-12	127, 127a, 128
MGMT	10q26	130b
hMSH2	2p22-21	130c
hMLH1	3p21-23	130d

pair deficiencies code for bifunctional proteins that also are engaged either in the regulation of gene expression or in transcription per se. The following discussion emphasizes recent advances that have been made in the area of transcription-coupled repair. There are currently two examples of genes that code for activators of transcription that also play an integral role in DNA repair. One example is the recently cloned gene ERCC6.[121,136] A mutated form of this nonvital gene is responsible for the human Cockayne syndrome, group B (CS-B) disorder. CS-B cells fail to carry out preferential repair, although overall genome repair in these cells is normal.[137] The ERCC6 gene product has helicase activity and is predicted to consist of 1493 amino acids.[136] The gene is homologous with certain yeast transcriptional activators, as well as a regulator of Drosophila homeotic genes.[137–139] Yeast genetics has shown that these related activators regulate the accessibility of particular genes to the transcriptional apparatus by regional modifications of chromatin structure (for review, see ref. 140). This class of regulator may activate gene expression by altering nucleosome packing, loop formation, DNA supercoiling, and/or matrix attachment. The other example is REF1 (also named APE and HAP1[127,127a,128]). This gene encodes the redox regulator of the transcriptional activators Fos/Jun. Interestingly, as discussed later in this chapter, the genes c-fos and c-jun are expressed in response to DNA damage. REF1 stimulates DNA binding by the Jun, homo-, and heterodimeric proteins, as well as several other transcriptional activators. The repair activity specific to REF1 is that of an apurinic/apyrimidinic endonuclease activity. This type of activity is associated with the repair of intrinsic or endogenous DNA damage that arises during metabolism.

Cloned human genes that complement certain XP cell lines also have provided insights into the functional linkage between DNA repair and mRNA transcription. An exciting recent discovery is that the product of the ERCC3 gene[117] (defective in XP-B cells) is a component of the transcription initiation factor TFIIH.[141] TFIIH serves as a basal transcription factor that is sensitive to template topology, and is recruited for transcription of class II promoters that contain TATA elements and other initiator DNA-binding elements.[142] The protein encoded by ERCC3, like that of the bacterial mfd gene, contains a helicase motif and a DNA-dependent ATPase domain. The 89-kDa protein derived from the human ERCC3 gene also has a protein kinase activity located at the carboxyl end. Additionally, the yeast RAD3 gene that shares homology with the human ERCC2 gene defective in XP-D cells is required for mRNA synthesis, and thermolabile mutants are inviable at the restrictive temperature.[142a] This result indicates that RAD3 is also an essential transcription factor. The dual functions of these gene products have been confirmed in experiments showing that both transcription and DNA repair in vitro require the ERCC2 and ERCC3 proteins as integral subunits of TFIIH.[142b] A dual repair function for other basic transcription factors can be envisioned, as well. For example, the cloned human ERCC5 gene (defective in XP-G) has a yeast homologue (RAD2).[143,144] The fact that RAD2 and other yeast repair

genes are essential for viability suggests that they also may be constituents of the transcriptional machinery.

Although not yet demonstrated to be involved in repair, the elongation factor TFIIS is predicted to play such a role. TFIIS transiently binds to RNA polymerase II in order to promote read-through by the elongation complex when the polymerase stalls at intrinsic stop sites in the template sequence.[145] TFIIS causes the reversal of the polymerase reaction by activating a $3' \rightarrow 5'$ ribonuclease activity and allowing the complex to translocate back 100 to 150 nucleotides. Hence, by facilitating the removal of the occluding complex, this factor may allow access to a damaged site by excision endonucleases. An understanding of the roles of eukaryotic transcription factors in initiation and elongation has been emerging over the past decade, but currently little is known about which factors or mechanisms operate in transcription-coupled DNA repair. Now that these two interests have merged, new insights are likely to develop at an accelerated pace.

Given the large size of typical mammalian genes (about 100 kb), it is clearly more efficient to couple DNA repair with transcription in order to prevent having to abort and restart a transcript because a single modified base is encountered during elongation. However, a consequence of this repair process is that lesions may persist on the nontranscribed strand of a gene and cause mutations during DNA replication. Strand-biased carcinogen-induced mutations are apparent in the model systems[39] discussed earlier in this chapter, as well as in the p53 gene detected in human lung cancers.[71,73–75] Moreover, in two model systems, a correlation between strand-biased mutations and transcription-coupled repair has been demonstrated.[146,147] Hence, finding this type of bias in altered oncogenes or tumor suppressor genes from human tumors is further evidence that these changes may have been induced by environmental agents.

Genomic Instability and Inducible Responses to DNA Damage

In multistage carcinogenesis, cells destined to become malignant contain mutations in cellular oncogenes and tumor suppressor genes, as well as chromosomal abnormalities. Numerous somatic changes accumulate in the genome during tumor progression. As shown in Table 4–6,[47,148–161] the genetic and epigenetic changes detected in human cancer are diverse in nature. Recent studies suggest that genomic instability resulting from defects in the control of the cell cycle may, in addition to DNA-damaging agents, play a critical role in driving the accumulation of mutations. Manifestations of genomic instability that appear to be increased in tumor cells include the ability to amplify DNA sequences[162] teleomeric associations by chromosomes,[163] and an apparent increased instability at simple repeat sequences. A consequence of this latter change is that expansions or contractions of simple repeat or iterated sequences (e.g., adenine or cytosine-adenine repeats) are seen at different chromosomal locations in a subset of human colon tumors.[153–155,164] There is evidence that one or all of these examples may represent a recessive genetic trait acquired early in the transformation process. Expression of this genetic instability trait may, in turn, promote the induction of further mutations. The recent discovery that alterations in the sizes of simple repeat sequences throughout the genomes of tumor cells from hereditary nonpolyposis colon cancer correlate with mutations in mismatch repair genes ($hMSH2$[130d] and $hMSLH1$[130d]) confirm findings in bacteria[164a] and yeast,[164b] namely that defects in this repair pathway produce a mutator phenotype which in initiated cells can drive cancer progression. This phenotype in cancer cells is termed RER$^+$.[164c]

Checkpoints control progression through the eukaryotic cell cycle and dictate a highly ordered sequence of events.[165,166] Thus, stimulation to enter the cell cycle requires that nonreplicating phase G_0 cells progress to phase G_1, which then is followed by the S, G_2, and M phases. Order is effected through the action of both positive and negative regulators that initiate or prevent entry into each of the successive phases of the cycle. Checkpoints halt progression to the following phase of the cycle until the error-free completion of earlier events has occurred. Studies with agents that cause DNA damage have revealed two checkpoints that lead to cell cycle arrest in phase G_1 or G_2. Additional checkpoints may be manifested by other effectors and act at the same or other stages of the cell cycle.

Studies on checkpoint control and DNA damage–inducible responses recently have merged and brought new insights to carcinogenesis research. Signal transduction pathways appear to be immediately activated in response to DNA damage, and these responses resemble in several respects the effects of mitogens and the activation of protein kinase C (PKC) by the tumor promoter TPA[167–169] (PKC and the effects of TPA are described in detail in "Multistage Carcinogenesis," later in this chapter). A hypothetical scheme of the events following DNA damage is diagrammed in Figure 4–2. Damage to DNA, and possibly other cellular targets, by unknown mechanisms leads to the activation of a protein kinase cascade that may include tyrosine kinases, PKC, Raf-1, and mitogen-activated protein kinase (MAPK), resulting in the transient expression of primary response genes, including the cellular oncogenes c-fos and c-jun. Their protein products are transcriptional activators that bind to specific sequence elements and activate a second wave of gene transcription. Genes induced in this phase collectively are termed "immediate early response genes." Some of these genes are involved in DNA metabolism and normally are induced in late phase G_1, in preparation for DNA synthesis in the S phase, but they may be induced in response to DNA damage to mediate DNA repair. An example of such a damage-inducible enzyme is ribonucleotide reductase that provides the four deoxyribonucleotides required for DNA synthesis.[169a,169b] The immediate early response also triggers the expression of other transcriptional activators (including $p53$) and the expression of downstream effector genes. Because the p53 protein regulates the expression of genes whose products are critically important for progression from G_1 to S, posttranslational modifications of this protein are relevant to events initiated by DNA dam-

TABLE 4–6. EXAMPLES OF GENETIC AND EPIGENETIC CHANGES IN CARCINOGENESIS

HERITABLE ALTERATION	GENE(S) AFFECTED	CONSEQUENCES	CANCER TYPE
Translocation[148]	bcl and abl	Fusion protein is an activated oncogene	Chronic myelogenous leukemia
Homozygous deletion[149]	NF1	Deregulated p21^{RAS}	Neurofibrosarcoma, pheochromocytoma, astrocytoma
Frameshift mutation ± 1 –5 bases[150,151]	APC	Null tumor suppressor gene	Colorectal carcinoma
Gene amplification[152]	EGFR	Autocrine activation by receptor tyrosine kinase overexpression	Glioma
Single base substitution[64]	$p53$	Loss of checkpoint control	Numerous
Simple repeat polymorphisms & hypermutability[153–156,129c,129d]	hMSH2 & hMLH1	Genetic instability	Colorectal carcinoma, Muir-Torre syndrome, small cell lung cancer
Minisatellite polymorphisms[156a]	Ha-ras	Cancer predisposition	Numerous
Teleomere reduction[157]	Numerous	Chromosomal deletions and/or loss	Colorectal carcinoma
Loss of genomic imprinting (parental allele-specific expression)[158,159]	IGF2 & H19	Gene dosage effects	Beckwith-Wiedemann syndrome & Wilm's renal tumor
Loss/gain of methylation[160,161]	Numerous	Altered gene expression, chromatin structure, replication timing (?)	Colorectal carcinoma

age. Phosphorylation at specific residues converts the p53 protein to either a proliferative or an antiproliferative form. After accumulating in the nucleus in response to stimuli elicited by DNA damage, p53 activates the expression of growth-arrest genes (*GADD* genes; see ref. 170), and presumably represses the expression of growth-promoting genes (e.g., c-*myc*). While *GADD* genes are associated with growth arrest, the gene putatively responsible for effecting *p53*-mediated G_1 arrest is *WAF1*, which encodes a 21 kDa inhibitor of cyclin-dependent kinases.[170a]

The induction of growth arrest in response to DNA damage permits repair to occur before replication (S phase) and is mediated by wild-type *p53* but not the mutant forms that frequently are found in tumor cells.[171] A signaling pathway that involves DNA repair genes and leads to transient growth arrest was reported by Kastan and coworkers.[172] They observed that exposure of normal cells to ionizing radiation caused the induction and nuclear accumulation of wild-type p53 protein, and that this response was reduced or nil in AT-C or AT-A cells, respectively.[172] At least one of the DNA damage-inducible genes, *GADD45*, also acted in this p53-mediated pathway because it was not induced in cells that contain either no p53 product or mutant forms. The authors claimed that AT gene products act upstream of p53 in this pathway, since *GADD45* also was not induced after irradiation of the AT cells. However, nuclear accumulation of p53 after X-ray or ultraviolet irradiation in repair-deficient XP-A, AT-A and -C, or 9/11 Bloom's syndrome primary fibroblasts was shown by Lu and Lane.[172a] In the latter study, no defects in the p53 response were noted in the case of the AT cells, although the kinetics were delayed. In order to explain the sensitivity of AT cells to ionizing radiation, it will be necessary to learn if elevated levels of p53 can inhibit progression to S phase. An efficient inducing signal for p53 nuclear accumulation is double-strand breaks in DNA, whereas other cell stresses, such as heat shock, do not induce p53.[172a] Induction of *GADD45* expression specifically requires genotoxic stress or growth arrest. Whereas the expression of immediate early genes (i.e., c-*jun*, tumor necrosis factor, collagenase, etc.) is inducible by TPA, *GADD45* expression is not.

In addition to its role in checkpoint control, *p53* is implicated in activating an alternative pathway leading to programmed cell death (apoptosis).[173] This pathway can be activated by treatment with physical or chemical agents (see ref. 174 for review). Hence, cell death is an important mechanism to minimize the mutagenic consequences that result from allowing the survival of heavily damaged cells. Interestingly, cells that bear mutant forms of *p53* exhibited markedly increased resistance to the lethal effects of radiation,[175] presumably because they escaped apoptosis and proliferated despite DNA damage. Another mechanism by which *p53* is involved in maintaining genomic stability relates to gene amplification. The potential for gene amplification in cultured cells was shown to accompany loss of wild-type *p53* function.[176,177] Consequently, the mutations in *p53* observed in a variety of human tumors may have the pernicious effect of engendering a tolerance to DNA damage and the promiscuous replication of aberrant cells that then allow further mutations to accumulate. However, it is now held that the function of this tumor suppressor gene is only one of possibly several necessary but not sufficient elements in the complex checkpoint pathways that suppress carcinogenesis. Supporting the view that defects in growth control substantially contribute to genomic instability are the finding that chromosomal abnormalities are rapidly observed in metaphase chromosomes in fibroblasts bearing an inducible Ha-*ras* oncogene when the inducer is present,[177a] and in keratinocytes expressing the E7 oncogene of human papilloma virus 16 that targets the RB protein.[177b] Other effectors that are involved in cell cycle control (e.g., cyclin genes and their regulators) are likely to affect the maintenance of genomic stability. Other effectors (perhaps cyclin genes) involved in cell cycle control are also likely to be involved in genome stability.

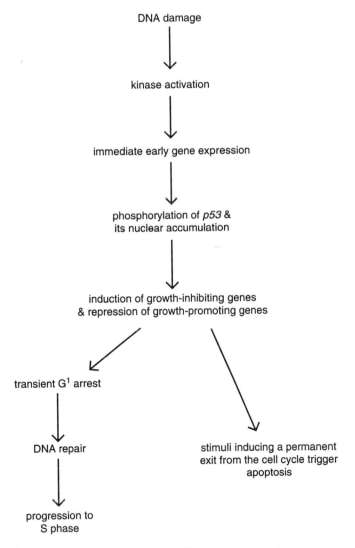

Figure 4–2. A hypothetical scheme illustrating the complex responses of mammalian cells to DNA damage by various agents. For additional details, see text and related references in "DNA Repair" and "Genomic Instability and Inducible Responses to DNA Damages."

Multistage Carcinogenesis

MULTIPLE FACTORS, MULTIPLE STAGES AND MULTIPLE GENETIC TARGETS

The development of a fully malignant tumor involves complex interactions between several factors, both exogenous (environmental) and endogenous (genetic, hormonal, immunologic, etc.). In addition, carcinogenesis often proceeds through multiple discernible stages (for review, see refs. 3,12,15,17,178,179). These include initiation, promotion (which leads to the appearance of benign tumors), and progression (the conversion of benign to malignant tumors and their further evolution to tumors with increasing degrees of malignancy). The overall process can occupy a major fraction of the life span of the individual. The transitions between successive stages can be enhanced or inhibited by different types of agents. Thus, it appears that the individual stages may involve qualitatively different mechanisms at the cellular and genetic levels. These aspects predict that the establishment and maintenance of a malignant tumor involves multiple factors, multiple cellular genes, and multiple types of changes in gene structure and function.[12]

As discussed earlier in this chapter, agents that initiate the carcinogenic process often do so by damaging cellular DNA. Hence, this has become an axiom in the field of chemical carcinogenesis. Because it is now apparent that successive mutation can occur throughout the multistage carcinogenic process,[17,67] it is likely that DNA-damaging carcinogens also act at later stages in the process. Hence, in experimental models DNA-damaging agents can enhance the process of tumor progression. It appears that tumor promoters act largely at the epigenetic level by altering signal transduction pathways, gene expression, and cellular differentiation, thus enhancing cell proliferation and the clonal expansion of previously mutated cells.[12,13,178] This aspect is discussed in greater detail later in this chapter. Detailed studies of human and rodent tumors indicate that the multistage process of carcinogenesis is associated with the successive occurrence of mutations and/or abnormal expression of at least three categories of genes; dominant acting proto-oncogenes; recessive tumor suppressor genes; and cyclin and related genes, which control the later phases of the cell cycle. These subjects have been mentioned briefly earlier in this chapter and are discussed in greater detail in Chapters 1, 2, 5, and 6, and at the end of this chapter.

Tumor Promotion and Progression and Multifactor Interactions

TUMOR PROMOTION

As mentioned earlier in this chapter, the evolution of a fully malignant tumor is a highly complex process that can involve multiple exogenous agents, multiple biochemical mechanisms, and multiple disturbances in cellular genes. Experimental studies have defined at least three distinct phases: initiation, promotion, and progression.

The most extensive studies on tumor promotion have been carried out on mouse skin. In this model, both initiation and promotion are required for the induction of benign papillomas (for review, see refs. 12,178). Each of these stages is elicited or inhibited by different types of agents and involves different biochemical mechanisms. The major difference is that initiation is an irreversible event that appears to involve DNA damage, whereas tumor promotion is reversible (at least at an early phase) and apparently involves epigenetic mechanisms. The two-stage mouse skin carcinogenesis system has served as a paradigm for studies on the multistage aspects of carcinogenesis in several other tissues and species. Studies in rodents indicate that induction of cancer in the liver, bladder, colon, and breast involves processes analogous to initiation and promotion on mouse skin, and there is reason to believe that similar processes occur during the development of certain human tumors.[12,178]

Tumor promoters can be defined as compounds that have very weak or no carcinogenic activity when tested alone but markedly enhance tumor yield when applied repeatedly following a low or suboptimal dose of a carcinogen (which is usually a DNA-damaging agent). The most detailed information on tumor promotion comes from studies on the potent phorbol ester tumor promoter 12-O-tetradecanoylphorbol-13-acetate (TPA). Early studies indicated that, in contrast to initiating agents, the phorbol ester tumor promoters do not bind to DNA but instead act by binding to membrane-associated receptors and thus produce their initial effects at the epigenetic level. Studies from several different laboratories revealed that TPA induces a number of phenotypic effects in cell culture systems that can be grouped into three categories: mimicry of the transformed phenotype, modulation (either inhibition or induction) of differentiation, and membrane effects.[12,178] Because it is likely that carcinogenesis involves major disturbances in differentiation, it is of interest that TPA is a highly potent modulator of gene expression and differentiation in a variety of cell systems.[12,178]

In 1982, it was discovered that TPA and related tumor promoters bind with high specificity to, and activate the function of, the enzyme PKC, a family of lipid-regulated serine and threonine protein kinases.[179] This and subsequent findings indicating that PKC plays a central role in signal transduction pathways, growth control, and differentiation, and in mediating the action of several growth factors and oncogenes, has merged research on tumor promotion with that on growth factors, signal transduction, and the action of specific oncogenes.[12,13,169–182] The role of PKC and other protein kinases in mediating the action of various growth factors, receptors, and signal transduction pathways that are involved in growth control, gene expression, and the action of cellular oncogenes is shown in Figure 4–2. The subject of growth factors and signal transduction is discussed further in Chapter 7. Because of the importance of PKC in tumor promotion and growth control, this enzyme system is described in greater detail.

RECENT RESEARCH ON PKC

PKC has two domains, a carboxyterminal catalytic domain, containing an ATP binding site and the region to which protein substrates bind, and an amino-terminal regulatory domain, which is controlled by allosteric cofactors, such as phospholipid, Ca^{2+}, diacylglycerol (DAG), and TPA.[180] The function of the regulatory domain is to maintain the enzyme in a folded and inactive conformation. It is thought that the binding of co-factors to the regulatory domain induces a conformational change that unfolds the enzyme, thus allowing substrates to bind to the catalytic domain and be phosphorylated. Cloning studies indicate that PKC belongs to a multigene family that encodes at least ten distinct isoforms.[180] They can be classified into three subgroups based on their sequence homologies and requirements for co-factors. Group 1 are termed cPKCs, which include α, β1, β2, and γ; group 2 are termed nPKCs and include ϵ, δ, and η; and group 3, termed aPKCs, include ζ and λ.[180] All of these isoforms require phosphatidylserine or other anionic lipids for activation. In addition, the cPKCs, but not the nPKCs or aPKCs, require Ca^{2+}. Diacylglycerol and TPA stimulate the activity of the cPKCs and nPKCs but not the aPKCs, apparently because the latter isoforms contain one rather than two cysteine-rich zinc finger motifs in their regulatory domain and, therefore, do not bind these agents. The requirement for Ca^{2+} by the cPKCs is associated with the presence of a specific amino acid sequence termed the C2 domain. Recent studies suggest that this domain acts in concert with the C1 domain and phospholipid to form a pocket to which Ca^{2+} binds, thus inducing a conformational change that activates the kinase activity of the catalytic domain (see ref. 183 and unpublished studies).

Normal tissues differ in terms of their profiles of expression of specific isoforms of PKC, and at the same time a single cell type can express multiple (often four to six) isoforms of PKC.[180,182] Although the nPKCs initially were thought to be "novel" isoforms, it is now apparent that they frequently are expressed at high levels in several different tissues and cell types. Because they do not require Ca^{2+} for activation, they may play important roles in signal transduction pathways that are not associated with increases in cytoplasmic levels of Ca^{2+} (i.e., pathways that do not specifically involve the agonist-induced hydrolysis of phosphatidylinositol-4,5-bisphosphate). The fact that individual isoforms of PKC differ in their intracellular localization and sensitivity to TPA-induced translocation from the cytosol to the membrane and particulate fractions of cells, and to TPA-induced down-regulation, also provides evidence of their specificity in signal transduction pathways. In cell culture systems, the expression of individual isoforms of PKC can change rather dramatically as a result of oncogene-induced cell transformation and the induction of differentiation.[182,184] Evidence is also accumulating that the profile of expression of isoforms of PKC changes during the process of tumor formation in vivo (see ref. 181 and unpublished studies). Thus, the family of PKC isoforms plays a complex and dynamic role in signal transduction and carcinogenesis.

The functions of individual isoforms of PKC have been studied by using gene transfer methods to obtain derivatives of rat fibroblasts that stably express high levels of either PKCβI, PKCα, or PKCε.[13,185-187] The cells that express high levels of PKCβI display several abnormalities in growth control, but this is not the case with cells that express similar high levels of PKCα.[186] A striking finding is that cells that overexpress PKCε are highly transformed by several criteria and are tumorigenic in nude mice.[187] Similar results have been obtained by other investigators with 3T3 murine fibroblasts.[188] Thus, when expressed at high levels, PKCε functions as an oncogene in rodent fibroblasts. These results provide direct evidence that individual isoforms of PKC play distinct roles in growth control, even in the same cell type. However, there is evidence that the function of a specific isoform of PKC also depends on the context of the cell in which it is expressed.[13,189] Studies are in progress to elucidate the events downstream of individual isoforms of PKC that account for their markedly different effects on growth control and cell transformation.

The evidence that specific isoforms of PKC play distinct roles in growth control and cell transformation, coupled with information on functional roles of specific domains in various isoforms of PKC, suggests that the development of agents that selectively activate or inhibit specific isoforms of PKC could provide novel strategies for cancer chemoprevention and/or the treatment of established tumors.[12,14]

As discussed earlier in this chapter, several other types of chemical agents (including phenobarbital, saccharine, and several halogenated organic compounds) act as tumor promoters in various organ systems in rodents.[31] It seems unlikely that all of these agents also act directly through the PKC system, but they may induce analogous changes in signal transduction pathways. This is an important area for future research in view of the evidence that a large number of agents that enhance tumor formation in rodent bioassays appear to act through nongenotoxic mechanism.[12,16] Alternatively, it is possible that some of these so-called nongenotoxic agents induce mutations in DNA through indirect effects, for example, the formation of activated forms of oxygen[19,24] or other events that lead to DNA damage.

TUMOR PROGRESSION

The causative factors and mechanisms that underlie the process of tumor progression (i.e., the conversion of benign tumors to malignant tumors) and the further evolution of these tumors into more malignant tumors that display increasing heterogeneity, autonomy, and drug resistance is poorly understood. In experimental systems, certain DNA-damaging agents enhance the conversion of benign to malignant tumors.[178] In experimental models of carcinogenesis and in human tumors, progression is associated with the progressive acquisition of mutations in oncogenes and tumor suppressor genes and gross chromosomal abnormalities, but in most cases the driving forces for these changes are not known. The possible role of genomic instability in tumor progression has been discussed earlier in this chapter. We also should emphasize that, although in some experimental models the stages of tumor initiation, promotion, and progression can be sharply defined, in the real world humans often are exposed simultaneously and repetitively to initiating agents and tumor-promoter mixtures (e.g., cigarette smoking and/ or exposures in the work place). Therefore, there may be repetitive rounds of DNA damage, tumor promotion, and clonal expansion.

CHEMICAL-VIRAL INTERACTIONS

There are numerous examples in experimental systems in which initiating carcinogens, tumor promoters, or other chemical and physical agents interact synergistically with viruses in the carcinogenic process, both in vivo and in cell culture.[190] It seems likely, therefore, that certain human cancers may be due to interactions between chemical agents and viruses that on their own have weak or no oncogenic potential. Thus, the high incidence of liver cancer in Africa and certain regions of Asia may be due to synergistic interactions between hepatitis B virus and aflatoxin, or other carcinogens in the diet.[22,190] Nasopharyngeal cancer in Asia and Burkitt's lymphoma in Africa might be due to an interaction between Epstein-Barr virus and nitrosamines in the diet or other environmental factors (not yet identified).[190] Cervical cancer may be due to an interaction between specific strains of human papillomavirus and carcinogens present in cigarette smoke or from other sources.[190] Thus, in future studies on the causation of specific human cancers, it is important to consider the likelihood of synergistic interactions between multiple types of environmental factors, including viruses. The subject of viral carcinogenesis is discussed in detail in Chapter 3.

Nutrition and Cancer

There is considerable evidence that dietary factors play a very important role in human cancer causation, although in most cases the precise factors and their mechanisms of action are not known with certainty. This subject has been reviewed in detail elsewhere.[14,191] Smoked, salted, and pickled foods have been implicated in the causation of gastric and esophageal cancers. The precise mechanisms are not known but appear to involve the production of nitrosamine carcinogens from nitrites and the stimulation of cell proliferation by a high salt concentration. Alcohol has been implicated in the causation of oral, esophageal, and gastric cancer, and possibly breast cancer, but the underlying mechanism is not known. As discussed in the previous section, the contamination of food by the carcinogen aflatoxin, in combination with chronic infection with hepatitis B virus, has been implicated in the causation of liver cancer in certain regions of Africa and Asia. Indeed, this provides an instructive example of synergy between a dietary factor and a virus in human cancer causation, and it is important to search for other possible examples in studies on nutrition and cancer. Dietary fat (especially saturated fat) is implicated in the causation of cancers of the colon, rectum, breast, and prostate, and increased body weight is associated with postmenopausal breast and endometrial cancer. In breast, endometrial, and prostate cancer hormonal factors have been implicated, but here too the precise mechanisms are not known. A possible mechanism for the role of dietary fat in colon cancer is discussed below. A diet rich in fruits and vegetables appears to be protective against several types of cancer, including cancers of the lung, colon, rectum, bladder, oral cavity, stomach, cervix, and esophagus. This may be due to the antioxidant effects of β-carotene, retinoids, and vitamins C and E, but other mechanisms have not been excluded; for example, it is well known that retinoids can modify gene expression through retinoid receptors. It should be stressed that in several cases there are conflicting data about the roles of these dietary factors and that, in general, precise cause-and-effect relations have not been established. Also, sufficient understanding is lacking at the mechanistic level on the role of dietary factors and cancer causation. This type of information is essential for a rational approach to dietary intervention studies.

Perhaps one of the most important associations in the fields of diet and cancer is that of dietary fat with colon cancer.[14,192] Experimental studies provide evidence that a high-fat diet enhances colon cancer by acting at the stage of tumor promotion.[14,31,191] Based on recent studies, a new theory has been proposed to explain the association between dietary fat and colon cancer.[14,191] The hypothesis is that the intestinal flora convert dietary lipids to DAG, which then enters the colonic epithelium and activates the enzyme PKC, thus enhancing cell proliferation and tumor promotion. Indeed, it has been found that, when bacteria obtained from normal human feces are incubated with [^{14}C]phosphatidylcholine, there is appreciable production of DAG.[192] Specific bile acids, whose levels are also increased in individuals on a high-fat diet, would be expected to enhance this process.[192] Assays for fecal DAG and PKC activity in biopsies of colonic epithelium therefore may be useful in future studies on dietary factors and human colon cancer.

Oxidant Stress and Other Endogenous Agents

It should be emphasized that various endogenous processes can result in DNA damage (for review, see refs. 3,19,20,193). These include: (1) the generation of activated forms of oxygen during normal metabolic processes, which can lead to the formation of oxidized bases in DNA, particularly 8-OH-dG; (2) spontaneous depurination of DNA; and (3) the deamination of 5-methylcytosine to yield thymidine, which can be enhanced by various chemicals. Some of these events can occur with high frequency and are known to be mutagenic in model systems. In addition, these types of DNA damage can be enhanced by various exogenous agents, especially agents that enhance the formation of activated forms of oxygen. Furthermore, nitroso carcinogens can be generated in the body from dietary nitrates and nitrites and from the endogenous production of nitric oxide by nitric oxide synthase.[194] The extent to which these mechanisms contribute to human cancer causation is not known at the present time. Alterations in the fidelity of DNA and chromosome replication and of DNA repair also might contribute to endogenous mechanisms that enhance tumor initiation and progression.

Inhibitors of the Multistage Carcinogenic Process

The human diet contains a number of naturally occurring substances that can inhibit cancer induction in experimental animals.[14,17,109,195,196] There are also several synthetic compounds that have these effects. These anticarcinogens appear to act at various stages of the carcinogenic process (Fig. 4–3). They include (1) chemicals that reduce the synthesis of carcinogens in the body, such as vitamin C, which inhibits nitrosamine formation in the stomach; (2) substances that reduce absorption of carcinogens, such as dietary fiber; (3) chemicals that alter the metabolism of carcinogens, such as benzyl isothiocyanate, which is present in cruciferous vegetables (e.g., cabbage), or selenium and β-carotene, and can act as antioxidants; (4) chemicals that inhibit the covalent binding of carcinogens to DNA, such as elagic acid or flavonoids, which are present in fruits and vegetables; (5) chemicals that inhibit tumor promotion, such as retinoids, β-carotene, and α-tocopherol, which are present in fruits and vegetables; and (6) substances that inhibit tumor formation by unknown mechanisms, such as organosulfur compounds in garlic and onions, curcumin in tumeric/curry, capsaicin in chili peppers, polyphenols in green tea, and various protease inhibitors.

The role of these compounds in human cancer is not known, but epidemiologic studies suggest that a diet rich in green and yellow vegetables decreases the risk of certain cancers.[14,191] Recent studies suggest, moreover, that retinoids are useful in cancer chemoprevention in humans.[195,197] In view of the association of breast and colon cancer with a high-fat diet, it seems likely that the incidence of these diseases also can be reduced by decreasing the consumption of fat.[14,191] It appears that some of the compounds listed in Figure 4–3 can act at more than one stage of the carcinogenic process. Further carcinogenesis studies should help to clarify the mechanism of action of these compounds and also suggest even more effective ones. For example, recent studies on nerolidal[195] and on limonene[198] indicate that these compounds may act by inhibiting posttranslational modification of the p21 *ras* protein by a farnesyl residue, thus providing a strategy to interfere with the action of an activated oncogene. We also should emphasize that, in certain experimental systems, some of the compounds shown in Figure 4–3 enhance rather than inhibit the carcinogenic process.[195] Thus, their use in clinical studies must be undertaken with caution and close surveillance. The subject of cancer chemoprevention is reviewed in detail elsewhere.[14,195,196]

MOLECULAR EPIDEMIOLOGY

Background

The concepts and methods emerging from research on molecular mechanisms of carcinogenesis provide new approaches for identifying potential human carcinogens and more precise approaches for risk assessment and extrapolation in the field of environmental carcinogenesis. They also provide methods for evaluating individual susceptibility to cancer in diverse human populations. Conventional approaches in cancer epidemiology have supplied a wealth of information, but they have serious limitations for identifying specific causal factors, particularly for those cancers that result from multifactor interactions. In addition, epidemiologic studies are largely retrospective rather than predictive, and, unless very large numbers of individuals are studied, they are quite insensitive to relatively small increases in risk. Animal bioassays and short-term laboratory tests for carcinogens are extremely useful for detecting potential human carcinogens, but it is often difficult to extrapolate quantitatively the results obtained to humans. To address this problem, a different approach has been developed based on biochemical, immunologic, and molecular assays of human tissues and biologic fluids, in combination with epidemiologic studies. This approach is known as "molecular cancer epidemiology." Highly sensitive and specific laboratory procedures are now available that can be used as biomarkers of specific factors related to (1) genetic and acquired host susceptibility, (2) metabolism and tissue levels of carcinogens, (3) levels of covalent adducts formed between carcinogens and DNA or other macromolecules, and (4) early cellular responses to carcinogen exposure. These methods now are being ap-

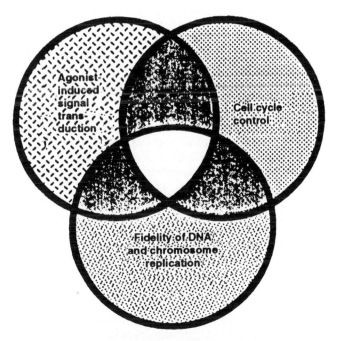

Figure 4–3. A holistic scheme of multistage carcinogenesis emphasizing the potential interactions between three types of control systems: (1) agonist-induced signal transduction and the control of gene expression, (2) cell cycle control, and (3) control of the fidelity of DNA and chromosome replication. All three of these systems interact, within each system and between the three systems, through complex cascades of protein phosphorylation and dephosphorylation, and cascades of gene expression. Exogenous agents (both genotoxic and nongenotoxic) and endogenous host factors (both inherited and acquired) can perturb all three systems, thus driving the multistage carcinogenic process. For additional details, see text and references in "New Frontiers in Molecular Carcinogenesis and Cancer Prevention" section.

plied in a broad spectrum of epidemiologic studies, and they offer great promise for expanding the scientific basis for cancer prevention. Some of these biomarkers are discussed briefly here (for detailed reviews of this subject, see refs. 199–204).

Biomarkers of Internal Dose

In conventional cancer epidemiology studies, exposure usually is assessed at the level of external source. Obviously, this approach has serious limitations with respect to precision and reliability. Highly sensitive analytic procedures and immunoassays now make it possible to measure the amounts of a chemical carcinogen or its metabolites in cells, tissues, or body fluids (saliva, blood, urine, or feces). These biomarkers of internal dose take into account individual differences in absorption or bioaccumulation of the compound in question and indicate the level of the compound within the body and in specific tissues or compartments. Examples include: assays for cotinine in serum or urine, resulting from cigarette smoke exposure; urinary levels of 1-hydroxypyrene, resulting from PAH exposure; aflatoxin levels in urine, from dietary or endogenous sources; and assays for dichlorodiphenyltrichloroethane (DDT) or polychlorinated biphenyls (PCBs) in serum or adipose tissue biopsies, from environmental contamination. An alternate method that is not specific to an individual chemical is the Ames *Salmonella typhimurium* mutagenesis assay, which measures the presence of mutagens in urine, reflecting exposure to cigarette smoke or other genotoxic environmental agents.

Biomarkers of Biologically Effective Dose

Although markers of internal dose are quite valuable, they do not indicate the extent to which a given compound has interacted with critical cellular targets. Therefore, assays of the "biologically effective dose" of a compound also have been developed. These assays measure the amount of a compound that has reacted with critical cellular macromolecules, usually DNA, or a protein such as hemoglobin in the blood.[201] DNA from the target tissue may not be readily available; therefore, surrogate tissues (e.g., placenta or peripheral blood cells) can be used instead. The relationship between the types and levels of adducts in these samples to those in the target tissue has not been well characterized in humans, but this relationship has been established for certain carcinogens in experimental animals. Another limitation is that levels of carcinogen-DNA adducts generally reflect recent exposure rather than distant past exposure.

Several sensitive and specific methods have been developed for detecting and quantitating carcinogen-DNA adducts in extracts of human peripheral blood cells and tissues. These include physical methods such as fluorescence spectroscopy and gas chromatography/mass spectrometry (GC/MS), the ^{32}P postlabeling procedure, immunoassays employing antisera to specific carcinogen-DNA adducts, and combinations of these

methods.[200,202] These methods are highly sensitive because, depending on the specific method, they can detect one carcinogen-DNA adduct per about 10^9 to 10^7 nucleotides, which is equivalent to about 1 or 100 adducts per cell, respectively. Detectable carcinogen-DNA adducts have been detected and quantitated in individuals exposed to putative carcinogens in occupational or environmental settings. Because of its relative ease and high sensitivity, the enzyme-linked immunosorbent assay (ELISA) procedure has been the most extensively employed method. For example, dramatic increases in PAH-DNA adduct levels were observed in workers occupationally exposed to high levels of PAHs. These included foundry, aluminum plant, and coke oven workers. PAH-DNA adducts and related markers have been linked to environmental exposure in individuals living in a highly polluted region of Poland.[203] Assays for protein (either hemoglobin or albumin) adducts in blood samples have proven to be very informative for certain chemical exposures. Such assays have been used to measure ethylene oxide, 4-aminobiphenyl, and tobacco-specific nitrosamines bound to human hemoglobin.[201]

Early Biologic Responses and Gene Mutations

The next category of biomarkers in the multistep sequence of carcinogenesis comprises markers of very early responses of cells to carcinogen DNA damage, especially responses that are thought to play a role in carcinogenesis. These effects can be measured in target tissues or a more convenient surrogate (e.g., peripheral white blood cells). Such biomarkers include assays for DNA single-strand breaks and assays for various cytogenic effects, including sister chromatic exchange, micronuclei, and chromosomal aberrations. Several methods now exist to detect mutations that have occurred in the intact human as a result of exposure to various environmental agents. These include mutations in the *HPRT* gene in peripheral blood T cells[205] and mutated forms of glycophorin proteins on the surface of red blood cells.[206] These assays have detected significant increases in somatic cell mutations in human populations exposed to ionizing radiation, patients on chemotherapy, and cigarette smokers.[204–206] The subject of mutational spectra was discussed earlier in this chapter.

Other Types of Biomarkers

Several chemicals enhance the carcinogenic process without forming covalent adducts with cellular DNA or proteins. These include certain tumor promoters (TPA and phenobarbital) and xenobiotics (e.g., tetrachlorodibenzodioxin [TCDD] and various PCBs), as well as hormones (including both natural and synthetic estrogens and androgens).[12,16,178] There is a need to develop assays for the biologically effective dose of these agents (i.e., assays at the cellular level). For specific hormones and TCDD, this effort might be directed toward assessing the extent of occupancy of their related high-affinity receptors. Because tumor promotion involves disturbances in signal transduction and gene expression, assays to evaluate levels of specific growth factors, growth factor receptors, second messengers such as cyclic AMP and DAG, protein kinases, specific phosphoproteins, and the expression of genes related to tumor promotion and cell proliferation can be incorporated into molecular epidemiology studies in the future. Immunocytochemical assays of PCNA, which is associated with replication and repair, or of other proteins associated with specific phases of the cell cycle (e.g., cyclins) also may prove to be useful.[14] Assays of various hormones, and their metabolites and receptors, have been used extensively in studies on human breast cancer and other endocrine-related tumors.[207] It would be of interest to utilize these types of biomarkers in parallel with some of the other markers mentioned above in future studies on the causation of human cancers of the breast, cervix, ovary, and prostate, because it seems likely that the causation of these tumors (like other tumors) results from the interaction of multiple factors. Thus far, biomarkers related to the various functions of the immune system have not been incorporated routinely into molecular cancer epidemiology studies. Biomarkers of an individual's immune status are also an important field for future development.

Because dietary histories have serious limitations in studies on nutrition and cancer, it is essential to have more objective markers. Assays have been used to measure the levels of various vitamins, minerals, and nutrients in human blood, tissues, and urine.[191] It would be useful, however, to develop biomarkers that monitor the biologic effects of various dietary factors in the intact individual, and their relevance to the carcinogenic process. For this and other purposes, biomarkers related to oxidative damage are of considerable importance. These include urinary levels of oxidized DNA bases; analyses of DNA samples for strand breaks or oxidized bases (thymine glycol, 8-hydroxyguanine, etc.); blood and tissue levels of malonaldehyde, an oxidized product of lipids; and markers of enzymes that detoxify activated forms of oxygen, such as catalase and superoxide dismutase.[19–21]

Markers of Individual Susceptibility

Mechanisms of carcinogenesis predict that individual susceptibility to cancer may result from several factors, including differences in the metabolism of carcinogenic chemicals (uptake, activation, and detoxification), DNA repair, inherited or acquired alterations in proto-oncogenes or tumor suppressor genes, nutritional status, hormonal factors, and immunologic factors. With respect to inter-individual variations in carcinogen metabolism, there appears to be an association between increased activity of a specific cytochrome P-450, CYP2D6,[208] plus increased inducibility of CYP1A1 (aryl hydrocarbon hydroxylase activity)[28] and lung cancer risk. However, decreases in phase II detoxifying enzymes might increase cancer risks. Examples include the association of decreased activity of the μ isozyme of glutathione-S-transferase with increased lung cancer risk,[208a,208b] and decreased activity of N-acetyltransferase (slow acetylator

phenotype) with increased bladder cancer risk.[209] Indeed, the clearance of low-dose carcinogens from individuals displaying this slow acetylator phenotype is decreased relative to individuals with the rapid one, suggesting the former may have an increased cancer risk.[209a] The cloning of the numerous genes that constitute the cytochrome P-450 gene family, and other genes involved in the metabolism and detoxification of various xenobiotics, will provide additional biomarkers of individual susceptibility to various exogenous chemical agents.

Acquired or inherited variations in the efficiency or fidelity of DNA repair also influence individual susceptibility to cancer. As discussed in "DNA Repair," earlier in this chapter, this principle is illustrated by the autosomal disease xeroderma pigmentosum. Apparent variations in DNA repair in the general population that appear to correlate with cancer risks have been reported.[3,210–212] The recent cloning of several human DNA repair genes (see Table 4–5) provides probes that can be used to monitor more precisely variations in DNA repair capacity and their relationship to cancer susceptibility. It will be interesting to learn if the loss of heterozygosity prevalent in specific types of cancer are coincident with the location of other DNA repair genes. Additionally, it will be important to identify individuals who are heterozygous by inheritance for specific DNA repair genes (e.g., hMSH2 and hMLH1, etc.) since their products maintain surveillance of the genome's integrity in somatic cells and are, in effect, tumor suppressors.

Most of the previously described markers of individual susceptibility relate mainly to DNA-damaging (genotoxic) agents. The multistage model of carcinogenesis predicts, however, that there also will be interindividual variation in susceptibility related to tumor promotion, cell proliferation, and tumor progression, but, as noted earlier in this chapter, biomarkers specific for these factors have not been well developed for routine use in molecular epidemiology studies.

Genetic predisposition to cancer also can be influenced by inherited mutations in tumor suppressor genes, as illustrated by the Li-Fraumeni syndrome, in which patients inherit mutations in one allele of the p53 gene, and by hereditary retinoblastoma, which involves the Rb gene. These diseases are discussed in detail in Chapter 5. It is of interest that inherited mutations in either of these tumor suppressor genes increase the susceptibility of individuals to certain radiation-induced tumors.[213] Inheritance of specific polymorphic alleles of the ras oncogene[214] and of the p53 gene[215] have been linked to lung cancer risk, but the significance of this association is not known. Moreover, inheritance of a specific polymorphism in a minisatellite sequence in the Ha-ras oncogene is correlated with increased risk of breast, colorectal, urinary bladder cancers, as well as acute leukemia.[156a] Current efforts to clone a gene on chromosome 17 that is associated with familial breast cancer[216] may provide a clue to genetic factors that influence breast cancer risks. Thus, in future studies in molecular epidemiology, it should be possible to monitor the complex interactions between both environmental and inherited factors in human cancer causation.

Future Directions in Molecular Epidemiology

The foregoing discussion indicates that remarkable progress has been made in a new approach to understanding human cancer causation. At the same time, further intensive research is required to validate existing biomarkers and to develop new ones. A key issue is the predictive value of specific markers; that is, when the marker is positive, does it truly predict an increased cancer risk and is there a dose-response relationship between increased level of the marker and cancer risk? There is accumulating evidence that there is a high degree of variability in biomarker levels among persons smoking the same number of cigarettes, among individuals working in the same industrial plant, and even among chemotherapy patients treated with standardized doses of chemotherapy agents.[200] As discussed earlier in this chapter, this is probably because of variability in metabolic processing of xenobiotics and/or in DNA repair, as well as errors in estimating individual exposure. Thus, the development and application of biomarkers has tremendous potential to increase the power of epidemiologic studies of cancer, because this approach has the capacity to assess objectively individual susceptibility.

An exciting recent trend that brings together cancer researchers interested in prevention with those interested in therapy is the fact that a number of the biomarkers being developed in the field of molecular epidemiology also may be applicable as early or intermediate endpoints in assessing the efficacy of various intervention trials (including chemoprevention) in the field of cancer prevention and also the efficacy of new forms of treatment in patients who have developed cancer. Thus, new bridges are being built between the fields of basic research on carcinogenesis, cancer epidemiology, cancer prevention, and therapy.[14]

NEW FRONTIERS IN MOLECULAR CARCINOGENESIS AND CANCER PREVENTION

In concluding this chapter, it is of interest to discuss briefly three relatively unexplored subjects that are critical to our understanding of the process of carcinogenesis and to the development of new approaches to cancer prevention and treatment. The first has to do with the phenomenon of inducible responses to DNA damage in mammalian cells. Although earlier in this chapter a sharp distinction was made between genotoxic carcinogens and tumor promoters, in terms of their mechanism of action (genetic versus epigenetic), as discussed in "Genomic Instability and Inducible Responses to DNA Damage," DNA-damaging agents (including radiation and chemicals) not only can cause mutations but also can induce cellular responses (yet to be defined) that apparently activate signal transduction pathways, thus leading to multiple alterations in gene expression. These changes include not only the induction of enzymes involved in DNA repair, but also some of the same early-response genes in-

duced by mitogens (e.g., c-*fos*, c-*myc*, plasminogen activator, ornithine decarboxylase, and growth factors). This may explain the fact that certain genotoxic carcinogens can act as complete carcinogens.[12] It also may explain some of the therapeutic effects and toxic side effects seen in patients treated with radiation or chemotherapy (e.g., changes in the differentiated state of tumors, pulmonary fibrosis).[12] The precise mechanism of how DNA damage, or damage to other cellular targets,[200a,200b] induces responses that overlap with those triggered through agonist-induced activation of signal transduction pathways is not known. Both the nature of the signal and response mechanism are important subjects for future studies related to carcinogenesis, as well as cancer therapy.

A second exciting new area of carcinogenesis has to do with the apparent ability of tumor cells to develop variants with a frequency greater than that of normal cells, which we have briefly reviewed in "Genomic Instability and Inducible Responses to DNA Damage," earlier in this chapter. Tumor heterogeneity represents one of the current major limitations of therapy. A given tumor can display mutations in at least five different loci (sometimes involving mutations in both alleles or multiple mutations in a single allele),[17,67] and additional genetic lesions still are being revealed in these tumors. Mechanistic studies are required to explain the frequency of these mutations, which include not only point mutations but also allelic loss, gene rearrangements, DNA amplification, and gross chromosomal abnormalities (Tables 4–3, 4–4, and 4–6). The recent finding of a high frequency of mutations in repetitive DNA sequences in a subset of human hereditary colon cancers[153–155,164] requires further study in these and other tumors. Very little is known about what "drives" these complex mutational events, and the relative roles of exogenous versus endogenous factors during the process of tumor progression. Genomic instability often is invoked, but, except in the case of studies on gene amplification,[162,176,177] this has not been precisely quantitated, and the underlying biochemical mechanisms are not known. Insights into these mechanisms might suggest therapeutic approaches that would block the generation of diversity in tumors.

Studies in yeast indicate that cells contain checkpoints in the cell cycle that monitor whether preceding events have occurred correctly and determine if progression of the cell cycle should proceed.[165,166] For example, the *RAD9* gene senses the occurrence of DNA damage and blocks entry into mitosis until repair corrects this damage. Tumor cells might lack such checkpoints, thus increasing the error frequency of replication, and it appears that the *p53* tumor suppressor gene normally plays this role in mammalian cells.[217] Alternatively, tumor cells may be aberrant with respect to the fidelity of DNA replication, genetic recombination, the synchrony or precise timing of replicon firing, or the mechanisms of chromosome replication and segregation. These events may operate via different mechanisms during development, and their ectopic reactivation in tumor cells may lead to the accumulation of genetic alterations. Thus, for example, there is possibly a window of time in development when certain mechanisms of replication or repair are distinct in rapidly dividing embryonic cells, but are reinstated in the cancer cell.

As discussed earlier in this chapter and in greater detail in Chapter 6, it appears that most of the oncogenes identified thus far code for components of signal transduction pathways that are involved in the responses of cells to external agonists (growth factors, hormones, etc.), and responses that frequently influence the G_0-to-G_1 transition and early events in the G_1 phase of the cell cycle. Recent research on cylcins and their related protein kinases and phosphatases that control later phases of the cell cycle has revealed another repertoire of genes that are potential targets for carcinogens (for review, see refs. 165,166,218 and Chapter 1). Mutations in these genes could have profound effects on carcinogenesis. Studies in yeast indicate that mutations in cyclin-related genes can influence the fidelity of chromosome replication and segregation.[218] It seems likely, therefore, that in higher organisms mutations in these genes also might play an important role in multistage carcinogenesis. Indeed, examples now exist of mutational changes in cyclins A, D1, and E genes in human cancers (for review, see refs. 218–221), and it seems likely that mutations in other cyclin-related genes, and/or abnormalities in their expression, will be found in human tumors. Indeed, a new tumor suppressor gene, *MTS1*, was recently identified as an inhibitor of cyclin-dependent kinase 4, one of the several cdks whose activity propels cells through the cell cycle.[221a] Mutations in this gene in various types of tumor cells appear to be as common as in *p53*. Thus, the repertoire of cellular genes that may be critical targets for carcinogens is even larger than previously anticipated.

A third frontier area of research, which is perhaps the one most poorly understood, has to do with the likelihood that multistage carcinogenesis involves not only mutational changes but also aberrations in epigenetic mechanisms that normally control gene expression and cell differentiation. There are several lines of evidence for implicating epigenetic mechanisms, in addition to gene mutations and chromosomal abnormalities, in carcinogenesis (for review, see refs. 12,222):

1. A variety of nongenotoxic agents can enhance tumor formation, apparently by acting through epigenetic mechanisms.

2. Tumors can be induced to differentiate or undergo reversion at very high frequency by nongenotoxic agents, indicating that a major portion of their phenotype is under epigenetic control.

3. Normal differentiation does not involve mutational changes (except in the immune system) and yet produces stable lineages and cell phenotypes. Aside from DNA methylation, the biochemical mechanisms that control the stability of differentiation are not well understood. Nevertheless, it seems reasonable to assume that distortions in these mechanisms also could produce abnormalities in cell phenotypes that are heritable in somatic cells. Indeed, there is evidence that carcinogenesis involves disturbances in DNA methylation, including both regions of hypomethylation and hypermethylation (for methylation changes, see ref. 160,161, and a review in ref. 224). Ab-

normalities in gene imprinting during the somatic development of tumors is another possible mechanism (for imprinting changes in cancer cells, see ref. 158,159, and a review in ref. 225). These alterations in DNA methylation could alter chromatin structure, thus affecting gene expression, the timing of replication of specific genes, and the occurrence of mutations.[222,224]

4. The high frequency of cell transformation induced by carcinogens in cell culture also suggests that epigenetic mechanisms might play an important role in carcinogenesis.[12]

These concepts are not new, but, in the intense race to identify the mutational changes in tumor cells, one should not ignore fundamental processes of cell determination and differentiation, and their potential contribution to the multistage carcinogenesis process. Research in this area is likely to provide new insights into the processes of tumor promotion and hormonal carcinogenesis, as well as new strategies for cancer prevention and treatment.

Figure 4–3 summarizes the foregoing discussion and displays a holistic view of multistage carcinogenesis. The diagram emphasizes potential interactions between three types of circuitry or control systems in eukaryotic cells: (1) agonist-induced signal transduction and the control of gene expression, (2) cell cycle control, and (3) control of the fidelity of DNA and chromosome replication. All three of these systems interact with each other through complex cascades of protein phosphorylation and dephosphorylation, and cascades of gene expression. Distortions in any one of these systems therefore can be transmitted to the other two systems. For example, distortions in signal transduction might drive cells from G_0 into G_1, and through G_1 into persistent cell cycling. Excessive expression of early-response genes also might place certain genes or chromosomes in jeopardy of mutational changes, because of the relationships between transcription, DNA repair, and DNA replication. Abnormalities in protein kinases that normally regulate signal transduction also might impair later steps in cell cycle control, for example, by aberrant protein phosphorylation. Abnormalities in cell cycle control during the G_0/G_1, S, G_2, and M phases could enhance the frequency of point mutations, DNA amplification, genetic recombination, or chromosomal aberrations, thus impairing the function of genes involved in either the positive or negative control of signal transduction pathways, or in cyclin-related functions that control various stages of the cell cycle. These combined events could result in error cascade, genomic instability, tumor progression, and tumor heterogeneity. The resulting disorders in gene expression would disrupt not only the internal machinery of the cell but also the expression of cell surface molecules and molecules destined for secretion, thus enhancing tumor invasion, metastasis, and angiogenesis. As discussed earlier in this chapter, these disorders might be due to mutations as well as distortions in epigenetic mechanisms that control gene expression and cell differentiation. The driving force for these changes can be certain exogenous chemical and physical agents, as well as the previously mentioned endogenous factors. Obviously, much more research is required to elucidate fully the details of these complex interactions. The findings obtained are likely to have a major impact on the design of more effective strategies for cancer prevention and treatment.

REFERENCES

1. Shimkin MB: Some classics of experimental oncology (NIH Publication No. 80-2150). Washington DC, National Institutes of Health, 1980
2. Weinstein IB: From chimney sweeps to oncogenes. Mol Carcinog 1:2, 1988
3. Harris CC: Chemical and physical carcinogenesis: Advances and perspectives for the 1990s. Cancer Res 51(suppl):5023S, 1992
4. Brugge J, Curran T, Harlow E, McCormick F (eds): Origins of Human Cancer: A Comprehensive Review. Plainview, NY, Cold Spring Harbor Laboratory Press, 1991
5. Bishop JM: Molecular themes in oncogenesis. Cell 64:235, 1991
6. Cantley LC, Auger KR, Carpenter C, et al: Oncogenes and signal transduction. Cell 64:281, 1991
7. Hunter T: Cooperation between oncogenes. Cell 64:249, 1991
8. Marshall C: Tumor suppressor genes. Cell 64:313, 1991
9. Weinberg R: Tumor suppressor genes. Science 254:1138, 1991
10. Boveri T: Zur Frage der eutstehung maligner Tumoren, vol. 1. Jena, Gustave Fischer Verlag, 1914
11. Miller E: Some current perspectives on chemical carcinogenesis in humans and experimental animals: Presidential address. Cancer Res, 38:1479, 1978
12. Weinstein IB: The origins of human cancer: Molecular mechanisms of carcinogenesis and their implications for cancer prevention and treatment. Cancer Res 48:4135, 1988
13. Weinstein IB, Borner CM, Krauss RS, et al: Pleiotropic effects of protein kinase C and the concept of carcinogenesis as a progressive disorder in signal transduction. In Brugge J, Curran T, Harlow E, McCormick F (eds): Origins of Human Cancer: A Comprehensive Review. Plainview, NY, Cold Spring Harbor Laboratory Press, 1991, pp 113–124
14. Weinstein IB: Cancer prevention: Recent progress and future opportunities. Cancer Res 51(suppl):508S, 1991
15. Weinstein IB: Chemical carcinogenesis; Fundamental mechanisms and implications for cancer prevention. In Calabresi P, Schein P (eds): Medical Oncology, 2nd ed. New York, McGraw-Hill, 1991, pp 107–120
16. Tomatis L, Aitio A, Wilbourn J, Shukar L: Human carcinogens so far identified. Jpn J Cancer Res 80:795, 1987
17. Sugimura T: Multistep carcinogenesis: A 1990s perspective. Science 258:603, 1992
18. Singer B, Grunberger D: Molecular Biology of Mutagens and Carcinogens. New York, Plenum, 1983
19. Cerutti PA, Trump BF: Inflammation and oxidative stress in carcinogenesis. Cancer Cells 3:1, 1991
20. Teebor GW, Boorstein RJ, Cadet J: The repairability of oxidative free radical mediated damage to DNA: A review. Int J Radiat Res 54:131, 1988
21. Pryor WA: Measurement of oxidative stress in humans. Cancer Epidemiol Biomarkers Prevention 2:289, 1993
22. Ross RK, Yuan J-M, Yu M, et al: Urinary aflatoxin biomarkers and risk of hepatocellular carcinoma. Lancet 339:943, 1992
23. Felton JS, Knize MG: Heterocyclic-amine mutagens/carcinogens in foods. In Cooper CS, Grover PL (eds): Chemical Carcinogenesis and Mutagenesis. Berlin, Springer-Verlag, 1990, pp 471–502
24. Ames BN, Gold LS: Too many rodent carcinogens: Mitogenesis increases mutagenesis. Science 249:970, 1990
25. Perera F, Boffetta P, Nisbet ICT: What are the major carcinogens in the etiology of human cancer? In DeVita VT, Hellman S, Rosenberg SA (eds): Important Advances in Oncology. Philadelphia, JB Lippincott Company, 1989, pp 237–247

26. Hoffmann D, Hecht SS: Nicotine-derived N-nitroamines and tobacco-related cancer: Current status and future direction. Cancer Res 45:935, 1985
27. Guengerich FP: Bioactivation and detoxification of toxic and carcinogenic chemicals. Drug Metab Dispos 21:1, 1993
28. Nebert DW: Role of genetics and drug metabolism in human cancer risk. Mutat Res 246:267, 1991
29. O'Handley SF, Sanford DG, Xu R, et al: Structural characterization of an N-acetyl-2-aminofluroene (AAF) modified DNA oligomer by NMR, energy minimization and molecular dynamics. Biochemistry 32:2481, 1993
30. Cosman M, de la Santos C, Fiala R, et al: Solution conformation of the $(+)$-cis-anti-[BP]dG adduct in a DNA duplex: Intercalation of the covalently attached benzo[a]pyrenyl ring into the helix and displacement of the modified deoxyguanosine. Biochemistry 16:4145, 1993
31. Kramer KH, Seidman MM: Use of supF, and Escherichia coli tyrosine suppressor tRNA gene, as a mutagenic target in shuttle-vector plasmids. Mutat Res 220:61, 1989
32. Basu AK, Essigman JM: Site-specifically modified oligodeoxynucleotides as probes for the structural and biological effects of DNA-damaging agents. Chem Res Toxicol 1:1, 1988
33. Yandell DW, Dryja TP, Little JB: Molecular genetic analysis of recessive mutations at a heterozygous autosomal locus in human cells. Mutat Res 229:89, 1990
34. Breimer L, Nalbantoglu J, Meuth M: Structure and sequence of mutations induced by ionizing radiation at selectable loci in Chinese hamster ovary cells. J Mol Biol 192:669, 1986
35. Waldren C, Jones C, Puck T: Measurement of mutagenesis in mammalian cells. Proc Natl Acad Sci USA 76:1358, 1979
36. Ashman CR, Jagadeeswaran P, Davidson RL: Efficient recovery and sequencing of mutant genes from mammalian chromosomal DNA. Proc Natl Acad Sci USA 83:3356, 1986
37. Wang Y, Maher VM, Liskay RM, McCormick JJ: Carcinogens can induce homologous recombination between duplicated chromosomal sequences in mouse L cells. Mol Cell Biol 8:196, 1988
38. Greenspan J, Xu F, Davidson RL: Molecular analysis of ethyl methanesulfonate-induced reversion of a chromosomally integrated mutant shuttle vector gene in mammalian cells. Mol Cell Biol 8:4185, 1988
39. Carothers AM, Mucha J, Grunberger D: DNA strand-specific mutations induced by $(\pm)$-3α,4β-dihydroxy-1α,2α-epoxy-1,2,3,4-tetrahydrobenzo[α]phenanthrene in the dihydrofolate reductase gene. Proc Natl Acad Sci USA 88:5749, 1991
40. Bardwell L: The mutagenic and carcinogenic effects of gene transfer. Mutagenesis 4:245, 1989
41. Craigie R: Hotspots and warm spots: Integration specificity of retroelements. TIG 8:187, 1992
42. Kitamura Y, HaLee YM, Coffin JM: Nonrandom integration of retroviral DNA in vitro: Effect of CpG methylation. Proc Natl Acad Sci USA 89:5532, 1992
43. Lichtenauer-Kaligis E, Thijssen J, den Dulk H, et al: Genome wide spontaneous mutation in human cells determined by the spectrum of mutations in hprt cDNA genes. Mutagenesis 8:207, 1993
44. Meuth M: The structure of mutation in mammalian cells. Biochim Biophys Acta 1032:1, 1990
45. Cohen J, Levinson A: A point mutation in the last intron responsible for increased expression and transforming activity of the c-Ha-ras oncogene. Nature 334:119, 1988
46. Carothers AM, Urlaub G, Mucha J, et al: Splicing mutations in the CHO DHFR gene preferentially induced by $(\pm)$-3α,4β-dihydroxy-1α, 2α-epoxy-1,2,3,4-tetrahydrobenzo[c]phenanthrene. Proc Natl Acad Sci USA 87:5464, 1990
47. LeClerc JE, Borden A, Lawrence CW: The thymine-thymine pyrimidine-pyrimidone (6-4) ultraviolet light photoproduct is highly mutagenic and specifically induces 3′ thymine-to-cytosine transitions in Escherichia coli. Proc Natl Acad Sci USA 88:9685, 1991
48. Reid TM, Loeb LA: Tandem double CC $\rightarrow$ TT mutations are produced by reactive oxygen species. Proc Natl Acad Sci USA 90:3904, 1993
49. Shibutani S, Takeshita M, Grollman AP: Insertion of specific

bases during DNA synthesis past the oxidation-damaged base 8-oxodG. Nature 349:431, 1991

50. Loeb LA, Preston BD: Mutagenesis by appurinic/apyrimidinic sites. Annu Rev Genet 20:201, 1986

51. Norman D, Abuaf P, Hingerty PE, et al: NMR and computational characterization of N-(deoxyguanosin-8-yl)aminofluorene adduct [(AF)G] opposite adenosine in DNA: (AF)G[syn]·A[anti] pair formation and its pH dependence. Biochemistry 28:7462, 1989

51a. Kouchakdjian M, Bodepudi V, Shibutani S, et al: NMR structural studies of the ionizing radiation adduct 7-hydro-8-oxo-deoxyguanosine (8-oxo-7H-dG) opposite deoxyadenosine in a DNA duplex, 8-oxo-7H-dG(syn)·dA(anti) alignment at lesion site. Biochemistry 30:1403, 1991

52. Burkhart-Schultz K, Thomas CB, Thompson CL, et al: Characterization of in vivo somatic mutations at the hypoxanthine phosphoribosyltransferase gene of a human control population. Environ Health Perspect 101(1):68, 1993

53. Gossen JA, de Leeuw WJF, Tan CHT, et al: Efficient rescue of integrated shuttle vectors from transgenic mice: A model for studying mutations in vivo. Proc Natl Acad Sci USA 86:7971, 1989

54. Sukumar S, Notario V, Martin-Zanca D, Barbacid M: Induction of mammary carcinomas in rats by nitroso-methyl urea involves malignant activation of H-ras-1 locus by single point mutations. Nature 306:658, 1983

55. Zarbl H, Sukumaar S, Arthur AV, et al: Direct mutagenesis of Ha-ras-1 oncogenes by N-nitro-N-methyl urea during initiation of mammary carcinogenesis in rats. Nature 315:382, 1985

56. Slaga TJ, Gleason GL, DiGiovanni J, et al: Potent tumor-initiating activity of the 3,4-dihydrodiol of 7,12-dimethylbenz[a]anthracene in mouse skin. Cancer Res 39:1934, 1979

57. Cheng SC, Prakash AS, Pigott MA, et al: A metabolite of the carcinogen 7,12 dimethylbenz[a]anthracene that reacts predominantly with adenine residues in DNA. Carcinogenesis 9:1721, 1988

58. Brown K, Buchmann A, Balmain A: Carcinogen-induced mutations in the mouse c-Ha-ras gene provide evidence of multiple pathways for tumor progression. Proc Natl Acad Sci USA 87:538, 1990

59. Quintanella M, Brown K, Ramsden M, Balmain A: Carcinogen-specific mutation and amplification of Ha-ras during mouse skin carcinogenesis. Nature 322:78, 1986

60. Bizub D, Wood AW, Skalka AM: Mutagenesis of the Ha-ras oncogene in mouse skin tumors induced by polycyclic aromatic hydrocarbons. Proc Natl Acad Sci USA 83:6048, 1986

61. Leon J, Kamino H, Steinberg JJ, Pellicer A: H-ras activation in benign and self-regressing skin tumors (keratocanthomas) in both humans and animal model system. Mol Cell Biol 8:786, 1988

62. Cardiff RD, Gumerlock PH, Soong M-M, et al: c-H-ras-1 expression in 7,12-dimethyl benzanthracene-induced Balb/c mouse mammary hyperplasia and their tumors. Oncogene 3:205, 1988

63. Hochwalt A, Solomon JJ, Garte SJ: Mechanism of H-ras oncogene activation in mouse squamous carcinoma induced by an alkylating agent. Cancer Res 48:556, 1988

64. de Fromentel CC, Soussi T: TP53 tumor suppressor gene: A model for investigating human mutagenesis. Genes Chromosom Cancer 4:1, 1992

65. Fearon ER, Hamilton SR, Vogelstein B: Clonal analysis of human colorectal tumors. Science 238:193, 1987

66. Vogelstein B, Fearon ER, Hamilton SR, et al: Genetic alterations during colorectal-tumor development. N Engl J Med 319:525, 1988

67. Fearon ER, Vogelstein B: A genetic model for colorectal tumorigenesis. Cell 61:759, 1990

68. Rodriguez NR, Rowan A, Smith MEF, et al: p53 mutations in colorectal cancer. Proc Natl Acad Sci USA 87:7555, 1990

69. Kikuchi-Yanoshita R, Konishi M, Ito S, et al: Genetic changes of both p53 alleles associated with the conversion from colorectal adenoma to early carcinoma in familial adenomatous polyposis and non-familial adenamatous polyposis patients. Cancer Res 52:3965, 1992

70. Nigro JM, Baker SJ, Preisinger AC, et al: Mutations in the p53 gene occur in diverse human tumor types. Nature, 342:705, 1989

71. Kupryjanczyk J, Thor AD, Beauchamp R, et al: p53 gene mutations and protein accumulation in human ovarian cancer. Proc Natl Acad Sci USA 90:4961, 1993

72. Sidransky D, Mikelsen T, Schwecheimer K, et al: Clonal expansion of p53 mutant cells is associated with brain tumor progression. Nature, 355:846, 1992

73. Iggo R, Gatter K, Bartek J, et al: Increased expression of mutant forms of p53 oncogene in primary lung cancer. Lancet 335:675, 1990

74. Chiba I, Takashi T, Nau MM, et al: Mutation in the p53 gene are frequent in primary, resected non-small cell lung cancer. Oncogene 5:1603, 1990

75. Kishimoto Y, Murakami Y, Shiraishi M, et al: Aberration of the p53 tumor suppressor gene in human non-small cell carcinomas of the lung. Cancer Res 52:4799, 1992

76. Bressac B, Kew M, Wands J, Ozturk M: Selective G to T-mutation of p53 gene in hepatocellular carcinoma from Southern Africa. Nature 350:429, 1991

77. Hsu IC, Metcalf RA, Sun T, et al: Mutational hotspot in the p53 gene in human hepatocellular carcinoma. Nature 350:427, 1991

77a. Unsal H, Yakicier C, Marçais C, et al: Genetic heterogeneity of hepatocellular carcinoma. Proc Natl Acad Sci USA 91:822, 1994

78. Prosser J, Thompson AL, Cranston G, Evans HJ: Evidence that p53 behaves as a tumor suppressor gene in sporadic breast tumors. Oncogene 5:1573, 1990

79. Coles C, Condie A, Chetty A, et al: p53 mutations in breast cancer. Cancer Res 52:5291, 1992

80. Mazars R, Spinardi L, BenCheikh M, et al: p53 mutations occur in aggressive breast cancer. Cancer Res 52:3918, 1992

81. Brash DE, Rudolph JA, Simon JA, et al: A role for sunlight in skin cancer UV-induced p53 mutations in squamous cell carcinoma. Proc Natl Acad Sci USA 88:10124, 1991

82. Ziegler A, Leffell DJ, Kunala S, et al: Mutation hotspots due to sunlight in the p53 gene of nonmelanoma skin cancers. Proc Natl Acad Sci USA 90:4216, 1993

83. Moles J-P, Moyret C, Guillot B, et al: p53 mutations in human epithelial skin cancers. Oncogene 8:583, 1993

83a. Nakazawa H, English D, Randell PL, et al: UV and skin cancer: Specific p53 gene mutation in normal skin as a biologically relevant exposure measurement. Proc Natl Acad Sci USA 91:360, 1994

84. Cooper DN, Krawczak M: The mutational spectrum of single base-pair substitutions causing human genetic disease: Patterns and predictions. Hum Genet 85:55, 1990

84a. Weitzman SA, Turk PW, Milkowski DH, Kozlowski K: Free radical adducts induce alterations in DNA cytosine methylation. Proc Natl Acad Sci USA 91:1261, 1994

84b. Smith S, Kan J, Baker J, et al: Recognition of unusual DNA structures by human DNA (cytosine-5) methyltransferase. J Mol Biol 217:39, 1991

85. Yang J-L, Chen R-H, Maher VM, McCormick JJ: Kinds and location of mutations induced by (±)-7β,8α-dihydroxy-9α,10α-epoxy-7,8,9,10-tetrahydrobenzo[a]pyrene in the coding region of the hypoxanthine guanine phosphoribosyltransferase gene in diploid human fibroblast. Carcinogenesis 12:71, 1991

85a. Malins DC, Haimanot R: Major alterations in the nucleotide structure of DNA in cancer of the female breast. Cancer Res 51:5430, 1991

86. Cheng KC, Cahill DS, Kasai H, et al: 8-Hydroxyguanine, an abundant form of oxidative DNA damage, causes G → T and A → C substitutions. J Biol Chem 267:166, 1992

86a. Carothers AM, Yuan W, Hingerty B, et al: Mutation and repair induced by the carcinogen 2-(hydroxyamino)-1-methyl-6-phenylimidazo[4,5-b]pyridine (N-OH-PhIP) in the dihydrofolate reductase gene of Chinese hamster ovary cells and conformational modeling of the dG-C8-PhIP adduct in DNA. Chem Res Toxicol 7:209, 1994

86b. Tornaletti S, Pfeifer GP: Slow repair of pyrimidine dimers at *p53* mutation hotspots in skin cancer. Science *263*:1436, 1994

87. Ito K, Inoue S, Yamamoto K, Kawanishi S: 8-Hydroxydeoxy-guanosine formation at the 5' site of 5'-GG-3' sequences in double-stranded DNA by UV radiation with riboflavin. J Biol Chem *268*:13221, 1993

87a. Magewu AN, Jones PA: Ubiquitous and tenacious methylation of the CpG site in codon 248 of the p53 gene may explain its frequent appearance as a mutational hot spot in human cancer. Mol Cell Biol *14*:4225, 1994

88. Sankaranarayanan K: Ionizing radiation and genetic risks. III, Nature of spontaneous and radiation-induced mutations in mammalian in vitro systems and mechanisms of induction of mutations by radiation. Mutat Res *258*:75, 1991

89. Evans HH: Cellular and molecular effects of radon and other alpha particle emitters. Adv Mutagenesis Res *3*:29, 1991

90. Vahakangas KH, Samet JM, Metcalf RA, et al: Mutations of p53 and *ras* genes in radon-associated lung cancer from uranium miners. Lancet *339*:576, 1992

91. Walker GC: Inducible DNA repair systems. Annu Rev Biochem *54*:425, 1985

92. Ruby SW, Szostak JW: Specific *Saccharomyces cerevisiae* genes are expressed in response to DNA-damaging agents. Mol Cell Biol *5*:75, 1985

93. Hickson ID, Harris AL: Mammalian DNA repair—use of mutants hypersensitive to cytotoxic agents. TIG *4*:101, 1988

94. Pegg AE, Byers TL: Repair of DNA containing O^6-alkylguanine. FASEB J *6*:2302, 1992

95. Tchou J, Grollman AP: Repair of DNA containing the oxidatively-damaged base, 8-oxoguanine. Mutat Res *299*:277, 1993

96. Todo T, Takemori H, Ryo H, et al: A new photoreactivating enzyme that specifically repairs ultraviolet light-induced (6-4) photoproducts. Nature *361*:371, 1993

96a. Lindahl T: DNA surveillance defect in cancer cells. Current Biology *4*:249, 1994

97. Huang J-C, Svoboda DL, Reardon JT, Sancar A: Human nucleotide excision nuclease removes thymine dimers from DNA by incising the 22nd phosphodiester bond 5' and the 6th phosphodiester bond 3' to the photodimer. Proc Natl Acad Sci USA *89*:3664, 1992

98. Covereley D, Kenny MK, Munn M, et al: Requirement for the replication protein SSB in human DNA excision repair. Nature *349*:538, 1991

99. Shivji MK, Kenny MK, Wood RD: Proliferating cell nuclear antigen is required for DNA excision repair. Cell *69*:367, 1992

100. Myles GM, Sancar A: DNA repair. Chem Res Toxicol *2*:197, 1989

101. Bohr VA: Gene specific DNA repair. Carcinogenesis *12*:1983, 1991

102. Felsenfeld G: Chromatin as an essential part of the transcriptional mechanism. Nature *355*:219, 1992

103. Lee DY, Hayes JJ, Pruss D, Wolffe AP: A positive role for histone acetylation in transcription factor access to nucleosomal DNA. Cell *72*:73, 1993

104. Carter KC, Bowman D, Carrington W, et al: A three-dimensional view of precursor messenger RNA metabolism within the mammalian nucleus. Science *259*:1330, 1993

105. Mellon I, Spivak G, Hanawalt PC: Selective removal of transcription-blocking DNA damage from the transcribed strand of the mammalian DHFR gene. Cell *51*:241, 1987

106. Leadon SA, Lawrence DA: Preferential repair of DNA damage on the transcribed strand of the human metallothionein gene requires RNA polymerase II. Mutat Res *255*:67, 1991

107. Selby CP, Sancar A: Transcription preferentially inhibits nucleotide excision repair of the template DNA strand *in vitro*. J Biol Chem *265*:21330, 1990

108. Chen Y-H, Matsumoto Y, Shibutani S, Bogenhagen DF: Acetylaminofluorene and aminofluorene adducts inhibit *in vitro* transcription of a *Xenopus* 5S RNA gene only when located on the coding strand. Proc Natl Acad Sci USA *88*:9583, 1991

109. Chen Y-H, Bogenhagen DF: Effects of DNA lesions on transcription elongation by T7 RNA polymerase. J Biol Chem *268*:5849, 1993

110. Gray PJ, Cullinane C, Phillips DR: In vitro transcription analysis of DNA alkylation by nitrogen mustard. Biochemistry *30*: 8036, 1991

111. Witkin EM: Mutation frequency decline revisited. Bioessays *16*: 437, 1994

112. Selby CP, Witkin EM, Sancar A: *Escherichia coli mfd* mutant deficient in "mutation frequency decline" lacks strand-specific repair: In vitro complementation with purified coupling factor. Proc Natl Acad Sci USA *88*:11574, 1991

113. Selby CP, Sancar A: Molecular mechanism of transcription-repair coupling. Science *260*:53, 1993

114. Hoeijmakers JHJ: Nucleotide excision repair II: From yeast to mammals. TIG *9*:212, 1993

115. Barnes DE, Kodama K-I, Tynan K, et al: Assignment of the gene encoding DNA ligase 1 to human chromosome 19q13.2-13.3. Genomics *12*:164, 1992

116. van Duin M, de Wit J, Odijk H, et al: Molecular characterization of the human excision repair gene ERCC-1:cDNA cloning and amino acid homology with the yeast DNA repair gene RAD10. Cell *44*:913, 1986

117. Weber CA, Salazar EP, Stewart SA, Thompson LH: ERCC2: cDNA cloning and molecular characterization of a human nucleotide excision repair gene with high homology to yeast RAD3. EMBO J *9*:1437, 1990

118. Weeda G, van Ham RCA, Masurel R, et al: Molecular cloning and biological characterization of the human excision repair gene ERCC-3. Mol Cell Biol *10*:2570, 1990

119. Liu P, Siciliano J, White B, et al: Regional mapping of human DNA excision repair gene ERCC4 to chromosome 16p13.13-p13.2 Mutagenesis *8*:199, 1993

120. Warburton D, Yu M-T, Richardson C, et al: Human excision repair gene ERCC5 maps to 13q32-q33 by in situ hybridization and also cross-hybridizes to 10q11, the site of ERCC6. Cytogenet Cell Genet *58*:1984, 1992

121. Troelstra C, Landsvater RM, Wiegant J, et al: Localization of the nucleotide excision repair gene ERCC6 to human chromosome 10q11-q21. Genomics *12*:745, 1992

122. Tanaka K, Miura N, Satokata I, et al: Analysis of a human DNA excision repair gene involved in group A xeroderma pigmentosum and containing a zinc-finger domain. Nature *348*:73, 1990

123. Gatti RA, Berkel I, Boder E, et al: Localization of an ataxia-telangiectasia gene to chromosome 11q22-23. Nature *336*: 577, 1988

124. Ziv Y, Rotman G, Frydman M, et al: The ATC lataxia telangiectasia complementation group C) locus localizes to 11q22-q23. Genomics *9*:373, 1991

125. Lambert C, Schultz RA, Smith M, et al: Functional complementation of ataxia-telangiectasia group D (AT-D) cells by microcell-mediated chromosome transfer and mapping of the AT-D locus to the region 11q22-23. Proc Natl Acad Sci USA *88*:5907, 1991

126. Legerski RJ, Liu P, Li L, et al: Assignment of xeroderma pigmentosum group C (XPC) gene to chromosome 3p25. Genomics *21*:266, 1994

127. Xanthoudakis S, Miao G, Wang F, et al: Redox activation of Fos-Jun DNA binding activity is mediated by a DNA repair enzyme. EMBO J *11*:3323, 1992

127a. Robson CN, Hickson ID: Isolation of cDNA clones encoding a human apurinic/apyrimidinic endonuclease that corrects DNA repair and mutagenesis defects in *E. coli xth* (exonuclease III) mutants. Nucleic Acids Res *19*:5519, 1991

128. Harrison L, Ascione AG, Meminger JC, et al: Human apurinic endonuclease gene (*APE*): Structure and genomic mapping (chromosome 14q11.2-12). Human Mol Genet *1*:677, 1992

129. Strathdee CA, Duncan AMV, Buchwald M: Evidence for at least four Fanconi anemia genes including *FACC* on chromosome 9. Nature Genetics *1*:196, 1992

130. McKinnon PJ: Ataxia-telangiectasia: An inherited disorder of ionizing radiation sensitivity in man; progress in the elucidation of the underlying biochemical defect. Hum Genet *75*: 197, 1987

130a. Chen DJ, Marrone BL, Nguyen T, et al: Regional assignment of a human DNA repair gene (XRCC5) to 2q35 by X-ray hybrid mapping. Genomics *21*:423, 1994

130b. Natarajan AT, Vermeulen S, Darroudi F, et al: Chromosomal localization of human O⁶-methyltransferase-DNA methyltransferase (MGMT) gene by *in situ* hybridization. Mutagenesis 7:83, 1992

130c. Fishel R, Lescoe MK, Rao MRS, et al: The human mutator gene homolog *MSH2* and its association with hereditary nonpolyposis colon cancer. Cell 75:1027, 1993

130d. Bronner CE, Baker SM, Morrison PT, et al: Mutation in the DNA mismatch repair gene homologue *hMLH1* is associated with hereditary non-polyposis colon cancer. Nature 368:258, 1994

131. Strathdee CA, Buchwald M: Molecular and cellular biology of Fanconi's anemia. Am J Pediatr Hematol Oncol 14:177, 1992

132. Lindahl T, Barnes DE: Mammalian DNA liases. Annu Rev Biochem 61:251, 1992

133. Strathdee CA, Gavish H, Shannon WR, Buchwald M: Cloning of cDNAs for Fanconi's anemia by functional complementation. Nature 356:763, 1992

134. Gatti RA: Localizating the genes for ataxia-telangiectasia; a human model for inherited cancer susceptibility. Adv Cancer Res 56:77, 1991

134a. Meyn MS: High spontaneous intrachromosomal recombination rates in Ataxia-Telangiectasis. Science 260:1327, 1993

135. Troelstra C, Odijk H, De Wit J, et al: Molecular cloning of the human DNA excision repair gene ERCC-6. Mol Cell Biol 10:5806, 1992

136. Venema J, Mullendeeers LHF, Natarajan AT, et al: The genetic defect in Cockayne syndrome is associated with a defect in repair of UV-induced DNA damage in transcriptionally active DNA. Proc Natl Acad Sci USA 87:4707, 1990

137. Peterson CL, Herskowitz I: Characterization of the yeast *SWI1, SWI2,* and *SWI3* genes, which encode a global activator of transcription. Cell 68:573, 1992

138. Davis JL, Kunisawa R, Thorner J: A presumptive helicase (*MOT1* gene product) affects gene expression and is required for viability in the yeast *Saccharomyces cerevisiae*. Mol Cell Biol 12:1879, 1992

139. Tamkun JW, Deuring R, Scott MP, et al: *brahma*: A regulator of *Drosophila* homeotic genes is structurally related to the yeast transcriptional activator SNF2/SWI2. Cell 68:561, 1992

140. Carlson M, Laurent BC: The SNF/SWI family of global transcriptional activators. Curr Biol 6:396, 1994

141. Schaeffer L, Roy R, Humbert S, et al: DNA repair helicase: A component of TBF2 (TFIIH) basic transcription factor. Science 260:58, 1993

142. Flores O, Lu H, Reinberg D: Factors involved in specific transcription by mammalian RNA polymerase II. J Biol Chem 267:2786, 1992

142a. Guzder SN, Qiu Hongfang, Sommers CH, et al: DNA repair gene *RAD3* of *S. cerevisiae* is essential for transcription by RNA polymerase II. Nature 367:91, 1994

142b. Drapkin R, Reardon JT, Ansari A, et al: Dual role of TFIIH in DNA excision repair and in transcription by RNA polymerase II. Nature 368:769, 1994

143. Scherly D, Nouspikel T, Corlet J, et al: Complementation of the DNA repair defect in xeroderma pigmentosum group G and rodent ERCC group 5. Nature 363:185, 1993

144. O'Donovan A, Wood RD: Identical defects in DNA repair in xeroderma pigmentosum group G and rodent ERCC group 5. Nature 363:185, 1992

145. Reines D: Elongation factor-dependent transcript shortening by template-engaged RNA polymerase II. J Biol Chem 267:3795, 1992

146. Chen R-H, Maher VM, Brouwer J, et al: Preferential repair and strand-specific repair of benzo[a]pyrene diol epoxide adducts in the *HPRT* gene of diploid human fibroblasts. Proc Natl Acad Sci USA 89:5413, 1992

147. Carothers AM, Zhen W, Mucha J, et al: DNA strand-specific repair of (±)-3α,4β-dihydrooxy-1α,2α-epoxy-1,2,3,4-tetrahydrobenzo[c]phenanthrene adducts in the hamster dihydrofolate reductase gene. Proc Natl Acad Sci USA 89:11925, 1992

148. Stam K, Heisterkamp N, Grosveld G, et al: Evidence of a new chimeric bcr/c-abl mRNA in patients with chronic myelocytic leukemia and the Philadelphia chromosome. N Engl J Med 313:1429, 1985

149. Wallace MR, Marchuk DA, Andersen LB, et al: Type 1 neurofibromatosis gene: identification of a large transcript disrupted in three NF1 patients. Science 249:181, 1990

150. Miyoshi Y, Ando H, Nagase H, et al: Germ-line mutations of the APC gene in *p53* familial adenomatous polyposis patients. Proc Natl Acad Sci USA 89:4452, 1992

151. Powell SM, Zilz N, Beazer-Barclay Y, et al: APC mutations occur early during colorectal tumorigenesis. Nature 359:235, 1992

152. Wong AJ, Ruppert JM, Bigner SH, et al: Structural alterations of the epidermal growth factor receptor gene in human gliomas. Proc Natl Acad Sci USA 89:2965, 1992

153. Peltomäki P, Aaltonen LA, Sistonen P, et al: Genetic mapping of a locus predisposing to human colorectal cancer. Science 260:810, 1993

154. Aaltonen LA, Peltomäki P, Leach FS, et al: Clues to the pathogenesis of familial colorectal cancer. Science 260:812, 1993

155. Thibodeau SN, Bren G, Schaid D: Microsatellite instability in cancer of the proximal bowel. Science 260:816, 1993

156. Honchel R, Halling KC, Schaid DJ, et al: Microsatellite instability in Muir-Torre syndrome. Cancer Res 54:1159, 1994

156a. Krontiris TG, Devlin B, Karp DD, et al: An association between the risk of cancer and mutations in the HRAS minisatellite locus. New Engl J Med 329:517, 1993

157. Hastie ND, Dempster M, Dunlop MG, et al: Teleomere reduction in human colorectal carcinoma and with aging. Nature 346:866, 1990

158. Rainer S, Johnson LA, Dobry CJ, et al: Relaxation of imprinted genes in human cancer. Nature 362:747, 1993

159. Ogawa O, Eccles MR, Szeto J, et al: Relaxation of insulin-like growth factor II gene imprinting implicated in Wilm's tumor. Nature 362:749, 1993

160. Goetz SE, Vogelstein B, Hamilton SR, Feinberg AP: Hypomethylation of DNA from benign and malignant human colon neoplasm. Science 228:187, 1985.

161. Makos M, Nelkin BD, Lerman MI, et al: Distinct hypermethylation patterns occur at altered chromosome loci in human lung and colon cancer. Proc Natl Acad Sci USA 89:1929, 1992

162. Tlsty TD, White A, Sanchez J: Suppression of gene amplification in human cell hybrids. Science 255:1425, 1992

163. Smith KA, Stark MB, Gorman PA, Stark GR: Fusion near teleomeres occurs very early in the amplification of *CAD* genes in Syrian hamster cells. Proc Natl Acad Sci USA 89:5427, 1992

164. Ionov Y, Peinado MA, Malkhosyan S, et al: Ubiquitous somatic mutations in simple repeated sequences reveal a new mechanism for colonic carcinogenesis. Nature 363:558, 1993

164a. Modrich P: Mechanisms and biological effects of mismatch repair. Annu Rev Genet 25:229, 1991

164b. Branch P, Aquillina G, Bignami M, Karran P: Defective mismatch binding and a mutator phenotype in cells tolerant to DNA damage. Nature 362:652, 1993

164c. Parsons R, Li G-M, Longley MJ, et al: Hypermutability and mismatch repair deficiency in RER⁺ tumor cells. Cell 75:1227, 1993

165. Hartwell L: Defects in cell cycle checkpoint may be responsible for the genomic instability of cancer cells. Cell 71:543, 1992

166. Weinert T, Lydall D: Cell cycle checkpoints, genetic instability and cancer. Semin Cancer Biol 4:129, 1993

167. Ronai AZ, Lambert ME, Weinstein IB: Identification of a UV-inducible protein that recognizes a TGACAACA sequence in the polyoma-virus regulatory region. Cancer Res 58:5374, 1990

168. Ronai ZA, Lambert ME, Weinstein IB: Inducible cellular responses to ultraviolet light irradiation and other mediators of DNA damage in mammalian cells. Cell Biol Toxicol 6:105, 1990

169. Herrlich P, Rahmsdorf HF: Transcriptional and post-transcriptional responses to DNA-damaging agents. Curr Biol 6:425, 1994

169a. Elledge SJ, Davis RW: DNA damage induction of ribonucleotide reductase. Mol Cell Biol 9:4932, 1989

169b. Hurta RA, Wright JA: Alterations in the activity and regulation of mammalian ribonucleotide reductase by chroambucil, a DNA damaging agent. J Biol Chem 267:7066, 1992

170. Fornace AJ: Mammalian genes induced by radiation; activation of genes associated with growth control. Annu Rev Genet 26:507, 1992

170a. El-Deiry WS, Tokino T, Velculescu VE, et al: WAF1, a potential mediator of p53 tumor suppression. Cell 75:817, 1993

171. Kuerbitz SJ, Plunkett BS, Walsh WV, Kastan MB: Wild-type p53 is a cell cycle checkpoint determinant following irradiation. Proc Natl Acad Sci USA 89:7491, 1992

172. Kastan MB, Zhan Q, El-Deiry WS, et al: A mammalian cell cycle checkpoint pathway utilizing p53 and GADD45 is defective in ataxia-telangiectasia. Cell 71:587, 1992

172a. Lu X, Lane DP: Differential induction of transcriptionally active p53 following UV or ionizing radiation: Defects in chromosome instability syndromes? Cell 75:765, 1993

173. Yonish-Rouach E, Grunwald D, Wilder S, et al: p53-mediated cell death: Relationship to cell cycle control. Mol Cell Biol 13:1415, 1993

174. Eastman A: Activation of programmed cell death by anticancer agents: Cisplatin as a model system. Cancer Cell 2:275, 1990

175. Lee JM, Bernstein A: p53 mutations increase resistance to ionizing radiation. Proc Natl Acad Sci USA 90:5742, 1993

176. Livingstone LR, White A, Sprouse J, et al: Altered cell cycle arrest and gene amplification potential accompany loss of wild-type p53. Cell 70:923, 1992

177. Yin Y, Tainsky MA, Bischoff FZ, et al: Wild-type p53 restores cell cycle control and inhibits gene amplification in cells with mutant p53 alleles. Cell 70:937, 1992

177a. Denko NC, Giaccia AJ, Stringer JR, Stambrook PJ: The human Ha-ras oncogene induces genomic instability in murine fibroblasts within one cell cycle. Proc Natl Acad Sci USA 91:5124, 1994

177b. Hashida T, Yasumoto S: Induction of chromosome abnormalities in mouse and human epidermal keratinocytes by the human papillomavirus type 16 E7 oncogene. J Gen Virol 72:1569, 1991

178. Diamond L: Tumor promoters and cell transformation. In Grunberger D, Goff S (eds): Mechanisms of Cellular Transformation by Carcinogenic Agents. Elmsford, NY, Pergamon Press, 1987, pp 731–734

179. Castagna M, Takai Y, Kaibuchi K, et al: Direct activation of calcium-activated phospholipid-dependent protein kinase by tumor-promoting phorbol esters. J Biol Chem 257:7847, 1992

180. Nishizuka Y: Intracellular signaling by the hydrolysis of phospholipids and activation of protein kinase C. Science 258:607, 1992

181. Rotenberg SA, Weinstein IB: Protein kinase C in neoplastic cells. In Pretlow TC, Pretlow TP (eds): Biochemical and Molecular Aspects of Selected Tumors. New York, Academic Press, 1990, pp 25–73

182. Borner C, Guadagno SN, Hsiao WW-L, et al: Expression of four protein kinase C isoforms in rat fibroblasts. II. Differential alterations in ras-, src-, and fos-transformed cells. J Biol Chem 247:12900, 1992

183. Luo J, Kahn S, O'Driscoll K, Weinstein IB: The regulatory domain of protein kinase Cβ1 contains phosphatidylserine and phorbol ester-dependent calcium binding activity. J Biol Chem 268:3715, 1993

184. Solomon DH, O'Driscoll K, Sosne G, et al: 1α,25-Dihydroxyvitamin D3-induced regulation of protein kinase C gene expression during HL-60 cell differentiation. Cell Growth Differ 2:187, 1991

185. Housey GM, Johnson MD, Hsiao W-L, et al: Overproduction of protein kinase C causes disordered growth control in rat fibroblasts. Cell 52:343, 1988

186. Borner C, Filipuzzi I, Weinstein IB, Imber R: Failure of wild-type or a mutant form of protein kinase C-α to transform fibroblasts. Nature 353:78, 1991

187. Cacace AM, Guadagno-Nichols S, Krauss R, et al: The epsilon isoform of protein kinase C is an oncogene when overexpressed in rat fibroblasts. Oncogene 8:2095, 1993

188. Mischak H, Goodnight J, Kolch W, et al: Overexpression of protein kinase C-δ and -ε in NIH 3T3 cells induces opposite effects on growth, morphology, anchorage dependence, and tumorigenicity. J Biol Chem 268:6090, 1992

189. Choi PM, Tchou-Wong KM, Weinstein IB: Overexpression of protein kinase C in HT29 colon cancer cells causes growth inhibition and tumor suppression. Mol Cell Biol 19:4650, 1990

190. Weinstein IB: Synergistic interactions between chemical carcinogens, tumor promoters, and viruses and their relevance to human liver cancer. Cancer Detect Prev 14:253, 1989

191. National Research Council Committee on Diet and Health: Implications for Reducing Chromic Disease Risk. Washington, DC, National Academy Press, 1989, pp 205–208

192. Morotomi M, Guillem JG, LGerfo P, Weinstein IB: Production of diacylglycerol, an activator of protein kinase C by intestinal microflora. Cancer Res 50:3595, 1990

193. Loeb L: Mutator phenotype may be required for multistage carcinogenesis. Cancer Res 51:3075, 1991

194. Nguyen T, Brunson D, Crespi CL, et al: DNA damage and mutation in human cells exposed to nitric oxide. Proc Natl Acad Sci USA 89:3030, 1992

195. Wattenberg LW: Inhibition of carcinogenesis by naturally occurring and synthetic compounds. In Kuroda Y, Shankel DM, Waters MD (eds): Antimutagenesis and Anticarcinogenesis, Mechanisms II. New York, Plenum Press, 1990, pp 155–166

196. Wattenberg L, Lipkin M, Boone CW, Kelloff G: Cancer Chemoprevention. Boca Raton, FL, CRC Press, 1993

197. Hong WK, Lippman SM, Itri LM, et al: Prevention of second primary tumors with isotretinoin in squamous cell carcinoma of the head and neck. N Engl J Med 323:785, 1990

198. Crowell PL, Chang RR, Gould MN: Inhibition of isoprenylation of p21 ras and other proteins by limonene. Proc Am Assoc Cancer Res 32:20, 1991

199. Perera F, Weinstein IB: Molecular epidemiology and carcinogen-DNA adduct detection: New approaches to studies of human cancer causation. J Chron Dis 35:581, 1982

200. Perera FP: Molecular epidemiology in cancer prevention. In Schottenfeld D, Fraumeni J (eds): Cancer Epidemiology and Prevention, 2nd edition. New York, Oxford University Press, 1993

200a. Devary Y, Rosette C, DiDonato JA, Karin M: NF-κB activation by ultraviolet light not dependent on a nuclear signal. Science 261:1442, 1993

200b. Engelberg D, Klein C, Martinetto H, et al: The UV response involving the Ras signaling pathway and AP-1 transcription factors is conserved between yeast and mammals. Cell 77:381, 1994

201. Skipper PL, Tannenbaum SR: Protein adducts in the molecular dosimetry of chemical carcinogens. Carcinogenesis 11:507, 1990

202. Santella RM: Application of new techniques for the detection of carcinogen adducts to human population monitoring. Mutat Res 205:271, 1988

203. Perera FP, Hemminki K, Grzybowska E, et al: Molecular damage from environmental pollution in Poland. Nature 360:256, 1992

204. Griffith J, Duncan RC, Goldsmith JR, Hulka BS: Biochemical and biological markers: Implications for epidemiologic studies. Arch Environ Health 44:375, 1989

205. Albertini RJ, Nicklas JA, O'Neill JP, Robison SG: In vivo somatic mutations in humans: Measurement and analysis. Annu Rev Genet 24:305, 1990

206. Langlois RG, Bigbee WL, Kgoizumi S, et al: Evidence for increased somatic cell mutations at the glycophorin A locus in atom bomb survivors. Science 236:445, 1987

207. Preston-Martin S, Malcolm PC, Ronald RK, et al: Increased cell division as a cause of cancer. Cancer Res 50:7415, 1990

208. Crespi CL, Penman BW, Gelvoin HV, Gonzales FJ: A tobacco smoke-derived nitrosamine, 4-(methylintrosamion)-1-(3-pyridyl)-1-butanone, is activated by multiple human cytochrome P450s including the polymorphic human cytochrome P4502D6. Carcinogenesis 12:1197, 1991

208a. Seidegard J, Pero RW, Miller DG, Beattie EJ: A glutathione transferase in human leukocytes as a marker for the susceptibility to lung cancer. Carcinogenesis 7:751, 1986

208b. Nazar-Stewart V, Motulsky AG, Eaton DL, et al: The glutathione S-transferase μ polymorphism as a marker for susceptibility to lung carcinoma. Cancer Res 53:2313, 1993

209. Karkaya AE, Cok L, Sardas S, et al: N-acetyltransferase phenotype of patients with bladder cancer. Hum Toxicol 5:333, 1986

209a. Vineis P, Bartsch H, Caporaso N, et al: Genetically based N-acetyltransferase metabolic polymorphism and low-level environmental exposure to carcinogens. Nature 369:154, 1994

210. Pero RW, Johnson DB, Markowitz M, et al: DNA repair synthesis in individuals with and without a family history of cancer. Carcinogenesis 10:6938, 1989

211. Schantz SP, Spitz MR, Hsu TC: Mutagen sensitivity in patients with head and neck cancers: A biologic marker for risk of multiple primary malignancies. J Natl Cancer Inst 82:1773, 1990

212. Wei Q, Matanoski G, Farmer ER, et al: DNA repair and aging in basal cell carcinoma: A molecular epidemiology study. Proc Natl Acad Sci USA 90:1614, 1993

213. Frebourg T, Friend SH: Cancer risks from germ line p53 mutations. J Clin Invest 90:1637, 1992

214. Weston A, Vineis P, Caporaso NE, et al: Racial variation in the distribution of H-ras-1 alleles. Mol Carcinog 4:265, 1991

215. Weston A, Perrin LS, Forrestes K, et al: Allelic frequency of a p53 polymorphism in human lung cancer. Cancer Epidemiol Biomarkers Prevent 1:481, 1992

216. King MC: Breast cancer genes: How many, where and who are they? Nature Genet 2:89, 1992

217. Norburg C, Nurse P: Animal cell cycles and their control. Annu Rev Biochem 61:441, 1992

218. Hunter T, Pines J: Cyclins and cancer. Cell 66:1071, 1991

219. Jiang W, Kahn SM, Tomita N, et al: Amplification and expression of the human cyclin D1 gene in esophageal cancer. Cancer Res 52:2980, 1992

220. Jiang W, Zhang Y-J, Kahn S, et al: Altered expression of the cyclin D1 and retinoblastoma genes in human esophageal cancer. Proc Natl Acad Sci USA 1993 (in press)

221. Keyomarsi K, Pardee AB: Redundant cyclin overexpression and gene amplification in breast cancer cells. Proc Natl Acad Sci USA 90:1112, 1993

221a. Kamb A, Gruis NA, Weaver-Feldhaus J, et al: A cell cycle regulator potentially involved in genesis of many tumor types. Science 264:436, 1994

222. Rubin H: Cancer development: The rise of epigenetics. Eur J Cancer 28:1, 1992

223. Hsiao WL-W, Gattoni-Celli S, Weinstein IB: Effects of 5-azacytidine on the expression of endogenous retrovirus-related sequences in C3H 10T1/2 cells. J Virol 57:1119, 1986

224. Baylin SB, Makos M, Wu J, et al: Abnormal patterns of DNA methylation in human neoplasia: Potential consequences for tumor progression. Cancer Cells 3:383, 1991

225. Tycko B: Genomic imprinting: Mechanism and role in human pathology. Amer J Pathol 144:431, 1994

5

TUMOR SUPPRESSOR GENES

ARNOLD J. LEVINE

HISTORICAL PERSPECTIVE: THE CONCEPT OF A TUMOR SUPPRESSOR GENE

Somatic Cell Genetics

The notion that one or more gene products could inhibit or suppress the proliferation of cells in a tumor derives from experiments first carried out using somatic cell genetics.[1] In these experiments, a cancerous cell, which was able to form a tumor in an animal, was fused with a nontumorigenic normal cell. The hybrid cells thus formed most often grew well in cell culture, and in most cases even retained many of the phenotypes of the cancerous parent cell, but these cells no longer produced tumors in animals. The hybrid between a tumorigenic and nontumorigenic cell was nontumorigenic, suggesting that a gene or genes from the normal cell were dominant and suppressed the tumorigenic potential of cancer cells. This result could be obtained with cancerous cells produced by chemical carcinogen treatment or by transformation by viral agents, or cells obtained from spontaneous tumors. These results also were independent of the tumor tissue types, so that epithelial cells, fibroblasts, or lymphocytes from cancers fused to normal cells usually failed to produce tumors when injected into animals.

As these studies progressed, it occasionally was observed that a hybrid cell line derived from a normal cell and a tumorigenic cell would produce a tumor in an animal. When the cells from these tumors were examined in more detail, it became clear that the tumorigenic hybrid cell had lost one or more chromosomes supplied by the normal parent. This approach was employed to identify the chromosomes that putatively carried a tumor suppressor gene or genes and conferred a normal phenotype on the hybrid cell. As the techniques used in somatic cell genetics became more sophisticated, it became possible to fuse a microcell, containing a single human chromosome

from a normal parent, to a cancerous cell, and the resultant hybrid no longer produced tumors in animals.[2] Based on these experiments, several different chromosomes from normal human cells were shown to carry putative tumor suppressor genes that were able to block tumor formation by the cancer cell. A list of these chromosomes and the cancerous cell types that were suppressed is presented in Table 5–1. These studies indicated that several distinct tumor suppressor genes existed and could suppress tumor formation, depending on the origin of the tumor-producing cells in the hybrid. The idea that the cancerous cells contained a mutant form of one or more of these tumor suppressor genes that was not functioning, and that different tumors contained different mutant tumor suppressor genes, was tested by experiments in which two different tumorigenic cell lines were fused to produce a hybrid cell. This hybrid cell no longer formed tumors in animals, suggesting that genetic complementation could explain these observations and that different tumor suppressor genes were genetically altered in different tumors.

Although the interpretation of these experiments is complicated by the transfer of entire chromosomes (alterations in gene dosages and the introduction of large amounts of genetic information) into cancerous cells, these results do serve to suggest an interesting concept. There exists a set of genes that can function in a dominant fashion to block the tumorigenic potential of cancer cells. The cancerous cells must sustain mutations in both alleles of these genes in order to gain the ability to produce tumors in the host or transplanted animals.

The Knudson Hypothesis

These ideas received considerable support from epidemiologic studies carried out by Knudson with retinoblastomas.[3] Retinoblastomas are tumors of the retinoblasts that occur in children up to the age of 7, after which the ret-

TABLE 5–1. TUMOR SUPPRESSION OBSERVED BY MICROCELL FUSION OF SINGLE NORMAL HUMAN CHROMOSMES

TUMORIGENIC CELL LINE	SUPPRESSING CHROMOSOME	REF.
Cervical carcinoma (HeLa)	11	2
Retinoblastoma	13	157
Renal cell carcinoma	3	158
Wilms' tumor	11	159
Colorectal carcinoma	5, 17, 18	152
Melanoma	6	160
Neuroblastoma	17	161
Fibrosarcoma	1, 11	162
Endometrial carcinoma	1, 6, 9	163

inoblast no longer divides. Knudson noted that about 40 per cent of these cancers occur in very young infants, with a mean age of about 14 months. These tumors were most commonly bilateral, occurring in both eyes, and such patients have an average of three independent tumors in both eyes. If the tumors are detected early and surgically removed, these patients then have a high incidence of osteogenic sarcoma later on in life (at 20 to 30 years of age). Some of these patients were from families with a history of retinoblastoma, indicating an inherited predisposition. The high incidence of multiple tumors in these patients also suggested an inherited component with these cancers. Knudson went on to note that 60 per cent of the retinoblastomas did not fit this pattern. In these cases, no family history could be detected and the first appearance of a retinoblastoma usually occurred in older children, with a mean age of 30 months. Tumors in this group were always unilateral (one eye) and only one tumor per patient was observed. Retinoblastomas fitting this description were quite rare, occurring in only 1 in every 30,000 live births. Knudson suggested a single hypothesis that explained both patterns of retinoblastomas.

He postulated that there was a genetic locus that later came to be called the retinoblastoma susceptibility gene (*Rb* gene). Patients in the first group, with early-presenting bilateral tumors, inherit one defective copy of this gene and one normal allele. With a very high frequency (a 95 per cent chance of occurrence), mutations arise in the normal allele (three independent mutations and tumors per patient) and these tumors arise very early in life. Patients in the second group, with a single unilateral tumor, inherit two normal or wild-type *Rb* alleles. Very rarely (1 in 30,000 people), two independent mutations occur in the same gene in the same retinoblast, destroying the *Rb* gene and resulting in cancer. In this manner, a single hypothesis could explain the two very different epidemiologic patterns of this cancer (Fig. 5–1).

Inherent in this postulate is the concept of a gene that normally prevents cancer or tumorous growth, and both copies of this gene must be lost to initiate a cancer. That is a tumor suppressor gene. A karyotypic analysis of some retinoblastoma cancer cells revealed a consistent deletion

in chromosome 13 in the region 13q14.[4] Cavenee et al.[5] employed several chromosome 13–specific DNA probes that mapped to the long arm of this chromosome to examine this genetic locus in normal and cancer cells from retinoblastoma patients. Several of these DNA probes detected polymorphisms in restriction enzyme sites in these DNA sequences on chromosome 13q. In some cases, the DNA from normal cells of these patients was heterozygous at a restriction enzyme site, with one chromosome containing DNA that was cut by a restriction enzyme while the other chromosome failed to have this cutting site. Using the Southern blotting technique to detect these differences, for several DNA probes, the DNA from the normal cells contained both alleles of this restriction fragment length polymorphism (RFLP). The DNA from the cancerous cells, however, lost this heterozygosity in the RFLP pattern, containing only one parental copy of this allele. This loss of heterozygosity or reduction to homozygosity in the cancer cells removed the normal or wild-type *Rb* allele and uncovered a recessive mutation in the *Rb* gene. The mechanism that produces this loss may be gene conversion (unequal recombination events or the copying of one sequence onto its opposite allele), or it may be a deletion and/or gene duplication at this locus. Most commonly, the paternal allele (from the father) remains in the cancerous cell, indicating that inherited mutations most commonly occur during spermiogenesis (arise independently each generation). Because a reduction to homozygosity may occur at a higher frequency than a spontaneous point mutation, the likelihood of disrupting the same gene twice in a single cell may well be higher than the likelihood of two independent point mutations arising in the same cell.

Thus, in the inherited form of retinoblastoma, the paternal allele containing a mutation is present in all cells of the patient, and a reduction to homozygosity in a retinoblast results in only the mutant allele, and a cancerous cell. In the spontaneous form of this cancer, a rare mutation arises in one allele of a retinoblast and then the reduction to homozygosity that uncovers this mutation must arise as a second independent event. The former mechanism has one inherited and one somatic mutation, whereas the latter has two somatic mutations or events (Fig. 5–1).

The *Rb* gene has now been isolated by molecular cloning[6] and shown to reside in 200 kb of DNA on chromosome 13. The availability of such DNA clones permitted a test of the Knudson hypothesis, which proved to be correct. Retinoblastomas have both alleles of the *Rb* gene altered by mutation or, more commonly, one allele is mutant with a reduction to homozygosity, providing only one mutation in the cancer cells. Individuals who have bilateral tumors and multiple cancers inherit one mutant allele, which can be isolated from their normal tissue, and this is the only allele present in the cancerous tissue. Patients with late-onset, unilateral retinoblastoma have two wild-type *Rb* alleles in the DNA extracted from normal tissues, but only mutant *Rb* alleles in their cancerous tissues.[7–15]

Studies employing somatic cell genetics have now introduced a normal chromosome 13 into a retinoblastoma cell (Table 5–1), producing a hybrid cell line that no longer initiated a tumor in an animal, consistent with the idea that the wild-type allele reverted this phenotype. The clearest evidence for this concept was obtained by the introduction of a wild-type *Rb* allele, in the absence of other chromosome 13 information, into a retinoblastoma or osteogenic sarcoma cell in culture using a retrovirus vector. The resulting clones of cells failed to produce tumors in animals, showing that a single gene, the *Rb* gene, could act as a tumor suppressor gene in these cell or tumor types.[16] This constituted a formal proof that the wild-type retinoblastoma gene product could act as a tumor suppressor for cells implanted into animals.

A Karyotypic Analysis of Cancer Cells

The third line of evidence that suggested the existence of tumor suppressor genes came first from an examination of the karyotypes of cancer cells (see Chapter 2). It is now well documented that cells derived from a tumor have reproducibly lost selected chromosomes or specific portions of chromosomes (deletions).[17] During the past 10 years, a large number of specific DNA probes have been isolated that cover a good deal of the human genome, and detect restriction site polymorphisms. This has permitted the documentation and mapping of reproducible specific deletions or altered DNA sequences in a wide variety of cancers. Examples of these types of deletions, loss of heterozygosity, or reproducible chromosomal aberrations are presented in Table 5–2. These data provide an indication that mutation followed by a reduction to homozygosity (via deletion) is common in many cancers and that multiple tumor suppressor genes may exist, depending on the tissue or tumor type. These observations are consistent with the somatic cell genetic analysis (Table 5–1) and reinforce the interpretation of these data.

DISTINCTIONS BETWEEN ONCOGENES AND TUMOR SUPPRESSOR GENES

Although the existence of both tumor suppressor genes[1,3] and oncogenes[18] (Chapter 6) first was postulated more than 20 years ago, evidence for the existence of oncogenes was obtained more rapidly[19] than evidence for the tumor suppressor genes.[6,20] In the decade between 1976 and 1986, the oncogenes held center stage in all attempts to explain the origins of cancer, and this yielded only a portion of the picture. The existence of tumor sup-

Chromosome 13

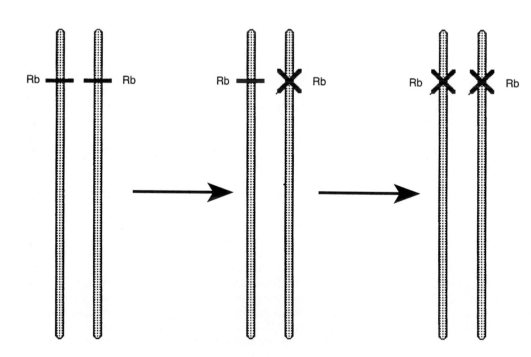

normal
1/30,000
single tumor/patient
presents late

inherited form
95% chance of cancer
multiple tumors
bilateral
presents early

1. cancerous
   retinoblast
2. common reduction
   to homozygosity

Figure 5–1. The retinoblastoma locus in normal, inherited predisposition, and cancerous cells. Normal individuals have the wild-type *Rb* gene in all cells and rarely (1/30,000) acquire two somatic mutations, which leads to a single tumor presenting at a late time after birth. An inherited mutation in one *Rb* allele has a very high (95 per cent) probability of resulting in cancer via a reduction to homozygosity at this locus. This results in an early presentation of multiple tumors in the infant.

TABLE 5–2. HUMAN TUMOR SUPPRESSOR LOCI MAPPED BY CYTOGENETIC OR RFLP ANALYSIS*

TUMOR	CHROMOSOME INVOLVED	KNOWN TUMOR SUPPRESSOR GENE(S)
Retinoblastoma	13q14	*Rb*
Wilms' tumor	11p13	*WT-1*
Beckwith-Wiedemann syndrome	11p15	Not known (*WT-2,?*)
Glioblastoma multiforme (astrocytoma)	17p13	*p53*
	9p, 10	Not known
Breast cancer	13p14	*Rb*
	17p13	*p53*
	1p, 1a, 11p, 13q	Not known
Small-cell lung cancer	13p14	*Rb*
	17p13	*p53*
	3p	Not known
Colorectal cancer	5q21	*APC, MCC*
	17p13	*p53*
	18q21	*DCC*
Neurofibroma	1p, 14q, 17	Not known
Neuroblastoma	1p, 14q, 17	Not known
Meningioma	1p, 14q, 17	Not known
	22	
Melanoma	1, 6q, 7, 10, 19	Not known
Myeloid leukemia	5q	Not known
Renal cell carcinoma	3p, 3q	Not known

* Each of these observations and assignments of tumor suppressor genes are discussed in detail by Stanbridge.[164]

pressor genes provided a clearer understanding of the inherited predispositions in cancer, the cell type or tissue specificity associated with some abnormal genes and their products, and the reproducible karyotypic abnormalities of certain cancers.

A number of distinctions now are recognized between the oncogenes (see Chapter 6) and tumor suppressor genes, and these are outlined in Table 5–3. The mutations that activate proto-oncogenes to oncogenes may reside in the structural gene and alter the protein product directly, or in some cases are found in the regulatory portion of a gene, leading to the overproduction of a normal protein product. In both of these cases, the altered gene products (the protein itself or the level of the protein) gain a function. This gain of function often results in a continuous signal or an abnormal signal for cell proliferation or growth. These types of mutations are dominant to the wild-type allele, and there is no further selection on this gene for the accumulation of mutations at this locus. In contrast, the tumor suppressor gene products act in some way to stop cell proliferation, even when abnormal signals for cell division are presented to the cell cycle regulatory machinery. Tumor suppressor gene products may be used to detect abnormal signals for proliferation or abnormal events during the cell cycle, such as DNA damage[21,22] or aberrant products of replication. In these circumstances, the tumor suppressors become negative regulators of proliferation or progression through the cell cycle. As negative regulators of cell proliferation, the loss of one allele via mutation is expected to have no impact on function of the second, wild-type allele, and so these mutations are loss-of-function mutations and act in a recessive fashion to the wild-type allele (in the case of *Rb*, for example). For this reason, both alleles of a tumor suppressor gene must sustain mutations to inactivate the function of these gene products. The most common way in which this oc-

TABLE 5–3. PROPERTIES OF ONCOGENES AND TUMOR SUPPRESSOR GENES

PROPERTY	PROTO-ONCOGENES	TUMOR SUPPRESSOR GENES
Number of mutational events required to contribute to the cancer	One	Two
Function of the mutant allele	Gain of function, acts in a dominant fashion	Loss of function, acts in a recessive fashion
Mutant allele may be inherited through the germ line	No examples at this time	Frequenty has an inherited form
Somatic mutation contributes to cancer	Yes	Yes
Tissue specificity of mutational event	Some, but can act in many tissues	Inherited form commonly has a tissue preference

curs is via a mutation in one allele followed by a reduction to homozygosity and the loss of the wild-type allele.

Because oncogene mutations act in a dominant fashion to contribute to abnormal proliferation, it is unlikely that a fetus that inherits such a mutation would survive normally to term. Such mutations are expected to be lethal in utero and rarely, if ever, are found in the germ line. However, the recessive mutations in tumor suppressor genes, in some cases at least, appear to have no developmental phenotype in the heterozygous state, and individuals with Rb[23] and $p53$[24–27] germ line mutations are born developmentally normal. In both cases, this predisposes these individuals to a high risk of specific cancers that often show a common tissue or cell type preference. Patients that inherit a single Rb mutation often (95 per cent of the time) develop retinoblastomas. If cured of this tumor, they are at high risk to develop osteogenic sarcoma later in life. Thus, inherited predispositions for developing cancers at the Rb and also the $p53$ locus result in a tissue or cell type preference for this disease. In these cases, this is not due to a tissue-restricted expression of these two proteins. Both Rb and p53 proteins can be detected in virtually all tissues of the body. Rather, the loss of functions of these gene products has a differential effect in different tissues. Some tissues may be solely dependent on these tumor suppressor genes to regulate cell proliferation (i.e., retinoblasts), whereas other tissue types may utilize additional redundant tumor suppressor genes as a buffer against abnormal cell proliferation. This tissue preference of tumor suppressor gene function is observed with some oncogenes (i.e., $bcr-abl$ in the Philadelphia chromosome of chronic myelogenous leukemia) but, by and large, many oncogenes are activated and function in cancers derived from a large number of tissue types ($ras, myc,$ etc.)

CANCER ARISES BY ACCUMULATION OF MUTATIONS IN ONCOGENES AND TUMOR SUPPRESSOR GENES

Cancer is predominantly a disease of the elderly, with the risk of acquiring this disease increasing with age. With regard to colorectal cancers, there are 150,000 new cases per year in the United States,[28] and it is estimated that a 50-year-old individual has a 5 per cent risk of developing this cancer by the age of 80.[29] This tumor appears to arise through a progression of events taking place over a period of years or decades.[30] The earliest recognizable change is the appearance of a small benign tumor or adenoma in the colonic mucosa. In some cases, a larger adenoma with increased malignant potential and an altered histologic appearance develops from the benign tumor. Some of these tumors progress to advanced metastatic cancer and are termed carcinomas at that time (Fig. 5–2).

Inherited genetic factors are thought to contribute to about 10 per cent of colorectal cancers. One of the most common genetic alterations is familial adenomatous polyposis (FAP), an autosomal dominant disease mapping on chromosome 5[31,32] that affects about 0.01 per cent of individuals in the United States, Great Britain, and Japan.[33] Patients with this genetic defect develop thousands of adenomatous polyps in the colon by 20 to 30 years of age. A small percentage of these polyps progress to carcinomas. The gene that gives rise to these inherited predispositions was localized to chromosome band 5q21 and identified by molecular cloning.[34,35] This gene, termed the ''adenomatous polyposis coli gene,'' or APC gene, was shown to be inherited in the heterozygous state, giving rise to FAP. In addition, sporadic colorectal cancers contain mutations in the APC gene,[35] and loss of heterozygosity at the 5q21 locus was observed in 35 to 45 per cent of tumor patients without inherited tendencies for colorectal cancer.[36,37] Thus, it appears that this gene and locus may be involved in the development of adenomas in both inherited and spontaneous colorectal cancers (see Tables 5–1 and 5–2), and a mutation in this critical gene leads to benign tumor growth. A second gene linked to APC on chromosome band 5q21, termed ''mutated in colorectal cancer'' or MCC, commonly was found to contain somatic mutations in sporadic colorectal cancers[35] and possibly contributes to the development of these cancers. Interestingly, benign adenomas are composed of clones of cells derived from a single progenitor cell.[38] This observation also suggests that the selection of a cell with a rare combination of mutations gives rise to the first stages of this benign tumor (Fig. 5–2).

About 50 per cent of colorectal carcinomas have a mutation (at codon 12 or 13) in the Ki-ras gene. Indeed, half the adenomas above 1 cm in size harbor these mutations,[30] and adenomas of this size are thought to have an increased risk of malignant transformation or conversion.[39] In comparison, small adenomas (under 1 cm) harbor few (less than 10 per cent) ras mutations, suggesting that such ras

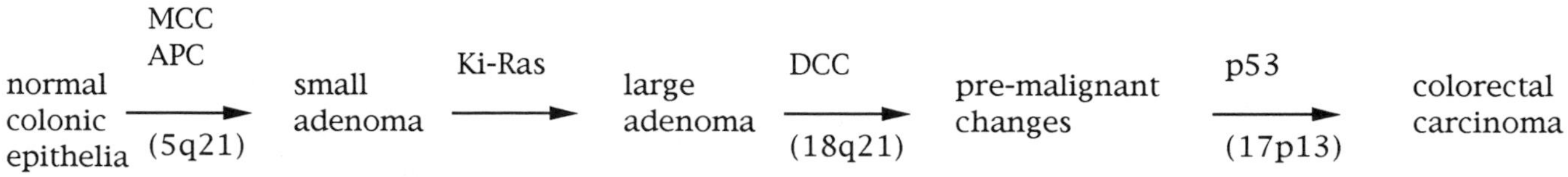

Figure 5–2. The multistep pathway to colorectal cancer. The accumulation of five to ten mutations in several tumor suppressor genes or oncogenes over a lifetime results in cancer. In some cases, an inherited mutation (APC) produces thousands of adenomas, which results in cancer at a younger age. MCC, mutated in colorectal cancer; APC, adenomatous polyposis coli, Ki-Ras, the Kirsten ras oncogene; DCC, deleted in colorectal cancer; p53, the $p53$ gene. (From Fearon ER: Genetic alterations underlying colorectal tumorigenesis. Cancer Survey 12:119, 1992, with permission of Oxford University Press.)

mutations may drive the next step in tumor progression. Occasionally, other oncogenes (*neu*, c-*myc*, *myb*) have been reported in amplified copies of colorectal carcinoma cells, but this is rare. More often elevated levels of c-*myc* and c-*src* activities are detected in colorectal cancers without any evidence of mutations in the structural or regulatory elements of these genes.[40] Whether this is due to mutations in *trans*-acting factors that regulate these genes, or even if this is an important observation, remains unclear.

As carcinomas develop from large adenomatous polyps, mutations at two additional loci often are observed—chromosome bands 17p13.1 and 18q21. The loss of heterozygosity at 17p13 occurs in over 75 per cent of colorectal carcinomas. These events rarely are observed in even large benign adenomas.[37] Nucleotide sequence analysis of the cDNAs derived from the *p53* gene (which resides at 17p13.1) in colorectal cancers showed common (70 to 80 per cent of the cases) missense mutations in the cancer cells.[41] A point mutation producing a faulty *p53* protein coupled with a reduction to homozygosity at that locus and the loss of the wild-type allele occurs very commonly.[30] A similar picture has emerged at the 18q21 chromosome locus. Allelic loss in this region of the chromosome has been observed in over 70 per cent of colorectal cancers. This is seen very infrequently in small adenomas, but approaches a 50 per cent frequency in the larger adenomas and a 70 per cent frequency in the carcinomas.[37] The gene involved has been identified by molecular cloning[42] and named "deleted in colorectal cancer," or *DCC*. About 15 per cent of the colorectal cancers surveyed had somatic *DCC* mutations (Fig. 5–2).

With mutations detected in colorectal carcinomas at the *APC* gene, the *MCC* gene, the *ras* oncogene, *p53*, and *DCC*, between five and ten genetic events (in some cases inherited, in most cases somatic) have been identified that may contribute to this disease (Fig. 5–2). This need to accumulate many mutations in a single cell may alone explain the late onset of carcinomas with the age of the population and why some individuals who inherit one or more of these mutant alleles may have an early-onset cancer. Clearly, both oncogenes (i.e., *ras*) and tumor suppressor genes (i.e., *p53*) contribute to the progression of this disease. More experimental evidence will be needed to clearly classify *APC, MCC,* and *DCC* in this scheme. With the identification of these genes and their products, several questions remain. First, what are the functions of these proteins in normal cells, and do they contribute a gain of function in cancer cells? Second, how do mutations in these genes arise, and are some subset of these mutations selected for in clonal populations of cells that go on to produce the cancer? Third, what is the relative contribution of each altered gene product to a particular stage in the development of the cancer, and do different combinations of mutant alleles in a cell contribute different prognostic capabilities to the neoplastic process? To begin answering some of these questions, the remainder of this chapter deals with the structure and function of the tumor suppressor gene products that have been identified to date.

Formal proof that a gene and its protein product act as a tumor suppressor comes from an experiment in which the wild-type allele is reintroduced into a tumorigenic cancer cell lacking the gene. If the resultant cell line no longer is able to initiate tumors in animals, then the gene can be properly classified a tumor suppressor gene. To date, this has only been accomplished with *Rb*[16] and *p53*.[43] However, there are a number of other genes that fulfill some of the criteria of tumor suppressor genes (Table 5–3), in which both alleles are lost or selected against in cancerous tissues (*APC, DCC*), or in which a mutation contributes to an inherited predisposition to a specific cancer in a dominant fashion (*WT-1, NF-1, APC*). The remainder of this chapter reviews all of these potential tumor suppressor genes and their products. However, first it will be informative to describe the oncogenes of several DNA tumor viruses, whose products interact with and alter *Rb* and *p53* activities.

DNA TUMOR VIRUSES: INTERACTIONS BETWEEN ONCOGENE PRODUCTS AND TUMOR SUPPRESSOR GENE PROTEINS

The DNA tumor viruses—simian virus 40 (SV40), some human adenoviruses, and some human papillomaviruses (HPV-16, HPV-18)—each encode one or more oncogene products that are responsible for the ability of these viruses to transform cells in culture or initiate tumors in animals.[44] The reason these viruses have evolved these gene products is to help promote the replication cycle of the virus. By and large, these viruses infect a resting cell of the body that is actively regulated so as not to enter the cell cycle and divide. The level of enzymes that synthesize nucleotide precursors for DNA synthesis is very low in such cells. The synthesis of histones (to package cellular and some of these viral DNA's) is not taking place in a resting cell. Enzyme activities needed for nucleotide polymerization are all at very low levels. These viruses have responded to this problem by producing oncogene products designed to interact with the major negative regulators of cell proliferation and force the cell into a DNA-synthetic or S phase. When cells receive conflicting signals, for proliferation from viral oncogene products and to remain at rest from cellular signals, they respond by stopping the progression through the cell cycle or preventing a cell from entering S phase. In some cases, abnormal signals for proliferation may even result in a commitment to a differentiated pathway or to cell death via apoptosis.[45–47] All of these cellular responses to the expression and activity of viral oncogenes in turn must be counteracted by the virus, so that the infected cell will enter the S phase and the virus will replicate efficiently. The protein-protein interactions of the viral-encoded oncogene products with Rb and p53 are precisely designed to overcome these cellular blocks to proliferation.

The oncogene product, the large tumor or T antigen of SV40, is a protein composed of 708 amino acids, and it is responsible for virtually all of the ability of this virus to transform cells or form tumors in animals.[48] This protein is composed of several domains, three of which contribute to the transformation of some cell types in cultures.[49,50] These three domains have been localized to (1) amino acid residues 1 through 75, (2) residues 105 through 114, and (3) residues 400 through 650. These same regions of this protein are responsible for transformation of cells in culture and bind to or interact with three cellular proteins: (1) residues 1 through 75 with a 300-kDa protein (Livingston, personal communication); (2) residues 105 through 114 with the Rb protein[51]; and (3) residues 400 through 670 with the p53 protein[52,53] (Table 5–4). Mutations in these regions of T antigen can result in a loss of the binding of a tumor suppressor gene product to T antigen and a simultaneous loss of the ability to transform some cell types in culture. Because tumor suppressor genes derived from human cancers are observed to contain mutations that are loss-of-function mutations, it has been assumed that the binding of T antigen to Rb or p53 results in a loss of Rb or p53 function. In at least some cases, which will be reviewed in more detail in a later portion of this chapter, this assumption appears correct. However, no evidence at present contradicts a possible gain of a new function that results from the binding of T antigen with Rb or p53 proteins.

Similarly, the adenovirus E1A protein (made from the 12S mRNA) is composed of 243 amino acid residues, and residues 1 through 80 and 121 through 139 have been shown to be critical and essential for transformation of cells in culture.[54,55] These two domains act as discrete functional elements because the 1 through 80 region mutants will complement the 121 through 139 region mutants in *trans*.[54] The amino acid residues between 1 and 80 bind to the 300-kDa protein (Table 5–4). Mutations in the E1A–300-kDa binding site can be complemented by SV40 T antigen, and this complementing activity maps to the 1 through 75 amino acid residues region that also binds the 300-kDa protein.[49] Residues 40 through 80 and 121 through 139 of E1A are responsible for binding to the Rb protein.[55]

The 300-kDa protein is a nuclear phosphoprotein that is heterogeneous in size on sodium dodecyl sulfate–polyacrylamide gels. Mutants of E1A deficient in binding 300-kDa protein fail to stimulate cellular DNA synthesis in resting cells[54] and fail to immortalize cells in culture.[56] Thus, the 300-kDa gene remains a candidate for an oncogene or tumor suppressor gene and this should become clear when this gene is molecularly cloned and characterized.

A second adenovirus protein, the E1B 55-kDa gene product, is required to transform cells in culture and has been shown to bind the *p53* tumor suppressor gene product.[57] Similarly, mutants in the E1B–55-kDa gene that fail to transform cells in culture fail to bind to p53 or fail to act on the function of p53.[58]

Finally, the HPVs, types 16 or 18, which are associated with a high risk for cervical cancers in humans (see Chapter 3), encode oncogene products E6 and E7, which bind to p53[59] and Rb.[60] The result of these interactions are reviewed in more detail in Chapter 3.

Thus, three distinct groups of DNA tumor viruses have evolved oncogene products that target Rb and p53 (see Table 5–4). The interaction of these oncogene products with Rb and p53 results in the stimulation of cell proliferation, cellular transformation, and/or tumorigenesis. Thus, Rb and p53 must be central players in maintaining cell stasis or responding to positive or abnormal signals for cell proliferation. The Rb binding sites on the SV40 T antigen, adenovirus E1A protein, and HPV E7 protein share a common amino acid residue motif[61] and so have evolved to recognize a specific site or set of amino acid residues in Rb protein. No such common motifs have been recognized for p53 protein binding to these viral oncoproteins.

RETINOBLASTOMA GENE AND PROTEIN

The *Rb* gene is located at chromosome band 13q14 and encompasses about 200 kb of DNA. The gene has 27 exons from which a primary transcript is spliced together to form a mRNA that is synthesized in virtually all cells of

TABLE 5–4. VIRAL ONCOGENE–TUMOR SUPPRESSOR GENE INTERACTIONS

VIRAL ONCOGENE	CELLULAR PROTEIN	REF.
SV40 large T antigen		
residues 1–75	300 kDa	62
residues 105–114	Rb	51
residues 400–650	p53	52
		53
Adenoviruses, type 5		
E1A proteins		
residues 1–80	300 kDa	55
residues 40—80		
and 121–139	Rb	165
E1B–55-kDa protein	p53	57
Human papillomaviruses types 16, 18		
E6	p53	59
E7	Rb	60

the body. The Rb protein is 105 to 110 kDa in size, depending on the species, and it is located in the nucleus of the cell. In addition to retinoblastomas, *Rb* mutations (in both alleles or with a reduction to homozygosity) have been detected in osteosarcomas, bladder carcinomas, prostate carcinomas, breast carcinomas, small-cell lung carcinomas, some types of leukemias, and cervical carcinomas. The frequency of *Rb* mutations in these cancers varies considerably among the different types of tumors. *Rb* mutations are found in all retinoblastomas and most small-cell lung carcinomas, suggesting that inactivation of Rb function may well be an obligatory step in the development of these cancers. Lower frequencies of *Rb* mutations have been recorded in bladder and mammary carcinomas (about 33 per cent of cases), suggesting that *Rb* mutations may be a contributing event, but cannot be considered an essential event in the ontogeny of these cancers.

Children with the inherited form of retinoblastoma do not suffer from these other tumors (bladder, mammary, small-cell lung) during the first year of life. This is in spite of the fact that these tissues must surely suffer mutations at the *Rb* locus because these same children average three *Rb* mutations in the retinal cells. Clearly additional factors are required for cancer to arise in other tissue types. When such children are cured of their retinoblastomas, they may suffer from additional cancers at a later age, and the tissue distribution of these cancers is also limited (mainly osteosarcomas). Small-cell lung, mammary, or bladder cancers either are not detected or are very rare in this group. Apparently something is different between germ line mutations and somatic mutations. This might simply be the age of the organism and associated hormonal or other changes, or this could be due to different cell cycle regulatory pathways in different tissues at different ages of the host. Certain cell types could have multiple or redundant mechanisms that maintain normal proliferation in the absence of Rb. Alternatively, the loss of Rb function could be lethal to some cell types and remains a possible explanation of these observations.

A wide variety of mutations have been documented that inactivate Rb functions in humans. Mutations in splice donor and acceptor sequences often result in the deletion of entire exons from the processed mRNA. Frameshift mutations and point mutations resulting in a stop codon produce fragments of Rb proteins that are most commonly unstable. Deletion mutations provide formal evidence that these mutants are true loss-of-function mutations. Most informative, however, are point mutations producing a missense mutant protein. These mutations cluster in two regions of the protein localized between amino acid residues 393 through 572 and 646 through 772. These two regions of the Rb protein form a binding site or pocket for the interactions of Rb protein with a variety of cellular and viral proteins that are regulated by or act on the Rb protein.[61-63] The viral-encoded proteins that bind to Rb in this pocket are the oncogene products of several DNA tumor viruses, and they result in the apparent inactivation of Rb function and progression of cells into the cell cycle, resulting in cell proliferation. Thus, the mutations that arise in the *Rb* gene in retinoblastomas result in a failure

of the Rb protein to bind to the viral-encoded oncogene products, the SV40 T antigen, the adenovirus E1A protein, and the E7 protein of HPV-16 or -18.[61-63] Clearly, these viruses are not present in retinoblastomas, so that the selection of such mutations must be for the loss of binding to cellular proteins that are similar to or function like the viral oncogene products. In this way, the viral oncogene products appear to bind to the Rb pocket or binding site and displace a cellular protein that previously occupied that site. The liberated cellular protein might now be free to function in the cell cycle events.

In resting cells, in phase G_0 or G_1, the Rb protein can be found in a complex with a cellular transcription factor called E2F.[64,65] E2F mediates the transcriptional activation of several viral genes[66] and cellular genes that produce enzymes that synthesize nucleotides and polymerize DNA (S-phase gene expression). When the Rb-E2F complex is exposed to the adenovirus E1A protein, Rb-E1A forms a complex, and E2F is released[64,67,68] with an increased ability of E2F to transcribe DNA from an E2F-responsive DNA sequence.[69] In this case, Rb acts to sequester a cellular transcription factor so that it will not act efficiently, and the viral oncogene product binds to Rb and releases E2F so it can now act to transcribe a set of genes presumably required for entry into the S phase of the cell cycle. Rb may regulate a number of other proteins or transcription factors in a similar fashion.[63] The Rb binding pocket has been shown to interact with additional cellular proteins.[70]

This model for the regulation of Rb function by the viral oncogene products does not lead to a clear understanding of how the Rb protein may be regulated when cells normally commit to cell division. Many cells that go on to divide have normal levels of the wild-type Rb protein throughout all stages of the cell cycle. What appears to change as a function of the cell cycle is the state of phosphorylation of the Rb protein. During the G_0 or G_1 phase of the cell cycle, the Rb protein either is not phosphorylated or is poorly phosphorylated. In late G_1 or early S phase, however, the Rb protein becomes progressively more phosphorylated at multiple sites in the protein.[71] The kinase that carries out these phosphorylation reactions is the cdk activity that is activated by a cyclin and regulates cell cycle events.[63,72] The level of Rb phosphorylation remains high until late in mitosis, when a phosphatase removes these groups and Rb is underphosphorylated in G_0/G_1.[73] These events tie Rb phosphorylation to other critical activities (cyclin-cdk) in the cell cycle and suggest that phosphorylation of Rb might regulate Rb activity and interaction with other proteins. This hypothesis is strongly supported by the observation that the SV40 large T antigen binds preferentially to the underphosphorylated form of Rb,[74] so that T antigen binds to and acts on Rb in G_0/G_1 when it is poorly phosphorylated. It would be reasonable to suggest that E2F binding to Rb might be regulated by phosphorylation, but this does not seem to be simply the case, and more information is required before this point can be clarified.

Thus, it appears that the function of Rb is to interact with transcription factors and to regulate their ability to act on a set of genes required for entry into the S phase of the cell cycle. Rb appears to be regulated at least in part by phosphorylation of multiple serine residues (the site is a serine-proline dipeptide in a context of basic amino acids) by a cell cycle–determining kinase, cdk activities, linking Rb activity to other events occurring in the cycle. Mutations in the Rb binding site release the transcription factors and no longer regulate their activities in the cell cycle. The E2F protein is now free in G_1 to stimulate the transcription of genes normally active in S phase, and this may aid the entry into the cell cycle. The viral oncogene products act in much the same fashion to bind to the Rb pocket (with a higher affinity than E2F) and release these transcription factors. Why this process shows a distinct tissue preference for cancers is not clear. What other functions are being regulated by the Rb protein now need to be determined.

p53 GENE AND PROTEIN

The *p53* gene in humans resides in 20 kb of DNA located on chromosome 17p13.1.[75] The gene is composed of 11 exons that produces a 2.2 to 2.5-kb mRNA that is expressed in almost all cell or tissue types of the body. The first exon (213 bases) is noncoding and forms a nontranslated mRNA leader sequence. Little is known about the transcriptional regulation of this gene, but the highest levels of *p53* mRNA are detected in the spleen and thymus[76] and lower levels are found in all other tissues. The protein is composed of 393 amino acid residues in humans and is a nuclear phosphoprotein. Based on the amino acid sequence of this protein, three domains or functional units may be recognized:

1. Amino acid residues 1 through 75 or 80 are very acidic and they are expected to be largely in an α-helical conformation. A number of serine residues in this domain (amino acid residues number 7, 9, 12, 18, 23, 37, and 58) are candidates for phosphorylation and are phosphorylated

by either casein kinase I and/or a DNA-dependent protein kinase.[72] These events add to the negative charge at the amino terminus of p53.

2. This domain, localized between residues 120 through 290, is responsible for binding to p53-specific DNA sequences. It cooperates with the N-terminal domain to promote transcription of a gene containing the p53 DNA binding site.[126,127]

3. The carboxy-terminal domain, consisting of residues 276 through 390 in mouse or 319 through 393 in humans, is very basic and may form an amphipathic helical structure. Amino acid residue 316 is phosphorylated by a cdk-activity[77] linking p53 to this central cell cycle kinase activity.[78] This site is quite close to the major nuclear localization signal (residues 319 through 323) for this protein.[79] The penultimate residue (389 in the mouse and 392 in the human) is phosphorylated, and it appears that casein kinase II may carry out this modification (a mitogen-stimulated kinase activity).

When *p53* genes are compared from sources as diverse as *Xenopus* through humans, they share good homology (56 per cent).[80] However, several regions of these proteins retain excellent homologies (90 to 100 per cent identity). These regions span residues 13 through 23, 117 through 142, 171 through 181, 236 through 258, and 270 through 286. The importance of these regions of high homology is reinforced by the common clustering in these very regions (except for residues 13 through 23) of point mutations found in human cancers[81,82] (Fig. 5–3).

p53 mutations have now been detected in a wide variety of carcinomas. Most commonly (87 per cent of the time) these mutations are missense mutations producing a faulty protein product, and the second allele in the cell is then lost, reducing the mutant allele to homozygosity.[83,84] Such mutations in humans have been demonstrated in tumors of the anus,[85] brain,[84] breast,[86–88] colon,[41] esophagus,[81,89] stomach,[90] liver,[91,92] lung (both small-cell and non–small-cell carcinomas),[93–96] lymphoid system,[97,98] ovary,[99] and

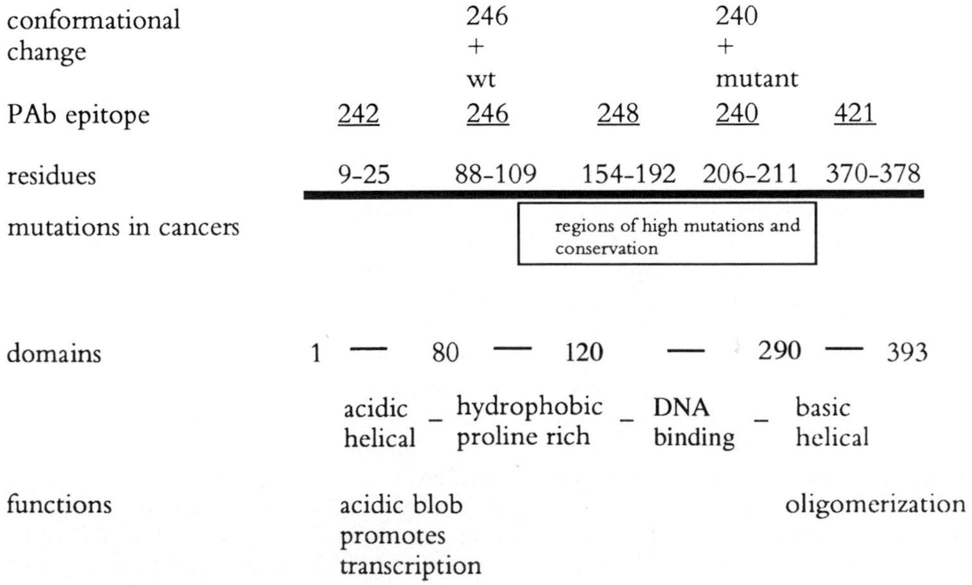

		246 + wt		240 + mutant		conformational change
PAb epitope	242	246	248	240	421	
residues	9-25	88-109	154-192	206-211	370-378	
mutations in cancers			regions of high mutations and conservation			
domains	1 —	80 —	120	— 290 —	393	
		acidic helical	hydrophobic proline rich	DNA binding	basic helical	
functions		acidic blob promotes transcription		oligomerization		

Figure 5–3. The organization of the p53 protein. PAb242, 246, 248, 240, and 421 monoclonal antibodies that recognize discrete epitopes given in amino acid number (1 to 393 amino acids). PAb246 recognizes the wild-type protein and PAb240 recognizes only the mutant protein. Functional and proposed structural domains in the proteins are indicated, and the regions of high mutations and conservation of amino acid sequences are given.

prostate.[100] The fact that these tumors contain missense mutations about 87 per cent of the time suggests the possibility that the altered or faulty protein may contribute to abnormal cell growth or proliferation. The position of these missense mutations in the faulty protein is nonrandom. Figure 5–4 presents the distribution of missense mutations from 191 independent carcinomas plotted as the frequency of occurrence of a mutation as a function of the codon in the gene. All the mutations cluster between amino acid residues 120 and 290, with most of these mutations in the regions of high amino acid sequence homology between p53 genes (compare Figs. 5–3 and 5–4). In addition, some mutations at specific codons occur or are selected for frequently (45 to 50 per cent of the time), and these map at codons 175, 248, 249, 273, and 282 (see Fig. 5–4). These hot spot mutations tend to be detected in different tissue types. For example, codon 249 mutations repeatedly (11/21 times, or 53 per cent of the cases examined) have been observed in liver cancers, especially from the regions of southern China and southern Africa, with a high incidence of hepatitis B virus and aflatoxin B.[91,92,101] Whether this distribution of hot spot mutations in the p53 gene reflects the function of specific mutant alleles being selected for promoting cell proliferation in a tissue-specific fashion, or it reflects the nature and activity of different mutagens in different tissues, remains to be tested. Recent results indicate that aflatoxin B-1 does indeed have the specificity to cause codon 249 mutations in the p53 gene. Thus, the nature of the mutations is determined by the mutagen. When lung and colon tumors are compared for the types of mutations detected in the p53 gene, the lung tumors contain both transition and transversion mutations, whereas the colon tumors are almost exclusively transition mutations. This would support the idea that the environmental mutagens that are present differ with different epithelial cell surfaces. The mutant codon might well depend on the nucleotide sequence context and the type of mutagen. In some cases, the change is observed to occur at a cytodylic-guanylic dinucleotide (CpG) (G:C $\rightarrow$ A:T changes). It is known that methylated cytosine residues in CpG dinucleotides have a mutation rate higher than nonmethylated cytosine. It therefore would be useful to examine whether methylated cytosine residues are present in a tissue-specific fashion in the p53 gene.

Whereas 87 per cent of the carcinomas with p53 mutations give rise to missense mutants with faulty p53 proteins, sarcomas and some lymphoid tumors most commonly contain deletions or gene rearrangements, resulting in loss of the p53 protein (Table 5–5). All osteosarcomas studied to date with p53 mutations[102,103] had gene rearrangements in intron I or homologous deletions. Similarly, six out of six p53 mutations observed in chronic myelogenous leukemias[97] had gene rearrangements in intron I or rearrangements in the 3' region of the gene. Several rhabdomyosarcomas,[103] leiomyosarcomas,[104] liposarcomas,[104] and a spindle cell sarcoma all had deletions or gene rearrangements as well. Unlike carcinomas, sarcomas appear to select for loss of the p53 protein, not for a faulty protein (also see the discussion of mdm2 and its role in sarcomas, later in this section).

Somatic p53 mutations are found in about 50 to 60 per cent of human cancers, and p53 mutations are also found in the germ line of some families. The Li-Fraumeni syndrome, originally defined by a family with a proband having a sarcoma at a young age and two first-degree relatives in the family with cancer,[105,106] has been shown to involve p53 mutations in the germ line.[24–27,107] The patients in these families most often have a proband with osteosarcoma and other relatives with adrenocortical carcinomas, breast cancers, and some brain tumors. Colon cancer, with very high levels of p53 somatic mutations (75 to 80 per cent) is not notably prevalent in these inherited p53 mutant families. The inherited mutations are both missense and stop codons, and they also are not randomly distributed over the gene. Members of these families also appear to be at risk for developing second independent malignancies during their life span. The presence of such missense or nonsense mutations in one p53 allele does not appear to result in any developmental abnormalities.

The introduction of a missense mutant p53 mouse allele into a transgenic mouse appears to produce a similar phenotype. In families of mice expressing a mutant p53 gene (one missense mutation and two wild-type alleles), cancer will develop at a frequency much higher than normal (20 per cent of the mice develop cancer at 6 to 9 months of age).[108] The time interval for developing cancer in these mice suggests the need for additional (mutagenic) events, and the fact that two wild-type p53 alleles do not prevent these cancers from developing suggests an active role for the missense p53 protein (enhancing the rate of other mutations), or that a gene conversion event eliminates the wild-type alleles.

Mice also have been produced that contain no p53 genes (eliminated by insertional mutagenesis and homologous recombination).[109] These animals progress through fetal development normally. The offspring, however, develop cancer early in life (3 to 6 months), with a variety of cancer tissue types observed. The most common cancer in such mice, however, is a lymphocytic lymphoma, which almost all of the mice develop. This is not commonly observed in Li-Fraumeni families, suggesting possible species differences. These sets of experiments demonstrate that, in the mouse, the p53 protein is not essential for normal cell cycle events or cell divisions. Rather, the protein acts as an oversight or checkpoint in the cell cycle, correcting events that may go wrong and stopping the cycle (a negative regulator) to permit repair or corrections of mistakes. Alternatively, the p53 protein in mice could be backed up by a second or redundant gene function in the cell cycle. Such a redundant feature may or may not need to be eliminated in the origins of murine cancers.

The phenotypes of p53 mutant genes and gene products result from one of three categories of mutational events. The first type of p53 mutation results in a loss of function. When the wild-type p53 allele is introduced into a transformed cell in culture and the p53 protein is overexpressed (an overexpression phenotype), cell division stops[110,111] and the cells are blocked in the G_1 phase of the cell cycle.[112,113] Similarly, when wild-type p53 alleles are introduced into a tumorigenic cell line, the cells now have a reduced ability to produce tumors in animals.[43] All of

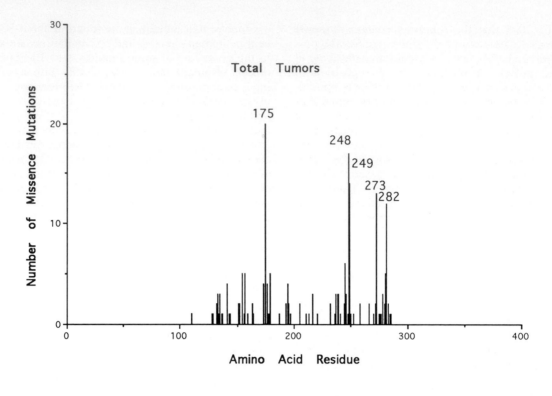

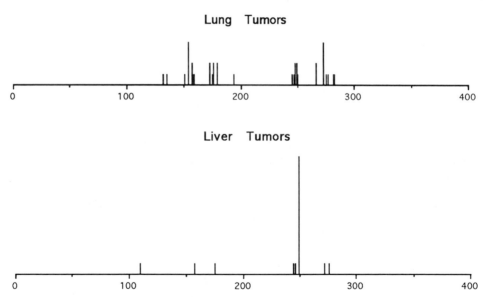

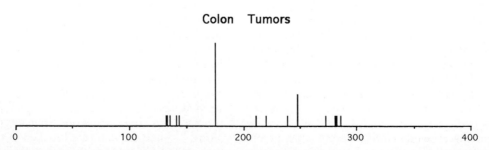

Figure 5–4. The distribution of mutations at each codon (amino acid residue) in the p53 protein. The number of missense mutations found in 191 independent carcinomas is given as a function of the codon in the *p53* gene or amino acid residue. The references for this are in the text.

the *p53* point mutations that have been tested for this growth-suppressing phenotype have lost this function.

At the same time, the *p53* missense mutations have gained a new function. When murine *p53* missense mutations were introduced into cells that contained no p53 proteins (deletion mutations in these cells), the altered or faulty p53 protein enhanced the tumorigenic potential of these cells.[43,114] Indeed, the human missense mutant alleles at hot spot codons 175, 248, and 273, when placed into mouse cells without endogenous *p53* genes, confer a new phenotype on these cells—the ability to produce tumors in nude mice (Dittmer, Teresky, and Levine, unpublished observations). Thus, the same mutation that confers a loss of function for growth suppression also confers a gain of function for promoting growth in tumors.

The third type of mutation observed to occur with the missense mutants in the *p53* gene is a dominant loss-of-function mutation or a *trans*-dominant mutation.[115] If a *p53* mutant allele is introduced into a primary rat embryo fibroblast, it enhances the plating efficiency of these cells sevenfold and enhances the rate of immortalization of these cells.[116] Similarly, mutant *p53* alleles, producing faulty proteins, can cooperate with the *ras* oncogene and transform these cells in culture.[115] The wild-type *p53* gene will not immortalize or transform these cells.[117] In all these cases, a mutant *p53* allele acts in a transformed cell that has endogenous wild-type *p53* alleles and proteins. The mutant allele appears to produce a protein that acts in a dominant fashion to overcome the effects of the endogenous wild-type protein in such cell lines in culture. The reason for this is that mutant and wild-type p53 proteins are found in oligomeric protein complexes in these cells.[118] If the faulty subunits in such a complex can inactivate the function of the wild-type subunit, then a mutant protein can act *trans*-dominant to the wild-type p53 protein.[115]

One of the reasons why mutant p53 proteins are so efficient in acting in a *trans*-dominant fashion and transforming cells in culture is that the stability of mutant p53 proteins is much greater than that of the wild-type p53 proteins. Wild-type p53 protein has a half-life in cells of only 20 minutes,[119] whereas all of the mutant *p53* alleles produce proteins with half-lives of hours.[120,121] This results in much higher concentrations of p53 proteins in transformed cells and even in tumor tissue.[95] Thus, the ratio of mutant to wild-type p53 protein in a cell could be an important variable in regulating cell division.

Given these complex phenotypes of p53 mutant proteins, what is the function of this protein? The available evidence suggests that p53 can act as a transcriptional activator or a transcription factor. When the first 75 amino acid residues of the p53 protein (the acidic blob) were fused to a known DNA-binding domain, the yeast Ga1–4 DNA binding protein, this fusion protein could promote transcription from a test gene regulated by Gal-4 DNA-binding sites.[122,123] Furthermore, the carboxy-terminal domain of p53 can bind to specific DNA sequences[124,125] and the p53 protein binds specifically to a known DNA consensus sequence[126,127]: 5'-Pu, Pu, Pu, C, A/T, T/A, G, Py, Py, Py-3', which can promote transcription of an adjacent test gene.[128] Thus, it has become clear that p53 can positively regulate a test gene when specific nucleotide sequences are placed upstream (even 3 kb upstream) from the gene.[129,130] p53 protein can act as a transcriptional activator.

Mutant forms of p53 protein fail to bind to DNA or have a reduced ability to bind to DNA.[125] Interestingly, in a mixture of mutant and wild-type proteins in solution,[128,129] mutant p53 proteins will act in a *trans*-dominant fashion to block the wild-type p53 proteins from binding to these specific DNA sequences. Similarly, the SV40 T antigen binds to wild-type p53 and blocks its ability to bind to these specific DNA sequences,[124] and the adenovirus E1B–55-kDa protein blocks the ability of p53 to stimulate the expression of a test gene regulated by p53-responsive sequences.[58] Mutant E1B–55-kDa alleles that fail to transform cells in culture all fail to block p53 from stimulating the transcription of such test genes.[58] Finally, the HPV-16 or -18 protein also blocks the ability of p53 to stimulate the expression of a test gene regulated by a p53-responsive promoter.[131] Thus, the p53 *trans*-dominant mutants act much like the oncogene products of the DNA tumor viruses in blocking the functional activity of the p53 protein.

TABLE 5–5. NATURE OF MUTATIONS IN THE *p53* GENE

TUMOR TYPE	MUTATIONS
Carcinomas	1. 87% missense mutations, 40% at codons 175, 248, 249, 273, 281 2. Some stop codons, deletions (13%)
Osteosarcomas	1. Most common gene rearrangements that produce no stable protein 2. Some wild-type *p53* gene and *mdm2* amplifications
Chronic myelogenous leukemia	1. Many gene rearrangements with no detectable protein 2. Some point mutations producing a missense protein and a reduction to homozygosity at blast crisis
Breast carcinomas	1. 30% missense mutations, little codon preference 2. About one third of the cancers with wild-type *p53* have *p53* localized in the cytoplasm (where it cannot function)

The available evidence therefore suggests that the p53 protein is most likely a transcription factor, but what gene or genes is this protein regulating in the cell? These genes are unlikely to be essential for entry into the cell cycle and proliferation, because the mouse with no p53 protein[109] duplicates all its cells normally throughout development. Rather, p53 levels are stimulated in response to DNA damage with ultraviolet light or γ-irradiation.[21,22] This induction appears to be due to a posttransitional stabilization of p53 protein in response to such damage. Cells that have wild-type p53 respond to such insults by blocking progression through the cell cycle, and pause in late G_1 to allow repair prior to DNA replication. Cells with mutant p53 proteins do not pause in G_1, and this may result in the accumulation of mutations and chromosomal rearrangements as well as cell death. Such events surely could lead to the rapid selection of cancerous cells. Abnormal signals for cell proliferation and/or DNA damage could activate p53 to mediate transcription of a set of genes leading to cell death or apoptosis[45,46] so as to minimize the creation of malignant clones of cells. Such a model, which is consistent with many of the facts, suggests that p53 acts as a transcription factor and a checkpoint protein in G_1 to modulate the cell cycle in response to damage or other signals of abnormal growth regulation.[132] This model does not yet explain the mode of action of p53 gain-of-function mutations, nor the obvious focus of the DNA tumor virus oncogenes on these p53 functions.

Whatever the functions of the p53 protein and the genes it regulates, it appears to be regulated itself not only by viral oncogene products but also by a cellular oncogene.[133] Both the mutant and wild-type p53 proteins in cells in culture form an oligomeric protein complex with a 90-kDa protein.[121] When this protein was purified and several peptides derived from it were sequenced, the 90-kDa protein was identified as an oncogene product called Mdm2.[134] Mdm2 was itself first identified as a gene amplified on double-minute chromosomes in Balb 3T3 cells in culture.[135] Because double-minute chromosomes contain no centromeres, the retention of these chromosomes suggests that they provide a selective growth advantage. These cell lines, unlike the parent Balb 3T3 cells, now are able to form tumors in nude mice.[134] The *mdm2* gene subsequently was cloned from these chromosomes and, when amplified and overproduced in Balb 3T3 cells, conferred an enhanced tumorigenic potential on these cells.[134] *mdm2*, a dominant oncogene when overexpressed in Balb 3T3 cells, produces a protein that binds to p53 protein, a tumor suppressor gene product.[133]

One hypothesis to explain these observations would be that high levels of Mdm2 would inactivate the p53 protein and its ability to transcribe a gene. This is in fact the case. High levels of Mdm2 will prevent wild-type p53 protein from promoting the transcription of a test gene containing a p53-responsive element.[133] Thus, Mdm2 negatively regulates p53. Whether this explains how Mdm2 enhances the tumorigenic potential of a cell by inactivating p53 directly, or whether mdm2 itself has an additional set of functions, remains to be determined. Mdm2 is a zinc finger protein, found in the cell nucleus, and could well act as a transcription factor by itself.

These observations, however, make an interesting prediction: There may well be some type of cancers that contain wild-type p53 proteins, but amplified copies of Mdm2. This is indeed the case.[136] Seven of 13 liposarcomas, 7/22 malignant fibrous histocytomas, and 3/11 osteosarcomas had 5- to 50-fold amplifications of the Mdm2 locus (see Table 5–5). Benign lipomas (5) and gastric and colorectal carcinomas (74 analyzed) did not have such amplifications.[136]

It is of some interest that the majority of carcinomas (missense mutations and faulty proteins) and sarcomas (deletions, gene rearrangements at the p53 locus, or Mdm2 amplifications) contain such different types of mutations (see Table 5–5), although it should be pointed out that some sarcomas with missense mutations are known and some carcinomas with deletions or stop codons have been observed. Whether this derives from the nature of the tissue, the mutagenic process, the functions of p53, or the selection of malignant clones of cells remains to be determined.

Thus, it appears that there are several mechanisms employed to inactivate the *p53* tumor suppressor gene product in cancers. The first and most common in human cancers is by mutation. The second is via the viral-encoded oncogene products such as the E6 protein of HPV-16 or -18 in cervical carcinomas. The third way is via the amplification of the *mdm2* gene, which is observed in several different human sarcomas. Recently, a fourth mechanism has been described[137] that results in the inactivation of p53 function even though the *p53* gene is normal or wild type in the cancer cells. In some breast cancers containing only the wild-type *p53* gene, the p53 protein is localized to the cell cytoplasm. Because p53 is a transcription factor, localizing this protein in the cell cytoplasm will not permit it to function as a tumor suppressor gene.[79] The nature of the mechanism that does not permit p53 to enter the cell nucleus, where it normally resides, remains unclear.

WILMS' TUMOR GENE AND PROTEIN

Wilms' tumor is a kidney cancer of children that, in some cases appears to have a genetic predisposition. This nephroblastoma occurs in about 1/10,000 children, and the tumor(s) may be bilateral (in 10 per cent of cases) and may be associated with congenital malformations of the urogenital tract. There is a good deal of evidence to suggest that several different loci may be involved in the genetic predisposition to Wilms' tumor. Chromosome 11 contains two loci associated with these tumors[138] that have been mapped to chromosome bands 11p13 and 11p15.

The first clue to identifying the putative tumor suppressor genes for Wilms' tumor came from an individual with a deletion in the short arm of chromosome 11 at band 13p.[139] Family members with this deletion had several abnormalities, including aniridia, genitourinary tract abnormalities, mental retardation, and a Wilms' tumor. Using the normal tissue and tumor tissue of this individual and

Wilms' tumors from other sources, Housman and his colleagues[140] isolated a gene, termed *WT-1*, that carried mutations in both alleles in several such tumors.

Patients with Beckwith-Wiedemann syndrome (see Table 5–2) develop a Wilms' tumor with few of the other symptoms and show chromosomal abnormalities at 11p15 but not at 11p13.[141,142] Furthermore, in rare familial Wilms' tumors not associated with either Beckwith-Wiedemann or aniridia, a third genetic locus appears to be involved. Clearly, several different genes or loci can contribute to Wilms' tumor, and the only gene in this complex isolated to date is *WT-1*.

The *WT-1* gene contains ten exons that span about 50 kb of DNA at chromosome band 11p13. The mRNA is about 3 kb in size, and several different spliced forms of this mRNA are known. The protein product is 46 to 49 kDa in size and is a zinc finger protein with four zinc finger motifs. The protein binds to a specific DNA sequence[143] and also contains a proline-glutamine–rich region, which is a common property of a number of transcription factors. In fact, WT-1 shares some amino acid sequence homology with several known transcription factors of yeast and mammalian cells. WT-1 has a limited spectrum of expression. The mRNA for WT-1 is detected in only kidney, spleen, gonads, and the uterus.[140] In the mouse, WT-1 is first expressed in fetal life, during the eighth day of gestation (the mouse has a 21-day gestation period). WT-1 mRNA levels continue to increase and peak at day 17 of gestation, followed by a decline to the low levels observed in adult kidneys. WT-1 is expressed in specific cell types of the developing gonads and kidney tissue, suggesting a role in developing of the organs. This is also consistent with the phenotypes of patients with defects in the *WT-1* gene.

The mutations in this gene are most commonly small deletions in the structural gene, although an occasional complete large deletion is found.[144] In most cases of the tumor, the normal wild-type allele is then lost, and so there appears to be selection against it and reason to expect that *WT-1* will be a tumor suppressor gene. In at least one well-documented case, however, the wild-type allele was present and expressed in the tumor tissue.[141] Additional studies and clearer functional tests, such as returning the *WT-1* gene into a cancerous cell, will be required to determine if this gene should be considered a tumor suppressor.

NEUROFIBROMATOSIS: *NF-1* GENE AND ITS PROTEIN

Von Recklinghausen's neurofibromatosis results from an abnormal proliferation of cells derived from the neural crest. In the mild form of this disease, abnormal growth of melanocytes result in café au lait spots throughout the body surface. More severe forms of this disease result in disfiguring neurofibromas composed of proliferating Schwann cells. This syndrome affects 1 in every 3500 people. In half of these cases, there is good evidence for an inherited defective allele. The inheritance pattern is dominant and acts like those observed with *Rb*, *p53*, and *WT-1*, suggesting the inheritance of one defective allele and the loss of the second allele giving rise to a cancer.

The gene that encodes the defect for this disease, *NF1*, has now been cloned[145] and mutations in this gene are detected in neurofibromas.[146,147] Interestingly, the amino acid sequence of the NF-1 protein contains a domain with very good homology to the GTPase-activating protein (GAP) that regulates the *ras* proto-oncogene.[148] The human NF-1 protein has its closest homology to two proteins from yeast called IRAs. These IRAs stimulate the GTPase activity of the yeast ras protein producing Ras-GDP. The Ras-GDP form of this protein no longer signals for proliferation of the yeast cells. Mutations in IRA, like tumor suppressor genes, act in a recessive fashion only and leave ras in the GTP-bound state for a longer time, resulting in stimulating cyclic AMP levels and prolonging the signal for cell division. In fact, NF-1 binds to the p21 *ras* proto-oncogene product from human cells and stimulates GTPase activity.[149] The binding of NF-1 to Ras is blocked by low levels of lipids, suggesting a regulatory role for these compounds.

NF-1 appears to be expressed in all cells and tissues of the body. Mutations in *NF-1*, however, have not been detected in tumors other than neurofibromas, indicating a tissue specificity similar to that seen with *Rb* and *p53* in their respective tissues. These observations may suggest a straightforward model for *NF-1* mutations contributing to cancer. In the absence of functional NF-1 protein, Ras remains in the Ras-GTP form and signals for growth of cells in an uncontrolled fashion. However, there are several observations that do not fit with this idea. First, the mutations observed in the *NF-1* gene to date all are located outside of the GTPase-activating domain of NF-1 and may not alter its activity or NF-1–Ras interactions. Second, in the Schwann cells that form neurofibromas, the Ras-GTP state is known to signal for growth arrest, not cell proliferation. This is the opposite of what the model would predict. Third, in many *NF-1* patients, the Schwann cells from the tumors often contain one *NF-1* mutant allele and one *NF-1* wild-type allele; there is no detectable reduction to homozygosity in these tumors. Clearly, there are some facts missing in understanding the role of *NF-1* in these tumors.

ADENOMATOUS POLYPOSIS COLI: *APC* GENE AND ITS PROTEIN

Familial adenomatous coli is observed in 1 in every 10,000 people and results in thousands of benign adenomatous polyps in the colon at 20 to 30 years of age. A small percentage of these polyps develop into colorectal carcinomas (see Fig. 5–2). The gene responsible for FAP first was identified and mapped to chromosome 5,[31] and then was isolated by molecular cloning using deletions at 5q21 found in two unrelated patients.[34,35,150] Yeast artificial chromosome vectors spanning this region of the genome indicated that these deletions spanned 100 to 200 kb and included three genes. One of those genes, the *APC* gene, was found to contain point mutations in the germ line from nine patients with FAP. Frameshift mutations, nonsense codons, and missense mutations are all found in this group. This same gene is also the target for somatic mutations in colorectal cancers, and reduction to homozygosity at this locus is common in these cancers (see Fig. 5–2).

The *APC* gene is large and encodes the information for a protein with 2843 amino acids. The primary sequence of amino acids in this protein provides no motifs or clues to a possible function or activity. The mRNA for this gene is expressed in a wide variety of tissue types, and so it is another example of ubiquitous gene expression that only produces tumors in a tissue-specific fashion when it is lost or inactivated.

The murine equivalent of the *APC* gene has been isolated, and defects in this gene result in the same phenotype, benign adenomatous polyps, in mice. This should provide an excellent experimental model for understanding the functions of this gene product.

OTHER CANDIDATE TUMOR SUPPRESSOR GENES

"Deleted in Colorectal Cancer" (*DCC*)

Reduction to homozygosity or allelic loss at chromosome 18q occurs in more than 70 per cent of colorectal carcinomas and in about 50 per cent of large benign adenomas. These chromosome alterations are rare in small early-stage adenomas.[37] Using restriction site polymorphisms, these allelic losses were mapped to chromosome 18q21 and the gene in question identified by walking across this region and molecular cloning techniques.[42] The gene, called *DCC*, covers 370 kb of DNA at that locus and encodes a protein with significant homologies to a neural cell adhesion protein, NCAM.[151] The DCC protein has a transmembrane domain with extracellular immunoglobulin-like domains, a fibronectin type III–like domain with repeated amino acid sequences, and a cytoplasmic tail. With a structure like this, it is possible that alterations in this protein could contribute to new adhesion and/or invasion properties of colorectal cancer cells. It is of some interest that returning chromosome 18 to a colorectal cancer cell in culture produces a cell line that no longer forms tumors in animals[152] (see Table 5–1). Most cell lines derived from colorectal cancers do not normally express DCC protein, whereas the normal colonic mucosa cells do express low levels of this gene product.[30]

"Mutated in Colorectal Cancer" (*MCC*)

Closely linked to the *APC* gene on chromosome 5q21 is a second putative tumor suppressor gene named *MCC*. It was found during the search for *APC* and detected by virtue of three independent examples of mutation in this gene from patients with sporadic colorectal cancer (rearranged gene and point mutations).[153] Further studies have

detected four additional examples of somatic mutation, but no evidence of germ line transmission exists.[30]

CONCLUSIONS: SOME TUMOR SUPPRESSOR GENES ACT AT CHECKPOINTS IN THE CELL CYCLE

With the very early experiments in somatic cell genetics (see Table 5–1) and the mapping of allelic loss or RFLP (see Table 5–2), it was clear that there were multiple examples of tumor suppressor genes. It even was clear that these gene products would behave differently in cancers of different cell or tissue types, having the ability to suppress tumor growth in some but not other cancers. The isolation of the two clearest examples of tumor suppressor genes, *Rb* and *p53*, has confirmed and extended these speculations. The best example of a pure (by definition) tumor suppressor gene is *Rb*, which sustains a true loss-of-function mutation in retinoblasts giving rise to a tumor, with little need to hypothesize additional genetic events. *p53* is clearly more complicated, with the true loss-of-function mutations (deletions, rearrangements) found preferentially in sarcomas, as are amplifications of Mdm2, which prevent p53 function.[133,136] Cervical carcinomas that express the HPV-16 or -18 E6 gene product promote the proteolysis of p53 in these cells, and so these are true loss-of-function events (although not mutations) as well. Carcinomas, in contrast, appear to select for missense mutations in *p53* and a gain of a new function as well as a loss of tumor suppressor activity. Unlike *Rb* in retinoblastomas, it appears that the loss of *p53* in most cancers, while necessary, is not sufficient for a cancer to arise. Additional mutagenic events are required and, in colorectal cancer (Fig. 5–2), there could be as many as ten such events or mutations. Some of these may well occur at a higher rate than simple point mutations via a reduction to homozygosity or through the creation of a mutator gene phenotype with the production of a *p53* missense mutant protein.

In recent years, the functions and events that regulate the cell cycle and cell proliferation have been elucidated by studies with yeast cells, *Xenopus* eggs, and cancerous tissues. It has become clear that the cell cycle is composed of two classes or categories of gene functions: (1) functions essential to the cycle that program for the duplication of all cellular components and the proper distribution of these components into two daughter cells, and (2) nonessential functions that negatively regulate the progression through the cell cycle and ensure the high fidelity of this process. These latter functions have come to be termed checkpoints in the cell cycle. Examples of essential functions for the cell cycle are the cyclins and the cdk activities, which signal for progression from G_1 to S or G_2 to M phases of the cycle. In the presence of active cyclin-cdk complex, the signal to progress through division is provided and so, in the absence of any control over these activities, the default pathway through the cell cycle progresses. The checkpoints provide a negative regulation on progress through the cycle. Typical checkpoints in the cell cycle are regulated by cell size, the availability of nutrients, cell-cell communication, or hormonal signaling. The integrity of the DNA template is tested in G_1 so as to be sure the template is ready for duplication without mistakes. If the DNA is damaged, the checkpoint control acts to hold up progression from G_1 to S or from G_2 to M so as to repair the breaks or altered templates prior to entry into the next phase of the cell cycle. Failure to repair this damage results in errors in segregation of chromosomes, gene amplifications, and other mutations.[154,155] These errors produce cell death or abnormal cells that permit the selection of cancerous clones of cells.

The Rb and p53 protein fit well into the definition of checkpoint proteins. Both of these proteins are nonessential for progression through the division cycle. Cells with no *Rb* or *p53* genes divide perfectly well (and even become cancerous). The *p53* gene is nonessential for even a normal round of cell division.[109] Both of these gene products negatively regulate progression through the cell cycle by blocking cells in the late G_1 phase of the cycle.[113,156] The levels of p53 protein are elevated in response to ultraviolet or γ-irradiation damage to the DNA.[21,22] Cells with a normal p53 protein pause in late G_1 for repair of DNA after irradiation. Cells with mutant p53 fail to pause, enter S phase, and have lower viability and presumably poor genomic stability.[22] Clearly, p53 protein acts as a late G_1 checkpoint, monitoring the integrity of the DNA template in S phase and ultimately genomic stability. The Rb protein bound to the transcription factor E2F blocks the expression of a number of genes that encode enzyme activities needed to synthesize deoxyribonucleoside triphosphates, the precursors of DNA replication. In the absence of Rb, the abnormal expression of such enzyme activities at the wrong stages of the cell cycle also could result in genomic instability and poor fidelity of duplication in the cell cycle. Thus, *Rb* and *p53*, the tumor suppressor genes, act much like checkpoint controls over the cell cycle. Failure of these genes to function is not lethal, but creates a mutator phenotype and cancer.

The communication between checkpoint controls and the essential elements for progression through the cell cycle, the cyclins and cdk activities, often are mediated by signal transduction pathways. Hormonal control of the cell cycle involves a receptor protein, linked to a G protein and/or a protein kinase. Proteases, phosphotases, and transcription factors communicate between the external stimuli and the cyclins or cdk activities. These signal transduction pathways often are composed of the proto-oncogene products that signal continuously for progression through the cell cycle in their mutant forms. It is likely that the tumor suppressor genes and proto-oncogenes produce proteins that are on the same pathway to regulate the functions of the cell cycle.

Thus, it appears that Rb regulates critical transcription factors in the cell cycle and p53 and WT-1 are themselves transcription factors. NF-1, at least in part, regulates Ras, a critical signal transducer for cell growth, and DCC is a transmembrane cell adhesion molecule. This diversity of functions follows the diversity of cancer cells and their properties and prognosis. Rb, p53, NF-1, and APC are all expressed in most adult tissues of the body, so it is not clear why mutations in each of these gene products result in a marked tissue preference for the tumors that arise. These observations suggest that different proteins can regulate the cell cycle in different tissue types.

These tumor suppressor genes now have provided a clearer understanding of the inherited basis of some cancers. These genes appear to be inherited as an autosomal dominant trait because of the very high probability of mutation or reduction to homozygosity in the remaining wild-type allele.

The evidence that *WT-1*, *NF-1*, *APC*, *DCC*, and *MCC* are tumor suppressor genes remains at this time incomplete. Each of these genes has features (see Table 5–3) that suggests that it is a tumor suppressor. In time, this will be resolved and new genes certainly will be added to this list. As this happens, we will understand the targets for mutation and the origins of cancer.

REFERENCES

1. Harris H, Miller OJ, Klein G, et al: Suppression of malignancy by cell fusion. Nature *223*:363, 1969
2. Saxon PJ, Srivatsan ES, Stanbridge EJ: Introduction of chromosome 11 via microcell transfer controls tumorigenic expression of HeLa Cells. EMBO J *5*:3461, 1986
3. Knudson AG Jr: Mutation and cancer: Statistical study of retinoblastoma. Proc Natl Acad Sci USA *68*:820, 1971
4. Yunis JJ, Ramsey N: Retinoblastoma and sub-band deletion of chromosome 13. Am J Dis Child *132*:161, 1978
5. Cavenee WK, Dryja TP, Phillips RA, et al: Expression of recessive alleles by chromosomal mechanisms in retinoblastoma. Nature *305*:779, 1983
6. Friend SH, Bernards R, Rogelj S, et al: A human DNA segment with properties of the gene that predisposes to retinoblastoma and osteosarcoma. Nature *323*:643, 1986
7. Fung YK, Murphree AL, T'Ang A, et al: Structural evidence for the authenticity of the human retinoblastoma gene. Science *236*:1657, 1987
8. Lee W-H, Bookstein R, Hong F, et al: Human retinoblastoma susceptibility gene: Cloning, identification, and sequence. Science *235*:1394, 1987
9. Dunn JM, Phillips RA, Becker AJ, et al: Identification of germ-line and somatic mutations affecting the retinoblastoma gene. Science *241*:1797, 1988
10. Canning S, Dryja TP: Short, direct repeats at the breakpoints of deletions of the retinoblastoma gene. Proc Natl Acad Sci USA *86*:5044, 1989
11. Dunn JM, Phillips RA, Zhu X, et al: Mutations in the RB1 gene and their effects on transcription. Mol Cell Biol *9*:4596, 1989
12. Horowitz JM, Yandell DW, Park S-H, et al: Point mutational inactivation of the retinoblastoma antioncogene. Science *243*: 937, 1989
13. Yandell DW, Campbell TA, Dayton SH, et al: Oncogenic point mutations in the human retinoblastoma gene: Their application to genetic counseling. N Engl J Med *321*:1689, 1989
14. Gallie BL, Dunn JM, Hamel PA, et al: Point mutations in retinoblastoma. N Engl J Med *322*:1397, 1990
15. Kaye FJ, Fratzke RA, Gerster JL, et al: A single amino acid substitution results in a retinoblastoma protein defective in phosphorylation and oncoprotein binding. Proc Natl Acad Sci USA *87*:6922, 1990
16. Huang HJS, Yee JK, Shew JY, et al: Suppression of the neoplastic phenotype by replacement of the Rb gene in human cancer cells. Science *242*:1563, 1988
17. Rowley JD: Consistent chromosomal rearrangements in human malignant disease and oncogene location. *In* Vande Woude GF et al (eds): Cancer Cells/2: Oncogenes and Viral Genes. Cold Spring Harbor, NY, Cold Spring Harbor Laboratory Press, 1984, p 221

18. Todaro GJ, Huebner RJ: The viral oncogene hypothesis: New evidence. Proc Natl Acad Sci USA 69:1009, 1972

19. Stehelin D, Varmus HE, Bishop JM, et al: DNA related to transforming gene(s) of avian sarcoma viruses is present in normal avian DNA. Nature 260:170, 1976

20. Friend SH, Horowitz JM, Gerber MR, et al: Deletions of a DNA sequence in retinoblastomas and mesenchymal tumors: Organization of the sequence and its encoded protein. Proc Natl Acad Sci USA 84:9059, 1987

21. Maltzman W, Czyzyk L: UV irradiation stimulates levels of p53 cellular tumor antigen in nontransformed mouse cells. Mol Cell Biol 4:1689, 1984

22. Kastan MB, Onyekwere O, Sidransky D, et al: Participation of p53 protein in the cellular response to DNA damage. Cancer Res 51:6304, 1991

23. Dryja TP, Mukai S, Petersen R, et al: Parental origin of mutations of the retinoblastoma gene. Nature 339:556, 1989

24. Malkin D, Li FP, Strong LC, et al: Germ line p53 mutations in a familial syndrome of breast cancer, sarcomas, and other neoplasms. Science 250:1233, 1990

25. Srivastava S, Zou Z, Pirollo K, et al: Germ-line transmission of a mutated p53 gene in a cancer-prone family with Li-Fraumeni syndrome. Nature 348:747, 1990

26. Malkin D, Jolly KW, Piraux NB, et al: Germline mutations of the p53 tumor suppressor gene in children and young adults with second malignant neoplasms. N Engl J Med 326:1309, 1992

27. Toguchida J, Yamaguchi T, Dayton SH, et al: Prevalence and spectrum of germline mutations of the p53 gene among patients with sarcoma. N Engl J Med 326:1301, 1992

28. Silverberg E, Boring CE, Squires TS: Cancer statistics, 1990. CA 40:9, 1990

29. Seidman H, Mushinski MH, Gelb E, et al: Probabilities of eventually developing or dying of cancer—United States. CA 35:36, 1985

30. Fearon ER: Genetic alterations underlying colorectal tumorigenesis. Cancer Surv 12:119–136, 1992

31. Bodmer WF, Bailey C, Bodmer J, et al: Localization of the gene for familial polyposis on chromosome 5. Nature 328:614, 1987

32. Leppert M, Dobbs M, Scambler P, et al: The gene for familial polyposis coli maps to the long arm chromosome 5. Science 238:1411, 1987

33. Utsunomiya J, Lynch HT (eds): Hereditary Colorectal Cancer. New York, Springer-Verlag, 1990.

34. Groden J, Thliveris A, Samowitz W, et al: Identification and characterization of the familial adenomatous polyposis coli gene. Cell 66:589, 1991

35. Nishisho I, Nakamura Y, Miyoshi Y, et al: Mutations of chromosome 5q21 genes in FAP and colorectal cancer patients. Science 253:665, 1991

36. Solomon E, Voss R, Hall V, et al: Chromosome 5 allele loss in human colorectal carcinomas. Nature 328:616, 1987

37. Vogelstein B, Fearon ER, Hamilton SR, et al: Genetic alterations during colorectal-tumor development. N Engl J Med 319:525, 1988

38. Fearon ER, Hamilton SR, Vogelstein B: Clonal analysis of human colorectal tumors. Science 238:193, 1987

39. Muto T, Bussey HJR, Morson BC, et al: The evolution of cancer of the colon and rectum. Cancer 36:2251, 1975

40. Astrin SM, Costanzi C: The molecular genetics of colon cancer. Semin Oncol 16:138, 1989

41. Baker SJ, Preisinger AC, Jessup JM, et al: p53 gene mutations occur in combination with 17p allelic deletions or late events in colorectal tumorigenesis. Cancer Res 50:7717, 1990

42. Fearon ER, Cho KR, Nigro JM, et al: Identification of a chromosome 18q gene that is altered in colorectal cancer. Science 247:49, 1990

43. Chen P-L, Chen Y, Bookstein R, et al: Genetic mechanisms of tumor suppression by the human p53 gene. Science 250:1576, 1990

44. Tooze J (ed): Molecular Biology of the Tumor Viruses. Cold Spring Harbor, NY, Cold Spring Harbor Laboratory Press, 1973, p 350

45. Yonish-Rouach E, Resnitzky D, Lotem J, et al: Wild-type p53 induces apoptosis of myeloid leukaemic cells that is inhibited by interleukin-6. Nature 352:345, 1991

46. Shaw P, Boucy R, Tardy S, et al: Induction of apoptosis by wild-type p53 in a human colon tumor-derived cell line. Proc Natl Acad Sci USA 89:4495, 1992

47. Rao L, Debbas M, Sabbatini P, et al: The adenovirus E1A proteins induce apoptosis which is inhibited by the E1B 19 Kd and Bcl proteins. Proc Natl Acad Sci USA 89:7742, 1992

48. Brinster RL, Chen HY, Messing A, et al: Transgenic mice harboring SV40 T antigen genes develop characteristic brain tumors. Cell 37:367, 1984

49. Pipas J: Common and unique features of T-antigens encoded by the polyoma virus group. J Virol 66:3979, 1992

50. Fanning E: Simian virus 40 large T antigen: The puzzle, the pieces and the emerging picture. J Virol 66:1289, 1992

51. DeCaprio JA, Ludlow JW, Figge J, et al: SV40 large tumor antigen forms a specific complex with the product of the retinoblastoma susceptibility gene. Cell 54:275, 1988

52. Linzer DIH, Levine AJ: Characterization of a 54K dalton cellular SV40 tumor antigen in SV40 transformed cells. Cell 17:43, 1979

53. Lane DP, Crawford LV: T antigen is bound to a host protein in SV40-transformed cells. Nature 278:261, 1979

54. Moran B, Zerler B: Interactions between cell growth-regulating domains in the products of the adenovirus E1A oncogene. Mol Cell Biol 8:1756, 1988

55. Whyte P, Williamson NM, Harlow E: Cellular targets for transformation by the adenovirus E1A proteins. Cell 56:67, 1989

56. Quinlan MP, White P, Grodzicker T: Growth factor induction by the adenovirus type 5 E1A 12S protein is required for immortalization of primary epithelial cells. Mol Cell Biol 8:1026, 1988

57. Sarnow P, Ho YS, Williams J, Levine AJ: Adenovirus E1B-58Kd tumor antigen and SV40 large tumor antigen are physically associated with the same 54Kd cellular protein in transformed cells. Cell 28:387, 1982

58. Yew PR, Berk AJ: Inhibition of p53 transactivation required for transformation by adenovirus E1B 55 Kd protein. Nature 357:82, 1992

59. Werness BA, Levine AJ, Howley PM: Association of human papillomavirus types 16 and 18 E6 proteins with p53. Science 248:76, 1990

60. Dyson N, Howley PM, Munger K, Harlow E: The human papillomavirus-16 E7 oncoprotein is able to bind to the retinoblastoma gene product. Science 243:934, 1989

61. Münger K, Scheffner M, Huibregtse JM, Howley P: The interactions of the HPV E6 and E7 oncoproteins with tumor suppressor gene products. Cancer Surv 12:197, 1992

62. Livingston DM: Functional analysis of the retinoblastoma gene product and of Rb-SV40 T antigen complexes. Cancer Surv 12:153, 1992

63. Dyson N, Harlow E: Adenovirus E1A targets key regulators of cell proliferation. Cancer Surv 12:161, 1992

64. Chellappan SP, Hiebert S, Mudryj M, et al: The E2F transcription factor is a cellular target for the TB protein. Cell 65:1053, 1991

65. Bandara L, Adamczewski J, Hunt T, LaThangue N: Cyclin A and the retinoblastoma gene product complex with a common transcription factor. Nature 352:249, 1991

66. Kovesdi I, Reichel R, Nevins JR: Identification of a cellular transcription factor involved in E1A trans-activation. Cell 45:219, 1986

67. Bandara LR, LaThangue NB: Adenovirus E1a prevents the retinoblastoma gene product from complexing with a cellular transcription factor. Nature 351:494, 1991

68. Bagchi S, Raychaudhuri P, Nevins J: Adenovirus E1A proteins can dissociate heteromeric complexes involved the E2F transcription factor: A novel mechanism for E1A trans-activation. Cell 62:659, 1990

69. Raychaudhuri P, Bagchi S, Neill S, Nevins JR: Activation of the E2F transcription factor in adenovirus infected cells involves an E1A-dependent stimulation of DNA binding activity and induction of cooperative binding mediated by an E4 gene product. J Virol 64:2702, 1990

70. DeFeo-Jones D, Huang PS, Jones RE, et al: Cloning of cDNAs for cellular proteins that bind to the retinoblastoma gene product. Nature 352:251, 1991

71. Buchkovich K, Duffy LA, Harlow E: The retinoblastoma protein is phosphorylated during specific phases of the cell cycle. Cell 58:1097, 1989

72. Lees-Miller SP, Anderson CW: The DNA activated protein kinase, DNA-PK: A potential coordinator of nuclear events. Cancer Cells 3:341, 1991

73. Ludlow JS, Shon J, Pipas JM, et al: The retinoblastoma susceptibility gene product undergoes cell cycle-dependent dephosphorylation and binding to and release from SV40 large T. Cell 60:387, 1990

74. Ludlow JW, DeCaprio JA, Huang CM, et al: SV40 large T antigen binds preferentially to an underphosphorylated member of the retinoblastoma susceptibility gene product family. Cell 56:57, 1989

75. Benchimol S, Lamb P, Crawford LC, et al: Transformation associated p53 protein is encoded by a gene on human chromosome 17. Somat Cell Mol Genet 11:505, 1985

76. Oren M: The p53 cellular tumor antigen: Gene structure, expression and protein properties. Biochim Biophys Acta 823:67, 1985

77. Bischoff JR, Friedman PN, Marshak DR, et al: Human p53 is phosphorylated by p60-cdc2 and cyclin B-cdc2. Proc Natl Acad Sci USA 87:4766, 1990

78. Stürzbecher HW, Maimets T, Chumakov P, et al: p53 interacts with p34^{cdc2} in mammalian cells: Implication for cell cycle control and oncogenesis. Oncogene 5:795, 1990

79. Shaulsky G, Goldfinger N, Rotter V: Alterations in tumor development in vivo mediated by expression of wild-type or mutant p53 proteins. Cancer Res 51:5232, 1991

80. Soussi T, Caron de Fromental C, Mechali M, et al: Cloning and characterization of a cDNA from Xenopus laevis coding for a protein homologous to human and murine p53. Oncogene 1:71, 1987

81. Hollstein MC, Peri L, Mandard AM, et al: Genetic analysis of human esophageal tumors from two high incidence geographic areas: Frequent p53 base substitutions and absence of ras mutations. Cancer Res 51:4102, 1991

82. Levine AJ, Quartin RS, Martinez J, et al: The p53 tumor suppressor gene. In Proceedings of the Yakult Symposium, Tokyo, Japan. 1991, p 65

83. Baker SJ, Fearon ER, Nigro JM, et al: Chromosome 17 deletions and p53 gene mutations in colorectal carcinoma. Science 244:217, 1989

84. Nigro JM, Baker SJ, Preisinger AC, et al: Mutations in the p53 gene occur in diverse human tumour types. Nature 342:705, 1989

85. Crook T, Wrede D, Tidy J, et al: Status of c-myc, p53 and retinoblastoma genes in human papillomavirus positive and negative squamous cell carcinomas of the anus. Oncogene 6:1251, 1991

86. Prosser J, Thompson AM, Cranston G, et al: Evidence that p53 behaves as a tumor suppressor gene in sporadic breast tumors. Oncogene 5:1573, 1990

87. Davidoff AM, Humphrey PA, Iglehart JK, et al: Genetic basis for p53 overexpression in human breast cancer. Proc Natl Acad Sci USA 88:5006, 1991

88. Varley JM, Brammar WJ, Lane DP, et al: Loss of chromosome 17p13 sequences and mutation of p53 in human breast carcinomas. Oncogene 6:413, 1991

89. Hollstein MC, Metcalf RA, Welsh JA, et al: Frequent mutation of the p53 gene in human esophageal cancer. Proc Natl Acad Sci USA 87:9958, 1990

90. Tamura G, Kihana T, Nomura K, et al: Detection of frequent p53 gene mutations in primary gastric cancer by cell sorting and polymerase chain reaction single-strand conformation polymorphism analysis. Cancer Res 51:3056, 1991

91. Bressac B, Kew M, Wands J, et al: Selective G to T mutations of p53 gene in hepatocellular carcinoma from Southern Africa. Nature 350:429, 1991

92. Hsu IC, Metcalf RA, Sun T, et al: Mutational hotspot in the p53 gene in human hepatocellular carcinoma. Nature 350:427, 1991

93. Takahashi T, Nau MM, Chiba I, et al: p53: A frequent target for genetic abnormalities in lung cancer. Science 246:491, 1989

94. Chiba I, Takahashi T, Nau MM, et al: Mutations in the p53 gene are frequent in primary resected non-small cell lung cancer. Oncogene 5:1603, 1990

95. Iggo R, Gatter K, Bartek J, et al: Increased expression of mutant forms of p53 oncogene in primary lung cancer. Lancet 1:675, 1990

96. Hensel CH, Xiang RH, Sakaguchi AY, Naylor SL: Use of the single strand conformation polymorphism technique and PCR to detect p53 gene mutations in small cell lung cancer. Oncogene 6:1067, 1991

97. Ahuja H, Bar-Eli M, Advani SH, et al: Alterations in the p53 gene and the clonal evolution of the blast crisis of chronic myelocytic leukemia. Proc Natl Acad Sci USA 86:6783, 1989

98. Gaidano G, Ballerini P, Gong JZ, et al: p53 mutations in human lymphoid malignancies: Association with Burkitt's lymphoma and chronic lymphocytic leukemia. Proc Natl Acad Sci USA 88:5413, 1991

99. Marks JR, Davidoff AM, Kerns BJ, et al: Overexpression and mutation of p53 in epithelial ovarian cancer. Cancer Res 51:2979, 1991

100. Isaacs WB, Carter BS, Ewing CM: Wild-type p53 suppressor growth of human prostate cancer cells containing mutant p53 alleles. Cancer Res 51:4716, 1991

101. Murakami Y, Hayashi K, Hirohashi S, et al: Aberrations of the tumor suppressor p53 and retinoblastoma genes in human hepatocellular carcinomas. Cancer Res 51:5520, 1991

102. Miller CW, Aslo A, Tsay C, et al: Frequency and structure of p53 rearrangements in human osteosarcoma. Cancer Res 50:7950, 1990

103. Mulligan LM, Matlashewski GJ, Scrable HJ, et al: Mechanisms of p53 loss in human sarcoma. Proc Natl Acad Sci USA 87:5863, 1990

104. Stratton MR, Moss S, Warren W, et al: Mutation of the p53 gene in human soft tissue sarcomas: Association with abnormalities of the RB1 gene. Oncogenes 5:1297, 1990

105. Li FP: Cancer families: Human models of susceptibility to neoplasia—The Richard & Hinda Rosenthal Foundation Award Lecture. Cancer Res 48:5381, 1988

106. Li FP, Fraumeni JF, Mulvihill JJ, et al: A cancer family syndrome in twenty-four kindreds. Cancer Res 48:5358, 1988

107. Iavarone A, Matthay KK, Steinkirchner TM, et al: Germ line and somatic p53 gene mutations in multifocal osteogenic sarcoma. Proc Natl Acad Sci USA 89:4207, 1992

108. Lavigueur A, Maltby V, Mock D, et al: High incidence of lung, bone, and lymphoid tumors in transgenic mice overexpressing mutant alleles of the p53 oncogene. Mul Cell Biol 9:3982, 1989

109. Donehower LA, Harvey M, Slagle BL, et al: Mice deficient for p53 are developmentally normal but susceptible to spontaneous tumours. Nature 356:215, 1992

110. Mercer WE, Shields MT, Amin M, et al: Negative growth regulation in a glioblastoma tumor cell line that conditionally expresses human wild-type p53. Proc Natl Acad Sci USA 87:6166, 1990

111. Diller L, Kassel J, Nelson CE, et al: p53 functions as a cell cycle control protein in osteosarcomas. Mol Cell Biol 10:5772, 1990

112. Michalovitz D, Halevy O, Oren M: Conditional inhibition of transformation and of cell proliferation by a temperature-sensitive mutant of p53. Cell 62:671, 1990

113. Martinez J, Georgoff I, Martinez J, Levine AJ: Cellular localization and cell cycle regulation by a temperature sensitive p53 protein. Genes Dev 5:151, 1991

114. Wolf D, Admon S, Oren M, Rotter V: Abelson murine leukemia virus-transformed cells that lack p53 protein synthesis express aberrant p53 mRNA species. Mol Cell Biol 4:552, 1984

115. Finlay CA, Hinds PW, Levine AJ: The p53 proto-oncogene can act as a suppressor of transformation. Cell 57:1083, 1989

116. Levine AJ, Finlay CA, Hinds PW: The p53 proto-oncogene and its product. In Villarreal LP (ed): Common Mechanisms of Transformation by Small DNA Tumor Viruses. Washington, DC, ASM Publications, 1989, pp 21–37

117. Hinds P, Finlay C, Levine AJ: Mutation is required to activate

the p53 gene for cooperation with the *ras* oncogene and transformation. J Virol *63*:739, 1989

118. Stürzbecher HW, Brain R, Addison C, et al: A C-terminal alpha helix plus basic motif is the major structural determinant of p53 tetramerization. Oncogene *7*:1513, 1992
119. Reich NC, Levine AJ: Growth regulation of a cellular tumor antigen, p53, in nontransformed cells. Nature *308*:199, 1984
120. Finlay CA, Hinds PW, Tan T-H, et al: Activating mutations for transformation by p53 produce a gene product that forms an hsc70-p53 complex with an altered half-life. Mol Cell Biol *8*: 531, 1988
121. Hinds PW, Finlay CA, Quartin RS, et al: Mutant p53 cDNAs from human colorectal carcinomas can cooperate with *ras* in transformation of primary rat cells: A comparison of the "hot spot" mutant phenotypes. Cell Growth Differ *1*:571, 1990
122. Fields S, Jang SK, et al: Presence of a potent transcription activating sequence in the p53 protein. Science *249*:1046, 1990
123. Raycroft L, Schmidt JR, Yoas K, Lozano G: Analysis of p53 mutants for transcriptional activity. Mol Cell Biol *11*:6067, 1991
124. Bargonetti J, Friedman PN, Kern SE, et al: Wild-type but not mutant p53 immunopurified proteins bind to sequence adjacent to the SV40 origin of replication. Cell *65*:1083, 1991
125. Kern SE, Kinzler KW, Bruskin A, et al: Identification of p53 as a sequence-specific DNA-binding protein. Science *252*:1708, 1991
126. Funk WD, Pak DJ, Karas RH, et al: A transcriptionally active DNA binding site for human p53 protein complexes. Mol Cell Biol *12*:2866, 1992
127. El-Deiry WS, Kern SE, Pietenpol JA, et al: Human genomic DNA sequences define a consensus binding site for p53. Nature Genet *1*:44, 1992
128. Farmer GE, Bargonetti J, Zhu H, et al: Wild-type p53 activates transcription in vitro. Nature *358*:83, 1992
129. Kern S, Pietenpol JA, Thiagalingam S, et al: Oncogenic forms of p53 inhibit p53-regulated gene expression. Science *256*: 827, 1992
130. Zambetti GP, Labow M, Levine AJ: A mutant p53 protein is required for the maintenance of the transformed cell phenotype in p53 plus *ras* transformed cells. Proc Natl Acad Sci USA *89*:3952, 1992
131. Scheffner M, Takahashi T, Huibregtse JM, et al: Interaction of the HPV16 E6 oncoprotein with wild-type and mutant p53 proteins. J Virol *66*:5100, 1992
132. Land D: Guardian of the genome. Nature *358*:15, 1992
133. Momand J, Zambetti GP, Olson DC, et al: The mdm-2 oncogene product forms a complex with the p53 protein and inhibits p53 mediated transactivation. Cell *69*:1, 1992
134. Fakharzadeh SS, Trusko SP, George DL: Tumorigenic potential associated with enhanced expression of a gene that is amplified in a mouse tumor cell line. EMBO J *10*:1565, 1991
135. Cahilly-Snyder L, Yang-Feng T, Francke U, et al: Molecular analysis and chromosomal mapping of amplified genes isolated from a transformed mouse 3T3 cell line. Somat Cell Mol Genet *13*:235, 1987
136. Oliner JD, Kinzler KW, Meltzer PS, et al: Amplification of a p53-associated gene in human sarcomas. Nature (London) *358*:80, 1992
137. Moll UM, Riou G, Levine AJ: Two distinct mechanisms alter p53 in breast cancer: Mutation and nuclear exclusion. Proc Natl Acad Sci USA *89*:7262, 1992
138. Haber DA, Housman DE: Rate-limiting steps: The genetics of pediatric cancers. Cell *64*:5, 1991
139. Riccardi VM, Sujansky E, Smith AC, Francke U: Chromosomal imbalance in the aniridia-Wilms' tumor association: 11p deletion. Pediatrics *61*:604, 1978
140. Call KM, Glaser T, Ito CY, et al: Isolation and characterization of a zinc finger polypeptide gene at the human 11 Wilms' tumor locus. Cell *60*:409, 1990
141. Haber DA, Housman DE: Role of the WT1 gene in Wilm's tumor. Cancer Surv *12*:105, 1992
142. Stanbridge EJ: Functional evidence for human tumor suppressor genes: Chromosome and molecular genetic studies. Cancer Surv *12*:5, 1992
143. Rauscher FJ, Morris JF, Tournay OE, et al: Binding of the Wilms' tumor zinc finger protein to the EGR1 consensus sequences. Science *250*:1259, 1990
144. Haber DA, Buckler AJ, Glaser T, et al: An internal deletion within an 11p13 zinc finger gene contributes to the development of Wilms' tumor. Cell *61*:1257, 1990
145. Cawthon RM, Weiss R, Xu G, et al: A major segment of the neurofibromatosis type 1 gene: cDNA sequence, genomic structure and point mutations. Cell *62*:192, 1990
146. Viskochil D, Buchberg AM, Xu G, et al: Deletions and a translocation interrupt a cloned gene at the neurofibromatosis type 1 locus. Cell *62*:187, 1990
147. Wallace MR, Marchuk DA, Anderson LB, et al: Type 1 neurofibromatosis gene: Identification of a large transcript disrupted in three NF1 patients. Nature *249*:181, 1990
148. Xu GF, Lin B, Tanaka K, et al: The catayltic domain of the neurofibromatosis type 1 gene product stimulates *ras* GTPase and complements IRA mutants of S. cerevisiae. Cell *63*:835, 1990
149. Martin GA, Viskochil D, Bollag G, et al: The GAP-related domain of the neurofibromatosis type 1 gene product interacts with *ras* p21. Cell *63*:843, 1990
150. Joslyn G, Carlson M, Thlweres A, et al: Identification of deletion mutations and three new genes at the familial polyposis locus. Cell *66*:601, 1991
151. Edelman GM: Morphoregulatory molecules. Biochemistry *27*: 3533, 1988
152. Tanaka K, Oshimura M, Kikuchi R, et al: Suppression of tumorigenicity in human colon carcinoma cells by introduction of normal chromosome 5 or 18. Nature *349*:340, 1991
153. Kinzler KW, Milbert MC, Vogelstein B, et al: Identification of a gene located at chromosome 5q21 that is mutated in colorectal cancers. Science *251*:1366, 1991
154. Brown M, Garvik B, Hartwell L, et al: Fidelity of mitotic chromosome transmission. Cold Spring Harb Symp Quant Biol *56*: 359, 1992
155. Schimke RT, Kung AL, Rush DR, Sherwood SW: Differences in mitotic control among mammalian cells. Cold Spring Harb Symp Quant Biol *56*:417, 1992
156. Weinberg RA: The retinoblastoma gene and gene product. Cancer Surv *12*:43, 1992
157. Stanbridge EJ: The genetic basis of tumor suppression. Ciba Found *142*:149, 1989
158. Shimizu M, Yokoto J, Mori N, et al: Introduction of normal chromosome 3p modulates the tumorigenicity of a human renal cell carcinoma cell line YCR. Oncogene *5*:185, 1990
159. Dowdy SF, Fashing CL, Araujo D, et al: Suppression of tumorigenicity in Wilms tumor by the p15.5-p14 region of chromosome 11. Science *253*:1, 1992
160. Trent JM, Stanbridge EJ, McBride HS, et al: Tumorigenicity in human melanoma cell lines controlled by introduction of human chromosome 6. Science *247*:568, 1990
161. Bader SA, Fasching C, Brodeur GM, et al: Dissociation of suppression of tumourigenicity and differentiation *in vitro* effected by transfer of single human chromosomes into human neuroblastoma cells. Cell Growth Diff *2*:245, 1991
162. Kugoh HM, Hashiba H, Shimizu M, et al: Suggestive evidence for functionally distinct, tumor suppressor genes on chromosomes 1 and 11 for a human fibrosarcoma cell line, HT1080. Oncogene *5*:1637, 1990
163. Yamada H, Wake N, Fujimoto S, et al: Multiple chromosomes carrying tumor suppressor activity for a uterine endometrial carcinoma cell line identified by microcell-mediated chromosome transfer. Oncogene *5*:1141, 1990
164. Stanbridge EJ: Human tumor suppressor gene. Annu Rev Genet *24*:615, 1990
165. Whyte P, Buchkovich KJ, Horowitz JM, et al: Association between an oncogene and an anti-oncogene; the adenovirus Ela proteins bind to the retinoblastoma gene product. Nature *334*: 124, 1988

6

ONCOGENES

NEAL ROSEN

Cancer is a disorder that results from a pleiotypic change of the state of the cell. The behavior of this transformed cell and the host response to its existence are responsible for all of the manifestations of the disease. Several key properties characterize the malignant cell: dysregulated cell division and differentiation, genomic instability, loss of normal senescence, and invasion into adjacent tissues.[1-4] One of the central questions of cancer research has been to explain the mechanism of this state change.

Although transformation as an inductive change induced by disordered host factors was an early, credible hypothesis, the weight of evidence indicates that cancer results from genetic changes in the cell. In this context, the question becomes whether malignancy results from many mutational events acquired over time in multiple genes, or whether mutations in a few key genes lead to specific cancers. This debate was fueled by disparate bodies of evidence and interpretation of data. On the one hand, cancer was associated with lifetime exposure to well-defined occupational chemical or physical mutagens, cancers in experimental animals could be induced by prolonged exposure to such mutagens, and the risk of most of the common adult malignancies increased markedly with age.[5-7] These data were taken as implying that mutations in many genes over time led to multiple defects that together created the cancer phenotype, as manifested by the transformed state. In its most extreme form, this "accumulation of errors" hypothesis states that eventually multiple lesions in the replicative, transcriptional, and translational apparatus render faithful DNA replication impossible and lead to progressively increased mutation rate and generation of variation.[8,9] The latter allows selection of the most rapidly growing cell, adapted to grow and spread into multiple environments within the host, and to resistance to host defenses and therapeutic manipulations.

Against this general picture, on the other hand, were the data obtained from the study of tumor viruses. Although the first of these was discovered in the first decade of the century, the implications of this phenomenon remained controversial for many years. In particular, the lack of convincing evidence for an infectious etiology for most human cancers and the difficulty in isolating human tumor viruses clouded the significance of the fact of viral oncogenesis.

The development of the principles and techniques of molecular virology led to the isolation and cloning of many examples of animal tumor viruses in the 1960s and 1970s.[10,11] Molecular characterization of these viruses revealed that they could be classified as having genomes comprised of DNA or RNA.[10,11] Studies on cells in culture showed that viruses induced transformation by directly affecting the cell and that the effect was caused by the viral genome.[10,11] Genetic experiments utilizing viruses with fairly simple genomes showed that, in some systems, cellular transformation was caused by the action of one or only a few viral genes.[12,13]

Thus, data accumulated from studies of viral oncogenesis suggested that the malignant phenotype could be induced by one or a few genetic events in particular genes, and that such genes could be transmitted by viruses. In this view, transformation results from the activation or mutation of key regulatory genes that encode products that have profound pleiotypic effects on cell growth and differentiation. The hypothetical viral or cellular genes responsible for inducing or maintaining the malignant phenotype were named "oncogenes."[14,21] The mass of data accumulated over the last 15 years confirms this idea, and many such oncogenes have been characterized functionally. The evolution of this idea and the nature of the oncogenes that have been found to be activated in human tumors are the subject of this chapter. However, it must be emphasized that the discordance between viral and tissue culture systems, in which relatively few hits involving well-defined pathways are sufficient to induce transformation, and chemical carcinogenesis systems and naturally occurring tumors, in which large numbers of hits occur, has not yet been explained completely.

ONCOGENE HYPOTHESIS

The isolation of tumor viruses led to the idea that these viruses encoded single genes that, alone or in combination with other such genes, were sufficient for inducing the transformed phenotype in infected cells.[11,15] This class of genes was given the name oncogene. Naturally occurring human tumors were thought to result from viral transmission of such genes or, alternatively, activation of functionally similar genes within the normal vertebrate genome. Tumor retroviruses have small RNA genomes.[11] Genetic analysis showed that, in many of these viruses, only one gene was sufficient to confer transforming capacity.[12,16] Molecular cloning of these viral oncogenes confirmed that they could, by themselves, cause tumors in animals and cellular transformation in tissue culture systems.[12,16,17] Similar results were obtained with DNA tumor viruses such as simian virus 40 (SV40) and polyomavirus, from which gene(s) were isolated that induced full transformation.[13,16,18] Conditional mutants for transformation were shown to map to the oncogenes.[19,20]

The concept of viral transformation as mediated by specific viral genes therefore became accepted. The problem of relating this phenomenon to human cancer remained. Despite the plethora of animal tumor viruses that were being isolated in the 1970s, it was difficult to characterize firmly any human tumor as infectious in mode of spread or viral in origin. It was possible that viral agents were difficult to isolate. Indeed, over the past 10 years, viruses have been shown to be important in the development of several human tumors (see Chapter 3, this volume). For the great majority of tumors, however, there is no evidence of a viral etiology. The possibility that latent oncogenes are present as a normal part of the vertebrate genome was considered.[21–23] Mutational activation of such oncogenes would be sufficient to induce the transformed phenotype, in a manner analogous to viral transduction of similar activated genes. Of course, it also was possible that oncogenes only played a role in viral oncogenesis, and that fundamentally different processes were involved in the ontogeny of most human tumors.

ONCOGENES AND PROTO-ONCOGENES

Initial attempts to identify functional or structural homologues of DNA tumor viruses in vertebrate genomes met with no success. However, in 1976, Stehlin and colleagues used solution hybridization techniques to determine that the oncogene responsible for the tumorigenicity of Rous sarcoma virus was represented by homologous sequences in the chicken genome.[24] Further work extended this finding to many other retroviral oncogenes.[4,14,16,23] Complete sequencing of multiple viral oncogenes and of their homologues in animal genomes revealed several important points. Most of the viral oncogenes had homologues in all of the vertebrate genomes analyzed.[16,23] Comparison of the cDNA sequences and intron-exon structure of the vertebrate genes made it clear that these genes were normal components of the genome and that the retrovirus had transduced them from these genomes, rather than the reverse.[16,23] Furthermore, whereas homologous genes from different organisms differed from each other in patterns consistent with evolutionary drift, with functionally important regions tending to display high degrees of conservation, their viral homologues often were altered or mutated substantially.[15,16,23] In some cases, the viral gene was altered during transduction, recombination having occurred during this process, yielding a fusion protein comprised of part of the oncogene and part of a viral protein (often the *gag* structural protein).[25,26] Multiple mutations also were identified.[16] The data suggested that oncogene-encoded proteins play a role in the physiology of normal cells, and that their mutation or changes in their regulation lead to transformation.[23] It further implied that mutational activation of the normal gene could occur by a variety of mechanisms not confined to those events associated with the retroviral life cycle.

The genes responsible for transformation in both naturally occurring and viral-induced tumors retained the designation *oncogene*. Their normal, unaltered forms were called *proto-oncogenes*.[14–16,26]

CONFIRMATION OF THE ONCOGENE HYPOTHESIS

It still remained to be proven that the mutations present in viral oncogenes were responsible for their transforming function and that proto-oncogenes in human tumors were altered and contributed to the transformed phenotype. This work was made easier by the development of in vitro assays and animal models with which transformation could be studied. A variety of criteria have been defined with which to assess whether cells growing in tissue culture display the malignant phenotype. These include characteristic morphologic changes,[27] immortalization in culture,[28] growth in low concentrations of serum or in the absence of serum,[29–31] changes in glucose transport and switch to anaerobic metabolism,[30] loss of contact inhibition associated with the continued growth and piling up of cells that have become confluent,[31] growth in soft agar (independence of the requirement for anchorage to the substratum),[32] and tumorigenicity in nude mice.[33,34] The operational correlate for malignant transformation in cell culture has become the ability of immortalized cells to grow in anchorage-independent fashion and to form tumors in nude mice.[34] To validate this definition, it has been shown that many, although by no means all, human tumor cells that have been adapted to cell culture display this phenotype.[35]

Several fibroblast cell lines from different vertebrate species have been selected to grow permanently, without becoming senescent, in cell culture.[36] These so-called immortalized cell lines are not fully transformed, however, because they are contact inhibited and they neither grow in soft agar nor form tumors in nude mice.[34,36] These cell lines can be transformed fully by infection with tumor viruses or when they are transfected with viral oncogenes.[16,31,34,37] Cell lines such as NIH 3T3 became useful systems for assessing the transforming potential of oncogenes with different structures.

Using such systems, it was found that, whereas the viral oncogenes *ras* and *src* (v-*ras* and v-*src*) could transform

NIH 3T3 cells in culture and could induce tumors in mice when encoded in retroviruses, the homologous proto-oncogenes from chickens or rodents did not have this capability or were much less efficient in conveying the phenotype.[38-41] Thus, the idea that oncogenes were activated forms of proto-oncogenes in regard to transformation capacity was given credence. The construction of recombinant chimeric *ras* genes comprised partly of the proto-oncogene and partly of the oncogene localized the region responsible for the transforming capacity of the protein to its amino-terminal region.[42,43] Sequencing of this region revealed that a single base pair change leading to a replacement of the glycine at codon 12 with a variety of other amino acids leads to the acquisition of transforming potential of the *ras* gene.[42,43] (Later work showed that mutations at positions 13, 59, and 61 were also oncogenic.)[43] Thus, the hypothesis that mutation of the proto-oncogene during recombination or viral transduction of the proto-oncogene is responsible for causing a gene that regulates normal cellular function to become a transforming gene was borne out. Other viral oncogenes, such as v-*src*, v-*raf*, and *erbB* later were shown to be activated by point mutations, deletions, or both.[15,39,44,45]

Mutations were not the only mechanisms found by which retroviral oncogenes became activated. In some cases, the viral *gag*-proto-oncogene product fusion protein was activated, either because the recombinatorial event resulted in the deletion of inhibitory sequences in the proto-oncogene product or because of activation by the *gag* sequence itself.[46] This sequence can cause the fusion protein to become compartmentalized to the membrane.[11]

In other cases, the viral oncogene was not mutated at all, or it was shown that the mutations were not necessary for oncogenic activation. In several of these instances, it was shown that transformation is dependent on juxtaposition of the proto-oncogene to the viral long terminal repeat (LTR), a strong promoter.[15] The result of the juxtaposition is overexpression or loss of appropriate transcriptional regulation of the protein. Thus, increase in the activity of the protein product of the gene, resulting either from changes in its structure or from its expression at high levels or at inappropriate times, leads to oncogenicity. In fact, this point was emphasized when retroviruses that induced tumors more slowly were analyzed.[11,47] These viruses induce few tumors, with a long latency of many months and cause only small numbers of tumors in infected animals, as opposed to the acutely transforming viruses, which have short latencies of weeks and induce many tumors. Oncogenes were identified fairly easily in the genomes of the acutely transforming viruses but were not found in those that transformed slowly. The mystery of how such viruses induced transformation was solved when it was shown that a "slow"-transforming virus, the avian leukosis virus, transformed cells when the provirus was integrated in the genome at a site upstream of the *myc* gene coding sequences.[47] The effect of this event was to place *myc* under the transcriptional control of the viral LTR. Thus, only those cells in which this integration site was used became transformed. In contrast, retroviruses containing the *myc* gene in which it is under the control of the viral LTR can transform cells without regard to integration site and are acutely transforming.[48]

ONCOGENES AND NATURALLY OCCURRING TUMORS

At this point, it was clear that the cell contained proto-oncogenes which encoded products that probably regulated normal cell division and differentiation and that many RNA tumor viruses transformed cells by activating these proto-oncogenes in the cell, either because mutated, activated proto-oncogenes were part of the viral genome that had been introduced into the cell or because the provirus was integrated near a cellular proto-oncogene and had activated its expression. The issue now became whether this mechanism was at all important in the genesis of human tumors.

Viruses are known to contribute to the etiology of only a few human tumors (see Chapter 3, this volume). The few retroviruses associated with the development of human T-cell malignancy (human T-cell leukemia viruses) or lymphomas and a variety of other tumors (human immunodeficiency viruses) are not acutely transforming and do not harbor obvious activated proto-oncogenes.[49,50] The mechanism by which they transform cells remains obscure. At any rate, a viral etiology has not been demonstrated for the great majority of human tumor types.

The initial evidence showing that activation of proto-oncogenes occurred in human tumors by non–viral-associated mechanisms and that this activation was important in their development came from several sources. It was reasoned that, if human tumors harbored activated oncogenes, introduction of human tumor DNA into normal cells could cause their transformation. The development of techniques for the transfection of high-molecular-weight DNA into animal cells[51] and the use of NIH 3T3 cells as recipients so that transformation could be assessed in vitro[52] enabled several investigators to determine whether activated proto-oncogenes were present in human tumor cell lines. Because introduction of cloned viral oncogenes such as v-*ras* and v-*src* into NIH 3T3 cells induces transformation that can be scored easily by the appearance of transformed foci, it was thought that, if activated oncogenes were present in human tumors cells, introduction of their genomic DNA into NIH 3T3 cells also would lead to transformation. This idea proved to be correct; introduction of genomic DNA purified from human bladder carcinoma cell lines into NIH 3T3 cells led to the formation of transformed foci at much greater frequency than observed when control DNA from normal cells or the recipient cell was used.[53,54] These foci, when isolated and propagated, were able to grow in soft agar and were tumorigenic in nude mice. Later the experiment was replicated with DNA derived from many other tumor cell lines and from tumor tissue.[4,43]

Thus, human tumor cells contained a gene or genes that could act like viral oncogenes in terms of their ability to transform immortalized fibroblasts in cell culture. The nature of these gene(s) was unknown. Human genes introduced into murine cells can be identified, isolated, and cloned by virtue of the existence of species-specific repetitive sequences.[55] However, large amounts of DNA are introduced into the genome when high-molecular-weight DNA is transfected. To get rid of human genes that were unassociated with the transformed phenotype, genomic DNA from NIH 3T3 transformants was transfected into NIH 3T3 cells.[55,56] Secondary transformants were isolated and the process was repeated. Any human DNA in the tertiary transfectants that resulted almost certainly would contain sequences required for transformation. It was striking, therefore, that, when the transferred gene was isolated, cloned, and identified, it turned out to be the homologue of the human Ha-*ras* gene.[57–59] Furthermore, the gene was mutated at codon 12, the activating mutation for the viral oncogene.[60–62] These findings confirmed the hypothesis that the fundamental processes involved in human carcinogesis and in retroviral carcinogenesis are similar and involve the activation of proto-oncogenes.

These data were reinforced with discoveries that had their origin in another field—cancer cytogenetics. Characteristic translocations, deletions, and other chromosomal lesions have been described for a variety of tumors.[2,63] These were postulated to represent changes that activated or inactivated particular genes responsible for the regulation of normal cellular growth.[63,64] Thus, the 9:22 Philadelphia translocation present in almost all cases of chronic myelogenous leukemia[65] and the 2;8, 8;14, and 14;18 translocations that together are present in most case of Burkitt's lymphoma[66] were believed to be translocations that caused genetic changes crucial to the development of these diseases.[63–66]

Advances in molecular biology allowed the cloning of these translocations and the identification of the genes present at their breakpoints. Strikingly, each of the three Burkitt's translocations involved a common gene on chromosome 14—the proto-oncogene c-*myc*.[66–69] Furthermore, the DNA sequences to which the c-*myc* gene had been juxtaposed on chromosomes 2, 8, and 18 all fell into the same class, transcriptional enhancers of immunoglobulin genes (kappa light chain, heavy chain, and lambda light chain, respectively).[66,69] These genes are transcriptionally active in B-cell lineages. So the c-*myc* gene becomes transcriptionally activated in Burkitt's lymphoma in a manner analogous to its activation by acutely transforming and slowly transforming retroviruses: it is juxtaposed to active transcriptional signals.

Similarly, when the Philadelphia translocation was cloned, it was shown that the translocated gene on chromosome 9 was the human proto-oncogene homologue of the transforming oncogene of the Abelson leukemia virus.[70] The translocation results in the deletion of the amino-terminal portion of the *abl* gene product and its replacement with the amino-terminal of the *bcr* (breakpoint cluster region) gene.[71,72] This fusion protein is activated in that its tyrosine kinase activity is elevated[73] and in that its introduction into murine bone marrow stem cells leads to a chronic myelogenous leukemia–like syndrome.[74,75] v-*abl* is activated in a similar manner, as the *gag-abl* fusion protein, with its amino-terminal portion replaced by *gag* sequences.[46] Thus, in both the Burkitt's and

Philadelphia chromosome translocations, the proto-oncogene homologue of a previously identified viral oncogene was identified at the breakpoint. Moreover, the mechanism whereby the translocation activated the proto-oncogene was analogous to that involved in activating the viral oncogene.

Another class of cytogenetic abnormalities specific to cancer cells are those due to somatic gene amplification.[63,76,77] This includes double minute chromosomes and homogeneously staining regions, which are the cytogenetic manifestations of tandemly repeated, multiple copies of DNA.[2,63,78] Such structures often are present in malignant cells and almost never on normal cells.[79] The amplified sequences of DNA they contain are assumed to confer a selective advantage to the cell. This was borne out by the first identification of genes present in double minute chromosomes in cancer cells, which revealed amplified copies of drug resistance genes such as that encoding dihydrofolate reductase.[80] In fact, cell lines grown in regular medium lost gene amplification over time.[81]

Some tumor cells contain amplified genes despite never having been exposed to drug.[63,76,77] This is especially common in cells derived from neuroblastoma or from small-cell lung cancer.[76,77,82,83] When the amplified genes in these tumors first were identified, they again turned out to be homologues of viral oncogenes, especially v-*myc*.[82,83] In this way, other members of the *myc* family (N-*myc* and L-*myc*) were discovered.[82,84] In some of these tumors, the amplified genes are carried on double minute chromosomes, which lack centromeres and are not evenly distributed between daughter cells at mitosis.[76–78] These structures tend to be lost from the cell if they do not carry genes that convey a selective advantage.[81] The finding that these cytogenetic abnormalities represented the amplification of proto-oncogenes enhanced the idea that activation of these genes by virtue of overexpression of their products was associated with carcinogenesis in human tumors. The stability in the tumor cell of the double minute chromosomes carrying these genes suggested that the amplified proto-oncogene product was necessary for maintaining the transformed phenotype.

Thus, it has been shown that viral oncogenes are activated homologues of proto-oncogenes present in the normal genome and that activation renders them oncogenic. Activated proto-oncogene homologues are present in human tumors as well and can be shown to be activated by structural or regulatory mutations that are analogous to those that activate viral oncogenes. Chromosomal abnormalities characteristically found in certain tumors represent structural lesions that activate proto-oncogenes. The presence of these lesions in each of the tumor cells and the persistence of double minute chromosomes in some tumors suggests that proto-oncogene activation is required for the maintenance of the transformed phenotype.

Taken together, these data suggest that human carcinogenesis, at least in part, results from activation of endogenous proto-oncogenes and that the mechanisms involved in the development of naturally occurring tumors have much in common with those that operate in viral oncogenesis. The hypothesis that cancer occurs because of activating mutations in genes that regulate normal growth and development and that mutated homologues transduced by retroviruses are viral oncogenes is supported strongly by these data. Furthermore, these data provide a unifying explanation for findings obtained in the disparate fields of cytogenetics, viral oncology, and the cell biology of transformed cells.

It should be noted, however, that the evidence for causality is circumstantial. Moreover, many instances of overexpression or elevated activity of proto-oncogene protein products for which no genetic mechanism is known have been described in human tumors.[26,29,85] In most of these cases, the biologic significance of the observation is unknown. Activation may be a result of transformation or a reflection of the differentiated state of the tissue of origin without significance in terms of the malignant phenotype. Alternatively, it may play an important role in regulating the transformed state.

WHAT DO ONCOGENES DO?

The genetic and biologic data that viral oncogenes and mutated proto-oncogenes are involved in carcinogenesis are compelling, but do not explain the mechanisms by which they induce transformation. The normal function of proto-oncogene products and the mechanism by which their activation leads to transformation have been the focus of an enormous amount of investigation over the past 15 years. This work has revealed that the idea that proto-oncogene products are involved in the regulation of normal cellular growth and differentiation is correct. In fact, the identification of transforming genes and suppressor genes and the search for their normal functions in vertebrates as well as in yeast and *Drosophila* have contributed strongly to the current picture of regulation of the normal cell growth.

This work is reviewed in detail in this volume in the chapters dealing with growth factors, signal transduction, suppressor genes, the cell cycle, and viral oncogenesis. When viral oncogene products first were characterized, several observations were made. Some oncogenes easily could transform NIH 3T3 cells, whereas others could not.[85,86] Two properties of transformation in vitro, morphologic transformation and immortalization in cell culture, had been defined as key to the transformed phenotype.[27,28] Because NIH 3T3 is immortalized, genes causing it to become fully transformed were thought to exert a function specific to morphologic transformation. Oncogenes incapable of transforming NIH 3T3 cells were believed to supply an immortalizing function, which would have been redundant in that context. The basis thereby was created for explaining multistep carcinogenesis in terms of oncogenes with varying functions that cause different aspects of the transformed phenotype and thus for defining proto-oncogenes in terms of complementation groups.

Oncogenes such as v-*src*, v-*raf*, and the middle T polyoma virus protein, as well as members of the *ras* family, fell into the family of genes that induced morphologic transformation.[34,85,86] v-*myc*, v-*myb*, and the large T poly-

oma antigen were immortalizing genes that did not transform NIH 3T3.[34,85,86] Before anything was known about the function of these proteins, their subcellular localization allowed them to be divided into to those that were bound to the membrane or confined to the cytosol and those that were nuclear. These two classes crudely correlated with the groups defined by transformation capacity; that is, the nuclear proteins had immortalizing function, and those in the membrane or cytosol effected morphologic transformation.[16,85,86]

The first clue as to the actual function of these proteins came from the discovery that many of the viral oncoproteins catalyzed the phosphorylation of proteins on tyrosine residues.[15,16,29,87] The level of phosphotyrosine in protein was elevated as much as 10- to 20-fold in cells transformed by these oncogenes.[87,88] Studies on v-*src*, the prototypic tyrosine kinase, showed that mutants that lost their tyrosine kinase activity were defective for transformation and that, in temperature-sensitive mutants, transforming capacity and kinase activity were linked closely.[19,39,88] Thus, this posttranslational modification, which accounts for less than 1 per cent of total cellular protein phosphorylation, perhaps led to changes in affected proteins that caused transformation. The association of tyrosine phosphorylation with transformation was given mechanistic significance with the finding that transmembrane growth factor receptors also had tyrosine kinase activity.[87,89] These include the receptors for epidermal growth factor (EGF), platelet-derived growth factor (PDGF), colony stimulating factor 1 (CSF-1), stem cell growth factor, insulin, and many others.[89] When the growth factor binds to the extracellular portion of this type of receptor, its tyrosine kinase domain, which is located in the cytoplasm, becomes activated.[29,89–91] This activation then leads to the tyrosine phosphorylation of a variety of protein substrates. These phosphorylations presumably cause regulatory changes in the substrate proteins that result in the stimulation of cell division.

Thus, activated tyrosine protein kinases were associated in one type of system with the transformed state and in another with stimulation of cellular growth. An obvious inference was that cell growth is stimulated or turned off by varying levels of ligand and thus receptor tyrosine kinase activity, as well as by regulating substrate phosphorylation and other events that follow tyrosine kinase activation.[29,41,89,91] If so, one class of proto-oncogenes might be those that encode products that are elements of the pathway that transduces the growth factor signal. Mutations that activate this pathway either by causing the constitutive elevation of receptor tyrosine kinase activity or of an element downstream of the receptor, or by overexpressing one of these proteins, could convert these proto-oncogenes into transforming genes.

The confirmation of this hypothesis initially came from three striking discoveries. The first was that the specific activity of the v-*src* oncoprotein tyrosine kinase was elevated compared to that of c-*src* and that this difference was shown to be integral to the ability of v-*src* to transform cells.[92,93] Eventually, similar findings were obtained for many of the other tyrosine kinase proto-oncogenes.[29,94] Second, the *sis* oncogene, the transforming gene of the simian sarcoma virus, was shown to be the homologue of the B chain of PDGF.[95,96] Overexpression of the oncogene or of the proto-oncogene in fibroblasts induces their transformation by activating the PDGF receptor.[97] Activating the growth signal cascade by constitutively overexpressing the ligand, therefore, can result in transformation. Finally, the *erbB* oncogene, which encodes a tyrosine kinase, was found to be the truncated homologue of the EGF receptor.[98] The oncogene encodes the transmembrane and cytoplasmic portions of the molecule, including the tyrosine kinase catalytic domain, but only a very short extracellular domain. The carboxy-terminal domain also contains several other mutations.[98–100] These changes cause activation of the tyrosine kinase activity of the protein.[99,101] Thus, a mutation leading to the ligand-independent activation of the receptor such that it is fixed in the active state causes it to become transforming. Moreover, it was shown subsequently that amplification of other tyrosine kinase receptors also leads to transformation via an increase in intracellular tyrosine kinase activity.[29] Members of the EGF receptor family (including HER-2*neu* and EGFR) have been shown to be amplified or overexpressed in individual cases of human tumors of several types, including lung cancer and breast cancer.[102,103] These data supported the hypothesis that at least one class of proto-oncogene is comprised of elements of the growth factor signal transduction pathway and that mutations that cause these proteins to become oncogenic cause this pathway to become activated in an unregulated way.

Of course, it is now known that regulation of mitogenic signal transduction is accomplished by a network of positive and negative elements.[4,26,85,91,94] Alteration of any of these potentially can lead to activation of the pathway and contribute to transformation, including loss of inhibitory elements. Genes encoding inhibitory elements have been called suppressor genes,[104] and are discussed in Chapter 5.

In some sense, too much is made of the distinction between oncogenes and suppressor genes on a biochemical, if not the genetic level. Mutations in these genes affect different elements of the same pathways.[29,85,89,94,104–107] It is now known that activation of the mitogenic signal transduction cascade that normally is induced by growth factors is a common occurrence during carcinogesis and is mediated by mutations in regulatory genes.[94] In normal cells, the first step in this cascade after receptor activation by ligand is tyrosine phosphorylation of multiple substrates.[94] The most prominent substrate is usually the receptor itself.[89,90] Other proteins then bind to these phosphotyrosines via so-called SH2 domains.[108] SH2-containing proteins then transmit many aspects of the signal. One pathway that appears to be common to transduction of the signal from many growth factors involves activation of the p21^{ras} protein.[41,43,91]

There is actually a family of three closely related *ras* proto-oncogenes (Ha-*ras*, Ki-*ras*, and N-*ras*) that encode GTP-binding proteins that are in the active state when bound to GTP and inactive when bound to GDP.[41,43,91] A nucleotide exchange factor protein catalyzes the exchange of GDP for GTP and thus activates Ras.[91] A class of docking proteins binds the phosphorylated growth factor re-

ceptor via an SH2 domain and, through another domain (SH3), binds to the exchange factor.[91,109] Thus, activation and autophosphorylation of the growth factor receptor leads to exchange factor activation of Ras.[41,91] The Ras protein has weak endogenous GTPase activity that is activated by a family of GTPase-activating proteins (GAPs).[10,110] Activated Ras is deactivated by stimulation of the conversion of Ras-GTP to Ras-GDP by GAP.[10,110,111]

Activated Ras binds to a serine protein kinase, Raf, which then causes the activation of members of a family of serine kinases, including those in the mitogen-activated protein (MAP) kinase family.[112,113] These kinases have multiple substrates, including some transcription factors.[114] This pathway is necessary for the stimulation of cell division induced by the growth factor. Interruption of the pathway with receptor antibodies, tyrosine kinase inhibitors, anti-p21^{ras} antibodies, or dominant negative mutants of the *ras* or *raf* genes prevents growth factor action.[41,112,115–119]

This is a cursory and oversimplified outline of what is known about the mechanism of growth factor induction of mitogenesis. Although the reality is much more complex, it is obvious that abnormal activation of this pathway might lead to the unregulated pattern of growth characteristic of transformation. Indeed, many elements of this pathway originally were described as viral oncogenes. These include the oncogenes *sis,* the homologue of the B chain of PDGF; *erbB* and *fms,* homologues of the EGF and CSF-1 receptors, respectively; other tyrosine kinases, such as *src, ras,* and *raf;* and transcription factors affected or induced by this pathway, such as *fos, jun,* and *myc.*[4,14–16,29,43,87,94,95,98] Thus, many of the activated proto-oncogenes function by causing constitutive mitogenic signal transduction.

How Is Transformation Induced?

How activation of this pathway induces transformation in NIH 3T3 cells is not fully understood. Cells transformed by *ras* or *src* grow abnormally, but also have altered morphology, cytoskeletal structure, and intercellular junctions, and respond abnormally to stimuli that induce differentiation.[27,33,120–122] Which of these changes are necessary for maintenance of the transformed phenotype is unclear, but it seems reasonable to infer that abnormal regulation of cellular proliferation plays a major role.

Many of the originally isolated oncogenes that fell into the membrane or cytosolic group turned out to encode elements of mitogenic signal transduction pathways. The other major group of viral oncogenes were homologues of proto-oncogenes that encoded nuclear proteins.[4,16,87] Many of these—*myc,*[123] *myb,*[124] *fos,*[125] *erbA,*[126] and members of the *ets* family[127]—later were shown to be transcription factors. Subsequently, cloning of translocations specific to a variety of tumors, especially lymphoid malignancies, and characterization of the involved genes identified many other transcription factors as putative proto-oncogenes that were activated by translocation.[128–130]

Presumably these factors function by altering the expression of key proteins or families of proteins that regulate aspects of the transformed phenotype. Although the DNA sequences to which many of these factors bind have been defined and genes that these factors regulate identified, the key proteins required for induction of transformation remain unknown. The idea that particular transcription factors may act as oncogenes when inappropriately expressed or activated is an attractive one in terms of explaining the pleiotropic changes that occur in the transformed cell. The programmed induction or repression of the expression of groups of proteins involved in DNA synthesis, mitosis, cellular migration, embryogenesis, wound healing, or differentiation occurs normally. Unregulated expression of these programs could lead to the multiple changes associated with the invasive, metastatic, or proliferative phenotypes of transformed cells.

Cell Cycle Deregulation

Ultimately, one aspect of the transformed state must, at some level, involve deregulation of the cell cycle. This subject is discussed in detail elsewhere in this volume. However, there are several points relevant to oncogene function that deserve to be emphasized. The cell cycle is controlled at several set points; a restriction point(s) in late G_1 determines whether a cell will synthesize DNA and traverse the cycle, arrest, differentiate, or undergo programmed cell death.[131] Cells that are starved or have damaged DNA may arrest here.[131–133] Another restriction point regulates passage from G_2 to M and is also sensitive to DNA damage as well as to the integrity of the mitotic apparatus.[131]

Passage through these restriction points and thus traversal of the cell cycle is positively controlled by a group of cell cycle–dependent serine kinases (cdks).[132,134,135] These kinases are regulated and activated by a set of proteins, cyclins, whose expression and activity vary in a cell cycle–dependent manner.[107,132,134] Cyclin B regulates cdks at G_2/M. Cyclins C, D, and E are expressed in early to mid-G_1; cyclin A expression increases in late G_1 and S. G_1-specific cdks may act, at least in part, by phosphorylating Rb, the protein encoded by the retinoblastoma suppressor gene, and consequently activating factors required for the transcription of proteins involved in DNA synthesis.[136–138]

It is clear that many oncogenes may act to deregulate this process, resulting in the inhibition of normal pathways involved in inducing differentiation or apoptosis or in stimulating traversal of the cell cycle. For instance, overexpression of transcription factors that normally bind to Rb might bypass cyclin-cdk control and lead to unregulated progression through the cell cycle. There is some evidence that this is the case for the Myc protein.[139] It also seems that the growth factor–activated signal transduction pathway must in some way regulate cyclin-cdk control mechanisms in order to induce proliferation. These mechanisms have not yet been defined.

It may be assumed that abnormalities in the cell cycle regulators themselves would lead to abnormal growth. So far, identified abnormalities have involved predominantly the loss of negative regulators of the cell cycle encoded by suppressor genes. These are discussed elsewhere in this volume and include lesions in the *p53* and *Rb* genes.[104,106] To date, genetic abnormalities in one G_1 cyclin have been reported in human tumor cells. The cyclin D1 gene is located on a segment of chromosome 11q13 that very often is amplified in several tumor types, including breast and esophageal carcinoma.[140,141] Cyclin D1 is overexpressed and amplified in these tumors. Furthermore, there is evidence that cyclin D1 is the oncogene present at the 11q13 breakpoint in parathyroid tumors and B-cell lymphomas.[142] Although there is no functional evidence, it is likely that increased levels of cyclin D1 contribute to the transformed phenotype in these cases via deregulation of cdks or interaction with the Rb protein.[107,137]

One aspect of cell cycle regulation concerns whether or not the cell will proliferate. Another is involved with the fate of cells that are arrested at a checkpoint. Such cells may remain viable at the checkpoint, but under normal conditions are more likely to go into a quiescent (G_0) state, to differentiate, or to undergo programmed cell death (apoptosis).[132,133,143] These are normally regulated processes, and their inhibition may play a role in carcinogenesis or in maintaining the transformed state. These mechanisms just now are being defined, and previously identified oncogenes and suppressor genes such as *myc* and *p53* probably play a role in their regulation.[133,143] *bcl-2* is a gene that was identified as present at the breakpoint in the common (14;18) translocation in follicular lymphomas.[144] When overexpressed, it acts to prevent the apoptosis associated with normal B-cell development, and thus leads to accumulation of a population of proliferating B cells.[145] The delineation of pathways that regulate the balance among cellular proliferation, differentiation, and apoptosis is currently an area of intense research interest. Mutations that upset this balance in favor of proliferation are probably fundamental to the development of most cancers.

MULTISTEP CARCINOGENESIS

Many proto-oncogenes now have been identified and some of the pathways that they regulate have begun to be characterized. A fundamental problem arises in the difference between viral oncogenesis and the development of human cancers. The former often seems to be a single- or two-hit phenomenon, with the one or two oncogenes encoded by the particular retrovirus both necessary and sufficient for the tumorigenesis. Moreover, single cloned viral oncogenes or their activated counterparts derived from human tumors are able to transform immortalized rodent cells in tissue culture, and their expression in these cells has been shown to be adequate for the activation of mitogenic signal transduction. In contrast, as pointed out earlier in this chapter, the kinetics of the development of human cancer is most consistent with a multihit process occurring over several years.[7] In addition, individual human tumors have been shown to harbor multiple genetic abnormalities, sometimes more than ten.[146]

The solution to this problem is the mass of experimental data that suggests that, in the great majority of cases, including those of viral oncogenesis, multiple genetic lesions are required for transformation, and that the lesions involved comprise the activation of proto-oncogenes and the inactivation of suppressor oncogenes.[87] This last is tautologic, because the definition of a proto-oncogene has become so loose as to be almost equivalent to "a genetic lesion present in all of the cells of a tumor." Be that as it may, many such lesions are homologous to or in the same family as previously described viral oncogenes.

Single oncogenes can, by themselves, transform NIH 3T3 cells, but not normal embryo fibroblasts.[86,147] The latter, it was discovered, can be transformed by combinations of oncogenes. Assay systems were developed in which rat embryo fibroblasts could be transformed with pairs of oncogenes such as polyoma large T and middle T, or myc and v-ras.[34,148] Such systems could be used to establish functional complementation groups. When this was done, one group was comprised of nuclear oncogenes such as myc, myb, fos, and polyoma large T, whereas the other group contained genes encoding activated tyrosine kinases and members of the ras family.[87,147] The two groups were almost exactly congruent with those defined above by cellular localization and presumed function, that is, immortalization genes complemented with "transforming" genes.[86,87,147] One can infer from these data that NIH 3T3 and other immortalized rodent "indicator" cells already had accumulated several oncogenic "hits" and therefore were susceptible to transformation by one oncogene. A corollary conclusion is that the molecular changes that already have occurred in NIH 3T3 cells strongly complement with activated ras, so that the high frequency of ras activation compared to other oncogenes in human tumors may be an artifact of the assay system.[149]

Experiments with transgenic mice also indicate that activation of single oncogenes is inadequate to induce cancer. Mice that carry activated ras, myc, or other oncogenes under the control of a strong, tissue-specific promoter do develop tumors, but the tumors are clonal and relatively rare, occurring after a latency period.[87,150,151] If expression of one activated oncogene were sufficient for tumorigenesis, all of the cells of the organ that express the oncogene would become transformed. Instead, the data suggest that, although expression of the oncogene increases the probability of transformation, additional events are required for its development. Indeed, mating of ras and myc transgenic mice yields an F1 generation with a greatly increased incidence of tumors.[152] Even so, these tumors are monoclonal, suggesting that, although myc and activated ras do act cooperatively, further events are needed for full transformation.

What, then, is the explanation for the rapid induction of tumors by retroviruses containing only one activated oncogene? The answer is not known, but one likely possibility is that the cells that become transformed are susceptible to the particular gene carried by the virus because they previously have accumulated other, complementary mutational "hits."

The cooperativity of oncogenes from different complementation groups in inducing transformation in model cell cultures and animal systems may be analogous to the multistep development of human tumors. However, despite the crude ability to ascribe common functional characteristics to members of the complementation groups, the mechanisms underlying the requirement for multiple genes and the absolute functional determinants of the complementation groups are unknown.

ONCOGENES AND HUMAN CANCER

Over the past several years, the knowledge acquired from model systems about the identity and nature of proto-oncogenes and suppressor genes has been applied to the study of the development of human tumors. Many of these data are reviewed in other chapters in this volume. There are some general points that should be made here.

As stated above, human tumors can be shown to contain mutations in many genes that in other contexts have been shown to regulate growth or differentiation. It generally has been concluded that each of these lesions is likely to have a selective effect on tumor survival or growth and therefore to be important in tumorigenesis or tumor progression. For the most part, the evidence for this is inferential and not direct. Only in very few cases has specific inhibition of activated oncogene products been shown to reverse transformation. Tyrosine kinase inhibitors and inhibitors of ras farnesylation have selective effects on tumors,[116] (N. Rosen and L. Sepp-Lorenzino, unpublished data), but the former lack specificity and the mechanism of action of the latter is not clear. Antibodies to growth factor receptors and antisense oligonucleotides have been used to reduce expression of proto-oncogene protein products and also have been shown to inhibit the growth or revert the transformed phenotype of specific human tumor cell lines.[153,154] Suggestive as these experiments are, they are almost all performed in cell lines, which clouds their interpetation. In addition, it is difficult to distinguish between antitumor effects and toxic effects because of the importance of the normal proto-oncogene product to the viability of the cell. In at least one case, homologous recombination techniques have been used to delete the mutated allele selectively from a colon carcinoma cell line that is heterozygous for mutated K-ras.[155] The cell retaining only the normal allele still could proliferate but no longer displayed the transformed phenotype.

Nevertheless, despite the paucity of data for causality, a mass of circumstantial data, summarized above, lead to the conclusion that many, perhaps most, of the genetic lesions present in all of the cells of the tumor contribute to its pathogenesis. These data include the activation of genes in human tumors that are homologous to viral oncogenes, the transforming capacity of activated genes isolated from human tumors in model tissue culture systems, the tumorigenic effect of these genes in transgenic animals, and the localization of these genes to chromosomal abnormalities peculiar to particular tumors.

Several themes seem to be emerging as more human tumors are analyzed on a molecular level. Activation of certain proto-oncogenes such as *ras* and *myc* seems to be involved commonly in human tumorigenesis, whereas genetic activation of others, such as *src*, seem to be rare events. Furthermore, it is not clear why some elements of signal transduction pathways, such as tyrosine kinase receptors, p21[ras] and some of the transcription factors often are found to be activated, but others (MAP kinases, exchange factors) have not been found to be involved. These observations may reflect profound differences in the biochemical and biologic consequences of activating these genes, or they may be merely artifacts of our assay systems and of which genes are studied most intensively.

Similarly, there is an emerging tissue specificity to the observed pattern of oncogene activation in human tumors. Amplification of the N-*myc* gene occurs very commonly in neuroblastoma and small-cell lung cancer but is extremely rare in other adult solid tumors.[82] The *bcr-abl* translocation almost always is present in chronic myelogenous leukemia and is peculiar to that disease and its variants.[65] Even a commonly activated gene such as *ras* is found to be mutated in high percentages of pancreatic, colorectal, and lung carcinomas, but almost never in esophageal, prostatic, or mammary carcinomas.[146,149,156] These findings almost certainly result from tissue-specific differences in the function of these genes and in mechanisms of transformation. The basis for these differences is almost entirely unknown. As discussed earlier, however, the differences sometimes may be due to observer artifact. For instance, it is not clear whether the frequent isolation of genes encoding transcription factors in translocations from T-cell malignancies reflects a peculiarity of the pathogenesis of these diseases or is an artifact of the relative ease of their detection in these cells.[143]

UNANSWERED QUESTIONS

An enormous amount has been learned about the pathogenesis of human tumors from the study of the molecular biology, cell biology, and biochemistry of oncogenes. We now broadly understand many of the mechanisms underlying tumor development and progression. However, much work remains before we have a detailed understanding of these processes. The work thus far has been reductionist (concentrated on the effects of single activated oncogenes), has stressed an understanding of the mechanism of the proliferative phenotype of the transformed cells, and has focused on useful but perhaps not universally applicable model systems.

Malignant transformation in the host requires uncontrolled proliferation and invasion into adjacent tissues, with subsequent metastasis. In the absence of the latter, the former results in a benign tumor. In model systems, certain oncogenes, such as *ras*, may contribute to both phenotypes.[122] The biochemical mechanisms underlying the effect of oncogenes on invasion and metastasis are largely unknown but now are being studied with increased interest (see Chapter 11, this volume).

As discussed earlier in this chapter, many molecular lesions have been described in human tumors, especially adult solid tumors of epithelial origin, and there is an emerging tissue specific pattern of activation. Virtually nothing is known about how combinations of lesions lead to aspects of the malignant phenotype or about the basis for tissue specificity. One of the problems in this regard is that studies of mechanism have utilized a few felicitous model systems—NIH 3T3 and Rat-1 rodent fibroblasts, the pheochromocytoma cell line PC-12, and mitogen- or antigen-activated T cells. There has not been much work on mechanism in model systems derived from the specific epithelial lineages from which most human tumors develop. We cannot disregard the possibility that lineage-specific mechanisms may be important in regulation of the transformed phenotype.

When these model systems are developed and studied, some attention must be paid to determining which molecular lesions are irrelevant or redundant, which were necessary for tumorigenesis but have become redundant for maintenance of transformation, and which are required for the tumor cell to continue to grow or invade. Many human tumor cells have multiple lesions in the same signal transduction pathway. For instance, tyrosine kinases are activated or overexpressed and *ras* is mutated in many colorectal and pancreatic cancer cell lines.[146,157] Whether this represents functional redundancy or synergy has not been studied. Determination of the molecular pathways required for maintenance of the transformed phenotype will be crucial for the development of effective specific therapies.

REFERENCES

1. Baserga R: The Biology of Cell Reproduction. Cambridge, MA, Harvard University Press, 1985
2. Heim S, Mitelman F: Primary chromosome abnormalities in human neoplasia. Adv Cancer Res 52:1, 1989
3. Fidler IJ, Hart IR: Biologic diversity in metastatic neoplasms—origins and implications. Science 217:998, 1982
4. Weinberg RA: Oncogenes, antioncogenes, and the molecular bases of multistep carcinogenesis. Cancer Res 49:3713, 1989
5. Doll R, Peto R: The Causes of Cancer: Quantitative Estimates of Avoidable Risks of Cancer in the United States Today. New York, Oxford University Press, 1981
6. Cooper C, Grover P (eds): Chemical Carcinogenesis and Mutagenesis I and II. Berlin, Springer-Verlag, 1990
7. Peto R, Roe FJC, Lee PN, et al: Cancer and aging in mice and men. Br J Cancer 32:411, 1975
8. Burnet FM: Cancer: A biological approach. BMJ 1:779, 1957
9. Cairns J: The origin of human cancers. Nature 289:353, 1981
10. Tooze J (ed): DNA Tumor Viruses. Cold Spring Harbor, NY, Cold Spring Harbor Laboratory Press, 1980
11. Weiss W, Teich N, Varmus H, Coffin J (eds): RNA Tumor Viruses. Cold Spring Harbor, NY, Cold Spring Harbor Laboratory Press, 1982
12. Copeland NG, Zelenetz AD, Cooper GM: Transformation by subgenomic fragments of Rous sarcoma virus DNA. Cell 19:863, 1980
13. Treisman RH, Novack V, Favalora J, Kamen R: Transformation of rat cells by an altered polyoma virus genome expressing only the middle T protein. Nature 292:595, 1981
14. Varmus H: An historical overview of oncogenes. In Weinberg RA (ed): Oncogenes and the Molecular Origins of Cancer. Cold Spring Harbor, NY, Cold Spring Harbor Laboratory Press, 1989, pp 3–44
15. Bishop JM: The molecular genetics of cancer. Science 235:305, 1987

16. Bishop JM: Viral oncogenes. Cell 42:23, 1985
17. Martin GS: Rous sarcoma virus: A function required for the maintenance of the transformed state. Nature 227:1021, 1970
18. Abrahams PJ, Mulder C, van de Voorde A, et al: Transformation of primary rat kidney cells by fragments of simian virus 40. J Virol 16:818, 1975
19. Sefton BM, Hunter T, Beemon K: Temperature-sensitive transformation by Rous sarcoma virus and temperature-sensitive protein kinase activity. J Virol 33:220, 1980
20. Schaffhausen BS, Silver JE, Benjamin TL: T-antigen(s) in cells productively infected by wild-type polyoma virus and mutant NG-18. Proc Natl Acad Sci USA 75:79, 1978
21. Huebner RJ, Todaro GJ: Oncogenes of RNA tumor viruses as determinants of cancer. Proc Natl Acad Sci USA 64:1087, 1969
22. Todaro GJ, Huebner RJ: The viral oncogene hypothesis: New evidence. Proc Natl Acad Sci USA 69:1009, 1972
23. Bishop JM, Varmus H. Functions and origins of retroviral transforming genes. In: Weiss W, Teich N, Varmus H, Coffin J (eds): RNA Tumor Viruses. Cold Spring Harbor, NY, Cold Spring Harbor Laboratory Press, 1982, pp 999–1108
24. Stehlin D, Varmus HE, Bishop JM, Vogt PK: DNA related to the transforming gene(s) of avian sarcoma viruses is present in normal avian DNA. Nature 260:170, 1976
25. Moelling K, Bunte T, Greiser-Wilke I, et al: Properties of the avian viral transforming proteins gag-myc, myc, and gag-mil. Cancer Cells 2:173, 1984
26. Bishop JM: Molecular themes in oncogenesis. Cell 64:235, 1991
27. Temin HM, Rubin H: Characteristics of an assay for Rous sarcoma virus and Rous sarcoma cells in tissue culture. Virology 6:669, 1958
28. Newbold RF: Multistep malignant transformation of mammalian cells by carcinogens: Induction of immortality as a key event. Carcinogenesis 9:17, 1985
29. Aaronson SA: Growth factors and cancer. Science 254:1146, 1991
30. Hatanaka M, Hanafusa H: Analysis of a functional change in membrane in the process of cell transformation by Rous sarcoma virus: Alteration in the characteristics of sugar transport. Virology 41:647, 1970
31. Risser R, Pollack R: A non-selective analysis of SV40 transformation of mouse 3T3 cells. Virology 59:477, 1974
32. Weiss R: Studies on the loss of growth inhibition in cells infected with Rous sarcoma virus. Int J Cancer 6:333, 1970
33. Shin S, Freedman VH, Risser R, Pollack R: Tumorigenicity of virus-transformed cells in nude mice is correlated specifically with anchorage independent growth in vitro. Proc Natl Acad Sci USA 72:4435, 1975
34. Land H, Parada HF, Weinberg RA: Tumorigenic conversion of primary embryo fibroblasts requires at least two cooperating oncogenes. Nature 304:596, 1983
35. Park JG, Oie HK, Sugarbaker PH, et al: Characteristics of cell lines established from human colorectal carcinoma. Cancer Res 47:6710, 1987
36. Todaro GJ, Green H: Quantitative studies of the growth of mouse embryo cells in culture and their development into established cell lines. J Cell Biol 17:299, 1963
37. Todaro GJ, Green H: An assay for cellular transformation by SV40. Virology 23:117, 1964
38. Kato JY, Takeya T, Grandori C, et al: Amino acid substitutions sufficient to convert the nontransforming p60c-src protein to a transforming protein. Mol Cell Biol 6:4155, 1986
39. Hunter T: A tale of two src's: Mutatis mutandis. Cell 49:1, 1987
40. Chang EH, Furth ME, Scolnick EM, Lowy DR: Tumorigenic transformation of mammalian cells induced by a normal human gene homologous to the oncogene of Harvey murine sarcoma virus. Nature 297:479, 1982
41. Medema RH, Bos JL: The role of p21ras in receptor tyrosine kinase signaling. Crit Rev Oncog 4:615, 1993
42. Papageorge A, Lowy D, Scolnick E: Comparative biochemical properties of p21 ras molecules coded for by viral and cellular ras genes. J Virol 44:509, 1982
43. Barbacid M: Ras genes. Ann Rev Biochem 56:779, 1987
44. Rapp UR, Goldsborough MD, Mark GE: Structure and biological activity of v-RAF, a unique oncogene transduced by a retrovirus. Proc Natl Acad Sci USA 80:4218, 1983
45. Downward J, Yarden Y, Mayes E, et al: Close similarity of epidermal growth factor receptor and v-erb-B oncogene protein sequences. Nature 307:521, 1984
46. Prywes R, Foulkes JG, Rosenberg N, et al: Sequences of the A-MuLV protein needed for fibroblast and lymphoid cell transformation. Cell 34:569, 1983
47. Hayward WS, Neel BG, Astrin SM: Activation of a cellular oncogene by promoter insertion in ALV-induced lymphoid leukosis. Nature 290:475, 1981
48. Lipsick JS, Boyle WJ, Lampert MA, Baluda MA: The oncogene of avian myeloblastosis virus is an altered proto-oncogene. Cancer Cells 2:143, 1984
49. Seika M, Eddy R, Shows TR, et al: Non-specific integration of the HTLV provirus genome into adult T-cell leukemia cells. Nature 309:640, 1984
50. McClure MO, Weiss RA: Human immunodeficiency virus and related viruses. Curr Top AIDS 1:95, 1987
51. Wigler M, Pellicer A, Silverstein S, Axel R: Biochemical transfer of single-copy eucaryotic genes using total cellular DNA as donor. Cell 14:725, 1978
52. Shih C, Shilo B-Z, Goldfarb MP, et al: Passage of phenotypes of chemically transformed cells via transfection of DNA and chromatin. Proc Natl Acad Sci USA 76:5714, 1979
53. Shih C, Padhy LC, Murray M, Weinberg RA: Transforming genes of carcinomas and neuroblastomas introduced into mouse fibroblasts. Nature 290:261, 1981
54. Krontiris TG, Cooper GM: Transforming activity of human tumor DNAs. Proc Natl Acad Sci USA 78:1181, 1981
55. Shih C, Weinberg RA: Isolation of a transforming sequence from a human bladder carcinoma cell line. Cell 29:161, 1982
56. Goldfarb M, Shimizu K, Perucho M, Wigler M: Isolation and preliminary characterization of a human transforming gene from T24 bladder carcinoma cells. Nature 296:404, 1982
57. Der CJ, Krontiris TG, Cooper GM: Transforming genes of human bladder and lung carcinoma cell lines are homologous to the ras genes of Harvey and Kirsten sarcoma viruses. Proc Natl Acad Sci USA 79:3637, 1982
58. Parada LF, Tabin CJ, Shih C, Weinberg RA: Human EJ bladder carcinoma oncogene is homologue of Harvey sarcoma virus ras gene. Nature 297:474, 1982
59. Santos E, Tronick SR, Aaronson S, et al: T24 human bladder carcinoma oncogene is an activated form of the normal human homologue of BALB- and Harvey-MSV transforming genes. Nature 298:343, 1982
60. Tabin CJ, Bradley SM, Bargmann CI, et al: Mechanism of activation of a human oncogene. Nature 300:143, 1982
61. Taparowsky E, Suard Y, Fasano O, et al: Activation of the T24 bladder carcinoma transforming gene is linked to a single amino acid change. Nature 300:762, 1982
62. Reddy EP, Reynolds RK, Santos E, Barbacid M: A point mutation is responsible for the acquisition of transforming properties by the T24 human bladder carcinoma oncogene. Nature 300:149, 1982
63. Solomon E, Borrow J, Goddard AD: Chromosome aberrations and cancer. Science 254:1153, 1991
64. Rowley JD: Recurring chromosome abnormalities in leukemia and lymphoma. Semin Hematol 27:122, 1990
65. De Klein A, Hagemeijer A: Cytogenetic and molecular analysis of the Ph^1 translocation in chronic myeloid leukemia. Cancer Surv 3:515, 1984
66. Leder P, Battey J, Lenoir G, et al: Translocations among antibody genes in human cancer. Science 222:765, 1983
67. Taub R, Kirsch I, Morton C, et al: Translocation of the c-myc gene into the immunoglobulin heavy chain locus in human Burkitt lymphoma and murine plasmacytoma cells. Proc Natl Acad Sci USA 79:7837, 1982
68. Dalla-Favera R, Bregni M, Erickson J, et al: Human c-myc oncogene is located on the region of chromosome 8 that is translocated in Burkitt lymphoma cells. Proc Natl Acad Sci USA 79:7824, 1982
69. Cesarman E, Dalla-Favera R, Bently D, et al: Mutations in the first exon are associated with altered transcription of c-myc in Burkitt lymphoma. Science 238:1272, 1987

70. De Klein A, van Kessel AG, Grosveld G, et al: A cellular oncogene is translocated to the Philadelphia chromosome in chronic myelocytic leukemia. Nature 300:765, 1982
71. McLaughlin J, Chianese E, Witte ON: In vitro transformation of immature hematopoietic cells by the p210 bcr/abl oncogene product of the Philadelphia chromosome. Proc Natl Acad Sci USA 84:6558, 1987
72. Kurzrock R, Gutterman JU, Talpaz M: The molecular genetics of Philadelphia chromosome-positive leukemias. N Engl J Med 319:990, 1988
73. Konopka JB, Watanabe SM, Witte ON: An alteration of the human c-abl protein in K562 leukemia cells unmasks associated protein tyrosine kinase activity. Cell 37:1035, 1984
74. Daley GQ, Van Etten RA, Baltimore D: Induction of chronic myelogenous leukemia in mice by the p210$^{bcr/abl}$ gene of the Philadelphia chromosome. Science 247:824, 1990
75. Sawyers CL, Denny CT, Witte ON: Leukemia and the disruption of normal hematopoiesis. Cell 64:337, 1991
76. Alitalo K, Schwab M: Oncogene amplification in tumor cells. Adv Cancer Res 47:235, 1986
77. Fukumoto M, Shevrin DH, Roninson IB: Analysis of gene amplification in human tumor cell lines. Proc Natl Acad Sci USA 85:6846, 1988
78. Cowell JK: Double minutes and homogeneously staining regions: Gene amplification in mammalian cells. Annu Rev Genet 16:21, 1982
79. Tlsty TD, Margolin BH, Lum K: Differences in the rates of gene amplification in nontumorigenic and tumorigenic cell lines as measured by Luria-Delbruck fluctuation analysis. Proc Natl Acad Sci USA 86:9441, 1989
80. Bertino JR, Carman MD, Weiner HL, et al: Gene amplification and altered enzymes as mechanisms for the development of drug resistance. Cancer Treat Rep 67:901, 1983
81. Curt GA, Carney DN, Cowan KH, et al: Unstable methotrexate resistance in human small cell carcinoma associated with double minute chromosomes. N Engl J Med 308:199, 1983
82. Schwab M, Varmus HE, Bishop JM: Chromosome localization in normal cells and neuroblastomas of a gene related to c-MYC. Nature 303:288, 1984
83. Little CD, Nau MM, Carney DN, et al: Amplification and expression of the c-MYC oncogene in human lung cell lines. Nature 306:194, 1983
84. Kawashima K, Shikama H, Imoto K: Close correlation between restriction fragment length polymorphism of the L-myc gene and metastasis of human lung cancer to the lymph nodes and other organs. Proc Natl Acad Sci USA 85:2353, 1988
85. Hunter T: Cooperation between oncogenes. Cell 64:249, 1991
86. Ruley HE: Transforming collaborations between ras and nuclear oncogenes. Cancer Cells 2:258, 1990
87. Hunter T: A thousand and one protein kinases. Cell 22:649, 1987
88. Sefton BM, Hunter T, Beemon K, Eckhart W: Evidence that the phosphorylation of tyrosine is essential for cellular transformation by Rous sarcoma virus. Cell 20:807, 1980
89. Ullrich A, Schlessinger J: Signal transduction by receptors with tyrosine kinase activity. Cell 61:203, 1990
90. Honegger AM, Kris RM, Ulrich A, Schlessinger J: Evidence that autophosphorylation of solubilized EGF-receptors is mediated by intermolecular cross phosphorylation. Proc Natl Acad Sci USA 86:925, 1989
91. Buday L, Downward J: Epidermal growth factor regulates p21ras through the formation of a complex of receptor, grb2 adapter protein, and sos nucleotide exchange factor. Cell 73:611, 1993
92. Iba H, Cross FR, Garber EA, Hanafusa H: Low level of cellular protein phosphorylation by nontransforming overproduced pp60^{c-src}. Mol Cell Biol 5:1058, 1985
93. Cooper JA, Howell B: The when and how of src regulation. Cell 73:1051, 1993
94. Cantley LC, Auger KR, Carpenter C, et al: Oncogenes and signal transduction. Cell 64:281, 1991
95. Robbins KC, Antoniades HN, Devare SG, et al: Structural and immunological similarities between simian sarcoma virus gene products and human platelet-derived growth factor. Nature 305:605, 1983
96. Johnsson A, Heldin C-H, Wasteson A, et al: The c-sis gene encodes a precursor of the B chain of platelet-derived growth factor. EMBO J 3:921, 1984
97. Josephs SF, Ratner L, Clarke MF, et al: Transforming potential of human c-sis nucleotide sequences encoding platelet-derived growth factor. Science 225:636, 1984
98. Downward J, Yarden Y, Mayes E, et al: Close similarity of epidermal growth factor receptor and v-erbB oncogene protein sequences. Nature 307:521, 1984
99. Ullrich A, Coussens L, Hayflick JS, et al: Human epidermal growth factor receptor cDNA sequence and aberrant expression of the amplified gene in A431 epidermoid carcinoma cells. Nature 309:418, 1984
100. Nilsen TW, Maroney PA, Goodwin RG, et al: C-erbB activation in ALV-induced erythroblastosis: Novel RNA processing and promoter insertion result in expression of an amino-truncated EGF receptor. Cell 41:719, 1985
101. Kris RM, Lax I, Gullick W, et al: Antibodies against a synthetic peptide as a probe for the kinase activity of the avian EGF receptor and v-erbB protein. Cell 40:619, 1985
102. Slamon DJ, Godolphin W, Jones LA, et al: Studies of the HER-2/NEU proto-oncogene in human breast and ovarian cancer. Science 244:707, 1989
103. Veale D, Ashcroft T, Marsh C, et al: Epidermal growth factor receptors in non-small cell lung cancer. Br J Cancer 55:513, 1987
104. Weinberg RA: Tumor suppressor genes. Science 254:1138, 1991
105. Laiho M, DeCaprio JA, Ludlow JW, et al: Growth inhibition by TGF-β linked to suppression of retinoblastoma protein phosphorylation. Cell 62:175, 1990
106. Marx J: How p53 suppresses cell growth. Science 262:1644, 1993
107. Sherr CJ: Mammalian G$_1$ cyclins. Cell 73:1059, 1993
108. Koch CA, Anderson D, Moran MF, et al: SH2 and SH3 domains: Elements that control interactions of cytoplasmic signaling proteins. Science 252:668, 1991
109. Lowenstein EJ, Daly RJ, Batzer AG, et al: The SH2 and SH3 domain-containing protein GRB2 links receptor tyrosine kinases to ras signaling. Cell 70:431, 1992
110. Marshall MS, Hill WS, Assunta SN, et al: A c-terminal domain of GAP is sufficient to stimulate ras p21 GTPase activity. EMBO J 8:1105, 1989
111. McCormick F: Ras GTPase activating protein: Signal transmitter and signal terminator. Cell 56:5, 1989
112. Wood KW, Sarnecki C, Roberts TM, Blenis J: Ras mediates nerve growth factor receptor modulation of three signal-transducing protein kinases: MAP kinase, Raf-1 and RSK. Cell 68:1041, 1992
113. Payne DM, Rossomando AJ, Martino P, et al: Identification of the regulatory phosphorylation sites in pp42/mitogen-activated protein kinase (MAP kinase). EMBO J 10:885, 1991
114. Howe LR, Leevers SJ, Gomez N, et al: Activation of the MAP kinase pathway by the protein kinase raf. Cell 71:335, 1992
115. Rodeck U, Williams N, Murthy U, Herlyn D: Monoclonal antibody 425 inhibits growth stimulation of carcinoma cells by exogenous EGF and tumor-derived EGF/TGF-α. J Cell Biochem 44:69, 1990
116. Qiu MS, Green SH: NGF and EGF rapidly activate p21^{ras} by distinct convergent pathways involving tyrosine phosphorylation. Neuron 7:937, 1991
117. Mulcahy LS, Smith MR, Stacey DW: Requirements for ras proto-oncogene function during serum-stimulated growth of NIH 3T3 cells. Nature 313:241, 1985
118. Medema RH, de Vries-Smits AMM, van der Zon GCM, et al: Ras activation by insulin and epidermal growth factor through enhanced exchange of guanine nucleotides on p21^{ras}. Mol Cell Biol 13:155, 1993
119. Kizaka-Kondoh, Sato SK, Tamura K, et al: Raf-1 protein kinase is an integral component of the oncogenic signal cascade shared by epidermal growth factor and platelet-derived growth factor. Mol Cell Biol 12:5078, 1992
120. Guan JL, Shalloway S: Regulation of focal adhesion-associated protein tyrosine kinase by both cellular adhesion and oncogenic transformation. Nature 358:690, 1992
121. Warren SL, Nelson WJ: Nonmitogenic morphoregulatory action

of pp60^{v-src} on multicellular epithelial structures. Mol Cell Biol 7:1326, 1987

122. Muschel RJ, Williams JE, Lowy DR, Liotta LA: Harvey *ras* induction of metastatic potential depends upon oncogene activation and the type of recipient cell. Am J Pathol *127*:1, 1985

123. Blackwell TK, Kretzner L, Blackwood EM, et al: Sequence-specific DNA binding by the c-Myc protein. Science *250*:1149, 1990

124. Sakura H, Kanei-Ishii C, Nasase T, et al: Delineation of three functional domains of the transcriptional activator encoded by the *c-myb* protooncogene. Proc Natl Acad Sci USA *86*:5758, 1989

125. Franza BR, Rauscher FJ, Josephs SF, Curran T: The Fos complex and Fos-related antigens recognize sequence elements that contain AP-1 binding sites. Science *239*:1150, 1988

126. Damm KC, Thompson CC, Evans RM: Protein encoded by *v-erbA* functions as a thyroid hormone receptor antagonist. Nature *339*:593, 1989

127. Nye JA, Peterson JM, Gunther CV, et al: Interaction of murine *ets-1* with GGA-binding sites establishes the ETS domain as a new DNA-binding motif. Genes Dev *6*:975, 1990

128. Levin B: Oncogenic conversion by regulatory changes in transcription factors. Cell *64*:303, 1991

129. Gutman A, Wasylyk B: Nuclear targets for transcription regulation by oncogenes. Trends Genet *7*:49, 1991

130. Cleary ML: Oncogenic conversion of transcription factors by chromosomal translocations. Cell *64*:619, 1991

131. Hartwell LH, Weinert TA: Checkpoints: Controls that ensure the order of cell cycle events. Science *246*:629, 1989

132. Pardee AB: G_1 events and regulation of cell proliferation. Science *246*:603, 1989

133. Lane DP: p53, guardian of the genome. Nature *358*:15, 1992

134. Norbury C, Nurse P: Animal cell cycles and their control. Annu Rev Biochem *61*:441, 1992

135. Minshull J, Golsteyn R, Hill CS, Hunt T: The A- and B-type cyclin associated cdc2 kinases in *Xenopus* turn on and off at different times in the cell cycle. EMBO J *9*:2865, 1990

136. Hinds PW, Mittnacht S, Dulic V, et al: Regulation of retinoblastoma protein functions by ectopic expression of human cyclins. Cell *70*:993, 1992

137. Kato J-Y, Matsushime H, Hiebert SW, et al: Direct binding of cyclin D to the retinoblastoma gene product (pRb) and pRb phosphorylation by the cyclin D-dependent kinase CDK4. Genes Dev *7*:331, 1993

138. Hiebert SW, Chellappan SP, Horowitz JM, Nevins JR: The interaction of RB with E2F coincides with an inhibiton of the transcriptional activity of E2F. Genes Dev *6*:177, 1992

139. Pietenpol JA, Munger K, Howley PM, et al: Factor-binding element in the human c-myc promoter involved in transcriptional regulation by transforming growth factor β1 and by the retinoblastoma gene product. Proc Natl Acad Sci USA *88*: 10227, 1991

140. Jiang W, Kahn SM, Tomita N, et al: Amplification and expression of the human cyclin D gene in esophageal cancer. Cancer Res *52*:2980, 1992

141. Kitagawa Y, Ueda M, Ando N, et al: Significance of *int-2/hst-1* coamplification as a prognostic factor in patients with esophageal squamous carcinoma. Cancer Res *51*:1504, 1991

142. Motokura T, Bloom T, Kim HG, et al: A novel cyclin encoded by a *bcl1*-linked candidate oncogene. Nature *350*:512, 1991

143. Williams GT, Smith CA: Molecular regulation of apoptosis: Genetic controls on cell death. Cell *74*:777, 1993

144. Tsujimoto Y, Croce CM: Analysis of the structure, transcripts and protein products of Bc1-2, the gene involved in human follicular lymphoma. Proc Natl Acad Sci USA *83*:5214, 1986.

145. McDonnell TJ, Deane N, Platt FM, et al: *Bc1-2*-immunoglobulin transgenic mice demonstrate extended B cell survival and follicular lymphoproliferation. Cell *57*:79, 1989

146. Fearon ER, Vogelstein B: A genetic model for colorectal tumorigenesis. Cell *61*:759, 1990

147. Weinberg RA: The action of oncogenes in the cytoplasm and the nucleus. Science *230*:770, 1985

148. Ruley HE: Adenovirus early region 1A enables viral and cellular transforming genes to transform primary cells in culture. Nature *304*:602, 1983

149. Bos JL: The *ras* family and human carcinogenesis. Mutat Res *195*:255, 1988

150. Stewart TA, Papengale PK, Leder P: Spontaneous mammary adenocarcinomas in transgenic mice that carry and express MMTV/*myc* fusion genes. Cell *38*:627, 1984

151. Hanahan D: Transgenic mice as probes into complex systems. Science *246*:1265, 1989

152. Sinn E, Muller W, Pattengale P, et al: Coexpression of MMTV/*v-H-ras* and MMTV/*c-myc* genes in transgenic mice: Synergistic action of oncogenes *in vivo*. Cell *49*:465, 1987

153. Masui H, Boman B, Hyman J, et al: Treatment with anti-EGF receptor monoclonal antibody causes regression of DiFi human colorectal carcinoma xenografts. Proc Am Assoc Cancer Res *32*:394, 1991

154. Daaka Y, Wickstrom E: Target dependence of antisense oligodeoxynucleotide inhibition of c-Ha-*ras* p21 expression and focus formation in T24-transformed NIH3T3 cells. Oncog Res *5*:267, 1990

155. Shirasawa S, Furuse M, Yokoyama N, Sasazuki T: Altered growth of human colon cancer cell lines disrupted at activated Ki-*ras*. Science *260*:85, 1993

156. Hollstein MC, Smits AM, Galiaia C, et al: Amplification of the epidermal growth factor receptor gene, but no evidence of *ras* mutation in primary esophageal squamous cancers. Cancer Res *48*:5119, 1988.

157. Rosen N, Sartor O, Foss F, Bolen JB: Altered expression of *src*-related tyrosine kinases in human colon cancer. Cancer Cells *7*:161, 1989

7

GROWTH FACTORS AND SIGNAL TRANSDUCTION

STEVEN R. TRONICK
STUART A. AARONSON

Intercellular communication is critical to embryonic development and tissue differentiation, as well as systemic responses to wounds and infections. These complex signaling networks are in large part mediated by growth factors. Such factors can influence cell proliferation in positive or negative ways, as well as inducing a series of differentiated responses in appropriate target cells. The interaction of a growth factor with its receptor by specific binding in turn activates a cascade of intracellular biochemical events ultimately responsible for the biologic responses observed. Cytoplasmic molecules that mediate these responses have been termed "second messengers." The transmission of these biochemical signals to the nucleus leads to the altered expression of a wide variety of genes involved in mitogenic and differentiation responses.

In the early 1980s, approaches aimed at identifying the functions of retroviral oncogenes converged with efforts to investigate normal mitogenic signaling by growth factors. Analysis of the predicted sequences of a number of retroviral oncogene products uncovered several with similarities to the prototype v-*src* product, whose enzymatic function as a protein kinase had been identified.[1] Unlike many protein kinases, which phosphorylated serine and/or threonine residues, the v-*src* product was a protein kinase capable of specifically phosphorylating tyrosine residues.[2]

Independent efforts to purify and sequence growth factors led to the discovery that the sequence of the platelet-derived growth factor (PDGF) B chain matched the predicted product of the transforming gene of simian sarcoma virus, designated v-*sis*.[3,4] The v-*erbB* product of avian erythroblastosis virus, predicted to encode a v-*src*–related protein tyrosine kinase, was then found to represent a truncated form of the epidermal growth factor (EGF) re-

ceptor.[5] Subsequent evidence demonstrated that EGF triggering of its receptor resulted in tyrosine autophosphorylation.[6] Thus, a direct link between growth factors, receptors with tyrosine kinase activity, and oncogenes was firmly developed, and more recent investigations have strengthened these ties. Present knowledge indicates that the constitutive activation of growth factor signaling pathways through genetic alterations affecting these genes contributes to the development and progression of most if not all human cancers. This chapter focuses on the families of growth factors that exert their effects through receptors possessing intrinsic protein tyrosine kinase activity and summarizes current knowledge of their "downstream" mitogenic signaling pathways. The proliferation, differentiation, functional activity, and survival of cells also are affected by a wide array of other cytokines that signal through transmembrane receptors that lack protein tyrosine kinase activity. Because these signaling systems also have been implicated in malignant transformation, they also are considered, but in less detail.

POLYPEPTIDE GROWTH FACTORS THAT ACT THROUGH PROTEIN TYROSINE KINASE RECEPTORS

Receptors

Membrane-spanning receptor protein tyrosine kinases (RPTKs) contain several discrete domains, including their extracellular ligand binding, transmembrane, juxtamembrane, protein tyrosine kinase, and carboxy-terminal tail domains[7,8] (Figs. 7–1 and 7–2). Interaction of a growth factor with its receptor at the cell surface leads to a tight association, so that growth factors are capable of mediating their activities at rather low nanomolar concentrations. There is substantial evidence that activation of the receptor tyrosine kinase is the trigger for the biochemical cascade of events that follows. It is possible that conformational changes induced by ligand binding to the receptor's external domain somehow are transmitted through the transmembrane domain to induce the conformational alterations of the receptor kinase, resulting in its activation. In an alternative model, ligand binding induces receptor dimer or oligomer formation.[7,8] By this latter mechanism, molecular interactions between adjacent cytoplasmic domains lead to activation of kinase function by either an intra- or intermolecular process.

In the case of growth factors such as EGF, a single growth factor interacts with a single receptor. In contrast, dimeric ligands such as PDGF appear to be bivalent such that a single growth factor molecule initiates dimerization of two receptors. Thus, available evidence strongly favors growth factor receptor dimerization in response to ligand binding,[7-9] and this property has been localized to the extracellular domains of at least some receptors.[7,8]

Most evidence indicates that the transmembrane domain does not directly influence signal transduction and is instead a passive anchor of the receptor to the membrane. It is important to note, however, that point mutations in the transmembrane domain of one receptor-like protein, the Neu/ErbB-2 protein, enhances its transforming properties.[10] The juxtamembrane sequence that

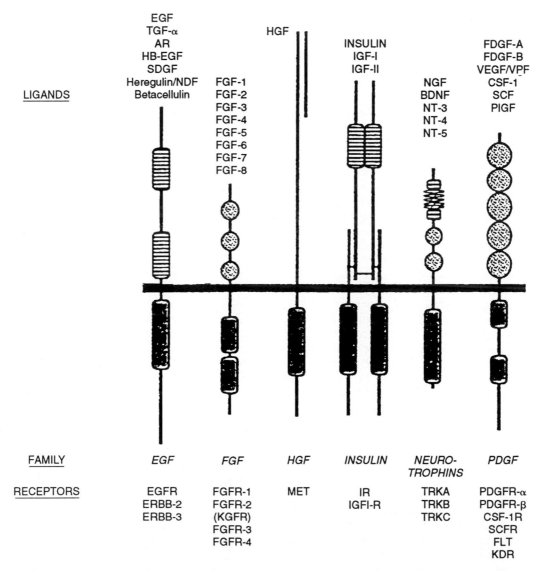

Figure 7–1. Structures of receptor protein tyrosine kinases. The horizontal bar represents the cytoplasmic membrane. Extracellular and intracellular environments are located above and below the membrane, respectively. Cysteine-rich domains = polygons with horizontal stripes; immunoglobulin-like (IG-L) loops = small stippled circles; leucine-rich motifs (LRMs) = larger ellipses; tyrosine kinase (TK) domains = shaded polygons. The insulin receptor extracellular domain also contains fibronectin type III repeats, but these have been omitted for clarity. The figure shows the members of each ligand and receptor family, but is not intended to indicate binding specificity. The EGF, insulin, PDGF, and FGF receptor families also have been classified as subclasses I, II, III, and IV, respectively.[7]

separates the transmembrane and cytoplasmic domains is not well conserved between different families of receptors. However, juxtamembrane sequences are highly similar among members of the same family, and studies indicate that this stretch plays a role in modulation of receptor function. For example, addition of PDGF to many types of cells causes a rapid decrease in high-affinity binding of EGF to its receptor. This has been shown to be a downstream effect of PDGF receptor activation in which protein kinase C, itself a serine protein kinase, is activated and, in turn, phosphorylates a site in the juxtamembrane domain of the EGF receptor.[7,8]

The tyrosine kinase is the most conserved domain, and its integrity is absolutely required for receptor signaling. For example, mutation of a single lysine in the ATP binding site, which blocks the ability of the receptor to phosphorylate tyrosine residues, completely inactivates receptor biologic function. Yet, such kinase mutants retain the ability to bind ligand with high affinity and exhibit normal internalization and down-regulation as well.[7,8]

The carboxy-terminal domain of the receptor is thought to play an important role in regulation of kinase activity. This region typically contains several tyrosine residues, which are phosphorylated by the activated kinase. In fact, the receptor itself is often the major tyrosine phosphorylated species observed following ligand stimulation. Tyrosine phosphorylation of the carboxy-terminal domain has been postulated to modulate kinase catalytic activity, and/or the ability of the kinase to interact with substrates. Thus, mutations that alter individual tyrosine sites or deletions of the carboxy-terminal domain have the effect of attenuating kinase function in those receptors so far analyzed.[7,8,11]

Growth Factors

EPIDERMAL GROWTH FACTOR FAMILY

EGF, purified from mouse submaxillary glands initially was found to promote precocious eyelid separation and early incisor eruption by enhancing epidermal growth and

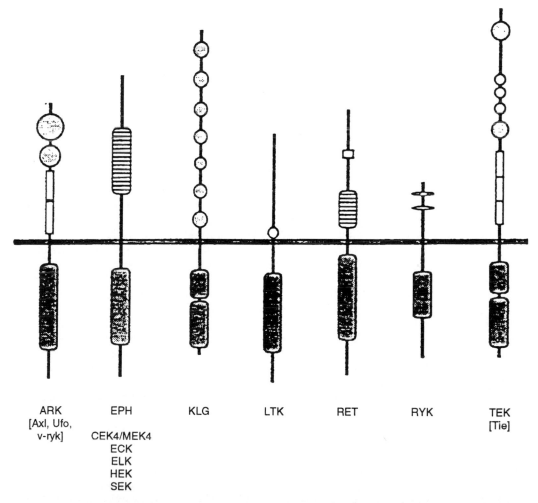

Figure 7–2. "Orphan" receptors. Open rectangles = fibronectin type III repeats; open circles = EGF-like repeats; open rectangle in RET = transmembrane-like domain. Other symbols are the same as in Figure 7–1. Isolates of the same receptor from the same or other species are bracketed. Known members of the EPH family are indicated.

keratinization while it induced early incisor eruption by enhancing the differentiation of the lips of treated animals.[12] The proliferative effects of EGF on epidermal cells in organ and tissue cultures derived from avian and mammalian species subsequently were established. Some years later, the discovery was made that urogastrone (URO), a hormone with gastric antisecretory activity, was identical to EGF.[12,13] The role of EGF/URO in inhibiting gastric secretion long remained a mystery until Wright et al.[14] reported the induction of novel EGF/URO-secreting cells by mucosal ulceration. Although EGF/URO was known to be a potent mitogen and differentiating agent for cells of the rat and human intestine, EGF/URO is not absorbed from the adult gut nor does it have an effect when given through the gut lumen. The new cells that form following ulceration of the human gastrointestinal tract eventually form a small gland that secretes EGF/URO, whose proliferative effects stimulate ulcer healing.

The EGF chain consists of 53 amino acids constrained by three internal disulfide bonds and is generated from a 1200-residue precursor with a remarkable structure[15,16] that includes eight units similar to EGF and a hydrophobic stretch near its carboxyl terminus, such as those found in integral membrane proteins. The precursor has been detected as a glycosylated membrane protein in cells transfected with a prepro-EGF precursor and retains biologic activity similar to that of EGF.[17]

The EGF family (for reviews, see refs. 18,19) includes transforming growth factor α (TGF-α); amphiregulin; poxvirus growth factor; heparin-binding EGF-like growth factor (HB-EGF)[20]; schwannoma-derived growth factor (SDGF), which may be the rodent homologue of amphiregulin[21], heregulin[22]/Neu differentiation factor (NDF)[23,24]; and betacellulin.[25] These proteins share sequence similarities as well as high binding affinity for the EGF receptor and mitogenic effects on EGF-responsive cells (except for heregulin/NDF). A distinct sequence motif (X_n-$CX_7CX_{2-3}GXCX_{10-13}CXCX_3YXGXRCX_4LX_n$) in each of these molecules is also present in diverse proteins found on the cell surface or extracellularly but that are not, however, ligands for the EGF receptor. Mature forms of these family members are generated by proteolysis of much larger transmembrane glycoproteins. Whereas EGF normally is expressed in kidney and submaxillary glands and is produced in response to gastrointestinal tract injury as well,[12,14,19] TGF-α appcars normally to be expressed by a variety of epithelial cells.[19,26] Amphiregulin transcripts have been detected in human placenta, ovarian, and breast tissue as well as in cells derived from squamous carcinomas and mammary adenocarcinomas.[27] SDGF was isolated from a rat Schwann cell tumor and also from a mouse mammary carcinoma[21,28]; however, little else is known regarding its tissue distribution. The betacellulin transcript is present in a wide variety of mouse tissues and is most abundant in lung, uterus, and kidney.[25]

A cDNA clone designated cripto[29] was found to contain an open reading frame of 188 codons derived from two unrelated genes that encodes a cysteine domain similar to those found in other EGF family members. However, the ability of the cripto protein to bind EGF family receptors has not been tested.

There are four known members of the EGF receptor gene family (see refs. 7,8,18 for reviews): EGF receptor (EGFR),[30-35] ERBB-2 (also designated neu and her),[36-38] ERBB-3[39] and ERBB-4.[39a] EGFR was identified and isolated by biochemical techniques, whereas the isolation of ERBB-2 and ERBB-3 was made possible by the use of low-stringency hybridization techniques using tyrosine kinase domain probes. In addition to those ligands that bind the EGFR, heregulin/NDF originally thought to be the ligand of the ERBB-2 receptor[22-24] binds ERBB-4.[39b] The ligands for ERBB-3 have not been reported. As discussed later in this chapter, EGFR family members frequently are overexpressed in human tumors.[39-41]

FIBROBLAST GROWTH FACTOR FAMILY

There are nine known members of the fibroblast growth factor (FGF) family. Because heparin can bind to and potentiate the biologic activity of these proteins, they also have been termed heparin-binding growth factors (HBGFs).[42] The members include acidic FGF (aFGF, FGF-1),[43] basic FGF (bFGF,FGF-2),[44] int-2 (FGF-3),[45] hst/KS3 (FGF-4),[46,47] FGF-5,[48] FGF-6,[49] keratinocyte growth factor (KGF, FGF-7),[50] androgen-induced growth factor (AIGF, FGF-8),[51] and glia-activating factor (GAF) FGF-9.[51a] FGFs are mitogenic for cells of mesenchymal, neuroectodermal, and epidermal origin, and their overexpression can lead to malignant transformation. In addition to these proliferative effects, certain FGFs support the survival of neurons from various parts of the nervous system, induce the differentiation of adipocytes and neuroepithelial precursor cells, and can inhibit the differentiation of muscle cells. The actions of FGFs also have been implicated in angiogenesis and in mesoderm induction during embryonal development in Xenopus (reviewed in refs. 52–54).

Basic FGF was the first family member isolated and was recognized in certain hormone preparations by its mitogenicity for mouse 3T3 cells and chondrocytes. It was later purified from bovine pituitary. Acidic FGF was purified independently from acidic extracts of bovine brain.[42] Both aFGF and bFGF are single-chain polypeptides of about 17,000 Da and share 55 per cent amino acid sequence identity. A striking feature of each of their structures, in contrast to those of other family members, is the lack of a consensus secretory signal peptide. This has generated a great deal of speculation regarding their mode of release from cells. Likely mechanisms include the liberation of FGF from cells by lysis or escort by other proteins out of intact cells.

Analysis of mammary tumors induced by mouse mammary tumor virus (MMTV) revealed that the viral genome frequently integrates within a genetic locus termed int-2, and thereby induction of expression of this gene by retroviral insertional mutagenesis has been linked to tumor induction.[55] The protein encoded by int-2 is predicted to be 245 amino acids long and highly similar to aFGF and bFGF. The normal expression of int-2 apparently is limited to embryonic tissues, and there is evidence from in vitro translation studies that it is a weak mitogen for mammary epithelial cells.[56] Recent transgenic mouse experiments have shown that int-2 expression leads to mammary gland hyperplasia in female mice and benign epithelial hyperplasia in the prostate of males.[57]

FGF-4 and FGF-5 were uncovered during searches for oncogenes in human tumor cells.[46-48] FGF-4 was isolated from both a human stomach tumor (hst)[46] and a Kaposi's sarcoma (KS3)[47] and is a mitogen for vascular endothelial cells, human melanocytes, and mouse NIH 3T3 fibroblasts. The FGF-5 gene also was isolated by DNA transfection of cells grown in chemically defined medium in which transformation was detected by the induction of proliferation in the absence of exogenous growth factors.[48] Thus, DNA from a human bladder carcinoma cell line induced morphologic transformation in the absence of FGF. FGF-5 was found to be activated by a DNA rearrangement that juxtaposed a retrovirus transcriptional enhancer upstream of its natural promoter. Partially purified FGF-5 preparations were found to be mitogenic for mouse fibroblasts and bovine heart endothelial cells.[48]

Isolation of additional members of gene families is sometimes possible by low-stringency molecular hybridization employing probes derived from the most highly conserved sequences among each gene. FGF-6 was isolated by this approach from a cosmid library prepared from a human lymphoblastoid cell line and was shown to act as a transforming gene for NIH 3T3 cells by transfection assays.[49] Other biologic activities of FGF-6 have yet to be demonstrated.

KGF (FGF-7) was isolated from media conditioned by a human embryonic lung fibroblast cell line. It was found to be a potent mitogen for epithelial cells (mouse keratinocytes) but lacked activity on fibroblasts or endothelial cells.[58] Thus, KGF is distinct in this regard not only from other members of the FGF family but from all other polypeptide growth factors as well. Molecular cloning and sequence analysis established it as a member of the FGF family whose predicted amino acid sequence is about 38 per cent identical to those of aFGF and bFGF.[50] KGF is expressed by stromal cells of many epithelial tissues, supporting the concept that this factor is important in the normal mesenchymal stimulation of epithelial cell growth.

AIGF[51] was isolated from media conditioned by a cell line derived from an androgen (testosterone)-dependent mammary carcinoma cell line. AIGF is approximately equidistantly related to the other FGFs. The target cell specificity of AIGF has not been determined, although it acts in an autocrine fashion to stimulate the growth of the mammary carcinoma cells from which it was derived.[51] GAF was purified from culture supernatants of a human glioma cell line. It lacks an identifiable signal sequence but was found to be efficiently secreted from cos cells transfected with GAF cDNA.[51a]

Four genes encoding FGF receptors have been identified, but they direct the synthesis of a larger number of receptor isoforms that display both unique and overlapping specificity for the various FGFs (see refs. 59–61 for reviews). The prototypes (and their various aliases) encoded by each gene are designated FGFR1 (mFR1, Flg, CEK1[62-68]), FGFR2 (BEK, CEK3, KGFR[65,69-72]), FGFR3,[70,73] and FGFR4.[74,75] The pattern of expression in normal and tumor cells can be highly complex in that the same cell can express more than one type of FGFR along with their respective structural variants.[61,76-80] Extracellular ligand-binding domains are characterized by three immunoglobulin-like (IG-like) loops and a stretch of acidic amino acid residues between the first and second loop. The juxtamembrane domain is longer than those of most other RPTKs (80 versus 60 residues), and the tyrosine kinase domain is "split" by 13 amino acids that show no similarity to tyrosine kinase domains of other RPTKs or nonreceptor tyrosine kinases.

One of the most striking examples of the functional consequences of the presence of alternate receptor forms comes from studies on the KGF receptor (KGFR). The KGF receptor binds both aFGF and KGF with about 10 to 20-fold higher affinity than bFGF.[81] Sequence analysis of the KGFR isolated by expression cDNA cloning techniques[71] revealed that it was identical to FGFR2 with the exception of 49 codons encompassing the carboxy-terminal region of IG-like loop III. In contrast, FGFR2 binds aFGF and bFGF equally well, but does not detectably bind KGF.[72] Polymerase chain reaction (PCR) analysis of genomic DNA demonstrated that FGFR2 and the KGFR are encoded by the same gene and are generated by alternative splicing.[72]

Two other distinct types of FGF receptors that lack protein tyrosine kinase activity also have been described. FGF can be covalently bound to heparan sulfate chains of a heparan/chondroitin sulfate proteoglycan (HSPG) called syndecan,[82] and there have been a number of studies suggesting that signaling by FGF is dependent on the presence of heparan sulfate.[64,76,83-86] Very recently, a cysteine-rich transmembrane protein designated CFR (cysteine-rich FGF receptor) was identified.[87] CFR binds FGF-1 -2, and -4 with dissociation constants of about 1 nM. It possesses a very short intracellular domain (13 amino acids) and is unrelated to any known sequence. Although the role of CFR in the diverse biologic effects of the FGFs is not known, it was found to be abundantly expressed in embryonic chick neuronal tissue.[87]

HEPATOCYTE GROWTH FACTOR

Studies on the mechanism of liver regeneration led to the identification of a hormone-like activity capable of stimulating hepatocyte proliferation.[88-90] The factor has been referred to as hepatocyte growth factor (HGF), hepatopoietin A, and hepatotropin (reviewed in ref. 91). Subsequent work revealed that HGF is mitogenic for melanocytes, renal tubular cells, and some endothelial and epithelial cells in culture.[92-95] HGF recently was shown to be identical[96,97] to scatter factor,[91,97,98] an agent that mediates the dispersion of certain epithelial and vascular endothelial cells. The relationship between HGF and scatter factor was not appreciated at first because scatter factor did not influence the growth of the indicator cell lines, and there were no reports that HGF affected cell motility.[91] HGF is encoded by a single transcript,[92,99-101] whose 728 amino acid–long product is processed by proteolytic cleavage into a dimer of 87 kDa formed by the disulfide bonding of heavy (~60kDa) and light (~30 kDa) chains.[88-90] The amino acid sequence of HGF is 38 per cent identical to plasminogen, including its serine protease domain, and HGF possesses disulfide bond–linked intrachain structures known as "kringles,"[102] which are typical of prothrombin, tissue plasminogen activator, urokinase, and coagulation factor XII. Neither plasminogen nor plasmin has HGF-like activity, and HGF is not likely to be a protease because the histidine and serine residues in the region corresponding to the catalytic site are replaced by other amino acids.[99]

HGF binds specifically to and induces the rapid tyrosine phosphorylation of a 145-kDa protein on the surface of a mammary epithelial cell line known to be particularly sensitive to the mitogenic effects of HGF.[103] The 145-kDa protein was similar in size to the β chain of the c-*met* proto-oncogene product,[104,105] and immunochemical and ligand cross-linking studies established that the c-*met* proto-oncogene product is the high-affinity cell surface receptor for HGF.[103] The viral oncogene *sea*[106] is closely related to *met* within its tyrosine kinase domain. However, it remains to be determined whether the *sea* proto-oncogene encodes a receptor for HGF or a related ligand.[106a]

THE INSULIN FAMILY

The diversity of metabolic effects of insulin has been studied intensively for decades.[107] Insulin's primary in vivo functions involve the regulation of rapid anabolic responses such as glucose uptake, lipogenesis, and amino acid and ion transport. Besides its effects on metabolism, insulin stimulates DNA synthesis and cell growth. The activities of insulin-like growth factors (IGF-I and IGF-II) first were recognized as serum factors that interacted with growth hormone in stimulating growth of skeletal tissues and were, as a result, termed somatomedins.[108] Somatomedin C is identical to IGF-I, and a polypeptide known as multiplication-stimulating factor (MSA) is homologous to IGF-II.

The IGFs are responsible for the insulin-like effects of serum on muscle and adipose tissue, but there are major differences between insulin and the IGFs. For example, whereas insulin levels fluctuate widely according to carbohydrate level, the IGFs are bound to carrier proteins and are maintained at steady concentrations in the blood stream. The major biologic effects of IGFs are to stimulate cell replication. The receptors for insulin and IGF-I are structurally related (see later) and possess tyrosine kinase activity. In contrast, the IGF-II receptor, which lacks this activity, is a single polypeptide chain and possesses only a very short cytoplasmic domain. At the structural level, IGF-I and insulin share 48 per cent of their amino acid sequences, whereas their similarity to IGF-II is 50 per cent.[109,110] Insulin is synthesized as a 109–amino acid precursor (preproinsulin) that is processed to a 6-kDa protein consisting of two chains (A and B) linked by two disulfide bonds. The structures of IGF-I and IGF-II are analogous but differ significantly from insulin in the region required for binding of carrier proteins.

In vivo studies indicate that IGF-I acts in an autocrine or paracrine mode, because infusion of IGF-I does not give rise to its growth-promoting actions.[108] Although it is not known whether overexpression of insulin family members can lead to transformation, a recent report indicated that addition of exogenous IGF-I or supraphysiologic levels of insulin to mouse NIH 3T3 cells overexpressing IGF-I receptors introduced by transfection induced morphologic transformation and enabled the cells to grow in soft agar and form tumors in nude mice.[111]

The mature insulin receptor is derived from precursor polypeptides, generated by alternative splicing of either 1370 or 1382 amino acids. These are cleaved to α (710 or 731 amino acids) and β (624 amino acids) subunits.[112,113] The chains associate to form a heterotetramer (α_2,β_2) in which the α subunits are extracellular and bind insulin, whereas the β subunits traverse the membrane and possess the tyrosine kinase activity.[114–116] The insulin receptor binds insulin with approximately 100-fold greater affinity than it does IGF-I and IGF-II (100 pM versus 10 nM).[115] The IGF-I receptor is closely related to the insulin receptor in sequence and structure[117] but binds IGF-I with highest affinity (100 pM), followed by IGF-II and insulin.[115] IGF-II is bound by another receptor that is 80 per cent similar to the mannose-6-phosphate receptor.[118,119] The IGF-II receptor binds IGF-II and IGF-I with high affinity but does not bind insulin,[115] and its role in IGF-II signaling is not known.[120]

The major in vivo roles of insulin and the IGFs are distinct (maintenance of metabolic homeostasis and growth and development, respectively), suggesting differences in the signaling pathways triggered by their respective receptors. There is evidence that under certain conditions the insulin and IGF-I receptors are functionally equivalent; however, other studies have indicated that the insulin receptor is intrinsically less mitogenic than the IGF-I receptor.[111,115,121] It is likely that identification of the substrates for each receptor will be required in order to define the molecular mechanisms leading to their distinct physiologic effects.

NEUROTROPHINS

The prototype neurotrophin (NT) is nerve growth factor (NGF),[122] which, as discussed earlier, was discovered over 40 years ago. NGF supports the survival and directs the differentiation of sensory and sympathetic neurons in the peripheral nervous system and influences the development and maintenance of cholinergic neurons of the basal forebrain.[122,123] It is not, as its name suggests, a mitogen for neurons.[122] The proliferative effect of NGF for fibroblasts was established only relatively recently following the discovery of its receptor, the *trk* proto-oncogene product.[124]

A number of studies pointed to the existence of additional discrete neurotrophic factors that would support the differentiation of other neuronal populations. The isolation of NGF from the mouse salivary gland required only a 100-fold purification, but it was estimated that, in order to purify it or related factors from normal target tissues, a 10^8-fold purification would be necessary.[125] Thus, the second neurotrophin, brain-derived neurotrophic factor (BDNF) was not characterized until 1982 and required a 10^6-fold purification after its identification in pig brain.[125] More recently, the use of modern molecular biology techniques quickly yielded NTs 3, 4, and 5.[126–129] The mature forms of neurotrophins, which are 50 to 66 per cent homologous,[129] consist of polypeptide chains of approximately 13 kDa.

Neurotrophins bind with high affinity to members of the *trk* family of RPTKs[124] as well as to a low-affinity receptor, designated p75[NGFR, 130,131] that is unrelated to RPTKs. *trk*A was discovered as a result of efforts to isolate oncogenes from human tumor cells.[132] The *trk (trk*A) proto-oncogene product[124] mediates the proliferative effects of NGF, NT-3, and NT-5, but not BDNF,[133] in fibroblasts. The other two *trk* family members (*trk*B and *trk*C) were isolated by screening mammalian cDNA libraries with *trk*A probes.[124] The product of the *trk*B gene binds BDNF, NT-3 or BDNF.[137] The role of p75[NGFR] in mediating the actions of neurotrophins is controversial. Some studies have suggested that p75[NGFR] forms the high-affinity neurotrophin receptor in concert with *trk* products, whereas others have indicated that *trk*-encoded receptors mediate proliferation and differentiation in the absence of p75[NGFR] (see ref. 138 for review). NGF mutants that lack the ability to bind p75[NGFR] have been reported to bind TrkA and stimulate cell proliferation as efficiently as NGF.[139] Nevertheless, studies of mice harboring a loss-of-function mutation in the p75[NGFR] gene[140] indicate that p75[NGFR] plays an important role in the development and function of the sensory neurons that innervate cutaneous tissues. Whether or not this function is dependent on binding neurotrophins in conjunction with *trk* gene products remains to be determined.

PLATELET-DERIVED GROWTH FACTOR FAMILY

A major mitogen for connective tissue cells is a markedly heat stable, cationic protein that consists of two related but nonidentical (36.7 per cent amino acid sequence identity) polypeptide chains designated A and B (also called PDGF-1 and PDGF-2).[3,4] PDGF molecules exist as AA and BB homodimers as well as an AB heterodimer.[141,142] Connective tissue and glial cells in culture are highly sensitive to the mitogenic effects of PDGF,[141,142] and it is these cells that express PDGF receptors. The α and β PDGF receptors are encoded by distinct genes,[143–146] and there is evidence that they exist as receptor subunits that differentially interact with the three dimeric PDGF ligands.[141,145,147] Thus, PDGF-AA can bind only the αα receptor dimer and PDGF-BB can interact with αα, αβ, and ββ receptor dimers. By this model, the PDGF-AB heterodimer interacts with and triggers αα and αβ receptors. This is an example of the fine degree of regulation that can evolve in the interactions of ligands with their receptors. Presumably, in the case of PDGF, this relates to quantitative regulation of responses based on differential availability in tissues of ligands and receptors, because there is evidence that the two PDGF receptors themselves each are capable of mediating the major known PDGF responses, including mitogenic signaling and chemotaxis.[148,149]

As noted earlier, the gene for the PDGF-B chain is the human homologue of the v-*sis* oncogene of simian sarcoma virus (SSV).[3,4] The transforming protein expressed by SSV shares close structural similarities with PDGF-B chain homodimers.[150,151] PDGF-B has been detected in human tumor cells[3,152,153] that also possess PDGF receptors. These findings, taken together with the demonstration that the normal PDGF-B gene can act as an oncogene when expressed at high levels,[152] suggest that PDGF-B plays a role in the development of certain human cancers. The PDGF-A chain frequently is expressed by human tumor cells, and AA homodimers are produced by osteosarcoma,[154] melanoma,[155] and glioblastoma[156] cells.

Efforts to identify factors that control angiogenesis led to the identification of a new growth factor that is a potent mitogen for vascular endothelial cells of small and large vessels, but has no effect on fibroblasts, lens epithelial cells, corneal endothelial cells, keratinocytes, or adrenal cortex cells. Vascular endothelial growth factor (VEGF) was isolated from the media of cultures of bovine pituitary follicular or folliculostellate cells and consists of two identical polypeptide chains of 23,000 Da.[157] At the same time, another group reported the cloning of a transcript encoding a protein termed "vascular permeability factor" (VPF), which also promotes endothelial cell growth and angiogenesis.[158] VPF was identified first in rodent tumor cells lines, but its purification and cDNA cloning were achieved by using the human histiocytic lymphoma cell line U937. Sequence comparisons revealed that VEGF and VPF are products of the same gene. VEGF/VPF share sequence similarity with the PDGF-A and PDGF-B chains (18 per cent identity). The eight cysteine residues in the PDGF-A and -B chains are all conserved, but VEGF/VPF possesses an additional eight cysteines within its carboxy-terminal domain. Like PDGF, VEGF/VPF is heat (boiling) and acid stable and shows heterogeneity in size and charge on electrophoretic analysis.

Another member of the PDGF/VEGF family was isolated accidentally in the course of attempts to obtain full-length cDNAs of an unrelated gene from a human placenta library.[159] Placenta growth factor (PlGF) is 53 per cent identical to VEGF/VPF within the region that is similar to PDGF. When expressed in COS cells, PlGF cDNA directed the synthesis of a secreted, glycosylated protein that stimulated the growth of an endothelial cell line. It is not known whether PlGF can form heterodimers with VEGF/VPF as do the PDGF-A and -B chains.

As indicated earlier in this chapter, a number of candidate receptors have been molecularly cloned by low-stringency hybridization techniques using sequences from known receptors as probes and by PCR techniques in which oligonucleotides representing tyrosine kinase domain consensus sequences are used as primers. Thus, de Vries et al.[160] found that the sequence of a clone isolated from a human placenta cDNA library was almost identical to that of a putative RPTK designated *flt*,[161] which was known to be most closely related to the PDGF receptors. COS cells transfected with the *flt*-related clone specifically bound VEGF/VPF with high affinity. Receptor-mediated signal transduction was demonstrated in *Xenopus laevis* oocytes injected with *flt* mRNA on the basis of induction of calcium efflux. Although tyrosine phosphorylation was not reported, it is likely that Flt mediates the biologic effects of VEGF/VPF in endothelial cells.

Terman et al.[162] identified a second VEGF/VPF receptor

in the same manner by screening a human endothelial cell cDNA library. The receptor encoded by this cDNA, designated KDR, is 43 per cent identical to Flt and binds VEGF/VPF with high affinity (75 pM), but signaling by VEGF/VPF through KDR was not demonstrated. Thus, many interesting questions remain to be answered, such as whether either Flt or KDR individually mediates mitogenic activity and/or cell permeability as homodimers or heterodimers and whether either or both receptor binds PlGF. Furthermore, two other genes related to *flt* have been isolated (*flt-3, flt-4*[163,164]) that encode putative receptors. Although neither of these genes is expressed in endothelial cells of blood vessels, the *flt-3* transcript is present in placenta and thus could be considered a candidate for the PlGF receptor.

"ORPHAN" GROWTH FACTORS AND RECEPTORS

The identification of new RPTKs implies the existence of new growth factors and, thus, there are several RPTKs awaiting assignment of their ligands. (Frequently, independent groups have isolated the same gene from the same or different species by various techniques and, therefore, the same gene has been designated differently. In what follows, the various isolates of the same gene are separated by slashes, in alphabetical order.) Putative RPTKs for yet-to-be-discovered growth factors include those encoded by the *ark/axl/ufo/v-ryk*,[165–168] *eph*,[169] *klg*,[170] *ltk*,[171] *ros*,[172] *ret*,[173] *sea*[106] (see earlier), *ryk*[174] (not the same as v-*ryk*), and *tek/tie*[175,176] genes (Fig. 7–2). The functional significance of Klg and Ryk proteins is not known because efforts to demonstrate their tyrosine kinase activity have not been successful.

The *ark* product is widely expressed, and three of the isolates (*axl, ufo,* and v-*ryk*) were isolated as transforming genes. The presence of two Ig-like loops at the amino-terminal region of the extracellular domain followed by two fibronectin type III repeats but no cysteine-rich domain distinguishes this receptor from its closest relatives, the insulin receptor and *eph* subclasses.[166] Its transcript has been detected in a wide variety of adult and embryonic mouse tissues,[167,177] particularly those of mesodermal origin.

The *eph* receptor, expressed most frequently in normal and malignant epithelial cells and first isolated from a hepatoma,[169] is the prototype of a family that includes the *cek4/mek4*,[178] *eck*,[179] *elk*,[180] *hek*,[181] and *sek*[182] genes. *Eph* transcripts are present in lung, liver, kidney, and testis,[183] whereas *cek4/mek4* transcripts are most abundant in adult and embryonic brain as well as in adult testis.[178] *Eck* is expressed primarily in lung, skin, ovary, and small intestine,[179] whereas *elk* expression is limited mainly to brain and testes.[180] *Hek* mRNA was detected only in certain human lymphoid tumor cell lines,[184] and *sek* is segmentally expressed in the developing mouse hindbrain.[182] Little is known about the specific cell types in which these *eph* family members are present, with the exception of *eck*, which is expressed predominantly in epithelial cells.[179] Recently, a protein designated B61, was shown to bind to, and induce autophosphorylation of *eck*.[182a] These results suggest that proteins related to B61, the product of

an early response gene induced by tumor necrosis factor-alpha 4, may serve as ligands for other members of the *eph* family.

The *ltk* gene is most closely related to the insulin receptor family, and its product was detected recently in human placenta and hematopoietic cell lines.[185] Analysis of the expression in mouse embryos of another insulin receptor–related gene, *ros*, which is the vertebrate homologue of the *Drosophila melanogaster* sevenless gene,[186–188] revealed a pattern restricted to kidney, intestine, and lung that coincided with phenotypic induction and proliferation of the epithelium in the kidney and intestine.

The *ret* gene is the only known member of a distinct subclass of receptors whose closest relatives are members of the FGFR family. Interest in *ret*, as mentioned earlier in this chapter, has focused mainly on its role in human tumors as an oncogene activated by recombination with an unrelated gene,[189,190] but there is little information on its normal function.

The *tek/tie* gene products contain two Ig-like loops in their extracellular domains, separated by three EGF-like domains. Three fibronectin type III repeats are located within the carboxy-terminal region of the extracellular domain.[176] The expression patterns of *tek* (mouse)[175] and *tie* (human)[176] were found to be similar in their respective species. In the mouse, *tek* transcripts were detected specifically in the endocardium, leptomeninges, and endothelial lining of the vasculature. The *tie* gene is expressed at high levels in endothelial cell lines and in fetal blood vessels as well as in some myeloid leukemia cell lines.[176] Thus, this receptor may be involved in the proliferation and survival of endothelial cells.

GROWTH FACTORS FOR HEMATOPOIETIC CELLS

The growth, differentiation, survival, and functional activation of hematopoietic cells is regulated by a diverse array of polypeptides (approximately 18), among which are the interleukins, colony-stimulating factors, and erythropoietin (for review, see refs. 191–199). Signaling by most of these molecules is mediated by members of the hematopoietin receptor superfamily, although two, macrophage colony-stimulating factor (macrophage growth factor) and *Steel* factor (stem cell factor), use RPTKs. Although the hematopoietin receptors lack intrinsic protein tyrosine kinase activity, there is evidence that some may signal through nonreceptor tyrosine kinases.[200–206] The following discussion focuses mainly on macrophage growth factor and *Steel* factor.

Colony-Stimulating Factor 1

Colony-stimulating factor 1 (CSF-1), also known as macrophage colony-stimulating factor (M-CSF), is synthesized by activated monocytes and macrophages as well as by fibroblasts and other mesenchymal cells.[207,208] CSF-1 mediates both the proliferation and differentiation of the precursors of mononuclear phagocytes and is required for the survival of mature monocytes and macrophages.[209] Alterations or deletions of CSF-1 were suspected to be involved in myelodysplastic syndrome and acute myeloid leukemia because the gene was mapped to the long arm of human chromosome 5,[210] which is nonrandomly deleted in the cells of patients suffering from these diseases. Furthermore, the genes for its receptor and several other cytokines are located at 5q23-31.[211] However, two independent groups recently found that CSF-1 actually maps to 1p13-21.[212,213] Mature CSF-1[209] is secreted as a disulfide-bonded homodimeric proteoglycan[214,215] with a molecular weight of 85,000. Larger proteoglycan forms (>200 kDa) also are secreted,[214,215] but their role in signaling is not known. Analysis of CSF-1 cDNAs[207,216–218] revealed that the primary transcript encodes a precursor of 554 amino acids containing a transmembrane domain and a short (35–amino acid) cytoplasmic tail. At least four other forms are generated by alternative splicing events that occur within a single exon (exon 6) that is downstream of the coding sequences (exons 1 through 5) required for mitogenic activity (reviewed in ref. 219). Thus the mature, secreted forms of CSF-1 are generated by proteolytic cleavage of a transmembrane precursor.[220,221] The structure of one alternatively spliced transcript predicts a membrane-bound protein, because the proteolytic cleavage site used for cleaving the precursor is spliced out.[218,222,223] The three-dimensional structure of dimeric human recombinant CSF-1, as revealed by x-ray crystallography,[224] resembles those of granulocyte-macrophage colony-stimulating factor (GM-CSF) and human growth hormone. Because the latter do not signal through RPTKs, the ligand-binding domains of otherwise highly diverse receptors are likely to share structural similarity.

The CSF-1 receptor (CSF-1R) (see refs. 191, 225 for review) is encoded by the c-fms proto-oncogene[226] and is considered a member of the PDGF family of growth factor receptors on the basis of primary sequence similarity, the presence of five Ig-like loops in its extracellular domain, and an insert within the tyrosine kinase domain.[7] CSF-1R expression is limited to monocytes, macrophages, and their progenitors.[227] This gene can become oncogenically activated by mutations within the extracellular domain that induce constitutive protein tyrosine kinase activity.[228,229] The v-fms retroviral oncogene also expresses a constitutively activated protein tyrosine kinase that contains point mutations throughout its sequence and is also carboxy-terminally truncated.[230]

Stem Cell Factor (Steel Factor, Mast Cell Growth Factor, Kit Ligand)

The various designations for this growth factor reflect its pleiotropic effects on a variety of cell types as uncovered by several independent groups of investigators.[231–235] Thus, stem cell factor (SCF) plays roles in melanogenesis, hematopoiesis, and gametogenesis.[236–238] Its discovery was the result of the convergence of independent studies on two mutations in mice (Sl, steel locus and W, white spotting locus) that led to similar phenotypes and the mapping of the c-kit proto-oncogene, which encodes an RPTK, to the W locus.[239] The defects in pigmentation, hematopoiesis, and fertility in W or Sl mice can be attributed to the derivation of the different cell types involved in these processes from migrating cells of the neural crest. For ex-

ample, the alterations in coat color in W or Sl mutants can be attributed to the chemotactic effect of SCF on melanocyte progenitors.[240] The conclusion that SCF is thought to play a role in the very early stages of hematopoiesis is supported by findings that it stimulates the proliferation of murine spleen colony-forming cells in vitro and that it synergizes with interleukin (IL)-1 or IL-3 in this system.[241–244] SCF also has been shown to increase the number and size of colonies from erythroid precursor cells (BFU-E) in conjunction with erythropoietin and to be required by mast cells for their survival, proliferation, and differentiation (see ref. 241 and references therein).

The human SCF mRNA encodes a 248-transmembrane protein with 189 and 42 amino acid–long extracellular and cystoplasmic domains, respectively.[232] SCF was purified from medium conditioned by various cell types[231,233,245] and also was demonstrated to be associated with the cell surface.[235,246] The 70,000- to 90,000-molecular weight secreted form is a noncovalently associated dimeric glycoprotein with an acidic isoelectric point resulting from the presence of sialic acid groups.[233,247] That the cell-associated form is critically important was indicated by analysis of the Sl product expressed by mice harboring the Dickie allele of Sl.[246,248] The affected mice are sterile and anemic and display the Sl coat color phenotype (black-eyed white) and only express a soluble form of SCF.

The similarities in phenotypes between the W and Sl mutations, taken together with the chromosomal localization of the c-kit proto-oncogene, led to the proposal that the c-kit product is the receptor for the Steel factor.[239,249] This hypothesis was proven in a series of studies by several groups.[231–235] The receptor encoded by c-kit is a member of the PDGF receptor family and was first recognized as the transforming gene of a feline sarcoma virus.[250] The defect in the c-kit product that gave rise to the original W mutation was the result of a deletion of a 78–amino acid stretch that includes the transmembrane domain.[251]

SIGNALING PATHWAYS OF TYROSINE KINASE RECEPTORS

Knowledge of the cascade of biochemical events triggered by ligand stimulation of tyrosine kinase receptors has increased rapidly in recent years and provides further evidence of the importance of these signaling pathways in cancer (Fig. 7–3). The PDGF system has served as the prototype for identification of the components of these systems. Certain molecules become physically associated and/or phosphorylated by the activated PDGF receptor kinase. Those identified to date include phospholipase C (PLC)-γ,[252,253] phosphatidylinositol-3′-kinase (PI-3K),[254] ras p21 GTPase-activating protein (GAP),[255–257] and src and src-like tyrosine kinases.[258,259] These molecules share so-called src homology (SH) regions 2 and 3, which are noncatalytic domains that appear to be important in binding interactions among tyrosine-phosphorylated proteins.[260] The raf proto-oncogene product also has been reported to become physically associated with the receptor and tyrosine phosphorylated as well,[261,262] although it lacks SH2 or SH3 domains.

PLC-γ is one of several PLC isoforms and is involved in the generation of two important second messengers, inositol triphosphate and diacylglycerol.[263,264] The former causes release of stored intracellular calcium and the latter activates protein kinase C (PKC). These second messengers appear rapidly in cells following stimulation by growth factors such as PDGF. The relative increase in their synthesis in vivo correlates reasonably well with the ability of a particular receptor kinase to induce tyrosine phosphorylation of PLC-γ.[252,253] In combination with recent evidence that tyrosine-phosphorylated PLC-γ exhibits increased catalytic activity in vitro,[265,266] it seems very likely that receptor-induced tyrosine phosphorylation activates this enzyme. The actions of a number of tumor promoters are thought to be mediated by PKC,[263,264] and PKC overexpression or gene alteration has been reported to increase cell proliferation in culture.[267,268]

PI-3K phosphorylates the inositol ring in PI in the 3′ position and becomes physically associated with a number of activated tyrosine kinases.[269] The 85-kDa subunit of the protein contains two SH2 domains as well as an SH3 domain and is tyrosine phosphorylated, but itself lacks PI-3K activity.[270–272] The catalytic domain likely is associated with a 110-kDa protein, which is part of a heterodimeric complex with the 85-kDa protein.[269] An argument for the role of this enzyme in transformation derives from evidence that the transforming ability of polyoma middle T mutants correlates tightly with PI-3K functional activity in complexes with pp60[c-src 273–275] Moreover, v-src and v-abl mutants that fail to associate with PI-3K are nontransforming.[276,277]

GAP is intimately involved in the function of the Ras proteins.[278] ras encodes a 21,000-Da guanine nucleotide binding protein (p21).[279] There is substantial evidence that ras is a critical component of intracellular mitogenic signaling pathways because oncogenically activated ras p21 induces DNA synthesis on microinjection of NIH 3T3 fibroblasts.[280] Mutations that cause ras oncogenic activation lead to accumulation of ras p21 GTP, the active form of the molecule.[279] GAP stimulates the GTPase activity inherent in ras p21,[279] and common oncogenic mutations in ras block the ability of GAP to down-regulate the ras p21 molecule to its inactive GDP-bound form.[279] GAP has been shown to act as a negative regulator of ras function.[281–183] There is also evidence that GAP may serve in a complex with ras p21 as an effector of its downstream signaling functions.[284] Thus, mutations that impair ras p21 interaction with GAP also block ras biologic function.

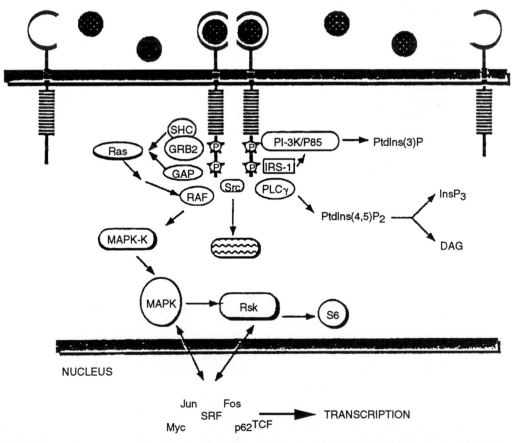

Figure 7–3. Summary of molecules involved in mitogenic signaling through RPTKs. This figure shows a dimerized and activated (tyrosine-phosphorylated) prototypical RPTK and illustrates some of the signaling molecules that associate (unshaded polygons) with receptors or reside further downstream (shaded polygons) in the pathway. The bidirectional arrows indicate cytoplasmic and nuclear localizations of MAP kinase and S6 kinase.

Stimulation of certain receptors results in physical interaction of GAP with the receptor kinase[135,256,257] as well as its cell membrane association, the known site of *ras* p21 function.[279] Tyrosine-phosphorylated GAP also is found to be associated in a complex with at least two other tyrosine-phosphorylated proteins (p62 and p190), which may modulate *ras* function.[285] There is also evidence that GAP complexed with p190 exhibits decreased ability to promote *ras* p21 GTPase activity in vitro.[286] PDGF stimulation leads to an increase in the level of GTP-bound *ras* p21,[287,288] consistent with the possibility that tyrosine phosphorylation of GAP and/or associated proteins transiently interrupts its negative regulation of *ras* p21 function. However, other *ras* p21 regulatory molecules, including a GTP exchange protein, have been identified in yeast,[289–291] and there is evidence for such activities in mammalian cells as well.[292–294] Thus, further studies are needed to establish firmly the mechanisms responsible for *ras* activation in growth factor–stimulated cells as well as the effector functions of this important signal transducer.

The ability of various receptor kinases to interact with known substrates differs markedly. For instance, the PDGF receptor kinase interacts with PLC-γ, PI-3K, and GAP, whereas the related CSF-1 receptor exhibits little if any activity with respect to PLC-γ or GAP.[295,296] The EGF receptor and *erbB*-2 also are relatively inefficient at GAP tyrosine phosphorylation.[297] The FGF receptors induce tyrosine phosphorylation of a prominent, as yet unidentified substrate, p90,[298,299] which is not phosphorylated in response to a number of other receptors. The insulin receptor signals uniquely through a protein designated IRS-1[300–302] that is unrelated to any known protein. IRS-1 is considered to be a "docking" protein because it is rapidly tyrosine phosphorylated by the insulin receptor following insulin stimulation and it then activates PI-3K by associating with the SH2 domains of the latter.[303]

Progress in identifying other components of mitogenic signaling cascades has been made recently through the use of a variety of techniques, including screening of cDNA libraries with nucleic acid probes representing SH2 domains[304,305] and using the tyrosine-phosphorylated carboxy-terminal domain of RPTKs as probes to select receptor binding proteins from expression libraries.[272,306] The identification of other signaling molecules has resulted from screening expression libraries with antibodies specific for proteins that become tyrosine phosphorylated shortly after growth factor triggering,[307] analyzing cellular or retroviral oncogenes containing SH2-related sequences,[308,309] and fortuitously as well.[310] The elucidation of a developmental pathway in the nematode (see later in this section) *Caenorhabditis elegans*[311] has provided important clues as to the placement of one of these putative signal transducers (GRB-2/ASH[305,312]) in signaling pathways.

A common feature of the so-called signaling proteins (i.e., those that are situated downstream of the receptor in the mitogenic signal transduction pathway) revealed by these studies is the presence of single or multiple copies of SH2 domains. Most, but not all, contain one or more SH3 domains (see refs. 8,313–315 for reviews). They can be classified into two groups[8,313]: I, proteins with enzymatic function; and II, proteins that serve as either "adaptors" or regulatory subunits of signaling proteins because they lack catalytic activity and/or similarity to proteins with known biochemical function. Members of group I include *src*, PLC-γ, GAP, the tyrosine phosphatase PTP1C, and the oncogene *vav*. Group II consists of the p85 subunit of PI-3K (also known as GRB1); c-*crk*, the cellular homologue of the viral oncogene v-*crk*; and *nck*, *shc*, and *sem5*/GRB2/ASH. As could be predicted by the oncogenicity of other members of their group, *nck* and *shc* have been shown to be potent transforming genes.[304,316]

The biochemical and molecular genetic studies on SH2 and SH3 domains, although elegant and persuasive, only indirectly implicated them as being important regulators of signal transduction. However, genetic analysis of the genes involved in vulval induction and in the migration of sex myoblasts in *C. elegans*, taken together with analysis of their mammalian counterparts, has provided very convincing evidence for such a role. The *let*-23 and *let*-60 gene products, homologues of the mammalian EGF receptor and Ras proteins, respectively, are required for signal transduction in vulval cells in *C. elegans*.[311] The *sem*-5 gene encodes a protein containing one SH2 and two SH3 domains and was shown to function immediately downstream of the *let*-23 product. A search for EGF receptor substrates using an expression cloning system yielded a gene designated *GRB2* (growth factor receptor binding), which was shown to be structurally and functionally equivalent to the *sem*-5 product.[312] Because the sequence of *sem*-5/*GRB2* does not predict a protein with catalytic function, it was postulated that it might act on another protein, perhaps a GDP-GTP exchange factor, to regulate the activity of a Ras GTPase. GRB2 can form a complex with Shc,[304] a class II SH2 signaling protein known to function upstream of Ras[317] in rat cells transformed by v-*src* or in growth factor–stimulated cells. This complex, rather than GRB2 alone, may function to regulate Ras exchange factors or even GAP.

Downstream Signaling Molecules

The mitogen-activated protein (MAP) kinases (for review see refs. 318–323) are very likely key intermediates in growth factor–triggered signaling pathways as well as in many other signal transduction pathways. Several investigators found that proteins of 41 to 45 kDa were rapidly and heavily phosphorylated on tyrosyl residues following growth factor treatment of cells or as a result of transformation by tyrosine kinase–encoding oncogenes.[323–327] The identity of these proteins as MAP kinases subsequently was established.[328,329] The MAP kinases have been referred to by a wide variety of designations, mainly based on in vitro substrates used to characterize their catalytic properties. Designations include ERT kinases (EGF-receptor threonine kinase), MAP-2 kinases (myelin basic protein kinase), and RSK kinases (ribosomal S6 protein kinase kinases). They also commonly are called ERKs (extracellular signal–regulated kinases).

Important features of the pathway for growth factor signaling through MAP kinases are becoming clear, although there are some uncertainties that must be resolved.[321,322] Perhaps one of the earliest events following growth factor triggering of its cognate receptor is activation of Ras p21.[330-336] Ras p21 directly or indirectly activates Raf serine/threonine kinase,[262,331,337-339] which is the product of the *raf* proto-oncogene.[340] Oncogenically activated forms of Raf resulting from deletions or mutations of its amino-terminal domain have been identified in tumors by gene transfer experiments, and accumulating evidence indicates that this domain normally serves to regulate the catalytic domain. Thus, *raf* oncogene products show constitutively increased serine-threonine kinase activity.[340] The Raf kinase is thought to phosphorylate the dual-specificity MAP kinase kinase (MAPKK), the direct activator of MAP kinase.[341-344] Gene transcription follows MAP kinase phosphorylation of the nuclear proto-oncogene product Jun, the transcription factor $p62^{TCF}$ and/or Myc.[345-348] MAP kinase is thought to reside at a branch point in the pathway because it phosphorylates RSK as well.[331,349,350] The substrate of RSK is the ribosomal S6 protein, but the nuclear proto-oncogene product Fos and a nuclear protein designated SRF also may be targets.[351]

Efforts to date have only begun to unravel the mysteries enshrouding the connections between biochemical signals emanating from primary receptor substrates that travel to the nucleus, resulting in the transcriptional activation of specific sets of genes and the inactivation of others. The nuclear proteins mentioned above are transcription factors that bind to DNA as homomeric or heteromeric dimers.[352-354] These molecules possess different types of sequence-specific DNA binding domains, and phosphorylation appears to modulate their functions as well.[355-358] A number, including *jun, fos, myc, myb, rel,* and *ets,* initially were identified as viral oncogenes (for review, see refs. 359,360) and subsequently were linked to mitogenic signaling pathways. For example, *jun* and *fos* are immediate early genes induced by a wide variety of growth factors in different cell types.[361] Moreover, inhibition of the induction of these genes by antibodies or antisense strategies blocks DNA synthesis.[362,363] There are also a number of *jun* and *fos* family members, and it has been shown that the transcription factor AP1, whose activity is induced by TPA via the PKC pathway, is composed of heterodimeric combinations of these molecules.[355-358] *myc* expression is induced by growth factor stimulation, and antisense experiments argue that *myc* function is also critical to normal cell proliferation.[361,364]

SIGNALING VIA OTHER RECEPTORS

Cytokines

Although it is not within the scope of this chapter to consider in detail all of the hematopoietic growth factors (see refs. 191–199,365,366), it is nevertheless important to briefly consider what is known about their signaling pathways. The receptors for hematopoietic growth factors are expressed at exceedingly low levels (100 to 1000 mol-

ecules per cell), and, because only *fms* and *kit* presented themselves to investigators conveniently packaged as retroviral oncogenes, it was not until relatively recently that the structures of most of these receptors were revealed. Thus, the receptors for (IL)-2, IL-3, IL-4, IL-5, IL-6, IL-7, IL-9, IL-12, erythropoietin (EPO), G-CSF, GM-CSF, growth hormone (GH), prolactin, leukemia inhibitory factor (LIF), and ciliary neurotrophic factor (CNTF) belong to a superfamily (hematopoietin cytokine receptors) lacking significant sequence similarity to PRTKs (Fig. 7–4).

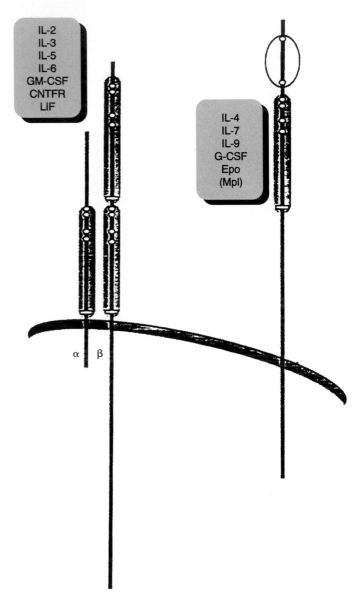

Figure 7–4. Representative structures of hematopoietin receptors. The two-chain and single-chain receptor structures are based on the sequences of the α and β chains of the GM-CSF and G-CSF receptors, respectively.[423] [425] (The IL-2α chain is unrelated to any known protein, but the γ chain is a member of the hematopoietin receptor family.) The small circles indicate cysteine residues highly conserved within the family, but, for clarity, not all cysteines are shown. The open rectangle indicates the position of the WSXWS motif and the elongated shaded ovals encompass the extracellular domain that typifies this receptor family. The ellipse at the amino-terminal region of the single-chain receptor represents an IG-L domain.

They share a common structural motif in their extracellular domains (about 200 amino acids) that includes amino-terminally conserved cysteine residues and the pattern WSXWS within the carboxy-terminal domain. Both extra- and intracellular portions of these receptors vary considerably in length (208 to 603 and 13 to 603 amino acids, respectively). The receptors for other cytokines, such as interferons α, β, and γ, IL-1, IL-8, tumor necrosis factor α (TNF-α) and lymphotoxin, are distinct, and the receptors for ILs 10 and 11 remain to be characterized. High-affinity ligand binding is achieved in some cases by the formation of receptor heterodimers. For example, IL-3, IL-5, and GM-CSF bind with high affinity to a receptor consisting of one unrelated α chain specific for the cognate ligand and a common β chain. The α chain alone binds ligand with only low affinity, whereas, depending on the species of origin, binding by the β chain is either weak or undetectable.

The biochemical pathways by which these receptors stimulate proliferation remain largely unexplored, although there are reports that triggering can lead to the appearance of tyrosine-phosphorylated proteins[200–206] as well as increased levels of GTP-bound *ras* p21.[287] Recent studies have linked activation of the *lck* tyrosine kinase to IL-2 stimulation of its receptor,[367] supporting the concept that *src* family members participate in signal transduction by this class of receptors. One example of oncogenic activation in this system involves in vitro mutations of the Epo receptor, which constitutively up-regulate its functional activity and cause transformation of appropriate hematopoietic target cells.[368] In another, erythroblastic leukemia induced by the spleen focus–forming virus is due to molecular mimicry of Epo by a recombinant *env* gene product of this defective retrovirus.[369,370] Another acute transforming retrovirus, myeloproliferative virus (MPLV),[371] infects a wide variety of hematopoietic progenitor cells and relieves them of factor dependence.[372,373] The MPLV transforming gene, v-*mpl*, is a truncated version, fused to viral *env* gene sequences, of a member of the hematopoietin receptor family.[374] Although the *mpl* proto-oncogene cDNA has been cloned, its ligand has not been identified,[375] nor is it known whether the *mpl* gene product represents an α or β receptor form. In human T-cell tumors associated with human T-lymphocyte virus 1 infection, viral gene products appear to stimulate proliferation of affected cells by up-regulating expression of both IL-2 and its receptor.[376]

Neurotransmitters

The transmission of signals generated by the reception of chemical and physical stimuli from the external and internal environments is mediated by a large variety of small molecules known as neurotransmitters. These molecules include acetylcholine; amino acid derivatives such as epinephrine, norepinephrine, serotonin, and dopamine; and peptides such as the angiotensins, β-endorphin, enkephalins, and somatostatin. Although neurotransmitters are known to be involved in controlling an enormous array of bodily functions, their role in stimulating cell pro-

liferation is just beginning to be appreciated. Early studies demonstrated that angiotensin was mitogenic for adrenocortical cells,[377] but it was not until the era of tumor DNA transfection experiments that the implications of these early observations with respect to growth control and cancer became more apparent. DNA isolated from a human epidermoid carcinoma induced tumors in nude mice in a cotransfection-tumorigenicity assay.[378,379] The oncogene responsible, designated *mas*, was found to encode a protein that possessed seven membrane-spanning regions characteristic of the G-protein–linked receptors, visual rhodopsin, and the α subunit of the acetylcholine receptor.[380] At about this same time, the sequences of additional neurotransmitter receptor genes were determined. Their structures were found to be closely related to *mas*, although overall amino acid sequence similarities were limited. These genes include the α_1-,[381] α_2-,[382] β_1-,[383,384] and β_2-[385] adrenergic receptors, the muscarinic acetylcholine receptors (mACHRs)[386–388] and the serotonin,[389] substance K,[390] and dopamine[391] receptors (Fig. 7–5).

Ashkenazi et al.[392] found that a stable acetylcholine analogue carbachol, was mitogenic via mACHRs in perinatal rat brain astrocytes and in brain-derived astrocytoma and neuroblastoma cell lines. When Chinese hamster ovary (CHO) cells were transfected with human mACHR genes, carbachol stimulated DNA synthesis in those cells expressing mACHR subtypes that are known to activate PI hydrolysis most efficiently (m1, m3, or m5), stimulate arachidonic acid release, and open Ca^{2+}-dependent potassium channels by coupling with a pertussis toxin–insensitive G protein, whereas the m2 and m4 mACHR subtypes couple to a pertussis toxin–sensitive G protein to inhibit adenylyl cyclase.[393–395] These data are consistent with the observations that acetylcholine stimulates phosphoinositide hydrolysis at peak levels in the brain during the perinatal period when certain glial cells proliferate and differentiate. Besides these proliferative effects, it has been pointed out that neurotransmitter/receptor systems

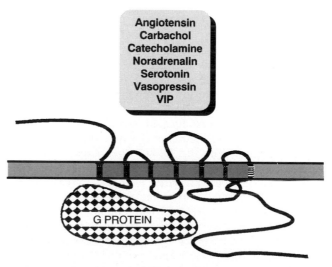

Figure 7–5. Mitogenic neurotransmitters. Receptors for neurotransmitters possess seven membrane-spanning domains and signal through small G proteins.

could act in other growth processes, such as stimulating hypertrophy of or inducing process extension in nondividing neurons.[396] Furthermore, carbachol was found to induce foci of transformation in cultures of NIH 3T3 cells transfected with either the m1, m3, or m5 but not the m2 and m4 mACHR subtypes.[397]

Serotonin (5-hydroxtryptamine, 5-HT) was shown to be mitogenic for smooth muscle cells[398] and subsequently for fibroblasts.[399] There are several receptor subtypes for serotonin, including those that couple either to signaling systems involving PLC activation (5-HT$_{1c}$ and 5-HT$_2$ receptors) or adenylate cyclase (5-HT$_{1a}$ and 5-HT$_{1b}$ receptors). Introduction of the 5-HT$_{1c}$ gene into mouse NIH 3T3 fibroblasts induced morphologic transformation that was dependent on receptor activation by serotonin.[400] In such cells, serotonin was shown to mobilize intracellular Ca^{2+} probably via PLC activation and production of inositol triphosphate. Because diacylglycerol also is released by the catalytic action of PLC, protein kinase C activation also may play a role in the induction of the transformed phenotype.

More recently, Allen et al.[401] demonstrated that the α_{1B}-adrenergic receptor, when introduced into either Rat-1 or NIH 3T3 cells, induced agonist-dependent (catecholamine) focus formation, and the transformed cells were tumorigenic in nude mice. Similar effects were achieved by overexpressing a mutant form of the receptor, but, in this case, transformation occurred in the absence of ligand stimulation.

Based on these studies and on the well-known oncogenic effects of mutated *ras* p21 proteins, a reasonable prediction could be made that perturbations of signaling pathways downstream of the transmitter-receptor interaction could lead to malignant transformation. Signal transmission through the β-adrenergic receptor to adenylyl cyclase is mediated by the G$_{\alpha s}$ subunit of the G protein G$_s$. A link between alterations of this signaling system and oncogenesis was uncovered by studies on two distinct groups within a subset of growth hormone–secreting human pituitary tumors.[402] In one group, G$_s$ was constitutively active, resulting in elevated adenylyl cyclase activity and growth hormone levels. The G$_{\alpha s}$ component was found to be activated by point mutations in either a site at which cholera toxin inactivates G$_s$ (Arg 201 → Cys/His) or at a residue equivalent to a GTPase-inhibiting mutation that causes malignant activation of *ras* p21 (Gln 227 → Arg). Because both mutations have the effect of destroying GTPase activity, G$_{\alpha s}$ (designated *gsp*) becomes constitutively activated in a manner analogous to the oncogenic activity of *ras* p21.

The two mutations are located in regions that are highly conserved among G$_\alpha$ proteins isolated from diverse eukaryotic species. With this knowledge, a search was conducted for tumors harboring GTPase-inhibiting mutations in genes of other G$_\alpha$ proteins.[403] In this survey, in 3/11 tumors of the adrenal cortex and 3/10 ovarian endocrine tumors, mutations of Arg 179 (the cognate of Arg 201 in G$_\alpha$) to Cys or His were found in the A chain of G$_{i2}$ (designated *gip2*). Additional *gsp* mutations were found in 18/42 growth hormone–secreting pituitary tumors. Subsequently it was shown that mutant forms of the α subunit of G$_{i2}$[404-407] as well the wild-type form of G$_{\alpha 12}$ (when overexpressed)[408] could transform rodent fibroblasts.

PROSPECTS FOR CANCER THERAPY

The rapidly expanding body of knowledge concerning growth factor–mediated mitogenic signaling pathways holds promise for the development of new cancer treatments. In considering the cascade of events that lead to the onset of growth factor–induced cell proliferation, the most obvious point of attack would seem to be the initial interaction between the growth factor and its cognate receptor at the cell surface of tumor cells whose growth is dependent on autocrine or paracrine mechanisms. Thus, specific antagonists could be developed based on the sequence of either the binding sites on the growth factor or receptors for one another. Such molecules have been found to be produced naturally, and presumably function physiologically to modulate growth factor signaling.[409,410] Another approach is based on the production of monoclonal antibodies that would specifically neutralize the activities of growth factors. Monoclonal antibodies directed toward the receptor would be useful in tumors in which, as discussed earlier, uncontrolled proliferation occurs as the result of receptor overexpression. For example, in tumors that overexpress either EGFR or *erbB*-2, their levels of expression often exceed that of normal cells by 50 to 100-fold. Promising results have been reported by investigators using experimental animal models in which administration of monoclonal receptor antibodies induced receptor down-regulation and impairment of tumor cell proliferation.[411-415] Another strategy utilizes receptor antibodies to deliver cytotoxic agents such as toxins or radioisotopes to tumor cells in a highly specific manner.[416]

Devising "molecular surgery"[417] for signaling reactions that occur inside the cell offers greater challenges. As indicated in this chapter, the number of known downstream signaling molecules is growing rapidly, potentially offering more targets for therapy. The tyrosine phosphorylation reaction is an attractive target, but the wide range of metabolic processes in which this protein modification is involved makes the design of a highly specific drug extremely difficult. Nevertheless, drugs termed "tyrphostins" have been found to block phosphorylation of tyrosine residues[418] and to inhibit cell proliferation in culture at concentrations exhibiting little toxicity.[418] The central role of *ras* p21 mitogenic signaling and its oncogenic activation in many tumors[279] has led to efforts to inhibit *ras* function. One target of such approaches is the posttranslational lipid modification of the p21 Ras molecule required for its membrane localization and essential for Ras function.[419-422] Recent efforts have led to purification of the farnesyl protein transferase responsible, and it has been possible to show that peptides as small as four amino acids can serve as substrates.[422] These findings raise the possibility that exogenously administered peptides or their analogues may act as inhibitors of p21 Ras by competing for this enzyme. Development of agents that interfere with the other types of signaling reactions considered here, such as receptor interactions with SH2/SH3 domain-containing proteins, threonine-serine–specific reactions mediated by MAP kinase, or oligomerization of components of transcription factors, could be envisioned as well. It is hoped that molecular biotherapeutics someday will replace or provide an important adjunct to present-day therapy for malignancies.

ACKNOWLEDGMENT: The authors thank Rose Windle and Matthias Kraus for help in preparing the manuscript and figures, respectively, and Jeffrey Rubin for sharing his unpublished review of the HGF literature.

REFERENCES

1. Collett MS, Erikson RL: Protein kinase activity associated with the avian sarcoma virus src gene product. Proc Natl Acad Sci USA 75:2021, 1978.
2. Hunter T, Sefton BM: Transforming gene product of Rous sarcoma virus phosphorylates tyrosine. Proc Natl Acad Sci USA 77:1311, 1980
3. Doolittle RF, Hunkapiller MW, Hood LE, et al: Simian sarcoma virus onc gene, v-sis, is derived from the gene (or genes) encoding a platelet-derived growth factor. Science 221:275, 1983
4. Waterfield MD, Scrace GT, Whittle N, et al: Platelet-derived growth factor is structurally related to the putative transforming protein p28sis of simian sarcoma virus. Nature 304:35, 1983
5. Downward J, Yarden Y, Mayes E, et al: Close similarity of epidermal growth factor receptor and v-erb-B oncogene protein sequences. Nature 307:521, 1984
6. Carpenter G, Cohen S. Epidermal growth factor. J Biol Chem 265:7709, 1990
7. Ullrich A, Schlessinger J: Signal transduction by receptors with tyrosine kinase activity. Cell 61:203, 1990
8. Schlessinger J, Ullrich A: Growth factor signaling by receptor tyrosine kinases. Neuron 9:383, 1992
9. Canals F: Signal transmission by epidermal growth factor receptor: Coincidence of activation and dimerization. Biochemistry 31:4493, 1992
10. Bargmann CI, Hung MC, Weinberg RA: Multiple independent activations of the neu oncogene by a point mutation altering the transmembrane domain of p185. Cell 45:649, 1986
11. Gill GN, Rosenfeld MG, Chen WS, et al: Analysis of functional domains in the epidermal growth factor receptor using site-directed mutagenesis. Adv Exp Med Biol 234:91, 1988
12. Cohen S, Epidermal growth factor. Biosci Rep 6:1017, 1986
13. Gregory H: Isolation and structure of urogastrone and its relationship to epidermal growth factor. Nature 257:325, 1975
14. Wright NA, Pike C, Elia G: Induction of a novel epidermal growth factor-secreting cell lineage by mucosal ulceration in human gastrointestinal stem cells. Nature 343:82, 1990
15. Gray A, Dull TJ, Ullrich A: Nucleotide sequence of epidermal growth factor cDNA predicts a 128,000-molecular weight protein precursor. Nature 303:722, 1983
16. Scott J, Urdea M, Quiroga M, et al: Structure of a mouse submaxillary messenger RNA encoding epidermal growth factor and seven related proteins. Science 221:236, 1983
17. Mroczkowksi B, Reich M, Chen K, et al: Recombinant human epidermal growth factor precursor is a glycosylated membrane protein with biological activity. Mol Cell Biol 9:2771, 1989
18. Prigent SA, Lemoine NR: The type 1 (EGFR-related) family of growth factor receptors and their ligands. Prog Growth Factor Res 4:1, 1992
19. Roberts AB, Sporn MB: Principles of molecular cell biology of cancer: growth factors related to transformation. In DeVita, VT, Hellman S, Rosenberg SA (eds): Cancer Principles and Practice of Oncology. Philadelphia, JB Lippincott Company, 1989, pp 67–80
20. Higashiyama S, Abraham JA, Miller J, et al: A heparin-binding growth factor secreted by macrophage-like cells that is related to EGF. Science 251:936, 1991
21. Kimura H, Fischer WH, Schubert D: Structure, expression and function of a schwannoma-derived growth factor. Nature 348:257, 1990
22. Holmes WE, Sliwkowski MX, Akita RW, et al: Identification of heregulin, a specific activator of p185erbB2. Science 256:1205, 1992
23. Peles E, Bacus SS, Koski RA, et al: Isolation of the neu/HER-2 stimulatory ligand: a 44 kd glycoprotein that induces differentiation of mammary tumor cells. Cell 69:205, 1992
24. Wen D, Peles E, Cupples R, et al: Neu differentiation factor: A transmembrane glycoprotein containing an EGF domain and an immunoglobulin homology unit. Cell 69:559, 1992
25. Shing Y, Christofori G, Hanahan D, et al: Betacellulin, A mitogen from pancreatic β cell tumors. Science 259:1604, 1993
26. Derynck R: Transforming growth factor alpha. Cell 54:593, 1988
27. Plowman GD, Green JM, McDonald VL, et al: The amphiregulin gene encodes a novel epidermal growth factor-related protein with tumor-inhibitory activity. Mol Cell Biol 10:1969, 1990
28. Sonoda H, Yamaguchi T, Watanabe S: Androgen-responsive expression and mitogenic activity of schwannoma-derived growth factor on an androgen-dependent shionogi mouse mammary carcinoma cell line. Biochem Biophys Res Commun 185:103, 1992
29. Ciccodicola A, Dona R, Obici S, et al: Molecular characterization of a gene of the 'EGF family' expressed in undifferentiated human NTERA2 teratocarcinoma cells. EMBO J 8:1987, 1989
30. Wrann MM, Fox CF: Identification of epidermal growth factor receptors in a hyperproducing human epidermoid carcinoma cell line. J Biol Chem 254:8083, 1979
31. Ullrich A, Coussens L, Hayflick JS, et al: Human epidermal growth factor receptor cDNA sequence and aberrant expression of the amplified gene in A431 epidermoid carcinoma cells. Nature 309:418, 1984
32. Carpenter G, King L Jr, Cohen S: Epidermal growth factor stimulates phosphorylation in membrane preparations in vitro. Nature 276:409, 1978
33. Ushiro H, Cohen S: Identification of phosphotyrosine as a product of epidermal growth factor-activated protein kinase in A-431 cell membranes. J Biol Chem 255:8363, 1980
34. Lin CR, Chen WS, Kruiger W, et al: Expression cloning of human EGF receptor complementary DNA: Gene amplification and three related messenger RNA products in A431 cells. Science 224:843, 1984
35. Xu YH, Ishii S, Clark AJ, et al: Human epidermal growth factor receptor cDNA is homologous to a variety of RNAs overproduced in A431 carcinoma cells. Nature 309:806, 1984
36. King CR, Kraus MH, Aaronson SA: Amplification of a novel v-erbB-related gene in a human mammary carcinoma. Science 229:974, 1985
37. Coussens L, Yang-Feng TL, Liao YC, et al: Tyrosine kinase receptor with extensive homology to EGF receptor shares chromosomal location with neu oncogene. Science 230:1132, 1985
38. Yamamoto T, Ikawa S, Akiyama T, et al: Similarity of protein encoded by the human c-erb-B2 gene to epidermal growth factor receptor. Nature 319:230, 1986
39. Kraus MH, Issing W, Miki T, et al: Isolation and characterization of ERBB3, a third member of the ERBB/epidermal growth factor receptor family: Evidence for overexpression in a subset of human mammary tumors. Proc Natl Acad Sci USA 86:9193, 1989
39a. Plowman GD, Green JM, Culouscou JM, et al: Heregulin induces tyrosine phosphorylation of HER4/p180erbB4. Nature 366:473, 1993
39b. Plowman GD, Culouscou JM, Whitney GS, et al: Ligand-specific activation of HER4/p180erbB4, a fourth member of the epidermal growth factor receptor family. Proc Natl Acad Sci USA 90:1746, 1993

40. DiFiore PP, Kraus MH: Mechanisms involving an expanding erbB/EGF receptor family of tyrosine kinases in human neoplasia. Cancer Treat Res *61*:139, 1992

41. Slamon DJ, Godolphin W, Jones LA, et al: Studies of the HER-2/neu proto-oncogene in human breast and ovarian cancer. Science *244*:707, 1989

42. Burgess WH, Maciag T: The heparin-binding (fibroblast) growth factor family of proteins. Annu Rev Biochem *58*:575, 1989

43. Gimenez-Gallego G, Rodkey J, Bennett C, et al: Brain-derived acidic fibroblast growth factor: Complete amino acid sequence and homologies. Science *230*:1385, 1985

44. Esch F, Baird A, Ling N, et al: Primary structure of bovine pituitary basic fibroblast growth factor (FGF) and comparison with the amino-terminal sequence of bovine brain acidic FGF. Proc Natl Acad Sci USA *82*:6507, 1985

45. Moore R, Casey G, Brookes S, et al: Sequence, topography and protein coding potential of mouse int-2: A putative oncogene activated by mouse mammary tumour virus. EMBO J *5*:919, 1986

46. Sakamoto H, Mori M, Taira M, et al: Transforming gene from human stomach cancers and a noncancerous portion of stomach mucosa. Proc Natl Acad Sci USA *83*:3997, 1986

47. Delli Bovi P, Curatola AM, Kern FG, et al: An oncogene isolated by transfection of Kaposi's sarcoma DNA encodes a growth factor that is a member of the FGF family. Cell *50*:729, 1987

48. Zhan X, Bates B, Hu XG, et al: The human FGF-5 oncogene encodes a novel protein related to fibroblast growth factors. Mol Cell Biol *8*:3487, 1988

49. Marics I, Adelaide J, Raybaud F, et al: Characterization of the HST-related FGF.6 gene, a new member of the fibroblast growth factor gene family. Oncogene *4*:335, 1989

50. Finch PW, Rubin JS, Miki T, et al: Human KGF is FGF-related with properties of a paracrine effector of epithelial cell growth. Science *245*:752, 1989

51. Tanaka A, Miyamoto K, Minamino N, et al: Cloning and characterization of an androgen-induced growth factor essential for the androgen-dependent growth of mouse mammary carcinoma cells. Proc Natl Acad Sci USA *89*:8928, 1992

51a. Miyamoto M, Naruo K, Seko C, et al: Molecular cloning of a novel cytokine cDNA encoding the ninth member of the fibroblast growth factor family, which has a unique secretion property. Mol Cell Biol *13*:4251, 1993

52. Goldfarb M: The fibroblast growth factor family. Cell Growth Differ *1*:439, 1990

53. Hearn MT: Structure and function of the heparin-binding (fibroblast) growth factor family. Baillieres Clin Endocrinol Metab *5*:571, 1991

54. Gospodarowicz D: Biological activities of fibroblast growth factors. Ann N Y Acad Sci *638*:1, 1991

55. Smith R, Peters G, Dickson C: Multiple RNAs expressed from the int-2 gene in mouse embryonal carcinoma cell lines encode a protein with homology to fibroblast growth factors. EMBO J *7*:1013, 1988

56. Dixon M, Deed R, Acland P, et al: Detection and characterization of the fibroblast growth factor-related oncoprotein INT-2. Mol Cell Biol *9*:4896, 1989

57. Muller WJ, Lee FS, Dickson C, et al: The int-2 gene product acts as an epithelial growth factor in transgenic mice. EMBO J *9*:907, 1990

58. Rubin JS, Osada H, Finch PW, et al: Purification and characterization of a newly identified growth factor specific for epithelial cells. Proc Natl Acad Sci USA *86*:802, 1989

59. Jaye M, Schlessinger J, Dionne CA: Fibroblast growth factor receptor tyrosine kinases: Molecular analysis and signal transduction. Biochim Biophys Acta *1135*:185, 1992

60. Givol D, Yayon A: Complexity of FGF receptors: Genetic basis for structural diversity and functional specificity. FASEB J *6*:3362, 1992

61. Johnson DE, Williams LT: Structural and functional diversity in the FGF receptor multigene family. Adv Cancer Res *60*:1, 1993

62. Reid HH, Wilks AF, Bernard O: Two forms of the basic fibroblast growth factor receptor-like mRNA are expressed in the developing mouse brain. Proc Natl Acad Sci USA *87*:1596, 1990

63. Safran A, Avivi A, Orr-Urtereger A, et al: The murine flg gene encodes a receptor for fibroblast growth factor. Oncogene *5*:635, 1990

64. Yayon A, Klagsbrun M, Esko JD, et al: Cell surface, heparin-like molecules are required for binding of basic fibroblast growth factor to its high affinity receptor. Cell *64*:841, 1991

65. Dionne CA, Crumley G, Bellot F, et al: Cloning and expression of two distinct high-affinity receptors cross-reacting with acidic and basic fibroblast growth factors. EMBO J *9*:2685, 1990

66. Ruta M, Howk R, Ricca G, et al: A novel protein tyrosine kinase gene whose expression is modulated during endothelial cell differentiation. Oncogene *3*:9, 1988

67. Lee PL, Johnson DE, Cousens LS, et al: Purification and complementary DNA cloning of a receptor for basic fibroblast growth factor. Science *245*:57, 1989

68. Pasquale EB, Singer SJ: Identification of a developmentally regulated protein-tyrosine kinase by using anti-phosphotyrosine antibodies to screen a cDNA expression library. Proc Natl Acad Sci USA *86*:5449, 1989

69. Kornbluth S, Paulson KE, Hanafusa H: Novel tyrosine kinase identified by phosphotyrosine antibody screening of cDNA libraries. Mol Cell Biol *8*:5541, 1988

70. Pasquale EB: A distinctive family of embryonic protein-tyrosine kinase receptors. Proc Natl Acad Sci USA *87*:5812, 1990

71. Miki T, Fleming TP, Bottaro DP, et al: Expression cDNA cloning of the KGF receptor by creation of a transforming autocrine loop. Science *251*:72, 1991

72. Miki T, Bottaro DP, Fleming TP, et al: Determination of ligand-binding specificity by alternative splicing: Two distinct growth factor receptors encoded by a single gene. Proc Natl Acad Sci USA *89*:246, 1992

73. Keegan K, Johnson DE, Williams LT, et al: Isolation of an additional member of the fibroblast growth factor receptor family, FGFR-3. Proc Natl Acad Sci USA *88*:1095, 1991

74. Partanen J, Makela TP, Eerola E, et al: FGFR-4, a novel acidic fibroblast growth factor receptor with a distinct expression pattern. EMBO J *10*:1347, 1991

75. Ron D, Reich R, Chedid M, et al: Fibroblast growth factor receptor 4 is a high affinity receptor for both acidic and basic fibroblast growth factor but not for keratinocyte growth factor. J Biol Chem *268*:5388, 1993

76. Bernard O, Li M, Reid HH: Expression of two different forms of fibroblast growth factor receptor 1 in different mouse tissues and cell lines. Proc Natl Acad Sci USA *88*:7625, 1991

77. Eisemann A, Ahn JA, Graziani G, et al: Alternative splicing generates at least five different isoforms of the human basic-FGF receptor. Oncogene *6*:1195, 1991 [published erratum appears in Oncogene *6*:2379, 1991]

78. Johnson DE, Lu J, Chen H, et al: The human fibroblast growth factor receptor genes: A common structural arrangement underlies the mechanisms for generating receptor forms that differ in their third immunoglobulin domain. Mol Cell Biol *11*:4627, 1991

79. Werner S, Duan DS, de Vries C, et al: Differential splicing in the extracellular region of fibroblast growth factor receptor 1 generates receptor variants with different ligand-binding specificities. Mol Cell biol *12*:82, 1992

80. Hattori Y, Odagiri H, Nakatani H, et al: K-sam, an amplified gene in stomach cancer, is a member of the heparin-binding growth factor receptor genes. Proc Natl Acad Sci USA *87*:5983, 1990

81. Bottaro DP, Rubin JS, Ron D, et al: Characterization of the receptor for keratinocyte growth factor: Evidence for multiple fibroblast growth factor receptors. J Biol Chem *265*:12767, 1990

82. Kiefer MC, Stephans JC, Crawford K, et al: Ligand-affinity cloning and structure of a cell surface heparan sulfate proteoglycan that binds basic fibroblast growth factor. Proc Natl Acad Sci USA *87*:6985, 1990

83. Klagsbrun M, Baird A: A dual receptor system is required for basic fibroblast growth factor activity. Cell *67*:229, 1991

84. Rapraeger AC, Krufka A, Olwin BB: Requirement of heparan sulfate for bFGF-mediated fibroblast growth and myoblast differentiation. Science 252:1705, 1991

85. Olwin BB, Rapraeger A: Repression of myogenic differentiation by a FGF, bFGF, and K-FGF is dependent on cellular heparan sulfate. J Cell Biol 118:631, 1992

86. Kan M, Wang F, Xu J, et al: An essential heparin-binding domain in the fibroblast growth factor receptor kinase. Science 259:1918, 1993

87. Burrus LW, Zuber ME, Lueddecke BA, et al: Identification of a cysteine-rich receptor for fibroblast growth factors. Mol Cell Biol 12:5600, 1993

88. Nakamura T, Nawa K, Ichihara A, et al: Purification and subunit structure of hepatocyte growth factor from rat platelets. FEBS Lett 224:311, 1987

89. Gohda E, Tsubouchi H, Nakayama H, et al: Purification and partial characterization of hepatocyte growth factor from plasma of a patient with fulminant hepatic failure J Clin Invest 81:414, 1988

90. Zarnegar R, Michalopoulos G: Purification and biological characterization of human hepatopoietin A, a polypeptide growth factor for hepatocytes. Cancer Res 49:3314, 1989

91. Gherardi E, Stoker M: Hepatocyte growth factor–scatter factor: mitogen, motogen, and met. Cancer cells 3:227, 1991

92. Rubin JS, Chan AM, Bottaro DP, et al: A broad-spectrum human lung fibroblast-derived mitogen is a variant of hepatocyte growth factor. Proc Natl Acad Sci USA 88:415, 1991

93. Kan M, Zhang GH, Zarnegar R, et al: Hepatocyte growth factor/hepatopoietin A stimulates the growth of rat kidney proximal tubule epithelial cells (RPTE), rat nonparenchymal liver cells, human melanoma cells, mouse keratinocytes and stimulates anchorage-independent growth of SV-40 transformed RPTE. Biochem Biophys Res Commun 174:331, 1991

94. Igawa T, Kanda S, Kanetake H, et al: Hepatocyte growth factor is a potent mitogen for cultured rabbit renal tubular epithelial cells. Biochem Biophys Res Commun 174:831, 1991

95. Matsumoto K, Tajima H, Nakamura T. Hepatocyte growth factor is a potent stimulator of human melanocyte DNA synthesis and growth. Biochem Biophys Res Commun 176:45, 1991

96. Furlong RA, Takehara T, Taylor WG, et al: Comparison of biological and immunochemical properties indicates that scatter factor and hepatocyte growth factor are indistinguishable. J Cell Sci 100:173, 1991

97. Weidner KM, Arakaki N, Hartmann G, et al: Evidence for the identity of human scatter factor and human hepatocyte growth factor. Proc Natl Acad Sci USA 88:7001, 1991

98. Rosen EM, Knesel J, Goldberg ID: Scatter factor and its relationship to hepatocyte growth factor and met. Cell Growth Differ 2:603, 1991

99. Nakamura T, Nishizawa T, Hagiya M, et al: Molecular cloning and expression of human hepatocyte growth factor. Nature 342:440, 1989

100. Tashiro K, Hagiya M, Nishizawa T, et al: Deduced primary structure of rat hepatocyte growth factor and expression of the mRNA in rat tissues. Proc Natl Acad Sci USA 87:3200, 1990

101. Miyazawa K, Tsubouchi H, Naka D, et al: Molecular cloning and sequence analysis of cDNA for human hepatocyte growth factor. Biochem Biophys Res Commun 163:967, 1989

102. Patthy L, Trexler M, Vali Z, et al: Kringles: Modules specialized for protein binding. Homology of the gelatin-binding region of fibronectin with the kringle structures of proteases. FEBS Lett 171:131, 1984

103. Bottaro DP, Rubin JS, Faletto DL, et al: Identification of the hepatocyte growth factor receptor as the c-met proto-oncogene product. Science 251:802, 1991

104. Tempest PR, Stratton MR, Cooper CS: Structure of the met protein and variation of met protein kinase activity among human tumour cell lines. Br J Cancer 58:3, 1988

105. Giordano S, DiRenzo MF, Ferracini R, et al: p145, a protein with associated tyrosine kinase activity in a human gastric carcinoma cell line. Mol Cell Biol 8:3510, 1988

106. Smith DR, Vogt PK, Hayman MJ: The v-sea oncogene of avian erythroblastosis retrovirus S13: Another member of the protein-tyrosine kinase gene family. Proc Natl Acad Sci USA 86:5291, 1989

106a. Huff JL, Jelinek MA, Borgman CA, et al: The protooncogene c-sea encodes a transmembrane protein-tyrosine kinase related to the Met/hepatocyte growth factor/scatter factor receptor. Proc Natl Acad Sci USA 90:6140, 1993

107. Espinal J: Mechanism of insulin action. Nature 328:574, 1987

108. Clemmons DR: Structural and functional analysis of insulin-like growth factors. Br Med Bull 45:465, 1989

109. Dull TJ, Gray A, Hayflick JS, et al: Insulin-like growth factor II precursor gene organization in relation to insulin gene family. Nature 310:777, 1984.

110. Ullrich A, Berman CH, Dull TJ, et al: Isolation of the human insulin-like growth factor I gene using a single synthetic DNA probe. EMBO J 3:361, 1984

111. Kaleko M, Rutter WJ, Miller AD: Overexpression of the human insulinlike growth factor I receptor promotes ligand-dependent neoplastic transformation. Mol Cell Biol 10:464, 1990

112. Ullrich A, Bell JR, Chen EY, et al: Human insulin receptor and its relationship to the tyrosine kinase family of oncogenes. Nature 313:756, 1985

113. Ebina Y, Ellis L, Jarnagin K, et al: The human insulin receptor cDNA: The structural basis for hormone-activated transmembrane signalling. Cell 40:747, 1985

114. Rosen OM: After insulin binds. Science 237:1452, 1987

115. Adamo M, Roberts CT, Jr, LeRoith D: How distinct are the insulin and insulin-like growth factor I signalling systems? Biofactors 3:151, 1992

116. Graves DT, Cochran DL, Mesenchymal cell growth factors. Crit Rev Oral Biol Med 1:17, 1990

117. Ullrich A, Gray A, Tam AW, et al: Insulin-like growth factor I receptor primary structure: Comparison with insulin receptor suggests structural determinants that define functional specificity. EMBO J 5:2503, 1986

118. Morgan DO, Edman JC, Standring DN, et al: Insulin-like growth factor II receptor as a multifunctional binding protein. Nature 329:301, 1987 [Published erratum appears in Nature 20:442, 1988]

119. MacDonald RG, Pfeffer SR, Coussens L, et al: A single receptor binds both insulin-like growth factor II and mannose-6-phosphate. Science 239:1134, 1988

120. Czech MP: Signal transmission by the insulin-like growth factors. Cell 59:235, 1989

121. Giorgino F, Belifiore A, Milazzo G, et al: Overexpression of insulin receptors in fibroblast and ovary cells induces a ligand-mediated transformed phenotype. Mol Endocrinol 5:452, 1991

122. Levi-Montalcini R: The nerve growth factor 35 years later. Science 237:1154, 1987

123. Ebendal T: Function and evolution in the NGF family and its receptors. J Neurosci Res 32461, 1192

124. Barbacid M, Lamballe F, Pulido D, et al: The trk family of tyrosine protein kinase receptors. Biochim Biophys Act 1072:115, 1991

125. Thoenen H: The changing scene of neurotrophic factors. Trends Neurosci 14:165, 1991

126. Hohn A, Leibrock J, Bailey K, et al: Identification and characterization of a novel member of the nerve growth factor/brain-derived neurotrophic factor family. Nature 344:339, 1990

127. Maisonpierre PC, Belluscio L, Squinto S, et al: Neurotrophin-3: A neurotrophic factor related to NGF and BDNF. Science 247:1446, 1990

128. Hallböök F, Ibáñez CF, Persson H: Evolutionary studies of the nerve growth factor family reveal a novel member abundantly expressed in Xenopus ovary. Neuron 6:845, 1991

129. Berkemeier LR, Winslow JW, Kaplan DR, et al: Neurotrophin-5: A novel neurotrophic factor that activates trk and trkB. Neuron 7:857, 1991

130. Johnson D, Lanahan S, Buck CR, et al: Expression and structure of the human NGF receptor. Cell 47:545, 1986

131. Radeke MJ, Misko TP, Hsu C, et al: Gene transfer and molecular cloning of the rat nerve growth factor receptor. Nature 325:593, 1987

132. Pulciani S, Santos E, Lauver AV, et al: Oncogenes in solid human tumours. Nature 300:539, 1982

133. Cordon-Cardo C, Tapley P, Jing SQ, et al: The trk tyrosine protein kinase mediates the mitogenic properties of nerve growth factor and neurotrophin-3. Cell 66:173, 1991

134. Klein R, Conway D, Parada LF, et al: The trkB tyrosine protein kinase gene codes for a second neurogenic receptor that lacks the catalytic kinase domain. Cell 61:647, 1990

135. Soppet D, Escandon E, Maragos J, et al: The neurotrophic factors brain-derived neurotrophic factor and neurotrophin-3 are ligands for the trkB tyrosine kinase receptor. Cell 65:895, 1991

136. Squinto SP, Stitt TN, Aldrich TH, et al: trkB encodes a functional receptor for brain-derived neurotrophic factor and neurotrophin-3 but not nerve growth factor. Cell 65:885, 1991

137. Lamballe F, Klein R, Barbacid M: trkC, a new member of the trk family of tyrosine protein kinases, is a receptor for neurotrophin-3. Cell 66:967, 1991

138. Meakin SO, Shooter EM: The nerve growth factor family of receptors. Trends Neurosci 15:323, 1992

139. Ibänez CF, Ebendal T, Barbany G, et al: Disruption of the low affinity receptor-binding site in NGF allows neuronal survival and differentiation by binding to the trk gene product. Cell 69:329, 1992

140. Lee KF, Li E, Huber LJ, et al: Targeted mutation of the gene encoding the low affinity NGF receptor p75 leads to deficits in the peripheral sensory nervous system. Cell 69:737, 1992

141. Heldin CH, Hammacher A, Nister M, et al: Structural and functional aspects of platelet-derived growth factor. Br J Cancer 57:591, 1988

142. Ross R, Raines EW, Bowen-Pope DR: The biology of platelet-derived growth factor. Cell 46:155, 1986

143. Claesson-Welsh L, Eriksson A, Westermark B, et al: cDNA cloning and expression of the human A-type platelet-derived growth factor (PDGF) receptor establishes structural similarity to the B-type PDGF receptor. Proc Natl Acad Sci USA 86:4917, 1989

144. Claesson-Welsh L, Hammacher A, Westermark B, et al: Identification and structural analysis of the A type receptor for platelet-derived growth factor: Similarities with the B type receptor. J Biol Chem 264:1742, 1989

145. Matsui T, Heidaran M, Miki T, et al: Isolation of a novel receptor cDNA establishes the existence of two PDGF receptor genes. Science 243:800, 1989

146. Yarden Y, Escobedo JA, Kuang WJ, et al: Structure of the receptor for platelet-derived growth factor helps define a family of closely related growth factor receptors. Nature 323:226, 1986

147. Hart CE, Forstrom JW, Kelly JD, et al: Two classes of PDGF receptor recognize different isoforms of PDGF. Science 240:1529, 1988

148. Matsui T, Pierce JH, Fleming TP, et al: Independent expression of human alpha or beta platelet-derived growth factor receptor cDNAs in a naive hematopoietic cell leads to functional coupling with mitogenic and chemotactic signaling pathways. Proc Natl Acad Sci USA 86:8314, 1989

149. Williams LT: Signal transduction by the platelet-derived growth factor receptor. Science 243:1564, 1989

150. Robbins KC, Antoniades HN, Devare SG, et al: Structural and immunological similarities between simian sarcoma virus gene product(s) and human platelet-derived growth factor. Nature 305:605, 1983

151. Robbins KC, Leal F, Pierce JH, et al: The v-sis/PDGF-2 transforming gene product localizes to cell membranes but is not a secretory protein. EMBO J 4:1783, 1985

152. Gazit A, Igarashi H, Chiu IM, et al: Expression of the normal human sis/PDGF-2 coding sequence induces cellular transformation. Cell 39:89, 1984

153. Igarashi H, Rao CD, Siroff M, et al: Detection of PDGF-2 homodimers in human tumor cells. Oncogene 1:79, 1987

154. Heldin CH, Johnsson A, Wennergren S, et al: A human osteosarcoma cell line secretes a growth factor structurally related to a homodimer of PDGF A-chains. Nature 319:511, 1986

155. Westermark B, Johnsson A, Paulsson Y, et al: Human melanoma cell lines of primary and metastatic origin express the genes encoding the chains of platelet-derived growth factor (PDGF) and produce a PDGF-like growth factor. Proc Natl Acad Sci USA 83:7197, 1986

156. Nister M, Hammacher A, Mellstrom K, et al: A glioma-derived PDGF A chain homodimer has different functional activities from a PDGF AB heterodimer purified from human platelets. Cell 52:791, 1988

157. Leung DW, Cachianes G, Kuang WJ, et al: Vascular endothelial growth factor is a secreted angiogenic mitogen. Science 246:1306, 1989

158. Keck PJ, Hauser SD, Krivi G, et al: Vascular permeability factor, an endothelial cell mitogen related to PDGF. Science 246:1309, 1989

159. Maglione D, Guerriero V, Viglietto G, et al: Isolation of a human placenta cDNA coding for a protein related to the vascular permeability factor. Proc Natl Acad Sci USA 88:9267, 1991

160. de Vries C, Escobedo JA, Ueno H, et al: The fms-like tyrosine kinase, a receptor for vascular endothelial growth factor. Science 255:989, 1992

161. Shibuya M, Yamaguchi S, Yamane A, et al: Nucleotide sequence and expression of a novel human receptor-type tyrosine kinase gene (flt) closely related to the fms family. Oncogene 5:519, 1990

162. Terman BI, Dougher-Vermazen M, Carrion ME, et al: Identification of the KDR tyrosine kinase as a receptor for vascular endothelial cell growth factor. Biochem Biophys Res Commun 187:1579, 1992

163. Rosnet O, Marchetto S, deLapeyriere O, et al: Murine Flt3, a gene encoding a novel tyrosine kinase receptor of the PDGFR/CSF1R family. Oncogene 6:1641, 1991

164. Pajusola K, Aprelikova O, Korhonen J, et al: FLT4 receptor tyrosine kinase contains seven immunoglobulin-like loops and is expressed in multiple human tissues and cell lines. Cancer Res 52:5738, 1992

165. Rescigno J, Mansukhani A, Basilico C: A putative receptor tyrosine kinase with unique structural topology. Oncogene 6:1909, 1991

166. O'Bryan JP, Frye RA, Cogswell PC, et al: axl, a transforming gene isolated from primary human myeloid leukemia cells, encodes a novel receptor tyrosine kinase. Mol Cell Biol 11:5016, 1991

167. Janssen JW, Schulz AS, Steenvoorden AC, et al: A novel putative tyrosine kinase receptor with oncogenic potential. Oncogene 6:2113, 1991

168. Jia R, Mayer BJ, Hanafusa T, et al: A novel oncogene, v-ryk, encoding a truncated receptor tyrosine kinase is transduced into the RPL30 virus without loss of viral sequences. J Virol 66:5975, 1992

169. Hirai H, Maru Y, Hagiwara K, et al: A novel putative tyrosine kinase receptor encoded by the eph gene. Science 238:1717, 1987

170. Chou YH, Hayman MJ: Characterization of a member of the immunoglobulin gene superfamily that possibly represents an additional class of growth factor receptor. Proc Natl Acad Sci USA 88:4897, 1991

171. Ben-Neriah Y, Bauskin AR: Leukocytes express a novel gene encoding a putative transmembrane protein-kinase devoid of an extracellular domain. Nature 333:672, 1988

172. Neckameyer WS, Wang LH: Nucleotide sequence of avian sarcoma virus UR2 and comparison of its transforming gene with other members of the tyrosine protein kinase oncogene family. J Virol 53:879, 1985

173. Takahashi M, Ritz J, Cooper GM: Activation of a novel human transforming gene, ret, by DNA rearrangement. Cell 42:581, 1985.

174. Hovens CM, Stacker SA, Andres AC, et al: RYK, a receptor tyrosine kinase-related molecule with unusual kinase domain motifs. Proc Natl Acad Sci USA 89:11818, 1992

175. Dumont DJ, Yamaguchi TP, Conlon RA, et al: tek, a novel tyrosine kinase gene located on mouse chromosome 4, is expressed in endothelial cells and their presumptive precursors. Oncogene 7:1471, 1992

176. Partanen J, Armstrong E, Makela TP, et al: A novel endothelial cell surface receptor tyrosine kinase with extracellular epidermal growth factor homology domains. Mol Cell Biol 12: 1698, 1992

177. Faust M, Ebensperger C, Schulz AS, et al: The murine ufo receptor: Molecular cloning, chromosomal localization and in situ expression analysis. Oncogene 7:1287, 1992

178. Sajjadi FG, Pasquale EB, Subramani S: Identification of a new eph-related receptor tyrosine kinase gene from mouse and chicken that is developmentally regulated and encodes at least two forms of the receptor. Nature New Biol 3:769, 1991

179. Lindberg RA, Hunter T: cDNA cloning and characterization of eck, an epithelial cell receptor protein-tyrosine kinase in the eph/elk family of protein kinases. Mol Cell Biol 10:6316, 1990

180. Lhotak V, Greer P, Letwin K, et al: Characterization of elk, a brain-specific receptor tyrosine kinase. Mol Cell biol 11: 2496, 1991

181. Boyd AW, Ward LD, Wicks IP, et al: Isolation and characterization of a novel receptor-type protein tyrosine kinase (hek) from a human pre-B cell line. J Biol Chem 267:3262, 1992

182. Gilardi-Hebenstreit P, Nieto MA, Frain M, et al: An Eph-related receptor protein tyrosine kinase gene segmentally expressed in the developing mouse hindbrain. Oncogene 7:2499, 1992

182a. Bartley TD, Hunt RW, Welcher AA, et al: B61 is a ligand for the eck receptor protein-tyrosine kinase. Nature 368:558, 1994

183. Maru Y, Hirai H, Yoshida MC, et al: Evolution, expression, and chromosomal location of a novel receptor tyrosine kinase gene, eph. Mol Cell Biol 8:3770, 1988

184. Wicks IP, Wilkinson D, Salvaris E, et al: Molecular cloning of HEK, the gene encoding a receptor tyrosine kinase expressed by human lymphoid tumor cell lines. Proc Natl Acad Sci USA 89:1611, 1992

185. Kozutsumi H, Toyoshima H, Hagiwara K, et al: Identification of the human ltk gene product in placenta and hematopoietic cell lines. Biochem Biophys Res Commun 190:674, 1993

186. Matsushime H, Shibuya M: Tissue-specific expression of rat c-ros-1 gene and partial structural similarity of its predicted products with sev protein of Drosophila melanogaster. J Virol 64:2117, 1990

187. Tessarollo L, Nagarajan L, Parada LF: c-ros: The vertebrate homolog of the sevenless tyrosine kinase receptor is tightly regulated during organogenesis in mouse embryonic development. Development 115:11, 1992

188. Chen JM, Heller D, Poon B, et al: The proto-oncogene c-ros codes for a transmembrane tyrosine protein kinase sharing sequence and structural homology with sevenless protein of Drosophila melanogaster. Oncogene 6:257, 1991

189. Grieco M, Santoro M, Berlingieri MT, et al: PTC is a novel rearranged form of the ret proto-oncogene and is frequently detected in vivo in human thyroid papillary carcinomas. Cell 60:557, 1990

190. Ishizaka Y, Ushijima T, Sugimura T, et al: cDNA cloning and characterization of ret activated in a human papillary thyroid carcinoma cell line. Biochem Biophys Res Commun 168: 402, 1990

191. Pierce JH: Oncogenes, growth factors and hematopoietic cell transformation. Biochim Biophys Acta 989:179, 1989

192. D'Andrea AD, Fasman GD, Lodush HF: A new hematopoietic growth factor receptor superfamily. Structural features and implications for signal transduction. Curr Opin Cell Biol 2: 648, 1990

193. Brizzi MF, Avanzi GC, Pegoraro L: Hematopoietic growth factor receptors. Int J Cell Cloning 9:274, 1991

194. Krystal G, Alai M, Cutler RL, et al: Hematopoietic growth factor receptors. Hematol Pathol 5:141, 1991

195. Williams ME, Quesenberry PJ: Hematopoietic growth factors. Hematol Pathol 6:105, 1992

196. Kaczmarski RS, Mufti GJ: The cytokine receptor superfamily. Blood Rev 5:193, 1991

197. Demetri GD: Hematopoietic growth factors: Current knowledge, future prospects. Curr Probl Cancer 16:177, 1992

198. Rowe JM, Rapoport AP: Hemopoietic growth factors: A review. J Clin Pharmacol 32:486, 1992

199. Taga T, Kishimoto T: Cytokine receptors and signal transduction. FASEB J 6:3387, 1992

200. Sorensen PH, Mui AL, Murthy SC, et al: Interleukin-3, GM-CSF, and TPA induce distinct phosphorylation events in an interleukin 3-dependent multipotential cell line. Blood 73: 406, 1989

201. Kanakura Y, Druker B, Cannistra SA, et al: Signal transduction of the human granulocyte-macrophage colony-stimulating factor and interleukin-3 receptors involves tyrosine phosphorylation of a common set of cytoplasmic proteins. Blood. 76: 706, 1990

202. Morla AO, Schreurs J, Miyajima A, et al: Hematopoietic growth factors activate the tyrosine phosphorylation of distinct sets of proteins in interleukin-3-dependent murine cell lines. Mol Cell Biol 8:2214, 1988

203. Kanakura Y, Druker B, Wood KW, et al: Granulocyte-macrophage colony-stimulating factor and interleukin-3 induce rapid phosphorylation and activation of the proto-oncogene Raf-1 in a human factor-dependent myeloid cell line. Blood 77:243, 1991

204. Isfort R, Huhn RD, Frackelton AR, Jr, et al: Stimulation of factor-dependent myeloid cell lines with interleukin 3 induces tyrosine phosphorylation of several cellular substrates. J Biol Chem 263:19203, 1988

205. Augustine JA, Schlager JW, Abraham RT: Differential effects of interleukin-2 and interleukin-4 on protein tyrosine phosphorylation in factor-dependent murine T cells. Biochim Biophys Acta 1052:313, 1990

206. Wang LM, Keegan AD, Paul WE, et al: Il-4 activates a distinct signal transduction cascade from IL-3 in factor-dependent myeloid cells. EMBO J 11:4899, 1992

207. Kawasaki ES, Ladner MB, Wang AM, et al: Molecular cloning of a complementary DNA encoding human macrophage-specific colony-stimulating factor (CSF-1). Science 230:291, 1985

208. Stanley ER, Heard PM: Factors regulating macrophage production and growth. Purification and some properties of the colony stimulating factor from medium conditioned by mouse L cells. J Biol Chem 252:4305, 1977

209. Stanley ER, Guilbert LJ, Tushinski RJ, et al: CSF-1—a mononuclear phagocyte lineage-specific hemopoietic growth factor. J Cell Biochem 21:151, 1983

210. Pettenati MJ, Le Beau MM, Lemons RS, et al: Assignment of CSF-1 to 5q33:1 Evidence for clustering of genes regulating hematopoiesis and for their involvement in the deletion of the long arm of chromosome 5 in myeloid disorders. Proc Natl Acad Sci USA 84:2970, 1987

211. Boulay JL, Paul WE: The interleukin-4-related lymphokines and their binding to hematopoietin receptors. J Biol Chem 267:20525, 1992

212. Morris SW, Valentine MB, Shapiro DN, et al: Reassignment of the human CSF-1 gene to chromosome 1p13-p21. Blood 78: 2013, 1991

213. Saltman DL, Dolganov GM, Hinton LM, et al: Reassignment of the human macrophage colony stimulating factor gene to chromosome 1p13–21. Biochem Biophy Res Commun 182: 1139, 1992

214. Price LK, Choi HU, Rosenberg L, et al: The predominant form of secreted colony stimulating factor-1 is a proteoglycan. J Biol Chem 267:2190, 1992

215. Suzu S, Ohtsuki T, Yanai N, et al: Identification of a high molecular weight macrophage colony-stimulating factor as a glycosaminoglycan-containing species. J Biol Chem 267: 4345, 1992

216. Wong GG, Witek JS, Temple PA, et al: Human GM-CSF: Molecular cloning of the complementary DNA and purification of the natural and recombinant proteins. Science 228:810, 1985

217. Cerretti DP, Wignall J, Anderson D, et al: Human macrophage-colony stimulating factor: Alternative RNA and protein processing from a single gene. Mol Immunol 25:761, 1988

218. Pampfer S, Tabibzadeh S, Chuan FC, et al: Expression of colony-stimulating factor-1 (CSF-1) messenger RNA in human

endometrial glands during the menstrual cycle: Molecular cloning of a novel transcript that predicts a cell surface form of CSF-1. Mol Endocrinol 5:1931, 1991

219. Kawasaki ES, Ladner MB: Molecular biology of macrophage colony-stimulating factor. Immunol Ser 49:155, 1990

220. Rettenmier CW, Roussel MF: Differential processing of colony-stimulating factor 1 precursors encoded by two human c-DNAs. Mol Cell Biol 8:5026, 1988

221. Manos MM: Expression and processing of a recombinant human macrophage colony-stimulating factor in mouse cells. Mol Cell Biol 8:5035, 1988

222. Rettenmier CW, Roussel MF, Ashmun RA, et al: Synthesis of membrane-bound colony-stimulating factor 1 (CSF-1) and downmodulation of CSF-1 receptors in NIH 3T3 cells transformed by cotransfection of the human CSF-1 and c-fms (CSF-1 receptor) genes. Mol Cell Biol 7:2378, 1987

223. Stein J, Borzillo GV, Rettenmier CW: Direct stimulation of cells expressing receptors for macrophage colony-stimulating factor (CSF-1) by a plasma membrane-bound precursor of human CSF-1. Blood 76:1308, 1990

224. Pandit J, Bohm A, Jancarik J, et al: Three-dimensional structure of dimeric human recombinant macrophage colony-stimulating factor. Science 258:1358, 1992

225. Sherr CJ: Mitogenic response to colony-stimulating factor 1. Trends Gen 7:398, 1991

226. Sherr CJ, Rettenmier CW, Sacca R, et al: The c-fms proto-oncogene product is related to the receptor for the mononuclear phagocyte growth factor, CSF-1. Cell 41:665, 1985

227. Woolford J, Rothwell V, Rohrschneider L: Characterization of the human c-fms gene product and its expression in cells of the monocyte-macrophage lineage. Mol Cell Biol 5:3458, 1985

228. Roussel MF, Downing JR, Rettenmier CW, et al: A point mutation in the extracellular domain of the human CSF-1 receptor (c-fms proto-oncogene product) activates its transforming potential. Cell 55:979, 1988

229. Woolford J, McAuliffe A, Rohrschneider LR: Activation of the feline c-fms proto-oncogene: Multiple alterations are required to generate a fully transformed phenotype. Cell 55:965, 1988

230. Roussel MF, Downing JR, Ashmun RA, et al: Colony-stimulating factor 1-mediated regulation of a chimeric c-fms/v-fms receptor containing the v-fms-encoded tyrosine kinase domain. Proc Natl Acad Sci USA 85:5903, 1988

231. Williams DE, Eisenman J, Baird A, et al: Identification of a ligand for the c-kit proto-oncogene. Cell 63:167, 1990

232. Martin FH, Suggs SV, Langley KE, et al: Primary structure and functional expression of rat and human stem cell factor DNAs. Cell 63:203, 1990

233. Zsebo KM, Williams DA, Geissler EN, et al: Stem cell factor is encoded at the Sl locus of the mouse and is the ligand for the c-kit tyrosine kinase receptor. Cell 63:213, 1990

234. Huang E, Nocka K, Beier DR, et al: The hematopoietic growth factor KL is encoded by the Sl locus and is the ligand of the c-kit receptor, the gene product of the W locus. Cell 63:225, 1990

235. Anderson DM, Lyman SD, Baird A, et al: Molecular cloning of mast cell growth factor, a hematopoietin that is active in both membrane bound and soluble form. Cell 63:235, 1990 [Published erratum appears in Cell 63:1112, 1990]

236. Bennett D: Developmental analysis of a mutant with pleiotropic effects in the mouse. J Morphol 98:199, 1956

237. Russell ES: Hereditary anemias of the mouse: A review for geneticists. Adv Genet 20:357, 1979

238. Poole TW, Silvers WK: Capacity of adult steel (Sl/Sld) and dominant spotting (W/Wv) mouse skin to support melanogenesis. Dev Biol 72:398, 1979

239. Chabot B, Stephenson DA, Chapman VM, et al: The proto-oncogene c-kit encoding a transmembrane tyrosine kinase receptor maps to the mouse W locus. Nature 335:88, 1988

240. Keshet E, Lyman SD, Williams DE, et al: Embryonic RNA expression patterns of the c-kit receptor and its cognate ligand suggest multiple functional roles in mouse development. EMBO J 10:2425, 1991

241. Williams DE, de Vries P, Namen AE, et al: The Steel factor. Dev Biol 151:368, 1992

242. de Vries P, Brasel KA, Eisenman JR, et al: The effect of recombinant mast cell growth factor on purified murine hematopoietic stem cells. J Exp Med 173:1205, 1991

243. Migliaccio G, Migliaccio AR, Valinsky J, et al: Stem cell factor induces proliferation and differentiation of highly enriched murine hematopoietic cells. Proc Natl Acad Sci USA 88:7420, 1991

244. Owaga M, Matsuzaki Y, Nishikawa S, et al: Expression and function of c-kit in hemopoietic progenitor cells. J Exp Med 174:63, 1991

245. Nocka K, Buck J, Levi E, et al: Candidate ligand for the c-kit transmembrane kinase receptor: KL, a fibroblast derived growth factor stimulates mast cells and erythroid progenitors. EMBO J 9:3287, 1990

246. Flanagan JG, Chan DC, Leder P: Transmembrane form of the kit ligand growth factor is determined by alternative splicing and is missing in the Sld mutant. Cell 64:1025, 1991

247. Arakawa T, Yphantis DA, Lary JW, et al: Glycosylated and unglycosylated recombinant-derived human stem cell factors are dimeric and have extensive regular secondary structure. J Biol Chem 266:18942, 1991

248. Brannan CI, Lyman SD, Williams DE, et al: Steel-Dickie mutation encodes a c-kit ligand lacking transmembrane and cytoplasmic domains. Proc Natl Acad Sci USA 88:4671, 1991

249. Geissler EN, Ryan MA, Housman DE: The dominant-white spotting (W) locus of the mouse encodes the c-kit proto-oncogene. Cell 55:185, 1988

250. Besmer P, Murphy JE, George PC, et al: A new acute transforming feline retrovirus and relationship of its oncogene v-kit with the protein kinase gene family. Nature 320:415, 1986

251. Nocka K, Tan JC, Chiu E, et al: Molecular bases of dominant negative and loss of function mutations at the murine c-kit/white spotting locus: W37, Wv, W41 and W. EMBO J 9:1805, 1990

252. Meisenhelder J, Suh PG, Rhee SG, et al: Phospholipase C-gamma is a substrate for the PDGF and EGF receptor protein-tyrosine kinases in vivo and in vitro. Cell 57:1109, 1989

253. Wahl MI, Olashaw NE, Nishibe S, et al: Platelet-derived growth factor induces rapid and sustained tyrosine phosphorylation of phospholipase C-gamma in quiescent BALB/c 3T3 cells. Mol Cell Biol 9:2934, 1989

254. Kaplan DR, Whitman M, Schaffhausen B, et al: Common elements in growth factor stimulation and oncogenic transformation: 85 kd phosphoprotein and phosphatidylinositol kinase activity. Cell 50:1021, 1987

255. Molloy CJ, Bottaro DP, Fleming TP, et al: PDGF induction of tyrosine phosphorylation of GTPase activating protein. Nature 342:711, 1989

256. Kaplan DR, Morrison DK, Wong G, et al: PDGF beta-receptor stimulates tyrosine phosphorylation of GAP and association of GAP with a signaling complex. Cell 61:125, 1990

257. Kazlauskas A, Ellis C, Pawson T, et al: Binding of GAP to activated PDGF receptors. Science 247:1578, 1990

258. Ralston R, Bishop JM: The product of the protooncogene c-src is modified during the cellular response to platelet-derived growth factor. Proc Natl Acad Sci USA 82:7845, 1985

259. Kypta RM, Goldberg Y, Ulug ET, et al: Association between the PDGF receptor and members of the src family of tyrosine kinases. Cell 62:481, 1990

260. Koch CA, Anderson D, Moran MF, et al: SH2 and SH3 domains: Elements that control interactions of cytoplasmic signaling proteins. Science 252:668, 1991

261. Morrison DK, Kaplan DR, Rapp U, et al: Signal transduction from membrane to cytoplasm: Growth factors and membrane-bound oncogene products increase Raf-1 phosphorylation and associated protein kinase activity. Proc Natl Acad Sci USA 85:8855, 1988

262. Morrison DK, Kaplan DR, Escobedo JA, et al: Direct activation of the serine/threonine kinase activity of Raf-1 through tyrosine phosphorylation by the PDGF beta-receptor. Cell 58:649, 1989

263. Berridge MJ, Irvine RF: Inositol phosphates and cell signalling. Nature 341:197, 1989

264. Kikkawa U, Kishimoto A, Nishizuka Y: The protein kinase C

family: Heterogeneity and its implications. Annu Rev Biochem 58:31, 1989

265. Nishibe S, Wahl MI, Hernandez-Sotomayor SM, et al: Increase of the catalytic activity of phospholipase C-gamma 1 by tyrosine phosphorylation. Science 250:1253, 1990

266. Goldschmidt-Clermont PJ, Kim, JW, Machesky LM, et al: Regulation of phospholipase C-gamma 1 by profilin and tyrosine phosphorylation. Science 251:1231, 1991

267. Hsiao WL, Housey GM, Johnson MD, et al: Cells that overproduce protein kinase C are more susceptible to transformation by an activated H-ras oncogene. Mol Cell Biol 9: 2641, 1989

268. Housey GM, Johnson MD, Hsiao WL, et al: Overproduction of protein kinase C causes disordered growth control in rat fibroblasts. Cell 52:343, 1988

269. Cantley LC, Auger KR, Carpenter C, et al: Oncogenes and signal transduction. Cell 64:281, 1991 [Published erratum appears in Cell 65:914, 1991]

270. Escobedo JA, Navankasattusas S, Kavanaugh WM, et al: cDNA cloning of a novel 85 kd protein that has SH2 domains and regulates binding of PI3-kinase to the PDGF beta-receptor. Cell 65:75, 1991

271. Otsu M, Hiles I, Gout I, et al: Characterization of two 85 kd proteins that associate with receptor tyrosine kinases, middle-T/pp60c-src complexes, and PI3-kinase. Cell 65:91, 1991

272. Skolnik EY, Margolis B, Mohammadi M, et al: Cloning of PI3 kinase-associated p85 utilizing a novel method for expression/cloning of target proteins for receptor tyrosine kinases. Cell 65:83, 1991

273. Whitman M, Kaplan DR, Schaffhausen B, et al: Association of phosphatidylinositol kinase activity with polyoma middle-T competent for transformation. Nature 315:239, 1985

274. Kaplan DR, Whitman M, Schaffhausen B, et al: Phosphatidylinositol metabolism and polyoma-mediated transformation. Proc Natl Acad Sci USA 83:3624, 1986

275. Courtneidge SA, Herber A: An 81 kd protein complexed with middle T antigen and pp60c-src: A possible phosphatidylinositol kinase. Cell 50:1031, 1987

276. Fukui Y, Hanafusa H: Phosphatidylinositol kinase activity associates with viral p60src protein. Mol Cell Biol 9:1651, 1989

277. Varticovski L, Daley GQ, Jackson P, et al: Activation of phosphatidylinositol 3-kinase in cells expressing abl oncogene variants. Mol Cell Biol 11:1107, 1991

278. McCormick F: ras GTPase activating protein: Signal transmitter and signal terminator. Cell 56:5, 1989

279. Barbacid M: ras genes. Annu Rev Biochem 56:779, 1987

280. Stacey DW, King HF: Transformation of NIH 3T3 cells by microinjection of Ha-ras p21 protein. Nature 310:508, 1984

281. Zhang K, DeClue JE, Vass WC, et al: Suppression of c-ras transformation by GTPase-activating protein [see comments]. Nature 346:754, 1990

282. Tanaka K, Matsumoto K, Toh-E A: IRA1, an inhibitory regulator of the RAS-cyclic AMP pathway in Saccharomyces cerevisiae. Mol Cell Biol 9:757, 1989

283. Ballester R, Michaeli T, Ferguson K, et al: Genetic analysis of mammalian GAP expressed in yeast. Cell 59:681, 1989

284. Yatani A, Okabe K, Polakis P, et al: ras p21 and GAP inhibit coupling of muscarinic receptors to atrial K^+ channels. Cell 61:769, 1990

285. Bouton AH, Kanner SB, Vines RR, et al: Transformation by pp60src or stimulation of cells with epidermal growth factor induces the stable association of tyrosine-phosphorylated cellular proteins with GTPase-activating protein. Mol Cell Biol 11:945, 1991

286. Moran MF, Polakis P, McCormick F, et alA: Protein-tyrosine kinases regulate the phosphorylation, protein interactions, subcellular distribution, and activity of p21ras GTPase-activating protein. Mol Cell Biol 11:1804, 1991

287. Satoh T, Nakafuku M, Miyajima A, et al: Involvement of ras p21 protein in signal-transduction pathways from interleukin 2, interleukin 3, and granulocyte/macrophage colony-stimulating factor, but not from interleukin 4. Proc Natl Acad Sci USA 88:3314, 1991

288. Gibbs JB, Marshall MS, Scolnick EM, et al: Modulation of guanine nucleotides bound to Ras in NIH3T3 cells by oncogenes, growth factors, and the GTPase activating protein (GAP). J Biol Chem 265:20437, 1990

289. Powers S, Gonzales E, Christensen T, et al: Functional cloning of BUD5, a CDC25-related gene from S. cerevisiae that can suppress a dominant-negative RAS2 mutant. Cell 65:1225, 1991

290. Chant J, Corrado K, Pringle JR, et al: Yeast BUD5, encoding a putative GDP-GTP exchange factor, is necessary for bud site selection and interacts with bud formation gene BEM1. Cell 65:1213, 1991

291. Jones S. Vignais ML, Broach JR: The CDC25 protein of Saccharomyces cerevisiae promotes exchange of guanine nucleotides bound to ras. Mol Cell Biol 11:2641, 1991

292. Huang YK, Kung HF, Kamata T: Purification of a factor capable of stimulating the guanine nucleotide exchange reaction of ras proteins and its effect on ras-related small molecular mass G proteins. Proc Natl Acad Sci USA 87:8008, 1990

293. Wolfman A, Macara IG: A cytosolic protein catalyzes the release of GDP from p21ras. Science 248:67, 1990

294. Downward J, Riehl R, Wu L, et al: Identification of a nucleotide exchange-promoting activity for p21ras. Proc Natl Acad Sci USA 87:5998, 1990

295. Downing JR, Margolis BL, Zilberstein A, et al: Phospholipase C-gamma, a substrate for PDGF receptor kinase, is not phosphorylated on tyrosine during the mitogenic response to CSF-1. EMBO J 8:3345, 1989

296. Reedijk M, Liu XQ, Pawson T: Interactions of phosphatidylinositol kinase, GTPasae-activating protein (GAP), and GAP-associated proteins with the colony-stimulating factor 1 receptor. Mol Cell Biol 10:5601, 1990

297. Fazioli F, Kim UH, Rhee SG, et al: The erbB-2 mitogenic signaling pathway: Tyrosine phosphorylation of phospholipase C-gamma and GTPase-activating protein does not correlate with erbB-2 mitogenic potency. Mol Cell Biol 11:2040, 1991

298. Coughlin SR, Barr PJ, Cousens LS, et al: Acidic and basic fibroblast growth factors stimulate tyrosine kinase activity in vivo. J Biol Chem 263:988, 1988

299. Bottaro DP, Rubin JS, Ron D, et al: Characterization of the receptor for keratinocyte growth factor: Evidence for multiple fibroblast growth factor receptors. J Biol Chem 265:12767, 1990

300. White MF, Maron R, Kahn CR: Insulin rapidly stimulates tyrosine phosphorylation of a Mr-185,000 protein in intact cells. Nature 318:183, 1985

301. Sun XJ, Rothenberg P, Kahn CR, et al: Structure of the insulin receptor substrate IRS-1 defines a unique signal transduction protein. Nature 352:73, 1991

302. Sun XJ, Miralpeix M, Myers MG Jr, et al: Expression and function of IRS-1 in insulin signal transmission. J Biol Chem 267: 22662, 1992

303. Myers MG Jr., Backer JM, Sun XJ, et al: IRS-1 activates phosphatidylinositol 3'-kinase by associating with src homology 2 domains of p85. Proc Natl Acad Sci USA 89:10350, 1992

304. Pelicci G, Lanfrancone L, Grignani F, et al: A novel transforming protein (SHC) with an SH2 domain is implicated in mitogenic signal transduction. Cell 70:93, 1992

305. Matuoka K, Shibata M, Yamakawa A, et al: Cloning of ASH, a ubiquitous protein composed of one Src homology region (SH) 2 and two SH3 domains, from human and rat cDNA libraries. Proc Natl Acad Sci USA 89:9015, 1992

306. Margolis B, Silvennoinen O, Comoglio F, et al: High-efficiency expression/cloning of epidermal growth factor-receptor-binding proteins with Src homology 2 domains. Proc Natl Acad Sci USA 89:8894, 1992

307. Fazioli F, Bottaro DP, Minichiello L, et al: Identification and biochemical characterization of novel putative substrates for the epidermal growth factor receptor kinase. J Biol Chem 267:5155, 1992

308. Bustelo XR, Ledbetter JA, Barbacid M: Product of vav proto-oncogene defines a new class of tyrosine protein kinase substrates. Nature 356:68, 1992

309. Margolis B, Hu P, Katzav S, et al: Tyrosine phosphorylation of

vav proto-oncogene product containing SH2 domain and transcription factor motifs. Nature 356:71, 1992 [see comments]

310. Lehmann JM, Riethmüller G, Johnson JP: Nck, a melanoma cDNA encoding a cytoplasmic protein consisting of the src homology units SH2 and SH3. Nucleic Acids Res 18:1048, 1990

311. Clark SG, Stern MJ, Horvitz HR: *C. elegans* cell-signalling gene sem-5 encodes a protein with SH2 and SH3 domains. Nature 356:340, 1992 [see comments]

312. Lowenstein EJ, Daly RJ, Batzer AG, et al: The SH2 and SH3 domain-containing protein GRB2 links receptor tyrosine kinases to ras signaling. Cell 70:431, 1992

313. Pawson T, Gish GD: SH2 and SH3 domains: From structure to function. Cell 71:359, 1992

314. Heldin CH: SH2 domains: Elements that control protein interactions during signal transduction. Trends Biochem Sci 16:450, 1991

315. Carpenter G: Receptor tyrosine kinase substrates: src homology domains and signal transduction. FASEB J 6:3283, 1992

316. Li W, Hu P, Skolnik EY, et al: The SH2 and SH3 domain-containing Nck protein is oncogenic and a common target for phosphorylation by different surface receptors. Mol Cell Biol 12:5824, 1992

317. Rozakis-Adcock M, McGlade J, Mbamalu G, et al: Association of the Shc and Grb2/Sem5 SH2-containing proteins is implicated in activation of the Ras pathway by tyrosine kinases. Nature 360:689, 1992

318. Thomas G: MAP kinase by any other name smells just as sweet. Cell 68:3, 1992

319. Blenis J: Growth-regulated signal transduction by the MAP kinases and RSKs. Cancer Cells 3:445, 1991.

320. Pelech SL, Sanghera JS: Mitogen-activated protein kinases: Versatile transducers for cell signaling. Trends Biochem Sci 17:233, 1992

321. Pelech SL, Sanghera JS: MAP kinases: Charting the regulatory pathways. Science 257:1355, 1992

322. Roberts TM: A signal chain of events. Nature 360:534, 1992

323. Cooper JA: Related proteins are phosphorylated at tyrosine in response to mitogenic stimuli and at meiosis. Mol Cell Biol 9:3143, 1989

324. Cooper JA, Sefton BM, Hunter T: Detection and quantification of phosphotyrosine in proteins. Methods Enzymol 99:387, 1983

325. Nakamura KD, Martinez R, Weber MJ: Tyrosine phosphorylation of specific proteins after mitogen stimulation of chicken embryo fibroblasts. Mol Cell Biol 3:380, 1983

326. Cooper JA, Sefton BM, Hunter T: Diverse mitogenic agents induce the phosphorylation of two related 42,000-dalton proteins on tyrosine in quiescent chick cells. Mol Cell Biol 4:30, 1984

327. Kohno M: Diverse mitogenic agents induce rapid phosphorylation of a common set of cellular proteins at tyrosine in quiescent mammalian cells. J Biol Chem 260:1771, 1985

328. Sturgill TW, Ray LB: Muscle proteins related to microtubule associated protein-2 are substrates for an insulin-stimulatable kinase. Biochem Biophys Res Commun 134:565, 1986

329. Sturgill TW, Wu J: Recent progress in characterization of protein kinase cascades for phosphorylation of ribosomal protein S6. Biochim Biophys Acta 1092:350, 1991

330. Thomas SM, DeMarco M, D'Arcangelo G, et al: Ras is essential for nerve growth factor- and phorbol ester-induced tyrosine phosphorylation of MAP kinases. Cell 68:1031, 1992

331. Wood KWW, Sarnecki C, Roberts TM, et al: ras mediates nerve growth factor receptor modulation of three signal-transducing protein kinases: MAP kinase, Raf-1, and RSK. Cell 68:1041, 1992

332. Alida MM, de Vries-Smits AM, Burgering BM, et al: Involvement of p21ras in activation of extracellular signal-regulated kinase 2. Nature 357:602, 1992

333. Robbins DJ, Cheng M, Zhen E, et al: Evidence for a Ras-dependent extracellular signal-regulated protein kinase (ERK) cascade. Proc Natl Acad Sci USA 89:6924, 1992

334. Pomerance M, Schweighoffer F, Tocque B, et al: Stimulation of mitogen-activated protein kinase by oncogenic Ras p21 in *Xenopus* oocytes: Requirement for Ras p21-GTPase-activating protein interaction. J Biol Chem 267:16155, 1992

335. Leevers SJ, Marshall CJ: Activation of extracellular signal-regulated kinase, ERK2, by p21ras oncoprotein. EMBO J 11:569, 1992

336. Hattori S, Fukuda M, Yamashita T, et al: Activation of mitogen-activated protein kinase and its activator by ras in intact cells and in a cell-free system. J Biol Chem 267:20346, 1991

337. Kolch W, Heidecker G, Lloyd P, et al: Raf-1 protein kinase is required for growth of induced NIH/3T3 cells. Nature 349:426, 1991

338. Williams NG, Roberts TM, Li P: Both p21ras and pp60v-src are required, but neither alone is sufficient to activate the Raf-1 kinase. Proc Natl Acad Sci USA 89:2922, 1992

339. Dickson B, Sprenger F, Morrison D, et al: Raf functions downstream of Ras1 in the Sevenless signal transduction pathway. Nature 360:600, 1992 [see comments]

340. Storm SM, Brennscheidt U, Sithanandam G, et al: raf oncogenes in carcinogenesis. Crit Rev Oncog 2:1, 1990

341. Adams PD, Parker PJ: Activation of mitogen-activated protein (MAP) kinase by a MAP kinase-kinase. J Biol Chem 267:13135, 1992

342. Kyriakis JM, App H, Zhang XF, et al: Raf-1 activates MAP kinase-kinase. Nature 358:417, 1992

343. Crews CM, Alessandrini A, Erikson RL: The primary structure of MEK, a protein kinase that phosphorylates the ERK gene product. Science 258:478, 1992

344. Rossomando A, Wu J, Weber MJ, et al: The phorbol ester-dependent activator of the mitogen-activated protein kinase p42mapk is a kinase with specificity for the threonine and tyrosine regulatory sites. Proc Natl Acad Sci USA 89:5221, 1992

345. Pulverer BJ, Kyriakis JM, Avruch J, et al: Phosphorylation of c-jun mediated by MAP kinases. Nature 353:670, 1991

346. Chou SY, Baichwal V, Ferrell JE Jr: Inhibition of c-Jun DNA binding by mitogen-activated protein kinase. Mol Biol Cell 3:1117, 1992

347. Gille H, Sharrocks AD, Shaw PE: Phosphorylation of transcription factor p62^{TCF} by MAP kinase stimulates ternary complex formation at c-*fos* promoter. Nature 358:414, 1992

348. Seth A, Gonzalez FA, Gupta S, et al: Signal transduction within the nucleus by mitogen-activated protein kinase. J Biol Chem 267:24796, 1992

349. Chung J, Pelech SL, Blenis J: Mitogen-activated Swiss mouse 3T3 RSK kinases I and II are related to pp44mpk from sea star oocytes and participate in the regulation of pp90rsk activity. Proc Natl Acad Sci USA 88:4981, 1991

350. Sturgill TW, Ray LB, Erikson E, et al: Insulin-stimulated MAP-2 kinase phosphorylates and activates ribosomal protein S6 kinase II. Nature 334:715, 1988

351. Chen RH, Sarnecki C, Blenis J: Nuclear localization and regulation of erk- and rsk-encoded protein kinases. Mol Cell Biol 12:915, 1992

352. Mitchell PJ, Tjian R: Transcriptional regulation in mammalian cells by sequence-specific DNA binding proteins. Science 245:371, 1989

353. Jones N: Transcriptional regulation by dimerization: Two sides to an incestuous relationship. Cell 61:9, 1990

354. Blackwood EM, Eisenman RN: Max: A helix-loop-helix zipper protein that forms a sequence-specific DNA-binding complex with Myc. Science 251:1211, 1991

355. Boyle WJ, Smeal T, Defize LH, et al: Activation of protein kinase C decreases phosphorylation of c-Jun at sites that negatively regulate its DNA-binding activity. Cell 64:573, 1991

356. Gonzalez GA, Montminy MR: Cyclic AMP stimulates somatostatin gene transcription by phosphorylation of CREB at serine 133. Cell 59:675, 1989

357. Ofir R, Dwarki VJ, Rashid D, et al: Phosphorylation of the C terminus of Fos protein is required for transcriptional transrepression of the c-fos promoter. Nature 348:80, 1990

358. Auwerx J, Sassone-Corsi P: IP-1: A dominant inhibitor of Fos/Jun whose activity is modulated by phosphorylation. Cell 64:983, 1991

359. Eisenman RN: In Oncogenes and the molecular origin of cancer, Cold Spring Harbor, NY, Cold Spring Harbor Laboratory Press, 1989, pp 175–221

360. Lewin B: Oncogenic conversion by regulatory changes in transcription factors. Cell 64:303, 1991

361. Rollins BJ, Stiles CD: Serum-inducible genes. Adv Cancer Res 53:1, 1989

362. Riabowol KT, Vosatka RJ, Ziff EB, et al: Microinjection of fos-specific antibodies blocks DNA synthesis in fibroblast cells. Mol Cell Biol 8:1670, 1988

363. Holt JT, Gopal TV, Moulton AD, et al: Inducible production of c-fos antisense RNA inhibits 3T3 cell proliferation. Proc Natl Acad Sci USA 83:4794, 1986

364. Spencer CA, Groudine M: Control of c-myc regulation in normal and neoplastic cells. Adv Cancer Res 56:1, 1991

365. Gordon MY: Hemopoietic growth factors and receptors: Bound and free. Cancer Cells 3:127, 1991

366. Miyajima A, Kitamura T, Harada N, et al: Cytokine receptors and signal transduction. Annu Rev Immunol 10:295, 1992

367. Hatakeyama M, Kono T, Kobayashi N, et al: Interaction of the IL-2 receptor with the src-family kinase p56lck: Identification of novel intermolecular association. Science 252:1523, 1991

368. Yoshimura A, Longmore G, Lodish HF: Point mutation in the exoplasmic domain of the erythropoietin receptor resulting in hormone-independent activation and tumorigenicity. Nature 348:647, 1990

369. Ruscetti SK, Janesch NJ, Chakraborti A, et al: Friend spleen focus-forming virus induces factor independence in an erythropoietin-dependent erythroleukemia cell line. J Virol 64:1057, 1990

370. Li JP, D'Andrea AD, Lodish HF, et al: Activation of cell growth by binding of Friend spleen focus-forming virus gp55 glycoprotein to the erythropoietin receptor. Nature 343:762, 1990

371. Wendling F, Varlet P, Charon M, et al: MPLV: A retrovirus complex inducing an acute myeloproliferative leukemic disorder in adult mice. Virology 149:242, 1986

372. Wendling F, Vigon I, Souyri M, et al: Factor-independent erythropoietic progenitor cells in leukemia induced by the myeloproliferative leukemia virus. Blood 73:1161, 1989

373. Wendling F, Vigon I, Souyri M, et al: Myeloid progenitor cells transformed by the myeloproliferative leukemia virus proliferate and differentiate in vitro without the addition of growth factors. Leukemia 3:475, 1989

374. Souyri M, Vigon I, Penciolelli JF, et al: A putative truncated cytokine receptor gene transduced by the myeloproliferative leukemia virus immortalizes hematopoietic progenitors. Cell 63:1137, 1990

375. Vigon I, Mornon JP, Cocault L, et al: Molecular cloning and characterization of MPL, the human homolog of the v-mpl oncogene: Identification of a member of the hematopoietic growth factor receptor superfamily. Proc Natl Acad Sci USA 89:5640, 1992

376. Wong-Staal F, Gallo RC, Human T-lymphotropic retroviruses. Nature 317:395, 1985

377. Gill GN, Ill CR, Simonian MH: Angiotensin stimulation of bovine adrenocortical cell growth. Proc Natl Acad Sci USA 74:5569, 1977

378. Blair DG, Cooper CS, Oskarsson MK, et al: New method for detecting cellular transforming genes. Science 218:1122, 1982

379. Fasano O, Birnbaum D, Edlund L, et al: New human transforming genes detected by a tumorigenicity assay. Mol Cell Biol 4:1695, 1984

380. Young D, Waitches G, Birchmeier C, et al: Isolation and characterization of a new cellular oncogene encoding a protein with multiple potential transmembrane domains. Cell 45:711, 1986

381. Cotecchia S, Schwinn DA, Randall RR, et al: Molecular cloning and expression of the cDNA for the hamster alpha 1-adrenergic receptor. Proc Natl Acad Sci USA 85:7159, 1988

382. Kobilka BK, Matsui H, Kobilka TS, et al: Cloning, sequencing, and expression of the gene coding for the human platelet alpha 2-adrenergic receptor. Science 238:650, 1987

383. Yarden Y, Rodriguez H, Wong SK, et al: The avian beta-adrenergic receptor: Primary structure and membrane topology. Proc Natl Acad Sci USA 83:6795, 1986

384. Frielle T, Collins S, Daniel KW, et al: Cloning of the cDNA for the human beta 1-adrenergic receptor. Proc Natl Acad Sci USA 84:7920, 1987

385. Kobilka BK, Frielle T, Dohlman HG, et al: Delineation of the intronless nature of the genes for the human and hamster beta 2-adrenergic receptor and their putative promoter regions. J Biol Chem 262:7321, 1987

386. Allard WJ, Sigal IS, Dixon RA: Sequence of the gene encoding the human M1 muscarinic acetylcholine receptor. Nucleic Acids Res 15:10604, 1987

387. Kubo T, Fukuda K, Mikami A, et al: Cloning, sequencing and expression of complementary DNA encoding the muscarinic acetylcholine receptor. Nature 323:411, 1986

388. Peralta EG, Winslow JW, Peterson GL, et al: Primary structure and biochemical properties of an M2 muscarinic receptor. Science 236:600, 1987

389. Fargin A, Raymond JR, Lohse MJ, et al: The genomic clone G-21 which resembles a beta-adrenergic receptor sequence encodes the 5-HT1A receptor. Nature 335:358, 1988

390. Masu Y, Nakayama K, Tamaki H, et al: cDNA cloning of bovine substance-K receptor through oocyte expression system. Nature 329:836, 1987

391. Bunzow JR, Van Tol HH, Grandy DK, et al: Cloning and expression of a rat D2 dopamine receptor cDNA. Nature 336:783, 1988

392. Ashkenazi A, Ramachandran J, Capon DJ: Acetylcholine analogue stimulates DNA synthesis in brain-derived cells via specific muscarinic receptor subtypes. Nature 340:146, 1989

393. Peralta EG, Ashkenazi A, Winslow JW, et al: Differential regulation of PI hydrolysis and adenylyl cyclase by muscarinic receptor subtypes. Nature 334:434, 1988

394. Jones SV, Barker JL, Buckley NJ, et al: Cloned muscarinic receptor subtypes expressed in A9 L cells differ in their coupling to electrical responses. Mol Pharmacol 34:421, 1988

395. Fukuda K, Higashida H, Kubo T, et al: Selective coupling with K^+ currents of muscarinic acetylcholine receptor subtypes in NG108-15 cells. Nature 335:355, 1988

396. Hanley MR: Mitogenic neurotransmitters. [news] Nature 340:97, 1989

397. Gutkind JS, Novotny EA, Brann MR, et al: Muscarinic acetylcholine receptor subtypes as agonist-dependent oncogenes. Proc Natl Acad Sci USA 88:4703, 1991

398. Nemecek GM, Coughlin SR, Handley DA, et al: Stimulation of aortic smooth muscle cell mitogenesis by serotonin. Proc Natl Acad Sci USA 83:674, 1986

399. Seuwen K, Magnaldo I, Pouyssegur J: Serotonin stimulates DNA synthesis in fibroblasts acting through 5-HT1B receptors coupled to a Gi-protein. Nature 335:254, 1988

400. Julius D, Livelli TJ, Jessell TM, et al: Ectopic expression of the serotonin 1c receptor and the triggering of malignant transformation. Science 244:1057, 1989

401. Allen LF, Lefkowitz RJ, Caron MG, et al: G-protein-coupled receptor genes as protooncogenes: Constitutively activating mutation of the alpha 1B-adrenergic receptor enhances mitogenesis and tumorigenicity. Proc Natl Acad Sci USA 88:11354, 1991

402. Landis CA, Masters SB, Spada A, et al: GTPase inhibiting mutations activate the alpha chain of Gs and stimulate adenylyl cyclase in human pituitary tumours. Nature 340:692, 1989

403. Lyons J, Landis CA, Harsh G, et al: Two G protein oncogenes in human endocrine tumors. Science 249:655, 1990

404. Pace AM, Wong YH, Bourne HR: A mutant alpha subunit of Gi2 induces neoplastic transformation of Rat-1 cells. Proc Natl Acad Sci USA 88:7031, 1991

405. Kalinec G, Nazarali AJ, Hermouet S, et al: Mutated alpha subunit of the Gq protein induces malignant transformation in NIH 3T3 cells. Mol Cell Biol 12:4687, 1992

406. Hermouet S, Merendino JJ, Jr, Gutkind JS, et al: Activating and inactivating mutations of the alpha subunit of Gi2 protein have opposite effects on proliferation of NIH 3T3 cells. Proc Natl Acad Sci USA 88:10455, 1991

407. Gupta SK, Gallego C, Lowndes JM, et al: Analysis of the fibroblast transformation potential of GTPase-deficient gip2 oncogenes. Mol Cell Biol 12:190, 1992

408. Chan AM, Fleming TP, McGovern ES, et al: Expression cDNA cloning of a transforming gene encoding the wild-type G alpha 12 gene product. Mol Cell Biol 13:762, 1993

409. Chan AM-L, Rubin JS, Bottaro DP, et al: Identification of a competitive HGF antagonist encoded by an alternative transcript. Science 254:1382, 1991

410. Duan D-SR, Werner S, Williams LT: A naturally occurring secreted form of fibroblast growth factor (FGF) receptor 1 binds basic FGF in preference over acidic FGF. J Biol Chem 267:16076, 1992

411. Kumar R, Shepard HM, Mendelsohn J: Regulation of phosphorylation of the c-erbB-2/HER2 gene product by a monoclonal antibody and serum growth factor(s) in human mammary carcinoma cells. Mol Cell Biol 11:979, 1991

412. Myers JN, Drebin JA, Wada T, et al: Biological effects of monoclonal antireceptor antibodies reactive with neu oncogene product, p185neu. Methods Enzymol 198:277, 1991

413. Hudziak RM, Lewis GD, Winget M, et al: p185HER2 monoclonal antibody has antiproliferative effects in vitro and sensitizes human breast tumor cells to tumor necrosis factor. Mol Cell Biol 9:1165, 1989

414. Kasprzyk PG, Song SU, Di Fiore PP, et al: Therapy of an animal model of human gastric cancer using a combination of anti-erbB-2 monoclonal antibodies. Cancer Res 52:2771, 1992

415. Arteaga CL: Interference of the IGF system as a strategy to inhibit breast cancer growth. Breast Cancer Res Treat 22:101, 1992

416. Pastan I, FitzGerald D: Recombinant toxins for cancer treatment. Science 254:1173, 1991

417. Roth JA: Molecular surgery for cancer. Arch Surg 127:1298, 1992

418. Levitzki A: Tyrphostins: Tyrosine kinase blockers as novel antiproliferative agents and dissectors of signal transduction. FASEB J 6:3275, 1992

419. Hara M, Akasaka K, Akinaga S, et al: Identification of Ras farnesyltransferase inhibitors by microbial screening. Proc Natl Acad Sci USA 90:2281, 1993

420. Reiss Y, Brown MS, Goldstein JL: Divalent cation and prenyl pyrophosphate specificities of the protein farnesyltransferase from rat brain, a zinc metalloenzyme. J Biol Chem 267:6403, 1992

421. Der CJ, Cox AD: Isoprenoid modification and plasma membrane association: Critical factors for ras oncogenicity. Cancer Cells 3:331, 1991

422. Reiss Y, Goldstein JL, Seabra MC, et al: Inhibition of purified p21ras farnesyl:protein transferase by Cys-AAX tetrapeptides. Cell 62:81, 1990

423. Gearing DP, King JA, Gough NM, et al: Expression cloning of a receptor for human granulocyte-macrophage colony-stimulating factor. EMBO J 8:3667, 1989

424. Hayashida K, Kitamura T, Gorman DM, et al: Molecular cloning of a second subunit of the receptor for human granulocyte-macrophage colony-stimulating factor (GM-CSF): Reconstitution of a high-affinity GM-CSF receptor. Proc Natl Acad Sci USA 87:9655, 1990

425. Larsen A, Davis T, Curtis BM, et al: Expression cloning of a human granulocyte colony-stimulating factor receptor: A structural mosaic of hematopoietin receptor, immunoglobulin, and fibronectin domains. J Exp Med 172:1559, 1990

SECTION

◼ II ◼

GROWTH AND SPREAD OF CANCER

CYTOKINETICS OF NEOPLASIA

◼

ADHESION MECHANISMS CONTROLLING CELL-CELL AND CELL-MATRIX INTERACTIONS DURING THE METASTATIC PROCESS

◼

TUMOR ANGIOGENESIS

◼

MOLECULAR MECHANISMS OF TUMOR CELL METASTASIS

8

CYTOKINETICS OF NEOPLASIA

TERESA GILEWSKI
LARRY NORTON

The statement that life is dynamic is a tautology. Cancer cells constantly are changing in three dimensions: in their intrinsic (internal) states, in their relationships with their cellular and chemical environment, and in their numbers. *Cytokinetics* is the study of the kinetics of cellular *proliferation* and tissue *growth,* two phenomena that relate to all three dimensions of change. Proliferation applies specifically to an increase in the number of cancer cells, which is now quantifiable by modern laboratory methods. Growth refers to increasing tumor volume, largely resulting from proliferation, but also from changes in cell size, edema, hemorrhage, and infiltration by normal host cells.

Cytokinetics is important because the features that define cancer—growth, invasion, and metastasis—are all dependent on the reproduction of cancer cells. Reproduction is, in turn, the ultimate expression of a complex chain of molecular events that also are linked to cell viability and function. Carcinogenesis is itself a kinetic process, fundamentally dependent on the proliferation of normal and preneoplastic target tissues. Once cancers are established, they frequently are described in kinetic terms: indolent growth, rapid growth, and slow or rapid regression in response to therapy. Anticancer drugs work in part by disrupting mitosis: Hence, cytokinetics relates both to therapeutic response and to toxic effects on host tissues that often are dividing more rapidly than the cancer cells themselves. Cytokinetics of clinical neoplasia also relates to prognostication, the design of treatment schedules, and the coordinated use of various modalities (surgery, radiation therapy, chemotherapy, hormonal therapy, and modern approaches to immunotherapy). For all of these reasons, studies of proliferation and growth are relevant both to the laboratory scientist and to the clinical oncologist.

PROLIFERATION KINETICS

Terminology

Normal somatic cells proliferate by *mitosis,* a sequence of biochemical and anatomic processes collectively called the *mitotic cycle, proliferative cycle,* or *cell cycle.* Many decades ago, the autoradiography of radioactively labeled deoxyribonucleic acids found that the cell cycle was divisible into four phases.[1,2] The four phases are defined in relationship to two key events—the synthesis of DNA (*synthesis phase* or *S phase*), and the division of the parent cell into two daughters (*mitosis phase* or *M phase*). M phase, the phase most popularly associated with cell division, contains the metaphase plate, which is visible microscopically. At the end of M phase, a normal mammalian somatic cell contains a diploid number of chromosomes, comprising a diploid (2N) cellular DNA content. Time gap number one, between M phase and S phase, is called G_1. Time gap number two, between S phase and M phase, is called G_2. Although the term *mitosis* often is used to refer specifically to M phase, the adjective *mitotic* refers generally to all cells in phases G_1, S, G_2, or M.

Nonmitotic cells are classified as belonging to special phases, distinguishable biochemically and often microscopically. The most common nonmitotic phase is G_0. Like G_1 cells, G_0 cells contain 2N DNA content, so they often are grouped together with G_1 cells. Rare nonmitotic cells may have progressed partially or completely through S phase prior to resting, so they contain more than 2N and less than or equal to 4N amounts of DNA.[3,4] Some very primitive or embryonic cells enter DNA synthesis immediately at the end of the M phase, so the G_1 duration is zero, but these are exceptions to the usual pattern. Yet the lengths of the G_0-G_1 phases are indeed highly variable, fitting a log-normal probability distribution that is skewed markedly to the right. The cells on the far right end of the distribution will never divide within the life span of the host. However, the distinction between G_0 and G_1 is biologic, not just stochastic. G_0 cells tend to be smaller than G_1 cells, have lower RNA and protein contents, and exhibit specific biochemical differences.[5–7] For example, the Ki-67 antigen, present in the G_1, S, G_2, and M phases, is absent from G_0 cells.[8] G_0 cells, having reduced mitochondrial activity[9] and active membrane pumps,[10] do not metabolize the cationic dye rhodamine. The ratio $G_1/(G_0 + G_1)$ defines the proportion of cells entering their next S phase.

During the G_0-G_1 phase, cells prepare to enter S by progressing through defined stages, dependent on protein synthesis, that are regulated by kinases and sensitive to extracellular growth factors and the supply of nutrients.[11] Cells in G_1 already have progressed through or bypassed several preliminary steps in G_0 to prepare for S phase. Many G_0 cells can be stimulated by external influences to enter G_1 and eventually S: This phenomenon is called *recruitment.* Cancer cells—by virtue of oncogene activation, suppressor gene deactivation, or loss of adhesion-dependent inhibition—are often less dependent on external signals and conditions than normal cells (hence, they can grow in suspension cultures free of extracellular matrix). As a consequence, cancer cells often are biased toward proliferation, and thence are recruited more easily into cycle than their normal counterparts.

The entry of G_1 cells into S may be restricted by a cyclic process in which the $p34^{cdc2}$ protein couples with different cyclin proteins to coordinate a cell's entry into S or M in an alternating pattern.[12] Abnormalities in this system could obstruct the normal block of re-replication (in which genes are replicated more than once during a single S phase), producing *aneuploidy,* or aberrant levels of DNA per neoplastic cell.[13] Progression through the S and G_2 phases is largely self-regulated, involving the completion of steps in strict sequence and indirect feedback loops.[14,15]

The S phase, less variable in length than G_0-G_1, lasts between 12 and 24 hours in mammalian cells, including cancer cells. Specific chromosomal regions replicate at specific times, in synchronous clusters, until DNA synthesis decelerates as the cellular DNA content approaches 4N.[16] G_2 usually lasts for about 3 hours in mammalian cells. It ends by a complex interplay of cyclins and other factors that initiate the *prophase* of the M phase, in which the cell becomes spherical.[17,18] Microtubules and cytoskeletal microfilaments rearrange, the Golgi apparatus degenerates into small vesicles, protein synthesis diminishes, and chromosomes become metabolically quiescent and condense into transportable units.[19] In *prometaphase,* these units orient themselves linearly toward opposite ends of the cell and migrate centrally to compose the *metaphase plate.* In *anaphase,* spindle fibers attached to kinetochores on each chromosome guide them toward centrosomes that have placed themselves at extreme opposite poles of the cell. The nuclei reform during *telophase,* the chromosomes disperse, and the cell halves, with one new nucleus per daughter cell. All of these complex processes take place in 1 hour, with little variability.

The total duration of the cell cycle in human cancers averages about 2 to 4 days. To put this in perspective, the cycle in *Drosophila* lasts minutes, and in mammalian embryos only hours. Many normal cells—hematopoietic progenitors and gastrointestinal mucosal cells—have comparable cycle times, indicating that cancer is more often a disease of persistant proliferation than of rapid proliferation.[20,21] The length of a cancer cell's cycle in vivo remains fairly constant over the life history of the tumor, although subtle changes occur in laboratory models grown to large size.[22,23] In contrast, phase lengths can shift significantly as cells are grown in vitro.[24]

Quantification

Cell cycle phases may be measured by many techniques. All of the older methods are based on light microscopy, which, although tedious, preserves the microanatomy of the specimen. This is advantageous because only cancer cells and not normal intermingled cells are evaluated. The most venerable of the older methods is the *mitotic index,* the counting of metaphase figures in histologic slides. Of late, this assay has been neglected because it is very labor intensive, which is unfortunate because it has a real and obvious biologic meaning.[25] The mitotic index may become more popular with technological advances in the automated counting of visually distinctive cells.[26,27] The *stathmokinetic index* is a historically important variant of the mitotic index in which a mitotic poison is applied prior to counting.[28]

The most classical of the older techniques is the *thymidine labeling index* (TLI), which is still in productive use.[29] Viable cells are exposed briefly in vitro to a radiolabeled precursor of DNA, usually tritium (^3H), but occasionally carbon-14. The percentage of tumor cells with autoradiographic grains over their nuclei estimates the fraction of cells that were in S phase during the period of thymidine exposure. Newer variants use monoclonal antibodies directed against proteins expressed during S phase.[8,30,31] Labeling indices have been used to generate graphs called *percentage of labeled mitoses (PLM) curves.* In this technique, the number of mitoses containing an S-phase label are counted as a function of time after exposure to the label. This measures the cells in M phase that had been in S phase at a specific point in time. The PLM method is the only procedure that directly estimates the durations of cell cycle phases. The theory is as follows: At time 0 only cells in S phase contain label. At time G_2 after exposure, the cells that were at the end of S phase at time 0 begin to enter the M phase. At a time equal to G_2 + M, all of the M-phase cells should contain label, but by time S + G_2 + M, all of the cells containing label should have passed through M phase. All M-phase cells should again show label when a time equivalent to the cell cycle time plus G_2 + M has passed. Were cell cycle phase lengths fixed and invariable, PLM curves would be sharp and precise and cycle durations could be derived by simple arithmetic. However, as mentioned above, cell cycle durations follow rather wide frequency distributions, so great variability is encountered, and the second peak of labeled mitoses is rarely sharp. Another difficulty with this method is that the pharmacokinetics of the label rarely assures labeling of all S-phase cells. Hence, many fewer than 100 per cent of M-phase cells contain label at any point in time. For this reason, it has proven necessary to use sophisticated mathematical models to estimate phase lengths.[32] This, plus the technical difficulties inherent in the method, plus the restrictions imposed by the use of radioisotopes, has limited the applications of PLM curves in recent times.

Modern techniques for kinetic measurements are based largely on the variation in cellular DNA content that occurs during the cell cycle. Such content can be measured rapidly by a collection of automated methods called *flow cytometry*.[33] The major disadvantage of automated techniques is that the cells being analyzed are not being visualized. Hence, normal stromal cells, normal blood cells, and tumor cells of various types all are being counted together. Cycle parameters often are not distributed homogeneously throughout the anatomy of a tumor mass. However, because DNA ploidy and proliferation activity now may be assessed by automated image analysis, this disadvantage may fade in the near future.[34,35] A more persistent disadvantage is that flow cytometry is technically delicate. It requires meticulous technique and constant attention to quality control. Despite these problems, by virtue of its speed and applicability to large-scale operations, flow cytometry has become the most widely applied cytokinetic assay.

The basic process involves automatically counting a suspension of individual cells by fluorescence-activated sorting by DNA content, RNA content, cell size, or antibody label, either alone or in combination.[36,37] Cells are obtained from fresh tissue—leukemias, tumor cells in effusions or ascites, or enzymatically dispersed solid tumors—or from paraffin-embedded archival material.[38,39] Although the primary use of flow cytometry is in the measurement of DNA content, the measurement of RNA content is helpful in distinguishing G_0 from G_1 cells. Also useful in this regard is labeling with the monoclonal Ki-67 antibody conjugated to a fluorescent dye.[8] This antibody binds to a proliferation-related nuclear antigen and thereby identifies cells in all cell cycle phases except G_0.[8] Ki-67 labeling therefore may be more sensitive than the TLI for determination of proliferative activity.[40] Other techniques include the exposure of viable cells to the pyrimidine analogues bromodeoxyuridine (BrdU) and iododeoxyuridine (IUDR). These reagents are incorporated into DNA during S phase, followed by reaction with an antibody tagged with a fluorescent dye. In addition to in vitro application, BrdU has been administered intravenously to patients several hours prior to obtaining specimens of solid tumors and leukemias.[41–47] The cancer cells so obtained then not only can be examined for S phase, but also can be exposed to tritiated thymidine. This provides a double label, which has been used to estimate

cycle phase durations.[48] BrdU labeling also has been employed for in vivo and in vitro analysis of proliferative activity without the use of flow cytometry.[47,49]

DNA content usually is quantified following reaction with intercalating or base-pair affinity dyes. A DNA *histogram* or *flow cytogram* shows the frequency distribution of cells with various complements of DNA per cell. On a DNA histogram, a diploid population will exhibit a high, relatively narrow peak at 2N, corresponding to G_0-G_1, and a wide, lower peak around 4N, reflecting the G_2-M cells. Standardization of the G_0-G_1 peak for DNA histograms uses normal diploid cells, commonly lymphocytes.[50] Cells with DNA content between 2N and 4N are called the *S-phase fraction* (SPF). The *proliferative index* is the fraction of cells that are in either S or G_2 or M.

DNA flow cytometry is particularly useful in identifying cells with abnormal amounts of DNA in their G_0-G_1 peak, termed *aneuploid*. Categories of ploidy include *near-diploid* (2N $\pm$ 10 per cent), *hypodiploid* (less than 2N), *simple hyperdiploid* (between 2N and 4N), *tetraploid* (4N), *near-tetraploid* (4N $\pm$ 10 per cent), *hypertetraploid* (greater than 4N), or combinations, called *multiploid*. Each aneuploid G_0-G_1 peak corresponds to a G_2-M peak with twice as much DNA. The *DNA index* is the ratio between the fluorescence channel of the malignant G_0-G_1 peak and that of the normal diploid G_0-G_1 peak. A DNA index of less than 0.9 or greater than 1.1 usually is considered abnormal (i.e., near-diploid is considered normal). The assessment of ploidy is a by-product of the use of flow cytometry to assess cell cycle parameters.[51] However, ploidy is important because the SPF is difficult to measure in cases of marked aneuploidy, because the diploid G_2-M peak can overlap with the aneuploid S curve. Yet recent improvements in experimental technique and, especially, analytic methods have made ploidy and SPF measurable in most solid tumor specimens.

It is of interest to note that flow cytometry can be used to measure variables other than DNA content. In particular, labeling with monoclonal antibodies has been used to detect proteins in the cell membrane and cytoplasm in both hematologic malignancies and solid tumors. This technique facilitates immunophenotyping of leukemias and lymphomas, and has been used to count hematopoietic progenitor cells of various degrees of differentiation.[52–54] Flow cytometry has been used to count, by sorting, cells with expression of multidrug resistance proteins,[55–57] estrogen and progesterone receptors,[52,58–60] cytokeratins,[61] oncogene products,[52,62] and other tumor-associated antigens.[63] A recent new application of flow cytometry involves fluorescence in situ hybridization (FISH), which can analyze multiple parameters, including oncogene RNA content.[53]

Mitotic Compartments

The above discussion implies that the cell cycle is a continuously dynamic process, with orderly progression through S, G_2, and M, followed by either mitotic quiescence (G_0) or biochemical steps (G_1) in preparation for S phase. A third possibility is cell death, which can occur at any time during the cycle. Although it is most proper to envision cell reproduction as such a continuous system, for practical purposes it is often expedient to classify the cells into compartments. For example, a cell in G_1, S, G_2, or M is a member of the *proliferative compartment,* also called the *proliferative fraction,* the *growth fraction,* or the *growth compartment.*[64] A cell in prolonged G_0 (or, less commonly, an arrested S phase, called S_0, or an arrested G_2) is in the *nonproliferative compartment, nonproliferative fraction, quiescent fraction,* or *quiescent compartment.*

The SPF as measured by flow cytometry correlates with but is not equivalent to the growth fraction. Indeed, the magnitude of the growth fraction is estimated by multiplying the TLI by the duration of the cell cycle divided by the duration of S phase.[65] The labeling index is used because the SPF includes S_0 cells that properly belong in the quiescent fraction. Hence, the SPF is usually larger than the TLI. About 2 to 20 per cent of cells in a typical cancer of the solid tumor type are in S at any one point in time. Because S phase occupies one quarter to one half of the cell cycle, the growth fraction is usually 4 to 80 per cent, with an average of less than 20 per cent.

Nonproliferative cells fall into three compartments. Some highly differentiated cells, such as neurons, are in the *immortal nonproliferative fraction.* These may survive for the whole life span of the organism. Most terminally differentiated cells, in distinction, do not divide but have a finite life span. An example of such a *mortal nonproliferative fraction* cell is the polymorphonuclear leukocyte. The third compartment is that of the *unstable nonproliferative fraction.* These are largely G_0 cells that may be recruited into G_1 by the proper environmental signal. An important class of cells of this latter type are *stem cells.* Stem cells may be proliferative cells or they may live quiescently, returning to cycle when needed to produce viable progeny.[66,67] They are relatively primitive cells that can replenish the whole spectrum of subtypes that constitute a mature organ or tumor. Stem cell recruitment is signaled by physiologic changes in the environment, induced by cell death, cell injury, drugs, or hormones. These cells are distinguished by their ability to form colonies in soft agar.[68] By this assay, it is estimated that only 0.1 to 1 per cent of the cells in a typical solid tumor have stem capacity. Yet these minority cells are the prime targets of anticancer therapy because they must be eradicated to preclude regrowth. This could be a common source of therapeutic failure because stem cells may remain in G_0 for long periods, and many anticancer drugs are toxic only to mitotic cells.[69]

Cells dying in any phase of their cell cycle collectively are termed the *cell loss fraction.*[70] Cell death is an important determinant of growth rate, which is the difference between cell production and cell loss. A tumor with a large cell loss fraction may appear to be growing slowly, when in fact the growth fraction also may be high. Because each mitotic cycle carries with it a finite probability of mutation,[71] the coincidence of high cell loss rates with high mitotic rates predisposes toward genetic lability.

Proliferation and Biologic Diversity

Diploidy is the common feature of wild-type normal cells. In contrast, about 70 per cent of cancers have at least a minor component of aneuploid cells. This has proven useful in cytologic screening for cancer, but has created more excitement because of its potential in prognostication. Aneuploidy, as evidence of aberrancy, is anticipated to correlate with deviation from normal behavior and hence clinical aggressiveness. The measurement of ploidy, however, is just a by-product of the kinetic assessment of cell cycle parameters. Of these parameters, SPF and TLI also have been evaluated as prognostic factors. Although in general the SPF in many cancers may be no higher than in some normal tissues, different patients with the same histologic type of cancer may have tumors with very different SPFs. Like aneuploidy, high SPF is frequently associated with greater malignancy. These observations raise the question of the reason for the association of aneuploidy with high SPF. It is possible that aneuploidy is a consequence of high mitotic activity as estimated by high SPF. Large growth fraction means many mitoses per unit of time, yielding more opportunities for mutations and other genetic events. Against this hypothesis is the observation that bone marrow and gastrointestinal epithelia have high SPFs but remain diploid. This raises the alternative possibility that a high SPF may not be the cause of aneuploidy, but rather the consequence of genetic aberrancy. The match is not universal because some clinically benign tumors are aneuploid. Yet aneuploidy is sufficiently associated with malignant behavior that the question of how fast mutations accumulate during growth is clinically relevant (see later in this chapter).

Spontaneous genetic change is an intrinsic property of cancer,[48,72] and may be based on loss of cell cycle control,[73] abnormalities in DNA repair,[74] or a propensity for recombination events. Most solid tumors,[75] including breast cancer,[76] exhibit nonrandom changes at meaningful loci. The clonal origin of tumors is well documented by several techniques, including glucose-6-phosphate dehydrogenase isotyping and cytogenetics.[77,78] From this clonal origin, cancers develop heterogeneity in morphology, behavior, immunogenicity, receptor content, and drug sensitivity.[79] Such characteristics frequently are correlated. For example, metastatic behavior is an acquired trait. Metastases tend to grow faster than the primary tumors from which they arise.[80,81] The relationship between ploidy and S phase may be similar. That is, both aneuploidy and high SPF may be the consequence of the same primary event, and occur together because they are linked by that common event, not because they are causally linked to each other.

In this context, the third determinant of growth rate, cell loss, also influences genetic lability, perhaps by increasing the opportunities for mutations. The evidence is strong. Carcinogenesis is a molecular genetic process that culminates a long process of preneoplasia.[82–85] Neoplastic transformation depends on high rates of cell turnover.[86] For example, thyroid carcinogenesis is promoted by elevated levels of thyroid-stimulating hormone, which stimulates growth.[87] Skin carcinogenesis is promoted by chronic thermal injury and solar damage, both of which cause compensatory hyperplasia.[88,89] Carcinogenesis in bone marrow is linked to the hyperproliferations of dysmyelopoiesis[90] and chronic granulocytic leukemia.[91] Colon carcinogenesis is associated with the hyperproliferations of inflammatory bowel disease and polyps.[92] Breast carcinogenesis in mice[93] and humans[94,95] also is rooted in hyperproliferation. Cancer cells respond to chronic drug treatment by high rates of cell turnover, which may predispose to genetically based drug resistance in Hodgkin's lymphoma[96] and gastrointestinal cancer.[97]

CYTOKINETICS OF CLINICAL NEOPLASIA

The clinical utility of cytokinetic measurements has been the subject of a plethora of published studies. An important, but relatively minor, use has been the flow-cytometric detection of aneuploidy as a supplement to classic histocytology in the search for malignant cells in clinical samples.[98,99] The larger role of cytokinetics has been in the prediction of prognosis and response to therapy.[100,101] Not unexpectedly, many of the data in this regard are conflicting. One source of discrepancy is an emphasis on patient subsets. This emphasis is dangerous because subset analysis often is driven retrospectively. If a data set shows a random, and hence biologically meaningless, difference between subsets, subset analysis will amplify the error. Indeed, it is very likely that some subsets within a data set will demonstrate differences by random error even when no true biologic differences exist. Hence, prospective corroboration of suspected differences between subsets is essential to the scientific process. Much of the confusion in the cytokinetics literature reflects the failure to insist on such validation. Another issue concerns the instability of positive findings when small samples are analyzed, especially if the effects of cytokinetics are relatively weak. That is, if cytokinetics imparts a weak advantage for one group over another, in some small trials this advantage will be apparent, whereas in others it will be lost in the noise of the data. For this reason, an overview approach may be helpful, either a formal statistical meta-analysis, which rarely is performed, or an informal gathering of the studies, taking care to include all of the published experience. This latter activity is dangerous because publication bias tends to emphasize positive studies, so false conclusions in the direction of positive results might be drawn.

Other sources of confusion are specific to the methods employed. As previously noted, flow cytometry is a multifaceted technique that has been used to measure DNA content, RNA content, and the presence of many antigens. Cancer is notoriously heterogeneous, so different parts of the same tumor can manifest significant cytokinetic differences.[102–105] In addition, many factors other than those rooted in true tumor biology can influence flow-cytometric data. The analysis of fresh tumor cells is not comparable with the analysis of cells obtained from paraffin sections, largely because of the greater amount of debris found in archival material.[102,106–110] Even if we restrict our attention to fresh samples, the various techniques used to disaggregate tumor cells—mechanical, enzymatic, and chemical—may yield preparations different enough to affect results.[109,111] In the cytometry process itself, an assortment of fluorescent stains that bind to DNA (ethidium bromide, propidium iodide, and several Hoechst dyes) are commonly in use.[112] These preparatory steps, and variability in the precision of the instruments used for measurement, contribute to variability in data. As an example, the National Cancer Institute's Flow Cytometry Network used mixtures of bladder carcinoma cell lines and peripheral blood lymphocytes to assess the variability within and among laboratories.[113,114] Although there were no major differences in the assays of mean DNA index, single specimens varied significantly in measurements of hyperdiploid fraction.

Other sources of variability in the analysis of DNA content by flow cytometry include: different definitions of ploidy based on DNA index, different selections of cells to be used as the diploid reference group, and inattention to the coefficient of variation, a quantification of the resolution and interpretability of the DNA histogram.[102] Attention to all of these points would allow for a more meaningful comparison of data between various laboratories, and would provide the reader with an assessment of the quality of the data. The general lesson is that the cytokinetics of human tumors is an evolving discipline, and caution must be used in interpretation of all data. Nevertheless, some important observations have been made regarding specific types of cancers, as well as neoplasia in general.

Genitourinary Cancer

PROSTATE CARCINOMA

Numerous studies have assessed DNA content by flow cytometry in prostate cancer.[100,115–120] The majority of these analyses indicate that ploidy provides prognostic information for localized prostate cancer: Aneuploid tumors recur more frequently than diploid tumors.[115,116,118,119] Aneuploidy tends to occur in more advanced stages of disease.[121,122] In a review article, Deitch et al. observed that DNA ploidy may predict tumor volume but does not predict who will profit from radiation therapy for localized disease.[122] Aneuploidy also has been found in benign tissue in close proximity to high-grade, large-volume disease.[122] Recently, SPF has been assessed by flow cytometry,[123] in vivo BrdU labeling,[124] and Ki-67 expression.[125]

RENAL CELL CARCINOMA

Conflicting data exist regarding the prognostic significance of DNA ploidy in renal cell carcinoma.[126–133] Recently, a retrospective univariate analysis of 381 paraffin blocks from 93 primary adenocarcinomas found that DNA ploidy and SPF were significantly associated with both tumor grade and survival.[134] However, when tumor grade was considered, the flow cytometry measurements were not of prognostic significance. The predictive significance of cytokinetics regarding response to therapy can be resolved only by prospective studies.

BLADDER CANCER

BrdU labeling has been used to assess the growth fraction in bladder cancer,[135] but most studies have used DNA flow cytometry. Walther has reviewed the role of ploidy in predicting and monitoring response to therapy and in screening urine samples for malignancy.[136] A number of studies have noted an association between DNA ploidy, tumor grade, and aggressiveness of bladder cancer.[136–141] However, it is not clear if cytokinetics provides any information superior to conventional clinical parameters.[142,143] A recent analysis of 448 paraffin specimens of transitional cell bladder cancer found that DNA ploidy was not an independent prognostic factor, although prognosis was predicted by SPF and mitotic index.[143]

TESTICULAR CARCINOMA

It has been reported recently that a high DNA index in nonseminomatous germ cell tumors of the testes is associated with advanced disease at presentation.[144] However, aneuploidy did not correlate with histology or vessel invasion.

Gynecologic Cancer

OVARIAN CANCER

Although DNA ploidy is not clearly associated with stage of ovarian cancer,[145,146] with some exceptions,[147] most studies have demonstrated that diploid tumors are associated with a better prognosis.[148–153] This association may be less apparent for patients with advanced disease.[154] The role of flow cytometry in analyzing ascitic fluid[155] and in monitoring treatment effects[150] is being explored. Assessment of SPF by Ki-67 staining,[156] flow cytometry,[152,153] and thymidine labeling[157–160] has produced variable results.

UTERINE CANCER

In endometrial carcinoma, with few exceptions,[161] aneuploidy has been associated with poorly differentiated tumors[162,163] and decreased survival.[162–164] Multiparametric analyses of response to hormonal therapy are ongoing.[165] Also of current interest are flow-cytometric determinations of levels of expression of epidermal growth factor receptors and c-erbB-2 oncoprotein.[166]

CERVICAL CARCINOMA

DNA ploidy and SPF have an unclear role as prognostic factors in cervical carcinoma,[167–172] although some studies have suggested that diploid or tetraploid tumors may have a worse prognosis.[173,174]

Gastrointestinal Cancer

COLORECTAL CARCINOMA

Although Ki-67 immunoreactivity has been used to measure proliferative activity in colorectal carcinoma,[175] most studies have used flow cytometry. Both retrospective and prospective data suggest that aneuploid colorectal carcinomas, particularly those in stages A, B, and C, have a worse prognosis.[101,176–183] However, this is not a universal finding.[184–186] Several analyses also have noted an increased frequency of aneuploidy in more advanced stages of disease.[101,182,187–189] Multivariate analyses have indicated that SPF or stage may be a better prognostic factor than ploidy.[190,191] Abnormal DNA content and high proliferative activity also have been noted in benign colonic mucosa adjacent to the primary tumor by some,[192] but not all,[193] investigators. Analysis of DNA ploidy as a means of identifying patients with ulcerative colitis at higher risk for developing colorectal cancer is an active area of investigation.[194]

PANCREATIC CARCINOMA

The cytokinetics of this disease has not been well studied. An analysis of 56 patients indicated that ploidy was an independent prognostic factor with a significant effect on survival.[195] In one small study, DNA ploidy did not predict the malignant behavior of insulinomas.[196] In another, ploidy did not differentiate benign serous cystadenomas from mucinous cystic cancers.[197]

HEPATOMA

The limited information concerning the prognostic importance of DNA flow cytometry for hepatocellular carcinoma is conflicting.[198] One retrospective multivariate analysis found a correlation between ploidy and overall and disease-free survival,[199] whereas another showed no association with survival.[200] The BrdU labeling index has been correlated with histologic findings from hepatocellular carcinomas and cirrhotic tissues.[201,202]

GASTRIC AND ESOPHAGEAL CARCINOMAS

There is very limited information about the cytokinetics of esophageal cancer.[203–206] However, for patients with gastric carcinoma, the most recent data have found that tumor aneuploidy is associated with decreased survival.[207–212] This finding is at variance with older studies that did not find this association.[213–215] Aneuploidy is present in a greater percentage of tumors of the gastroesophageal junction and cardia than in those of the body and antrum.[208,209] Lymph node involvement is also more common in aneuploid tumors.[208,209,216] Assessment of proliferative activity by thymidine or BrdU labeling also may be of prognostic significance.[210,211,217,218]

Cancer of the Respiratory Tract

HEAD AND NECK CANCER

There is disagreement in the literature regarding the prognostic significance of DNA ploidy in squamous cell carcinoma of the head and neck.[219,220] Some studies identified a more favorable prognosis for aneuploid tumors,[221–223] whereas others found a better outcome for diploid tumors.[224] One analysis found no significant association between DNA ploidy and response to chemotherapy.[225] Several studies have reported increased radiosensitivity for aneuploid lesions.[219] An evaluation of 110 patients with oral cavity lesions noted an increased likelihood of aneuploidy in poorly differentiated and larger tumors.[226] Only limited studies with BrdU and thymidine have been performed.[227–229] A retrospective examination of 45 patients with adenoid cystic carcinomas of the salivary glands, a tumor type of low malignant potential, found that the majority of tumors were diploid.[230]

LUNG CARCINOMA

Numerous studies of non–small-cell lung carcinoma have found an association between aneuploidy and shorter survival times.[231–238] However, other analyses have not confirmed this observation.[239,240] In several studies, ploidy was found to be of prognostic significance for squamous cell carcinomas, but not for non–squamous cell tumors.[231,232] Aneuploidy also has been correlated with phenotypic heterogeneity in non–small-cell lung cancer.[241] It remains unclear if the TLI is of prognostic significance, although increased p170 glycoprotein expression has been noted in tumors with low proliferative activity.[242,243] Limited data are available concerning the prognostic significance of ploidy in small-cell lung cancer.[244,245] The ability of flow cytometry to detect bone marrow micrometastases in patients with small-cell lung cancer is being investigated.[246]

Brain Cancer

BrdU labeling was found to convey prognostic information in several studies of primary brain malignancies.[247–249] A prospective study of 174 patients with intracranial gliomas found the BrdU labeling index to be an important predictor of survival for low-grade astrocytomas. This index, in conjunction with the patient's age, was also predictive of survival for glioblastomas and malignant astrocytomas.[249] BrdU labeling studies have found that cell proliferation increases after in vitro administration of exogenous growth factors to cultured primary glioma cells.[250] Flow cytometry has been used to assess ploidy in meningiomas[251] as well as in stereotactic brain biopsies of several types of lesions.[252] In gliomas, aneuploidy has been associated with high histologic grade and poor outcome.[248,253–255] However, aneuploid medulloblastomas may be more sensitive to treatment.[256]

Thyroid Cancer

There is no definite role for DNA ploidy as a prognostic factor in thyroid cancer.[257–259] Aneuploidy has been noted in both malignant[260–262] and benign[263,264] thyroid lesions.

Thymomas

Aneuploidy has been associated with more advanced disease, increased tumor recurrence, and the existence of myasthenia gravis.[265]

Sarcomas

There is limited information on the role of DNA analysis for soft tissue and bone sarcomas.[266–268] The presence of diploid or near-diploid tumors may be associated with a more favorable prognosis for chondrosarcomas and osteosarcomas.[269,270] Although most malignant tumors are aneuploid,[271,272] benign tumors (including schwannomas) may be aneuploid as well.[273] Aneuploid gastric leiomyosarcomas appear to have a worse prognosis.[274] Flow cytometry also has been used to assess ploidy in Kaposi's sarcoma[275] and chromosomal abnormalities in Ewing's sarcoma cell lines.[276]

Pediatric Tumors

Several studies have noted an unfavorable prognosis for diploid neuroblastomas.[277–281] Amplification of the N-*myc* oncogene also has been associated with these diploid tumors.[282–284] Recent analysis reveals a correlation between high SPF and near-diploid/near-tetraploid DNA content, N-*myc* amplification, and more advanced disease.[285] DNA content of neuroblastomas also may correlate with response to therapy.[286] There are few data regarding DNA ploidy and Wilms' tumors[287] or nephroblastomas.[288]

Most rhabdomyosarcomas are aneuploid. Although DNA content has been correlated with age[289] and clinical stage,[290] there is no definite evidence that ploidy is of important prognostic significance.

Melanoma

Numerous analyses of patients with primary melanoma indicate a correlation between aneuploidy and higher recurrence rates and/or shorter survival.[291–295] For metastatic melanoma, aneuploidy has been associated with both a more favorable prognosis[296,297] and a worse outcome.[293] Evaluation of SPF by flow cytometry is also of prognostic significance for Stage III[295] and metastatic disease.[297] For Stage II melanoma, slow proliferation as measured by thymidine labeling indicates a significant advantage in relapse-free and overall survival.[298] Experimentally, flow cytometry has been used to assess the effect of an autocrine-secreted melanoma growth-inhibiting activity on the cytokinetics of tumor cells.[299]

Hematologic Malignancies

HODGKIN'S DISEASE

The few studies of Hodgkin's disease that have been reported have noted a low incidence of aneuploidy.[300-303] This may be the result of the difficulty encountered in isolating malignant cells from a large population of benign cells of similar composition.[304] A recent retrospective analysis of 137 patients with Hodgkin's disease found no correlation between aneuploidy and other prognostic factors, or with survival.[304] Although tumors with a high SPF had a less favorable outcome, this prognostic factor was not independent of others.

NON-HODGKIN'S LYMPHOMA

Non-Hodgkin's lymphoma is such a heterogeneous collection of diseases that it is not surprising that the role of DNA flow cytometry remains ill defined, with many conflicting data.[305,306] Nevertheless, it is clear that aneuploidy is more common in lesions of high-grade or of B-cell lineage.[303,307] As a prognostic factor, however, ploidy is neither strong nor independent.[308-310] In contrast, most,[311-315] but not all,[316] studies have shown that SPF or other measures of proliferative activity are useful prognostically. SPF has been used to evaluate clinical course[317] and to augment histologic classification.[318] In this regard, kinetic labeling with IUDR and BrdU[319,320] and flow-cytometric analysis using a monoclonal antibody to an S-phase protein[321] are under investigation. Scant data are available regarding the cytokinetics of such uncommon lymphomas as mycosis fungoides,[322] nonendemic Burkitt's lymphoma,[323] and gastric lymphoma.[324]

MULTIPLE MYELOMA AND MONOCLONAL GAMMOPATHIES

Aneuploidy frequently is found in cases of multiple myeloma, but it also has been found in benign monoclonal gammopathies,[325,326] so it is not an unequivocally distinguishing feature. One recent analysis found aneuploidy in bone marrow cells of 54 per cent of 46 patients with untreated multiple myeloma.[327] Only 1 of 15 patients with benign monoclonal gammopathy had aneuploid cells, and this patient progressed to multiple myeloma 34 months later. In these cases DNA content did not predict survival. Several other studies of malignant disease have noted an association between aneuploidy and decreased survival[328-330]; others have not.[331] Hence, a larger number of patients will need to be assessed in this regard. Labeling of bone marrow cells with BrdU and the monoclonal antibody Ki-67 can be used to determine proliferative activity in patients with multiple myeloma and monoclonal gammopathies.[332]

LEUKEMIAS

Flow-cytometric analysis of leukemias has been used primarily for immunophenotypic classification, cytogenetic studies, and the determination of gene rearrangements.[333] Regarding the prognostic significance of DNA content, several studies of childhood acute lymphoblastic leukemia (ALL) have noted that the presence of hyperdiploid blasts conveys a more favorable outcome and a better response to therapy.[334,335] Also, lower DNA content in the ALL blasts in children has been associated with a greater frequency of late relapses.[336] However, in one trial the TLI of blasts before treatment was of no prognostic significance.[337] Flow cytometry could be used to monitor residual disease in certain subgroups of ALL.[338] Measurement of S-phase activity by BrdU has been employed to assess the sensitivity of ALL cells to cytosine arabinoside. Results have been mixed.[339] In ALL in adults, aneuploidy has been associated with a worse outcome.[340]

Although several studies have used a variety of techniques to assess the cell kinetics of acute nonlymphocytic leukemia (ANLL) and chronic granulocytic leukemia, the prognostic value of these measurements remains unclear.[337,341-348] Some have found that aneuploidy predicts a more favorable prognosis, as it does in childhood ALL.[340] BrdU labeling of leukemic promyelocytes revealed a lower labeling index and longer cell cycle than in other types of ANLL.[349] These results were thought to be secondary to the marked expression of transforming growth factor β. One recent analysis of ANLL found that a high proliferative activity, as measured by BrdU labeling and proliferative cell nuclear antigen staining, was a positive prognostic factor for those receiving S-phase–specific drugs prior to anthracyclines.[350]

Breast Cancer

Breast neoplasms have been the major subject of cytokinetic analysis for several decades. As early as 1980, a retrospective analysis found that patients with diploid tumors survived longer than those with aneuploid tumors.[351] Subsequent data over the last two and a half decades, however, have been conflicting, for all of the reasons cited in the introduction to this section: heterogeneity of sampling[352-354] and sample preparation (fresh tissue versus paraffin-embedded specimens), differences in clinical stage, variations in estrogen receptor status, heterogeneity in patient age distribution and in the tumor, differences in the type of treatment administered, and variations in analytic techniques.[355-358]

One important question concerns the stability of proliferative activity in primary disease (in the breast) and in metastatic locations.[359] Similarly, in patients with locally advanced disease, the tritiated TLI of primary cancers and of metastatic lesions in the axilla did correlate, albeit with wide variation.[360]

Too few studies have examined the value of cytokinetics in predicting response to drug therapy. Some have concluded that aneuploid tumors may be more sensitive to chemotherapy or hormone therapy.[361-363] This finding might well be artifactual, because aneuploid tumors might relapse more quickly than diploid cancers; thus, a difference between patients who have or have not received drug treatment will emerge more quickly in aneuploid cases, but might still exist in those with diploid tumors but take longer to document. Cytokinetics also may be of prognostic significance for locally recurrent tumors in patients treated with lumpectomy and radiation therapy.[364] Most of the activity in the field of breast cancer cytokinetics has focused on prognostication in the absence of drug treatment. Because of the volume and complexity of the results, the data are best viewed from the perspective of the various techniques employed.

PLOIDY

DNA content has been evaluated extensively in breast cancer. In spite of promising initial reports,[365-367] the preponderance of evidence does not support an association between DNA ploidy and lymph node status.[368-373] Only 4 of 17 studies demonstrated a statistically significant correlation between axillary nodal status and ploidy.[374] The majority of reports also indicate no correlation between DNA ploidy and patient age, menopausal status, tumor size or hormone receptor content.[374] A few studies have found that aneuploidy is more frequent among estrogen receptor–negative tumors, so this association may be real but weak, and therefore lost in random variation among other studies of small size.[365,367,368,375,376] Special histologic types of tumors—which tend to have a good prognosis—such as mucinous, tubular, and papillary, are often diploid.[374] Lobular carcinomas also tend to be diploid. Medullary carcinomas are usually aneuploid, even when they are small and do not involve axillary lymph nodes, and thereby have a low incidence of metastatic involvement.[377] There is a consistent correlation between DNA ploidy and tumor grade, with aneuploidy more common among the less differentiated tumors.[374,378-381] In addition, most studies indicate a strong relationship between aneuploidy and high SPF.[374,378,379]

Because of the association of aneuploidy and poor differentiation and, possibly, low estrogen receptor content, it has been expected that ploidy would be of prognostic significance in primary breast cancer. This has been analyzed in patients whose axillary lymph nodes contained metastatic tumor cells (*node positive*) and in those without such involvement (*node negative*). In node-positive patients, several studies with at least 5 years of follow-up have noted statistically significant differences in relapse-free survival[365] and overall survival[382] in favor of diploid versus aneuploid tumors. However, because ploidy correlates with other known prognostic factors, few multivariate analyses have found that ploidy is of independent significance.[382] In addition, other studies have found no significant difference in relapse-free or overall survival based on ploidy status,[383,384] so no firm conclusion can be drawn. Early reports that patients with diploid node-negative cancers remain disease free and survive longer than those with aneuploid tumors was met with great excitement.[382,385,386] Indeed, several multivariate analyses found that ploidy may be an independent prognostic factor.[382,385,387,388] However, several other evaluations did not confirm these findings.[389-394] In general, for analyses of node-negative and node-positive disease, the literature is ambiguous, with defenders[395-399] and opponents[374,400-404] of ploidy as a prognostic marker. One multi-subset analysis found in favor of ploidy, but admitted that SPF was a more powerful factor.[405] Another subset analysis found prognostic significance with a combination of ploidy and estrogen receptor content.[406] A consensus review of the usefulness of DNA index found that ploidy is a weak prognostic factor, which is not of independent value in multivariate analysis.[407]

S-PHASE FRACTION

Most analyses have not demonstrated an association between SPF and axillary nodal status, tumor size, or menopausal status,[374] although some studies have found that high SPF values are present more frequently in tumors in patients younger than 50 years.[389,408,409] Nevertheless, there is strong evidence that SPF is lower in estrogen and progesterone receptor–positive tumors,[367,372,374,408] in those with more normal differentiation,[374] and in those with diploid DNA content.[384,389,392,400,408] Most of the available data support the prognostic significance of SPF. Several studies with median follow-up of at least 4 years of node-negative breast cancer have found that low SPF is an independent predictor of lower relapse rate or longer survival.[386,389-393,409-411] For example, a recent retrospective analysis of 195 samples from patients with node-negative disease found that, in those with tumors over 1 cm in diameter, the relapse-free rate was 78 per cent for cases with SPF of 10 per cent or less but 52 per cent for others.[390] Although similar data exist for node-positive cases, SPF does not emerge consistently as an independent factor in multivariate analyses.[365,384] In addition, the value of SPF as a prognostic factor sometimes has been limited to subgroups,[400,402,403,405,412-416] raising the possibility of multi-subset errors, as discussed earlier. Also, the validity of multivariate analysis to confirm the independence of a prognostic factor depends on which variables are included in the analysis: If an important variable is not included in the process—a variable correlated with SPF—then the independence of SPF could be artifactual. It is of concern in this regard that most studies identify an association between DNA ploidy and grade and between ploidy and SPF,[417] because grade—inexpensively determined by light microscopy—is a time-honored prognostic factor. It is confusing that the majority of analyses have found that ploidy is not of independent prognostic value, whereas SPF is.[409] A consensus review of published data found that SPF is associated with tumor grade as well as relapse and survival in node-negative and node-positive disease.[407] It remains a strong prognostic factor in multivariate analysis.

TRITIATED THYMIDINE LABELING INDEX

The technique of thymidine labeling has been applied extensively to human breast cancer.[418-420] An analysis of 9200 primary tumors from 1973 through 1992 found that the TLI was independent of lymph node status and tumor size, but that there was a trend for increased proliferative activity in lesions over 5 cm in size.[421] A higher TLI also was noted for estrogen and progesterone receptor–negative tumors versus others. In patients with node-positive disease who were treated with adjuvant chemotherapy, those with tumors with low TLI relapsed less rapidly and lived longer.[422] In multivariate analysis, TLI seemed to be an independent factor. Concordantly, TLI seemed to be the most important predictor of recurrence in patients with node-negative disease who were not treated with adjuvant systemic therapy.[423] It is interesting, and somewhat confusing, that in this study SPF by flow cytometry was not of prognostic value, although ploidy was, because others have found a correlation between TLI and SPF.[372]

Locally advanced breast cancer usually is treated by chemotherapy prior to surgical removal of the tumor. In elderly patients with this presentation, there was an association of high TLI, negative estrogen receptor status, and aneuploidy.[424] One study noted a divergence between clinical behavior and TLI in pretreatment biopsies of locally advanced tumors.[425] TLI in this and other studies[360] did not correlate simply with response to chemotherapy. Another study with follow-up in excess of 8 years failed to find an association between TLI and survival.[426]

OTHER TECHNIQUES

Both in vitro and in vivo labeling experiments have been performed with the thymidine analogue BrdU. One study using the in vivo technique failed to find an association between normal breast tissue and that of the tumor.[427] However, they noted greater proliferation of normal cells in premenopausal patients than in older women. BrdU labeling has correlated positively with high TLI, large tumor size, poor differentiation, aneuploidy, and high SPF,[428,429] but not estrogen receptor status.[429,430] Strong staining with Ki-67 has been found in cancers with poor estrogen receptor content, aneuploidy, high nuclear grade, short disease-free survival, and young age.[431] There is no clear association yet between Ki-67 staining and tumor size or histologic grade.[431,432] Overexpression of the proto-oncogene c-erbB-2 (HER2/neu), a growth factor receptor of the epidermal growth factor family, has been correlated with high SPF and with aneuploidy in node-positive breast cancer,[433,434] but not clearly associated with high TLI.[435,436] c-erbB-2 expression and SPF have been found to be independent prognostic factors for node-positive disease,[437] although not all data are confirmatory.[438,439] In preinvasive in situ carcinoma, high TLI and c-erbB-2 expression have been associated,[440] which is curious because the prognosis for this form of breast cancer is so favorable. Regarding other prognostic factors (each of which must be regarded as putative[441]), cathepsin D expression does not correlate well with TLI and other proliferative factors.[442,443] The correlation of epidermal growth factor receptor content with SPF, ploidy, or Ki-67 staining is unclear.[444,445] Investigation of p53 protein[446–449] and proliferative cell nuclear antigen expression in comparison with other measurements of cytokinetics[450–452] is ongoing.

GROWTH KINETICS

The previous discussion focuses on the evidence that cytokinetic parameters are predictive of some clinical characteristics of cancers. These characteristics include virulence, metastatic potential, and drug resistance. Because such characteristics all are founded in the process of tumor progression,[453] measures of cell proliferation may measure the rate of generation of tumor heterogeneity. Cell proliferation, of course, has a more direct influence on clinical behavior, in that it is the obvious mechanism for tumor growth. Hence, growth and heterogeneity are linked by proliferation. In addition, anticancer therapy is fundamentally antiproliferative, and is manifested by tumor volume regression, the opposite of growth. Growth and volume regression are described by a class of mathematical functions called *growth curves*. Because growth and tumor heterogeneity are linked, growth curves both summarize clinical course and relate to the generation of clinically significant mutations.

In this section, we discuss growth curves with a particular emphasis on the one tumor characteristic that is most clinically relevant in the modern era: resistance to anticancer drugs. The two most popular curves are the *exponential curve* and the *Gompertzian curve*. These two curves are not too dissimilar mathematically, even though they have very different implications regarding carcinogenesis, clinical course, and response to treatment. Further theoretical developments are described briefly, and the relevance of these concepts to the molecular scientist are indicated.

Exponential Model

EXPONENTIAL GROWTH

Most of the pioneering work on tumor growth kinetics was based on the transplantable leukemia L1210 in BDF_1 or DBA mice. This cancer grows exponentially to a lethal volume of 10^9 cells, which is about 1 cm^3 of packed cells.[454] Exponential growth means that the percentage of cells dividing—about 90 per cent every 12 to 13 hours—is the same for tiny tumors of 10^2 or 10^3 cells as for tumors close to the lethal volume. As a consequence, the *doubling time* is always constant. If it takes 11 hours for 10^2 cells to grow into 2×10^2 cells, it will take 11 hours for 10^6 cells to grow into 2×10^6 cells. Because it takes 40 hours for 10^3 cells to grow into 10^4 cells (an increase by a factor of ten), it would take 40 hours for 10^7 cells to grow into 10^8 cells.

The general equation for exponential growth is

$$V_T = \alpha V_0 \qquad \text{(Eq. 8–1)}$$

where V_T is the tumor size at a fixed time T after time 0, V_0 is the tumor size at time 0, and α is a constant. In the case of L1210, the cell number N is equivalent to the tumor volume V, because a leukemia is a free-floating mass without stroma. In the above example, when $T = 11$ hours, $\alpha = 2$.

Exponential growth curves are clinically meaningful by virtue of the concept of the doubling time, which is the value of T for $\alpha = 2$.[78] There is great divergence among different histologic types of cancer in their doubling times, at least in the range of tumor sizes found in the clinic.[455]

Human testicular cancers and choriocarcinomas, which tend to be responsive to anticancer drugs and radiation, tend to have doubling times of less than 1 month. Cancers that are somewhat less responsive, such as squamous cell cancer of the head and neck, double in size about every 2 months. Colon adenocarcinomas, which do not respond well to treatment, tend to double each 3 months. It long has been assumed that this clinical observation relates to the relatively higher chemosensitivity of proliferating cells. This may be because mitotic cells are more sensitive, or because slow growth is due to high cell loss fraction, increasing the rate of mutation toward drug resistance.

SKIPPER-SCHABEL-WILCOX MODEL

The original growth curve in clinical oncology is the Skipper-Schabel-Wilcox model, frequently termed the *log kill model*.[456,457] These investigators observed that, when an exponential tumor that is homogeneous in drug sensitivity is treated with anticancer drugs, the fraction of cells killed is always the same regardless of the number of cells present at the moment of drug administration. If a certain dose of a drug reduces 10^6 cells to 10^5, the same therapy would reduce 10^4 cells to 10^3. By Equation 8–1, this means that α has become negative. Both 10^6 to 10^5 and 10^4 to 10^3 are examples of a *one-log kill,* meaning a 90 per cent decrease in cell number. Log kill often increases with increasing dose.[458,459] If two or more drugs are used, the log kills are multiplicative. For example, if a dose of drug A would kill 90 per cent of X cells (a one-log kill), leaving 10 per cent alive, and if a dose of drug B also would kill 90 per cent of X cells, then drug A plus drug B would kill 99 per cent of X cells (a two-log kill), because A would leave 10 per cent alive, and B would kill 90 per cent of that 10 per cent, leaving 1 per cent. If we add a dose of drug C, which also can kill by one log, only 0.1 per cent of cells would survive, a log kill of three. From these roots, the concept of combination chemotherapy was born, and was of major importance in the design of effective regimens for childhood leukemia.[460]

Great optimism resulted from the application of the concept of fractional kill to the postoperative adjuvant treatment of micrometastases.[461,462] In part this excitement was due to the laboratory observation that very small solid tumors contain a higher percentage of actively dividing cells than larger cancers of the same histology.[22,23] If chemotherapy preferentially damages mitotic cells, micrometastases should suffer huge cell kills in the clinic. Unfortunately, this concept has not translated well to real life. For example, adjuvant chemotherapy of primary breast cancer prolongs life and life without cancer, but does so to a modest degree.[463,464]

Much of the activity in the study of cancer growth has concentrated on the reasons for the clinical failure of the log kill model. Skipper and colleagues have catalogued many reasons for this divergence of theory and practice. The first possibility is that the chemotherapy is adequate to cure, but is not being continued for long enough to eradicate all cells. In many situations this is untenable. For example, in the adjuvant chemotherapy of primary breast cancer, durations of treatment beyond 4 to 6 months are not superior to shorter therapies.[464] Another possibility is that a fraction of cells in the tumor are completely, permanently resistant to the drugs that we commonly employ. Such resistance would have to arise spontaneously as the cancer grows from its inception (the carcinogenic event) to clinically appreciable size. Indeed, the generation of such resistance would be associated with the growth kinetics of the cells, and should be correlated with other acquired atypias, such as aneuploidy and metastatic potential. Were this true, cure would be impossible in most cases with current treatments. This hypothesis has been the driving force behind much of the cytokinetic literature of recent years, and underlies the extensive science of drug resistance.

DELBRUCK-LURIA CONCEPT

It long has been assumed that failure to cure with anticancer drugs is largely due to cellular drug resistance.[465] We later reexamine this assumption, but before we turn to that discussion, let us examine the implications of the concept of randomly acquired drug resistance. In the above description of proliferation kinetics, we asserted that proliferation underlies mutation. If resistance is acquired by tumor progression while a cancer grows, the only way to guarantee the absence of resistant cells is to initiate therapy at a tumor size too small to have allowed mutations to occur. Hence, for practical purposes—if we assume that this concept is valid—we must determine when in the time course of growth resistance develops. The concept leads us to believe that only by diagnosing tumors before this time point will we be able to start drug treatment when the tumor is still curable.[466]

Quantitative models of the emergence of drug resistance have been developed to address these issues. In 1943, Luria and Delbruck found that isolated bacterial cultures developed mutations resistant to bacteriophage infection at random (and hence variable) times.[467] Actual exposure to the viruses was not needed, except to select out the resistant bacteria. If a culture had experienced a mutation early in its growth history, it would have time for this clone to become a significant fraction of all bacteria present. A restatement of the model is as follows. The probability of a bacterium not mutating to bacteriophage resistance during one mitosis is $(1 - x)$ also not mutating in $(N - 1)$ mitoses is $(1 - x)^{(N - 1)}$. If each of these $N - 1$ mitoses produces two viable cells (i.e., no cell loss), N cells will result. Because $\log_e (1 - x) \approx -x$ for small x, the probability of finding no resistant bacterium in a culture of N bacteria is

$$\exp[-x(N - 1)] \qquad \text{(Eq. 8–2)}$$

This same mathematical pattern soon was found to apply to the emergence of methotrexate resistance in L1210 cells.[468] Hence, drug resistance seemed to be a random trait acquired spontaneously during cancer cell proliferation. This concept supported the development of modern combination chemotherapy[469]: If a cancer could develop resistance to a drug to which it had not yet been exposed, then only combinations of drugs could possibly eradicate all cancer cells.[470]

GOLDIE-COLDMAN HYPOTHESIS

Although the concept of drug resistance was highly influential in a qualitative sense at the very dawn of the chemotherapy era, the Delbruck-Luria model first was applied quantitatively to human cancer starting in the 1970s.[471–473] Equation 8–2 predicts that, at a tenable mutation rate of $x = 10^{-6}$, the probability of no mutants to any one drug in 10^5 cells is about 90 per cent.[474] However, the probability of no such mutants in 10^7 cells is only 0.0045 per cent. Hence, incurability can arise quickly as a tumor grows from 10^5 to 10^7 cells. The mutation rate of 10^{-6} could apply to other types of acquired genetic traits, such as metastatic ability. The approximate volume of 10^7 densely packed cells is 0.01 cm^3. Because tumor cells usually are packed more loosely together with benign host tissue—stromal cells, blood and lymph and their vessels, colloid, collagen, and extracellular fluid—these same 10^7 cells could occupy a volume of 0.1 to 1.0 cm^3, or a spherical tumor mass 0.58 to 1.24 cm in diameter. It is therefore probably not a coincidence that this happens to be a critical size in human oncology. For example, it is at about 1 cm in diameter that breast cancers frequently become node positive (i.e., develop metastatic potential).[475] It is also at this size that node-negative breast cancers frequently demonstrate a rapidly increasing chance of producing distant metastases.[377,476]

The difficulty arises when we recognize that the strict interpretation of the model would suggest that cancers larger than 0.1 to 1.0 cm^3 in size should always be incurable with any single agent, but that smaller cancers should be cured in at least 90 per cent of cases. This predicts major advantage to, for example, the perioperative or even preoperative chemotherapy of primary breast cancer. In any case, once treatment is started, as many effective drugs as possible should be applied as soon as possible, lest cells that are already resistant to one drug mutate to resistance to others, and the tumor becomes incurable. If combination chemotherapy is impossible because of toxicity,[477] then the strict alternation of two or more regimens would be the best approach.[478]

CRITIQUE OF THE EXPONENTIAL MODEL

In examining these concepts, we must first question the assumption that all chemotherapeutic failure is rooted in absolute drug resistance. Indeed, much of our clinical experience challenges this idea. For example, lymphomas and leukemias frequently are treated to complete remission, meaning disappearance of all signs and symptoms of disease, yet they often relapse later with visible disease, indicating that some cells remained viable after treatment. When these recurrent cancers are treated with the same chemotherapy that accomplished the first remission, they frequently respond again, sometimes with complete remission.[479] If the cells that remained at the first remission were not eradicated because they were drug resistant, they would have had to regain their drug sensitivity over the disease-free interval between the first remission and the relapse. This might occur for some drugs (i.e., methotrexate), but not most. Hence, the greater likelihood is that drug-sensitive cells somehow escaped effective therapy.

A similar observation has been made for breast cancers, which frequently respond to chemotherapy after they relapse from prior postoperative adjuvant chemotherapy. In one trial, patients received cyclophosphamide, Adriamycin and 5-fluorouracil (CAF) with or without tamoxifen as their first treatment for advanced (metastatic) breast cancer.[480] Some of these patients had had prior adjuvant chemotherapy, but the response rate, response duration, and overall survival were unaffected by this history. In another trial, patients with progressive disease after adjuvant cyclophosphamide, methotrexate, and 5-fluorouracil (CMF) responded as well to CMF for advanced disease as those who previously had been randomized to not receive adjuvant CMF.[481] Hence, breast cancer cells that regrow after exposure to adjuvant CMF are not universally resistant to CMF.[482]

Clinical extrapolations of the exponential model are strongly dependent on the concept of stable drug resistance, which we now recognize as an indefensible simplification. It already has been mentioned that one of the conclusions of the exponential model is that cancers larger than 1.0 cm in diameter cannot be cured with single drugs. Again, clinical experience is not confirmatory. Gestational choriocarcinoma and non–acquired immunodeficiency syndrome Burkitt's lymphoma, two rapidly growing cancers, have been cured with single drugs even when therapy is initiated at tumor sizes much larger than 1.0 cm^3.[483]

Although it is reasonable to believe that mutations develop as a consequence of proliferation, the mathematics linking growth rate to the probability of mutations is clearly more complex than Equation 8–2 would suggest. We may examine, as another illustration, the phenomenon of acquired metastatic ability. Until the 1890s, primary breast cancers were usually left to grow in the breast, because no effective therapies were then in use. In these cases, breast cancers always became metastatic.[484] Almost all patients died of metastatic disease within 16 years from the appearance of the lump in the breast. Hence, metastatogenic cells always will develop by random mutation by the time breast cancers reach large size. The implementation of radical mastectomy at about the turn of the century (now, fortunately, supplanted by simple mastectomy or lumpectomy, axillary dissection and radiotherapy with no loss of efficacy) changed the natural history of this disease. A large number of patients have been followed for more than 30 years after radical mastectomy, and more than 30 per cent seem to be cured of their disease.[485,486] The mortality rate is about 10 per cent per year in the first year, dropping monotonically to about 2 per cent per year by year 25.[487] After 30 years, the rate of mortality is indistinguishable from that of the general population.[488,489] Hence, although all breast cancers have the potential for developing metastases, not all have already done so by the time of the first clinical appearance in the breast. Many metastatogenic cells must develop between the first breast lump and the advanced local disease that would result from no local therapy. But it is not at all clear that these cells develop rapidly as Equation 8–2 would imply. In one key trial, some patients with primary disease were treated by lumpectomy without radiotherapy.[490] The local relapse rate was high, consistent with the understanding that viable cancer resided in the nonirradiated breast. Yet patients so undertreated did not have a higher metastatic rate than patients treated adequately by lumpectomy plus immediate radiotherapy. Hence, cancer can grow in the breast without developing metastatogenic cells rapidly.

We therefore have reason to question both the concept that all chemotherapeutic failure is due to drug resistance and the assertion that such drug resistance arises rapidly over a short space of time. We therefore should not be surprised that the most famous contention of the Goldie-Coldman hypothesis—that chemotherapy must be started as soon as possible after diagnosis to be effective—is not consistent with clinical data. An early trial discovered that acute leukemia responded to an antimetabolite as readily if that drug were used as first chemotherapy or after prior chemotherapy with a different antimetabolite.[470] A randomized trial in node-positive breast cancer found equal efficacy in 7 months of chemotherapy starting within 36 hours of surgery as in 6 months of chemotherapy starting 1 month after surgery.[491] A trial in stage B nonseminomatous testicular cancer randomized patients after retroperitoneal lymph node dissection to either two cycles of cisplatin combination chemotherapy or observation.[492] Few patients randomized to adjuvant chemotherapy relapsed, compared to half of patients randomized to observation. Yet the chemotherapeutic response of relapsing cases was excellent, so there was no significant difference in survival between the two approaches. Hence, breast cancer, testicular cancer, and leukemia cells do not mutate rapidly to drug resistance in clinical circumstances, so it is not necessary to rush to treatment.

Indeed, delayed therapy in certain circumstances may have its advantages. In one trial, node-positive patients with primary breast cancer were treated after mastectomy with 8 months of an adjuvant regimen (CMFVP, or CMF plus vincristine and prednisone) followed by either more CMFVP or 6 months of vinblastine, doxorubicin, thiotepa, and the androgen fluoxymesterone (VATH).[493,494] Patients receiving VATH experienced better disease-free survival. Hence, total VATH resistance did not develop rapidly in the cancer cells residual after treatment with CMFVP.

Alternating chemotherapy regimens have been proposed as a way of delivering drugs sooner, "before drug resistance develops." That is, if one has two regimens A and B, the use of ABABAB etc. will deliver B sooner than AAABBB. Alternating chemotherapy regimens have been used in patients with small-cell lung cancer, with little or no benefit.[495] In the treatment of diffuse aggressive non-Hodgkin's lymphoma, a ProMACE-MOPP hybrid, which delivered eight drugs during each monthly cycle, was not better than a plan delivering a full course of ProMACE (prednisone, methotrexate, Adriamycin, cyclophosphamide, etoposide) followed by a full course MOPP (mechlorethamine, vincristine, procarbazine, prednisone).[496] In advanced Hodgkin's disease, ABVD (doxorubicin, bleomycin, vinblastine, and dacarbazine) is superior to MOPP alternating with ABVD.[497–500] Also in this disease, there is no advantage to MOPP alternating with lomustine, Adriamycin, bleomycin, and streptozocin over MOPP alone.[501] In patients with advanced breast cancer, there is no advantage to CMFVP alternating with VATH over CAF or VATH alone.[502] In patients with primary node-positive breast cancer, four 3-week courses of adjuvant doxorubicin (A) followed by eight 3-week courses of intravenous CMF (C), symbolized as AAAACCCCCCCC, was superior to two courses of CMF alternated with one course of doxorubicin four times for a total of 12 courses, symbolized as CCACCACCACCA.[503]

Hence, a major conclusion of the exponential model—the superiority of alternating chemotherapy regimens—is not supported by experimental evidence. It is not clear that we can yet enumerate all of the reasons for the divergence of sensible theory and actual practice. Next, we reconsider one key assumption, that cancers grow exponentially. We examine the possibility that some of the divergence may be explained by the possibility that human cancers grow by a growth pattern that differs from simple exponential growth. However, it would be incorrect to state that Gompertzian growth—the nonexponential model that is probably more realistic than the exponential model—can explain all of the phenomena that we have cited above.

It also would be improper to leave this discussion of exponential growth without noting that the log kill model never said that total, permanent drug resistance was the only possible cause of chemotherapeutic failure. Indeed, Skipper and colleagues long have noted that much drug resistance is relative rather than absolute. Relative drug resistance depends on the dose level of the drug. One tumor may experience a log kill of two (99 per cent reduction in cell number) when it is exposed to the same dose and duration of treatment that causes a log kill of one (90 per cent shrinkage) in another tumor of identical histology. However, if the second tumor is treated with an increased dose intensity of chemotherapy, more cells possibly could be killed.[504,505] Dose intensity is not just the total amount of drug received, nor is it just the amount of drug received per unit of time, but rather a mathematical combination of both. Let D stand for a certain number of milligrams of a drug and M for a certain time duration. As a ratio, D/M is equivalent to $2D/2M$, but $2D/2M$ might be superior therapy. It is possible that $2D/M$ would be even better, but this must be proven. If D/M is equal to $2D/2M$ in efficacy, it must be proven that $D/2M$ is inferior to D/M. In many,[506] but not all,[507] clinical examples, $2D/M$ is the best approach. In randomized trials in childhood acute lymphoblastic leukemia,[508] adult germ cell tumors,[509] and advanced breast cancers,[510] the higher dose regimen has proven superior. Retrospective analyses are also compelling.[511] For the adjuvant chemotherapy of breast cancer, durations of treatment of 12 to 24 months (i.e., $2D/2M$ to $4D/4M$) are not superior to those giving the same dose/time ratio for 6 months (D/M).[464]

Hence, clinical treatment failure within the exponential model—as within the Gompertzian model discussed next—might be the consequence of insufficient dose intensity. A tumor may fail to be cured because some of its cells, relatively but not absolutely insensitive to the agents applied, are not exposed to enough drug to be eradicated. A danger here, as in the treatment of infectious diseases with antibiotics, is that underdosing might give surviving cells many opportunities for mitosis, increasing the odds of mutation toward biochemical resistance by Equation 8–2. A corollary is that it is possible that increased dose intensity could improve clinical results.[506,512] This latter possibility depends on the shape of the dose-response curve for each agent for each disease and on the shape of the curve of tumor volume regression, which is considered further next.

Gompertzian Model

GOMPERTZIAN GROWTH

The log kill model and its later developments were based on exponential growth. Exponential growth is a common pattern in laboratory models. In addition, estimated volumes of nodular pulmonary metastases and, occasionally, those of measurable lesions in other sites, fit exponential curves for short periods relative to the tumors' whole growth history.[513–515] Doubling times of lung lesions range from 1 week to 1 year, with a median of 1 to 3 months. These doubling times correlate with histologic type of cancer, growth fraction, and cell loss fraction.

However, many, if not all, human and animal cancers do not exhibit a constant doubling time.[516–521] In 1825, Benjamin Gompertz presented an alternative growth curve[516]:

$$V_T = \alpha V_0 \beta \qquad \text{(Eq. 8–3)}$$

Whereas in exponential growth β equals 1, in Gompertzian growth β is less than 1 but greater than 0. This of course means that the doubling time is not fixed, but increases as the tumor gets larger. For example, let $\alpha = 2$ and $\beta = 0.9$. $V_0 = 1$ will grow into $V_T = 2$ in T units of time, but $V_0 = 25$ will take about $2T$ units of time to reach 50 and $V_0 = 100$ will take more than $3T$ units of time to double. The assumption that a clinical cancer is exponential would tend to overestimate the doubling time during the preclinical phase of growth.[522] That is, preclinical cancers may grow more rapidly than we would predict from observations of clinical cancers. At the other extreme, as V_0 grows very large, the doubling time approaches infinity. That is, the tumor mass approaches a plateau size V_∞. Whole animals and all normal organs follow Gompertzian kinetics, with V_∞ being our adult size. For cancers, however, the plateau size is incompatible with the life of the host. The larger the plateau size, the more lethal the cancer.

SPEER-RETSKY MODEL

Speer, Retsky, and colleagues derived a modified Gompertzian model using an extensive data set: survival histories for patients who received no therapy for their breast cancers,[484] growth histories of mammographic shadows,[523] and data for disease-free survival following mastec-

tomy.[524] They used a computer model in which tumors grow in randomly increasing steps of Gompertzian plateaus, with an overall pattern that resembles a Gompertzian curve.[525] The validity of the model has been challenged because the temporary plateaus that are predicted have never actually been observed.[526] These authors recommended that postsurgical adjuvant chemotherapy of breast cancer should be applied intermittently over a prolonged duration so as to coincide with presumed growth spurts. This approach was tested clinically and was found to be ineffective.[527] At the heart of the Speer-Retsky model is the assumption that all breast cancers start along the same growth path, with heterogeneity developing in random steps over time. The same clinical data can be fit more parsimoniously, and with greater accuracy, by a family of simple Gompertzian curves with nascent heterogeneity.[518] A family of exponential curves could not be fit to these data because the predicted time from relapse to death would be too short. Hence, there are insufficient data at present to abandon the Gompertzian curve, or close relatives, as a useful description of human malignant growth.

NORTON-SIMON MODEL

Norton and Simon extended the Skipper-Schabel-Wilcox model to cases of Gompertzian growth. As in the original model, the Norton-Simon model conceptualizes both tumor growth and tumor regression in response to chemotherapy. We already have considered that the rate of tumor regression may be positively related to the dose intensity of chemotherapy. Experimental and clinical data also indicate that the rate of tumor regression may be positively related to the growth rate of the unperturbed tumor at the moment of treatment.[454,528,529] In exponential growth, the growth rate is always proportional to tumor size. Hence, a rate of regression proportional to growth rate also would be proportional to tumor size, resulting in a constant proportional (or ''log'') kill. The distinction between the Skipper-Schabel-Wilcox model and the Norton-Simon model is that, in Gompertzian growth, unlike exponential growth, the growth rate of the unperturbed tumor is always changing. Hence, the log kill will change as well. Indeed, the log kill will be greater for small tumors than for large tumors. However, the regrowth rate will be greater for small tumors also, so the overall impact of treatment will be modest, unless the tumor is eradicated.

This latter conclusion would not be very different from the Skipper-Schabel-Wilcox model were the tumor homogeneous in drug sensitivity. However, if the cancer had different sublines, with different growth rates and different sensitivities to treatment, the Norton-Simon model would predict that it would be more difficult to eradicate the tumor than if simple exponential kinetics were in force. Eradicating some sublines would leave others to grow, sometimes with different growth kinetics than the sublines that were eradicated. Because the residual sublines may regrow rapidly (following the rule that small tumors have shorter doubling times than their larger counterparts), large increases in log kill could translate to only small increases in disease-free survival in the clinic. The pessimistic aspect of this conclusion is that more aggressive chemotherapy in the clinic may produce little real survival benefit. However, more optimistically, this model suggests that current adjuvant chemotherapies for diseases such as breast cancer actually might be bringing us closer to total cellular eradication than we might otherwise be led to suspect.

According to this model, the eradication of all sublines in a cancer heterogeneous in Gompertzian growth rates would require eliminating slowly growing, slowly regressing populations as well as the rapidly growing cells that are easier to kill.[530] Slower growing cells should be in the minority by the time of diagnosis because by then they should have been overgrown by faster growing cells. Slow-growing cells also may result from the sublethal action of chemotherapy.[531] The Norton-Simon model suggests that the best way to cure this heterogeneous population is to treat the dominant, faster growing cells as efficiently as possible, and then to treat the numerically inferior, slower growing cells as efficiently as possible.[532] Pending the development of better therapeutic approaches, efficiency means dose intensity as discussed above. Goldie and Coldman's prediction of the superiority of alternating chemotherapy was dependent on the assumption of "symmetry": sublines with equal numbers of cells, equal growth rates, and equal mutation rates. Recently, Day reconsidered the Goldie-Coldman model, but performed computer simulations of mutation to drug resistance under asymmetrical conditions.[533] He formulated a rule that is quite similar to that of the Norton-Simon model in that it predicted the inferiority of an alternating plan.[534]

Confirming these theoretical predictions, the cure of 10^{11} L1210 cells requires induction with cytosine arabinoside plus 6-thioguanine for two or three courses, followed by one high-dose treatment with cyclophosphamide plus carmustine.[535] In the treatment of the M5076 tumor in BDF$_1$ mice, the addition of one dose of L-phenylalanine mustard (l-PAM)—a drug that by itself is weakly active—after four doses of methyl-lomustine doubles the complete remission rate and the median survival.[536] Indeed, this model explains the superiority of AAAACCCCCCCC, giving eight cycles of CMF over 33 weeks, and four cycles of doxorubicin over 9 weeks, over CCACCAC-CACCA, giving eight cycles of CMF over 30 weeks and four cycles of Adriamycin over 33 weeks.[537] In the AAAACCCCCCCC plan, the dose intensity of the doxorubicin was superior. Similarly, in the adjuvant chemotherapy of resected osteosarcoma, doxorubicin alone was superior to doxorubicin alternating with high-dose methotrexate because the dose intensity of the superior agent doxorubicin was impaired by the alternation.[538] A classic trial in the treatment of ALL in children demonstrated that induction by vincristine plus prednisone facilitates the anticancer activity of crossover methotrexate.[539]

In the adjuvant chemotherapy of breast cancer, a plan giving dose-intense doxorubicin followed by dose-intense cyclophosphamide has been piloted successfully, and the prospective determination of comparative efficacy with a more traditional combination chemotherapy is in progress.[540] For patients with diffuse large-cell lymphoma, standard chemotherapy was inferior to induction with doxorubicin, vincristine, and prednisone followed by sequential high-dose cyclophosphamide, then methotrexate (plus vincristine), then etoposide, then l-PAM, then total body irradiation.[541] These plans, and others of their type, exploit the ability of hematopoietic growth factors and other means of hematopoietic reconstitution[542–544] to permit dose intensification.

CRITIQUE OF THE GOMPERTZIAN MODEL

A consideration of Gompertzian kinetics extends the basic ideas derived from exponential kinetics, but it is still dependent on some concepts of tumor growth and response that might be too primitive to move cancer therapeutics rapidly into a more promising future. One key element of both models is the assumption that more rapidly growing cells are more sensitive to chemotherapy because they are more rapidly proliferating. That is, that mitotic cells respond best to treatment because drug interference with their DNA synthesis is lethal.[545] We may call this statement the *mitotoxicity hypothesis*. There is evidence in support of the mitotoxicity hypothesis. For example, stimulation of MCF-7 cells in vitro with estradiol or epidermal growth factor increases both cell proliferation and cell kill from Adriamycin.[546] Also, estradiol administration enhances the cytotoxicity of melphalan in hormone-responsive cell lines.[547] In the clinic, hormone recruitment of locally advanced breast cancer has resulted in high local response rates.[548,549]

However, an unquestioned acceptance of the mitotoxicity hypothesis leaves several enigmas unresolved. The advantages of recruitment are moot in the treatment of metastatic breast cancer.[550–552] Also, tamoxifen—a proliferation-inhibiting estrogenic drug—can cause a G_1-S arrest in sensitive cells, but it antagonizes the cytotoxicity of melphalan and 5-fluorouracil at dose levels insufficient to accomplish this action.[547] Tamoxifen actually enhances the cytotoxicity of doxorubicin and the alkylating agent 4-hydroxycyclophosphamide.

Mitotoxicity has never been an adequate explanation for the chemotherapeutic response of clinical breast cancer. Only about 5 per cent of the cells in an average breast cancer are in S phase. Hence, even with drugs that kill G_1 and G_2 cells, only about 15 to 20 per cent of the tumor mass possibly could be killed by a single treatment. Yet regressions greater than one log frequently are seen after single treatments with high-dose chemotherapy.[544] The TLI of breast cancer does not predict chemosensitivity either in locally advanced disease[425] or in the adjuvant setting.[553] Normal tissues—bone marrow, hair follicles, alimentary mucosa—with higher growth fractions than many tumors can recover from the influence of chemotherapy, whereas many cancers—acute leukemias, malignant lymphomas, choriocarcinomas, and germ cell cancers—often do not.

As we search for a better model, some possibilities will need to be explored. One is that chemotherapy could damage G_0 cells that die as they are recruited into cycle. Another concerns growth factors, which are known to be important in a variety of tumors. Malignant transformation frequently alters gene expression for growth factors, their receptors, and intracellular signal transduction proteins.[554] Leukemogenic alkylating agents cause cytogenetic abnormalities at loci coding for growth factors and related proteins.[555] We will need to explore the possibility that chemotherapy could share with hormonal therapy an action on growth factor loop disruption.[556] Cytokinetic analysis of MCF-7 cells exposed to low levels of Adriamycin does not show an immediate S-phase reduction but rather an accumulation of cells in late S, G_2, and M phases starting 2 days after treatment.[557] Chemotherapy is now known to kill cells by inducing *apoptosis,* an orderly process of programmed cell death. When hematopoietic cells are deprived of essential growth factors, they too die by apoptosis.[558–560] In the laboratory, chemotherapy can influence growth factor loops. Doxorubicin, for example, may upregulate epidermal growth factor receptors in HeLa and 3T3 cells.[561] Activation of the intracellular signal protein kinase C increases cell kill by cisplatin without increasing drug uptake.[562] In the treatment of human cancer xenografts, antibodies to growth factor receptors, which can by themselves inhibit growth, synergize with a variety of chemotherapeutic agents.[563] Hence, the cytotoxic effects of chemotherapy might transcend simple mitotoxicity.

Another issue is the biologic basis for Gompertzian growth. An old concept is that a solid tumor "outgrows" its supply of nutrients, and therefore cannot sustain unimpeded exponential growth, which otherwise would be its natural tendency. This has been challenged by evidence that even small tumors, with rich blood supply, follow Gompertzian patterns, and that large tumors, with relatively slow growth rates, often have adequate vascularity. Indeed, the ability to induce neovascularization is a hallmark of malignancy.[564] In addition, the progressive slowing of Gompertzian growth may be more the result of decreased cell production than increased cell loss.[22,23]

What is needed, then, is a more sophisticated model. In this regard, abnormal growth, as well as invasion and metastasis, may be dependent on the relationship between the cancer cell and its local environment. Loss of stromal restraint on mitosis would be tumorigenic, loss of stromal anatomic barriers would permit invasion, and loss of the inhospitality of distant stromal sites would provide for the viability of metastases. In primary breast cancer, stromal cells make growth factors,[565,566] proteinases,[567] and other essential substances,[568,569] perhaps in reaction to signals from the cancer cells.[570] In hereditary gastrointestinal cancer, the stroma itself may be abnormal.[571]

The geometric relationship between cancer cells and their stroma is complex. Most cancerous masses are composed of repeating elements—such as branching tree patterns or multiple nodules—that are self-similar over various scales of size. The most common arrangement, the branching pattern, is reminiscent of a tissue's vascular supply, and is the normal structure of glandular organs. The breast, for example, is composed of lobules and ducts organized into branching tubes. As a fractal geometric pattern, this means that the number of cells is proportional to the tumor volume raised to a power less than or equal to 1, that power being a function of the packing ratio of the cells and the average size of the basic unit (such as

the duct).[572,573] Packing ratio refers to the number of cells per unit of volume in the basic unit. Low packing ratios produce low power constants and therefore low ratios of number of cells per volume of tumor. Such tumors, with relatively few cells per microscopic field, tend to be more benign, whereas cancers with densely packed cancer cells and little intervening stroma tend to be more malignant.[574]

An interesting observation is that the power constant relates to a tumor's pattern of growth. Equation 8–2 concerns tumor volume V, which is comprised of N cancer cells plus $(V - N)$ stroma (expressing V in units of cell volume). Both exponential and Gompertzian growth occur when a new volume V_T is proportional to the number of cells N_0 in the old volume V_0:

$$V_T = \alpha N_0 \qquad \text{(Eq. 8–4)}$$

Because N_0 is proportional to V_0 raised to the power constant, exponential growth occurs when the power constant is 1, and Gompertzian growth occurs when the power constant is between 0 and 1. As described above, much of the malignant behavior of the Gompertzian tumor is determined by its plateau size, V_∞. The plateau size is very dependent on the power constant in a surprising way. V_∞ is very small over a very wide range of power constants. Hence, even if the power constant changes markedly, a tumor can remain at a benign size. However, if the power constant increases greater than a certain threshold, V_∞ rapidly becomes very large, creating a key attribute of malignancy. By this model, a normal tissue can sustain considerable genotypic-phenotypic change toward a larger power constant without becoming malignant (i.e., a long process of an evolving preneoplasia). However, a precancerous mass suddenly can become malignant with just a small additional increment in the power constant over a threshold. Because the power constant is dependent on the packing ratio, this means that tumors with widely varying packing ratios can be benign, but, once a population is close to a boundary of tight packing, a further small change in geometry toward increased packing could be associated with malignant transformation. The most extreme case, when the cancer cells are contiguous so that the packing ratio is 1, would be identified with the most malignant growth, exponential growth.

How does clonal expansion relate to invasion and metastasis? Let us consider the hypothesis that the primary defect is loss of constraint by the stroma, which is equivalent to autonomy from the stroma. This may be because the cancer cells are independent of growth-promoting stromal influences, or still dependent but so sensitive to growth-promoting chemicals that they are stimulated by minute amounts (humoral or mediated by contact). If stromal chemicals are inhibitory rather than stimulatory, cancer cells also might become independent by losing the ability to be inhibited by the stromal influences, as has been observed in melanoma[575] and carcinoma[576] cell lines. As cancer cells gain autonomy, they may escape from anatomic constraints (i.e., become invasive). Because they no longer require admixture with stroma, they increase their packing ratio. As the packing ratio increases, the power constant increases, and, when it crosses a critical threshold, a dramatic increase in V_∞ occurs. Thus, growth and invasion are linked. Relative autonomy from stroma also would permit metastasis to anatomic locations that produce, normally or in response to the cancer cells, the growth factors on which the cancer cells are partially dependent or to which the cancer cells are inordinately sensitive.[577] Thus, growth and metastatic behavior are linked: In breast cancer, as in most solid tumors, metastatic potential is a direct function of tumor size.[578] Total autonomy (acrine growth or infinite sensitivity) would mean that the cancer cells could grow anywhere in the host, and might even grow exponentially via a packing ratio of 1 (no stromal cells present).

CONCLUSION

This brief review of the ever-changing field of cytokinetics should serve to indicate that this branch of experimental science addresses all three dynamics of neoplasia: changes in internal biochemical states, changes in the relationships between cancer cells and their cellular and chemical environment, and changes in cancer cell numbers. These dynamics are indeed the determinants of carcinogenesis, growth, invasion, metastasis, and response to therapy. As the field matures, it is hoped that our understanding of the kinetics of cancer will add to our ability to eradicate or, even better, prevent all malignant proliferation and growth.

REFERENCES

1. Howard A, Pelc SR: Nuclear incorporation of ^{32}P as demonstrated by autoradiographs. Exp Cell Res 2:178, 1951
2. Lajtha LG, Oliver R, Ellis F: Incorporation of ^{32}P and adenine ^{14}C into DNA by human bone marrow cells in vitro. Br J Cancer 8:367, 1954
3. Gelfant S: Cycling-noncycling cell transitions in tissue aging, immunological surveillance, transformation and tumor growth. Int Rev Cytol 70:1, 1981
4. Darzynkiewicz Z: Metabolic and kinetic compartments of the cell cycle distinguished by multiparameter flow cytometry. In Skehan P, Friedman SJ (eds): Growth, Cancer and the Cell Cycle. Clifton, NJ, Humana Press, 1984, pp 249–278
5. Ling MR, Kay JE: Lymphocyte Stimulation. Elsevier, New York, 1965
6. Baserga R: Growth in size and cell DNA replication. Exp Cell Res 151:1, 1984
7. Darzynkiewicz Z, Traganos F, Melamed MR: New cell cycle compartments identified by multiparameter flow cytometry. Cytometry 1:98, 1980
8. Gerdes J, Lemke H, Baisch H, et al: Cell cycle analysis of a cell proliferation: Associated human nuclear antigen defined by the monoclonal antibody Ki-67. J Immunol 133:1710, 1984
9. Johnson LV, Walsh ML, Chen LB: Localization of mitochondria in living cells with rhodamine 123. Proc Natl Acad Sci USA 77:990, 1980
10. Chaudhary PM, Roninson IB: Expression and activity of P glycoprotein, a multidrug efflux pump, in human hematopoietic stem cells. Cell 66:85, 1991
11. Pardee AB: G, events and regulation of cell proliferation. Science 246:603, 1989
12. Broek D, Bartlett R, Crawford K, Nurse P: Involvement of P34^{cdc2} in establishing the dependency of S phase on mitosis. Nature 349:388, 1991
13. Murray AW: Remembrance of things past. Nature 349:367, 1991
14. Hartwell LH, Weinert TA: Checkpoints: Controls that ensure the order of cell cycle events. Science 246:629, 1989
15. Murray AW, Kirschner MW: Dominoes and clocks: The union of two views of the cell cycle. Science 246:614, 1989
16. Laskey RA, Fairman MP, Blow JJ: S phase of the cell cycle. Science 246:609, 1989
17. O'Farrell PH, Edgar BA, Lakich D, Lehner CF: Directing cell division during development. Science 246:635, 1989
18. Folkman J, Moscona A: Role of cell shape in growth control. Nature 273:345, 1978
19. McIntosh JR, Koonce MP: Mitosis. Science 246:622, 1989
20. Hoffman J, Post J: In vivo studies of DNA synthesis in human normal and tumor cells. Cancer Res 27:898, 1967
21. Quastler H, Sherman FG: Cell population kinetics in the intestinal epithelium of the mouse. Exp Cell Res 17:420, 1959
22. LaLa PK: Age-specific changes in the proliferation of Ehrlich ascites tumor cells grown as solid tumors. Cancer Res 32:628, 1972
23. Watson JV: The cell proliferation kinetics of the EMT6/M/AC mouse tumor at four volumes during unperturbed growth in vivo. Cell Tissue Kinet 9:147, 1976
24. Baserga R: The Biology of Cell Reproduction. Cambridge, MA, Harvard University Press, 1985
25. Baak JPA: Mitosis counting in tumors. Hum Pathol 21:683, 1990
26. Kaman EJ, Smeulders AWN, Verbeek PW, et al: Image processing for mitoses in sections of breast cancer: A feasibility study. Cytometry 5:244, 1984
27. Schipper NW, Smeulders AW, Baak JP: Automated estimation of epithelial volume in breast cancer sections: A comparison with the image processing steps applied to gynecological tumors. Pathol Res Pract 186:737, 1990
28. Frei E III, Whang J, Scoggins RB, et al: The stathmokinetic effect of vincristine. Cancer Res 24:1918, 1964
29. Steel GG: Autoradiographic analysis of the cell cycle: Howard and Pelc to the present day. Int J Radiat Biol 49:227, 1986
30. Alama A, Nicolin A, Conte PF, Drewinko B: Evaluation of growth fractions with monoclonal antibodies to human alpha-DNA polymerase. Cancer Res 47:1892, 1987
31. Crocker J: Proliferation indices in malignant lymphomas. Clin Exp Immunol 77:299, 1989
32. Simon RM, Stroot MT, Weiss GH: Numerical inversion of Laplace transforms with application to percent labelled mitoses experiments. Comput Biomed Res 5:596, 1972
33. Dressler LG, Bartow SA: DNA flow cytometry in solid tumors: Practical aspects and clinical applications. Semin Diagn Pathol 6:55, 1989
34. Ghali VS, Liau S, Teplitz C, et al: A comparative study of DNA ploidy in 115 fresh-frozen breast carcinomas by image analysis versus flow cytometry. Cancer 70:2668, 1992
35. Dawson AE, Norton JA, Weinberg DS: Comparative assessment of proliferation and DNA content in breast carcinoma by image analysis and flow cytometry. Am J Pathol 136:1115, 1990
36. Kamensky LA, Melamed MR: Instrumentation for automated examination of cellular specimens. Proc IEEE 57:2007, 1969
37. VanDilla MA, Trujillo TT, Mullaney PF, Coulter JR: Cell microfluorometry: A method for rapid fluorescence measurement. Science 169:1213, 1969
38. Hedley DW, Freidlander MD, Taylor IW, et al: Method for analysis of cellular DNA content of paraffin-embedded pathological material using flow cytometry. J Histochem Cytochem 31:1333, 1983
39. Pallavicini MG: Solid tissue dispersal for cytokinetic analyses. In Gray JW, Darzyniewicz Z (eds): Techniques for Analysis of Cellular Proliferation. Clifton, NJ, Humana Press, 1986, pp 139–162
40. Deshmukh P, Ramsey L, Garewal HS: Ki-67 labelling index is a more reliable measure of solid tumor proliferative activity than tritiated thymidine labeling. Am J Clin Pathol 94:192, 1990
41. Shimomatsuya T, Tanigawa N, Muraoka R: Proliferative activity of human tumors: Assessment using bromodeoxyuridine and flow cytometry. Jpn J Cancer Res 82:357, 1991
42. Giordano M, Riccardi A, Danova M, et al: Cell proliferation of human leukemia and solid tumors studied with in vivo bro-

modeoxyuridine and flow cytometry. Cancer Detect Prev *15*: 391, 1991

43. Wilson GD: Assessment of human tumor proliferation using bromodeoxyuridine—current status. Acta Oncol *30*:903, 1991

44. Riccardi A, Danova M, Dionigi P, et al: Cell kinetics in leukaemia and solid tumors studied with *in vivo* bromodeoxyuridine and flow cytometry. Br J Cancer *59*:898, 1989

45. Kawamoto K, Wada Y, Kumazawa H, et al: Experimental and clinical evaluation by flow cytometry for the mechanism of combination therapy (Cisplatin and peplomycin). Cytometry *13*:307, 1992

46. Latt SA: Fluorometric detection of DNA synthesis: Possibilities for interfacing bromodeoxyuridine dye techniques with flow fluorometry. J Histochem Cytochem *25*:913, 1977

47. Meyer JS, Nauert J, Koehm S, Hughes J: Cell kinetics of human tumors by *in vitro* bromodeoxyuridine labeling. J Histochem Cytochem *37*:1449, 1989

48. Raza A, Yasin Z, Grande C: A comparison of the rate of DNA synthesis in myeloblasts from peripheral blood and bone marrows in patients with acute nonlymphocytic leukemia. Exp Cell Res *176*:13, 1988

49. Miller MA, Mazewski CM, Yousuf N, et al: Simultaneous immunohistochemical detection of IUdR and BrdU infused intravenously to cancer patients. J Histochem Cytochem *39*:407, 1991

50. Hiddeman WH, Schumann J, Andreeff M, et al: Convention on nomenclature for DNA cytometry. Cytometry *5*:445, 1984

51. Herman CJ: Cytometric DNA analysis in the management of cancer: Clinical and laboratory considerations. Cancer *69*: 1553, 1992

52. Stewart CC: Clinical applications of flow cytometry: Immunologic methods for measuring cell membrane and cytoplasmic antigens. Cancer *69*:1543, 1992

53. Giorgi JV, Hurtubise PE, Cram LS, et al: Clinical applications of cytometry: 6th annual meeting. Cytometry *13*:445, 1992

54. Hanson CA: Immunophenotyping of hematologic malignant conditions: To flow or not to flow? Am J Clin Pathol *96*:295, 1991

55. Gheuens EE, van Bockstaele DR, van der Keur M, et al: Flow cytometric double labeling technique for screening of multidrug resistance. Cytometry *12*:636, 1991

56. Funato T, Bando Y, Kato H, et al: Analysis of P-glycoprotein in patients with acute leukemias by flow cytometry. Rinsho Byori *37*:899, 1989

57. Van Dijk J, Tsuruo T, Segal DM, et al: Bispecific antibodies reactive with the multidrug-resistance-related glycoprotein and CD3 induce lysis of multidrug-resistant tumor cells. Int J Cancer *44*:738, 1989

58. Butler JA, Trezona T, Vargas H, State D: Value of measuring hormone receptor levels of regional metastatic carcinoma of the breast. Arch Surg *124*:1131, 1989

59. Graham ML, Bunn RA, Jewett PB, et al: Simultaneous measurement of progesterone receptors and DNA indices by flow cytometry: Characterization of an assay in breast cancer cell lines. Cancer Res *49*:3934, 1989

60. Graham ML, Dalquest KE, Horwitz KB: Simultaneous measurement of progesterone receptors and DNA indices by flow cytometry: Analysis of breast cancer cell mixtures and genetic instability of the T47D line. Cancer Res *49*:3943, 1989

61. Leader M, Patel J, Makin C, Henry K: An analysis of the sensitivity and specificity of the cytokeratin marker CAM 5.2 for epithelial tumors: Results of a study of 203 sarcomas, 50 carcinomas, and 28 malignant melanomas. Histopathology *10*: 1315, 1986

62. Stewart CC: Flow cytometric analysis of oncogene expression in human neoplasia. Arch Pathol Lab Med *113*:634, 1989

63. van Dam PA, Watson JV, Lowe DG, et al: Tissue preparation for simultaneous flow cytometric quantitation of tumor associated antigens and DNA in solid tumors. J Clin Pathol *43*:833, 1990

64. Mendelsohn ML: The growth fraction: A new concept applied to neoplasia. Science *132*:1496, 1960

65. Killman SA: Acute leukemia: The kinetics of leukemic blast cells in man. Series Hematol *1*:38, 1968

66. Bruce WR, Valeriote FA: Normal and malignant stem cells and

chemotherapy. *In* The Proliferation and Spread of Neoplastic Cells, University of Texas MD Anderson Hospital and Tumor Institute at Houston, 21st Annual Symposium on Fundamental Cancer Research 1967. Baltimore, Williams & Wilkins, 1968, pp 409–422

67. Till JE, McCulloch GA, Phillips RA, Siminovitch L: Aspects of the regulation of stem cell function. *In* The Proliferation and Spread of Neoplastic Cells, 21st Annual Symposium on Fundamental Cancer Research 1967. University of Texas MD Anderson Hospital and Tumor Institute at Houston, Baltimore, Williams & Wilkins, 1968, pp 235–244

68. Hamburger A, Salmon SE: Primary bioassay of human myeloma stem cells. J Clin Invest *60*:846, 1977

69. Look AT, Douglass EC, Meyer WH: Clinical importance of near-diploid tumor stem lines in patients with osteosarcoma of an extremity N Engl J Med *318*:1567, 1988

70. Steel GG: Cell loss as a factor in the growth rate of human tumors. Eur J Cancer *3*:381, 1967

71. Novick A, Szilard L: Experiments with the chemostat on spontaneous mutations of bacteria. Proc Natl Acad Sci USA *36*: 708, 1950

72. Foulds L: The histologic analysis of mammary tumors of mice. II. The histology of responsiveness and progression. The origins of tumors. J Natl Cancer Inst *17*:713, 1956

73. Hartwell L: Defects in cell cycle checkpoint may be responsible for genomic instability of cancer cells. Cell *71*:543, 1992

74. Kastan MB, Zhan Q, el-Deiry WS, et al: A mammalian cell cycle checkpoint pathway utilizing p53 and GADD45 is defective in ataxia-telangiectasia. Cell *71*:587, 1992

75. Lasko D, Cavenee W, Nordenskjold M: Loss of constitutional heterozygosity in human cancer. Annu Rev Genet *25*:281, 1991

76. Gould MN: Cellular and molecular aspects of the multistage progression of mammary carcinogenesis in humans and rats. Semin Cancer Biol *4*:161, 1993

77. Iannaccone PM, Weinberg WC, Dearaut FD: On the clonal origin of tumors: A review of experimental models. Int J Cancer *39*: 778, 1987

78. Frei E III: Models and the clinical dilemma. *In* Fidler IJ, White RJ (eds): Design of Models for Testing Therapeutic Agents. New York, Van Nostrand Reinhold, 1982, pp 248–259

79. Fidler IJ: Tumor heterogeneity and the biology of cancer invasion and metastases. Cancer Res *38*:2651, 1978

80. Charbit A, Malaise EP, Tubiana M: Relation between the pathological nature and the growth rate of human tumors. Eur J Cancer *7*:307, 1971

81. Simpson-Herren L, Sanford AH, Holmquist JP: Cell population kinetics of transplanted and metastatic Lewis lung carcinoma. Cell Tissue Kinet *7*:349, 1974

82. Varmus H: An historical overview of oncogenes. *In* Weinberg RA (ed): Oncogenes and the Molecular Origins of Cancer. Cold Spring Harbor, NY, Cold Spring Harbor Laboratory Press, 1989, pp 3–44

83. Vogelstein B, Kinzler KW: The multi-step nature of cancer. Trends Genet *9*:138, 1993

84. Weinberg RA: Oncogenes, antioncogenes and the molecular basis of multistep carcinogenesis. Cancer Res *49*:3713, 1989

85. Knudson AG: Hereditary cancers: Clues to mechanisms of carcinogenesis. Br J Cancer *59*:661, 1989

86. Ryser HJP: Chemical carcinogenesis. N Engl J Med *285*:721, 1971

87. Wegelin C: Malignant disease of the thyroid gland and its relations to goitre in man and animals. Cancer Rev *3*:297, 1928

88. Neve EF: Kangri-burn cancer. Br Med J *2*:1255, 1923

89. Graham JH, Helvig EB: *In* Graham JH, Johnson WC, Helvig EB (eds): Dermal Pathology. New York, Harper and Row, 1972, pp 561–581

90. Greenberg PL, Mara B: The preleukemic syndrome: Correlation of *in vitro* parameters of granulocytopoiesis with clinical features. Am J Med *66*:951, 1979

91. Peterson LC, Bloomfield CD, Brunning RD: Blast crisis as an initial or terminal manifestation of chronic myeloid leukemia. Am J Med *60*:209, 1976

92. Parks TG, Bussey HJR, Lockhart-Mummery HE: Familial po-

lyposis coli associated with extracolonic abnormalities. Gut *11*:323, 1970

93. De Ome KB, Medina D: A new approach to mammary tumorigenesis in rodents. Cancer *24*:1255, 1969

94. Davis HH, Simons M, Davis JB: Cystic disease of the breast: Relationship to carcinoma. Cancer *17*:957, 1964

95. Sandison AT: An autopsy study of the adult human breast: With special reference to the proliferative epithelial changes of importance in the pathology of the breast. Natl Cancer Inst Monogr *8*:1, 1962

96. Glicksman AS, Pajak TF, Gottlieb AJ, et al: Second malignant neoplasms in patients successfully treated for Hodgkin's disease: A Cancer and Leukemia Group B study. Cancer Treat Rep *66*:1035, 1982

97. Boice JD Jr, Greene MH, Killen JY Jr, et al: Leukemia and preleukemia after adjuvant treatment of gastrointestinal cancer with semustine (methyl-CCNU). N Engl J Med *309*:1079, 1983

98. Fuhr JE, Kattine AA, Sullivan TA, Nelson HS: Flow cytometric analysis of pulmonary fluids and cells for the detection of malignancies. Am J Pathol *141*:211, 1992

99. Rijken A, Dekker A, Taylor S, et al: Diagnostic value of DNA analysis in effusions by flow cytometry and image analysis: A prospective study on 102 patients as compared with cytologic examination. Am J Clin Pathol *95*:6, 1991

100. Koss LG, Czerniak B, Herz F, Wersto RP: Flow cytometric measurements of DNA and other cell components in human tumors: A critical appraisal. Hum Pathol *20*:528, 1989

101. Seckinger D, Sugarbaker E, Frankfurt O: DNA content in human cancer. Arch Pathol Lab Med *113*:619, 1989

102. Wersto RP, Liblit RL, Koss LG: Flow cytometric DNA analysis of human solid tumors: A review of the interpretation of DNA histograms. Hum Pathol *22*:1085, 1991

103. Carey FA, Lamb D, Bird CC: Intratumoral heterogeneity of DNA content in lung cancer. Cancer *65*:2266, 1990

104. Carey FA, Lamb D, Bird CC: Importance of sampling method in DNA analysis of lung cancer. J Clin Pathol *43*:820, 1990

105. Hiddemann W, von Bassewitz DB, Kleinemeier H-J, et al: DNA stemline heterogeneity in colorectal cancer. Cancer *58*:258, 1986

106. Frierson HF: Flow cytometric analysis of ploidy in solid neoplasms: Comparison of fresh tissues with formalin-fixed paraffin-embedded specimens. Hum Pathol *19*:290, 1988

107. Yauner D, Weinberg D, Lage J: Flow cytometric analysis of DNA from ovarian and endometrial tumors: Fresh vs. fixed tissues [abstr]. Mod Pathol *2*:107, 1989

108. Klemi PJ, Joensuu H: Comparison of DNA ploidy in routine fine needle aspiration biopsy samples and paraffin-embedded tissue samples. Anal Quant Cytol Histol *10*:195, 1988

109. Bach BA, Knape WA, Edinger MG, Tubbs RR: Improved sensitivity and resolution in the flow cytometric DNA analysis of human solid tumor specimens. Am J Clin Pathol *96*:615, 1991

110. Joensuu H, Kallioniemi OP: Different opinions on classification of DNA histograms produced from paraffin-embedded tissue. Cytometry *10*:711, 1989

111. van Dam PA, Watson JV, Lowe DG, et al: Comparative evaluation of fresh, fixed, and cryopreserved solid tumor cells for reliable flow cytometry of DNA and tumor associated antigen. Cytometry *13*:722, 1992

112. Shapiro HM: Flow cytometry of DNA content and other indicators of proliferative activity. Arch Pathol Lab Med *113*:591, 1989

113. Coon JS, Deitch AD, de Vere White RW, et al: Check samples for laboratory self-assessment in DNA flow cytometry. Cancer *63*:1592, 1989

114. Wheeless LL, Coon JS, Cox C, et al: Precision of DNA flow cytometry in inter-institutional analyses. Cytometry *12*:405, 1991

115. Blute ML, Nativ O, Zincke H, et al: Pattern of failure after radical retropubic prostatectomy for clinically and pathologically localized adenocarcinoma of the prostate: Influence of tumor deoxyribonucleic acid ploidy. J Urol *142*:1262, 1989

116. Fordham MVP, Burdge AH, Matthews J, et al: Prostatic carcinoma cell DNA content measured by flow cytometry and its relation to clinical outcome. Br J Surg *73*:400, 1986

117. Haugen OA, Mjlnerd O: DNA-ploidy as prognostic factor in prostatic carcinoma. Int J Cancer *45*:224, 1990

118. Montgomery BT, Nativ O, Blute ML, et al: Stage B prostate adenocarcinoma: Flow cytometric nuclear DNA ploidy analysis. Arch Surg *125*:327, 1990

119. Nativ O, Winkler HZ, Raz Y, et al: Stage C prostatic adenocarcinoma: Flow cytometric nuclear DNA ploidy analysis. Mayo Clin Proc *64*:911, 1989

120. Ritchie AWS, Dorey F, Layfield LJ, et al: Relationship of DNA content to conventional prognostic factors in clinically localised carcinoma of the prostate. Br J Urol *62*:254, 1988

121. Tribukait B: DNA flow cytometry in carcinoma of the prostate for diagnosis, prognosis and study of tumor biology. Acta Oncol *30*:187, 1991

122. Deitch AD, deVere White RW: Flow cytometry as a predictive modality in prostate cancer. Hum Pathol *23*:352, 1992

123. Tinari N, Natoli C, Angelucci D, et al: DNA and S-phase fraction analysis by flow cytometry in prostate cancer. Cancer *71*:1289, 1993

124. Nemoto R, Hattori K, Uchida K, et al: S-phase fraction of human prostate adenocarcinoma studied with *in vivo* bromodeoxyuridine labeling. Cancer *66*:509, 1990

125. van Weerden WM, Moerings EPCM, van Kreuningen A, et al: Ki-67 expression and BrdUrd incorporation as markers of proliferative activity in human prostate tumor models. Cell Prolif *26*:67, 1993

126. Blute ML, Tsushima K, Farrow GM, et al: Transitional cell carcinoma of the renal pelvis: Nuclear deoxyribonucleic acid ploidy studied by flow cytometry. J Urol *140*:944, 1988

127. Banner BF, Brancazio L, Bahnson RR, et al: DNA analysis of multiple synchronous renal cell carcinomas. Cancer *66*:2180, 1990

128. Tachibana M, Deguchi N, Baba S, et al: Bromodeoxyuridine and deoxyribonucleic acid bivariate analysis in human renal cell carcinoma: Does flow cytometric determination predict malignant potential or prognosis of patients with renal cell carcinoma? Am J Clin Pathol *97*(suppl 1):S38, 1992

129. Al-Abadi H, Nagel R: Prognostic relevance of ploidy and proliferative activity of renal cell carcinoma. Eur Urol *15*:271, 1988

130. Rainwater LM, Hosaka Y, Farrow GM, Lieber MM: Well differentiated clear cell renal carcinoma: Significance of nuclear deoxyribonucleic acid patterns studied by flow cytometry. J Urol *137*:15, 1987

131. Ekfors TO, Lipasti J, Nurmi MJ, et al: Flow cytometric analysis of the DNA profile of renal cell carcinoma. Pathol Res Pract *182*:58, 1987

132. Currin SM, Lee SE, Walther PJ: Flow cytometric assessment of deoxyribonucleic acid content in renal adenocarcinoma: Does ploidy status enhance prognostic stratification over stage alone? J Urol *143*:458, 1990

133. Ljungberg B, Forsslund G, Stenling R, Zetterberg A: Prognostic significance of the DNA content in renal cell carcinoma. J Urol *135*:422, 1986

134. Masters JRW, Camplejohn RS, Parkinson MC, et al: Does DNA flow cytometry give useful prognostic information in renal parenchyma adenocarcinoma? Br J Urol *70*:364, 1992

135. Nemoto R, Hattori K, Uchida K, et al: Estimation of growth fraction *in situ* in human bladder cancer with bromodeoxyuridine labelling. Br J Urol *65*:27, 1990

136. Walther PJ: The role of flow cytometry in the management of bladder cancer. Hematol Oncol Clin North Am *6*:81, 1992

137. Gustafson H, Tribukait B, Esposti PL: DNA pattern, histological grade and multiplicity related to recurrence rate in superficial bladder tumours. Scand J Urol Nephrol *16*:135, 1982

138. Tribukait B, Gustafson H, Esposti PL: The significance of ploidy and proliferation in the clinical and biological evaluation of bladder tumours: A study of 100 untreated cases. Br J Urol *54*:130, 1982

139. Blomjous ECM, Schipper NW, Baak JPA, et al: The value of morphometry and DNA flow cytometry in addition to classic prognosticators in superficial urinary bladder carcinoma. Am J Clin Pathol *91*:243, 1989

140. Tribukait B: Flow cytometry in assessing the clinical aggressiveness of genitourinary neoplasms. World J Urol *5*:108, 1987

141. Jacobsen AB, Lunde S, Ous S, et al: T2/T3 bladder carcinomas treated with definitive radiotherapy with emphasis on flow cytometric DNA ploidy values. Int J Radiat Oncol Biol Phys 17: 923, 1989

142. Lipponen PK, Collan Y, Eskelinen MJ, et al: Comparison of morphometry and DNA flow cytometry with standard prognostic factors in bladder cancer. Br J Urol 65:589, 1990

143. Lipponen PK, Nordling S, Eskelinen MJ, et al: Flow cytometry in comparison with mitotic index in predicting disease outcome in transitional-cell bladder cancer. Int J Cancer 53:42, 1993

144. de Graaff WE, Sleijfer DT, de Jong B, et al: Significance of aneuploid stem lines in nonseminomatous germ cell tumors. Cancer 72:1300, 1993

145. Kuhn W, Kaufmann M, Feichter GE, et al: DNA flow cytometry, clinical and morphological parameters as prognostic factors for advanced malignant and borderline ovarian tumors. Gynecol Oncol 33:360, 1989

146. Friedlander ML, Taylor IW, Russell P, et al: Ploidy as a prognostic factor in ovarian cancer. Int J Gynecol Pathol 2:55, 1983

147. Redman CWE, Finn C, Ward K, et al: Tumour cell activity markers in epithelial ovarian cancer: Are biochemical and cytometric indices complementary? Br J Cancer 61:755, 1990

148. Rodenburg CJ, Cornelisse CJ, Heintz PA, et al: Tumor ploidy as a major prognostic factor in advanced ovarian cancer. Cancer 59:317, 1987

149. Iversen O-E: Prognostic value of the flow cytometric DNA index in human ovarian carcinoma. Cancer 61:971, 1988

150. Braly PS, Klevecz RR: Flow cytometric evaluation of ovarian cancer. Cancer 71:1621, 1993

151. Drescher CW, Flint A, Hopkins MP, Roberts JA: Prognostic significance of DNA content and nuclear morphology in borderline ovarian tumors. Gynecol Oncol 48:242, 1993

152. Kallioniemi O, Punnonen R, Mattila J, et al: Prognostic significance of DNA index, multiploidy, and S-phase fraction in ovarian cancer. Cancer 61:334, 1988

153. Barnabei VM, Miller DS, Bauer KD, et al: Flow cytometric evaluation of epithelial ovarian cancer. Am J Obstet Gynecol 162: 1584, 1990

154. Friedlander ML, Hedley DW, Swanson C, Russell P for the Gynecologic Oncology Group of the Clinical Oncology Society of Australia: Prediction of long-term survival by flow cytometric analysis of cellular DNA content in patients with advanced ovarian cancer. J Clin Oncol 6:282, 1988

155. Rotmensch J, Atcher RW, Schwartz JL, Grdina DJ: Analysis of ascites from patients with ovarian carcinoma by cell flow cytometry. Gynecol Oncol 44:10, 1992

156. Huettner PC, Weinberg DS, Lage JM: Assessment of proliferative activity in ovarian neoplasms by flow and static cytometry: Correlation with prognostic features. Am J Pathol 141: 699, 1992

157. Alama A, Muttini MP, Merlo F, et al: Survival predictors in relapsed ovarian cancer: Performance status and cell kinetics [abstr]. Proc Am Assoc Cancer Res 31:188, 1990

158. Silvestrini R, Daidone MG, Bolis G, et al: Cell kinetics: A prognostic marker in epithelial ovarian cancer. Gynecol Oncol 35: 15, 1989

159. Silvestrini R, Daidone MG, Valentinis B, et al: Potentials of cell kinetics in the management of patients with ovarian cancers. Eur J Cancer 28:386, 1992

160. Conte PF, Alama A, Rubagotti A, et al: Cell kinetics in ovarian cancer: Relationship to clinicopathologic features, responsiveness to chemotherapy, and survival. Cancer 64:1188, 1989

161. Geisinger KR, Homesley HD, Morgan TM, et al: Endometrial adenocarcinoma: A multiparameter clinicopathologic analysis including the DNA profile and the sex steroid hormone receptors. Cancer 58:1518, 1986

162. Lindahl B, Alm P, Ferno M, et al: Prognostic value of flow cytometrical DNA measurements in stage I-II endometrial carcinoma: Correlations with steroid receptor concentration, tumor myometrial invasion, and degree of differentiation. Anticancer Res 7:791, 1987

163. Rosenberg P, Wingren S, Simonsen E, et al: Flow cytometric measurements of DNA index and S-phase on paraffin-embedded early stage endometrial cancer: An important prognostic indicator. Gynecol Oncol 35:50, 1989

164. Iversen OE: Flow cytometric deoxyribonucleic acid index: A prognostic factor in endometrial carcinoma. Am J Obstet Gynecol 155:770, 1986

165. Nguyen HN, Sevin BU, Averette HE, et al: Determination of hormonal response in uterine cancer cell lines by the ATP bioluminescence assay and flow cytometry. Gynecol Oncol 46: 55, 1992

166. van Dam PA, Lowe DG, Watson JV, et al: Multiparameter flow-cytometric quantitation of epidermal growth factor receptor and c-erbB-2 oncoprotein in normal and neoplastic tissues of the female genital tract. Gynecol Oncol 42:256, 1991

167. Miller B, Dockter M, El Torky M, Photopulos G: Small cell carcinoma of the cervix: A clinical and flow-cytometric study. Gynecol Oncol 42:27, 1991

168. Strang P, Stendahl U, Bergstrom R, et al: Prognostic flow cytometric information in cervical squamous cell carcinoma: A multivariate analysis of 307 patients. Gynecol Oncol 43:3, 1991

169. Leminen A, Paavonen J, Vesterinen E, et al: Deoxyribonucleic acid flow cytometric analysis of cervical adenocarcinoma: Prognostic significance of deoxyribonucleic acid ploidy and S-phase fraction. Am J Obstet Gynecol 162:848, 1990

170. Jakobsen A: Ploidy level and short-time prognosis of early cervix cancer. Radiother Oncol 1:271, 1984

171. Jakobsen A: Prognostic impact of ploidy level in carcinoma of the cervix. Am J Clin Oncol 7:475, 1984

172. Dyson JED, Joslin CAF, Rothwell RI, et al: Flow cytofluorometric evidence for the differential radioresponsiveness of aneuploid and diploid cervix tumours. Radiother Oncol 8:263, 1987

173. Rutgers DH, van der Linden PM, van Peperzeel HA: DNA-flow cytometry of squamous cell carcinomas from the human uterine cervix The identification of prognostically different subgroups. Radiother Oncol, 7:249, 1986

174. Atkin NB, Richards BM: Clinical significance of ploidy in carcinoma of cervix: Its relation to prognosis. BMJ 2:1445, 1962

175. Shepherd NA, Richman PI, England J: Ki-67 derived proliferative activity in colorectal adenocarcinoma with prognostic correlations. J Pathol 155:213, 1988

176. Wolley RC, Schreiber K, Koss LG, et al: DNA distribution in human colon carcinomas and its relationship to clinical behavior. J Natl Can Inst 69:15, 1982

177. Kokal WA, Gardine RL, Sheibani K, et al: Tumor DNA content in resectable, primary colorectal carcinoma. Ann Surg 209: 188, 1989

178. Jones DJ, Moore M, Schofield PF: Refining the prognostic significance of DNA ploidy status in colorectal cancer: A prospective flow cytometric study. Int J Cancer 41:206, 1988

179. Quirke P, Dixon MF, Claydens AD, et al: Prognostic significance of DNA aneuploidy and cell proliferation in rectal adenocarcinomas. J Pathol 151:285, 1987

180. Scott NA, Wieand HS, Moertel CG, et al: Colorectal cancer: Duke's stage, tumor site, preoperative plasma CEA level, and patient prognosis related to tumor DNA ploidy pattern. Arch Surg 122:1375, 1987

181. Schutte B, Reynders MMJ, Wiggers T, et al: Retrospective analysis of the prognostic significance of DNA content and proliferative activity in large bowel carcinoma. Cancer Res 47: 5494, 1987

182. Scivetti P, Danova M, Riccardi A, et al: Prognostic significance of DNA content in large bowel carcinoma: A retrospective flow cytometric study. Cancer Lett 46:213, 1989

183. Bosari S, Lee AKC, Wiley BD, et al: Flow cytometric and image analyses of colorectal adenocarcinomas: A comparative study with clinical correlations. Am J Clin Pathol 99:187, 1993

184. Melamed MR, Enker WE, Banner P, et al: Flow cytometry of colorectal carcinoma with three-year follow-up. Dis Colon Rectum 29:184, 1986

185. Fisher ER, Siderits RH, Sass R, Fisher B: Value of assessment of ploidy in rectal cancers. Arch Pathol Lab Med 113:525, 1989

186. Offerhaus GJA, De Feyter EP, Cornelisse CJ, et al: The relation-

ship of DNA aneuploidy to molecular genetic alterations in colorectal carcinoma. Gastroenterology 102:1612, 1992

187. Scott NA, Rainwater LM, Wieand HS, et al: The relative prognostic value of flow cytometric DNA analysis and conventional clinicopathologic criteria in patients with operable rectal carcinoma. Dis Colon Rectum 30:513, 1987

188. Jass JR, Mukawa K, Goh HS, et al: Clinical importance of DNA content in rectal cancer measured by flow cytometry. J Clin Pathol 42:254, 1989

189. Meling GI, Rognum TO, Clausen OPF, et al: Association between DNA ploidy pattern and cellular atypia in colorectal carcinomas: A new clinical application of DNA flow cytometric study? Cancer 67:1642, 1991

190. Bauer KD, Lincoln ST, Vera-Roman JM, et al: Prognostic implications of proliferative activity and DNA aneuploidy in colonic adenocarcinomas. Lab Invest 57:329, 1987

191. Wiggers T, Arends JW, Schutte B, et al: A multivariate analysis of pathologic prognostic indicators in large bowel cancer. Cancer 61:386, 1988

192. Ngoi SS, Staiano-Coico L, Godwin TA, et al: Abnormal DNA ploidy and proliferative patterns in superficial colonic epithelium adjacent to colorectal cancer. Cancer 66:953, 1990

193. Wersto RP, Greenebaum E, Deitch D, et al: Deoxyribonucleic acid ploidy and cell cycle events in benign colonic epithelium peripheral to carcinoma. Lab Invest 58:218, 1988

194. Meling GI, Clausen OPF, Bergan A, et al: Flow cytometric DNA ploidy pattern in dysplastic mucosa, and in primary and metastatic carcinomas in patients with longstanding ulcerative colitis. Br J Cancer 64:339, 1991

195. Porschen R, Remy U, Bevers G, et al: Prognostic significance of DNA ploidy in adenocarcinoma of the pancreas: Flow cytometric study of paraffin embedded specimens. Cancer 71:3846, 1993

196. Graeme-Cook F, Bell DA, Flotte TJ, et al: Aneuploidy in pancreatic insulinomas does not predict malignancy. Cancer 66:2365, 1990

197. Unger PD, Danque POV, Fuchs A, Kaneko M: DNA flow cytometric evaluation of serous and mucinous cystic neoplasms of the pancreas. Arch Pathol Lab Med 115:563, 1991

198. Fujimoto J, Okamoto E, Yamanaka N, et al: Nuclear DNA analysis of hepatocellular carcinoma. J Jpn Surg Soc 90:1568, 1989

199. Chiu H, Kao HL, Wu LH, et al: Prediction of relapse or survival after resection of human hepatomas by DNA flow cytometry. J Clin Invest 89:539, 1992

200. Nagasue N, Yamanoi A, Takemoto Y, et al: Comparison between diploid and aneuploid hepatocellular carcinomas: A flow cytometric study. Br J Surg 79:667, 1992

201. Tarao K, Shimizu A, Harada M, et al: In vitro uptake of bromodeoxyuridine by human hepatocellular carcinoma and its relation to histopathologic findings and biologic behavior. Cancer 68:1789, 1991

202. Tarao K, Shimizu A, Harada M, et al: Difference in the in vitro uptake of bromodeoxyuridine between liver cirrhosis with and without hepatocellular carcinoma. Cancer 64:104, 1989

203. Dorman AM, Walsh TN, Droogan O, et al: DNA quantification of squamous cell carcinoma of the oesophagus by flow cytometry and cytophotometric image analysis using formalin fixed paraffin embedded tissue. Cytometry 13:886, 1992

204. Edwards JM, Jones DJ, Wilkes SJL, et al: Ploidy as a prognostic indicator in oesophageal squamous carcinoma and its relationship to various histological criteria. J Pathol 159:35, 1989

205. Matsuura H, Sugimachi K, Uro H, et al: Malignant potential of squamous cell carcinoma of the oesophagus predictable by DNA analysis. Cancer 57:1810, 1986

206. Sugimachi K, Hirako I, Takeshi O, et al: Cytophotometric DNA analysis of mucosal and submucosal carcinoma of the oesophagus. Cancer 53:2683, 1984

207. Bronzo R, Heit P, Weissman G, et al: Implications of flow cytometry in malignant conditions of the stomach. Am J Gastroenterol 84:1065, 1989

208. Nanus DM, Kelsen DP, Niedzwiecki D, et al: Flow cytometry as a predictive indicator in patients with operable gastric cancer. J Clin Oncol 7:1105, 1989

209. Johnson H, Belluco C, Masood S, et al: The value of flow cytometric analysis in patients with gastric cancer. Arch Surg 128:314, 1993

210. Ohyama S, Yonemura Y, Miyazaki I: Prognostic value of S-phase fraction and DNA ploidy studied with in vivo administration of bromodeoxyuridine on human gastric cancers. Cancer 65:116, 1990

211. Yonemura Y, Ooyama S, Sugiyama K, et al: Retrospective analysis of the prognostic significance of DNA ploidy patterns and S-phase fraction in gastric carcinoma. Cancer Res 50:509, 1990

212. Yoshino H: A study of DNA ploidy patterns of gastric cancers. J Jpn Surg Soc 89:522, 1988

213. Odegaard S, Hostmark J, Skagen DW, et al: Flow cytometric DNA studies in human gastric cancer and polyps. Scand J Gastroenterol 22:1270, 1987

214. Macartney JC, Camplejohn RS, Powell G: DNA flow cyotmetry of histological material from human gastric cancer. J Pathol 148:273, 1986

215. Deinlein E, Schmidt H, Riemann JF, et al: DNA flow cytometric measurements in inflammatory and malignant human gastric lesions. Virchows Arch (A) 402:185, 1983

216. Korenaga D, Okamura T, Saito A, et al: DNA ploidy is closely linked to tumor invasion, lymph node metastasis, and prognosis in clinical gastric cancer. Cancer 62:309, 1988

217. Kamata T, Yonemura Y, Sugiyama K, et al: Proliferative activity of early gastric cancer measured by in vitro and in vivo bromodeoxyuridine labeling. Cancer 64:1665, 1989

218. Amadori D, Bonaguri C, Volpi A, et al: Cell kinetics and prognosis in gastric cancer. Cancer 71:1, 1993

219. Joensuu H: DNA flow cytometry in the prediction of survival and response to radiotherapy in head and neck cancer. Acta Oncol 29:513, 1990

220. Tytor M, Franzen G, Olofsson J: DNA ploidy in oral cavity carcinomas with special reference to prognosis. Head Neck 11:257, 1989

221. Lampe HB, Flint A, Wolf GT, et al: Flow cytometry: DNA analysis of squamous cell carcinoma of the upper aerodigestive tract. J Otolaryngol 16:371, 1987

222. Goldsmith MM, Cresson DH, Arnold LA, et al: DNA flow cytometry as a prognostic indicator in head and neck cancer. Otolaryngol Head Neck Surg 96:307, 1987

223. Goldsmith MM, Cresson DH, Postma DS, et al: Significance of ploidy in laryngeal cancer. Am J Surg 152:396, 1986

224. Sickle-Santanello BJ, Farrar WB, Dobson JL, et al: Flow cytometric analysis of DNA content as a prognostic indicator in squamous cell carcinoma of the tongue. Am J Surg 152:393, 1986

225. Campbell BH, Schemmel JC, Hopwood LE, Hoffmann RG: Flow cytometric evaluation of chemosensitive and chemoresistant head and neck tumors. Am J Surg 160:424, 1990

226. Hemmer J, Kreidler J: Flow cytometric DNA ploidy analysis of squamous cell carcinoma of the oral cavity: Comparison with clinical staging and histologic grading. Cancer 66:317, 1990

227. Browman GP, Daya D, Booker L, et al: Comparison of bromodeoxyuridine (BRDU), tritiated thymidine (T) and tritiated deoxyuridine (DU) for assessing DNA synthesis labeling index (LI) in tumor fragments of squamous carcinoma of the head and neck (SCHN). Proc Am Assoc Cancer Res 29:26, 1988

228. Forster G, Cooke TG, Cooke LD, et al: Tumour growth rates in squamous carcinoma of the head and neck measured by in vivo bromodeoxyuridine incorporation and flow cytometry. Br J Cancer 65:698, 1992

229. Hirano T, Zitsch R, Gluckman JL: Cell kinetics study of upper aerodigestive tract squamous cell carcinoma using bromodeoxyuridine. Ann Otol Rhinol Laryngol 102:42, 1993

230. Greiner TC, Robinson RA, Maves MD: Adenoid cystic carcinoma: A clinicopathologic study with flow cytometric analysis. Am J Clin Pathol 92:711, 1989

231. Sahin AA, Ro JY, El-Naggar AK, et al: Flow cytometric analysis of the DNA content of non-small cell lung cancer: Ploidy as a significant prognostic indicator in squamous cell carcinoma of the lung. Cancer 65:530, 1990

232. Isobe H, Miyamoto H, Shimizu T, et al: Prognostic and thera-

peutic significance of the flow cytometric nuclear DNA content in non-small cell lung cancer. Cancer 65:1391, 1990

233. Zimmerman PV, Bint MN, Hanson GAT, Parsons PG: Ploidy as a prognostic determinant in surgically treated lung cancer. Lancet 2:530, 1987

234. Bunn PA, Carney DN, Gazdar AF, et al: Diagnostic and biologic implications of flow cytometric DNA content analysis in lung cancer. Cancer Res 43:5026, 1983

235. Volm M, Drings P, Mattern J, et al: Prognostic significance of DNA patterns and resistance-predictive tests in non-small cell lung carcinoma. Cancer 56:1396, 1985

236. Volm M, Hahn EW, Mattern J, et al: Five-year follow-up study of independent clinical and flow cytometric prognostic factors for the survival of patients with non-small cell lung carcinoma. Cancer Res 48:2923, 1988

237. Volm M, Mattern J, Muller T, Drings P: Flow cytometry of epidermoid lung carcinomas: Relationship of ploidy and cell cycle phases to survival. A five-year follow up study. Anticancer Res 8:105, 1988

238. Tirindelli-Danesi D, Teodori L, Mauro F, et al: Prognostic significance of flow cytometry in lung cancer: A 5 year study. Cancer 60:844, 1987

239. Van Bodegom PC, Baak JPA, Stroet-van Galen S, et al: The percentage of aneuploid cells is significantly correlated with survival in accurately staged patients with stage I resected squamous cell lung cancer and long-term follow up. Cancer 63:143, 1989

240. Ten Velde GPM, Schutte B, Vermeulen A, et al: Flow cytometric analysis of DNA ploidy level in paraffin embedded tissue of non-small cell lung cancer. Eur J Cancer Clin Oncol 24:455, 1988

241. Pujol JL, Simony J, Laurent JC, et al: Phenotypic heterogeneity studied by immunohistochemistry and aneuploidy in non-small cell lung cancers. Cancer Res 49:2797, 1989

242. Alama A, Repetto L, Vaira F, et al: Analysis of tumor kinetics in non small cell lung cancer (NSCLC): Comparison with clinical variables. Proc Am Assoc Cancer Res 29:231, 1988

243. Volm M, Mattern J, Samsel B: Relationship of inherent resistance to doxorubicin, proliferative activity and expression of p-glycoprotein 170 and glutathione s-transferase in human lung tumors. Cancer 70:764, 1992

244. Abe S, Makimura S, Itabashi K, et al: Prognostic significance of nuclear DNA content in small cell carcinoma of the lung. Cancer 56:2025, 1985

245. Oud PS, Pahlplatz MMM, Beck JLM, et al: Image and flow DNA cytometry of small cell carcinoma of the lung. Cancer 64:1304, 1989

246. Vredenburgh JJ, Davis B, Ball ED: The detection of low percentages of small cell carcinoma of the lung (SCCL) or breast cancer cells in the bone marrow by two-color flow cytometry. Proc Am Soc Clin Oncol 9:7, 1990

247. Fujimaki T, Matsutani M, Nakamura O, et al: Correlation between bromodeoxyuridine-labeling indices and patient prognosis in cerebral astrocytic tumors of adults. Cancer 67:1629, 1991

248. Nishizaki T, Orita T, Furutani Y, et al: Flow-cytometric DNA analysis and immunohistochemical measurement of Ki-67 and BUdR labeling indices in human brain tumors. J Neurosurg 70:379, 1989

249. Hoshino T, Ahn D, Prados MD, et al: Prognostic significance of the proliferative potential of intracranial gliomas measured by bromodeoxyuridine labeling. Int J Cancer 53:550, 1993

250. Engebraaten O, Bjerkvig R, Pedersen PH, Laerum OD: Effects for EGF, bFGF, NGF and PDGF(bb) on cell proliferative, migratory and invasive capacities of human brain-tumour biopsies in vitro. Int J Cancer 53:209, 1993

251. Spaar FW, Ahyai A, Blech M: DNA-fluorescence-cytometry and prognosis (grading) of meningiomas: A study of 104 surgically removed tumors. Neurosurg Rev 10:35, 1987

252. Franzini A, Broggi G, Giorgi C, et al: Predictive accuracy of cell kinetics data in glial tumors investigated by serial stereotactic biopsy. J Neurosurg Sci 33:43, 1989

253. Spaar FW, Blech M, Ahyai A: DNA-flow fluorescence-cytometry of ependymomas: Report on ten surgically removed tumours. Acta Neuropathol (Berl) 60:153, 1986

254. Darona M, Riccardi A, Mazzini G, et al: Ploidy and proliferative activity of human brain tumors: A flow cytofluorometric study. Oncology 44:102, 1987

255. Zaprianov Z, Christov K: Histological grading, DNA content, cell proliferation, and survival of patients with astroglial tumors. Cytometry 9:380, 1988

256. Tomita T, Yasue M, Engelhard HH, et al: Flow cytometric DNA analysis of medulloblastoma: Prognostic implication of aneuploidy. Cancer 61:744, 1988

257. Cusick EL, MacIntosh CA, Krukowski ZH, et al: Comparison of flow cytometry with static densitometry in papillary thyroid carcinoma. Br J Surg 77:913, 1990

258. Klemi PJ, Joensuu H, Eerola E: DNA aneuploidy in anaplastic carcinoma of the thyroid gland. Am J Clin Pathol 89:154, 1988

259. Rainwater LM, Farrow GM, Hay ID, Lieber MM: Oncocytic tumours of the salivary gland, kidney, and thyroid: Nuclear DNA patterns studied by flow cytometry. Br J Cancer 53:799, 1986

260. Joensuu H, Klemi P, Eerola E, et al: Influence of cellular DNA content on survival in differentiated thyroid cancer. Cancer 58:2462, 1986

261. Tangen KO, Lindmo T, Sorbinho-Simoes M, et al: A flow cytometric DNA analysis of medullary thyroid carcinoma. Am J Clin Pathol 79:172, 1983

262. Johannessen JV, Sobrinho-Simoes M, Tangen KO, et al: A flow cytometric deoxyribonucleic acid analysis of papillary thyroid carcinoma. Lab Invest 45:336, 1981

263. Greenebaum E, Koss LG, Elequin F, et al: The diagnostic value of flow cytometric DNA measurements in follicular tumors of the thyroid gland. Cancer 56:2011, 1985

264. Cusick EL, Ewen SWB, Krukowski, Matheson NA: DNA aneuploidy in follicular thyroid neoplasia. Br J Surg 78:94, 1991

265. Davies SE, Macartney JC, Camplejohn RS, et al: DNA flow cytometry of thymomas. Histopathology 15:77, 1989

266. Helio J, Karaharju E, Nordling S: Flow cytometric determination of DNA content in malignant and benign bone tumours. Cytometry 6:165, 1985

267. Kreicbergs A, Silfversward C, Tribukait B: Flow DNA analysis of primary bone tumors: Relationship between cellular DNA content and histopathologic classification. Cancer 53:129, 1984

268. Alvegard TA, Berg NO, Baidetorp B, et al: Cellular DNA content and prognosis of high-grade soft tissue sarcoma: The Scandinavian Sarcoma Group experience. J Clin Oncol 8:538, 1990

269. Alho A, Connor JF, Mankin HJ, et al: Assessment of malignancy of cartilage tumors using flow cytometry: A preliminary report. J Bone Joint Surg 65:779, 1983

270. Look AT, Douglass EC, Meyer WH: Clinical importance of near-diploid tumor stem lines in patients with osteosarcoma of an extremity. N Engl J Med 318:1567, 1988

271. Bauer HCF, Kreicbergss A, Silfversward C, Triubukait B: DNA analysis in the differential diagnosis of osteosarcoma. Cancer 61:1430, 1988

272. Xiang J, Spanier SS, Benson NA, Brayalan RC: Flow cytometric analysis of DNA in bone and soft tissue tumors using nuclear suspensions. Cancer 59:1951, 1987

273. Agarwal V, Greenebaum E, Wersto R, Koss LG: DNA ploidy of spindle cell soft tissue tumors and its relationship to histology and clinical outcome. Arch Path Lab Med 115:558, 1991

274. Tsushima K, Rainwater LM, Goeilner JR, et al: Leiomyosarcomas and benign smooth muscle tumors of the stomach: Nuclear DNA patterns studied by flow cytometry. Mayo Clinic Proc 62:275, 1987

275. El-Jabbour J, Wilsin G, Henry K, et al: A flow cytometric (FCM) study of 35 Kaposi's sarcomas (KS) from HIV+ve patients. J Pathol 168(suppl): 113A, 1992.

276. Boschman GA, Rens W, Manders EMM, et al: Detection of recurrent chromosome abnormalities in Ewing's sarcoma and peripheral neuroectodermal tumor cells using bivariate flow karyotyping. Genes Chromosom Cancer 5:375, 1992

277. Gansler T, Chatten J, Varello M, et al: Flow cytometric DNA analysis of neuroblastoma: Correlation with histology and clinical outcome. Cancer 58:2453, 1986

278. Taylor SR, Blatt J, Constantino JP, et al: Flow cytometric DNA

analysis of neuroblastoma and ganglioneuroma: A 10-year retrospective study. Cancer 62:749, 1988

279. Oppedal BR, Storm-Mathisen I, Lie SO, Brandtzaeg P: Prognostic factors in neuroblastoma: Clinical, histopathologic, and immunohistochemical features and DNA ploidy in relation to prognosis. Cancer 62:772, 1988

280. Bourhis J, DeVatharie F, Wilson GD, et al: Combined analysis of DNA ploidy index and N-muc genomic content in neuroblastoma. Cancer Res 51:33, 1991

281. Brenner DW, Barranco SC, Winslow BH, Shaeffer J: Flow cytometric analysis of DNA content in children with neuroblastoma. J Pediatr Surg 24:204, 1989

282. Bourhis J, Dominici C, McDowell H, et al: N-myc genomic content and DNA ploidy in stage IVS neuroblastoma. J Clin Oncol 9:1371, 1991

283. Dominici C, Negroni A, Romeo A, et al: Association of near-diploid DNA content and N-myc amplification in neuroblastomas. Clin Exp Metastasis, 7:201, 1989

284. Hayashi Y, Kanda N, Inaba T, et al: Cytogenetic findings and prognosis in neuroblastoma with emphasis on marker chromosome. Cancer 63:126, 1989

285. Dominici C, Negroni A, Romeo A, et al: Flow cytometric and molecular analysis of proliferative activity and DNA content in neuroblastoma: Presence of stationary cells in S-phase. Anticancer Res 12:59, 1992

286. Look AT, Hayes FA, Nitschke R, et al: Cellular DNA content as a predictor of response to chemotherapy in infants with unresectable neuroblastoma. N Engl J Med 311:231, 1984

287. Rainwater LM, Hosaka Y, Farrow GM, et al: Wilms tumors: Relationship of nuclear deoxyribonucleic acid ploidy to patient survival. J Urol 138:974, 1987

288. Schmidt D, Wiedemann B, Keil W, et al: Flow cytometric analysis of nephroblastomas and related neoplasms. Cancer 58:2494, 1986

289. Dias P, Kumar P, Marsden HB, et al: Prognostic relevance of DNA ploidy in rhabdomyosarcomas and other sarcomas of childhood. Anticancer Res 12:1173, 1992

290. Kowal-Vern A, Gonzalez-Crussi F, Turner J, et al: Flow and image cytometric DNA analysis in rhabdomyosarcoma. Cancer Res 50:6023, 1990

291. von Roenn JM, Kheir SM, Wolter JM, et al: Significance of DNA abnormalities in primary malignant melanomas and nevi, a retrospective flow cytometric study. Cancer Res 46:3192, 1986

292. Kheir SM, Bines SD, Vonroenn JH, et al: Prognostic significance of DNA aneuploidy in stage I cutaneous melanoma. Ann Surg 207:455, 1988

293. Sondergaard K, Larsen JK, Moller U, et al: DNA ploidy-characteristics of human malignant melanoma analysed by flow cytometry and compared with histology and clinical course. Virchows Arch (B) 42:43, 1983

294. Bartkowiak D, Schumann J, Otto FJ, et al: DNA flow cytometry in the prognosis of primary malignant melanoma. Oncology 48:39, 1991

295. Karlsson M, Boeryd B, Carstensen J, et al: DNA ploidy and S-phase in primary malignant melanoma as prognostic factors for stage III disease. Br J Cancer 67:134, 1993

296. Muhonen T, Pyrhönen S, Laasonen A, et al: DNA aneuploidy and low S-phase fraction as favourable prognostic signs in metastatic melanoma. Br J Cancer 64:749, 1991

297. Muhonen T, Pyrhönen S, Laasonen A, et al: Tumour growth rate and DNA flow cytometry parameters as prognostic factors in metasatic melanoma. Br J Cancer 66:528, 1992

298. Costa A, Silvestrini R, Mezzanotte G, et al: Cell kinetics: An independent prognostic variable in stage II melanoma of the skin. Br J Cancer 62:826, 1990

299. Weilbach FX, Bogdahn U, Poot M, et al: Melanoma-inhibiting activity inhibits cell proliferation by prolongation of the S-phase and arrest of cells in the G₂ compartment. Cancer Res 50:6981, 1990

300. Joensuu GH, Klemi PJ, Korkeila E: Prognostic value of DNA ploidy and proliferative activity in Hodgkin's disease. Am J Clin Pathol 90:670, 1988

301. Morgan KG, Quirke P, O'Brien CJ, Bird CC: Hodgkin's disease: A flow cytometric study. J Clin Pathol 41:365, 1988

302. Anastasi J, Bauer KE, Variakojis D: DNA aneuploidy in Hodgkin's disease: A multiparameter flow-cytometric analysis with cytologic correlation. Am J Pathol 128:573, 1987

303. Diamond LW, Nathwani BN, Rappaport H: Flow cytometry in the diagnosis and classification of malignant lymphoma and leukemia. Cancer 50:1122, 1982

304. Erdkamp FL, Breed WP, Schouten HC, et al: DNA aneuploidy and cell proliferation in relation to histology and prognosis in patients with Hodgkin's disease. Ann Oncol 4:75, 1993

305. Macartney JC, Camplejohn RS: DNA flow cytometry of non-Hodgkin's lymphomas. Eur J Cancer 26:635, 1990

306. Braylan RC: Flow-cytometric DNA analysis in the diagnosis and prognosis of lymphoma. Am J Clin Pathol 99:374, 1993

307. Wain SL, Braylan RC, Borowitz MJ: Correlation of monoclonal antibody phenotyping and cellular DNA content in non-Hodgkin's lymphoma; the Southeastern Cancer Study Group experience. Cancer 60:2403, 1987

308. Young GA, Hedley DW, Rugg CA, Iland HJ: The prognostic significance of proliferative activity in poor histology non-Hodgkin's lymphoma: A flow cytometry study using archival material. Eur J Cancer Clin Oncol 23:1497, 1987

309. Cowan RA, Harris M, Jones M, Crowther D: DNA content in high and intermediate grade non-Hodgkin's lymphoma—prognostic significance and clinicopathological correlations. Br J Cancer 60:904, 1989

310. Lehtinen T, Aine R, Lehtinen M, et al: Flow cytometric DNA analysis of 199 histologically favourable or unfavourable non-Hodgkin's lymphomas. J Pathol 157:27, 1989

311. Costa A, Silvestrini R, Giardini R, et al: Contribution of ³H-thymidine labelling index and flow cytometric S-phase in predicting survival of patients with non-Hodgkin's lymphoma. Br J Cancer 66:680, 1992

312. Lindh J, Jonsson H, Lenner P, Roos G: Fraction of S-phase cells in blood mononuclear cells in non-Hodgkin's lymphomas—correlation with clinical features and prognosis. Eur J Haematol 42:331, 1989

313. Christensson B, Tribukait B, Linder IL, et al: Cell proliferation and DNA content in non-Hodgkin's lymphoma. Cancer 58:1295, 1986

314. Christensson B, Lindemalm C, Johansson B, et al: Flow cytometric DNA analysis: A prognostic tool in non-Hodgkin's lymphoma. Leuk Res 13:307, 1989

315. Silvestrini R, Costa A, Giardini R, et al: Prognostic implications of cell kinetics, histopathology and pathologic stage in non-Hodgkin's lymphomas. Hematol Oncol 7:411, 1989

316. Cavalli C, Danova M, Gobbi PG, et al: Ploidy and proliferative activity measurement by flow cytometry in non-Hodgkin's lymphomas: Do speculative aspects prevail over clinical ones? Eur J Cancer Clin Oncol 25:1755, 1989

317. Joensuu H, Klemi PJ, Jalkanen S: Biologic progression in non-Hodgkin's lymphomas: A flow cytometric study. Cancer 65:2564, 1990

318. Joensuu H, Klemi PJ, Söderström KO, Jalkanen S: Comparison of S-phase fraction, working formulation, and Kiel classification in non-Hodgkin's lymphomas. Cancer 68:1564, 1991

319. Yanik G, Yousuf N, Miller M, et al: In vivo determination of cell cycle kinetics of non-Hodgkin's lymphomas using iododeoxyuridine and bromodeoxyuridine. J Histochem Cytochem 40:723, 1992

320. Witzig TE, Gonchoroff NJ, Greipp PR, et al: Rapid S-phase determination of non-Hodgkin's lymphomas with the use of an immunofluorescence bromodeoxyuridine labeling index procedure. Am J Clin Pathol 91:298, 1989

321. Krauss JS, Pantazis CG, Chandler FW: The proliferative fraction in lymph nodes: A comparison of proliferating cell nuclear antigen morphometry to flow cytometry. Ann Clin Lab Sci 22:189, 1992

322. Bunn PA Jr, Whang-Peng J, Carney DN, et al: DNA content analysis by flow cytometry and cytogenetic analysis in mycosis fungoides and Sezary's syndrome. J Clin Invest 65:1440, 1980

323. Lehtinen T, Lehtinen M, Aine R, et al: Nuclear DNA content of non-endemic Burkitt's lymphoma. J Clin Pathol 40:1201, 1987

324. Joensuu H, Söderström K-O, Klemi PJ, et al: Nuclear DNA con-

tent and its prognostic value in lymphoma of the stomach. Cancer 60:3042, 1987

325. Latreille J, Barlogie B, Johnston D, et al: Ploidy and proliferative characteristics in monoclonal gammopathies. Blood 59:43, 1982

326. Montecucco C, Riccardi A, Merlini G, et al: Plasma cell DNA content in multiple myeloma and related paraproteinemic disorders: Relationship with clinical and cytokinetic features. Eur J Cancer Clin Oncol 20:81, 1984

327. Tienhaara A, Pelliniemi TT: Flow cytometric DNA analysis and clinical correlations in multiple myeloma. Am J Clin Pathol 97:322, 1992

328. Morgan RJ, Gonchoroff NJ, Katzmann JA, et al: Detection of hypodiploidy using multi-parameter flow cytometric analysis: A prognostic indicator in multiple myeloma. Am J Hematol 30:195, 1989

329. Barlogie B, Alexanian R, Gehan EA, et al: Marrow cytometry and prognosis in myeloma. J Clin Invest 72:853, 1983

330. Bunn PA, Krasnow S, Makuch RW, et al: Flow cytometric analysis of DNA content of bone marrow cells in patients with plasma cell myeloma: Clinical implications. Blood 59:528, 1982

331. Tafuri A, Meyers J, Lee BJ, Andreeff M: DNA and RNA flow cytometric study in multiple myeloma. Cancer 67:449, 1991

332. Girino M, Riccardi A, Luoni R, et al: Monoclonal antibody Ki-67 as a marker of proliferative activity in monoclonal gammopathies. Acta Haematol 85:26, 1991

333. Geisler CH, Larsen JK, Hansen NE, et al: Prognostic importance of flow cytometric immunophenotyping of 540 consecutive patients with B-cell chronic lymphocytic leukemia. Blood 78:1795, 1991

334. Look AT, Roberson PK, Williams DL, et al: Prognostic importance of blast cell DNA content in childhood acute lymphoblastic leukemia. Blood 65:1079, 1985

335. Barlogie B, McLaughlin P, Alexanian R: Characterization of hematologic malignancies by flow cytometry. Anal Quant Cytol Histol 9:147, 1987

336. Pui CH, Dodge RK, Look AT, et al: Risk of adverse events in children completing treatment for acute lymphoblastic leukemia: St Jude total therapy studies VIII, IX, and X. J Clin Oncol 9:1341, 1991

337. Murphy SB, Aur RJA, Simone JV, et al: Pretreatment cytokinetic studies in 94 children with acute leukemia: Relationship to other variables at diagnosis and to outcome of standard treatment. Blood 49:683, 1977

338. Tsurusawa M, Kaneko Y, Katano N, et al: Flow cytometric evidence for minimal residual disease and cytological heterogeneities in acute lymphoblastic leukemia with severe hypodiploidy. Am J Hematol 32:42, 1989

339. Katano N, Tsurusawa M, Niwa M, Fujimoto T: Flow cytometric determination with bromodeoxyuridine/DNA assay of sensitivity of S-phase cells to cytosine arabinoside in childhood acute lymphoblastic leukemia. Am J Pediatr Hematol Oncol 11:411, 1989

340. Barlogie B, Stass S, Dixon D, et al: DNA aneuploidy in adult acute leukemia. Cancer Genet Cytogenet 28:213, 1987

341. Raza A, Preisler HD, Day R, et al: Direct relationship between remission duration in acute myeloid leukemia and cell cycle kinetics. Blood 76:2191, 1990

342. Raza A, Preisler H, Lampkin B, et al: Biological significance of cell cycle kinetics in 128 standard risk newly diagnosed patients with acute myelocytic leukaemia. Br J Haematol 79:33, 1991

343. Hiddemann W, Buchner T, Andreeff M, et al: Cell kinetics in acute leukemia: A critical reevaluation based on new data. Cancer 50:250, 1982

344. Dosik GM, Barlogie B, Smith TL, et al: Pretreatment flow cytometry of DNA content in adult acute leukemia. Blood 55:474, 1980

345. Riccardi A, Giordano M, Danova M, et al: Cell kinetics with in vivo bromodeoxyuridine and flow cytometry: Clinical significance in acute non-lymphoblastic leukaemia. Eur J Cancer 27:882, 1991

346. Giordano M, Danova M, Pellicciari C, et al: Proliferating cell nuclear antigen (PCNA)/cyclin expression during the cell cycle in normal and leukemic cells. Leukemia Res 15:965, 1991

347. Hart JS, George SL, Frei E, et al: Prognostic significance of pretreatment proliferative activity in adult acute leukemia. Cancer 39:1603, 1977

348. Ogawa M, Fried J, Sakai Y, et al: Studies of cellular proliferation in human leukemia: The proliferative activity, generation time, and emergence time of neutrophilic granulocytes in chronic granulocytic leukemia. Cancer 25:1031, 1970

349. Raza A, Yousuf N, Abbas A, et al: High expression of transforming growth factor-β long cell cycle times and a unique clustering of S-phase cells in patients with acute promyelocytic leukemia. Blood 79:1037, 1992

350. Giordano M, Danova M, Mazzini G, et al: Cell kinetics with in vivo bromodeoxyuridine assay, proliferating cell nuclear antigen expression and flow cytometric analysis: Prognostic significance in acute nonlymphoblastic leukemia. Cancer 71:2739, 1993

351. Auer GU, Caspersson TO, Wallgren AS: DNA content and survival in mammary carcinoma. Anal Quant Cytol 2:161, 1980

352. Fuhr JE, Frye A, Kattine AA, et al: Flow cytometric determination of breast tumor heterogeneity. Cancer 67:1401, 1991

353. Vielh P, Magdelenat H, Mosseri V, et al: Immunocytochemical determination of estrogen and progesterone receptors on 50 fine-needle samples of breast cancer. Am J Clin Pathol 97:254, 1992

354. Daidone M, Orefice S. Mastore M, et al: Comparing core needle to surgical biopsies in breast cancer for cell kinetic and ploidy studies. Breast Cancer Res Treat 19:33, 1991

355. Sigurdsson H, Baldetorp B, Borg A, et al: Flow cytometry in primary breast cancer: Improving the prognostic value of the fraction of cells in the S-phase by optimal categorization of cut-off levels. Br J Cancer 62:786, 1990

356. Kallioniemi O, Joensuu H, Klemi P, et al: Inter-laboratory comparison of DNA flow cytometric results from paraffin-embedded breast carcinomas. Breast Cancer Res Treat 17:59, 1990

357. Fernö M, Baldetorp B, Ewers S, et al: One or multiple samplings for flow cytometric DNA analyses in breast cancer—prognostic implications? Cytometry 13:241, 1992

358. Visscher DW, Shaheen C, Drozdowicz S, Crissman JD: Image cytophotometric DNA histogram heterogeneity in adenocarcinoma of the breast. Anal Quant Cytol Histol 15:206, 1993

359. Meyer JS, McDivitt RW: Reliability and stability of the thymidine labeling index of breast carcinoma. Lab Invest 54:160, 1986

360. Daidone MG, Silvestrini R, Valentinis B, et al: Proliferative activity of primary breast cancer and of synchronous lymph node metastases evaluated by ³H-thymidine-labeling index. Cell Tissue Kinet 23:401, 1990

361. Brifford M, Spyratos F, Tubiana-Hulin M, et al: Sequential cytopunctures during preoperative chemotherapy for breast cancer: Cytomorphologic changes, initial tumor ploidy and tumor regression. Cancer 63:631, 1989

362. Baildam AD, Zaloudik J, Howell A, et al: DNA analysis by flow cytometry, response to endocrine treatment, and prognosis in advanced carcinoma of the breast. Br J Cancer 55:553, 1987

363. Stuart-Harris R, Hedley DW, Taylor IW, et al: Tumor ploidy, response and survival in patients receiving endocrine therapy for advanced breast cancer. Br J Cancer 51:573, 1985

364. Haffty BG, Toth M, Flynn S, et al: Prognostic value of DNA flow cytometry in the locally recurrent, conservatively treated breast cancer patient. J Clin Oncol 10:1839, 1992

365. Hedley DW, Rugg CA, Gelber RD: Association of DNA index and S-phase fraction with prognosis of node positive early breast cancer. Cancer Res 47:4729, 1987

366. Cornelisse CJ, van de Velde CJH, Caspers RJC, et al: DNA ploidy and survival in breast cancer patients. Cytometry 8:225, 1987

367. Dressler LG, Seamer LC, Owens MA, et al: DNA flow cytometry and prognostic factors in 1331 frozen breast cancer specimens. Cancer 61:420, 1988

368. Meckenstock G, Bojar H, Wort W: Differentiated DNA analysis in relation to steroid receptor status, grading, and staging in human breast cancer. Anticancer Res 7:749, 1987

369. Owainati AAR, Robins RA, Hinton C, et al: Tumor aneuploidy, prognostic parameters and survival in primary breast cancer. Br J Cancer 55:449, 1987

370. Dowle CS, Owainati A, Robins A, et al: Prognostic significance of the DNA content of human breast cancer. Br J Surg 74:133, 1987

371. Fallenius AG, Franzen SA, Auer GU: Predictive value of nuclear DNA content in breast cancer in relation to clinical and morphologic factors. Cancer 62:521, 1988

372. McDivitt RW, Stone KR, Craig RB, et al: A proposed classification of breast cancer based on kinetic information. Cancer 57:269, 1986

373. Remvikos Y, Magdelenat H, Zajdela A: DNA flow cytometry applied to fine needle sampling of human breast cancer. Cancer 61:1629, 1988

374. Frierson HF: Ploidy analysis and S-phase fraction determination by flow cytometry of invasive adenocarcinomas of the breast. Am J Surg Pathol 15:358, 1991

375. Baildam AD, Zaloudik J, Howell A, et al: DNA analysis by flow cytometry, response to endocrine treatment and prognosis in advanced carcinoma of the breast. Br J Cancer 55:553, 1987

376. Horsfall DJ, Tilley WD, Orell SR, et al: Relationship between ploidy and steroid hormone receptors in primary invasive breast cancer. Br J Cancer 53:23, 1986

377. Rosen PP, Groshen S, Kinne DW, Norton L: Factors influencing prognosis in node-negative breast carcinoma: Analysis of 767 T1N0M0/T2N0M0 Patients with long-term follow-up. J Clin Oncol 11:2090, 1993

378. O'Reilly SM, Camplejohn RS, Barnes DM, et al: DNA index, S-phase fraction, histological grade and prognosis in breast cancer. Br J Cancer 61:671, 1990

379. Feichter GE, Mueller A, Kaufmann M, et al: Correlation of DNA flow cytometric results and other prognostic factors in primary breast cancer. Int J Cancer 41:823, 1988

380. Lawry J, Rogers K, Duncan JL, Potter CW: The identification of informative parameters in the flow cytometric analysis of breast carcinoma. Eur J Cancer 29A:719, 1993

381. Frierson HF: Grade and flow cytometric analysis of ploidy for infiltrating ductal carcinomas. Hum Pathol 24:24, 1993

382. Kallioniemi O-P, Blanco G, Alavaikko M, et al: Tumour DNA ploidy as an independent prognostic factor in breast cancer. Br J Cancer 56:637, 1987

383. Kute TE, Muss HB, Cooper MR, et al: The use of flow cytometry for the prognosis of stage II adjuvant treated breast cancer patients. Cancer 66:1810, 1990

384. Witzig TE, Ingle JN, Schaid DJ, et al: DNA ploidy and percent S-phase as prognostic factors in node-positive breast cancer: Results from patients enrolled in two prospective randomized trials. J Clin Oncol 11:351, 1993

385. Lewis WE: Prognostic significance of flow cytometric DNA analysis in node-negative breast cancer patients. Cancer 65:2315, 1990

386. Sigurdsson H, Baldetorp B, Bord A, et al: Indicators of prognosis in node-negative breast cancer. N Engl J Med 322:1045, 1990

387. Clark GM, Dressler LG, Owens MA, et al: Prediction of relapse or survival in patients with node-negative breast cancer by DNA flow cytometry. N Engl J Med 320:627, 1989

388. Balslev I, Christensen J, Bruun Rasmussen B, et al: Flow cytometric DNA ploidy defines patients with poor prognosis in node-negative breast cancer. Int J Cancer 56:16, 1994

389. Muss HB, Kute, TE, Case LD, et al: The relation of flow cytometry to clinical and biologic characteristics in women with node negative primary breast cancer. Cancer 64:1894, 1989

390. O'Reilly SM, Camplejohn RS, Barnes DM, et al: Node-negative breast cancer: Prognostic subgroups defined by tumor size and flow cytometry. J Clin Oncol 8:2040, 1990

391. Dressler LG, Eudey L, Gray R, et al: Prognostic potential of DNA flow cytometry measurements in node-negative breast cancer patients: Preliminary analysis of an intergroup study (INT 0076). J Natl Cancer Inst Monogr 11:167, 1992

392. Clark GM, Mathieu M, Owens MA, et al: Prognostic significance of S-phase fraction in good-risk, node-negative breast cancer patients. J Clin Oncol 10:428, 1992

393. Merkel DE, Winchester DJ, Goldschmidt RA, et al: DNA flow cytometry and pathologic grading as prognostic guides in axillary lymph node-negative breast cancer. Cancer 72:1926, 1993

394. Keyhani-Rofagha S, O'Toole RV, Farrar WB, et al: Is DNA ploidy an independent prognostic indicator in infiltrative node-negative breast adenocarcinoma? Cancer 65:1577, 1990

395. van der Lindon JC, Lindeman J, Baak JPA, et al: The multivariate prognostic index and nuclear DNA content are independent prognostic factors in primary breast cancer patients. Cytometry 10:56, 1989

396. Beerman H, Kluin M, Hermans J, et al: Prognostic significance of DNA-ploidy in a series of 690 primary breast cancer patients. Int J Cancer 45:34, 1990

397. Aaltomaa S, Lipponen P, Papinaho S, et al: Nuclear morphometry and DNA flow cytometry as prognostic factors in female breast cancer. Eur J Surg 158:135, 1992

398. Gnant MFX, Blijham G, Reiner A, et al: DNA ploidy and other results of DNA flow cytometry as prognostic factors in operable breast cancer: 10 year results of a randomised study. Eur J Cancer 28:711, 1992

399. Gnant MFX, Blijham GH, Reiner A, et al: Aneuploidy fraction but not DNA index is important for the prognosis of patients with stage I and II breast cancer—10-year results. Ann Oncol 4:643, 1993

400. Fisher B, Gunduz N, Costantino J, et al: DNA flow cytometric analysis of primary operable breast cancer. Cancer 68:1465, 1991

401. Toikkanen S, Joensuu H, Klemi P: Nuclear DNA content as a prognostic factor in $T_{1-2}N_0$ breast cancer. Am J Clin Pathol 93:471, 1990

402. Ewers S, Attewell R, Baldetorp B, et al: Flow cytometry DNA analysis and prediction of loco-regional recurrences after mastectomy in breast cancer. Acta Oncol 31:733, 1992

403. Stanton PD, Cooke TG, Oakes SJ, et al: Lack of prognostic significance of DNA ploidy and S phase fraction in breast cancer. Br J Cancer 66:925, 1992

404. Joensuu H, Toikkanen S, Klemi PJ: DNA index and S-phase fraction and their combination as prognostic factors in operable ductal breast cancer. Cancer 66:331, 1990

405. Fernö M, Baldetorp B, Borg Å, et al: Flow cytometric DNA index and S-phase fraction in breast cancer in relation to other prognostic variables and to clinical outcome. Acta Oncol 31:157, 1992

406. Ewers SB, Attewell R, Baldetorp B, et al: Prognostic significance of flow cytometric DNA analysis and estrogen receptor content in breast carcinomas—a 10 year survival study. Breast Cancer Res Treat 24:115, 1992

407. Hedley DW, Clark GM, Cornelisse CJ, et al: Consensus review of the clinical utility of DNA cytometry in carcinoma of the breast. Cytometry 14:482, 1993

408. Stål O, Brisfors A, Carstensen J, et al, and members of the South-East Sweden Breast Cancer Group: Interrelations between cellular DNA content, S-phase fraction, hormone receptor status and age in primary breast cancer. Acta Oncol 31:283, 1992

409. Dressler LG: Are DNA flow cytometry measurements providing useful information in the management of the node-negative breast cancer patient? Cancer Invest 10:477, 1992

410. Winchester DJ, Duda RB, August CZ, et al: The importance of DNA flow cytometry in node-negative breast cancer. Arch Surg 125:886, 1990

411. Arnerlöv C, Emdin SO, Lundgren B, et al: Mammographic growth rate, DNA ploidy and s-phase fraction analysis in breast carcinoma. Cancer 70:1935, 1992

412. Stål O, Carstensen J, Hatschek T, et al: Significance of S-phase fraction and hormone receptor content in the management of young breast cancer patients. Br J Cancer 66:706, 1992

413. Ottestad L, Pettersen EO, Nesland JM, et al: Flow cytometric DNA analysis as prognostic factor in human breast carcinoma. Pathol Res Pract 189:405, 1993

414. Hatschek T, Fagerberg G, Stål O, et al: Cytometric characterization and clinical course of breast cancer diagnosed in a population-based screening program. Cancer 64:1074, 1989

415. Ewers S-B, Attewell R, Baldetorp B, et al: Prognostic potential of flow cytometric S-phase and ploidy prospectively deter-

mined in primary breast carcinomas. Br Cancer Res Treat 20: 93, 1991

416. Bosari S, Lee AKC, Tahan SR, et al: DNA flow cytometric analysis and prognosis of axillary lymph node-negative breast carcinoma. Cancer 70:1943, 1992

417. Batsakis JG, Sneige N, El-Naggar AK: Flow cytometric (DNA content and S-phase fraction) analysis of breast cancer. Cancer 71:2151, 1993

418. Meyer JS: Cell kinetics in selection and stratification of patients for adjuvant therapy of breast carcinoma. Natl Cancer Inst Monogr 1:25, 1986

419. Meyer JS, Coplin MD: Thymidine labeling index, flow cytometric S-phase measurement, and DNA index in human tumors. Am J Clin Pathol 59:586, 1988

420. Tubiana M, Pejovic MH, Koscielny S, et al: Growth rate, kinetics of tumor cell proliferation and long-term outcome in human breast cancer. Int J Cancer 44:17, 1989

421. Silvestrini R, Daidone MG, Mastore M, et al: Cell kinetics of 9200 human breast cancers: Consistency of basic and clinical results. Proc Am Assoc Cancer Res 33:238, 1992

422. Silvestrini R, Daidone MG, Valagussa P, et al: ³H-Thymidine-labeling index as a prognostic indicator in node-positive breast cancer. J Clin Oncol 8:1321, 1990

423. Silvestrini R, Daidone MG, Del Bino G, et al: Prognostic significance of proliferative activity and ploidy in node-negative breast cancers. Ann Oncol 4:213, 1993

424. Valentinis B, Silvestrini R, Daidone MG, et al: ³H-Thymidine-labeling index, hormone receptors, and ploidy in breast cancers from elderly patients. Breast Cancer Res Treat 20:19, 1991

425. Daidone M, Silvestrini R, Valentinis B, et al: Changes in cell kinetics induced by primary chemotherapy in breast cancer. Int J Cancer 47:380, 1991

426. Cooke TG, Stanton PD, Winstanley J, et al: Long-term prognostic significance of thymidine labelling index in primary breast cancer. Eur J Cancer 28:424, 1992

427. Christov K, Chew KL, Ljung B, et al: Proliferation of normal breast epithelial cells as shown by in vivo labeling with bromodeoxyuridine. Am J Pathol 138:1371, 1991

428. Remvikos Y, Vielh P, Padoy E, et al: Breast cancer proliferation measured on cytological samples: A study by flow cytometry of S-phase fractions and BrdU incorporation. Br J Cancer 64: 501, 1991

429. Meyer JS, Koehm S, Hughes JM, et al: Bromodeoxyuridine labeling for S-phase measurement in breast carcinoma. Cancer 71:3531, 1993

430. Goodson WH, Waldman F, Ljung B, et al: Bromodeoxyuridine labelling of human breast cancer: Preliminary results and inverse association with progesterone receptor content. Proc Am Soc Clin Oncol 9:50, 1990

431. Brown RW, Allred DC, Clark GM, et al: Prognostic significance and clinical-pathological correlations of cell-cycle kinetics measured by KI-67 immonocytochemistry in axillary node-negative carcinoma of the breast. Breast Cancer Res Treat 16: 192, 1990

432. Gasparini G, Dal Fior S, Pozza F, et al: Correlation of growth fraction by Ki-67 immunohistochemistry with histologic factors and hormone receptors in operable breast carcinoma. Breast Cancer Res Treat 14:329, 1989

433. Anbazhagan R, Gelber RD, Bettelheim R, et al: Association of c-erbB-2 expression and S-phase fraction in the prognosis of node positive breast cancer. Ann Oncol 2:47, 1991

434. Slamon DJ, Clark GM, Wong SG, et al: Human breast cancer: Correlation of relapse and survival with amplification of the Her-2 neu oncogene. Science 235:177, 1987

435. Tommasi S, Paradiso A, Mangia A, et al: Biological correlation between Her-2/neu and proliferative activity in human breast cancer. Anticancer Res 11:1395, 1991

436. French D, Pizzi C, De Marchis L, et al: Proliferative activity and genetic alterations in breast carcinoma. Proc Am Assoc Cancer Res 34:517, 1993

437. O'Reilly SM, Barnes DM, Camplejohn RS, et al: The relationship between c-erbB-2 expression, S-phase fraction and prognosis in breast cancer. Br J Cancer 63:444, 1991

438. Babiak J, Hugh J, Poppema S: Significance of c-erB-2 amplification and DNA aneuploidy: Analysis in 78 patients with node-negative breast cancer. Cancer 70:770, 1992

439. Noguchi M, Koyasaki N, Ohta N, et al: Internal mammary nodal status is a more reliable prognostic factor than DNA ploidy and c-erb B-2 expression in patients with breast cancer. Arch Surg 128:242, 1993

440. Barnes DM, Meyer JS, Gonzalez JG, et al: Relationship between c-erbB-2 immunoreactivity and thymidine labeling index in breast carcinoma in situ. Breast Cancer Res Treat 18:11, 1991

441. Clark GM, Wenger CR, Beardslee S, et al: How to integrate steroid hormone receptor, flow cytometric, and other prognostic information in regard to primary breast cancer. Cancer 71: 2157, 1993

442. Paradiso A, Mangia A, Correale M, et al: Cytosol cathepsin-D content and proliferative activity of human breast cancer. Breast Cancer Res Treat 23:63, 1992

443. Isola J, Weitz S, Visakorpi T, et al: Cathepsin D expression detected by immunohistochemistry has independent prognostic value in axillary node-negative breast cancer. J Clin Oncol 11: 36, 1993

444. Gasparini G, Reitano M, Bevilacqua P, et al: Relationship of the epidermal growth factor-receptor to the growth fraction (Ki-67 antibody) and the flow cytometric S-phase as cell kinetics parameters, in human mammary carcinomas. Anticancer Res 11:1597, 1991

445. Charpin C, Devictor B, Bonnier P, et al: Epidermal growth factor receptor in breast cancer: Correlation of quantitative immunocytochemical assays to prognostic factors. Br Cancer Res Treat 25:203, 1993

446. Allred DC, Clark GM, Elledge R, et al: Association of p53 protein expression with tumor cell proliferation rate and clinical outcome in node-negative breast cancer. J Natl Cancer Inst 85: 200, 1993

447. Silvestrini R, Benini E, Daidone MG, et al: p53 as an independent prognostic marker in lymph node-negative breast cancer patients. J Natl Cancer Inst 85:965, 1993

448. H Ji, Lipponen P, Aaltomaa S, Syrjänen S, et al: c-erbB-2 oncogene related to p53 expression, cell proliferation and prognosis in breast cancer. Anticancer Res 13:1147, 1993

449. Elledge RM, Fuqua SAW, Clark GM, et al: Prognostic significance of p53 gene alterations in node-negative breast cancer. Breast Can Res Treat 26:225, 1993

450. Visscher DW, Wykes S, Kubus J, et al: Comparison of PCNA/cyclin immunohistochemistry with flow cytometric S-phase fraction in breast cancer. Breast Cancer Res Treat 22:111, 1992

451. Gillett CE, Barnes DM, Camplejohn RS: Comparison of three cell cycle associated antigens as markers of proliferative activity and prognosis in breast carcinoma. J Clin Pathol 46: 1126, 1993

452. Klijn JGM, Berns EMJJ, Bontenbal M, Foekens J: Cell biological factors associated with the response of breast cancer to systemic treatment. Cancer Treat Rev 19:45, 1993

453. Poste G, Fidler IJ: The pathogenesis of cancer metastases. Nature 283:139, 1980

454. Norton L, Simon R: Growth curve of an experimental solid tumor following radiotherapy. J Natl Cancer Inst 58:1735, 1977

455. Shackney SE, McCormack GW, Cuchural GJ Jr: Growth rate patterns of solid tumors and their relation to responsiveness to therapy: An analytical review. Ann Intern Med 89:107, 1978

456. Skipper HE, Schabel FM Jr, Wilcox WS: Experimental evaluation of potential anticancer agents XIII: On the criteria and kinetics associated with "curability" of experimental leukemia. Cancer Chemother Rep 35:1, 1964

457. Skipper HE: Laboratory models: The historical perspective. Cancer Treat Rep 70:3, 1986

458. Goldin A, Venditti JM, Humphreys SR, Mantel N: Influence of the concentration of leukemic innoculum on the effectiveness of treatment. Science 123:840, 1956

459. Roosa R, Weaver CF, DeLamater ED: Importance of transplant size in chemotherapeutic assay with the use of the Gardner lymphosarcoma. Proc Am Assoc Cancer Res 2:243, 1957

460. Holland JF: Clinical studies of unmaintained remissions in acute

lymphocytic leukemia. *In* The Proliferation and Spread of Neoplastic Cells, 21st Annual Symposium on Fundamental Cancer Research 1967. Baltimore, Williams & Wilkins, 1968, pp 453–462

461. Schabel FM: Concepts for the systemic treatment of micrometastases. Cancer *35*:15, 1975

462. Shapiro DM, Fugmann RA: A role for chemotherapy as an adjunct to surgery. Cancer Res *17*:1098, 1957

463. Early Breast Cancer Trialists' Collaborative Group: Systemic treatment of early breast cancer by hormonal, cytotoxic, or immune therapy. Lancet *339*:1, 1992

464. Early Breast Cancer Trialists' Collaborative Group: Systemic treatment of early breast cancer by hormonal, cytotoxic, or immune therapy. Lancet *339*:71, 1992

465. DeVita VT: Principles of chemotherapy. *In* DeVita VT Jr, Hellman S, Rosenberg SA (eds): Cancer: Principles and Practice, 3rd ed. Philadelphia, JB Lippincott Company, 1988, p 279

466. DeVita VT: The relationship between tumor mass and resistance to treatment of cancer. Cancer *51*:1209, 1983

467. Luria SE, Delbruck M: Mutations of bacteria from virus sensitivity to virus resistance. Genetics *28*:491, 1943

468. Law LW: Origin of resistance of leukaemic cells to folic acid antagonists. Nature *169*:628, 1952

469. Burchenal JH, Cramer MA, Williams BS, Armstrong RA: Sterilization of leukemic cells in vivo and in vitro. Cancer Res *11*:700, 1951

470. Frei E III, Freireich EJ, Gehan E, et al: Studies of sequential and combination antimetabolite therapy in acute leukemia: 6-mercaptopurine and methotrexate. Blood *18*:431, 1961

471. Goldie JH, Coldman AJ: A mathematic model for relating the drug sensitivity of tumors to their spontaneous mutation rate. Cancer Treat Rep *63*:1727, 1979

472. Goldie JH, Coldman AJ: Application of theoretical models to chemotherapy protocol design. Cancer Treat Rep *70*:127, 1986

473. Goldie JH: Scientific basis for adjuvant and primary (neoadjuvant) chemotherapy. Semin Oncol *14*:1, 1987

474. Kendal WS, Frost P: Metastatic potential and spontaneous mutation rates: Studies with two murine cell lines and their recently induced metastatic variants. Cancer Res *46*:6131, 1986

475. National Cancer Institute (USA): Surveillance, Epidemiology and End Results (SEER) Program, Cancer Statistics Review 1973–1990. Bethesda, MD, 1993

476. Rosen PP, Groshen S, Kinne DW: Survival and prognostic factors in node-negative breast cancer: Results of long-term follow-up studies. Natl Cancer Inst Monogr *11*:159, 1992

477. DeVita VT, Young RC, Cannellos GP: Combination vs. single agent chemotherapy: A review of the basis for selection of drug treatment of cancer. Cancer *35*:98, 1975

478. Coldman AJ, Goldie JH: A mathematical model of drug resistance in neoplasms. *In* Bruchovsky N, Goldie JH (eds): Drug and Hormone Resistance in Neoplasia. Boca Raton, FL, CRC Press, 1982, pp 55–78

479. Fisher RI, DeVita VT, Hubbard SM, et al: Prolonged disease-free survival in Hodgkin's disease with MOPP reinduction after first relapse. Ann Intern Med *90*:761, 1979

480. Kardinal CG, Perry MC, Korzun AH, et al: Responses to chemotherapy or chemohormonal therapy in advanced breast cancer patients treated previously with adjuvant chemotherapy: A subset analysis of CALGB study 8081. Cancer *61*:415, 1988

481. Valagussa P, Tancini G, Bonadonna G: Salvage treatment of patients suffering relapse after adjuvant CMF chemotherapy. Cancer *58*:1411, 1986

482. Valagussa P, Brambilla C, Zambetti M, Bonadonna G: Salvage treatment after first relapse of breast cancer: A review. *In* Proceedings of the Third International Conference on Adjuvant Therapy of Primary Breast Cancer, St. Gallen, Switzerland, 1988, p 9

483. Iversen OH, Iversen U, Ziegler JL, Bluming AZ: Cell kinetics in Burkitt's lymphoma. Eur J Cancer *10*:155, 1974

484. Bloom H, Richardson M, Harris B: Natural history of untreated breast cancer (1804–1933): Comparison of treated and untreated cases according to histological grade of malignancy. BMJ, *2*:213, 1962

485. Adair F, Berg J, Joubert L, Robbins GF: Long-term follow-up of breast cancer patients: The 30-year report. Cancer *33*:1145, 1974

486. Ferguson DJ, Meier P, Karrison T, et al: Staging of breast cancer and survival rates: An assessment based on 50 years experience with radical mastectomy. JAMA *248*:1337, 1982

487. Harris JR, Hellman S: Observations on survival curve analysis with particular reference to breast cancer. Cancer *57*:925, 1986

488. Brinkley D, Haybittle JL: The curability of breast cancer. Lancet *2*:95, 1975

489. Rutqvist LE, Wallgren A, Nilsson B: Is breast cancer a curable disease? A study of 14,731 women with breast cancer from the Cancer Registry of Norway. Cancer *53*:1793, 1984

490. Fisher B, Redmond C, Poisson R, et al: Eight-year results of a randomized clinical trial comparing total mastectomy and lumpectomy with or without irradiation in the treatment of breast cancer. N Engl J Med *320*:822, 1989

491. Ludwig Breast Cancer Study Group: Combination adjuvant chemotherapy for node positive breast cancer. N Engl J Med *319*:677, 1988

492. Williams S, Stablein D, Einhorn L, et al: Immediate adjuvant chemotherapy versus observation with treatment at relapse in pathological stage II testicular cancer. N Engl J Med *317*:1433, 1987

493. Perloff M, Norton L, Korzun A, et al: Advantage of an Adriamycin combination plus halotestin after initial CMFVP for adjuvant therapy of node-positive stage 11 breast cancer. Proc Am Soc Clin Oncol *70*:273, 1986

494. Korzun A, Norton L, Perloff M, et al: Clinical equivalence despite dosage differences of two schedules of cyclophosphamide, methotrexate, 5-fluorouracil, vincristine and prednisone (CMFVP) for adjuvant therapy of node-positive stage II breast cancer. Proc Am Soc Clin Oncol *7*:12, 1988

495. Wampler GL, Heim WJ, Ellison NA, et al, for the Mid-Atlantic Oncology Program: Comparison of cyclophosphamide, doxorubicin, and vincristine with an alternating regimen of methotrexate, etoposide, and cisplatin/cyclophosphamide, doxorubicin, and vincristine in the treatment of extensive-disease small-cell lung cancer. J Clin Oncol *9*:1438, 1991

496. Longo DL, DeVita VT Jr, Duffey PL, et al: Superiority of ProMACE-CytaBOM over ProMACE-MOPP in the treatment of advanced diffuse aggressive lymphoma: Results of a prospective randomized trial. J Clin Oncol *9*:25, 1991

497. Bonadonna G, Santoro A: ABVD chemotherapy in the treatment of Hodgkin's disease. Cancer Treat Rev *9*:21, 1982

498. Santoro A, Bonfante V, Viviani S, et al: Salvage chemotherapy in relapsing Hodgkin's disease. Proc Am Soc Clin Oncol *3*:254, 1984

499. Bonadonna G, Valagussa P, Santoro A: Alternating noncross-resistant combination chemotherapy or MOPP in stage IV Hodgkin's disease. Ann Intern Med *104*:739, 1986

500. Valagussa P, Santoro A, Boracchi P, et al: 9-year results of two randomized studies with MOPP and ABVD in Hodgkin's disease: Multiple regression analysis. Proc Am Soc Clin Oncol *8*:976, 1989

501. Longo DL, Duffey PL, DeVita VT Jr, et al: Treatment of advanced-stage Hodgkins disease: Alternating noncrossresistant MOPP/CABS is not superior to MOPP. J Clin Oncol *9*:1409, 1991

502. Aisner J, Korsun A, Perloff M, et al: A randomized comparison of CAF, VATH, and VATH alternating with CMFVP for advanced breast cancer, a CALGB study. Proc Am Soc Clin Oncol *7*:27, 1988

503. Buzzoni R, Bonadonna G, Valagussa P, Zambetti M: Adjuvant chemotherapy with doxorubicin plus cyclophosphamide, methotrexate, and fluorouracil in the treatment of resectable breast cancer with more than three positive axillary nodes. J Clin Oncol *9*:2134, 1991

504. Bruce WR, Meeker BE, Valeriote FA: Comparison of the sensitivity of normal hematopoietic and transplanted lymphoma colony-forming cells to chemotherapeutic agents administered in vivo. J Natl Cancer Inst *37*:233, 1966

505. Griswold OP Jr, Trader MW, Frei E III, et al: Response of drug-sensitive and resistant L1210 leukemias to high dose chemotherapy. Cancer Res *47*:2323, 1987

506. Frei E III, Canellos GP: Dose: A critical factor in cancer chemotherapy. Am J Med 69:585, 1980

507. Tattersall MHN, Parker LM, Pitman SW, Frei E III: Clinical pharmacology of high-dose methotrexate. Cancer Chemother Rep Part 3, 6:25, 1975

508. Pinkel C, Hernandez K, Borella L, et al: Drug dosage and remission duration in childhood lymphocytic leukemia. Cancer 27:247, 1971

509. Samson MK, Rivlin SE, Jones SE, et al: Dose-response and dose-survival advantage for high- vs. low-dose Cisplatin combined with vinblastine and bleomycin in disseminated testicular cancer. Cancer 53:1029, 1984

510. Tannock IF, Boyd NF, DeBoer G, et al: A randomized trial of two dose levels of cyclophosphamide, methotrexate, and fluorouracil chemotherapy for patients with metastatic breast cancer. J Clin Oncol 6:1377, 1988

511. Crown JPA, Norton L: Issues in Chemotherapy: Breast Cancer. New York, Triclinica, 1993

512. DeVita VT Jr: Dose-response is alive and well. J Clin Oncol 4:1157, 1986

513. Collins V, Loeffler RK, Tivey H: Observations on growth rates of human tumors. Am J Roentgenol 76:988, 1956

514. Steel GG: Growth Kinetics of Tumours—Cell Population Kinetics in Relation to the Growth and Treatment of Cancer. Oxford, England, Clarendon Press, 1977, pp 46–52

515. Tubiana M: Tumor cell proliferation kinetics and tumor growth rate. Acta Oncol 28:113, 1989

516. Laird AK: Dynamics of growth in tumors and in normal organisms. Natl Cancer Inst Monogr 30:15, 1969

517. Sullivan PW, Salmon SE: Kinetics of tumor growth and regression in IgG multiple myeloma. J Clin Invest 51:1697, 1972

518. Norton L: A Gompertzian model of human breast cancer growth. Cancer Res 48:7067, 1988

519. Spratt JA, Von Fournier D, Spratt JS, Weber EE: Decelerating growth and human breast cancer. Cancer 71:2013, 1993

520. Spratt JS, Greenberg RA, Hauser LS: Geometry, growth rates and duration of cancer and carcinoma in situ of the breast before detection by screening. Cancer Res 46:970, 1986

521. Demicheli R: Growth of testicular neoplasm lung metastases: Tumor-specific relation between two Gompertzian parameters. Eur J Cancer 16:1603, 1980

522. Norton L: Mathematical interpretation of tumor growth kinetics. In Greenspan EM (ed): Clinical Interpretation and Practice of Cancer Chemotherapy. New York, Raven, 1982, pp 53–70

523. Heuser L, Spratt J, Polk H: Growth rates of primary breast cancer. Cancer 43:1888, 1979

524. Fisher B, Slack N, Katrych D, Wolmark N: Ten-year follow-up results in patients with carcinoma of the breast in a cooperative clinical trial evaluating surgical adjuvant chemotherapy. Surg Gynecol Obstet 140:528, 1975

525. Speer JF, Petrovsky VE, Retsky MW, Wardwell RH: A stochastic numerical model of breast cancer that simulates clinical data. Cancer Res 44:4124, 1984

526. Norton L: Reply to letter to the Editor. Cancer Res 49:6444, 1989

527. Fisher B, Brown AM, Dimitrov NV, et al: Two months of doxorubicin-cyclophosphamide with and without interval reinduction therapy compared with 6 months of cyclophosphamide, methotrexate, and fluorouracil in positive-node breast cancer patients with tamoxifen-nonresponsive tumors: Results from the National Surgical Adjuvant Breast and Bowel Project B-15. J Clin Oncol 8:1483, 1990

528. Norton L, Simon R: Tumor size, sensitivity to therapy, and the design of treatment schedules. Cancer Treat Rep 61:307, 1977

529. Hill RP, Stanley JA: Pulmonary metastases of the Lewis lung tumor—cell kinetics and response to cyclophosphamide at different sizes. Cancer Treat Rep 61:29, 1977

530. Norton L, Simon R: The Norton-Simon hypothesis revisited. Cancer Treat Rep 70:163, 1986

531. Ross DW, Capizzi RL: Differentiation vs. cytoreduction during remission induction in acute nonlymphoblastic leukemia treated with sequential high-dose araC and asparaginase. Cancer 53:1651, 1984

532. Norton L: Implications of kinetic heterogeneity in clinical oncology. Semin Oncol 12:231, 1985

533. Day RS: Treatment sequencing, asymmetry, and uncertainty: Protocol strategies for combination chemotherapy. Cancer Res 46:3876, 1986

534. Norton L, Day R: Potential innovations in scheduling in cancer chemotherapy. In DeVita VT, Hellman S, Rosenberg SA (eds): Important Advances in Oncology. Philadelphia, JB Lippincott Company, 1991, pp 57–72

535. Skipper HE: Analyses of multiarmed trials in which animals bearing different burdens of L1210 leukemia cells were treated with two, three, and four drug combinations delivered in different ways with varying dose intensities of each drug and varying average dose intensities. South Res Inst Booklet 7, 42:87, 1986

536. Griswold DP, Schabel FM Jr, Corbett TH, Dykes DJ: Concepts for controlling drug-resistant tumor cells. In Fidler IJ, White RJ (eds): Design of Models for Testing Cancer Therapeutic Agents. New York, Van Nostrand Reinhold, 1982, pp 215–224

537. Buzzoni R, Bonadonna G, Valagussa P, et al: Adjuvant chemotherapy with doxorubicin and cyclophosphamide, methotrexate and fluorouracil in the treatment of resectable breast cancer with more than three positive axillary nodes. J Clin Oncol 9:2134, 1994

538. Cortes EP, Necheles TF, Holland JF, et al: Adjuvant chemotherapy for primary osteosarcoma: A Cancer and Leukemia Group B experience. In Salmon SE, Jones SE (eds): Adjuvant Chemotherapy of Cancer III. New York, Grune & Stratton, 1981, pp 201–210

539. Selawry OS, Hananian J, Wolman IJ, et al: New treatment schedule with improved survival in childhood leukemia. JAMA 194:187, 1965

540. Hudis C, Lebwohl D, Crown J, et al: Dose-intensive sequential crossover adjuvant chemotherapy for women with high risk node-positive primary breast cancer. In Salmon SE (ed): Adjuvant Therapy of Cancer IV. Philadelphia, JB Lippincott Company, 1993, pp 214–219

541. Gianni AM, Bregni M, Siena S, et al: Prospective randomized comparison of MACOP-B vs. rhGM-CSF-supported high-dose sequential myeloablative chemoradiotherapy in diffuse large cell lymphoma. Proc Am Soc Clin Oncol 10:951, 1991

542. Gabrilove JL: Colony-stimulating factors: Clinical status. In DeVita VT, Hellman S, Rosenberg SA (eds): Important Advances in Oncology. Philadelphia, JB Lippincott Company, 1991, pp 215–237

543. Frei E III, Antman K, Teicher B, et al: Bone marrow anutotransplantation for solid tumor prospects. J Clin Oncol 7:515, 1989

544. Peters WP: High dose chemotherapy and autologous bone marrow support for breast cancer. In DeVita VT, Hellman S, Rosenberg SA (eds): Important Advances in Oncology. Philadelphia, JB Lippincott Company, 1991, pp 135–150

545. Valeriote F, van Putten L: Proliferation-dependent cytotoxicity of anticancer agents: A review. Cancer Res 35:2619, 1975

546. Hug V, Johnston D, Finders M, Hortobagyi G: Use of growth-stimulating hormones to improve the in vitro therapeutic index of doxorubicin for human breast cancer. Cancer Res 46:147, 1986

547. Osborne CK, Kitten L, Arteaga CL: Antagonism of chemotherapy-induced cytotoxicity for human breast cancer cells by antiestrogens. J Clin Oncol 7:710, 1989

548. Conte PF, Alama A, Bertelli G, et al: Chemotherapy with estrogenic recruitment and surgery in locally advanced breast cancer: Clinical and cytokinetic results. Int J Cancer 40:490, 1987

549. Swain SM, Sorace RA, Bagley CS, et al: Neoadjuvant chemotherapy in the combined modality approach of locally advanced nonmetastatic breast cancer. Cancer Res 47:3889, 1987

550. Conte PF, Pronzato P, Rubagotti A, et al: Conventional vs. cytokinetic polychemotherapy with estrogenic recruitment in metastatic breast cancer: Results of a randomized cooperative trial. J Clin Oncol 5:339, 1987

551. Lippman ME: Hormonal stimulation and chemotherapy for breast cancer (editorial). J Clin Oncol 5:331, 1987

552. Lippman ME, Cassidy J, Wesley M, Young RC: A randomized attempt to increase the efficacy of cytotoxic chemotherapy in metastatic breast cancer by hormonal synchronization. J Clin Oncol 2:28, 1984

553. Dressler LG: DNA flow cytometry measurements have significant prognostic impact in the node negative breast cancer patient: An intergroup study (INT 0076). *In* Treatment of Early Stage Breast Cancer: Program and Abstracts, NIH Consensus Development Conference. Washington, DC, National Institutes of Health, 1990, pp 99–101

554. Weinberg RA, Bishop JM, Minna JD, Sharp PA: Gene regulation and oncogenes: AACR Special Conference in Cancer Research. Cancer Res *49*:2188, 1989

555. Rowley JD, Golomb AM, Vardiman JW: Nonrandom chromosomal abnormalities in acute leukemia and dysmyelopoietic syndromes in patients with previously treated malignant disease. Blood *58*:759, 1981

556. Norton L: Biology of residual breast cancer after therapy: A kinetic interpretation. *In* Ragaz J, Simpson-Herren L, Lippman ME, Fisher B (eds): Effects of Therapy on Biology and Kinetics of the Residual Tumor, Part A: PreClinical Aspects. New York, Wiley-Liss, 1990, pp 109–132

557. Bontenbal M, Siewerts AM, Klijn JGM, et al: Effect of hormonal manipulation and doxorubicin administration on cell cycle kinetics of human breast cancer cells. Br J Cancer *60*:688, 1989

558. Koury MJ, Bondurant MC: Erythropoietin retards DNA breakdown and prevents programmed death in erythroid progenitor cells. Science *248*:378, 1990

559. Williams GT, Smith CA, Spooncer E, et al: Haemopoietic colony stimulating factors promote cell survival by suppressing apoptosis. Nature *343*:76, 1990

560. Barry MA, Behnke CA, Eastman A: Activation of programmed cell death (apoptosis) by cisplatin, other anticancer drugs, toxins and hyperthermia. Biochem Pharmacol *40*:2353, 1990

561. Zuckiet G, Tritton TR: Adriamycin causes up-regulation of epidermal growth factor receptors in actively growing cells. Exp Cell Res *148*:155, 1983

562. Isonishi S, Andrews PA, Howell SB: Increased sensitivity to cis-diamminedichloroplatinum (11) in human ovarian carcinoma cells in response to treatment with 12-0-tetradecanoylphorbol-13-acetate. J Biol Chem *265*:3623, 1990

563. Baselga J, Mendelsohn J: The epidermal growth factor receptor as a target for therapy in breast carcinoma. Breast Cancer Res Treat *29*:127, 1994

564. Folkman J, Shing Y: Angiogenesis. J Biol Chem *267*:10931, 1992

565. Yee D, Paik S, Lebovic G, et al: Analysis of IGF-I gene expression in malignancy—evidence for a paracrine role in human breast cancer. Mol Endocrinol *3*:509, 1989

566. Cullen KJ, Smith HS, Hill S, et al: Growth factor messenger RNA expression by human breast fibroblasts from benign and malignant lesions. Cancer Res *51*:4978, 1991

567. Basset P, Bellocq JP, Wolf C: A novel metalloproteinase gene specifically expressed in stromal cells of breast carcinomas. Nature *348*:699, 1990

568. Garin-Chesa P, Old LJ, Rettig WJ: Cell surface glycoprotein of reactive stromal fibroblasts as a potential antibody target in human epithelial cancers. Proc Natl Acad Sci *87*:7235, 1990

569. Smith HS, Stern R, Liu E, Benz C: Early and late events in the development of human breast cancer. Basic Life Sci *57*:329, 1991

570. Shekhar PV, Aslakson CJ, Miller FR: Molecular events in metastatic progression. Semin Cancer Biol *4*:193, 1993

571. Paraskeva C, Williams AC: Promotability and tissue specificity of hereditary cancer genes: Do hereditary cancer patients have a reduced requirement for tumor promotion because all their somatic cells are heterozygous at the predisposing locus? Mol Carcinog *5*:4, 1992

572. Onoda G, Toner J: Fractal dimensions of model particle packing having multiple generations of agglomerates. J Am Ceram Soc *69*:C278, 1986

573. Norton L: Introduction to Clinical Aspects of Preneoplasia: A Mathematical Relationship between Stromal Paracrine Autonomy and Population Size. Ares-Serono Symposia. *In* Marks PA, Türler H, Weil R (eds): Precancerous lesions: A multidisciplinary approach. Ares-Serono Symposia Publications, Milan, Italy, Vol 1, 1993, pp 269–276

574. McDivitt RW, Boyce W, Gersell D: Tubular carcinoma of the breast: Clinical and pathological observations concerning 135 cases. Am J Surg Pathol *6*:401, 1982

575. Lu C, Vickers MF, Kerbel RS: Interleukin 6: A fibroblast-derived growth inhibitor of human melanoma cells from early but not advanced stages of tumor progression. Proc Natl Acad Sci *89*:9215, 1992

576. Frixen U, Behrens J, Sachs M, et al: E-cadherin mediated cell-cell adhesion prevents invasiveness of human carcinoma cell lines. J Cell Biol *117*:173, 1991

577. Nicolson GL: Cancer progression and growth: Relationship of paracrine and autocrine growth mechanisms to organ preference of metastases. Exp Cell Res *204*:171, 1993

578. Koscielny S, Tubiana M, Le MG: Breast cancer: Relationship between the size of the primary tumour and the probability of metastatic dissemination. Br J Cancer *49*:709, 1984

9

ADHESION MECHANISMS CONTROLLING CELL-CELL AND CELL-MATRIX INTERACTIONS DURING THE METASTATIC PROCESS

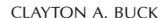

CLAYTON A. BUCK

The metastatic cascade commences with the dislodgment of cells from the primary tumor mass and terminates in the establishment of tumors at secondary sites in the body. It is schematically summarized in Figure 9–1. Each step in the cascade involves the establishment and termination of adhesive interactions. These interactions involve families of receptors whose program of expression is as complex as the metastatic cascade itself. The purpose of this chapter is to examine these adhesive interactions at the molecular level, identifying the receptors most likely to be involved at each step along the way, describing the molecular organization required for adhesive interactions, showing how these adhesive events can be regulated, and, finally, discussing how closely the information obtained from experimental systems reflects what is known from examining patient material. Specific experimental paradigms are used to illustrate the possible role for each adhesion receptor in the metastatic cascade.

Many of the models designed to explain tumor cell movement through the circulatory system and subsequent lodgment at specific, reproducible sites draw heavily on what we know of the molecular events occurring during inflammation and during lymphocyte trafficking. Thus, many of the same inflammatory agents, cytokines, and receptor-ligand interactions that are important to white cell–endothelial cell adhesion also may be relevant to the interaction of circulating tumor cells with the microvas-

cular endothelium. Similarly, much of our understanding of adhesion receptor function in metastatic systems comes from our knowledge of how these same molecules function during morphogenetic events occurring during embryonic development. Thus, to understand the molecular basis of receptor function involved in tumor formation and metastasis, it is necessary to examine how these receptors function and how they are regulated under normal physiologic conditions.

ORGANIZATION OF ADHESION RECEPTORS: GENERAL CONSIDERATIONS

A typical adhesion complex is illustrated in Figure 9–2. In this case, the receptors demonstrated are heterodimers known as integrins. An intact receptor consists of an α subunit noncovalently associated with a β subunit. Adhesion receptors, whether made up of a single protein or several proteins, consist of an extracellular (usually amino-terminal) domain, a hydrophobic transmembrane domain, and a cytoplasmic domain of variable length. The extracellular domain interacts with the appropriate ligand, either the extracellular matrix or a molecule on an adjacent cell. The cytoplasmic domain interacts with cytoskeletal elements of the cell that provide the scaffolding required for assembly of the adhesive complex. Thus, receptors serve as transmembrane anchors between cells or between a cell and the extracellular matrix. This provides strength and structural stability to tissue, and allows the establishment of polarity required for the vectoral movement of material across various epithelial sheets, as in the kidney or the gut.

Adhesion receptors also serve to transmit information between the extracellular environment and the cell, providing information required for the cell to determine its position within the organism as well as its state of differentiation. In other words, the receptors serve as conduits through which information from the extracellular environment is transmitted into the cell, triggering the organiza-

tion of molecular complexes or activating specific genetic programs.[1] This is referred to as signal transduction. It is the result of subtle structural changes that accompany ligand-receptor interactions, initiating a series of secondary messages, usually through the activation of protein kinases or G proteins. The molecules involved in transducing the signals initiated by receptor-ligand interactions are organized either within the membrane or just beneath the membrane in close juxtaposition with the various adhesion receptors, as illustrated by the two tyrosine kinases, c-Src and FAK, in Figure 9–2. These molecules activate other protein kinases, phosphatases, and phospholipases, the products of which activate proteins required to amplify intracellular signals necessary for gene regulation and cy-

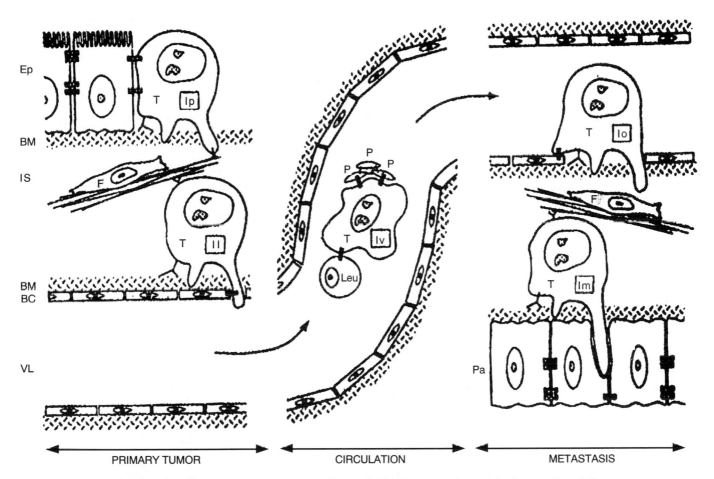

Figure 9–1. Metastatic cascade. Metastasis likely is initiated by a genetic event leading to, among other things, changes in the expression of adhesion receptors on the tumor cell surface that facilitate a morphologic transition from epithelial-like to a more motile, fibroblastic cell (epithelial-mesenchymal transformation) incapable of responding to the environmental cues required for its continued function as an epithelial cell. The metastatic cell now can migrate through the extracellular matrix into a nearby capillary bed utilizing receptors of the integrin family required for cell migration. Once in the circulatory system, the cells may form complexes with platelets or white cells that may lodge in the capillary bed, be destroyed by circulating immune cells, or themselves interact with tissue-specific receptors on the surface of capillary endothelial cells. This latter event requires the coordinated expression and function of diverse groups of receptors, including the integrins, selectins, members of the immunoglobulin superfamily, and proteoglycan-binding proteins. As a result of tumor cell adhesion, the endothelial cells will retract, exposing the underlying extracellular matrix, through which the cell may migrate and establish a secondary tumor. This requires the activation of receptors again including other members of the integrin family, proteoglycans, cytokines, and chemotactic factors released from the extracellular matrix. T, tumor cell; Ep, epithelium; BM, basement membrane; F, fibroblastic mesenchymal cell; ED, endothelial cells; VL, vascular lumen; Leu, leukocyte; P, platelet; Pa, parenchyma at site of metastatic nodule formation. (From Van Roy F, Mareel M: Tumor invasion: Effects of cell adhesion and motility. Trends Cell Biol 2:163, 1992, with permission.)

toskeletal organization. Clearly, an equally complex series of events must be initiated from within the cell in order for a cell to change shape, dedifferentiate, or move from one place to another. Again, the end result of these signals from within the cell is a structural change in the receptor, allowing it to change ligand specificity, release a particular ligand, or interact with a different set of cytoskeletal proteins.

ADHESION RECEPTORS AND THE METASTATIC PROCESS—THEORIES, PARADIGMS, AND MODELS: GENERAL CONSIDERATIONS

Historically, two different explanations for the organ-specific hematogenous spread of tumor cells were proposed. The first, originally articulated by Paget in 1889,[2] explained the tendency of different tumors to metastasize to distinct sites on the basis of there being something about that site that made it the right place for cells derived from a particular tumor to lodge and grow. This was known as the "seed and soil" hypothesis. At the time of the proposal, distinguishing characteristics of a particular site were not known. However, the use of the metaphor of seeds growing only on fertile soil suggests that Paget had in mind factors in the environment that contributed to the proliferation of the tumor cells. At that time, the concept of tissue-specific receptors directing cell movement and cell interactions had not evolved.

The seed and soil hypothesis was challenged in a treatise on tumors published 40 years later.[3] It was argued that the nonrandom colonization of tumors could be accounted

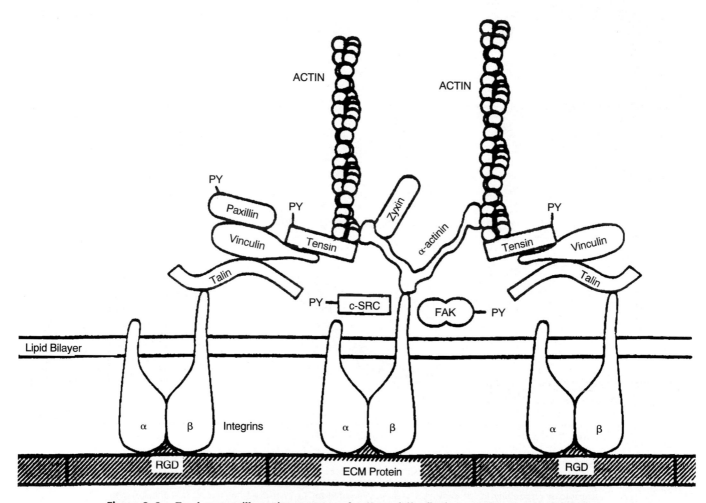

Figure 9–2. Focal contact illustrating structure of a "generic" adhesion complex. A typical adhesion structure consists of the following elements organized at a specific site on the cell surface: (1) the ligand or counterreceptor with which adhesion receptors bind to either the extracellular matrix or the molecules on adjacent cells; (2) a group of membrane-spanning adhesion receptors; (3) a complex of cytoskeletal-associated molecules serving as links between the receptors and the filamentous cytoskeleton (actin microfilaments, microtubules, etc.); and (4) a group of regulatory elements required for transducing information from the external environment into the cell, and from the cell to the receptor (these include protein kinases, phosphatases, G proteins, and phospholipases). In this example, the ligand(s) are molecules in the extracellular matrix (ECM); the receptors are members of the integrin family that are heterodimers each consisting of an α and a β subunit; the cytoskeletal-associated molecules linking the integrins to the actin-containing microfilaments are a group of interacting molecules (talin, vinculin, paxillin, tensin, zyxlin, and α-actinin[161]); and the regulatory elements include two phosphotyrosine kinases, c-Src, and FAK. (From Schwartz MA: Signaling by integrins: Implications for tumorigenesis. Cancer Res 53:1503, 1993, with permission.)

for by the direction of blood flow away from the primary tumor mass. According to this argument, the first capillary bed encountered by the tumor cells would be the site of arrest of the largest number of cells and therefore the site of establishment of secondary tumors. Tumor spread was accounted for entirely by the mechanical trapping of cells within the closest capillary bed and required nothing special about the tissue to account for the successful establishment of secondary tumors. There is probably some truth in this hypothesis. For example, many tumors initially establish secondary growths in draining lymph nodes. The liver is a common site for metastasis, and tumor cells can aggregate with platelets or with one another in circulation and become mechanically lodged in capillary beds. However, we now know that growth at these sites probably depends on the appropriate extracellular matrix as well as the release of cytokines and angiogenic factors sequestered within the surrounding matrix,[4] as proposed in the seed and soil hypothesis. Several excellent reviews discuss these ideas in detail.[5-8]

Current theories of nonrandom metastasis are based on our knowledge of specific adhesion receptors and cell trafficking. They postulate that adhesion receptors expressed on tumor cells facilitate their movement from the primary tumor mass to a secondary site, the location of which is determined by the presence of unique ligands on the capillary endothelial cells. The appeal of this theory accounts for recent attempts to identify such receptors or ligands. Their identification would be extremely valuable in tumor detection, prognosis, and treatment. Unfortunately, despite all the evidence for the function of such molecules in embryonic development and normal cell trafficking, none has been found that is unique to any population of tumors.

LYMPHOCYTE-ENDOTHELIUM INTERACTIONS PROVIDING INSIGHTS INTO THE MOLECULAR EVENTS REQUIRED FOR METASTATIC SPREAD

Lymphocytes cross regularly from the vascular lumen to the interstitium of lymph nodes.[9,10] Lymphocyte trafficking to specific nodes is controlled by the interaction of receptors on the lymphocyte, operationally defined as "homing receptors," that recognize specific ligands or counterreceptors presented on the surface of high endothelial venules (HEV) of lymph nodes. Thus, as might be the case for the hematogenous spread of tumor cells, circulating lymphoid cells recognize specific receptors and undergo a series of interactions required for adhesion to the endothelial lining and subsequent movement into the surrounding tissue.

In the case of the inflammatory response, receptors are expressed or activated on postcapillary venules in response to inflammatory stimuli.[11-13] These receptors bind ligands or counterreceptors constitutively expressed on circulating neutrophils, delaying their movement through a particular capillary bed and allowing a series of receptor-ligand interactions to occur that are necessary for the cells to move across the capillary endothelium into the

surrounding tissue. Lymphocyte trafficking and neutrophil infiltration are thought to occur by similar mechanisms, which likely differ only in the receptors involved in the initial endothelial cell interactions.

The interaction of circulating white cells and vascular endothelium involves four families of adhesion molecules. These are the selectins, members of the immunoglobulin superfamily, the integrins, carbohydrate-rich proteins referred to as gly-CAMs (glycosylation-dependent cell adhesion molecules)[14-16] and CD44, each of which is discussed in detail later in this chapter.

The inflammatory cascade, as summarized in Figure 9–3, is initiated by the release of histamines, interleukin 1, tumor necrosis factor, or transforming growth factor β (TGF-β) by mast cells and macrophages responding to various stimuli, including bacterial infections. This causes an immediate expression of carbohydrate-binding receptors on the surface of endothelial cells known as selectins. P-selectin (platelet selectin) stored in Weible-Palade bodies on endothelial cells, is immediately expressed on their surface, where it is available for binding to carbohydrate residues on circulating neutrophils. This provides a transient interaction between the white cell and endothelium, but does not provide tight adhesion, accounting for the rolling of white cells along the surface of the endothelium of vessels near inflammatory stimuli (Fig. 9–3B). This slowing is thought to keep the white cell in the inflamed area long enough for it to respond to local cytokines required for the up-regulation of other receptors. This initial interaction is important because it can occur under conditions of blood flow. In its absence, the subsequent steps either do not occur or are delayed.[17] Within a matter of minutes, the P-selectin is lost from the endothelial cell surface, to be replaced by E-selectin (endothelial selectin) that has been synthesized in response to the inflammatory stimuli and will remain on the endothelial cell surface for 1 to 2 hours. Both L-selectin (leukocyte selectin) and E-selectins bind to the highly glycosylated molecules (gly-CAMS or mucins) on the surface of the interacting cells.[14,18,19] Subsequently, the immunoglobulin superfamily molecules such as intercellular adhesion molecule (ICAM)-1, ICAM-2, and vascular cell adhesion molecule (VCAM)-1 are being expressed on the endothelial cell surface and the rolling white cells have responded to cytokines and chemotactic factors in the region by activating the integrins on their surface (Fig. 9–3C). The integrins and immunoglobulin superfamily receptors interact with one another, providing a more stable adhesion of the white cell to the endothelium. At this point, the rolling ceases and the white cells are anchored firmly to the endothelial cell surface. This is thought to stimulate the endothelial cells to retract, exposing the underlying matrix. The white cells, possibly in response to other soluble factors in the environment or to the binding of the integrins with their counterreceptors, begin shedding the integrins responsible for cell-cell interactions and initiate the expression of other integrins that serve as adhesion receptors for extracellular matrix molecules and facilitate the movement of the neutrophils into the surrounding tissue (Fig. 9–3D). The chemotactic stimuli required for this directed migration are provided by inflammatory factors and proteolytic

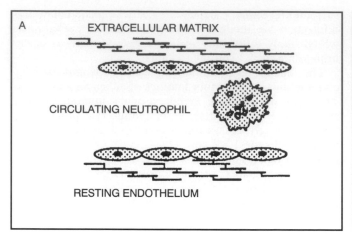

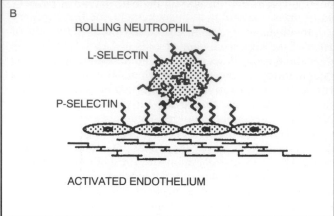

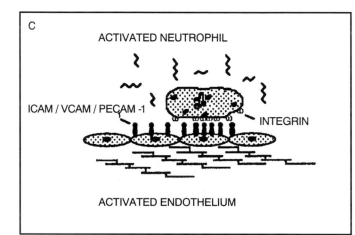

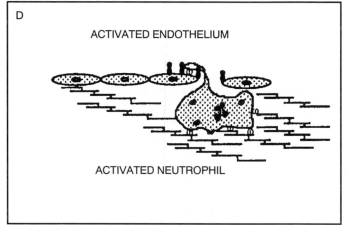

Figure 9–3. Inflammatory cascade as a model for extravasation of metastatic cells. The inflammatory process may provide mechanistic paradigms for the local extravasation of metastatic cells. Like metastasis, it involves circulating cells, adhesion to a specific capillary bed, movement of cells across the endothelial lining, and invasion of the surrounding matrix. These events in turn require the programmed expression of cell surface adhesion receptors designed to facilitate each step in the inflammatory cascade. *A*, A neutrophil moving unencumbered through a microvascular bed. There is no interaction between the circulating neutrophil and endothelium. *B*, Results of specific receptor expression by the endothelial cells of a capillary in the vicinity of tissue damage resulting from infection or injury. Histamines or inflammatory cytokines stimulate the expression of receptors known as selectins by endothelial cells of a local microvascular bed. The endothelial selectins (P-selectin, later E-selectin) interact with carbohydrates presented on the surface of selectins or other carbohydrate-containing proteins, such as gly-CAMs on the circulating neutrophil, resulting in the "rolling" interaction between the neutrophil and the activated endothelium. *C*, Results of the up-regulation of a second set of receptors on the rolling neutrophil, as well as on the activated endothelial cell in response to local inflammatory cytokines, chemotactic factors, and neutrophil–endothelial cell adhesion. This second set of receptors is required for a stable interaction between the activated neutrophil and the activated endothelium. The selectins, no longer required to maintain adhesion, are shed from both cells. The receptors for more avid binding of circulating cells and the endothelium include members of the integrin family as well as members of the immunoglobulin superfamily. *D*, Process of cell movement across the endothelium. This involves the retraction of the endothelium in response to neutrophil adhesion, the turnover of receptors from the cell surface, and activation of receptors (integrins and glycosaminoglycan-binding receptors [CD44]) required for the movement of cells into the surrounding extracellular matrix. Unlike the neutrophil, at this point the successful metastatic tumor cell will replicate, forming a small angiogenic tumor mass that eventually will enlarge and itself give rise to new metastatic cells.

peptide fragments released as the cell moves through the matrix.

The model of inflammatory white cell–endothelial cell interaction provides insights into the molecular processes required for cells to move from the circulation into tissue. Organotypic specificity is not provided within this model. Its isolated occurrence is due strictly to localized changes in the endothelium induced by inflammatory agents. It therefore does not address completely the idea of organ-specific metastasis through specific receptors expressed in different capillary beds. However, the process of lympho-cyte homing does suggest that such a possibility exists.

Lymphocytes continuously circulate from the blood to the lymph, extravasating either through the HEVs of lymph nodes (naive T cells) or through the afferent lymph (memory T cells). In both instances, receptors on endo-thelial cells must engage counterreceptors on lympho-cytes, facilitating their movement across the endothelial lining. There is some specificity involved, because lym-phocytes show a tendency to recirculate through specific lymph nodes. This is known as lymphocyte homing.[20] The receptors on the circulating lymphocytes are "homing re-ceptors." Their counterreceptors on HEVs are known as "addressins." There are at least three distinct populations of HEVs involved in this more specific form of lympho-cyte trafficking: those found in the peripheral lymph nodes, those found in Peyer's patch lymph nodes, and those controlling lymphocyte movement into the synov-ium. These HEVs can be distinguished by the addressins displayed on their surface,[9,20,21] which are thought to pro-vide the specificity required for the admission of only se-lected populations of lymphocytes into the appropriate lymph nodes. The molecular basis of lymphocyte-HEV adhesion has not been studied in as much detail as that of the inflammatory process, but it does support the idea that adhesive mechanisms exist to provide specificity at the molecular level that might facilitate nonrandom metastasis.

CADHERINS AND THE METASTATIC CASCADE

Lymphocyte trafficking and white cell movement across the vascular endothelium provide insights into how tumor cells might obtain access to other regions of the body. However, before any of this can take place, the subpo-pulation of tumor cells capable of forming secondary tu-mors must leave the original tumor mass and move into the blood stream. This separation implies a breakdown in normal intercellular adhesion responsible for the mainte-nance of tissue integrity. In the case of epithelial cells, the cell of origin of most human tumors, this involves a breakdown in the function of members of the cadherin superfamily of adhesion molecules.

Cadherins are a superfamily of molecules required for cell-cell recognition, tissue morphogenesis, and mainte-nance of tissue integrity in both vertebrates and inverte-brates.[22–24] Members of the superfamily were given names according to the tissue from which they were first isolated.

That is, E-cadherin was expressed in epithelial cells, and N-cadherin was expressed in neuronal cells. A summary of the more recently described cadherins is presented in Table 9–1.

The typical mammalian cadherin is a transmembrane glycoprotein consisting of 723 to 748 amino acids, the fully mature forms of which have a molecular mass of approximately 120 kDa (Fig. 9–4A). The extracellular portion consists of four repeating units of approximately 110 amino acids each, within which are Ca^{2+} binding do-mains,[25] explaining the Ca^{2+} dependence of cadherin ac-tivity.[26] Cadherins have only four cysteine residues found near the transmembrane region of the extracellular do-main. The cytoplasmic domain is fairly large, having a molecular mass of approximately 14 kDa, and shows the highest degree of amino acid homology among cadher-ins,[25] reflecting its common function as a linker to the cytoskeletal system of the cell. Most cadherins contain a hydrophobic sequence anchoring them within the membrane. A single exception is T-cadherin, identified in neuronal tissue, that contains no cytoplasmic domain and is anchored in the membrane via a glycosylphosphatidy-linositol glycan linkage.[27]

Molecular Organization of Cadherins at the Cell Surface

There are many subfamilies of molecules within the cadherin superfamily. Some are found as part of complex adhesive structures known as desmosomes,[24] and others appear to be involved primarily in histogenic cell-cell ad-hesion and are located in less complex structures such as adherens junctions. They promote cell-cell adhesion by a homophilic Ca^{2+}-dependent mechanism, as illustrated in Figure 9–4B. That is, the interaction of two identical cad-herin molecules (homophilic) on adjacent cells of the same tissue type (homotypic) in the presence of Ca^{2+} re-sults in the cadherin-mediated aggregation of the two cells. Experimentally, the adhesive capacity and specific-ity of cadherins is demonstrated most easily by transfect-ing cells that normally produce no cadherins with vectors carrying cDNA coding for specific cadherins. If mouse L cells, which grow nicely in suspension, are transfected with cDNA coding for E-cadherin, they will aggregate with one another. This aggregation can be blocked by monoclonal antibodies specific for E-cadherin, but not with antibodies specific for other cadherins. The trans-fected L cells will aggregate only with other L cells ex-pressing E-cadherin and not with nontransfected cells or cells transfected with cDNA coding for a different cad-herin. In fact, if L cells expressing two different cadherins are mixed together, the cells will form mixed aggregates in which cells expressing like cadherins are adjacent to each other, in much the same manner as might occur dur-ing normal histogenesis.

There appear to be two regions of the molecule that control ligand specificity. One is within the first 113 amino-terminal amino acids, and involves nonconserved residues on either side of a common His-Ala-Val se-quence.[28] The second is located nearer the cysteine-con-

TABLE 9–1. THE CADHERIN FAMILY

	CADHERIN	SPECIES	T	F	L
Embryonal and epithelial cadherins	Uvomorulin/E-Cad	Mouse	Early embryo and epithelia	+	8
	CAM 120/80	Human	MCF-7	+	
	Arc-1	Dog	MDCK	+	16
	rr-1	Dog	MDCK	+	
	gp 140 K/E-cad	*Xenopus*	Early embryo and epithelia	+	
	XB-cad	*Xenopus*	Early embryo and epithelia	+	
	U-cad	*Xenopus*	Early embryo and epithelia	+	
	EP-cad	*Xenopus*	Early embryo and epithelia		*
	L-CAM	Chicken	Liver	+	
	B-cad/K-CAM	Chicken	Neuronal cells		*
Neuronal and mesodermal cadherins	N-cad/A-CAM/N-Cal-CAM	Chicken	Neuronal and mesodermal cells	+	18
	N-cad	Human	Neuronal and mesodermal cells	+	
	N-cad				
	M-cad	*Xenopus*	Neuronal and mesodermal cells		
	T-cad				
	R-cad	Bovine	Endothelium		
	Cad 4	Mouse	Myoblast	+	
		Chicken	Neuronal cells		
		Chicken	Retina		
		Rat	Brain tissue		
Desmosomal cadherins	Desmocollin DG II/III	Human	Epithelial cells	+	9
	Desmoglein DGI	Human	Epithelial cells		18
	PVA	Human	Epidermis		18
Unclassified cadherins	P-cad	Mouse	Placenta	+	8
		Human	Placenta	+	16
	V-cad	Bovine	Endothelial cells	+	
	Cad 5-11	Rat	Brain tissue		
	Fat protein	*Drosophila*	Larval imaginal discs		

From Kemler R: Classical cadherins. Semin Cell Biol *3*:149, 1992, with permission.

*Abbreviations: T, tissue or cell type where the cadherin was identified; F, the adhesive function has been demonstrated (+); L, chromosomal localization of the gene (asterisks indicate a tandem arrangement of these genes).

taining regions adjacent to the transmembrane domain. These two regions are widely separated on a linear peptide map, leading to the suggestion that ligand binding requires that cadherins be folded in such a manner as to bring these two regions in close apposition.

The cytoplasmic domain of cadherins is highly conserved and regulates the interaction between cytoskeletal elements and the receptor itself. Deletion analysis has revealed that cytoskeletal interactions require the last carboxy-terminal 72 amino acids. Deleting portions of this region of the molecule completely inactivates it so far as adhesion-promoting activity is concerned.

As with many other adhesion receptors, cadherins interact with the actin-containing microfilaments via intermediate cytoskeletal-associated molecules. In this case, this interaction involves three different proteins called catenins (Fig. 9–4A). The catenins are designated α, β, and γ, and range in molecular size from 83 to 102 kDa. α-Catenin is a vinculin-like protein,[29] whereas the other two catenins seem to be members of the plakoglobin family,[30] representatives of which are found in desmosomes and adherens junctions in vertebrate cells.

There is evidence for some differences between catenins from various tissues. The α-catenin found in epithelial cells that interacts with E-cadherin is distinct from, but related to, a similar α-catenin expressed primarily in neural tissue.[31] These observations suggest that there may be differences in how the cadherin-cytoskeleton interactions are organized and regulated in various tissues.

Evidence for the association of catenins with cadherins is both direct and indirect. Immunolocalization studies show that cadherins and catenins are found in the same adhesion complexes, leading to the suggestion that they were somehow engaged in organizing or regulating receptor-cytoskeleton interactions. Immunoprecipitation data show that the two sets of molecules are co-precipitated with antibodies specific for the cadherins. Physical biochemical studies show that the complexes of cadherins (E-cadherin) and catenins can be isolated and characterized.[32] Such complexes contain all three catenins, with β-catenin being most firmly associated with the cadherin molecule itself. Cells in which a single catenin is missing fail to adhere to one another,[31] and cadherins will only form complexes with globular actin in the presence of all three catenins.[33] Thus, the catenins are required for cadherin function; they associate with the cytoplasmic domain of the receptor-forming complexes that mediate the interaction of the cadherins with the actin-containing cytoskeletal network of the cell.

Cadherins as Mediators of Morphogenetic Events

That cadherins mediate homophilic cell-cell adhesion (Fig. 9–4B) has been demonstrated by cell aggregation experiments. Evidence that they have the same function in situ is more difficult to come by, but nevertheless exists.

Immunolocalization data show cadherins to be localized to cell-cell borders or, in the case of desmosomes and adherens junctions,[34] to specific junctional complexes.

Cadherin expression is modulated during morphogenesis in the developing embryo. During gastrulation, cells of the epiblast, which initially express E-cadherin (L-CAM in the chick), cease expressing it and begin expressing N-cadherin as they become part of the mesoderm.[26,35] Similarly, as cells from the neural plate separate from the overlying ectoderm to form the neural tube, they switch from E-cadherin expression to N-cadherin expression. Changes in cadherin expression are associated with morphogenetic movements. As neural crest cells migrate from the neural ridge, cadherin expression is lost, only to be regained once they become part of the peripheral nervous system. This also occurs as cells from the tightly compacted somites begin to migrate. In this case, the cells cease to express N-cadherin prior to migration.

In general, during morphogenesis, cells move from one cell layer to become part of another. This movement is accompanied by a loss of cadherin expression and subsequent reexpression, usually of a different cadherin, at the time the cell is integrated into new tissue. This has led to the proposal that programmed cadherin expression is a fundamental part of the morphogenetic process.[36,37] Supporting this idea is the observation that inappropriate cadherin expression,[38,39] or the administration of anti-cadherin antibodies at times of maximum histogenesis in the developing embryo, results in the formation of abnormal tissue, or the failure of cells to separate from the initial embryonic site.[40]

Thus, the cadherins function as anchors holding cells together, as well as morphoregulatory molecules that help determine cell position within the body. Cell movement, at least within the developing embryo, is accompanied by loss of cadherin expression, perhaps required to free the cell from the tissue of origin. Cadherins then are reexpressed as cells become incorporated into new tissues. These properties of cadherins raise the possibility that changes in cadherin expression could play a role in tumor development and metastasis.

Expression of Cadherins Suppresses Cell Invasion: Studies with Cultured Cells

Insights into the possible role of cadherins in tumorigenesis have come from studies of a canine epithelial cell line termed MDCK (Madin-Darby canine kidney). Work with this cell line has revealed the importance of the cadherins for maintaining the polarity of epithelial cells and the integrity of epithelial sheets. MDCK cells express E-cadherin and form typical cobblestone-like monolayers in culture. They maintain epithelial cell polarity and transport properties[41,42] to the point of forming small dome-like bugles in the monolayer as a result of directional fluid transport. If these cells are plated in low Ca^{2+}–containing medium, they fail to form cell-cell junctions, and they fail to organize into sheets of polarized columnar epithelial cells. This is due to the inability of E-cadherins on adjacent cells to interact effectively with one another in low-calcium medium. Similarly, if MDCK cells or certain human breast cancer cells are grown in the presence of antibodies to E-cadherin, the cells become fibroblastic[43-45] and fail to assemble into a polarized epithelial sheet.

Based on the above observations and the fact that down-regulation of cadherin expression accompanies tissue separation and cell migration during embryonic development, it has been postulated that a loss of cadherin expression or a failure of cadherin function could facilitate tumor cell invasion. Experimental support for this concept

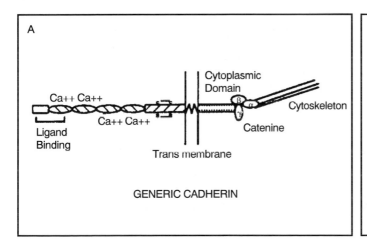

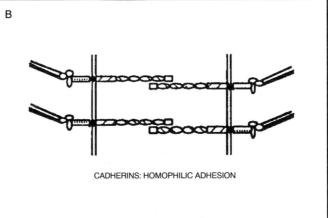

Figure 9–4. Schematic summary of cadherin structure and function in homophilic adhesion. This schematic model demonstrates the major properties of cadherins. *A*, The amino-terminal region is of major importance for the homophilic interactions (ligand binding). The cadherin domain structure with the Ca^{2+} binding motifs (ovals) is thought to stabilize the protein conformation. The carboxy-terminal region in the cytoplasm is complexed with the catenins (α, β, γ), which regulate the connections with the cytoskeletal elements of the cell. *B*, Cadherins promote Ca^{2+}-dependent, homophilic adhesion. This involves primarily the amino-terminal portion of the molecule, but the structural integrity of the disulfide linked region (S—S) near the transmembrane domain (*A*) appears also to be required.

comes from several observations,[46,47] with the most convincing evidence being generated using tumors derived from MDCK cells and mouse mammary glands.[47,48] Tumor cell lines used in these experiments were highly invasive in two in vitro assays. One involved the co-culture of tumor cells with pieces of embryonic chick heart. The tumor cells attached to fragments of the heart and invaded the myocardial tissue. The other involved plating cells on top of collagen gels and microscopically monitoring the invasion of the cells into the gel. Each invasive cell line failed to express E-cadherin. In both assays, nontumorigenic MDCK cells employed as controls were noninvasive. If the tumor cells were transfected with cDNA coding for E-cadherin, they lost their invasive phenotype. That is, they did not migrate into collagen gels, nor did they invade the myocardial fragments. If the transfected cells expressing E-cadherin were plated in the presence of antibodies that inhibited the cadherin-binding activity, they were once again invasive. When transfected and control cells were injected into nude mice, cells that continued to express E-cadherin formed well-differentiated, noninvasive tumors, whereas the nontransfected controls remained highly invasive. These observations are consistent with other reports in which invasiveness was inversely correlated with the level of E-cadherin expression in tumor cell lines.[49]

The correlation between cadherin expression and loss of the invasive phenotype extends to many experimental tumors. In general, cells remaining epitheloid in nature continue to express cadherins and are noninvasive when injected into animals. In contrast, cells from carcinomas with fibroblastoid phenotypes that are not expressing E-cadherin give rise to undifferentiated, highly invasive tumors.[50]

Members of the Cadherin Superfamily Are Tumor Suppressors in *Drosophila*

Further support for a regulatory role of cadherins is found in *Drosophila*.[51] Recessive lethal mutations of the *fat* locus result in hyperplasia of imaginal disc cells during larval development. Mitotic recombination within clones of cells results in overgrowth of cells and subsequent protrusions of patches of mutated tissue from the body of the fly. These areas of hyperplasia are surrounded by normal tissue, suggesting that the effect is limited to cells carrying the mutation and is not due to any secreted molecules. Thus, the inactivation of a cadherin gene can cause hyperplastic growth of epithelial-like cells in *Drosophila*, suggesting that cadherins not only may function to control cell adhesion, but also may regulate cell growth.

Cadherin Expression in Invasive Carcinomas

The obvious clinical corollary to the above observations in flies and mammalian cells is that highly differentiated, noninvasive, and nonmetastatic carcinomas will continue to express functional levels of cadherins, whereas poorly differentiated, highly invasive tumors will not. This correlation has been found to exist for squamous cell carcinomas of the head and neck.[52] Well-differentiated tumors continued to express E-cadherin at levels equal to that of surrounding, noninvolved stratified epithelium as determined by immunofluorescence and immunoblotting of tumor extracts. Tumors showing an intermediate phenotype (i.e., moderately differentiated tumors) were heterogeneous, showing reduced E-cadherin expression. Undifferentiated tumors as well as a lymph node metastasis all showed no signs of E-cadherin expression.

An examination of other tumors, however, shows a less precise correlation between tumor progression and E-cadherin expression. As in the previous example, the intensity of E-cadherin expression in a study of 44 human prostate tumors was inversely correlated with tumor grade,[53,54] the least well-differentiated tumors showed no E-cadherin expression, and tumors of intermediate grade showed heterogeneity in E-cadherin expression. However, metastatic lesions exhibited a variety of phenotypes with respect to E-cadherin expression. Two exhibited normal levels of expression; five were heterogeneous with tumors containing both E-cadherin–positive and E-cadherin–negative cells within the same lesion; and only one was completely E-cadherin negative.

Similarly, studies of tumors of the female reproductive tract also suggest that a loss of E-cadherin expression may not be a prerequisite for metastasis.[55] An examination of tumors of the uterus, cervix, and vagina indicated that all tumors continued to express E-cadherin at cell-cell borders at levels equivalent to those seen in normal tissue. This was not true of mesenchymal tumors, an observation that is consistent with that seen in epithelial cell lines, in which a change to fibroblastoid morphology was dependent on a loss of cadherin expression. Also, less well-differentiated areas of each of the tumors examined expressed lower levels of E-cadherin. However, in ten sets of primary and metastatic tumors examined, all the metastatic nodules expressed E-cadherin in a manner characteristic of the original tumor.

Analysis of cadherin expression in several other types of tumors also fails to show an absolute correlation between a loss of E-cadherin expression and metastasis. Studies including a series of 103 human gastric tumors[56] revealed that E-cadherin expression was maintained at either normal levels (42 per cent of tumors) or slightly reduced levels (58 per cent of tumors) in all tumors. Large, poorly differentiated, highly invasive, metastatic tumors, however, mostly exhibited reduced levels of cadherin expression, although some tumors of this type continued to express normal levels of E-cadherin. Tumors of the esophagus, stomach, and breast,[57] another series of gastric tumors,[58,59] and a group of 44 lung tumors,[60] as well as a variety of others,[59,61] showed the same trend. That is, cadherin expression was variable, ranging from nearly normal to absent. However, cadherin expression tended to be more reduced in the least well-differentiated tumors. Likewise, a careful comparison of tumor grade and E-cadherin expression by 120 different breast tumors revealed a strong correlation between the loss of E-cadherin expression or change in distribution within the cell and increased tumor invasiveness. Over 70 per cent of all lymph node metastases, and 85 per cent of distant metastases, showed a significant change in E-cadherin expression.[62]

A change in E-cadherin expression by a majority of epithelial tumors would appear to be an indication of increased metastatic potential. Even in those instances when surface expression of cadherins is normal, it is possible that cadherin function is compromised. Thus, whereas a loss of cadherin expression by various carcinomas is a strong indication of increased invasiveness, the continued, apparently normal expression, is not, in itself, a strong indicator of a less aggressive phenotype. Possible explanations for this are found in certain experimental tumors. For example, PC 9, a human lung carcinoma cell line, was found to express E-cadherin at normal levels, but the cell line was fibroblastic in morphology and exhibited an invasive phenotype. A careful examination of this line showed that it failed to make α-catenin, one of the cytoskeletal-associated molecules required for cadherin-cytoskeleton interactions. Thus, even though these cells produced E-cadherin, it could not function.[63] Interestingly, invasive gastric carcinomas have been described that continue to express E-cadherin but fail to express α-catenin,[63] possibly explaining their invasive phenotype.

Cadherin function may be affected by modifications of the receptor itself as well as the associated proteins. Examples of this are found in the response of epithelial cells or epitheloid tumors to various factors that induce cell proliferation, cell migration, and matrix invasion.[64,65] These factors include autocrine motility factor (AMF), migration-stimulating factor (MSF), scatter factor or hepatocyte growth factor (SF/HGF), and other growth factors, including epidermal growth factor (EGF), transforming growth factor α (TGF-α), insulin-like growth factor II (IGF-II), and acidic fibroblast growth factor (aFGF).[64] The effect of these factors on cell behavior has been studied in considerable detail using NBT-II rat bladder carcinoma cells[66] and MDCK cells.[67] Both lines undergo epithelial/mesenchymal transition and become fibroblastic, invasive, and highly motile on exposure to SF/HGF or aFGF. Although there is an internalization of desmosomes during this process, there is no change in E-cadherin expression, but rather a redistribution of cadherins.[67] In fact, transfection of NBT-II cells with E-cadherin cDNA and the subsequent overproduction of E-cadherin had no effect on the ability of aFGF to induce the invasive behavior of NBT-II cells.[68] Thus, cells can be made to behave as highly invasive tumor cells while continuing to express cadherins. The cadherins are, in these instances, clearly not functioning either to promote cell-cell adhesion or to suppress the invasive phenotype. How these cadherins are being functionally inactivated is not known at the present time. It is interesting, however, that many of these motility-inducing factors are ligands for transmembrane protein tyrosine kinases.[64] It may be, therefore, that the function of cadherins can be affected by phosphorylation of either the cadherin itself or other cadherin-interactive proteins, such as the catenins. In fact, cadherin-mediated cell-cell interactions can be perturbed by phosphorylation of tyrosines within the cadherin-catenin complex.[69]

INTEGRINS

Once a cell has broken from the tumor mass, perhaps as a result of a loss of functional cadherins and a disruption of regulatory cell-cell interactions, it must move beyond a basement membrane, traverse the interstitium, and enter the blood stream. This involves the activity of extracellular proteinases and cell surface molecules that are capable of recognizing interstitial extracellular matrix (see Fig. 9–1). The receptors for these extracellular matrix molecules are members of an adhesion receptor family called the integrins (Fig. 9–5).

The integrins are a recently recognized family of receptors expressed on the surface of most cells.[70] Integrins serve as receptors for extracellular matrix molecules required for the interaction of cells with basement membranes and for the migration of cells through the interstitium.[71] They also serve as receptors engaged in cell-cell adhesion during lymphocyte homing, white cell–endothelial cell interactions, and T-cell killing.[12] They are important in blood clotting and include the platelet receptor glycoprotein IIb-IIIa, which, when mutated as in the case of patients with Glanzmann's thrombasthenia, results in bleeding disorders. Mutations involving the integrins expressed on white cells, as in patients with leukocyte adhesion deficiency (LAD), result in the loss of the ability of neutrophils to bind to endothelial cells at sites of inflammation.[72,73] The life of such patients is compromised by recurring infections.

Integrins are the targets of therapeutic interventions in inflammation-based pathologic conditions such as ischemia, arthritis, and asthma. They are thought to be important in vascular disorders such as atherosclerosis, and are absolutely required for normal morphogenesis during embryonic development[74] as well as wound healing and endometrial function.[75] They even serve as receptors for certain echoviruses.[76] Thus, integrins play a central role in many important biologic phenomena and, as is discussed later in this chapter, are probably important in tumor invasion and metastasis.

The Integrin Receptor Family

Integrins are heterodimers consisting of an α subunit, noncovalently associated with a β subunit (Fig. 9–5). To date, there are eight known β subunits and 14 α subunits, not including alternatively spliced forms.[1] These are organized into 20 different integrins in mammalian systems. This does not include the homologues of mammalian integrins in such diverse species as fruit flies[77,78] and frogs.[79,80]

Given the diversity and ever-increasing number of integrins being discovered, the development of a workable nomenclature has been something of a problem. A solution to this problem was suggested once it was realized, through gene cloning and immunologic studies, that several groups were working with related receptors, and that receptor variety was created by the interaction of various β subunits with several different α subunits. This resulted in the grouping of integrins into subfamilies each sharing a common β subunit[70] (Fig. 9–5). According to this nomenclature, the different β subunits are distinguished by a numerical subscript (i.e. β_1, β_2, β_3, etc.). The α subunits are distinguished by either a numerical subscript or a subscript letter indicating ligand specificity. The β_1 integrins include those primarily involved in cell-matrix adhesion, serving as receptors for laminin, collagen, and fibronectin. The β_2 integrins are limited exclusively to white cells and include integrins involved in white cell–endothelial cell interactions as well as T-cell killing. The β_3 integrins are found primarily on platelets and include the platelet glycoprotein IIb-IIIa, now designated $\alpha_{IIb}\beta_3$. Figure 9–5 contains a listing of all known integrins grouped according to major subfamilies.[1]

A few general principles can be gleaned from examining Figure 9–5. Many of the β subunits can combine with a number of different α subunits. There is selectivity, however, and a β subunit can only combine with certain α subunits. Thus, although β_1 can combine with α_1 through α_8, it is never found in association with α_L or α_{IIb}. Some β subunits, however, are more restricted in their α subunit repertoire, being limited to a single subunit.

Ligand specificity is determined by a particular αβ pair. The β_1 subunit combined with the α_5 subunit constitutes a fibronectin receptor, but in combination with α_6 it forms a laminin receptor. The molecular basis of α subunit selection is not understood. It is clear, however, that neither subunit can function by itself.[81]

There are α subunits that can combine with more than

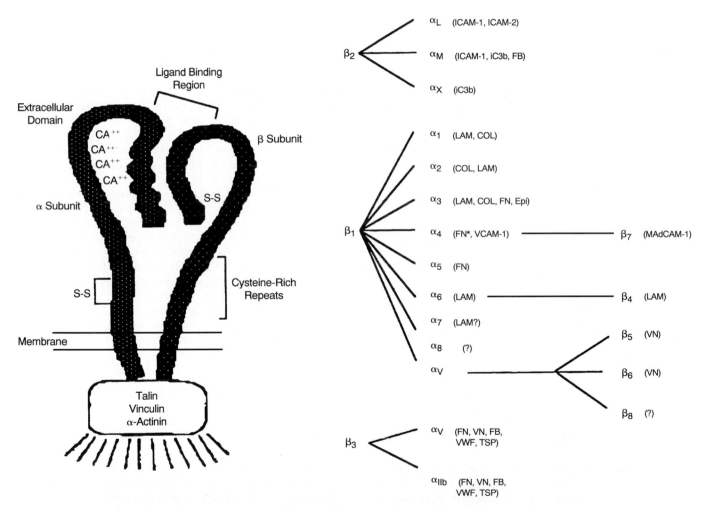

Figure 9–5. Schematic summary of integrin structure and ligand specificity. Integrins are composed of two noncovalently associated subunits designated α and β. Both subunits are integral membrane proteins. The extracellular domains contain the ligand-binding region. The α subunit contains amino acid sequences that coordinate divalent cation binding (Ca^{++}). The β subunit contains four cysteine-rich repeats within the stem of the "question mark" model shown here. The large loop in the amino terminus of the extracellular domain of the β subunit is stabilized by intrachain disulfide bonding (S—S). The cytoplasmic domains of both subunits are relatively small. Cytoskeletal-associated proteins (talin, vinculin, α-actinin) link the integrins via the cytoplasmic domain of the β subunit to the actin-containing cytoskeleton. Known αβ heterodimer pairs are joined by lines. The ligands are designated in parentheses. iC3b, complement-binding fragment; FB, fibrinogen; LAM, laminin; COL, collagen; FN, fibronectin; FN*, cell-binding domain; Epi, epiligrin; MadCAM-1, mucosal addressin; VN, vinculin; VWF, von Willebrand factor; TSP, thrombospondin; others are as in the text.

one β subunit. Probably the most promiscuous α subunit is α_v, originally described as part of the vitronectin receptor. This α subunit is found in combination with five different β subunits. Each α_v-containing integrin has different properties. For example, $\alpha_v\beta_3$ can serve as a receptor for a wide variety of ligands, including fibrinogen, fibronectin, vitronectin, thrombospondin, osteopontin, and collagens. In contrast, $\alpha_v\beta_5$ is strictly a vitronectin receptor. The molecular basis of this difference is not known because we do not have a complete idea of the molecular configuration of the ligand-binding site.

Integrins can serve as receptors for multiple ligands. Although this is not always the case, at least half of the known integrins interact with more than one ligand. This has led to a search for common binding domains within various ligands because, for the most part, the integrin ligands are large, complex molecules. Interestingly, the recognition domains on many ligands have been reduced to sequences of as little as three to six amino acids. The paradigm for this has been work involving the fibronectin receptor $\alpha_5\beta_1$. By analyzing the effect of fibronectin peptides of ever-decreasing size on cell attachment to fibronectin and on receptor-ligand binding, it was found that the interaction of this receptor with its ligand could be blocked by a tripeptide consisting of the amino acids arginine, glycine, and aspartic acid (RGD).[82–84] Experiments in which exposure to this tripeptide disrupted embryonic development,[85,86] cell adhesion and migration,[87] and tumor metastasis[88,89] emphasized even further the role of domains containing this sequence in receptor ligand recognition.

Interestingly, it was also found that the binding affinity of the fibronectin receptor for its ligand became weaker as the size of the peptide fragment was decreased. This observation suggested that, whereas integrin-fibronectin recognition may involve the RGD sequence, the actual receptor ligand binding involved other domains within the fibronectin molecule that acted synergistically to stabilize the molecular complex.[90] This emphasizes the fact that ligand recognition occurs within the context of the three-dimensional structure of the molecule.

Because the RGD sequence can be found in many molecules, it was thought that this might represent a universal recognition sequence for integrins that attach to the various extracellular matrix molecules.[83] This did not turn out to be the case. There are a number of integrins that do not recognize RGD sequences on their ligands. Even among integrins that recognize fibronectin, they do not all interact exclusively with the RGD-containing region of the molecule. For example, $\alpha_4\beta_1$ recognizes a domain on fibronectin that does not include the RGD-binding site.[91–93]

The ligands (counterreceptors) for integrins involved in cell-cell recognition include receptors that are members of the immunoglobulin superfamily. In instances when both members of an adhesion complex have been independently described as receptors (immunoglobulin superfamily molecules were independently identified as receptors involved in lymphocyte trafficking and diapodesis), the intercellular adhesive event is considered the result of a receptor-counterreceptor interaction.

The ligand recognized by a particular integrin may be influenced by the cell in which it is expressed.[94] This suggests that the molecular microenvironment on the cell surface can influence integrin function. This could include proteins such as the integrin-associated proteins,[95] as well as the composition of the lipid bilayer.[96] Both the kind and concentration of divalent cations in the surrounding medium can influence integrin-ligand binding.[97–99] More recently, the possibility of integrin modifications through changes in glycosylation,[100,101] phosphorylation,[102–104] or amino acid composition resulting from alternative mRNA splicing[105–111] have been shown to affect integrin function.

There are multiple integrins for many ligands. Why a cell would require more than one receptor for collagen or laminin, for example, is not clear. It has been demonstrated that integrins transmit signals across the membrane into the cell,[112–117] and different integrins may transmit different messages. Thus, if integrins are capable of regulating cell behavior, physiology, or morphology, it may be that each of these different integrins plays a separate role in these processes, and a cell requires multiple receptors for this purpose.

Integrin Structure-Function Correlations

Most of our knowledge of integrin structure-function relationships has come from work with platelet glycoprotein $\alpha_{IIb}\beta_3$,[118] and from the fact that the complete cDNAs for all the known integrin subunits have been isolated for both sequencing and experimental purposes. The first β subunit to be sequenced was the avian β_1 subunit.[119] The characteristics of β subunits deduced from this information could be generalized to all presently known β subunits with the exception of β_4. The β subunits range in size from 90 to 120 kDa. They can be divided into three domains: a large, approximately 75-kDa amino-terminal extracellular domain; a hydrophobic transmembrane domain; and a short, approximately 50–amino acid, cytoplasmic carboxy-terminal domain. It is in this region that the β_4 subunit differs from all others. This subunit has an extremely large cytoplasmic domain consisting of over 1000 amino acids, which brings its total size to approximately 180 kDa.[120,121]

The β subunits are highly disulfide–cross-linked molecules, containing up to 56 cysteine residues. Although there is some variability in the total number of cysteine residues, they are located in homologous positions on all β subunits.[122] Most of these residues are found in four cysteine-rich repeats on the extracellular domain of the subunit. The conserved positioning of these cysteines suggests that all β subunits are folded into a homologous tertiary structure and that the precision of this structure is essential for integrin function. Careful chemical analyses of the platelet β_3 subunit have revealed that, for the most part, these cysteine residues pair with their nearest neighbor.[123,124] There are, however, two important long-range disulfide bonds. One links the first cysteine (C1) at position 7 with C16 at position 445. The result is that the molecule is folded into a "question mark"–like configuration, shown in Figure 9–5. The second long-range disulfide bond is thought to be between C14 at position 415 and C54 at position 672,[124] theoretically resulting in a more globular structure. The existence of this second long-range bond has been questioned, because such folding is inconsistent with electron micrographs of purified integrins,[125–127] and these cysteines are among those missing in integrins with fewer than 56 cysteines.

Evidence for the function of specific regions of the extracellular domain of the subunit has come from studying naturally occurring mutations found in Glanzmann's thrombasthenia patients,[128] the mutated β_2 subunits found in LAD patients,[73,129] and chemical cross-linking.[130,131] These examples suggest that the ligand-binding domain of this subunit rests somewhere within the first 200 amino acids of the extracellular domain. A single amino acid mutation at position 119 within this region renders $\alpha_{IIb}\beta_3$ incapable of ligand binding,[132] and a mutation at the corresponding position in the β_1 subunit has a similar effect.[133] The epitopes of monoclonal antibodies that block platelet aggregation have been mapped to this region of both the β_3[134] and β_1[135] subunits. Consistent with these observations is the fact that a 19–amino acid peptide found in this region of the molecule and conserved among all β subunits blocks $\alpha_{IIb}\beta_3$ binding to von Willebrand factor and to vitronectin.[136] Whether other regions of the subunit are involved in ligand binding has not been determined, but it should be noted that the epitopes of two other adhesion-perturbing monoclonal antibodies were mapped to a more distal region of the β_1 subunit.[135] This region also could be involved directly in ligand binding, or it could represent a "regulatory" domain of the molecule that can affect ligand binding secondarily. This is supported by the observation that among the monoclonal antibodies whose epitopes map to this region is one that activates laminin binding by β_1 integrins.[137]

It should be noted that this molecule is rather "malleable" in that structural changes in the β subunit have been observed in response to ligand binding. These changes can be seen as an expression of new antibody-binding sites following receptor-ligand interactions in platelets.[138–140] Similarly, antibodies are capable of activating or changing the ligand specificity of the β_3,[141,142] β_2[143] and β_1[137,144,145] subunits. This undoubtedly occurs as a result of antibody-induced conformational changes in the molecule itself.

The transmembrane domains of the β subunits apparently serve as membrane insertion sequences because this region of two different subunits can be interchanged without any effect on receptor function as measured by ligand binding, participation in cell substratum adhesion, or α subunit selection.[146]

As with the cadherins, the integrins not only interact with extracellular ligands, they also interact with cytoskeletal elements. Direct evidence for this initially was obtained by equilibrium gel filtration experiments in which it was shown that purified integrins could bind fibronectin or laminin[147] as well as the cytoskeletal-associated protein talin.[148] It also was shown that integrins would interact with vinculin, a second cytoskeletal-associated protein, only after talin was bound, providing the first evidence to support the model of integrin organization and function, shown schematically in Figure 9–5. Integrins also bind to a second cytoskeletal-associated protein termed "α-actinin."[149,150]

It was not until vectors carrying β_1 cDNA with deleted cytoplasmic domains were available that it became possible to show directly that the cytoplasmic domain of the β subunit interacted with cytoskeletal-associated proteins.[151–153] A detailed mutational analysis of this domain has suggested that there is considerable structure within this region of the subunit that must be maintained for it to interact with the cytoskeleton.[152,153]

The cytoplasmic domain of the β subunit appears itself sufficient to determine the distribution of integrins within the cell. Evidence for this comes from experiments in which a chimeric receptor was constructed consisting of the interleukin-2 receptor carrying the cytoplasmic domain of either the β_1 subunit or the α_5 subunit.[154] If the chimeric receptor carried the β_1 cytoplasmic domain, it was localized to focal contacts, the points of interaction between cultured cells and the extracellular matrix, in the absence of any ligand. If the receptor carried the α_5 cytoplasmic domain, it remained diffusely distributed throughout the surface membrane. The chimeric receptor carrying the β_1 cytoplasmic domain therefore behaved as if it were a ligand-occupied receptor. Thus, for the most part, the β subunit cytoplasmic domain appears to play an important role in mediating integrin interactions with the microfilament system of the cell.

The α subunits, which make up the other part of an integrin heterodimer, are usually slightly larger than the accompanying β subunit, running in size between 120 and 140 kDa, with the exception of α_1, which is about 180 kDa.[155,156] As with the β subunits, integrin α subunits are transmembrane molecules with the amino terminus making up the extracellular domain, followed by a transmembrane domain and finally a short cytoplasmic domain (Fig. 9–5). In certain instances, the extracellular domain is posttranslationally cleaved into a short (25 to 30 kDa) membrane-associated fragment that is disulfide bonded to the remaining 100-kDa amino-terminal fragment. The functional significance of this cleavage is not clear because many α subunits are not modified in this manner. A further modification found in the α subunits associated with β_2 integrins, as well as α_2 and α_4, is the presence of an additional insert termed "I." The functional significance of this additional domain is not known, but it may be involved in divalent cation binding and, in the case of α_2, echovirus attachment.

Unlike the β subunits, the cytoplasmic domains of each α subunit are significantly different from one another. This difference is sufficiently marked that antibodies against cytoplasmic domain peptides can be used to distinguish one α subunit from another. The function of the α cytoplasmic domain is not clear, but evidence suggests that it may be regulatory in nature, controlling the distribution of the receptor as well as certain functions. For example, a heterodimer made up of an intact β subunit and α subunit with a truncated cytoplasmic domain is swept to focal contacts even in the absence of a ligand.[157] The α subunit cytoplasmic domain appears to regulate negatively the positioning of integrins, keeping them distributed throughout the cell surface. This regulation apparently is released on ligand binding, allowing the integrin to become part of an adhesive complex. This cytoplasmic domain also can influence the function of the integrin once it has bound to a particular ligand.[158]

The cytoplasmic domain of the α subunit appears to regulate certain aspects of receptor function. These include ligand binding, cell migration, and extracellular matrix modification. For example, $\alpha_{IIb}\beta_3$ receptors in which the cytoplasmic domain of the α_{IIb} subunit has been deleted show an increased binding affinity for fibrinogen as well as the ability to bind to an activation-dependent monoclonal antibody.[159] Such a receptor therefore behaves as an activated receptor. Replacement of the α_{IIb} cytoplasmic domain with the original cytoplasmic domain, but not with the cytoplasmic domain of α_5, restored normal receptor-binding properties.

The cytoplasmic domain of the α subunit also determines the behavior of the cell following ligand binding. Cells attach to collagen gels via the $\alpha_2\beta_1$ collagen receptor. After a period of time, the collagen gels are retracted as a result of the adhesive interaction between the cells and the collagen. If cells expressing a chimeric α_2 subunit carrying an α_5 or α_4 cytoplasmic domain are similarly plated on collagen gels, the cells are no longer capable of remodeling the collagen gel even though they can adhere to and spread perfectly well on the collagen matrix. They are unable to apply the contractual force necessary to cause the collagen gel to retract, presumably because of the absence of the appropriate cytoplasmic domain.[160] Interestingly, cells expressing integrins consisting of a chimeric α_2 subunit carrying an α_4 cytoplasmic domain migrated more freely on collagen than did cells expressing wild-type $\alpha_2\beta_1$ or the α_2 chimeric subunit carrying an α_5 cytoplasmic domain. The mechanism whereby the various α subunit cytoplasmic domains affect integrin function is not known, but it appears that each α cytoplasmic domain may influence integrins in different ways. Consistent with this is the fact that, except for a short sequence of amino acids near the site of insertion into the cell membrane, each α subunit possesses a distinctly different cytoplasmic domain that is conserved throughout many species.

Figure 9–2 is a schematic summation of integrin organization within a focal contact. Focal contacts are adhesive organelles[161] in which integrins, extracellular matrix molecules, cytoskeletal molecules,[162] and various regulatory molecules such as protein kinases[102,163] are concentrated. They are responsible for the tight adhesive interaction between cells and the extracellular matrix. The formation of focal contacts is initiated by receptor-ligand binding, which probably stimulates the generation of a series of signals required for the molecular rearrangements leading to receptor clustering. It is thought that cell migration requires the constant assembly and disassembly of focal contact–like structures.

In Situ Integrin Function

Most of our knowledge of integrin function has come from cell culture experiments in which cell-matrix inter-actions are blocked by reagents known to interfere with receptor ligand binding.[1,71] The results of such experiments have been confirmed genetically and in vivo using similar reagents. Genetically, it already has been pointed out that the bleeding disorder Glanzmann's thrombasthenia and the leukocyte function disorder LAD are the result of mutations in the β subunit of two different subfamilies of integrins. In the former case, point mutations within the β_3 subunit impair platelet aggregation and clot formation. In the latter case, point mutations within the β_2 subunit result in the failure of α subunit pairing and lack of integrin expression on the cell surface. In this case, the severity of the phenotype can be quite variable, ranging from mild to severe depending on how severely $\alpha\beta$ subunit association has been compromised.

Integrins are expressed in *Drosophila*, where they are known as position-specific (PS) antigens[77,164] because they are expressed in specific locations at specific times during early fly development. Loss of the PS antigens is lethal because they are found at the site of muscle insertion and, the first time muscle contraction occurs in the young embryo, the muscles are pulled from the points of insertion and the embryo dies. By delaying expression or limiting it to specific tissues, it has been shown that integrins are required for adhesion of the cell layers making up the wing.[78] Further delays in mutation expression have shown that integrins also are required for appropriate orientation of facets within the developing eye of the insect.[165] These experiments directly demonstrate the requirement of integrins in organ formation.

Within mammalian systems, it has been demonstrated that anti-integrin antibodies interfere with neural crest outmigration and muscle formation in the developing avian embryo.[166–169] Similarly, integrins have been shown to be required for neuronal development in the bird. In this case, retrovirus vectors carrying antisense integrin sequences were generated in cells using retrovirus vectors to suppress the β_1 subunit. There was a significant reduction in integrin mRNA as well as expression of the β_1 subunit. This resulted in altered neuroblast migration.[170]

Less direct evidence for integrin requirements for histogenesis and the anchoring of cells in position in tissues comes from the fact that there appear to be tissue-specific profiles of integrin expression. For example, epithelial cells express a different combination of integrins than endothelial cells, and large vessel endothelium expresses different integrins than capillary endothelium.[171–173] These profiles change during both normal and disease processes. During wound healing, the pattern of integrin expression by epithelial sheets is changed.[174–176] Among the changes is the up-regulation of the $\alpha_5\beta_1$ fibronectin receptor, which is not expressed in adult resting epithelial cells. During embryonic development, the pattern of integrin expression changes or is modulated with time in most tissues, not taking on the adult repertoire until histogenesis is complete,[177,178] further suggesting that there is a program of integrin expression that is required at specific times during tissue formation and repair. Direct proof of this hypothesis will require the creation of mouse models in which the function of various integrin subunits is compromised or lost.

Integrin Regulation and Signal Transduction

The foregoing observations are particularly important in light of the fact that evidence is accumulating that integrins clearly participate in transmitting signals from the outside to the inside of the cell. These signals affect cell physiology, shape, and differentiation, and hence add another dimension to the role integrins may play in the cell. Signal transduction through the fibronectin receptor has been shown to induce proteolytic enzymes such as collagenase and stromelysin, required for basement membrane penetration and cell migration.[179] It also has been shown that ligand binding by β_1 integrins is required for myoblast differentiation.[180]

The mechanisms by which integrins influence these processes have not yet been determined. However, it recently has been shown that integrin clustering[104,112,113] or integrin-mediated cell-matrix interactions[117,163,181–184] result in the phosphorylation of integrins and integrin-associated proteins thought to mediate integrin-cytoskeleton interactions. It is clear, given the fact that many cells cannot replicate unless they are in contact with a solid surface, that integrin-ligand interactions also might transmit signals required to initiate DNA synthesis and subsequent mitosis. Signal transduction pathways may involve Src kinase and a newly described protein tyrosine phosphokinase found in focal adhesions, termed FAK.[163,185–187] Other signal transduction pathways, including those involving phospholipases, and phosphatidylinositol turnover also have been implicated in signal transduction via integrin clustering or ligand binding.[104] The rapid elevation of intracellular pH and Ca^{2+} [188] is particularly significant, because these changes can be correlated with anchorage-independent growth, again suggesting that integrin occupancy can play a role in controlling cell division.

In addition to participating in signal transduction from the outside of the cell in, integrins also participate in signal transduction from the inside out. In this case, the signal transduction results in integrin activation. The presence of integrins on the cell surface does not necessarily mean that they are functional. Perhaps the best example of this involves platelets that express the integrin $\alpha_{IIb}\beta_3$ on their surface, and yet aggregate and participate in clot formation only when appropriate. This is because this particular integrin is capable of being activated; that is, the receptor undergoes a structural change as a result of signals being transmitted from within the cell that somehow increases its ligand-binding activity. These signals are generated as a result of platelet activation by agonists such as collagen or thrombin.

The signal pathways involved with integrins include the activation of G proteins, changes in intracellular pH and divalent cation concentration, turnover of phosphatidylinositol and protein kinase activation.[104] The integrins on white cells undergo activation as a result of cytokine stimulation, phorbol ester treatment, and exposure to inflammatory mediators.[1,12] They also can be activated as a result of antigen stimulation[189,190] or the binding of ligands to other receptors such as the platelet–endothelial cell adhesion molecule (PECAM-1)[191,192] found on the surface of certain T cells. As in the case of platelets, this activation

results in an antibody-detectable change in the structure of integrins already present on the cell surface and not the synthesis of a new receptor.

The organization of integrins into adhesive structures also must involve intercellular communication between different receptors. This is suggested by experiments in which fibroblasts plated on fibronectin fail to form focal contacts unless they are expressing glycosaminoglycans on the cell surface.[193] Focal contact formation can be blocked with small glycosaminoglycan fragments.[194] This effect may be mediated via heparan sulfate proteoglycan on the cell surface binding to the appropriate domain on fibronectin and may require message transduction via systems involving protein kinase C.[195]

Integrin expression on cells is subject to regulation. As pointed out earlier, integrins on white cells are *functionally* up-regulated in response to inflammatory cytokines. However, integrins on other cells, such as fibroblasts[196] and tumor cells,[197] also respond to cytokines such as TGF-β. This response involves the biosynthesis and transport of new integrins to the cell surface rather than the activation of existing integrins. The integrins of the endometrial epithelium also appear to respond to changes in hormones during the normal menstrual cycle[75] by expressing the vitronectin receptor $\alpha_v\beta_3$ as well as the collagen receptor $\alpha_1\beta_1$. Interestingly, the vitronectin receptor expression corresponds to the time of implantation, suggesting a role for integrins in the initial events of trophoblast-endometrium interaction. These examples may be relevant to tumor cell behavior, particularly in tumor cells that respond either to cytokines or to steroid hormones.

Integrins clearly are involved in regulatory events within the cell. Not only can integrins serve to generate signals that control cell behavior, they themselves respond to signals required to regulate their function, expression, and organization within the cell. They participate in a cascade of signaling events required for the maintenance of normal cell behavior. A breakdown of events anywhere within this complex pattern of intermolecular communication could result in abnormal cell movement or replication, either of which could possibly lead to unregulated cell growth and metastasis.

Integrin Expression by Tumors and Homologous Normal Tissue

With the availability of monoclonal antibodies specific for integrin α subunits, it has been possible to compare, by immunohistochemistry, integrin expression in both primary and metastatic tumors as well as in surrounding normal tissue. These comparisons have been made for carcinomas of the lung, gut, breast, and prostate, as well as for lymphomas, leukemias, melanomas, glioblastomas,[198] and neuroblastomas (reviewed in refs. 199–201). In all cases, the pattern of integrin expression was different from that of surrounding normal tissue.

The integrins found primarily in normal epithelium of the adult are the collagen/laminin receptors $\alpha_2\beta_1$, $\alpha_3\beta_1$, and $\alpha_6\beta_1$. In general, the less well-differentiated the tumor, the more different from normal the integrin expression pattern is found to be. Poorly differentiated carcinomas of the skin,[202,203] colon,[204] breast,[205,206] pancreas,[207] and lung[208,209] tend to show a general loss of integrin expression, with no particular pattern emerging. In more highly differentiated tumors, or regions of the tumor still contacting the basement membrane, the pattern of integrin expression tends to be more nearly normal. These data suggest that contact with an intact basement membrane might influence the integrin profile and hence the behavior of the tumor.

To date, the only tumor system in which a consistent, reproducible, and predictable change in integrin expression is correlated with tumor progression is the melanoma.[210] Integrin expression during the progression from melanocyte to highly metastatic melanoma has been followed by examining the integrin profile of normal melanocytes, melanocytes in preneoplastic nevi, and melanocytes from primary and metastatic tumors from the same individual. In all cases, the integrin profile of melanocytes from skin and nevi as well as tumor cells within a primary, nonmetastatic melanoma show the same integrin profile as epithelial cells. However, melanomas exhibit a change in integrin profile concomitant with a change in growth pattern from the radial growth phase (RGP), in which they form invasive but localized tumors, to the vertical growth phase (VGP), in which they become highly metastatic.[211,212] At this point, the cells begin expressing the vitronectin receptor $\alpha_v\beta_3$.[210] This receptor is also found in all the metastases derived from the original VGP melanomas. Other new integrins also are expressed by the more malignant melanomas. These include $\alpha_4\beta_1$,[210] the receptor for fibronectin, and the immunoglobulin superfamily receptor VCAM-1, as well as the platelet receptor $\alpha_{IIb}\beta_3$.[213] Expression of these integrins is not, however, consistently correlated with the metastatic potential.

The significance of changes in integrin expression on tumor cell behavior has been examined in three different ways. Investigators have attempted to block the establishment of metastatic lesions with specific agents (antibodies or peptides) that perturb integrin-ligand interaction. Alternatively, mutant cell lines have been established that fail to express a particular receptor in an attempt to correlate the change of the integrin expression with changes in metastatic potential. Finally, tumor cells have been transfected with full-length cDNAs coding for various integrin subunits and the effect of the expression of a new integrin on their metastatic properties has been evaluated.

In experiments using a murine B16-F10 melanoma, it was found that simultaneous administration of RGD-containing peptides would diminish greatly the number of lung metastatic nodules.[88] These experiments were confirmed by others using cyclic peptides containing the RGD sequence, which have a longer half-life in vivo and are more effective competitive inhibitors,[214] or RGD-mimicking reagents from snake venoms, named "dysintegrins," that are far more effective than most RGD-containing peptides in interfering with integrin-ligand binding.[215] These experiments have been interpreted to support a role for integrins in the establishment of metastatic nodules.

The vitronectin receptor $\alpha_v\beta_3$ has been implicated in tumor invasion and metastasis in experiments in which cells were selected for properties consistent with increased tumorigenicity. A subpopulation of cells was selected from a melanoma for their ability to adhere to the vascular endothelium of frozen sections of lymph nodes. These cells showed increased metastatic capacity and consistently expressed $\alpha_v\beta_3$.[216] Conversely, $\alpha_v\beta_3$-negative cells were selected from a population of metastatic human melanoma cells.[217] When these cells were injected subcutaneously into nude mice, they were found to have lost their ability to form tumors and metastasize, again pointing to a role for the vitronectin receptor in the metastatic process. However, when these cells were transfected with cDNA coding for the α_v subunit, thereby restoring the synthesis of the vitronectin receptor, they once again could form tumors, but these tumors did not metastasize. In this case, it would appear that $\alpha_v\beta_3$ could be involved in the regulation of cell growth or adhesion, but not directly in metastasis.

The interpretation of the role of integrins in tumor invasion or metastasis is more complicated than would be expected if these receptors are merely serving to promote adhesion. For example, treatment of melanoma cells with antibodies specific for the vitronectin receptor *stimulated* invasion through basement membrane matrices in vitro.[218] This occurred whether cells were treated with antibodies that block the binding of this receptor to its ligand or with antibodies having no functional effect on the integrins. In fact, the inclusion of vitronectin in the basement membrane matrix also increased the invasive behavior of the cells. Receptor occupancy by either the natural ligand, vitronectin, or by antibodies promoted movement of cells into the matrix. This increased matrix invasion was attributed to the increased production of collagenase resulting from vitronectin receptor occupancy, further stressing the role of integrins as signal transducers as well as adhesion receptors.

The effect of integrin expression on tumor cell behavior has been examined in other systems. Chinese hamster ovary (CHO) cells selected for low expression of the fibronectin receptor $\alpha_5\beta_1$ were more tumorigenic in nude mice; that is, they grew faster when injected subcutaneously than did cells expressing $\alpha_5\beta_1$.[219] Consistent with this observation is the fact that transfection of these CHO cells with cDNA coding for the α_5 subunit resulted in a loss of the cells' ability to grow in soft agar as well as a loss of tumorigenicity in nude mice.[220] In this respect, the $\alpha_5\beta_1$ fibronectin receptor appeared to suppress the tumorigenic phenotype of CHO cells. In contrast, rhabdomyosarcoma cells became metastatic after transfection with cDNA coding for the α_2 subunit of the collagen receptor.[221] The mechanisms accounting for these changes and their relevance to in situ development of metastases are not clear.

The role of integrins in cell movement over and through three-dimensional matrices in vitro has been examined as a model for tumor invasiveness. Tumor cells will migrate over the matrix and into a three-dimensional gel. Monoclonal antibodies and synthetic peptides that inhibit integrin-mediated adhesion to fibronectin or laminin will inhibit this activity.[222–225] Reagents that block the function of β_1 integrins are particularly effective when applied to human fibrosarcoma cells, bladder carcinoma cells, and virus-transformed cells.[222] Thus, integrins that interact with extracellular matrix molecules facilitate cell movement through the extracellular matrix, one of the initial requirements of tumor invasive activity.

The β_2 integrins, such as $\alpha_L\beta_2$, found primarily on lymphocytes and white cells, have been implicated in lymphoma metastasis to the liver. In experimental systems, it was shown that antibodies to this integrin could block lymphoma cell adhesion to hepatocytes,[226] and lymphomas not expressing $\alpha_L\beta_1$ failed to establish metastases in the liver.[227] Others have failed to find any significant correlation between the expression of this particular integrin and the hematogenous spread of lymphomas.

In summary, there is to date no predictably consistent correlation between the expression of an integrin or combination of integrins and tumorigenicity or metastatic potential, with the single exception of $\alpha_v\beta_3$ expression in VGP and metastatic melanomas. There is, however, an apparent down-regulation of integrin expression by most carcinomas in situ. What this means in terms of tumor cell behavior is not yet known. Experimental evidence suggests that integrins can control tumor growth, promote tumor cell migration and invasion through basement membranes, and facilitate the metastatic process. The fact that integrins serve regulatory functions within cells affecting cell behavior, cell replication, and cell differentiation, suggests that meaningful correlations between integrin expression and tumor cell behavior may require a combinatorial analysis of the integrin repertoire in a given cell, as the combination of integrins expressed by a cell may be more important than the presence or absence of a single receptor.

ADHESION RECEPTORS AND VASCULAR DISSEMINATION OF METASTATIC CELLS

At this point, we have examined adhesion receptors that are likely involved in the disruption of cell-cell interactions, leading to uncontrolled cell growth, eventual destruction of basement membranes, and cell movement through the interstitium and across the vascular endothelium into the circulatory system. Once within the circulation, tumor cells may establish metastatic nodules at various sites throughout the body. To accomplish this, cells must interact with the vascular endothelium, and move across the endothelial lining and into the vascular bed as described earlier. Among the major adhesion molecules likely to be involved in this cascade are the selectins[15,228]; members of the immunoglobulin superfamily,[12,205,229,230] including VCAM-1, ICAM-1, ICAM-2, and ICAM-3, carcinoembryonic antigen (CEA), PECAM-1, and "deleted in colorectal carcinoma" (DDC), mucosal addressin cell adhesion molecule (MAdCAM-1)[21]; integrins; CD44,[231] a glycoprotein found on lymphocytes[232] having sequence homologies with members of the cartilage link protein family[233]; and organ-specific endothelial cell adhesion molecules such as Lu-ECAM-1 (lung–endothelial cell adhesion molecule).[234]

Selectins: Oligosaccharide-Recognizing Molecules Mediating Cellular Interactions with the Vascular Endothelium

The interaction of lymphocytes with the high endothelium of lymph node vessels, or of neutrophils and monocytes with activated endothelial cells at sites of inflammation, requires that cells bind to the endothelium under conditions of flow, attach firmly, move between endothelial cells, cross the basement membrane, and enter the surrounding stroma. These initial interactions could involve receptors with properties like the selectins, characterized in Table 9–2. At present three have been identified. They are named for the cell on which they were initially described.

L-selectin (leukocyte selectin) is expressed on lymphocytes, neutrophils, macrophages, and monocytes. It originally was identified on mouse cells using the monoclonal antibody MEL-14 that blocked lymphocyte adhesion to high endothelium exposed on frozen sections of lymph nodes,[235] and was known as the murine lymph node homing receptor. The human equivalent was designated Leu-8[236] or LAM-1.[237]

E-selectin (endothelial selectin) like L-selectin, was identified with the aid of a monoclonal antibody.[238] It is found on endothelial cells and previously was referred to as endothelial cell–leukocyte adhesion molecule 1 (ELAM-1).[239] It is not expressed on lymphocytes. E-selectin is expressed by endothelial cells only following induction by cytokines such as interleukin-1, tumor necrosis factor and γ interferon.[240] This is in contrast to L-selectin which is constitutive on the surface of lymphocytes. Its expression is transient, reaching a maximum a few hours after induction and then rapidly declining. Its adhesive function was demonstrated by showing that an antibody against it could inhibit white cell attachment to activated human umbilical vein endothelial cells.[239]

The third known selectin, P-selectin (platelet selectin), was originally isolated from platelets. It has also been known by several other names including granule membrane protein 140 (GMP-140)[241] and platelet activation-dependent granule-external membrane protein (PADGEM).[242] It is rapidly expressed on the surface of platelets following activation. It is also expressed on the surface of endothelial cells following activation by histamine, interleukin 8 and oxidizing agents. Unlike E-selectin, P-selectin expression does not require protein synthesis as it is released from preformed α-granules in platelets and Weible-Palade bodies in endothelial cells. It mediates the adhesion of neutrophils to platelets[243,244] as well as to endothelial cells.[245]

The genes for all three selectins have been cloned (reviewed in refs. 15, 228). The extracellular portion of each selectin consists of three domains. At the amino terminus is a 120 amino acid sequence homologous with the carbohydrate recognition domain on C-type or Ca^{2+}-dependent animal lectins. The lectin domain is followed by a 35 to 40 amino acid EFG-like sequence. This is followed by two to nine repeated sequences of about 60 amino acids each that are homologous to complement-binding protein domains. Finally, there is a short hydrophobic transmembrane region followed by a cytoplasmic tail of 17 to 35 amino acids.

As would be predicted from their structure, the ligand for each selectin includes carbohydrates. L-selectin-mediated lymphocyte binding to HEV can be inhibited with mannose-6-phosphate rich polysaccharides and fucoidin, a sulfated fucose polymer. Removal of the sialic acid from the surface of lymphocytes and endothelial cells abolishes their ability to bind to one another either in vitro or in vivo, suggesting that sialic acid is an important constituent of the carbohydrate ligand recognized by selectins. Antibodies to a cell surface oligosaccharide, termed sialyl Lewis^x, block E-selectin mediated adhesion of neutrophils, and purified sialyl Lewis^x can block neutrophil-endothelial cell adhesion as well as bind directly to purified selectins. Sialyl Lewis^x is a tetrasaccharide with the structure N-acetyl-D-neuraminic acid-α(2,3)-D-galactose-β(1,4)-[D-fucose-α(1,3)]-N-acetyl-D-glucosamine. Removal of the fucose or the sialic acid renders the sialyl Lewis^x inactive as far as blocking E-selectin–mediated adhesion is concerned. Removal of sialic acid reduces, but does not abolish, its blocking activity against P-selectin.

The interaction of P-selectin with sialyl Lewis^x is of low affinity. This may be because the complete ligand expressed on neutrophils or endothelial cells is a glycosylated protein and high-affinity binding requires the presentation of the carbohydrate ligand in the context of the polypeptide backbone.[246] In this way, carbohydrate binding to selectins is analogous to RGD peptide binding to integrins. The affinity is much higher for the complete molecule. The oligosaccharide may provide specificity for these adhesive events.

Using the monoclonal antibody MECA79, which interferes with the adhesion of peripheral lymphocytes to lymph node HEVs,[14,247] it was possible to isolate the mucoproteins from endothelial cells that appear to be the ligands for L-selectin. These isolated mucoproteins will bind lymphocytes and purified L-selectin. Interestingly, L-selectin can serve as a ligand for E-selectin,[248,249] suggesting that, as cell surface glycoproteins, selectins can present oligosaccharides in such a way as to bind selectins on opposing cells. There must be some selectivity, however, or there would be self-binding of selectins on the same cell or aggregation of lymphocytes that are constitutively presenting L-selectin on their cell surface.

The selectins are the first molecules to be engaged during an inflammatory response or as lymphocytes interact with HEVs. It has been found that selectins are responsible for the rolling interaction between white cells and the endothelium. Although cells are capable of adhering to any number of ligands under static conditions, under the conditions of blood flow, only selectins interacting between the circulating cell and the endothelium can slow the cell down sufficiently to allow the other receptors to be presented to their respective ligands. This has been demonstrated both in vitro and in vivo. If various receptors are used to coat lipid bilayers on the surface of two apposing glass surfaces and fluid is pumped between the two surfaces at a rate equal to blood flow, lymphocytes added to the moving solution slow down and "roll" over the surface if it is coated with P-selectin, but not if it is coated with ICAM-1, the ligand for β_2 integrins. Rolling is blocked by antibodies against the selectin.[250] In contrast, if the plates are coated with a lipid bilayer carrying both P-selectin and ICAM-1, the lymphocytes will roll over the surface until an inflammatory cytokine is added that upregulates the β_2 integrins on the rolling lymphocyte. At this point, the rolling lymphocyte comes to a halt and sticks firmly to the plate. Similar results are noted in vivo

TABLE 9–2. THE SELECTINS

STRUCTURE*	NAME	LOCATION	EXPRESSION	ADHERENT CELL TYPES	PROPOSED FUNCTION
	L-selectin	Leukocytes (constitutive)	Decreases on cell activation	PLN endothelium Endothelium adjacent to inflammatory sites (rolling)	Lymphocyte recirculation through PLN Neutrophil (+ other leukocyte?) inflammation
	E-selectin	Endothelium (transcriptionally activated)	Increases on inflammatory activation (IL-1, TNF, LPS) (~hours)	Monocytes Neutrophils (rolling) T cell subsets (cutaneous?)	Leukocyte inflammation
	P-selectin	Platelets (α granules) Endothelium (Weibel-Palade bodies)	Increases on thrombin activation, histamine, substance P, peroxide (~minutes)	Monocytes Neutrophils (rolling) T cell subsets (cutaneous?)	Leukocyte inflammation

From Laskey K: Selectins: Interpreters of cell-specific carbohydrate information during inflammation. Science *258*:964, 1992, with permission.
*Abbreviations: L, lectin; E, epidermal growth factor-like; C, complement-binding protein-like; PLN, peripheral lymph node.

when vital blood flow is monitored in microvessels.[251] Thus, it appears that selectins are used to retard the movement of cells across a surface in order to enable them to interact with cytokines or other factors that are present in specific capillary beds as a result of injury or inflammation or in the normal process of lymphocyte trafficking through the lymph nodes.

The fact that these receptors recognize sialylated-fucosylated oligosaccharides is perhaps significant to the metastatic process in light of the well-established observation that a great majority of tumor cells show elevated levels of sialylated-fucosylated glycoproteins on their surface when compared to control cells.[252–254] The increased presence of these oligosaccharides could, in certain instances, provide the ligands for initial tumor cell–endothelial cell interactions once the metastatic cell has entered the circulatory system. This could be particularly relevant to the initial lodging of many metastatic cells in draining lymph nodes. Significantly, a careful study of highly metastatic versus poorly metastatic human colon carcinoma cell lines has revealed an increased expression of sialyl Lewis[x] structures at the end of terminal polylactosaminyl side chains on the surface of the metastatic cell lines,[255] making it possible that selectin-mediated adhesion could facilitate the interaction of the tumor cells with the vascular endothelium.

Support for a possible role of selectins in the spread of metastatic cells comes from observations using soluble forms of both P-selectin and E-selectin.[256] In this case, the selectins were presented as soluble immunoglobulin chimeras that could be used for immunohistochemical localization in much the same manner as antibodies. It was found that P-selectin would bind to a variety of human carcinomas, including colon, lung, and breast. In contrast, E-selectin was more specific, binding to only colon carcinomas. Neither selectin chimera reacted with melanomas. Thus, the more metastatic forms of several carcinomas were found to carry ligands for selectins that might facilitate the spread of blood-borne metastases.

That selectins may well play a role in adhesion of metastatic cells to the endothelium has been demonstrated indirectly by the fact that prevention of the formation of O-glycosyl linkages in tumor cells results in the loss of the ability of cells to bind platelets or to adhere to monolayers of activated endothelial cells.[257] It is entirely plausible that, under conditions of flow, blood-borne tumor cells may use selectins to initiate their interaction with endothelial cells or perhaps to facilitate aggregation with platelets.

CD44: Representative of a Second Receptor Family Facilitating Interactions with Endothelial Cells and Implicated in Metastasis

CD44, a member of the collagen link family of proteins,[233] is expressed in many different isoforms that are correlated with the metastatic potential of various tumors.[258–260] CD44 originally was thought to be required for the attachment of lymphocytes to HEVs and their subsequent movement into the lymph node.[233,261] Evidence now suggests that this may not be the case in every instance of white cell extravasation.[262,263] However, CD44's ability to bind hyaluronic acid may facilitate extravasation of tumor cells following their binding to microvascular or lymph node high endothelium either by functioning cooperatively with other receptors in stabilizing cell-cell interactions or by facilitating cell migration.

CD44, also known as Pgp-1, Ly-24, ECMIII, and gp90[Hermes],[261] is present in at least ten different isoforms,[264] all of which are capable of binding hyaluronic acid. As with other receptors, CD44 can be divided into three domains: the external, amino-terminal domain; a transmembrane domain; and a cytoplasmic domain through which it interacts directly with elements of the cytoskeleton, most likely ankyrin.[265] The molecular mass of CD44 is quite variable, ranging from 80 to as high as 200 kDa. The most common forms of the receptor are the 90-kDa form found on lymphocytes and the 180-kDa form found on epithelial cells. The wide variation in size is due to the variability in the amount of glycosylation on each form, and the synthesis of alternatively spliced isoforms.[266,267] Alternative splicing occurs within one region of the extracellular domain of the molecule, and involves any combination of ten different exons within the CD44 gene.[267]

Strong evidence exists to support the idea that alternatively spliced forms of CD44 are important to cell behavior and can, in fact, bestow a metastatic phenotype onto nonmetastatic cells.[268,269] For example, two different isoforms of CD44 were identified on a metastatic rat pancreatic carcinoma cell line. Nonmetastatic clones did not express these alternatively spliced forms. Transfection of cDNA encoding either of these isoforms restored the metastatic properties to these cells. This same CD44 isoform, as well as others, have been identified in lung, breast, and colon carcinomas.[14] Although the expression of various CD44 isoforms is a property of many normal epithelial cells, the homologues of the ''metastatic'' rat CD44 isoform were found only on tumor cells and early adenomatous polyps.

In a second set of experiments based on the observation that high expression of CD44 in human non-Hodgkin's lymphomas is associated with aggressive growth and wide dissemination,[270] human lymphoma cells were transfected with CD44 (the lymphocyte form) and injected intravenously into nude mice, either alone or in the presence of a soluble form of the same CD44 isoform. The soluble CD44 significantly reduced tumor formation in the animals, presumably as a result of competitive inhibition with CD44 on the cell surface and its ligand within the animal.[271]

The alternatively spliced forms of CD44 appear to have different functions, because transfection of a B cell line that contained no CD44 receptors with cDNA coding for the 90-kDa lymphocyte form enabled these cells to bind to rat lymph node high endothelial cells in culture. Transfection of these same cells with cDNA coding for the 180-kDa epithelial form did not promote adhesion to the lymph node endothelial cells.[266]

The expression of various combinations of alternatively

spliced isoforms of CD44 may be used to distinguish metastatic from nonmetastatic forms of lung, colon, or breast tumors.[272] Indeed, the absence of certain CD44 isotypes from mammary carcinomas has been correlated with a higher 5-year survival rate. As pointed out earlier, metastatic forms of non-Hodgkin's lymphoma appear to express higher levels of CD44 than tumors that fail to metastasize,[270] and increased levels of CD44 expression have been correlated with increased metastatic potential of human melanoma variants.[273,274]

The contribution of CD44 to increased metastatic potential may be due to the fact that different isoforms appear to have different adhesive potentials.[266,275,276] Increased avidity of metastatic cells for molecules expressed in large quantities on HEVs or other endothelial cells would likely facilitate metastatic spread. Also, like the integrins, CD44 has been found to facilitate signal transduction within the cell[277,278] as well as movement through the extracellular matrix.[279] This also could potentiate metastatic spread by regulating the expression of other receptors, growth factors, or proteases by the tumor cell.

Tumor Cell–Endothelium Interactions: Immunoglobulin Superfamily Receptors

If metastasizing cells behave as neutrophils during an inflammatory response or as lymphocytes trafficking through lymph nodes, and are slowed as they pass through capillary beds by selectins and perhaps CD44, then the next phase of the process would be a more firm attachment of cells to the endothelium and subsequent movement into the stroma of a particular organ. During lymphocyte trafficking or an inflammatory response, this occurs through the interaction of integrins with their appropriate ligands on the endothelial cells. The integrins, in the case of white cells, are primarily those of the β_2 superfamily and perhaps $\alpha_4\beta_1$ or $\alpha_4\beta_7$. These integrins, as well as their immunoglobulin superfamily counterreceptors, are up-regulated by inflammatory cytokines.[205,230,280]

The immunoglobulin superfamily is one of the most diverse families of receptors known. It includes not only immunoglobulins, but the major histocompatibility receptors, T-cell receptors, and molecules associated with various neoplasias, such as CEA[281]; DCC,[282] a molecule altered in colorectal cancers thought to act as a tumor suppressor affecting normal cellular interactions; and cell-cell recognition molecules, such as neural cell adhesion molecule (NCAM).[283] The more prominent immunoglobulin superfamily members in terms of cell trafficking include ICAM-1,[284] ICAM-2,[285] ICAM-3,[286] VCAM-1,[287,288] and possibly PECAM-1.[289,290]

Members of the immunoglobulin superfamily are distinguished by the presence of immunoglobulin homology units in the extracellular domain, as illustrated schematically for the ICAMs and VCAM-1 in Figure 9–6A. An immunoglobulin superfamily member may contain any

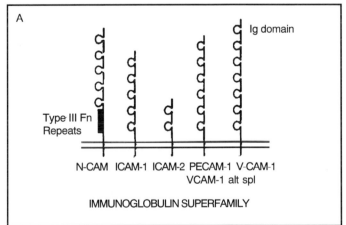

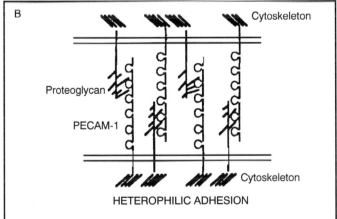

Figure 9–6. Schematic presentation of selected members of the immunoglobulin superfamily illustrating binding domains and alternatively spliced regions. *A,* Members that serve as receptors/counterreceptors for integrins involved in the inflammatory response. This shows the difference between alternatively spliced forms of VCAM-1 as well as the location of the binding domains for two different integrins on ICAM-1. Each loop represents an immunoglobulin homology unit or immunoglobulin (Ig) domain. NCAM is representative of immunoglobulin superfamily members carrying domains homologous to portions of other proteins, in this case type III fibronectin (Fn) repeats (filled rectangles). The Ig domains vary in both number and amino acid composition depending on the receptor. Thus, even though two receptors have the same number of Ig domains, they recognize different ligands (counterreceptors) as a result of differences in amino acid composition. *B,* Heterophilic adhesion as typified by human PECAM-1. In this case, cell adhesion is facilitated by two different molecules interacting with one another (immunoglobulin superfamily member PECAM-1 with a glycosaminoglycan-presenting proteoglycan on the participating cell). Both interacting molecules are organized via cytoskeletal elements into clusters of receptors and counterreceptors, providing the adhesive strength required to maintain the cell-cell contact. VCAM-1 alt spl, alternatively spliced isoform.

number of immunoglobulin domains (Fig. 9–6A). In general, these units are made of up 70 to 110 amino acids organized into seven to nine β-pleated strands. These strands each contain 5 to 10 amino acids folded into a sandwich-like structure made up of two layers of β strands arranged in an antiparallel manner. This conformation is stabilized by hydrophobic interactions between the two juxtaposed layers of β strands, thereby positioning the hydrophilic side chains of the constituent amino acids to the exterior of the molecule.[205,229]

Most members of the immunoglobulin superfamily exist as transmembrane molecules and interact with the cytoskeletal elements of the cell. Also associated with the cytoplasmic domain of immunoglobulin superfamily receptors are certain protein kinases that may serve to regulate the activity of the receptor, or initiate a chain of second message reactions that result in the activation of other receptors or result in the initiation of cell division.[192,291,292] As has been noted for other receptors, the ligand-induced clustering of immunoglobulin superfamily receptors on the cell surface probably provides the initial stimulus to trigger second message pathways.

The structure of immunoglobulin superfamily molecules allows for considerable functional diversity. Within an individual receptor, each homology unit may serve as the binding domain for a counterreceptor. In addition, the same immunoglobulin superfamily molecule may function as a viral receptor or may pair with other members of the superfamily to form highly diverse receptor complexes characterized by the T-cell receptor or major histocompatibility complex (MHC) receptor.[12]

ICAM-1 expression is induced by inflammatory cytokines such as interferon γ, tumor necrosis factor α, and interleukin 1, as well as lipopolysaccharides. This may facilitate the movement of white cells and lymphocytes into the surrounding tissue. ICAM-2 expression seems to be constitutive, not being affected by inflammatory mediators.[12,293,294] All three ICAMs function as counterreceptors for $\alpha_L\beta_2$, and ICAM-1 also acts as a counterreceptor for $\alpha_M\beta_2$.

The other member of the immunoglobulin superfamily functioning as an integrin counterreceptor is VCAM-1. VCAM-1 exists in two isoforms differing from one another on the basis of the number of immunoglobulin homology units, the more common form having seven and the alternatively spliced form six (Fig. 9–6). VCAM-1 is cytokine inducible and is found primarily on endothelial cells.[287,288] It is a counterreceptor for $\alpha_4\beta_1$ and $\alpha_4\beta_7$,[295] and is involved in lymphocyte homing to Peyer's patch lymph nodes[296] and perhaps the seeding of bone marrow stroma with hemopoietic stem cells.[297,298]

For the most part, the interaction of immunoglobulin superfamily adhesion receptors with their respective ligands is Ca^{2+} dependent and is heterophilic in nature. That is, the immunoglobulin superfamily receptor interacts with a different molecule on an adjacent cell. This is illustrated in Figure 9–6B. Human PECAM-1 mediates aggregation of PECAM-1–transfected L cells by binding to oligosaccharides presented by proteoglycans on the surface of participating cells.[299] In fact, human PECAM-1–producing L cells can aggregate with nontransfected L

cells in just this manner. In contrast, certain members may promote both homophilic and heterophilic adhesion and also may participate in Ca^{2+}-independent adhesion. NCAM is such an adhesion molecule. NCAM originally was described as a neural cell adhesion molecule. It subsequently has been discovered on many types of cells. Its expression is highly regulated during embryonic development and it is thought to play a central role in muscle innervation.[283,300] It exists in several isoforms formed as a result of alternatively spliced mRNA, proteolytic cleavage, or oligosaccharide heterogeneity.[283,301] These modifications can affect the binding properties of NCAM,[302] particularly modifications in the oligosaccharides.[303] NCAM exists in an adult and an embryonic form. The difference in the two forms involves the number of variable-length homopolymers of α-2,8-linked sialic acid. The embryonic form contains more sialic acid than the adult form. It has been demonstrated that NCAM carrying the more highly sialylated embryonic form adheres less avidly than the adult form.[302–304] It has been postulated that the less adhesive embryonic form allows the plasticity of cell recognition and movement required for histogenesis during embryonic development.[305]

NCAM is one of the few immunoglobulin superfamily molecules involved in homophilic interactions; that is, NCAM on one cell interacts with NCAM on an adjacent cell. This also occurs in a Ca^{2+}-independent manner.[304] However, there is also evidence that NCAM can participate in heterophilic adhesive events involving heparan- or heparan sulfate–containing proteoglycans.[306,307] In this case, heparan and heparan sulfate both have been shown to block NCAM-mediated retinal cell aggregation and adhesion to NCAM-coated substrates. Similarly, peptides corresponding to the presumptive heparan-binding domain of NCAM block cell adhesion to NCAM, and forms of NCAM produced without the heparan-binding domain fail to promote adhesion.[306,307] In each case, reagents targeted at proteoglycan-facilitated NCAM adhesive events do not reduce adhesion completely to background, suggesting that both proteoglycan-dependent and -independent interactions may be important to NCAM function.

PECAM-1 also appears to facilitate both homophilic and heterophilic adhesive interactions. It appears that PECAM-1 can mediate endothelial cell–endothelial cell adhesive events by a homophilic interaction of PECAM-1 on one cell with PECAM-1 on an adjacent cell.[290] In contrast, the aggregation of PECAM-1–transfected L cells[308] appears to require heparin or heparan sulfate proteoglycans.[309,310] In this case, aggregation can be shown to be sensitive to enzymes that degrade proteoglycans and to be blocked by heparan and to a lesser extent chondroitin sulfate, but not dextran sulfate or hyaluronic acid. Interestingly, like NCAM, PECAM-1 also contains a consensus proteoglycan-binding site[311] that can be mutated with a subsequent loss of ability to promote L cell aggregation. Polypeptides homologous with the proteoglycan-binding sequence block PECAM-mediated cell aggregation.

PECAM-1 has several postulated functions, including promoting endothelial cell-cell adhesion, serving as a trigger molecule on lymphocytes responsible for up-regulating integrins on the cell surface,[192] and perhaps serving as a receptor on endothelial cells that facilitates the transmigration of cells across the endothelium.[312–314] Because it has been shown to bind to proteoglycans as well as other PECAM molecules, it may serve in much the same capacity as CD44 or the selectins to facilitate the capture of circulating cells into the microvasculature of tissues or lymph nodes.

IMMUNOGLOBULIN SUPERFAMILY ADHESION RECEPTORS AND TUMOR CELL BEHAVIOR

The immunoglobulin superfamily adhesion receptors of most interest in tumor cell metastasis are those that are likely to be involved in tumor cell–endothelial cell interactions. These would include the ICAMs, VCAM-1, and PECAM-1. It is perhaps not so much the expression of these molecules on the tumor cells themselves that is of significance, but their function in the context of facilitating the interaction of cells with the endothelium. Nevertheless, both the ICAMs and VCAM-1 have been identified on tumor cells; PECAM-1 has not. The frequency of ICAM-1 expression is low on most tumors except for melanomas and certain squamous cell carcinomas.[201,315] Melanoma tumor progression and increased risk of metastasis has been correlated with ICAM-1 expression.[316] However, in experimental systems, there is no clear evidence that ICAM-1 expression contributes significantly to tumor progression.[315] In fact, it might be postulated that ICAM-1 expression would put a tumor cell at a disadvantage because lymphocytes interact with target cells through ICAM-1–mediated pathways,[12] and melanoma cells not expressing ICAM-1 have been shown to be relatively resistant to T-cell lysis.[317] Nevertheless, there is no positive correlation between metastasis of melanomas or breast tumors and the expression of ICAM-1.[315]

VCAM-1 expression on vascular endothelial cells in culture has been shown to promote the adhesion of melanoma cells.[318–320] This is undoubtedly through the interaction of $\alpha_4\beta_1$ integrin on the melanoma cell. It should be pointed out that $\alpha_4\beta_1$ frequently has been detected on metastatic melanomas in situ. However, loss of VCAM-1 expression by melanoma cells appears to be associated with tumor progression toward metastasis. A comparative study showed VCAM-1 expression on 79 per cent of benign nevi, 62 per cent of primary melanomas less than 1.5 mm in depth, 6 per cent of deeper melanomas, and 14 per cent of lymph node metastases.[321]

CEA, also known as oncofetal protein, has been associated with tumors of the gut and lung.[322] In fact, historically, it is one of the best known tumor markers used to follow the progression of colorectal carcinomas.[322] CEA constitutes a family of related molecules within the immunoglobulin superfamily.[322] Six members of this family have been described. One of the major differences among the members of this family is the way they are anchored to the cell surface. CEA itself is anchored via a phosphatidylinositol linkage and has no cytoplasmic domain, whereas others are anchored via typical hydrophobic transmembrane amino acid sequences and possess cytoplasmic domains of varying lengths. The function of CEA is not clear. Only recently has it been shown to promote cell aggregation in a homophilic, Ca^{2+}-independent manner[281] reminiscent of NCAM. This, combined with the fact that CEA is found at intercellular locations in intestinal cells of both adult and developing embryos, suggests that it may play a role in cell-cell adhesion. There is some experimental evidence that cells producing CEA show increased metastasis to the liver, and more specifically to the hepatic sinusoids.

As with CEA, a change in expression of NCAM has been correlated with certain tumors. Immunohistochemistry has revealed NCAM on neural and neuroendocrine tumors, including Wilms' tumor, pituitary adenomas, pheochromocytomas, and small-cell carcinomas of the lung.[323] In each case, it is the embryonic, less avidly adhesive, form of the molecule that is associated with these tumors. Expression of NCAM on tumor cells has been correlated with significantly reduced survival times.

How NCAM might relate to tumor phenotype is not clear. It is possible, however, that the expression of the less adhesive form of the molecule results in an increased propensity of cells to break from the tumor mass and move elsewhere in the body. However, it must be kept in mind that NCAM, and any other adhesive molecule for that matter, must function in the context of other adhesive molecules on the surface of the tumor cell as well as on the surface of other cells within the tissue. It is therefore hard to see how a change in expression of one surface receptor would have a dominant, "deadhesive" effect at the site of the original tumor.

We have seen evidence that the cadherins can act, under certain conditions, as if they are tumor suppressors. Indeed, in *Drosophila,* there is genetic evidence supporting this position (see discussion earlier in this chapter). There is also genetic evidence for a tumor suppressor gene in normal epithelial cells of the colon. This is based on the observation that 70 per cent of colorectal tumors and 50 per cent of adenomas show an allelic loss involving chromosome 18q.[324] The region lost in colorectal tumors carries a gene termed "deleted in colorectal carcinomas" (*DCC*), which codes for a protein that is homologous to NCAM and, hence, is a member of the immunoglobulin superfamily. It has been postulated that DCC may function in growth control, as described earlier for other adhesion receptors, and that a diminution of DCC on the cell surface could result in increased growth and clonal expansion of cells carrying an inactive *DCC* allele.[324]

ADHESION RECEPTORS MEDIATING ORGAN-SPECIFIC TARGETING OF TUMOR CELLS

Evidence for organ-specific, or nonrandom, metastasis comes from both clinical and experimental observations.[6,7] In general, melanomas tend to metastasize to the liver, and bone is the major metastatic site for neuroblastomas and carcinomas of the breast, thyroid, prostate, and kidney. Tumors arising from the breast, kidney, gastrointestinal tract, and lung also frequently are observed to metastasize to the brain. Experimentally, organ-specific metastatic tumors have been selected by serially passaging human or murine tumor cells through mice and selecting for growth in specific organs.[325-327] One of the most frequently used model systems involves the murine B16 melanoma. In this case, cells are injected intravenously, bypassing an initial step in metastasis—the separation of potentially metastatic cells from the primary tumor mass. However, this system has been useful in attempting to analyze the molecular mechanism of organ-specific homing of blood-borne cells.

An in vitro selection of B16 melanomas that preferentially homed to the lung was accomplished using a system originally developed to demonstrate nodal preference in lymphocyte homing.[328,329] B16 melanoma cells that preferentially adhered to frozen sections of lung showed an enhanced frequency of metastasis to the lung as compared to brain on reinjection into mice.[330] These experiments suggested that there may well be specific adhesion receptors in the target organ that allow for the preferential adhesion of tumor cells similar to those noted within the lymph nodes that allowed selective trafficking of lymphocytes.[9] Further support for this idea came from the demonstration that melanoma cells selected for their ability to home to the lung would aggregate with crude membrane vesicles prepared from the target organ, but not from other organs.[331]

A direct demonstration that endothelial cells might be involved in organ-specific metastasis came from experiments utilizing cultured endothelial cells. In this instance, capillary endothelial cells were cultured from various organs. Tumor cells were added to the monolayers and assayed for their ability to adhere to the underlying endothelial cells. Metastatic cells were found to adhere to capillary endothelial cells and not large-vessel endothelium,[332] providing in vitro evidence for what pathologists had known for some time—that is, micrometastases always were found in capillary beds. It was further shown that murine melanoma lines that homed to the lung showed a preference for adherence to lung microvessel endothelial cells and those homing to the brain showed a preference for brain microvessel endothelial cells.[333] Similar observations were made using a murine lymphoma line, MB6A, that displayed preferential adherence to isolated liver endothelial cells, and a human melanoma that showed preferential adherence to lung rather than liver endothelium.[7] It should be pointed out that these experiments showed quantitative, not qualitative, differences in preferential adhesion of tumor cells to organ-specific capillary endothelium. That is, the preference was not absolute. The tumor cells could adhere to other capillary endothelial cells, but showed a preference for cells isolated from the targeted organ. This suggested that there may not be absolutely organ-specific receptors, but that there may be different amounts or different combinations of receptors expressed on the targeted endothelial cells. This is perhaps not surprising given the history of the search for organ-specific adhesion receptors. So far, no receptor has been described that is restricted to only one cell type. More often, the receptor is present on several different cells and its expression may vary with the cell type, the state of growth of the cell, or the presence of specific matrix molecules or cytokines.

The next question to arise concerns the nature of the adhesion receptors, on both the tumor cell and the endothelial cell, that might be responsible for the preferred adhesion to one capillary bed over another. Several approaches have been taken to this question. Gluteraldehyde-fixed tumor cells have been used in an attempt to adsorb specific molecules from extracts of endothelial cells. A variety of proteins were adsorbed to the tumor cells and analyzed by polyacrylamide gel electrophoresis. Different proteins were isolated from lung endothelial cell extracts when compared to extracts of other endothelial cells. Alternatively, extracts from endothelial cells have been subjected to polyacrylamide gel electrophoresis, and the separated proteins electroeluted onto nitrocellulose membranes. Proteins that would support tumor cell adhesion were identified by overlaying the membrane with radioactive or biotinylated tumor cells and locating the regions on the membrane to which the cells adhered.[7] Tumor cells tended to adhere to five polypeptides ranging in size from 18 to 32 kDa, with different tumor cells showing a preference for different bands. These proteins, designated ECAM-1 through -5 for endothelial common adhesion molecule, have been isolated by lectin affinity chromatography. Antibodies prepared against three of these glycoproteins show reactivity with microvascular endothelial cells in several organs but no clear organ specificity. These proteins have not been further characterized, but it is clear, on the basis of size, that they are not cadherins, integrins, or members of the immunoglobulin superfamily. Whether or not they are involved in any aspect of the metastatic process has yet to be demonstrated.

To date, the only clearly identified and characterized endothelial cell components shown to promote endothelial cell–tumor cell adhesion in vitro are those previously characterized as being required for lymphocyte homing or white cell–endothelial cell interactions during the inflammatory process. VCAM-1 is particularly interesting because it was found to mediate melanoma cell adhesion to endothelial cell monolayers that were exposed to cytokines.[318,319] Similar experiments have suggested that selectins might mediate tumor cell–endothelial cell adhesion.[256,257] It is not clear, however, that VCAM-1, E-selectin, or ICAM-1 are required to mediate tumor cell–endothelial cell adhesion, because there are experiments suggesting that adhesive interactions can occur in the presence of antibodies specific for these receptors.[334] These molecules are not likely to provide any type of organ-specific signals because they are found on all cytokine-stimulated microvascular endothelial cells.

A molecule that may be organ specific has been described recently. This is a 90-kDa glycoprotein called Lu-ECAM-1 that is expressed on bovine endothelial cells cultured on matrix material extracted from lungs. The approach used to identify Lu-ECAM-1 was based on the fact that the composition of the extracellular matrix can influence the properties of cultured endothelial cells to the point that they can be induced to form tubules or capillary-like structures in the presence of the appropriate extracellular matrix.[335] It was observed that bovine aortic endothelial cells (BAECs) plated on extracellular matrix material extracted from different organs would exhibit organ-specific binding activity when exposed to various metastatic cell lines. That is, BAECs grown on matrix extract from lung would preferentially bind B16 melanoma cells that homed to the lung rather than those that homed to the brain.[336] Similarly, liver metastatic tumor cell lines selectively adhered to BAECs grown on matrix extracted from liver. This property of organotypic adhesion of metastatic cell lines was acquired only after prolonged growth of BAECs on the appropriate substrata and was lost if the cells were grown in the absence of the matrix material. The activity within the matrix extract that induced tumor-specific binding has been called TAMs for tumor cell attachment modulators. These have not been further characterized.

Lu-ECAM-1 was characterized using monoclonal antibodies prepared against vesicles formed by perfusing isolated rat lungs with a buffer containing formaldehyde and the reducing agent dithiothreitol.[337] These vesicles would bind preferentially to melanoma cells that metastasized to the lung. Similar vesicles prepared from leg vessels showed no organotypic binding preference. Interestingly, the treatment of these vesicles with neuraminidase to remove sialic acid from the surface-exposed glycoproteins eliminated their binding activity in a manner reminiscent of that seen for selectin-mediated adhesion (see earlier in this chapter). Monoclonal antibodies were prepared using these vesicles as immunogens.[338] Two hybridomas were isolated that produced monoclonal antibodies that would react only with BAECs grown on lung matrix and that selectively recognized endothelia from small and medium-sized bovine lung venules. They did not react with endothelial cells from other organs. One of these antibodies also could block the organotypic adhesion of metastatic cells to BAECs grown on the appropriate matrix and also could reduce lung colonization by melanoma cells injected into the tail vein of mice.[234] Using this monoclonal antibody, it was possible to isolate Lu-ECAM-1 from nonionic detergent extracts of mouse lung and BAEC cultured on lung TAMs by immunoaffinity chromatography.

That Lu-ECAM-1 was capable of mediating organotypic tumor cell binding was confirmed by demonstrating that purified Lu-ECAM-1, when coated on plastic culture dishes, could selectively promote the Ca^{2+}-dependent adhesion of lung-specific melanoma cells as compared to nonmetastatic control tumor cells. This adhesion could be blocked by the anti–Lu-ECAM-1 monoclonal antibody as well as by soluble Lu-ECAM-1.[339] In addition, mice immunized with Lu-ECAM-1 showed reduced metastasis when challenged with lung-specific metastasizing B16-F10 melanoma cells. Similar results were obtained when the anti–Lu-ECAM-1 monoclonal antibody was administered to mice along with the tumor cell challenge.[339] Lu-ECAM-1 was found not to promote adhesion or metastasis of other lung-specific metastasizing tumors, suggesting that the effect is specific for melanomas and not tumors originating from other sources.

ENTRAPMENT OF TUMOR CELLS IN CAPILLARY BEDS

It is not necessary to explain all nonrandom, organ-preferred metastasis by the presence of specific receptors or groups of receptors. It is equally possible that tumor cells may be trapped within a given capillary bed, and survive based entirely on the presence of appropriate cytokines or matrix molecules in the vicinity. However, in this case, adhesion receptors are likely to be required for the formation of tumor cell aggregates and subsequent invasion of the surrounding stroma.

There is evidence that tumor cell entrapment within a capillary bed may form the basis of initial tumor cell–endothelium interaction.[340–342] Probably the first indication that this might be the case came from early studies showing that tumor cells could induce platelet aggregation and that agents, including neuraminidase, that prevented platelet aggregation reduced the formation of metastatic lesions in mice.[343–345] These studies included B16 murine melanomas as well as a metastatic colon adenocarcinoma. Although these studies did not get at the mechanism of tumor-induced platelet aggregation, they suggest that oligosaccharides may be an important element, pointing to a possible role of the selectins in entrapment. These receptors had not been defined at that time, however. More recent investigations into other systems suggest that tumor cell–platelet aggregation may be mediated by the integrin $\alpha_{IIb}\beta_3$ found on platelets and acting as a receptor for fibronectin, fibrinogen, von Willebrand factor, and so forth (see Fig. 9–5). Antibodies specific for this integrin, as well as the RGD-containing peptides that block the binding of $\alpha_{IIb}\beta_3$ to its various ligands, reduced platelet tumor cell aggregation in vitro and tumor metastasis in vivo.[346–349] This is supported by the observation that exposure of melanoma cells, human colon carcinoma cells, and murine colon and lung carcinomas to thrombin increased the platelet-binding activity on the tumors and increased the number of experimental pulmonary metastases.[350] Thrombin activation of $\alpha_{IIb}\beta_3$ on tumor cells could enhance the binding of ligands such as von Willebrand factor, vitronectin, fibrinogen, and so forth, which subsequently would interact with circulating platelets, resulting in a bolus of cells capable of lodging in any capillary bed. Because these receptors also will promote the adhesion of tumor cells to matrix molecules such as fibronectin, their activation could enhance the ability of the tumor cells to adhere to the surrounding stroma. This possibility is supported by the discovery of the presence of the integrins $\alpha_{IIb}\beta_3$[351–353] and $\alpha_v\beta_3$[198,216,217,354] on the surface of many tumors, including metastatic human melanomas in situ.[210]

It is evident, both from experimental models and cumulative observations of tumors originating from various organs, that the dissemination of metastatic cells to secondary sites can be both a random and nonrandom process. In the latter case, there is experimental support for the idea that this occurs as a result of the interaction of adhesion receptors on the tumor cells with counterreceptors expressed by different capillary beds. The receptors on endothelial cells may distinguish one capillary bed from another. However, one need not necessarily postulate specific adhesion receptors on endothelial cells to account for apparent nonrandom metastasis. The aggregation of tumor cells with platelets could result in lodging of a cluster of cells in any capillary bed. If this results in retraction of endothelial cells and exposure of underlying basement membrane,[355] the tumor cells then will adhere to the exposed constituents of the basement membrane via their integrins. Subsequently, the matrix material will be exposed to the proteolytic enzymes known to be concentrated at sites of tumor cell–matrix adhesion. Subsequent migration of the tumor into the surrounding stroma then could be triggered either by motility factors produced by the tumors themselves[356] or by proteolytic fragments generated as a result of local proteolysis of the extracellular matrix.[357] Interestingly, tumor cells tend to respond to factors released from ''target'' tissues more readily than to factors released from organs in which they do not usually establish metastatic growth. In addition, the proteolytic degradation of matrix also can lead to the release of active cytokines that will stimulate tumor cell replication in the area. In this manner, nonrandom metastasis could be a consequence of factors other than merely organ-specific adhesion receptors, and possibly could be initiated by nonspecific entrapment of clusters of tumor cells and platelets.

The nonrandom nature of metastatic spread may occur more often through the lymphatics than through hematogenous circulation.[6] It also may be enhanced by injury to the vasculature, because it has been demonstrated that vascular trauma, particularly in the lungs, will lead to increased metastasis in experimental systems.[358,359] Microvascular injury resulting from exposure to chemotherapeutic drugs (cyclophosphamide), environmental toxins (including hyperoxia), and bleomycin results in greatly increased incidence of metastatic growth in microvascular beds of lungs, kidney, and liver. Exposure to these agents also can cause the release of chemotactic factors to which tumor cells can respond. The adhesion receptors involved in tumor cell attachment under these conditions have not been evaluated. It is likely that they could include receptors such as integrins and CD44, which have the ability to bind to extracellular matrix molecules exposed as a result of vascular injury, as well as the inducible immunoglobulin superfamily receptors such as VCAM-1 and the ICAMs, displayed on endothelial cells as a result of activation by inflammatory cytokines.[318,319] Injection of cytokines will increase the incidence of metastasis of experimental tumors to nontargeted organs[360,361] as well as increase the incidence of spread of non-Hodgkin's lymphoma.[362]

CONCLUDING COMMENTS

The past 5 years have been particularly productive in terms of the identification of cell surface adhesion receptors. New families of receptors have been recognized, new members of previously known receptor families have been discovered, and the molecular basis of their adhesive activities has been established thanks to cloning the cDNAs as well as the increasing number of structures that have been analyzed crystallographically.[363–365] The analysis of both naturally occurring and laboratory-produced mutations, as well as the construction of hybrid molecules, has allowed us to dissect the functional domains of the receptors. We have come to realize that these molecules not only serve an anchoring function, but communicate information from the external environment that is essential for cell replication and for regulating cellular behavior and morphogenesis. The activity of surface receptors is dynamically regulated. Existing receptors can be activated and inactivated in response to cytokines, chemotactic peptides, and hormones. Their expression changes in an ordered fashion during embryonic development and during tissue repair.

In the context of cell adhesion and the biology of cell behavior, no adhesion receptor functions alone. They function in conjunction with other adhesion receptors, some providing specificity, some providing transient adhesive interactions, and some providing more permanent anchors. Their ligands include other adhesion receptors, proteoglycans, proteins, and carbohydrates. The ligands may be found on other cells or they may be found as part of the extracellular matrix. With the use of highly specific monoclonal antibodies, we are becoming aware of the role of individual receptors in numerous biologic processes.[366]

It may be overly simplistic to explain the tendency of certain tumors to metastasize to specific organs on the basis of a single, organ-specific receptor. It is more likely that individual organs or endothelial beds express combinations of receptors that are relatively unique but not absolutely specific. This receptor profile may be variable depending on the growth state of the cell, the presence of cytokines or chemotactic molecules, or perhaps even injury. Organ-preferred metastasis then would be the result of a combination of receptors on the circulating tumor cell being presented with a compatible combination of counterreceptors on the microvascular endothelium of the targeted tissue. This model resembles that postulated to account for specific cellular interactions during embryonic development. That is, cells produce a complex series of receptors, each of which is required to facilitate cell-cell and cell-matrix interactions as well as cell movement. The combination of receptors expressed by a cell is both time and place dependent, and changes in response to environmental conditions as required for histogenesis and cell differentiation. Thus, specificity for the assembly of cells into a particular tissue derives from this carefully programmed presentation of combinations of receptors, rather than the presentation of a single, organ-specific molecule.[305,367,368] It may be that the changes in gene regulation accompanying neoplastic transformation and finally the development of a malignancy include the presentation of different sets of receptors on the cell surface. It is also possible that there is a combination of receptors characteristic of metastatic clones of various tumors, and that this combination would vary depending on the tissue of origin and the grade of the tumor. This combination of receptors might most nearly be complementary to counterreceptors expressed on specific capillary beds, thus increasing the tendency of particular tumors to metastasize to a limited number of sites.

A combination of genetics, cellular, molecular, and structural biology has led to more sophisticated insights into the role of adhesion molecules in normal and pathologic processes. Our understanding of the molecular basis of cancer cell behavior has profited greatly from this. As we proceed to discover new adhesion molecules and to understand more about the functions of existing ones, we may well be able to manipulate these receptors at the genetic level, as well as at the functional level, in a manner that will specifically target tumor cells. There is hope for this because it is clear that actively growing cells, cells migrating through the extracellular matrix, or cells otherwise activated express different sets of receptors than the majority of cells in a more quiescent state in adult tissue. The rapid advances in the field of gene therapy may soon make it possible to stop cell growth or induce tumor cell death based upon our knowledge of molecular consequences of cell-cell and cell-matrix adhesion.[369,370]

ACKNOWLEDGMENTS: The author wishes to thank Dr. Steve Albelda for many helpful discussions, Ms. Marie Lennon for her tireless patience in preparation of the manuscript, and Ms. Irene Crichton for her patient assistance in editing and organizing the final draft. Supported by NIH grants CA19144, CA10815, HL39023, and HL47670.

REFERENCES

1. Hynes RO: Integrins: Versatility, modulation, and signaling in cell adhesion. Cell 69:11, 1992
2. Paget S: The distribution of secondary growths in cancer of the breast. Lancet 1:571, 1889
3. Ewing J: A treatise on tumors, Philadelphia, WB Saunders Company, 1928
4. Klagsbrun M: Regulators of angiogenesis: Stimulators, inhibitors, and extracellular matrix. J Cell Biochem 47:199, 1991
5. Nicolson GL: Metastatic tumor cell interactions with endothelium, basement membrane and tissue. Curr Opin Cell Biol 1:1009, 1989
6. Zetter BR: The cellular basis of site-specific tumor metastasis. In Flier JS, Underhill LH (eds): Seminars in Medicine of the Beth Israel Hospital. Boston, Beth Israel Hospital, 1990, p 605
7. Belloni PN, Tressler RJ: Microvascular endothelial cell heterogeneity: Interactions with leukocytes and tumor cells. Cancer Metastasis Rev 8:353, 1990
8. Pauli BU, Augustin-Voss HG, El-Sabban ME, et al: Organ-preference of metastasis. Cancer Metastasis Rev 9:175, 1990
9. Berg EL, Goldstein LA, Jutila MA, et al: Homing receptors and vascular addressins: Cell adhesion molecules that direct lymphocyte traffic. Immunol Rev 108:5, 1989
10. Butcher EC: Leukocyte-endothelial cell adhesion as an active, multi-step process: A combinatorial mechanism for specificity and diversity in leukocyte targeting. Adv Exp Med Biol 323:181, 1992
11. Smith CW: Molecular determinants of neutrophil adhesion. Am J Respir Cell Mol Biol 2:487, 1990
12. Springer TA: Adhesion receptors of the immune system. Nature 346:425, 1990
13. Butcher EC: Leukocyte-endothelial cell recognition: Three (or more) steps to specificity and diversity. Cell 67:1033, 1991
14. Lasky LA, Singer MS, Dowbenko D, et al: An endothelial ligand for L-selectin is a novel mucin-like molecule. Cell 69:927, 1992
15. Lasky LA: The selectins: Interpreters of cell-specific carbohydrate information during inflammation. Science 258:964, 1992
16. Bevilacqua MP: Endothelial-leukocyte adhesion molecules. Annu Rev Immunol 11:767, 1993
17. Mayadas TN, Johnson RC, Rayburn H, et al: Leukocyte rolling and extravasation are severely compromised in P selectin-defecient mice. Cell 74:541, 1993
18. Imai Y, Lasky LA, Rosen SD: Sulphation requirement for GlyCAM-1, an endothelial ligand for L-selectin. Nature 361:555, 1993
19. Shimizu Y, Shaw S: Mucins in the mainstream. Nature 366:630, 1993
20. Butcher EC: Cellular and molecular mechanisms that direct leukocyte traffic. Am J Pathol 136:3, 1990
21. Briskin MJ, McEvoy LM, Butcher EC: MAdCAM-1 has homology to immunoglobulin and mucin-like adhesion receptors and to IgA1. Nature 363:461, 1993
22. Takeichi M: Cadherin cell adhesion receptors as a morphogenetic regulator. Science 251:1451, 1991
23. Kemler R: Classical cadherins. Semin Cell Biol 3:149, 1992
24. Buxton RA, Magee AI: Structure and interactions of desmosomal and other cadherins. Semin Cell Biol 3:157, 1992
25. Hatta K, Nose A, Nagafuchi A, Takeichi M: Cloning and expression of cDNA encoding a neural calcium-dependent cell adhesion molecule: Its identity in the cadherin gene family. J Cell Biol 106:873, 1988
26. Takeichi M: The cadherins: Cell-cell adhesion molecules controlling animal morphogenesis. Development 102:639, 1988
27. Ranscht B, Dours-Zimmermann MT: T-cadherin, a novel cadherin cell adhesion molecule in the nervous system lacks the conserved cytoplasmic region. Neuron 7:391, 1991
28. Ozawa M, Horshutzky H, Herrenknecht K, Kemler R: A possible new adhesive site in the cell-adhesion molecule uromorulin. Mech Dev 33:49, 1990
29. Nagafuchi A, Takeichi M, Tsukita S: The 102 kd cadherin-associated protein: Similarity to vinculin and posttranscriptional regulation of expression. Cell 65:849, 1991
30. Knudsen KA, Wheelock MJ: Plakoglobin, or an 83-kD homologue distinct from β-catenin, interacts with E-cadherin and N-cadherin. J Cell Biol 118:671, 1992
31. Hirano S, Kimoto N, Shimoyama Y, et al: Identification of a neural α-catenin as a key regulator of cadherin function and multicellular organization. Cell 70:293, 1992
32. Ozawa M, Kemler R: Molecular organization of the uvomorulin-catenin complex. J Cell Biol 116:989, 1992
33. Ozawa M, Ringwald M, Kemler R: Uvomorulin-catenin complex formation is regulated by a specific domain in the cytoplasmic region of the cell adhesion molecule. Proc Natl Acad Sci USA 87:4246, 1990
34. Volk T, Geiger B: A 135-kd membrane protein of intercellular adherens junctions. EMBO J 3:2249, 1984
35. Thiery J-P, Delouvee A, Gallin W, et al: Ontogenic expression of cell adhesion molecules: L-CAM is found in epithelia derived from the three primary germ layers. Dev Biol 102:61, 1984
36. Edelman GM: Morphoregulation. Dev Dyn 193:2, 1992
37. Takeichi M: Cadherins: A molecular family important in selective cell-cell adhesion. Annu Rev Biochem 59:237, 1990
38. Fujimore T, Miyatani S, Takeichi M: Ectopic expression of N-cadherin perturbs histogenesis in Xenopus embryos. Development 110:97, 1990
39. Detrick R, Dickey D, Kintner CR: The effects of N-cadherin misexpression on morphogenesis in Xenopus embryos. Neuron 4:493, 1990
40. Matsunaga M, Hatta K, Takeichi M: Role of N-cadherin cell adhesion molecules in the histogenesis of neural retina. Neuron 1:289, 1988
41. Rodriguez-Boulan E, Nelson WJ: Morphogenesis of the polarized epithelial cell phenotype. Science 245:718, 1989

42. Wollner DA, Krzeminski KA, Nelson WJ: Remodeling the cell surface distribution of membrane proteins during the development of epithelial cell polarity. J Cell Biol 116:889, 1992

43. Damsky CH, Richa J, Solter D, et al: Identification and purification of a cell surface glycoprotein mediating intercellular adhesion in embryonic and adult tissue. Cell 34:455, 1983

44. Gumbiner B, Simons K: A functional assay for proteins involved in establishing an epithelial occluding barrier: Identification of a uvomorulin-like polypeptide. J Cell Biol 102:457, 1986

45. Behrens J, Birchmeier W, Goodman SL, Imhof BA: Dissociation of Madin-Darby canine kidney epithelial cells by the monoclonal antibody anti-Arc-1: Mechanistic aspects and identification of the antigen as a component related to uvomorulin. J Cell Biol 101:1307, 1989

46. Van Roy F, Mareel M: Tumour invasion: Effects of cell adhesion and motility. Trends Cell Biol 2:163, 1992

47. Behrens J, Frixen U, Schipper J, et al: Cell adhesion in invasion and metastasis. Semin Cell Biol 3:169, 1992

48. Vleminckx K, Vakaet L Jr, Mareel M, et al: Genetic manipulation of E-cadherin expression by epithelial tumor cells reveals an invasion suppressor role. Cell 66:107, 1991

49. Navarro P, Gómez M, Pizzaro A, et al: A role for the E-cadherin cell-cell adhesion molecule during tumor progression of mouse epidermal carcinogenesis. J Cell Biol 115:517, 1991

50. Frixen UH, Behrens J, Sachs M, et al: E-cadherin-mediated cell-cell adhesion prevents invasiveness of human carcinoma cells. J Cell Biol 113:173, 1991

51. Mahoney PA, Weber U, Onofrechuk P, et al: The fat tumor suppressor gene in Drosophila encodes a novel member of the cadherin gene superfamily. Cell 67:853, 1991

52. Schipper JH, Frixen UH, Behrens J, et al: E-cadherin expression in squamous cell carcinomas of head and neck: Inverse correlation with tumor dedifferentiation and lymph node metastasis. Cancer Res 51:6328, 1991

53. Umbas R, Schalken JA, Aalders TW, et al: Expression of the cellular adhesion molecule E-cadherin is reduced or absent in high-grade prostate cancer. Cancer Res 52:5104, 1992

54. Giroldi LA, Schalken JA: Decreased expression of the intercellular adhesion molecule E-cadherin in prostate cancer. Biological significance and clinical implications. Cancer Metastasis Rev 12:29, 1993

55. Inoue M, Ogawa H, Miyata M, et al: Expression of E-cadherin in normal, benign, and malignant tissues of female genital organs. Am J Clin Pathol 98:76, 1992

56. Oka H, Shiozaki H, Kobayashi K, et al: Immunohistochemical evaluation of E-cadherin adhesion molecule expression in human gastric cancer. Virchows Archiv A Pathol Anat 421:149, 1992

57. Shiozaki H, Tahara H, Oka H, et al: Expression of immunoreactive E-cadherin adhesion molecules in human cancers. Am J Pathol 139:17, 1991

58. Shimoyama Y, Hirohashi S: Expression of E- and P-cadherin in gastric carcinomas. Cancer Res 51:2185, 1991

59. Matsuura K, Kawanishi J, Fujii S, et al: Altered expression of E-cadherin in gastric cancer tissues and carcinomatous fluid. Br J Cancer 66:1122, 1992

60. Shimoyama Y, Hirohashi S, Hirano S, et al: Cadherin cell-adhesion molecules in human epithelial tissues and carcinomas. Cancer Res 49:2128, 1989

61. Eidelman S, Damsky C, Wheelock M, Damjanov I: Expression of the cell-cell adhesion glycoprotein cell-CAM 120/80 in normal human tissues and tumors. Am J Pathol 135:101, 1989

62. Oka H, Shiozaki H, Kobayashi K, et al: Expression of E-cadherin cell adhesion molecules in human breast cancer tissues and its relationship to metastasis. Cancer Res 53:1696, 1993

63. Shimoyama Y, Nagafuchi A, Fujita S, et al: Cadherin dysfunction in a human cancer cell line: Possible involvement of loss of α-catenin expression in reduced cell-cell adhesiveness. Cancer Res 52:5770, 1992

64. Jouanneau J, Tucker GC, Boyer B, et al: Epithelial cell plasticity in neoplasia. Cancer Cells 3:525, 1991

65. Vallés AM, Boyer B, Tucker GC, et al: The epithelial to mesenchymal transition of rat bladder carcinoma cells: An in vitro model system to study the initial steps of cancer dissemination. Beitr Onkol 44:49, 1992

66. Menter DG, Cavanaugh PG, Nicolson GL: Adhesion and growth properties of metastatic tumor cells that colonize specific organ sites. Beitr Onkol 44:60, 1992

67. Weidner KM, Behrens J, Vandeker J, Birchmeier W: Scatter factor: Molecular characteristics and effect on the invasiveness of epithelial cells. J Cell Biol 111:2097, 1990

68. Boyer B, Dufour S, Thiery JP: E-cadherin expression during the acidic FGF-induced dispersion of a rat bladder carcinoma cell line. Exp Cell Res 201:347, 1992

69. Matsuyoshi N, Hamaguchi M, Taniguchi S, et al: Cadherin-mediated cell-cell adhesion is perturbed by v-src tyrosine phosphorylation in metastatic fibroblasts. J Cell Biol 118:703, 1992

70. Hynes RO: Integrins, a family of cell surface receptors. Cell 48:549, 1987

71. Albelda SM, Buck CA: Integrins and other cell adhesion molecules. FASEB J 4:2868, 1990

72. Anderson DC, Springer T: Leukocyte adhesion deficiency: An inherited defect in the Mac-1, LFA-1 and p150,95 glycoproteins. Annu Rev Med 38:175, 1987

73. Arnaout MA, Dana N, Gupta SK, et al: Point mutations impairing cell surface expression of the common β subunit (CD18) in a patient with leukocyte adhesion molecule (Leu-Cam) deficiency. J Clin Invest 85:977, 1990

74. Yang JT, Rayburn H, Hynes R: Embryonic mesodermal defects in α5 integrin-deficient mice. Development 119:1093, 1993

75. Lessey BA, Damjanovich L, Coutifaris C, et al: Integrin adhesion molecules in the human endometrium; correlation with the normal and abnormal menstrual cycle. J Clin Invest 90:188, 1992

76. Bergelson JM, Shepley MP, Chan BMC, et al: Identification of the integrin VLA-2 as a receptor for Echovirus 1. Science 255:1718, 1992

77. Leptin M, Aebersold R, Wilcox M: Drosophila position-specific antigens resemble the vertebrate fibronectin-receptor family. EMBO J 6:1037, 1987

78. Wilcox M: Genetic analysis of the Drosophila PS integrins. Cell Differ Dev 32:391, 1990

79. DeSimone DW, Hynes RO: Xenopus laevis integrins: Structural conservation and evolutionary divergence of integrin β subunits. J Biol Chem 263:5333, 1988

80. Howard JE, Hirst EMA, Smith JC: Are β1 integrins involved in Xenopus gastrulation? Mech Dev 38:109, 1992

81. Buck CA, Shea E, Duggin K, Horwitz A: Integrin, the CSAT antigen: Functionality requires oligomeric integrity. J Cell Biol 103:2421, 1986

82. Pierschbacher MD, Ruoslahti E: Cell attachment activity of fibronectin can be duplicated by small synthetic fragments of the molecule. Nature 309:30, 1984

83. Yamada KM, Kennedy DW: Dualistic nature of adhesive protein function: Fibronectin and its biologically active peptide fragments can autoinhibit fibronectin function. J Cell Biol 99:29, 1984

84. Ruoslahti E, Pierschbacher MD: New perspectives in cell adhesion: RGD and integrins. Science 238:491, 1987

85. Naidet C, Semeriva M, Yamada KM, Thiery JP: Peptides containing the cell-attachment recognition signal Arg-Gly-Asp prevent gastrulation in Drosophila embryos. Nature 325:348, 1987

86. Boucaut JC, Darribere T, Poole TJ, et al: Biological active synthetic peptides as probes of embryonic development: A competitive peptide inhibitor of fibronectin function inhibits gastrulation in amphibian embryos and neural crest cell migration in the avian embryo. J Cell Biol 99:1822, 1984

87. Neff NT, Lowrey C, Decker C, et al: Monoclonal antibody detaches embryonic skeletal muscle from extracellular matrices. J Cell Biol 95:654, 1982

88. Humphries MJ, Olden K, Yamada K: A synthetic peptide from fibronectin inhibits experimental metastasis of murine melanoma cells. Science 233:467, 1986

89. Humphries MJ, Yamada KM, Olden K: Investigation of the biological effects of anti-cell adhesion synthetic peptides that inhibit experimental metastasis of B16-F10 murine melanoma cells. J Clin Invest 81:782, 1988

90. Mould AP, Komoriya A, Yamada K, Humphries M: The CS5 peptide is a second site in the IIICS region of fibronectin recognized by the integrin $\alpha_4\beta_1$. J Biol Chem 266:3579, 1991

91. Wayner EA, Kovach NL: Activation-dependent recognition by hematopoietic cells of the LDV sequence in the V region of fibronectin. J Cell Biol 116:489, 1992

92. Nojima Y, Humphries MJ, Mould AP, et al: VLA-4 mediates CD3-dependent CD4+ T cell activation via the CS1 alternatively spliced domain of fibronectin. J Exp Med 172:1185, 1990

93. Guan J-L, Hynes RO: Lymphoid cells recognize an alternatively spliced segment of fibronectin via the integrin receptor $\alpha_4\beta_1$. Cell 60:53, 1990

94. Hemler ME, Elices MJ, Chan BMC, et al: Multiple ligand binding functions for VLA-2 ($\alpha^2\beta_1$) and VLA-3 ($\alpha^3\beta_1$) in the integrin family. Cell Differ Dev 32:229, 1990

95. Brown E, Hooper L, Ho T, Gresham H: Integrin-associated protein: A 50-kD plasma membrane antigen physically and functionally associated with integrins. J Cell Biol 111:2785, 1990

96. Smyth SS, Hillery CA, Parise LV: Fibrinogen binding to purified platelet glycoprotein IIb-IIIa (integrin $\alpha_{IIb}\beta_3$) is modulated by lipids. J Biol Chem 267:15568, 1992

97. Gailit J, Ruoslahti E: Regulation of the fibronectin receptor affinity by divalent cations. J Biol Chem 263:12927, 1988

98. Kirchhofer D, Gailit J, Ruoslahti E, et al: Cation-dependent changes in the binding specificity of the platelet receptor GPIIb/IIa. J Biol Chem 265:18525, 1990

99. Elices MJ, Urry LA, Hemler ME: Receptor functions for the integrin VLA-3: Fibronectin, collagen, and laminin binding are differently influenced by ARG-GLY-ASP peptide and by divalent cations. J Cell Biol 112:169, 1991

100. Kim LT, Ish S, Lee C-C, et al: Altered glycosylation and cell surface expression of β_1 integrin receptors during keratinocyte activation. J Cell Sci 103:743, 1992.

101. Kawano T, Takasaki S, Tao T-W, Kobata A: Altered glycosylation of β_1 integrins associated with reduced adhesiveness to fibronectin and laminin. Int J Cancer 53:91, 1993

102. Hirst R, Horwitz A, Buck CA, Rohrschneider L: Phosphorylation of the fibronectin receptor complex in cells transformed by oncogenes that encode tyrosine kinases. Proc Natl Acad Sci USA 83:6470, 1986

103. Valmu L, Autero M, Siljander P, et al: Phosphorylation of the β-subunit of CD11/CD18 integrins by protein kinase C correlates with leukocyte adhesion. Eur J Immunol 21:2857, 1991

104. Shattil SJ, Brugge JS: Protein tyrosine phosphorylation and the adhesive functions of platelets. Curr Opin Cell Biol 3:869, 1991

105. van Kuppevelt T, Languino L, Gailit J, et al: An alternative cytoplasmic domain of the integrin β_3 subunit. Proc Natl Acad Sci USA 86:5415, 1989

106. DeSimone DW, Norton PA, Hynes RO: Identification and characterization of alternatively spliced fibronectin mRNAs expressed in early Xenopus embryos. Dev Biol 149:357, 1992

107. Languino L, Ruoslahti E: An alternative form of the integrin β_1 subunit with a variant cytoplasmic domain. J Biol Chem 267:7116, 1992

108. Altruda F, Cervella P, Tarone G, et al: A human integrin β_1 subunit with a unique cytoplasmic domain generated by alternative mRNA processing. Gene 95:261, 1990

109. Tamura RN, Cooper HM, Collo G, Quaranta V: Cell type-specific integrin variants with alternative α chain cytoplasmic domains. Proc Natl Acad Sci USA 88:10183, 1991

110. Hogervorst F, Admiraal LG, Niessen C, et al: Biochemical characterization and tissue distribution of the A and B variants of the integrin α_6 subunit. J Cell Biol 121:179, 1993

111. Hierck B, Thorsteinsdottir S, Niessen C, et al: Variants of the $\alpha_6\beta_1$ laminin receptor in early murine development: Distribution, molecular cloning and chromosomal localization of the mouse integrin α_6 subunit. Cell Adhesion and Communication 1:33, 1993

112. Kornberg LJ, Earp HS, Turner CE, et al: Signal transduction by integrins: Increased protein tyrosine phosphorylation caused by clustering of β_1 integrins. Proc Natl Acad Sci USA 88:8392, 1991

113. Kornberg L, Juliano RL: Signal transduction from the extracellular matrix: The integrin-tyrosine kinase connection. Trends Pharmacol Sci 13:93, 1992

114. Yamada A, Kaneyuki T, Torimoto Y, et al: Signaling from LFA-1 contributes signal transduction through CD2 alternative pathway in T cell activation. Cell Immunol 142:145, 1992

115. Schwartz MA: Signaling by integrins: Implications for tumorigenesis. Cancer Res 53:1503, 1993

116. Huang M-M, Lipfert L, Cunningham M, et al: Adhesive ligand binding to integrin $\alpha_{IIb}\beta_3$ stimulates tyrosine phosphorylation of novel protein substrates before phosphorylation of pp125^{FAK}. J Cell Biol 122:473, 1993

117. Guan J-L, Trevithick JE, Hynes RO: Fibronectin/integrin interaction induces tyrosine phosphorylation of a 120-kDa protein. Cell Regul 2:951, 1991

118. Ginsberg MH, Loftus JC, Plow EF: Common and ligand-specific integrin recognition mechanisms. Chem Immunol 50:75, 1991

119. Tamkun JW, DeSimone DW, Fonda D, et al: Structure of integrin, a glycoprotein involved in the transmembrane linkage between fibronectin and actin. Cell 46:271, 1986

120. Suzuki S, Naitoh Y: Amino acid sequence of a novel integrin β_4 subunit and primary expression of the mRNA in epithelial cells. EMBO J 9:757, 1990

121. Hogervorst F, Kuikman I, von dem Borne AEGR, Sonnenberg A: Cloning and sequence analysis of beta-4 cDNA: An integrin subunit that contains a unique 118 kd cytoplasmic domain. EMBO J 9:765, 1990

122. Yee G, Hynes RO: A novel, tissue-specific integrin subunit, β_v, expressed in the midgut of Drosophila melanogaster. Development 118:845, 1993

123. Beer J, Coller BD: Evidence that platelet glycoprotein IIIa has a large disulfide-bonded loop that is susceptible to proteolytic cleavage. J Biol Chem 264:17564, 1989

124. Calvete JJ, Henschen A, González-Rodriguez J: Assignment of disulphide bonds in human platelet GPIIIa: A disulphide pattern for the β-subunits of the integrin family. Biochem J 274:63, 1991

125. Parise LV, Phillips DR: Platelet membrane glycoprotein IIb-IIIa complex incorporated into phospholipid vesicles. J Biol Chem 260:1750, 1985

126. Carrell NA, Fitzgerald LA, Steiner B, et al: Structure of human platelet membrane glycoproteins IIb and IIIa as determined by electron microscopy. J Biol Chem 260:1743, 1985

127. Nermut MV, Green NM, Eason P, et al: Electron microscopy and structural model of human fibronectin receptor. EMBO J 7:4093, 1988

128. Newman PJ: Platelet GP IIb-IIIa: Molecular variations and alloantigens. Thromb Haemost 66:111, 1991

129. Wardlaw AJ, Hibbs ML, Stacker SA, Springer TA: Distinct mutations in two patients with leukocyte adhesion deficiency and their functional correlates. J Exp Med 172:335, 1990

130. D'Souza SE, Ginsberg M, Burke T, et al: Localization of an Arg-Gly-Asp recognition within an integrin adhesion receptor. Science 242:91, 1988

131. Smith JW, Cheresh DA: The Arg-Gly-Asp-binding domain of the vitronectin receptor. J Biol Chem 263:18726, 1988

132. Loftus JC, O'Toole TE, Plow EF, et al: A β_3 integrin mutation abolishes ligand binding and alters divalent cation-dependent conformation. Science 249:915, 1991

133. Takada Y, Ylänne J, Mandelman D, et al: A point mutation of integrin β_1 subunit blocks binding of $\alpha_5\beta_1$ to fibronectin and invasion but not recruitment to adhesion plaques. J Cell Biol 119:913, 1992

134. Ramsamooj P, Lively MO, Hantgan RR: Evidence that the central region of glycoprotein IIIa participates in integrin receptor function. Biochem J 276:725, 1991

135. Shih D-T, Edelman JM, Horwitz AF, et al: Structure/function analysis of the integrin β_1 subunit by epitope mapping. J Cell Biol 122:1361, 1993

136. Andrieux A, Rabiet M-J, Chapel A, et al: A highly conserved sequence of the Arg-Gly-Asp-binding domain of the integrin β_3 subunit is sensitive to stimulation. J Biol Chem 266:14202, 1991

137. Neugebauer KM, Reichardt LF: Cell-surface regulation of β_1-integrin activity on developing retinal neurons. Nature 350:68, 1991

138. Coller BS: A new murine monoclonal antibody reports an activation-dependent change in the conformation and/or microenvironment of the platelet glycoprotein IIb/IIIa complex. J Clin Invest 76:101, 1985

139. Shattil SJ, Hoxie JA, Cunningham M, Brass LF: Changes in the platelet membrane glycoprotein IIb-IIIa complex during platelet activation. J Biol Chem 260:11107, 1985

140. Frelinger AL III, Du X, Plow EF, Ginsberg MH: Monoclonal antibodies to ligand-occupied conformers of integrin $\alpha_{IIb}\beta_3$ (glycoprotein IIb-IIIa) alter receptor affinity, specificity, and function. J Biol Chem 266:17106, 1991

141. Anderson GP, Van de Winkel JGJ, Anderson CL: Anti-GPIIb/IIIa (CD41) monoclonal antibody-induced platelet activation requires Fc receptor-dependent cell-cell interaction. Br J Haematol 79:75, 1991

142. Frojmovic MM, O'Toole TE, Plow EF, et al: Platelet glycoprotein II$_b$-III$_a$ ($\alpha_{IIb}\beta_3$ integrin) confers fibrinogen- and activation-dependent aggregation on heterologous cells. Blood 78:369, 1991

143. Altieri DC, Edgington TS: A monoclonal antibody reacting with distinct adhesion molecules defines a transition in the functional state of the receptor CD11b/CD18. J Immunol 141:2656, 1988

144. Masumoto A, Hemler ME: Multiple activation states of VLA-4. Mechanistic differences between adhesion to CS1/fibronectin and to vascular cell adhesion molecule-1. J Biol Chem 268:228, 1993

145. Weitzman JB, Pasqualini R, Takada Y, Hemler ME: The function and distinctive regulation of the integrin VLA-3 in cell adhesion, spreading, and homotypic cell aggregation. J Biol Chem 268:8651, 1993

146. Solowska J, Edelman JM, Albelda SM, Buck CA: Cytoplasmic and transmembrane domains of integrin β_1 and β_3 subunits are functionally interchangeable. J Cell Biol 114:1079, 1991

147. Horwitz AF, Duggan K, Greggs R, et al: The CSAT antigen has properties of a receptor for laminin and fibronectin. J Cell Biol 101:2134, 1985

148. Horwitz AF, Duggan K, Buck CA, et al: The CSAT antigen is a dual receptor for talin and fibronectin. Nature 320:531, 1986

149. Otey C, Pavalko F, Burridge K: An interaction between α-actinin and the β_1 integrin subunit in vitro. J Cell Biol 111:721, 1990

150. Pavalko FM, Otey CA, Simon KO, Burridge K: α-Actinin: A direct link between actin and integrins. Biochem Soc Trans 19:1065, 1991

151. Solowska J, Guan JG, Marcantonio E, et al: Expression of normal and mutant avian integrin subunits in rodent cells. J Cell Biol 109:853, 1989

152. Marcantonio EE, Guan J-L, Trevithick JE, Hynes RO: Mapping of the functional determinants of the integrin β_1 cytoplasmic domain by site-directed mutagenesis. Cell Regulation 1:597, 1990

153. Hayashi Y, Haimovich B, Reszka A, et al: Expression and function of chicken integrin β_1 subunit and its cytoplasmic domain mutants in mouse NIH 3T3 cells. J Cell Biol 110:175, 1990

154. LaFlamme SE, Akiyama SK, Yamada KM: Regulation of fibronectin receptor distribution. J Cell Biol 117:437, 1992

155. Hemler M, Ware C, Strominger J: Characterization of a novel differentiation antigen complex recognized by a monoclonal antibody (A1A5): Unique activation-specific molecular forms on stimulated T cells. J Immunol 131:334, 1983

156. Hemler ME: VLA proteins in the integrin family: Structures, functions, and their role on leukocytes. Annu Rev Immunol 8:365, 1990

157. Ylanne J, Chen Y, O'Toole T, et al: Distinct functions of integrin α and β subunit cytoplasmic domains in cell spreading and formation of focal adhesions. J Cell Biol 122:223, 1993

158. McMahon AP, Bradley A: The Wnt-1 (int-1) proto-oncogene is required for development of a large region of the mouse brain. Cell 62:1073, 1990

159. O'Toole TE, Mandelman D, Forsyth J, et al: Modulation of the affinity of integrin $\alpha_{IIb}\beta_3$ (GPIIb-IIIa) by the cytoplasmic domain of α_{IIb}. Science 254:845, 1991

160. Chan BMC, Kassner PD, Schiro JA, et al: Distinct cellular functions mediated by different VLA integrin α subunit cytoplasmic domains. Cell 68:1051, 1992

161. Burridge K, Fath K, Kelly T, et al: Focal adhesions: Transmembrane junctions between the extracellular matrix and the cytoskeleton. Annu Rev Cell Biol 4:487, 1988

162. Damsky CH, Knudsen KA, Bradley D, et al: Distribution of the cell-substratum attachment (CSAT) antigen on myogenic and fibroblastic cells in culture. J Cell Biol 100:1528, 1985

163. Lipfert L, Haimovich B, Schaller MD, et al: Integrin-dependent phosphorylation and activation of the protein tyrosine kinase pp125^{FAK} in platelets. J Cell Biol 119:905, 1992

164. Wilcox M, DiAntonio A, Leptin M: The function of PS integrins in *Drosophila* wing morphogenesis. Development 107:891, 1989

165. Zusman S, Grinblat Y, Yee G, et al: Analyses of PS integrin functions during *Drosophila* development. Development 118:737, 1993

166. Bronner-Fraser M: Alterations in neural crest migration by a monoclonal antibody that affects cell adhesion. J Cell Biol 101:610, 1985

167. Bronner-Fraser M: An antibody to a receptor for fibronectin and laminin perturbs cranial neural crest development in vivo. Dev Biol 117:528, 1986

168. Jaffredo T, Horwitz AF, Buck CA, et al: Myoblast migration specifically inhibited in the chick embryo by grafted CSAT hybridoma cells secreting an anti-integrin antibody. Development 103:431, 1988

169. Rosen GD, Sanes JR, LaChance R, et al: Roles for the integrin VLA-4 and its counter receptor VCAM-1 in myogenesis. Cell 69:1107, 1992

170. Galileo DS, Majors J, Horwitz AF, Sanes JR: Retrovirally introduced antisense integrin RNA inhibits neuroblast migration in vivo. Neuron 9:1117, 1992

171. Buck CA, Albelda S, Damjanovich L, et al: Immunohistochemical and molecular analysis of β_1 and β_3 integrins. Cell Differ Dev 32:189, 1990

172. Albelda SM: Endothelial and epithelial cell adhesion molecules. Am J Respir Cell Mol Biol 4:195, 1991

173. Albelda SM, Solowska J, Edelman JM, et al: The role of integrins in development: Structure, function, and tissue specific expression. *In* LeDouarin N, Dieterlen-Lievre F, Smith J (eds): The Avian Model in Developmental Biology: From Organism to Genes. Paris, Edition du CNRS, 1991, p 261

174. Cheresh DA: Integrins in thrombosis, wound healing and cancer. Biochem Soc Trans 19:835, 1991

175. Murakami J, Nishida T, Otori T: Coordinated appearance of β_1 integrins and fibronectin during corneal wound healing. J Lab Clin Med 120:86, 1992

176. Hertle MD, Kubler M-D, Leigh IM, Watt FM: Aberrant integrin expression during epidermal wound healing and in psoriatic epidermis. J Clin Invest 89:1892, 1992

177. Muschler JL, Horwitz AF: Down-regulation of the chicken $\alpha_5\beta_1$ integrin fibronectin receptor during development. Development 113:327, 1991

178. Bronner-Fraser M, Artinger M, Muschler J, Horwitz AF: Developmentally regulated expression of α_6 integrin in avian embryos. Development 115:197, 1992

179. Werb Z, Tremble P, Behrendtsen O, et al: Signal transduction through the fibronectin receptor induces collagenase and stromelysin gene expression. J Cell Biol 109:877, 1989

180. Menko AS, Boettiger D: Occupation of the extracellular matrix receptor, integrin, is a control point for myogenic differentiation. Cell 51:51, 1987

181. Nojima Y, Rothstein DM, Sugita K, et al: Ligation of VLA-4 on T cells stimulates tyrosine phosphorylation of a 105-kD protein. J Exp Med 175:1045, 1992

182. Guan J-L, Shalloway D: Regulation of focal adhesion-associated protein tyrosine kinase by both cellular adhesion and oncogenic transformation. Nature 358:690, 1992

183. Hanks SK, Calalb MB, Harper MC, Patel SK: Focal adhesion protein-tyrosine kinase phosphorylated in response to cell attachment to fibronectin. Proc Natl Acad Sci USA 89:8487, 1992

184. Burridge K, Turner CE, Romer LH: Tyrosine phosphorylation of paxillin and pp125^FAK accompanies cell adhesion to extracellular matrix: A role in cytoskeletal assembly. J Cell Biol 119: 893, 1992

185. Kanner SB, Reynolds LAB, Vines RR, Parsons JT: Monoclonal antibodies to individual tyrosine-phosphorylated protein substrates of oncogene-encoded tyrosine kinases. Proc Natl Acad Sci USA 87:3328, 1990

186. Kornberg L, Earp HS, Parsons JT, et al: Cell adhesion or integrin clustering increases phosphorylation of a focal adhesion-associated tyrosine kinase. J Biol Chem 267:23439, 1992

187. Zachary I, Rozengurt E: Focal adhesion kinase (p125^FAK): A point of convergence in the action of neuropeptides, integrins and oncogenes. Cell 71:891, 1992

188. Schwartz MA, Ingber DE, Lawrence M, et al: Multiple integrins share the ability to induce elevation of intracellular pH. Exp Cell Res 195:533, 1991

189. Shimizu Y, Van Seventer G, Horgan K, Shaw S: Regulated expression and binding of three VLA (β₁) integrin receptors on T cells. Nature 345:250, 1990

190. Chan BMC, Wong J, Rao A, Hemler M: T cell receptor-dependent, antigen-specific stimulation of a murine T cell clone induces a transient, VLA protein-mediated binding to extracellular matrix. J Immunol 147:398, 1991

191. Tanaka Y, Shaw S: T cell adhesion cascades: General considerations and illustration with CD31. Adv Exp Med Biol 323: 157, 1992

192. Tanaka Y, Albelda SM, Horgan KJ, et al: CD31 expressed on distinctive T cell subsets is a preferential amplifier of β₁ integrin-mediated adhesion. J Exp Med 176:245, 1992

193. LeBaron RG, Esko JD, Woods A, et al: Adhesion of glycosaminoglycan-deficient Chinese hamster ovary cell mutants to fibronectin substrata. J Cell Biol 106:945, 1988

194. Bidanset DJ, LeBaron R, Rosenberg L, et al: Regulation of cell substrate adhesion: Effects of small galactosaminoglycan-containing proteoglycans. J Cell Biol 118:1523, 1992

195. Woods A, Couchman JR: Protein kinase C involvement in focal adhesion formation. J Cell Sci 101:277, 1992

196. Cheifetz S, Weatherbee JA, Tsang ML, et al: The transforming growth factor β system, a complex pattern of cross-reactivity with ligands and receptors. Cell 48:409, 1987

197. Heino J, Massague J: Transforming growth factor-β switches the pattern of integrins expressed in MG-63 human osteosarcoma cells and causes a selective loss of cell adhesion to laminin. J Biol Chem 264:21806, 1989

198. Gladson CL, Cheresh DA: Glioblastoma expression of vitronectin and the αᵥβ₃ integrin: Adhesion mechanism for transformed glial cells. J Clin Invest 88:1924, 1991

199. Dedhar S: Integrins and tumor invasion. BioEssays 12:583, 1990

200. Muroi K, Toya K, Suzuki T, et al: Expression of CD11B, CD14 and CD36 antigens by B-cell lymphoma. Br J Haematol 80: 126, 1992

201. Albelda SM: The role of integrins and other cell adhesion molecules in tumor progression and metastasis. Lab Invest 68:4, 1993

202. Peltonen J, Larjave H, Jaakkola S, et al: Localization of integrin receptors for fibronectin, collagen and laminin in human skin. J Clin Invest 84:1916, 1989

203. Stamp GWH, Pignatelli M: Distribution of β₁, α₁, α₂ and α₃ integrin chains in basal cell carcinomas. J Pathol 163:307, 1991

204. Pignatelli M, Bodmer WF: Integrin cell adhesion molecules and colorectal cancer. J Pathol 162:95, 1990

205. Williams AF, Barclay AN: The immunoglobulin superfamily—domains for cell surface recognition. Annu Rev Immunol 6: 381, 1988

206. Zutter MM, Krigman HR, Santora SA: Altered integrin expression in adenocarcinoma of the breast. Am J Pathol 142:1439, 1993

207. Weinel RJ, Rosendahl A, Neumann K, et al: Expression and function of VLA-α₂, -α₃, -α₅ and α₆-integrin receptors in pancreatic carcinoma. Int J Cancer 52:827, 1992

208. Zutter MM, Mazoujian G, Santoro SA: Decreased expression of integrin adhesive protein receptors in adenocarcinoma of the breast. Am J Pathol 137:863, 1990

209. Damjanovich L, Albelda SM, Mette SA, Buck CA: Distribution of integrin cell adhesion receptors in normal and malignant lung tissue. Am J Respir Cell Mol Biol 6:197, 1992

210. Albelda SM, Mette SA, Elder DE, et al: Integrin distribution in malignant melanoma: Association of the β₃ subunit with tumor progression. Cancer Res 50:6757, 1990

211. Clark W, Elder D, Guerry D, et al: A study of tumor progression: The precursor lesions of superficial spreading and nodular melanoma. Hum Pathol 15:1147, 1984

212. Clark W, Elder D, Guerry D, et al: Model predicting survival in stage 1 melanoma based on tumor progression. J Natl Cancer Inst 81:1893, 1989

213. McGregor B, McGregor JL, Weiss LM, et al: Presence of cytoadhesins (IIb-IIIa-like glycoproteins) on human metastatic melanomas but not on benign melanocytes. Am J Clin Pathol 92:495, 1989

214. Kumagai H, Tajima M, Ueno Y, et al: Effect of cyclic RGD peptide on cell adhesion and tumor metastasis. Biochem Biophys Res Commun 177:74, 1991

215. Soszka T, Knudsen KA, Beviglia L, et al: Inhibition of murine melanoma cell-matrix adhesion and experimental metastasis by albolabrin, an RGD-containing peptide isolated from the venom of Trimeresurus albolabris. Exp Cell Res 196:6, 1991

216. Nip J, Shibata H, Loskutoff DJ, et al: Human melanoma cells derived from lymphatic metastases use integrin αᵥβ₃ to adhere to lymph node vitronectin. J Clin Invest 90:1406, 1992

217. Felding-Habermann B, Mueller BM, Romerdahl CA, Cheresh DA: Involvement of integrin αᵥ gene expression in human melanoma tumorigenicity. J Clin Invest 89:2018, 1992

218. Seftor REB, Seftor EA, Gehlsen KR, et al: Role of the αᵥβ₃ integrin in human melanoma cell invasion. Proc Natl Acad Sci USA 89:1557, 1992

219. Schreiner C, Fisher M, Hussein S, Juliano RL: Increased tumorigenicity of fibronectin receptor deficient Chinese hamster ovary cell variants. Cancer Res 51:1738, 1991

220. Giancotti FG, Ruoslahti E: Elevated levels of the α₅β₁ fibronectin receptor suppress the transformed phenotype of Chinese hamster ovary cells. Cell 60:849, 1990

221. Chan BMC, Matsuura N, Takada Y, et al: In vitro and in vivo consequences of VLA-2 expression on rhabdomyosarcoma cells. Science 251:1600, 1991

222. Yamada K, Kennedy DW, Yamada SS, et al: Monoclonal antibody and synthetic peptide inhibitors of human tumor cell migration. Cancer Res 50:4485, 1990

223. Gehlsen KR, Argraves WS, Pierschbacher MD, Ruoslahti E: Inhibition of in vitro tumor cell invasion by Arg-Gly-Asp-containing synthetic peptides. J Cell Biol 106:925, 1988

224. Skubitz APN, McCarthy JB, Zhao Q, et al: Definition of a sequence, RYVVLPR, within laminin peptide F-9 that mediates metastatic fibrosarcoma cell adhesion and spreading. Cancer Res 50:7612, 1990

225. Gehlsen KR, Sriramarao P, Furcht LT, Skubitz APN: A synthetic peptide derived from the carboxy terminus of the laminin A chain represents a binding site for the α₃β₁ integrin. J Cell Biol 117:449, 1992

226. Roos E, Roossien F: Involvement of leukocyte function-associated antigen-1 (LFA-1) in the invasion of hepatocyte cultures by lymphoma and T-cell hybridoma cells. J Cell Biol 105:553, 1987

227. Roossien F, de Rijk D, Bikker A, Roos E: Involvement of LFA-1 in lymphoma invasion and metastasis demonstrated with LFA-1 deficient mutants. J Cell Biol 108:1979, 1989

228. Vestweber D: Selectins: Cell surface lectins which mediate the binding of leukocytes to endothelial cells. Semin Cell Biol 3: 211, 1992

229. Hunkapiller T, Hood L: Diversity of the immunoglobulin gene superfamily. Adv Immunol 44:1, 1989
230. Buck CA: Immunoglobulin superfamily: Structure, function and relationship to other receptor molecules. Semin Cell Biol 3: 179, 1992
231. Culty M, Miyake M, Kincade PW, et al: The hyaluronate receptor is a member of the CD44 (H-CAM) family of cell surface glycoproteins. J Cell Biol 111:2765, 1990
232. Haynes BF, Telen MJ, Hale LP, Denning SM: CD44—a molecule involved in leukocyte adherence and T-cell activation. Immunol Today 10:423, 1989
233. Stamenkovic I, Amiot M, Pesando JM, Seed B: A lymphocyte molecule implicated in lymph node homing is a member of the cartilage link protein family. Cell 56:1057, 1989
234. Zhu D, Cheng C-F, Pauli BU: Mediation of lung metastasis of murine melanomas by a lung-specific endothelial cell adhesion molecule. Proc Natl Acad Sci USA 88:9568, 1991
235. Gallatin WM, Weissman IL, Butcher EC: A cell surface molecule involved in organ-specific homing of lymphocytes. Nature 304:30, 1983
236. Camerini D, James SP, Stamenkovic I, Seed B: Leu8/TQ1 is the human equivalent of the MEL-14 lymph node homing receptor. Nature 342:78, 1989
237. Tedder TF, Isaacs CM, Ernst TJ, et al: Isolation and chromosomal localization of cDNAs encoding a novel human lymphocyte cell surface molecule LAM-1. J Exp Med 170:123, 1989
238. Pober JS, Lapierre LA, Stolpen AH, et al: Activation of cultured human endothelial cells by recombinant lymphotoxin: Comparison with tumor necrosis factor and interleukin 1 species. J Immunol 138:3319, 1987
239. Bevilacqua MP, Pober JA, Mendrick DL, et al: Identification of an inducible endothelial-leukocyte adhesion molecule. Proc Natl Acad Sci USA 84:9238, 1987
240. Pober JS, Gimbrone MA Jr, Lapierre LA, et al: Overlapping patterns of activation of human endothelial cells by interleukin 1, tumor necrosis factor, and immune interferon. J Immunol 137:1893, 1986
241. Stenberg PE, McEver RP, Shuman MA, et al: A platelet alpha-granule membrane protein (GMP-140) is expressed on the plasma membrane after activation. J Cell Biol 101:880, 1985
242. Berman CL, Yeo EC, Wenzel-Drake JD, et al: A platelet alpha-granule membrane protein that is associated with plasma membrane after activation. J Clin Invest 78:130, 1986
243. Larsen E, Celli A, Gilbert GE, et al: PADGEM protein: A receptor that mediates the interaction of activated platelets with neutrophils and monocytes. Cell 59:305, 1989
244. Hamburger SA, McEver RP: GMP-140 mediates adhesion of stimulated platelets to neutrophils. Blood 75:550, 1990
245. Geng JG, Bevilacqua MS, Moore KL, et al: Rapid neutrophil adhesion to activated endothelium mediated by GMP-140. Nature 343:757, 1990
246. Moore KL, Varki A, McEver RP: GMP-140 binds to a glycoprotein receptor on human neutrophils: Evidence for a lectin-like interaction. J Cell Biol 112:491, 1991
247. Imai Y, Singer MS, Fennie C, et al: Identification of a carbohydrate-based endothelial ligand for a lymphocyte homing receptor. J Cell Biol 113:1213, 1991
248. Kishimoto TK, Warnock RA, Jutila MA, et al: Antibodies against human neutrophil LECAM-1 (LAM-1/Leu-8/DREG-56 antigen) and endothelial cell ELAM-1 inhibit a common CD18-independent adhesion pathway in vitro. Blood 78:805, 1991
249. Picker LJ, Warnock RA, Burns AR, et al: The neutrophil selectin LECAM-1 presents carbohydrate ligands to the vascular selectins ELAM-1 and GMP-140. Cell 66:921, 1991
250. Lawrence MB, Springer TA: Leukocytes roll on a selectin at physiologic flow rates: Distinction from and prerequisite for adhesion through integrins. Cell 65:859, 1991
251. Ley K, Gaehtgens P, Fennie C, et al: Lectin-like cell adhesion molecule 1 mediates leukocyte rolling in mesenteric venules in vivo. Blood 77:2553, 1991
252. Buck CA, Glick MC, Warren L: A comparative study of the glycoproteins from the surface of control and Rous sarcoma virus transformed hamster cells. Biochemistry 9:4567, 1970
253. Buck CA, Glick MC, Warren L: Glycopeptides from the surface of control and virus-transformed cells. Science 172:169, 1971
254. Warren L, Fuhrer JP, Buck CA: Surface glycoproteins of normal and transformed cells: A difference determined by sialic acid and a growth-dependent sialyl transferase. Proc Natl Acad Sci USA 69:1838, 1972
255. Saito O, Want W-C, Lotan R, Fukuda M: Differential glycosylation and cell surface expression of lysosomal membrane glycoproteins in sublines of a human colon cancer exhibiting distinct metastatic potentials. J Biol Chem 267:5700, 1992
256. Aruffo A, Dietsch M, Wan H, et al: Granule membrane protein 140 (GMP140) binds to carcinomas and carcinoma-derived cell lines. Proc Natl Acad Sci USA 89:2292, 1992
257. Kojima N, Handa K, Newman W, Hakomori S: Inhibition of selectin-dependent tumor cell adhesion to endothelial cells and platelets by blocking O-glycosylation of these cells. Biochem Biophys Res Commun 182:1288, 1992
258. Hofmann M, Rudy W, Gunthert U, et al: A link between ras and metastatic behavior of tumor cells: ras induces CD44 promoter activity and leads to low-level expression of metastasis-specific variants of CD44 in CREF cells. Cancer Res 53:1516, 1993
259. Heider K-H, Hofmann M, Hors E, et al: A human homologue of the rat metastasis-associated variant of CD44 is expressed in colorectal carcinomas and adenomatous polyps. J Cell Biol 120:227, 1993
260. Carpenter G: Receptor tyrosine kinase substrates: src homology domains and signal transduction. FASEB J 6:3283, 1992
261. Underhill C: CD44: The hyaluronan receptor. J Cell Sci 103:293, 1992
262. Camp RL, Scheynius A, Johansson C, Puré E: CD44 is necessary for optimal contact allergic responses but is not required for normal leukocyte extravasation. J Exp Med 178: 497, 1993
263. Yang H, Binns RM: CD44 is not directly involved in the binding of lymphocytes to cultured high endothelial cells from peripheral lymph nodes. Immunology 79:418, 1993
264. Aruffo A, Stamenkovic I, Melnick M, et al: CD44 is the principal cell surface receptor for hyaluronate. Cell 61:1303, 1990
265. Bourguignon LYW, Lokeshwar VB, He J, et al: CD44-like endothelial cell transmembrane glycoprotein (GP116) interacts with extracellular matrix and ankyrin. Mol Cell Biol 12:4464, 1992
266. Stamenkovic I, Aruffo A, Amiot M, Seed B: The hematopoietic and epithelial forms of CD44 are distinct polypeptides with different adhesion potentials for hyaluronate-bearing cells. EMBO J 10:343, 1991
267. Tölg C, Hofmann M, Herrlich P, Ponta H: Splicing choice from ten variant exons establishes CD44 variability. Nucleic Acids Res 21:1225, 1993
268. Gunthert U, Hofmann M, Rudy W, et al: A new variant of glycoprotein CD44 confers metastatic potential to rat carcinoma cells. Cell 65:13, 1991
269. Rudy W, Hofmann M, Schwartz-Albiez R, et al: The two major CD44 proteins expressed on a metastatic rat tumor cell line are derived from different splice variants: Each one individually suffices to confer metastatic behavior. Cancer Res 53: 1262, 1993
270. Horst E, Meijer CJLM, Radaszkiewicz T, et al: Adhesion molecules in the prognosis of diffuse large cell lymphoma: Expression of a lymphocytic homing receptor (CD44), LFA-1 (CD11a/CD18) and ICAM-1 (CD54). Leukemia 4:595, 1990
271. Sy M-S, Guo Y-J, Stamenkovic I: Inhibition of tumor growth in vivo with a soluble CD44-immunoglobulin fusion protein. J Exp Med 176:623, 1992
272. Matsumura Y, Tarin D: Significance of CD44 gene products for cancer diagnosis and disease evaluation. Lancet 340:1053, 1992

273. Birch M, Mitchell S, Hart IR: Isolation and characterization of human melanoma cell variants expressing high and low levels of CD44. Cancer Res 51:6660, 1991

274. Hart IR, Mitchell S, Birch M: Cell adhesion receptors and melanoma dissemination. Beitr Onkol 44:250, 1992

275. Brown TA, Bouchard T, St John T, et al: Human keratinocytes express a new CD44 core protein (CD44E) as a heparan-sulfate intrinsic membrane proteoglycan with additional exons. J Cell Biol 113:207, 1991

276. Camp RL, Kraus TA, Pure E: Variations in the cytoskeletal interaction and posttranslational modification of the CD44. J Cell Biol 115:1283, 1991

277. Shimizu Y, Van Seventer G, Siraganian R, et al: Dual role of the CD44 molecule in T-cell adhesion and activation. J Immunol 143:2457, 1989

278. Koopman G, Van Kooyk Y, De Graaff M, et al: Triggering of the CD44 antigen on T lymphocytes promotes T cell adhesion through the LFA-1 pathway. J Immunol 145:3589, 1990

279. Zambruno G, Marchisio PC, Melchiori A, et al: Expression of integrin receptors and their role in adhesion, spreading and migration of normal human melanocytes. J Cell Sci 105:179, 1993

280. Dustin ML, Springer TA: Role of lymphocyte adhesion receptors in transient interactions and cell locomotion. Ann Rev Immunol 9:27, 1991

281. Benchimol S, Fuks A, Jothy S, et al: Carcinoembryonic antigen, a human tumor marker, functions as an intercellular adhesion molecule. Cell 57:327, 1989

282. Fearon ER, Cho KR, Nigro JM, et al: Identification of a chromosome 18q gene that is altered in colorectal cancers. Science 247:49, 1990

283. Cunningham BA, Hemperly JJ, Murray BA, et al: Neural cell adhesion molecule: Structure, immunoglobulin-like domains, cell surface modulation, and alternative RNA splicing. Science 236:799, 1987

284. Bastiani MJ, Harrelson AJ, Snow PM, Goodman CS: Expression of fasciclin I and II glycoproteins on subsets of axon pathways during neuronal development in the grasshopper. Cell 48:745, 1987

285. Staunton D, Dustin ML, Springer T: Functional cloning of ICAM-2, a cell adhesion ligand for LFA-1 homologous to ICAM-1. Nature 339:61, 1989

286. De Fougerolles AR, Springer T: ICAM-3, a third adhesion counter-receptor for LFA-1 on resting lymphocytes. J Exp Med 175:185, 1992

287. Rice GE, Munto JM, Bevilacqua MP: Inducible cell adhesion molecule 110 (INCAM-110) is an endothelial receptor for lymphocytes. J Exp Med 171:1369, 1990

288. Osborn L, Hession C, Tizard R, et al: Direct expression cloning of vascular cell adhesion molecule 1, a cytokine-induced endothelial protein that binds to lymphocytes. Cell 59:1203, 1989

289. Newman PG, Berndt MC, Gorsky J, et al: PECAM-1 (CD31): Cloning and relation to adhesion molecules of the immunoglobulin gene superfamily. Science 247:1219, 1990

290. Albelda SM, Oliver P, Romer L, Buck CA: EndoCAM: A novel endothelial cell-cell adhesion molecule. J Cell Biol 110:1227, 1990

291. Klausner RD, Samelson LE: T cell antigen receptor activation pathways: The tyrosine kinase connection. Cell 64:875, 1991

292. Shimizu Y, Newman W, Gopal TV, et al: Four molecular pathways of T cell adhesion to endothelial cells: Roles of LFA-1, VCAM-1, and ELAM-1 and changes in pathway hierarchy under different activation conditions. J Cell Biol 113:1203, 1991

293. Nortamo P, Li R, Renkonen R, et al: The expression of human intercellular adhesion molecule-2 is refractory to inflammatory cytokines. Eur J Immunol 21:2629, 1991

294. Sanchez-Madrid F, Corbi AL: Leukocyte integrins: Structure, function and regulation of their activity. Semin Cell Biol 3:199, 1992

295. Elices MJ, Osborn L, Takada Y, et al: VCAM-1 on activated endothelium interacts with the leukocyte integrin VLA-4 at a site distinct from the VLA-4/fibronectin binding site. J Immunol 60:577, 1990

296. Holzmann B, Weissman IL: Integrin molecules involved in lymphocyte homing to Peyer's patches. Immunol Rev 108:45, 1989

297. Miyake K, Weissman IL, Greenberger JS, Kincade PW: Evidence for a role of the integrin VLA-4 in lympho-hemopoiesis. J Exp Med 173:599, 1991

298. Miyake K, Medina K, Ishihara K, et al: A VCAM-like adhesion molecule on murine bone marrow stromal cells mediates binding of lymphocyte precursors in culture. J Cell Biol 114:557, 1991

299. Delisser HM, Yan HC, Newman PJ, et al: Platelet/endothelial cell adhesion molecule-1 (CD31)-mediated cellular aggregation involves cell surface glycosaminoglycans. J Biol Chem 268:16037, 1993

300. Shin J, Dunbrack RL Jr, Lee S, Strominger JL: Phosphorylation-dependent down-modulation of CD4 requires a specific structure within the cytoplasmic domain of CD4. J Biol Chem 266:10658, 1991

301. Blanchard DK, Hall RE, Djeu JY: Role of CD18 in lymphokine activated killer (LAK) cell-mediated lysis of human monocytes: Comparison with other LAK targets. Int J Cancer 45:312, 1990

302. Sadoul R, Hirn M, Deagostini-Bazin H, et al: Adult and embryonic mouse neural cell adhesion molecules have different binding properties. Nature 304:347, 1983

303. Acheson A, Sunshine JL, Rutishauser U: NCAM polysialic acid can regulate both cell-cell and cell-substrate interactions. J Cell Biol 114:143, 1991

304. Hoffman S, Edelman GM: Kinetics of homophilic binding by embryonic and adult forms of neural cell adhesion molecule. Proc Natl Acad Sci USA 80:5762, 1983

305. Edelman GM, Crossin KL: Cell adhesion molecules: Implications for a molecular histology. Annu Rev Biochem 60:155, 1991

306. Cole GJ, Loewy A, Glaser L: Neuronal cell-cell adhesion depends on interactions of NCAM with heparin-like molecules. Nature 320:445, 1986

307. Reyes A, Akeson R, Brezina L, Cole GJ: Structural requirements for neural cell adhesion molecule-heparin interaction. Cell Regul 1:567, 1990

308. Albelda SM, Muller WA, Buck CA, Newman PJ: Molecular and cellular properties of PECAM-1 (endoCAM/CD31): A novel vascular cell-cell adhesion molecule. J Cell Biol 114:1059, 1991

309. Delisser HM, Muller WA, Newman PJ, Albelda SM: PECAM-1 (CD31) mediates heterophilic cell-cell adhesion. J Cell Biol 115:70a, 1991

310. Delisser HM, Yan HC, Newman PJ, et al: Platelet/endothelial cell adhesion molecule-1 (CD31)-mediated cellular aggregation involves cell surface glycosaminoglycans. J Biol Chem 268:16037, 1993

311. Cardin AD, Weintraub HJR: Molecular modeling of protein-glycosaminoglycan interactions. Arteriosclerosis 9:21, 1989

312. Bogen SA, Watkins SC, Abbas AK: CD31 is associated with lymphocyte recruitment and vascular transmigration following antigenic stimulation. Unpublished manuscript, 1991

313. Bogen SA, Baldwin HS, Watkins SC, et al: Association of murine CD31 with transmigrating lymphocytes following antigenic stimulation. Am J Pathol 141:843, 1992

314. Muller WA, Weigl SA, Deng X, Phillips DM: PECAM-1 is required for transendothelial migration of leukocytes. J Exp Med 178:449, 1993

315. Leppa S, Mali M, Miettinen HM, Jalkanen M: Syndecan expression regulates cell morphology and growth of mouse mammary epithelial tumor cells. Proc Natl Acad Sci USA 89:932, 1992

316. Johnson JP, Stade BG, Holzmann B, et al: De novo expression of intercellular adhesion molecule-1 in melanoma correlates with increased risk of metastasis. Proc Natl Acad Sci USA 86:641, 1989

317. Braakman E, Goedegebuure P, Vreugdenhil R, et al: ICAM⁻ melanoma cells are relatively resistant to CD3-mediated T-cell lysis. Int J Cancer 46:475, 1990

318. Rice GE, Bevilacqua M: An inducible endothelial cell surface

glycoprotein mediates melanoma adhesion. Science *246*:1303, 1989

319. Dejana E, Bertocchi F, Bortolami M, et al: Interleukin 1 promotes tumor cell adhesion to cultured human endothelial cells. J Clin Invest *82*:1466, 1988

320. Jonjic N, Marìn-Padura I, Pollicino T, et al: Regulated expression of vascular cell adhesion molecule-1 in human malignant melanoma. Am J Pathol *141*:1323, 1992

321. Denton KJ, Stretch JR, Gatter KC, Harris AL: A study of adhesion molecules as markers of progression in malignant melanoma. J Pathol *167*:187, 1992

322. Thomas P, Toth C, Saini K, et al: The structure, metabolism and function of the carcinoembryonic antigen gene family. Biochim Biophys Acta *1032*:177, 1990

323. Kibbelaar RE, Moolenaar KEC, Michalides RJAM, et al: Neural cell adhesion molecule expression, neuroendocrine differentiation and prognosis in lung carcinoma. Eur J Cancer *27*:431, 1991

324. Fearon ER, Vogelstein B: A genetic model for colorectal tumorigenesis. Cell *61*:759, 1990

325. Fidler IJ, Nicolson G: Organ selectivity for implantation, survival, and growth of B16 melanoma variant tumor lines. J Natl Cancer Inst *57*:1100, 1976

326. Brunson K, Beatty G, Nicolson G: Selection and altered tumor cell properties of brain colonizing metastatic melanoma. Nature *272*:543, 1978

327. Fidler IJ: Selection of successive tumor line for metastasis. Nature New Biol *242*:148, 1973

328. Stemper HB Jr, Woodruff JJ: Lymphocyte homing into lymph nodes: In vitro demonstration of the selective affinity of recirculating lymphocytes to high endothelial venules. J Exp Med *144*:828, 1976

329. Butcher EC, Scollay R, Weissman I: Lymphocyte adherence to high endothelial venules: Characteristics of a modified in vitro assay and examination of the binding of syngeneic and allogeneic lymphocyte populations. J Immunol *123*:1996, 1979

330. Netland P, Zetter B: Metastatic potential of B16 melanoma cells after in vitro selection for organ-specific adherence. J Cell Biol *101*:720, 1985

331. Nicolson G, Winkelhake J: Organ specificity of blood-borne tumour metastasis determined by cell adhesion? Nature *255*:230, 1975

332. Auerbach R, Lu WC, Pardon E, et al: Specificity of adhesion between murine tumor cells and capillary endothelium: An *in vitro* correlate of preferential metastasis *in vivo*. Cancer Res *47*:1492, 1987.

333. Nicolson G: Organ specificity of tumor metastasis: Role of preferential adhesion invasion and growth of malignant cells at specific secondary sites. Cancer Met Rev *7*:143, 1988

334. Lee KH, Lawley TJ, Xu Y, Swerlick RA: VCAM-1-, ELAM-1-, and ICAM-1-independent adhesion of melanoma cells to cultured human dermal microvascular endothelial cells. J Invest Dermatol *98*:79, 1992

335. Folkman J, Shing Y: Angiogenesis. J Biol Chem *267*:10931, 1992

336. Pauli B, Lee C: Organ preference of metastasis: The role of organ-specifically modulated endothelial cells. Lab Invest *58*:379, 1988

337. Johnson RC, Augustin-Voss HG, Zhu D, Pauli BU: Endothelial cell membrane vesicles in the study of organ preference of metastasis. Cancer Res *51*:394, 1991

338. Zhu D, Pauli BU: Generation of monoclonal antibodies directed against organ-specific endothelial cell surface determinants. J Histochem Cytochem *39*:1137, 1991

339. Zhu D, Cheng C-F, Pauli BU: Blocking of lung endothelial cell adhesion molecule-1 (Lu-ECAM-1) inhibits murine melanoma lung metastasis. J Clin Invest *89*:1718, 1992

340. Jackson AM, Alexandrov AB, Prescott S, et al: Expression of adhesion molecules by bladder cancer cells: Modulation by interferon-gamma and tumour necrosis factor-alpha. J Urol *148*:1583, 1992

341. Gralnick HR: von Willebrand factor, integrins, and platelets: Their role in cancer. J Lab Clin Med *119*:444, 1992

342. Chammas R, Brentani R: Integrins and metastases: An overview. Tumor Biol *12*:309, 1991

343. Gasic G, Gasic T, Stewart C: Antimetastatic effects associated with platelet reduction. Proc Natl Acad Sci USA *61*:46, 1968

344. Gasic G, Gasic T, Galanti N, et al: Platelet-tumor cell interactions in mice: The role of platelets in the spread of malignant disease. Int J Cancer *11*:704, 1973

345. Pearlstein E, Ambrogio C, Karpatkin S: Effect of anti-platelet antibody on the development of pulmonary metastases following injection of CT26 colon adenocarcinoma, Lewis lung carcinoma and B16 amelanotic melanoma tumor cells into mice. Cancer Res *44*:3884, 1984

346. Karpatkin S, Pearlstein E, Ambrogio C, Coller B: Role of adhesive proteins in platelet tumor interactions in vitro and metastasis formation in vivo. J Clin Invest *81*:1012, 1988

347. Sugimoto Y, Watanabe M, Oh-hara T, et al: Suppression of experimental lung colonization of a metastatic variant of murine colon adenocarcinoma 26 by a monoclonal antibody 8F11 inhibiting tumor cell-induced platelet aggregation. Cancer Res *51*:921, 1991

348. Boukereche H, BerthierVergnes O, Tabone E, et al: Platelet-melanoma cell interaction is mediated by the glycoprotein IIb-IIIa complex. Blood *74*:658, 1989

349. Chen YQ, Gao X, Timar J, et al: Identification of the $\alpha_{IIb}\beta_3$ integrin in murine tumor cells. J Biol Chem *267*:17314, 1992

350. Nierodzik MLR, Kajumo F, Karpatkin S: Effect of thrombin treatment of tumor cells on adhesion of tumor cells to platelets *in vitro* and tumor metastasis *in vivo*. Cancer Res *52*:3267, 1992

351. Grossi I, Hatfield J, Fitzgerald L, et al: Role of tumor cell glycoproteins immunologically related to glycoproteins Ib and IIb/IIIa in tumor cell-platelet and tumor cell-matrix interactions. FASEB J *2*:2385, 1988

352. Chang YS, Chen YQ, Timar J, et al: Increased expression of $\alpha_{IIb}\beta_3$ integrin in subpopulations of murine melanoma cells with high lung-colonizing ability. Int J Cancer *51*:445, 1992

353. Honn KV, Chen YQ, Timar J, et al: $\alpha_{IIb}\beta_3$ Integrin expression and function in subpopulations of murine tumors. Exp Cell Res *201*:23, 1992

354. Leavesley DI, Ferguson GD, Wayner EA, Cheresh DA: Requirement of the integrin β_3 subunit for carcinoma cell spreading or migration on vitronectin and fibronectin. J Cell Biol *117*:1101, 1992

355. Crissman J, Hatfield J, Menter D, et al: Morphological study of the interaction of intravascular tumor cells with endothelial cells and subendothelial matrix. Cancer Res *48*:4065, 1988

356. Liotta L, Schiffmann E: Tumour motility factors. Cancer Surv *7*:631, 1988

357. Hujanen E, Terranova V: Migration of tumor cells to organ-derived chemoattractants. Cancer Res *45*:3517, 1985

358. Lafrenie R, Shaughnessy SG, Orr FW: Cancer cell interactions with injured or activated endothelium. Cancer Metastasis Rev *11*:377, 1992

359. Weiss L, Orr F, Honn K: Interactions of cancer cells with the microvasculature during metastasis. FASEB J *2*:12, 1988

360. Giavazzi R, Garofalo A, Bani M: Interleukin 1-induced augmentation of experimental metastases from a human melanoma in nude mice. Cancer Res *50*:4771, 1990

361. Bani M, Garofalo A, Scanziani E, Giavazzi R: Effect of interleukin-1-beta on metastasis formation in different tumor systems. J Natl Cancer Inst *83*:119, 1991

362. Ruco LP, Pomponi D, Pigott R, et al: Cytokine production (IL-1α, IL-1β, and TNFα) and endothelial cell activation (ELAM-1 and HLA-DR) in reactive lymphadenitis, Hodgkin's disease, and in non-Hodgkin's lymphomas: An immunocytochemical study. Am J Pathol *137*:1163, 1990

363. Erbe DV, Wolitzky BA, Presta LG, et al: Identification of an E-selectin region critical for carbohydrate recognition and cell adhesion. J Cell Biol *119*:215, 1992

364. Kolatkar PR, Oliveira MA, Rossmann MG, et al: Preliminary X-ray crystallographic analysis of intercellular adhesion molecule-1. J Mol Biol *225*:1127, 1992

365. Graeme W, Air GM, Webster RG, Smith-Gill S: Epitopes on protein antigens: Misconceptions and realities. Cell *61*:553, 1990
366. Carlos TM, Harlan JM: Membrane proteins involved in phagocyte adherence to endothelium. Immunol Rev *114*:5, 1990
367. Edelman GM, Cunningham BA: Place-dependent cell adhesion, process retraction, and spatial signaling in neural morphogen-

esis. Cold Spring Harb Symp Quant Biol *55*:303, 1990
368. Edelman GM: Morphoregulation. Dev Dyn *193*:2, 1992
369. Morsy MA, Mitani K, Clemens P, et al: Progress toward human gene therapy. JAMA *270*:2338, 1993
370. McKusick VA: Medical genetics. A 40-year perspective on the evolution of a medical specialty from basic science. JAMA *270*:2351, 1993

10

TUMOR ANGIOGENESIS

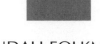

JUDAH FOLKMAN

It is now widely recognized that the ability of a tumor to induce the proliferation of new blood vessels from its host has a profound effect on tumor growth and metastasis. The onset of angiogenic activity permits rapid expansion of a tumor population and increases the risk of metastasis. In contrast, primary or metastatic tumor cells that are not angiogenic generally are prevented from enlarging to a population size that is clinically detectable. Absence of angiogenic activity limits tumor implants or spontaneous in situ tumors to a few million cells in a volume of a few cubic millimeters. This new understanding of tumor biology is based on a series of incremental discoveries made over the past 25 years. These laboratory findings now have been translated to clinical application and have led to novel diagnostic and therapeutic approaches in the management of patients with cancer. This chapter attempts to organize our current knowledge about tumor angiogenesis and its clinical applications.

TUMORS ARE ANGIOGENESIS DEPENDENT: A HYPOTHESIS

The idea that tumor growth is dependent on induction of neovascularization originated in the early 1960s from experiments in which tumors were grown in isolated perfused organs.[1] Prior to this series of reports, the conventional wisdom was that the hyperemia and increased vascularity commonly associated with tumors was mainly due to simple *dilation* of preexisting host vessels.[2,3] This vasodilation was thought to be a side effect of tumor metabolites and necrotic tumor products. Certain terms such as ''inflammatory'' carcinoma, still used today, are based on this earlier misconception. However, one report in 1939 and another in 1945 suggested that tumor hyperemia could be the result of *new* vessel proliferation, rather than vasodilation.[4,5] Despite these reports, a debate continued in the literature for the next two decades about whether tumors were supplied by existing vessels or by *neo*vascularization.[6] Those few investigators who had begun to

accept the notion that tumors might induce neovascularization still assumed that this vascular response was an inflammatory reaction—that is, a host defense against the tumor and of no importance for the growth of the tumor.[7]

Tumors in Isolated Perfused Organs: Absence of Angiogenesis

In the 1960s, a new view of the role of blood vessels in tumor growth originated from experiments in which neovascularization was *prevented*. When tumor cells were inoculated into isolated perfused organs, complete absence of angiogenesis was associated with restriction of tumor growth to small spheroids of 1 mm^3 or less.[8-10] This was the first time that viable tumor had been grown as a three-dimensional mass in a tissue without neovascularization. When the tiny tumor was transferred to the mouse strain from which it originated, it became *neo*vascularized and grew to more than 1000 times its maximal size in the isolated organ.

Hypothesis: The Necessity of Neovascularization

From these experiments, a hypothesis was proposed that tumor growth is angiogenesis dependent, and in 1971 the idea first was advanced that inhibition of angiogenesis could be therapeutic.[10] In its simplest terms, the hypothesis states: ''Once tumor take has occurred, every further increase in tumor cell population must be preceded by an increase in new capillaries which converge upon the tumor.''[11]

Evidence That Tumors Are Angiogenesis Dependent

Subsequent studies provided supporting evidence for this hypothesis, mainly of an indirect or correlative nature.

Experiments carried out in the past 4 years have provided direct evidence. Taken together, these data provide a firm scientific basis for the hypothesis.

INDIRECT EVIDENCE

Indirect evidence in support of the hypothesis was derived during the 1970s mainly from experiments in which a tumor mass was separated from its vascular bed. Other indirect evidence was based on observations of tumors that were still in the prevascular stage:

1. Tumors implanted in subcutaneous transparent chambers grow very slowly before vascularization, and tumor volume increases linearly. After vascularization, tumor growth is rapid and tumor volume may increase exponentially.[5]

2. Tumor growth in the avascular rabbit cornea proceeds slowly and at a linear rate, but switches to exponential growth after vascularization.[12]

3. Tumors suspended in the aqueous fluid of the anterior chamber of the rabbit eye remain viable, avascular, and limited in size (<1 mm^3). These tumors induce neovascularization of iris vessels, but are too remote from these vessels to be invaded by them. Once a tumor spheroid is implanted contiguous to the proliferating iris vessels, the tumor can enlarge up to 16,000 times its original volume within 2 weeks.[13]

4. Tumors grown in the vitreous of the rabbit eye remain viable but attain diameters of less than 0.50 mm for as long as 100 days. Once such a tumor reaches the retinal surface, it becomes neovascularized and within 2 weeks can undergo a 19,000-fold increase in volume over the avascular tumor.[14] Cross-sectional histology of the avascular tumor reveals proliferating cells in the outer portion of the tumor and dying cells in the interior.

5. Human retinoblastomas that have metastasized to the vitreous are viable, avascular, and growth restricted.[15]

6. Within a solid tumor, the ^{3}H-thymidine labeling index of tumor cells decreases with increasing distance from the nearest open capillary. The mean labeling index for certain tumors is correlated with the labeling index of the vascular endothelial cells in that tumor.[16]

7. Tumors implanted on the chorioallantoic membrane of the chick embryo are restricted in growth during the avascular phase but enlarge rapidly once they are vascularized.[17]

8. Tumors implanted on the chorioallantoic membrane in successively older embryos grow at slower rates corresponding to the reduced rates of endothelial turnover with age.[17]

9. Vascular casts of metastases in the rabbit liver reveal that tumors of up to 1 mm in diameter are usually avascular, but beyond that size are vascularized.[18]

10. Carcinoma of the human ovary metastasizes to the peritoneal membrane as tiny avascular seeds. These implants rarely grow beyond a limited diameter of a few millimeters, until after vascularization.

11. In transgenic mice that develop carcinomas of the beta cells in the pancreatic islets, large tumors arise from a subset of preneoplastic hyperplastic islets that have become vascularized.[19]

12. In another experiment, neoplastic cells injected subcutaneously developed into tumors that became vascularized at about 0.4 mm^3. As tumor size increased, blood vessels continued to proliferate and were enveloped by encroaching tumor. The vessels eventually occupied up to 1.5 per cent of the tumor volume. This is a 400 per cent increase in vascular density over normal subcutaneous tissue.[20]

13. In rat colon tumors arising spontaneously after administration of a carcinogen, the vascular phase can be divided further into two distinct stages.[21] In the early stage (<3.5-mm diameter), the tumor is supplied by preexisting host microvessels that are dilated and widened. Some of this dilation may result from proliferation and lateral migration of endothelial cells in postcapillary venules. In a later stage (>5.7-mm diameter), new capillary vessels sprout and proliferate to produce a greater microvessel density than normal. All of these studies are summarized in a recent review.[22]

DIRECT EVIDENCE

Direct evidence that supports the hypothesis that neovascularization is necessary for tumor growth is based on five recent reports:

1. An angiogenesis inhibitor, AGM-1470, a synthetic analogue of fumagillin, potently inhibits tumor growth in vivo but not in vitro.[23] It inhibits proliferating endothelial cells in vitro and in vivo.

2. Basic fibroblast growth factor (bFGF) is mitogenic for vascular endothelial cells (as well as for other cell types) and is strongly angiogenic (see later in this chapter). It is produced by endothelial cells and they also have receptors for it. A human colon carcinoma that lacks high-affinity receptors for bFGF and for which bFGF is not mitogenic in vitro was grown in nude mice.[24] Systemic injection of bFGF stimulated an increase in the density and branching of blood vessels in the tumor as well as a twofold increase in tumor size. Receptor autoradiography of histologic tumor sections demonstrated the presence of bFGF receptors on the vascular endothelium. When the tumor-bearing mice received neutralizing monoclonal antisera against bFGF, tumor growth was retarded significantly. This study shows that changes in growth rate of tumor blood vessels directly govern tumor growth.

3. In another experiment, the cDNA for human bFGF hybridized to a signal sequence was transfected into normal mouse fibroblasts.[25] The transfected fibroblasts became tumorigenic, exported bFGF, and also were highly angiogenic. They formed large lethal tumors when implanted into mice. The angiogenesis was mediated mainly by the bFGF released from these tumors. Furthermore, the structure of the bFGF had been modified by site-specific mutagenesis so that two serines had been substituted for cysteines. Thus, the bFGF released by the tumor could be neutralized by a specific antibody that had no effect on natural bFGF. When this antibody was administered to the tumor-bearing mice, there was dramatic reduction in neovascularization and in tumor volume.

4. In a similar experiment, a different angiogenic pep-

tide, vascular endothelial growth factor (VEGF), was blocked by neutralizing antibody. The antibody was administered to mice whose tumors produced VEGF as their only mediator of angiogenesis.[26] Tumor growth was inhibited by more than 90 per cent. The receptor for VEGF functions mainly on vascular endothelial cells.[27]

5. The growth of a brain tumor in nude mice was inhibited significantly or prevented when tumor angiogenesis was suppressed by a strategy in which a dominant-negative mutant of the receptor (Flk-1) for the angiogenic peptide VEGF was introduced into host endothelial cells (carried by a retrovirus). This signaling-defective receptor mutant formed an inactive dimer with the native Flk-1 receptor on endothelial cells and prevented them from forming new capillary blood vessels in response to the release of VEGF by the tumor.[28]

The hypothesis that tumor growth is angiogenesis dependent is consistent with the observation that angiogenesis is necessary but not sufficient for continued tumor growth. Although the absence of angiogenesis will limit tumor growth severely, the onset of angiogenic activity in a tumor permits, but does not guarantee, continued expansion of the tumor population. For example, adrenal adenomas are benign tumors that are highly neovascularized. Their tumor cells, however, lack the growth potential to take advantage of the new blood vessels they have induced. Thus, angiogenesis does not always correlate with malignancy.[29] Furthermore, angiogenesis may not be necessary for certain tumor cells that can grow as a flat sheet between membranes (i.e., gliomatosis in the meninges).

Evidence That Metastasis Is Angiogenesis Dependent

Recent evidence suggests that metastasis is also an angiogenesis-dependent process. For a tumor cell to me-tastasize successfully, it must breach several barriers and be able to respond to specific growth factors.[30–33] Thus, tumor cells must gain access to the vasculature in the primary tumor, survive the circulation, arrest in the microvasculature of the target organ,[34,35] exit from this vasculature,[36] grow in the target organ, and induce angiogenesis.[37,38] Angiogenesis is necessary at the beginning as well as at the end of the metastatic cascade (Fig. 10–1). In experimental animals, tumor cells rarely shed into the circulation before a primary tumor is vascularized, but can appear in the circulation continuously after neovascularization.[39,40] In this animal study, the number of cells shed from the primary tumor correlated with the density of tumor blood vessels as well as with the number of lung metastases observed later. Tumor cells can enter the circulation by penetrating through proliferating capillaries, which have fragmented basement membranes and are leaky.[41,42] Furthermore, increased levels of collagenases and plasminogen activator are produced by the migrating, invading endothelial cells at the tip of a new capillary vessel.[43] When endothelial cell chemotaxis is stimulated in vitro by an angiogenic factor, there is a significant increase in cell-associated enzymatic activity capable of degrading both type IV and type V collagen.[44]

These degradative enzymes may facilitate the entry of tumor cells into the circulation. An interesting experiment that supports this concept is the injection of India ink into the rabbit cornea interposed between an implant of carcinoma and the limbal edge of the cornea. As new blood vessels enter the cornea and grow toward the tumor, they first encounter the India ink. The inferior border of the India ink becomes fragmented, presumably as a result of the liquefaction of cornea by neovascularization. The opposite border of the India ink, contiguous to the avascular tumor, remains intact. In the absence of neovascularization, India ink remains in the cornea indefinitely like a tattoo.[45] Because of the clonal origin of metastases,[38,46] it is more likely that a primary tumor containing a high pro-

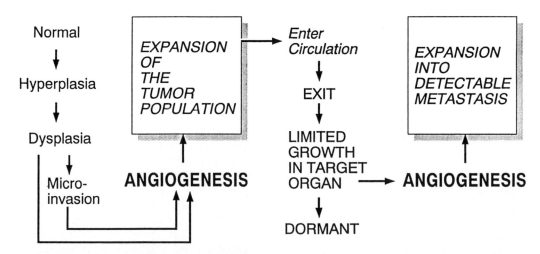

Figure 10–1. Model of role of angiogenesis in metastasis. At the beginning of the metastatic cascade, angiogenesis permits expansion of the primary tumor and provides increased vascular surface area for escape of tumor cells into the circulation. At the end of the metastatic cascade, angiogenesis permits expansion of the metastatic implant. (From Folkman J: Tumor angiogenesis. *In* Holland JF, Frei E, Bast RC, et al [eds]: Cancer Medicine, 3rd ed. Philadelphia, Lea & Febiger, 1993, pp 153–170, with permission.)

portion of angiogenic cells will generate metastases that are already angiogenic when they arrive at the target tissue.

Metastases also are suppressed by angiogenesis inhibitors administered to tumor-bearing animals, despite the fact that the tumor cells are not inhibited in vitro by these drugs.[47,48]

Two types of clinical studies indicate that metastasis depends on angiogenesis. Cutaneous melanomas less than 0.76 mm thick rarely metastasize and are rarely lethal.[49] Melanomas with a thickness of 1.0 mm or greater have an increasing metastatic and lethal potential.[50] The relationship between tumor thickness and metastatic risk can be explained by the fact that thin melanomas usually are contained entirely above the basement membrane that separates the avascular epithelium from the normally vascularized dermis. These lesions rarely are vascularized. Thicker melanomas usually are associated with angiogenesis in the dermis[50] and eventually with tumor envelopment of new capillary blood vessels. It is likely that the increased tumor thickness and the increased metastatic potential *both* result from neovascularization.[51]

Neovascularization now can be quantitated in human tumors by staining histologic sections with an antibody that specifically identifies endothelial cells, such as factor VIII–related antigen (see section on Clinical Applications of Angiogenesis Research). This method also reveals a significant direct correlation between the highest density of microvessels in a histologic section of invasive breast cancer and the occurrence of future metastasis.[37] Microvessel counts in other tumors also have been correlated with metastatic risk and clinical outcome.

Angiogenesis and Lymph Node Metastasis

Metastasis to lymph nodes also may depend on neovascularization of the primary tumor. Tumors do not induce new lymphatic vessels, and lymphatics are rarely if ever found within tumors.[52] Thus, lymph fluid that escapes from intratumoral capillaries flows toward the tumor surface and is carried away by host lymphatics, which become engorged. Human lymph node metastases may arise from a neovascularized primary tumor, but are rarely if ever associated with prevascular in situ tumors. The rabbit cornea model is again instructive. India ink injected into a neovascularized cornea appears rapidly in the ipsilateral lymph node, but ink is retained indefinitely in an avascular cornea.[45] This experiment suggests that tumor neovascularization per se may increase the pressure and flow of lymph from a tumor toward regional lymph nodes.

Angiogenesis and Invasion

Tumor invasion may occur in the presence or absence of neovascularization. For example, in histologic sections of breast cancer with microvessels highlighted by antibody to factor VIII–related antigen, microinvasion may be observed in carcinomas in situ before they have become neovascularized.[37] A thin file of tumor cells breaches the basement membrane of a duct filled with tumor. However, after neovascularization has occurred, invasion into adjacent connective tissue is extensive along a broad front, and tumor cords may follow the path of new blood vessels.[53]

TUMORS SWITCH TO THE ANGIOGENIC PHENOTYPE

Prevascular and Vascular Phases of Tumor Growth

Whereas virtually all solid tumors are neovascularized by the time they are detected in animals or humans, spontaneously arising tumor cells are not usually angiogenic. Therefore, angiogenic activity must be switched on during tumor progression. The term "switch" indicates that the onset of angiogenic activity in a tumor is usually focal in nature and relatively sudden. Experimental and clinical data indicate that most tumors arise without angiogenic activity, exist in the in situ stage without neovascularization for a long period of time (months to years), and then become neovascularized when a *subset* of cells within the tumor switches to the angiogenic phenotype.

In certain cases, the switch to the angiogenic phenotype may occur *before* the full development of tumor (i.e., in the preneoplastic or the preinvasive stage).[54] For example, hyperplastic preneoplastic lesions of the mouse and human breast are angiogenic when transplanted to the rabbit eye, whereas normal breast epithelium is not.[55,56] Preneoplastic bladder epithelium is angiogenic in the rabbit eye, but normal bladder epithelium is not.[57] In a transgenic mouse model that develops carcinomas of the beta cells of the pancreatic islets, the switch to angiogenesis occurs in a subset of hyperplastic islets before they become neoplastic, and at a frequency that correlates with tumor development.[19] In transgenic mice that develop fibrosarcomas, angiogenesis appears first in premalignant and then in malignant lesions. It is mediated mainly by bFGF, which can be detected as a secreted form only in vascularized tumors.[58] The first demonstration of the switch to the angiogenic phenotype in a naturally occurring human preinvasive lesion was reported recently for cervical dysplasia.[59] A region of neovascularization developed along the basement membrane beneath cervical dysplasia or cervical intraepithelial neoplasia (CIN), both of which are premalignant precursors to cervical cancer (Fig. 10–2). Therefore, the switch to the angiogenic phenotype appears to behave independently of other activities that arise during tumorigenesis. It may occur before or concomitant with the transformation to neoplasia (as defined by histologic criteria).

Prevascular Phase

In a Primary Tumor

During the prevascular phase, when angiogenic activity is absent or insufficient, tumors remain small, with volumes measured in a few cubic millimeters. Growth of the whole tumor is slow, and doubling times for the whole tumor may be years. However, this does not mean that the tumor cells are proliferating slowly. Experimental evidence demonstrates that tumor cells in a prevascular neoplasm may have as high a [H^3]-thymidine labeling index as a large vascularized tumor, but that the prevascular tumor has reached a steady state in which generation of new tumor cells is balanced by tumor cell death.[19]

Most prevascular neoplasms are difficult to detect unless they are visible on an external surface, such as the skin, oral cavity, or cervix. Thus, in the cervix, preneoplastic cervical dysplasia or CIN overlies an intact basement membrane beneath which there may be normal nonproliferating capillary blood vessels or an increased number of new microvessels.[59,60] The prevascular phase of bladder cancer is similar,[61] as is the prevascular phase of cutaneous melanoma.[62,63] These lesions are thin or flat, slowly growing, stable for months to years, usually asymptomatic, and rarely metastatic. For the majority of tumors, however, the prevascular stage is clinically undetectable and can be observed only microscopically. For

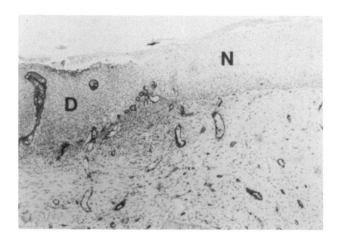

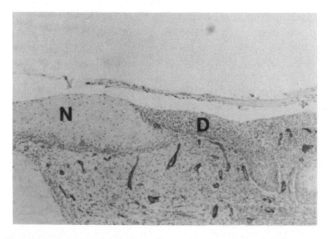

Figure 10–2. Immunohistochemical staining of factor VIII–related antigen in the cervix. Both examples show the transition between normal (N) and dysplastic (D) cervical epithelium in the preneoplastic stage of cervical carcinoma and demonstrate the abrupt appearance of angiogenesis adjacent to the lesion. (From Brem S, Jensen HM, Guillino PM: Angiogenesis as a marker of preneoplastic lesions of the human breast. Cancer 41:239, 1978, with permission.)

example, in breast and prostate cancer, carcinomas in situ *before* neovascularization and *after* neovascularization can be observed in the same specimen.[37,64,65]

IN A METASTASIS: TUMOR DORMANCY

The steady state achieved in a prevascular tumor, in which generation of new tumor cells is balanced by dying tumor cells, also may take place in a micrometastasis that has not become vascularized. The evidence for this concept first was derived from human retinoblastoma cells, which metastasize to the vitreous chamber of the eye.[15] There they grow into small spheroidal tumors unable to become vascularized because of their distance from the retinal vascular bed. These metastatic implants rarely grow beyond 1 mm in diameter. Histology reveals outer layers of proliferating tumor cells with dying cells in the center.[15] A similar pattern is observed in tumor spheroids grown in animal models or in vitro. Animal models have been developed by implanting V2 carcinoma into the vitreous or the aqueous of the rabbit eye[14]; in vitro models employ the culture of tumor spheroids in soft agar.[66] In all of these systems, three-dimensional aggregates of tumor cells are restricted in their total volume, but the replication rate of a subpopulation of tumor cells remains high and is offset by dying cells. The prevascular phase of a spontaneous tumor of the beta cells in pancreatic islets of transgenic mice shows the same pattern.[19]

Therefore, at least one mechanism by which micrometastases may lie ''dormant'' for years (as, for example, in the lung of patients with breast cancer) is that they remain in the prevascular phase. The onset of neovascularization would permit rapid expansion of the rapidly replicating portion of the metastasis. This mechanism has been advanced as a hypothesis to explain dormancy of metastases.[67] Recent experimental evidence supports this hypothesis (L. Holmgren, M. O'Reilly and J. Folkman, unpublished data). In mice treated with an angiogenesis inhibitor, microscopic lung metastases form perivascular cuffs (of less than 0.5-mm diameter) around preexisting pulmonary vessels but do not stimulate neovascularization. However, the rate of DNA synthesis [by bromodeoxyuridine (BrdU) labeling] is 30 per cent or greater. Five days after discontinuing antiangiogenic therapy, the microscopic metastases have been invaded by new capillaries and have grown to more than twice the diameter of the prevascular metastases, but the BrdU labeling index is the same. The important difference between the two lesions is that the incidence of cell death by apoptosis in the prevascular lesions is 7.0 per cent and that in the vascularized tumor is 2.0 per cent.

Vascular Phase

Human tumors that have undergone neovascularization may enter a phase of rapid growth, intensified invasion, and increased metastatic potential. Vascularized tumors are the major cause of accumulating symptoms in cancer patients.[37]

PERFUSION EFFECTS OF NEOVASCULARIZATION ON TUMOR GROWTH

Neovascularization permits rapid tumor growth because it temporarily solves the problem of exchange of nutrients, oxygen, and wastes by a crowded three-dimensional cell population for which simple diffusion of these molecules across its outer surface has become inadequate.[66,68,69]

PARACRINE EFFECTS OF NEOVASCULARIZATION ON TUMOR GROWTH

It has been recognized recently that the contribution of neovascularization to tumor growth lies not only in *perfusion* of the tumor, but also in the *paracrine* effects of vascular endothelial cells on tumor cells.[53,70–72] Endothelial cells release growth factors that stimulate tumor cells.[71] Endothelial cells that line the myriads of new vessels induced by a tumor also may contribute growth factors such as bFGF, platelet-derived growth factor (PDGF), insulin-like growth factor (IGF) type 1, IGF-2,[74] and cytokines such as interleukins (ILs) IL-1, IL-6,[75] and IL-8[76] and granulocyte-macrophage colony-stimulating factor (GM-CSF),[77] which can augment tumor growth. Tumor cells grow preferentially along endothelial channels in vitro in the absence of blood flow.[53] Thus, a bidirectional paracrine relationship emerges in which tumor cells and endothelial cells stimulate the proliferation of each other (Fig. 10–3). Furthermore, the hypoxic conditions that arise in some areas of a tumor as a result of vascular compression may up-regulate endothelial receptors for specific angiogenic peptides such as vascular permeability factor (VPF)/VEGF.[78,79]

INCREASE OF METASTATIC POTENTIAL BY NEOVASCULARIZATION

In addition to the increased hydrostatic pressure and increased leakiness of tumor vessels (as discussed earlier),

neovascularization of a primary tumor also expands the replicating population of tumor cells. This increases the chance of generating metastatic variants that produce the appropriate enzymes and growth factors to penetrate a target organ and survive. The amplification of a proliferating tumor cell population may be one of the more dangerous aspects of the onset of neovascularization. Tumor cells that induce new vessels within a primary tumor not only are presented with more vascular channels in which to enter the circulation but, on arrival at a target organ, are already angiogenic. Thus, they have an increased chance of becoming a detectable metastasis.[72]

ASSOCIATION OF NEOVASCULARIZATION WITH INCREASED SYMPTOMS

Neovascularization is responsible for some of the new symptoms that appear after a tumor has switched to the angiogenic phenotype. Blood in the urine, in the sputum, or between menstrual periods may signify the presence of a vascularized tumor in the bladder, bronchus, or cervix. When ovarian carcinoma has metastasized to the peritoneal lining or to the omentum, tiny implants of a few millimeters in diameter may remain white, avascular, and nearly uniform in size. When some of these lesions become neovascularized, the ascites fluid in the peritoneal cavity becomes bloody and rarely returns to its previous straw color. Local edema is another cause of symptoms related to the onset of angiogenesis. Many of the early symptoms of brain tumors arise from local brain edema and protein leakage from highly permeable new capillary blood vessels.[41,80,81]

Of the known angiogenic molecules,[82] VPF was identified first in tumor ascites.[83] VPF subsequently was found to be identical to VEGF when it was isolated and purified from pituitary glands.[84]

Increased vascular premeability together with a virtual absence of lymphatics within a tumor contribute to ele-

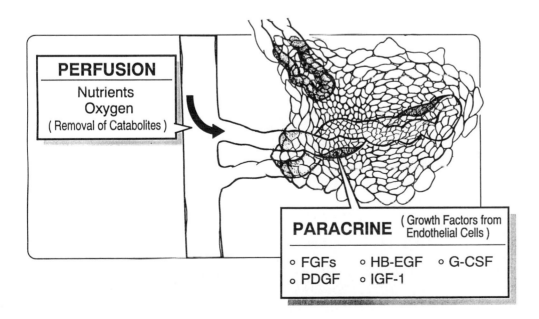

PERFUSION

Nutrients
Oxygen
(Removal of Catabolites)

PARACRINE (Growth Factors from Endothelial Cells)

○ FGFs   ○ HB-EGF   ○ G-CSF
○ PDGF   ○ IGF-1

Figure 10–3. Tumor neovascularization. Diagram to illustrate the concept that the onset of tumor angiogenesis not only *perfuses* the tumor with nutrients as well as providing for removal of waste catabolites, but that capillary endothelial cells produce growth factors that can stimulate tumor cells in a *paracrine* fashion. Nicosia's studies[53] suggest that the subendothelial matrix also may stimulate adhesion and growth of tumor cells selectively.

vated interstitial pressure. Vessels are compressed and occluded in the central areas of a tumor as a result of high interstitial pressure. This pattern can be observed experimentally[85,86] and clinically. For example, angiography may reveal that the center of a tumor is poorly perfused because radiopaque dye cannot enter the compressed vessels. These necrotic areas may lead to tumor rupture or hemorrhage, a not uncommon occurrence in tumors with a large necrotic center, such as Wilms' tumor. Vessel compression also interferes with the optimal delivery of therapeutic agents.[52] These compressed areas become ischemic, and necrosis follows. It is inaccurate to say that these areas are "avascular" or that a tumor "outgrew its blood supply."

Certain clinical signs and symptoms associated with the onset of neovascularization are unique to specific tumor types. For example, retinoblastomas in the back of the eye induce iris neovascularization in the front. Certain brain tumors induce angiogenesis in remote areas of the brain. Bone pain in metastatic prostate cancer may be related in part to neovascularization. A problem in the diagnosis of a primary bone tumor is that, if the biopsy specimen contains only the neovascular response at the periphery of the tumor, it may be mistaken for granulation tissue or inflammation.

A variety of cancer syndromes, such as inappropriate hormonal activities, hypercoagulation states, and cachexias, are secondary to biologically active peptides released into the circulation from vascularized tumors.

The angiogenesis induced by cervical cancer may be observed by colposcopy,[60] the appearance of "telangiectasia" or "vascular spiders" in a mastectomy scar may herald local recurrence of tumor, color Doppler can detect neovascularization in breast cancer[87] and other tumors, bladder carcinoma is detected by cystoscopy based in part on its vascularization, and mammography often reveals the vascularized rim of a breast tumor. In fact, a wide range of radiologic signs of cancer are based on "enhancement" of lesions by radiopaque dyes trapped in the neovasculature of a tumor. Furthermore, in some tumors large central areas cannot be penetrated by radiopaque dyes because of vascular compression, a situation that is unusual in prevascular tumors.

Finally, harmful effects of tumor neovascularization, in addition to pathologic symptoms and signs, also result from the potential for rapid expansion of variant tumor cells that may have higher metastatic potential, more rapid proliferative capacity, and higher levels of drug resistance. All of these effects of neovascularization are important reasons for considering the potential benefit of long-term antiangiogenic therapy (see later in this chapter).

Heterogeneity of Angiogenic Activity in Tumors

The neovascularization of a tumor usually originates in a subset of its cells. Furthermore, even a highly vascularized tumor contains focal areas of high microvessel density as well as areas of low microvessel density.[37] Vascularized tumors also contain a mixture of angiogenic and nonangiogenic tumor cells, as demonstrated experimentally.[72] For example:

1. In islet cell tumors arising spontaneously in transgenic mice, about 10 per cent of the preneoplastic islets become angiogenic at 6 to 7 weeks of age.[19] The angiogenic clusters of tumor cells then give rise to large vascularized tumors.

2. When multifocal fibrosarcomas arise spontaneously in transgenic mice, angiogenic activity is switched on after thin tumors have been present for a few months, but only in a subset of lesions.[58] The angiogenic tumors undergo rapid expansion, whereas the nonangiogenic lesions remain flat and pale.

3. When individual tumor cells are isolated from animal tumors (such as sarcoma 180) and grown in vitro, some cells are strongly mitogenic for capillary endothelial cells and other tumor cells produce little or no growth factor activity for endothelium.

4. In human tumors that are visible throughout their development (e.g., cutaneous melanomas), the onset of angiogenic activity appears after several years, but only in a local area of a thin preangiogenic nevus. Neovascularization rarely envelops the entire melanoma at once.

5. As already pointed out, in breast cancer and in prostate cancer, non-neovascularized as well as neovascularized carcinomas in situ can be observed in the same histologic section.

These observations further support the concept that only a subset of tumor cells acquire angiogenic activity. The new vessels that are recruited apparently then contribute to the growth of nonangiogenic tumor cells.

MOLECULAR MEDIATORS OF ANGIOGENESIS

Positive Regulators

The switch to the angiogenic phenotype is mediated by a balance between positive and negative regulators of microvessel growth. Positive regulators include the angiogenic peptides listed in Table 10–1. Several nonpeptide molecules also have been reported to be angiogenic. These include 1-butyryl glycerol,[88] the prostaglandins (PGs) E_1 and E_2[89–91] nicotinamide,[92] adenosine,[93] certain degradation products of hyaluronic acid,[94] and the tripeptide glycine-histidine-lysine (especially when it is complexed to copper).[95] At this writing, however, bFGF and VPF/VEGF are the angiogenic peptides that have been studied the most extensively in animal and human tumors.

bFGF is distributed widely in normal and neoplastic tissues. Its expression has been reported in a variety of different human tumors.[96,97] It lacks a signal peptide and is mainly cell associated, but it is also localized in basement membranes of diverse tissues,[98,99] where its high affinity for heparin appears to be responsible for its binding to heparan sulfate proteoglycans. An unsolved problem is how bFGF is exported from tumor cells in the absence of a signal sequence. In spontaneous tumors in transgenic mouse models, beta cell tumors that have become neo-vascularized release diffusible angiogenic activity into in vitro collagen gels (VEGF and acidic fibroblast growth factor [aFGF]), or into conditioned medium. Angiogenic fibrosarcomas arising in transgenic mice release bFGF into the conditioned medium.[58] These peptides are not exported by preangiogenic tumors. Furthermore, bFGF is found to be elevated abnormally in the serum and urine of patients with a wide variety of human cancers (see section on Clinical Applications of Angiogenesis Research). The source of these high levels of circulating and urinary bFGF is unknown. In an animal tumor transfected with a mutated bFGF that contained a signal peptide, virtually all of the urinary bFGF was exported from the tumor itself.[100] However, in cancer patients, in addition to the export of bFGF from tumor cells, bFGF also may be mobilized from extracellular matrix by tumor-derived heparinases or collagenases.[98,101] bFGF and other angiogenic peptides also could be released from host cells, such as macrophages, recruited into the tumor.[102] Another puzzle is why bFGF remains elevated in serum of tumor patients when it normally is cleared within minutes after intravenous injection.[103] The normal clearance mechanisms for bFGF[104] may be saturated or disturbed in some cancer patients. Abnormal levels of circulating bFGF may be detrimental because endothelial cell proliferation could be accelerated in micrometastases, as has been demonstrated in animal tumors.[24] bFGF also is elevated abnormally in the cerebrospinal fluid of patients with different types of brain tumors.[105]

bFGF is one of the most potent of the known angiogenic peptides and is a strong mitogen and chemotactic factor for vascular endothelial cells. It is also a mitogen for fibroblasts and smooth muscle cells and for some epithelial cells in vitro. An unresolved puzzle is that histologic sections of tumors usually reveal a predominance of capillary endothelial cell proliferation, with little fibroblast and smooth muscle proliferation. A transfected mouse sarcoma that secretes human bFGF containing a signal peptide stimulates predominately vascular endothelial cells in vivo.[25] It is not clear how such a pleiotrophic growth factor as bFGF can be so relatively selective as an endothelial stimulator during tumor angiogenesis. Possible (but untested) explanations are that the tumor releases endogenous inhibitors of smooth muscle and fibroblast proliferation, or exports unusual isoforms of bFGF, or that its bFGF mobilizes VPF/VEGF.

For VPF/VEGF, the mechanisms of export and selective stimulation of endothelial cell growth are not as problematic as for bFGF. VPF/VEGF is a secreted growth factor. It is mitogenic specifically for endothelial cells in vitro, and it is angiogenic in vivo.[106–108] Expression of VPF/VEGF and its receptor correlates well with blood vessel growth during embryogenesis[109–112] and with angiogenesis in the female reproductive tract[113] and in tumors.[73,108] The receptor for VPF/VEGF is restricted mainly to endothelium of blood vessels.[73,78,79,109] VPF/VEGF is also a heparin-binding protein but, in contrast to bFGF, only two of its four forms have high heparin affinity. Of the four forms, 121, 165, 189, and 206 amino acids in length, the two higher molecular weight forms have high affinity for heparin and are not secreted. They may in fact be trapped by heparan sulfate proteoglycans on the cell surface and in the basement membrane. The two smaller forms have low heparin affinity and are secreted from tumor cells.[114] The 120–amino acid form has the lowest heparin affinity and is almost completely exported as a soluble peptide, whereas the 165–amino acid form of VPF/VEGF has slightly higher heparin affinity and about 50 to 70 per cent of it is bound to putative heparin-containing cell surface or subcellular sites in the matrix.[109] Thus, a signal peptide may be necessary but not sufficient for export of VPF/VEGF. The peptide also may have to pass through a heparan sulfate "cage" at the cell surface. In this way, certain tumor cells that elaborate heparinases may be able to mobilize VPF/VEGF from cell surfaces and/or basement membranes. VPF/VEGF and bFGF also stimulate endothelial mitosis and chemotaxis synergistically in vitro.[116,117] Thus, tumors that export bFGF may amplify angiogenesis further by potentiating VPF/VEGF.

TABLE 10–1. PURIFIED ANGIOGENIC FACTORS

GROWTH FACTOR	MOLECULAR WEIGHT	ENDOTHELIAL MITOGEN IN VITRO	REFS.
Fibroblast growth factors			
Basic	18,000	+	285
Acidic	16,400	+	325
Angiogenin	14,100	o	326
Transforming growth factor α	5,500	+	327
Transforming growth factor β*	25,000	−	328
Tumor necrosis factor α	17,000	−	329
Vascular endothelial growth factor	45,000	+	84, 330–332
Platelet-derived endothelial growth factor	45,000	DNA synthesis	333
Granulocyte colony-stimulating factor	17,000	+	334
Placental growth factor	25,000	+	335
Interleukin 8	40,000	+	336
Hepatocyte growth factor	92,000	+	337, 338

*TGF-β inhibits endothelial proliferation in vitro, but a focal injection in vivo stimulates angiogenesis, possibly by recruiting active macrophages and possibly by mobilizing VPF/VEGF from extracellular matrix.

VPF/VEGF expression also is up-regulated by hypoxia.[78,79] Furthermore, hypoxia appears to up-regulate receptors for VPF/VEGF.[118,119] Because ischemic areas usually appear during the vascular phase of tumor growth (as a result of vessel compression),[52] the hypoxic stimulus to angiogenesis may be responsible for cyclic periods of angiogenesis.

VPF/VEGF mRNA and protein are induced in fibroblastic and epithelial cells by transforming growth factor β (TGF-β).[115] In contrast, mRNA for placental growth factor, which is related to VEGF, is not induced by TGF-β. These recent findings suggest that the angiogenic effect of TGF-β is mediated in part by its induction of VEGF in tissues.

At this writing, we are just beginning to be able to detect abnormally elevated levels of VPF/VEGF in the serum of some breast cancer patients (J. Folkman, unpublished data). It remains to be seen whether certain tumors will be associated predominantly with elevated levels of bFGF or VPF/VEGF.

Of interest is that two angiogenic factors, angiogenin and platelet-derived endothelial cell growth factor (PD-ECGF) are enzymes. Both are chemotactic for endothelial cells in vitro and angiogenic in vivo, but not mitogenic in vitro. Angiogenin has a unique ribonucleolytic activity that appears to be essential for its angiogenic activity.[120,121] Angiogenin stimulates endothelial cells to form diacylglycerol and to secrete prostacyclin by activating phospholipase C and phospholipase A2 respectively.[122,123] PD-ECGF has thymidine phosphorylase activity; 120 amino acids of human thymidine phosphorylase are identical to the sequence of PD-ECGF.[124,125] Thymidine phosphorylase and 2-deoxy-D-ribose (one of the degradation products of thymidine by thymidine phosphorylase) are both chemotactic to endothelial cells in vitro and angiogenic in vivo.[126]

Negative Regulators

The onset of angiogenic activity in a tumor cannot be explained simply by increased expression, increased export, or mobilization of angiogenic factors. These positive mediators of capillary blood vessel growth must overcome a variety of negative regulators that, under normal conditions, *defend* vascular endothelium from stimulation. Certain of these negative regulators in fact are themselves diminished during the switch to the angiogenic phenotype.

Under normal conditions, angiogenesis is a rare event that occurs for a few days each month in the reproductive organs of the female and rarely in the male. Even wound-healing angiogenesis in the male or female is short lived. In contrast to bone marrow cells, which are rapidly replicating at approximately 6×10^9 cell divisions per hour and have a turnover time of approximately 5 days, turnover times for endothelial cells usually exceed 1000 days.[127,128] However, during angiogenesis, endothelial cells are capable of replicating as rapidly as bone marrow cells. Furthermore, DNA synthesis is only one component of the angiogenic process. Many other components of capillary vessel formation (e.g., endothelial migration) are held in

check under normal conditions. In an x-irradiated rabbit cornea in which DNA synthesis is completely blocked, new capillary blood vessels can grow for at least 4 days, forming normal branches and sustaining blood flow.[129] At this early stage of neovascularization, endothelial migration is essential but replication is not. (Thus, endothelial DNA synthesis does not always correlate with intensity of angiogenesis.)

Other Mechanisms of Regulating Angiogenesis

STORAGE OF GROWTH FACTORS

One mechanism that restricts endothelial growth is that certain endothelial mitogens such as aFGF and bFGF lack a signal peptide and remain cell associated. Endothelial mitogens also are made inaccessible to endothelial cells by being sequestered in basement membrane or on the surface of producer cells themselves. The greater the heparin affinity of an angiogenic peptide, the more likely it is to be retained in basement membrane or on the cell surface.

STORAGE OF ANGIOGENESIS INHIBITORS

A specific low-molecular-weight oligosaccharide derived from heparan sulfate, with the sequence –[GlcA-β 1,4-GlcNAc-α 1,4]n–, inhibits angiogenesis in the chick embryo and is not potentiated by the addition of hydrocortisone.[130] Thus, heparan sulfate proteoglycans on the endothelial cell surface may contain antiangiogenic fragments that restrict endothelial growth.

CELL SHAPE

Another mechanism of growth control is that endothelial cell proliferation is tightly controlled by endothelial cell *shape*.[131-133] Thus, bFGF is switched from a potent mitogen for vascular endothelial cells to a nonmitogenic differentiation factor when these cells are foreshortened (to 500 to 700 μm^2) from a prior elongated configuration (>3000 μ^2) in vitro. This partly may explain why early vessel dilation appears to be a prerequisite for DNA synthesis during formation of coronary collaterals, in retinal vessels of the diabetic, and in the postcapillary venules that give rise to neovascularization in a tumor bed.

CELL-CELL INTERACTIONS

A third mechanism of endothelial growth control is inhibition by close contact with other cells. In two cell types that have been studied to date, the suppressor cells elaborate endothelial inhibitor peptides that act over short distances.

Pericytes appear to inhibit endothelial proliferation by TGF-β. Co-cultures of pericytes and capillary endothelial cells demonstrate that both cell types release a latent form of TGF-β into the medium. However, close contact of the cells activates TGF-β which inhibits proliferation of endothelial cells.[134–136] It is not clear whether this mechanism operates in vivo. However, diabetic retinal neovascularization often is associated with pericyte dropout. Angiogenesis in some tumors also is accompanied by a paucity of pericytes, but other tumors induce capillaries rich in pericytes.[137]

Fibroblasts in certain tissues appear to inhibit endothelial growth by releasing β-interferon (β-IFN). Fidler[138] showed that human renal carcinomas or colon carcinomas would grow poorly or not at all when transplanted to subcutaneous tissue of athymic mice, but would produce large tumors when transplanted to the kidney capsule or the colon wall, respectively. He discovered that the success of "orthotopic" tumor transplantation[139] was due to the fact that skin fibroblasts produced large quantities of β-IFN but little or no IFN was produced by kidney or colon fibroblasts. Fidler further found[138,342] that α- and β-IFN down-regulated mRNA and protein synthesis of aFGF and bFGF in human tumor cells. He showed that FGF-producing human tumors transplanted subcutaneously were growth inhibited and not neovascularized. In contrast, tumors in the kidney subcapsule or in the colon grew rapidly and were highly neovascularized. α-IFN previously has been shown to inhibit endothelial migration in vitro[140] and angiogenesis in vivo.[141,142] Thus, fibroblasts may be heterogeneous for IFN production depending on their tissue location.

CIRCULATING ENDOTHELIAL CELL INHIBITORS

Several proteins in the circulation inhibit endothelial cell proliferation and may contribute to restriction of endothelial cell growth, despite their low concentrations in the circulation. These include platelet factor 4 (PF4),[143,168] thrombospondin,[144–149] TGF-β, tissue inhibitors of metalloproteinases (TIMP),[150–152] α-IFN, and possibly a 16-kDa fragment of prolactin.[153] Certain angiostatic steroids, such as tetrahydrocortisol, a nonglucocorticoid, nonmineralocorticoid metabolite of cortisol, also circulate.[154] Tetrahydrocortisol is lipid soluble and may be taken up by endothelial cells together with other lipids.

TUMOR-DERIVED ENDOTHELIAL INHIBITORS

In the conditioned medium of angiogenic tumor cells from transgenic mice, stimulators and inhibitors of endothelial proliferation were found together. Furthermore, a transplanted mouse tumor (Lewis lung carcinoma) was found to release endothelial mitogens in the tumor bed, but also to release an inhibitor of endothelial cell proliferation into the circulation.[156] Thus, our preliminary evidence suggests that the onset of angiogenesis in the tumor bed depends on the presence of positive regulators of angiogenesis in excess of negative regulators. However, in the serum, the negative regulator(s) may accumulate in excess of positive regulators, because of the accelerated clearance of most endothelial mitogens from the circulation. We propose that, in those primary tumors that suppress the growth of their metastases,[157,158] circulating inhibitors of angiogenesis may be responsible for inhibiting metastatic growth.[156] Indeed, Noel Bouck and her colleagues first reported that, during transformation of hamster cells to angiogenic tumor cells, the production of thrombospondin, an angiogenesis inhibitor, was down-regulated.[144,159]

ANGIOGENESIS SUPPRESSOR GENES

Bouck et al. further proposed that thrombospondin normally may be under the control of the *p53* tumor suppressor gene.[72,160] Bouck studied fibroblasts from cancer-prone patients with the Li-Fraumeni syndrome. These fibroblasts contain only one allele of *p53*. The cells are not tumorigenic or angiogenic in vivo. After repeated passage in culture, they lose the remaining allele of *p53* and become angiogenic and tumorigenic, with concomitant down-regulation of thrombospondin synthesis to approximately 4 per cent of the parental cells. The cells could be rescued from the angiogenic phenotype by transfection with *p53* or with thrombospondin. Bouck et al. concluded that wild-type *p53,* in addition to its many other functions,[161,341] may regulate angiogenic activity negatively in Li-Fraumeni cells by ensuring that they produce a high level of antiangiogenic thrombospondin.[72] In a similar study by different investigators, a glioblastoma cell line was made conditionally inducible for *p53*. When wild-type *p53* was expressed in this cell line, it elaborated an inhibitor of angiogenesis that was not thrombospondin.[162] It is known that the α-IFN gene complex is deleted in certain cancers of the bladder,[163] in some leukemias,[164] in melanoma, and in other tumors. Because α-IFN is an angiogenesis inhibitor, we can ask whether the α-IFN gene complex may be acting as an angiogenesis suppressor gene, similarly to *p53*.

ANGIOGENESIS INHIBITORS

The possible existence of specific angiogenesis inhibitors was predicted in 1971,[10,165] the first reported antiangiogenic activity was found in cartilage in 1973,[166,167] and the first angiogenesis inhibitors of known structure, protamine and PF4, were identified in 1982.[168] Currently more than 25 inhibitors have been reported that interfere with angiogenesis itself or with some component of the angiogenic process.

The general strategy of antiangiogenic therapy is to return a focal area of abnormally persistent and intense capillary blood vessel growth to its physiologically quiescent state. This strategy is also applicable to a variety of diseases in which angiogenesis is the dominant pathology, including neovascularization in the eye, skin, joints, and tumors. Thus, in principle, an angiogenesis inhibitor specific for proliferating capillaries should have few side effects and a wide therapeutic window. PF4 illustrates that such a goal in fact can be accomplished—it has no median lethal dose in animals and as yet shows virtually no toxicity in phase I/II clinical trials. Nevertheless, many drugs and biologic modifiers that inhibit angiogenesis also have other activities and are not purely antiangiogenic. In fact, their antiangiogenic activity may be limited by toxicities unrelated to inhibition of blood vessel growth. An example is α-IFN, which is an effective angiogenesis inhibitor for infants with life-threatening hemangiomas. α-IFN is tolerated well by infants and young children, but less well by elderly adults. Furthermore, these inhibitors are not equally effective in blocking angiogenesis at a given site (i.e., in a tumor), because some block only the source of a particular angiogenic peptide, others interfere with the endothelial target of angiogenic peptides, and still others block inflammatory cells, but not tumor cells, from releasing angiogenic peptides. The problem of comparing potency of different angiogenesis inhibitors remains unsolved, in part because none of the currently available in vitro bioassays, including a recently developed quantitative assay in the chick embryo,[169] accurately predicts antiangiogenic activity in vivo. Nevertheless, the available in vitro bioassays have been valuable to identify novel angiogenesis inhibitors. It should be noted that antiangiogenic therapy differs from antivascular therapy,[170] which is based on pharmacologic occlusion of vessels in a tumor bed.

All of the known angiogenesis inhibitors cannot be discussed here. However, a most recent and comprehensive review is that by Auerbach and Auerbach.[171] Other important reviews on antiangiogenic therapy also have been published recently.[38,172–181] I here outline only a few of the known angiogenesis inhibitors in order to provide representative examples of different pharmacologic mechanisms by which angiogenesis can be suppressed, and to illustrate the types of angiogenesis inhibitors that have entered clinical trial.

Antiangiogenic Protease Inhibitors

Cartilage was the first source from which antiangiogenic activity was identified,[166,167,182–185] and it now is known to contain inhibitors both of angiogenesis and of endothelial proliferation. One antiangiogenic protein, cartilage-derived inhibitor (CDI), recently has been purified completely from bovine cartilage and partially sequenced.[150] It has a molecular weight of 27.6 kDa, and inhibits angiogenesis in vivo and capillary endothelial proliferation and migration in vitro. It is also a collagenase inhibitor. Other molecules that inhibit endothelial proliferation are present in cartilage.[186–188] Of interest is an angiogenesis inhibitor isolated from the conditioned medium of a human chondrosarcoma cell line[189] that has not yet been purified completely. In addition to bovine cartilage, shark cartilage also contains angiogenesis-inhibitory molecules.[190–192] However, the commercial use of crude extracts of shark cartilage for administration into the human gastrointestinal tract as a source of antiangiogenic activity remains questionable. This is an unproven and unapproved therapy for which there is no evidence of efficacy from any controlled trial reported in the medical literature at this writing.

Minocycline is a semisynthetic tetracycline antimicrobial that inhibits collagenase activity in the synovial fluid of patients with rheumatoid arthritis[193] and in the cornea.[194]

Medroxyprogesterone is a synthetic steroid that inhibits collagenolysis and tumor-induced angiogenesis in the rabbit cornea when the steroid is implanted in the cornea.[195] It also inhibits plasminogen activator produced by endothelial cells. Plasminogen activator–mediated proteolytic activity can release bFGF from endothelial cells.[196] Thus, both of these properties may play a role in the antitumor effect of medroxyprogesterone acetate when it is used to treat patients with advanced or recurrent endometrial cancer.[197] The binding affinities of medroxyprogesterone and its analogues to receptors for glucocorticoids, progesterone, and androgen are unrelated to its angiostatic activity.[198] In this study, the analogue 6,6'-dehydromedroxyprogesterone was inactive. Of interest is that the angiostatic activity of medroxyprogesterone was completely abolished by mefipristone (RU486).

Chitin is a homogeneous polysaccharide composed of *N*-acetylglucosamine residues. A chemically modified chitin derivative into which 6-*O*-sulfate and 6-*O*-carboxymethyl groups are introduced (e.g., SCM-chitin) is an inhibitor of type IV collagenase and heparanase.[199] SCM-chitin inhibits tumor-induced angiogenesis and tumor growth in mice when the polysaccharide is injected into the tumor.[199]

Angiogenesis Inhibitors Associated with Heparin

PLATELET FACTOR 4

Protamine was shown to be an angiogenesis inhibitor,[168] but cumulative toxicity from prolonged administration and a narrow window of angiostatic efficacy[200] prevented its consideration for clinical use or further animal study. PF4 first was tested for antiangiogenic activity because it could bind and neutralize heparin similarly to protamine.[168,201] It inhibited angiogenesis in the chick embryo, but there was insufficient material for testing in other systems. Recently, recombinant human PF4 (rHuPF4) has been produced[143]; it specifically inhibits endothelial proliferation and migration in vitro.[202] The inhibitory activities are associated with the carboxy-terminal region of the molecule. The growth of human colon carcinoma in athymic mice and the growth of murine melanoma are markedly inhibited by intralesional injections, whereas tumor cells are completely insensitive to rHuPF4 in vitro at levels that inhibit normal endothelial cell proliferation. The dose levels of rHuPF4 for systemic administration in tumor-bearing mice have not yet been optimized, but may be high because of rapid inactivation and clearance of the peptide. Addition of heparin abolishes the antiangiogenic activity of PF4.[143] However, an analogue of PF4 that does not bind heparin, rHuPF4-241, still inhibits angiogenesis.[203]

THROMBOSPONDIN

This heparin-binding protein is constitutively secreted by certain types of normal cells. It inhibits endothelial cell proliferation in vitro and also inhibits angiogenesis in the cornea.[144,145,159] During malignant transformation of these hamster cells, expression of the inhibitor, which appears to be under the control of a cancer-suppressor gene, is down-regulated. Of interest is that thrombospondin is a heparin-binding protein that also is stored in extracellular matrix. Its effect as an antitumor agent has not been tested. Thrombospondin appears to be a specific inhibitor of proliferation of endothelial cells from different tissues.[204,205] Thrombospondin also appears to destabilize contacts between endothelial cells.[206] Heparin interferes with the binding of thrombospondin to endothelial cells. Accumulating evidence suggests that, for most tumors, the switch to the angiogenic phenotype depends on the outcome of a balance between angiogenic stimulators and angiogenic inhibitors, both of which may be produced by tumor cells and by certain host cells.[179] Thrombospondin may be one of the natural angiogenesis suppressors that is down-regulated in a tumor during the switch to the angiogenic phenotype, as first suggested by Bouck.[149] Thrombospondin also may be down-regulated in psoriatic keratinocytes as they up-regulate interleukin 8 to become angiogenic.[207] It is not clear whether this balance also is operating in activated angiogenic macrophages, which secrete significantly higher amounts of thrombospondin than their nonactivated counterparts.[208]

ANGIOSTATIC STEROIDS

Cortisone or hydrocortisone have little or no antiangiogenic activity by themselves, but can be converted to potent angiogenesis inhibitors by administration with heparin.[154,201,209] Neither the glucocorticoid nor the mineralocorticoid function of these steroids is necessary for antiangiogenic activity,[154,210] but specific structure-activity relationships are critical (for review, see ref. 211). Thus, pregnenolone, progesterone, and estrone have no antiangiogenic activity, whereas tetrahydrocortisol and other "angiostatic steroids" have high antiangiogenic activity (with heparin). The anticoagulant function of heparin is not necessary for its antiangiogenic activity with steroids. Angiostatic steroids administered with heparin fragments that lack anticoagulant activity inhibit angiogenesis in the chick embryo and the rabbit cornea. These steroid-heparin combinations also inhibit tumor growth[201] and metastasis[210,212] in some tumor-bearing mice. Certain tumors are potently inhibited or regress when treated with cortisone-heparin mixtures but not with cortisone alone, whereas other tumors are refractory.[201,213] The explanation for this difference is unknown, but may lie in differences in output of angiogenic activity or differences in degradation of steroids or of heparin by different types of tumors. Furthermore, if exogenous heparin is omitted, angiostatic steroids can be potentiated equally well by a synthetic arylsulfatase inhibitor that protects endogenous heparin-like molecules from desulfation.[214] Synthetic sulfated cyclodextrins also can substitute for heparin.[215] β-Cyclodextrin tetradecasulfate is 100 to 1000 times more potent than heparin as a potentiator of angiostatic steroids. A critical ratio of cyclodextrin to steroid is necessary for optimum angiostatic activity. This observation, taken together with other experimental results,[215] suggests that the steroid enters the hydrophobic cavity of β-cyclodextrin to form a complex. In fact, the complex inhibits chemokinesis of capillary endothelial cells,[216] whereas the steroid and the polysaccharide alone are ineffective.

The mechanism of action of angiostatic steroids is not understood completely.[217] However, in the presence of steroid-heparin combinations, the basement membranes of growing capillaries undergo rapid dissolution.[218] Basement membrane of nongrowing capillaries or of larger vessels is not degraded. Angiostatic steroids also up-regulate endothelial plasminogen activator inhibitor (PAI),[219] and thus help to prevent degradation of basement membrane.[175,220]

Angiostatic steroids are currently in clinical trial for topical application to treat corneal neovascularization refractory to conventional therapy. It is possible that neovascularization in mast cell–rich inflammatory lesions or in hemangiomas sometimes is suppressed by corticosteroids alone, because of the high levels of endogenous heparin.

PENTOSAN POLYSULFATE

Pentosan polysulfate is a negatively charged polysaccharide that, in combination with hydrocortisone, inhibits endothelial cell motility and tubule formation in vitro and inhibits angiogenesis in the chick embryo chorioallantoic membrane. Its antitumor activity against a variety of animal tumors may in part be due to its antiangiogenic activity.[221]

Bacteria-Derived Angiogenesis Inhibitors

A sulfated polysaccharide-peptidoglycan complex derived from the bacterial wall of an *Arthrobacter* species inhibited angiogenesis in the chorioallantoic membrane and also inhibited the growth of sarcoma 180 tumor in mice.[222] The effect was potentiated greatly by corticosteroids. Other sulfated polysaccharides, including dextran sulfates, were relatively ineffective.

Fungus-Derived Angiogenesis Inhibitors

The synthesis of a family of novel angiogenesis inhibitors that are analogues of fumagillin, a naturally secreted antibiotic of *Aspergillus fumigatus fresenius,* has been reported recently.[23,223] One of these "angioinhibins," AGM-1470 [angiogenesis modulator 1470, also known as TNP-470 (Takeda Neoplastic Product)], inhibits proliferation and migration of capillary endothelial cells and inhibits angiogenesis in the chick embryo. It also suppresses growth of a wide variety of mouse tumors, with treated/control (T/C) ratios of 0.30 to approximately 0.50, and with little or no toxicity to the host.

Other "antibiotic" angiogenesis inhibitors include herbimycin,[224] eponemycin,[225] erbstatin,[226] and staurosporine.[227]

DRUGS THAT INTERFERE WITH BASEMENT MEMBRANE TURNOVER

As described earlier in this chapter, basement membrane synthesis and degradation are among the essential steps in the process of angiogenesis.[228] After it was learned that dissolution of basement membrane of growing capillaries is one mechanism by which angiostatic steroids inhibit angiogenesis,[218,220] other specific modulators of matrix metabolism were examined.[228–230] Regression of growing capillaries in the chick embryo was induced by proline analogues such as L-azetidine-2-carboxylic acid, cis-hydroxyproline, dL-3,4,dehydroxyproline, and thioproline. These compounds and a,a-dipyridyl, an inhibitor of prolyl hydroxylase, all interfere with triple helix formation and prevent collagen deposition. β-Aminopropionitrile, an inhibitor of collagen cross linking, was also antiangiogenic, although β-methyl-d-xyloside, an inhibitor of glycosaminoglycan deposition, was not.[218,220] Co-administration of suboptimal doses of collagen modulators with angiostatic steroids and/or heparin potentiated inhibition of angiogenesis. These general inhibitors of collagen formation also inhibited tumor growth in mice, but were too toxic for long-term safe administration. Nevertheless, recent reports suggest that it may be possible to design collagen modulators that are more specific inhibitors of type IV collagen deposition, but are less toxic.

D-Penicillamine and Gold Thiomalate

Two drugs employed in the treatment of arthritis have been found to inhibit angiogenesis. D-Penicillamine, a copper chelator, inhibits endothelial cell proliferation in vitro.[231] It also inhibits angiogenesis in the rabbit cornea at serum concentrations that are similar to the serum levels of this drug in treated patients. D-Penicillamine may play an important role in suppressing neovascularization in the joints of patients with rheumatoid arthritis. It is not clear whether the mechanism of antiangiogenesis depends on the ability of D-penicillamine to act as a copper chelator. However, it is interesting that copper depletion in rats and rabbits treated with penicillamine and fed a copper-deficient diet suppressed tumor-induced angiogenesis and tumor growth in the brain.[232] Gold thiomalate and other gold derivatives have been used effectively to ameliorate the symptoms of arthritis. These gold compounds now are known to inhibit endothelial cell proliferation in vitro[233] and to block the release of angiogenic activity by activated macrophages.[234] The mechanism of action of gold compounds remains to be elucidated, but other macrophage functions are not suppressed when angiogenic activity is blocked.

Vitamin D₃ Analogues

The active metabolite of vitamin D_3, 1α,25-dihydroxyvitamin D_3, and a synthetic analogue, 22-oxa-1α,25-dihydroxyvitamin D_3, which has little or no effect on calcium metabolism, inhibit angiogenesis in the chick embryo chorioallantoic membrane.[235] Vitamin D_3 itself is not effective.

Interferon Alfa-2a

The antiproliferative activity of IFN against human tumors first was demonstrated in the 1960s with partially purified α-IFN by Strander at the Karolinska Institute (for review, see ref. 236). IFN therapy delayed recurrent growth of tumor in osteogenic sarcoma after surgery. Subsequently, α-IFN was shown to be effective for other tumors, including lymphomas[237] and hairy-cell leukemia[238] (for review, see ref 239). Recently, recombinant interferon alfa-2a (rIFN alfa-2a) was discovered to have antiangiogenic activity. This began with the finding that a mixture of IFNs inhibited the migration of capillary endothelial cells in vitro[140] and lymphocyte-induced angiogenesis in vivo,[142] as well as tumor angiogenesis.[141] Based on these studies, a child with pulmonary capillary hemangiomatosis was treated successfully with rIFN alfa-2a.[240] This rare disease, with excessive growth of capillary blood vessels in the lung, carries a high mortality. The cause of this neovascularization is unknown. Nevertheless, long-term administration (months) of rIFN alfa-2a at 3 million units/m^2/day subcutaneously caused regression of the pulmonary hemangiomas, an unprecedented outcome for this disease.[241] As a result of this report, rIFN alfa-2a recently has been used to treat life-threatening systemic hemangiomatosis in infants whose lesions have failed to respond to steroid therapy.[242–246,340]

Carboxyaminoimidazole

An imidazole derivative, carboxyaminoimidazole (CAI), which is a novel inhibitor of signal transduction and which blocks ligand-stimulated calcium influx, has been found to inhibit bFGF-stimulated endothelial cell proliferation, tube formation in vitro, and angiogenesis in the chick embryo chorioallantoic membrane.[247]

Thalidomide

Thalidomide is a sedative introduced in Europe in the 1950s. In 1961, it was reported that maternal usage of thalidomide was associated with severe limb defects and other anomalies in babies.[248,249] Although humans were found to be exquisitely sensitive to the teratogenic effects of thalidomide, experiments in rodents failed to reveal similar effects.[250,251] However, teratogenic effects could be reproduced experimentally by the oral administration of thalidomide to rabbits.[252,253] Over the past 30 years, the mechanism of thalidomide's teratogenicity has been studied extensively but has remained unknown.[254] We have shown recently that orally administered thalidomide is an inhibitor of angiogenesis induced by bFGF in the rabbit cornea.[255] These results suggest a mechanism for the teratogenicity of thalidomide and hold promise for its potential use as an orally administered drug for the treatment of pathologic angiogenesis, for example, in ocular neovascularization. Because the drug is not metabolized in rodents, it is not known if thalidomide has antitumor activity.

Antiangiogenic Antibodies

Short-term administration of antibodies directed against specific angiogenic peptides, such as bFGF[25] or VEGF,[26] has produced profound inhibition of tumor growth in animals when the tumors were dependent on a single angiogenic peptide. The integrin $\alpha v \beta 3$ is the endothelial cell receptor for von Willebrand factor, fibrinogen, and fibronectin.[256] This integrin initiates a calcium-dependent signaling pathway leading to endothelial cell migration,[257] and therefore may play a central role in vascular cell biology.[258] The integrin appears to be expressed selectively on growing blood vessels and is up-regulated during angiogenesis, for example, in human wound granulation tissue and in the growing chick chorioallantoic membrane. A monoclonal antibody directed against $\alpha v \beta 3$ blocked angiogenesis induced by bFGF, tumor necrosis factor α, and human melanoma fragments in the chick embryo chorioallantoic membrane assay, but had no effect on preexisting vessels.[258]

CLINICAL APPLICATIONS OF ANGIOGENESIS RESEARCH

Current clinical applications of angiogenesis research can be grouped into three categories: (1) stimulation of angiogenesis by administration of angiogenic peptides to accelerate healing of wounds or peptic ulcers, (2) diagnostic and prognostic applications based on quantitation of angiogenesis in tumors and of angiogenic peptides in tumor patients, and (3) inhibition of angiogenesis. This section summarizes current clinical studies in cancer patients based on the latter two categories.

Diagnostic and Prognostic Applications

QUANTITATION OF TUMOR ANGIOGENESIS IN HISTOLOGIC SECTIONS

It is becoming clear that determination of the intensity of angiogenesis in a given tumor at the time of the initial diagnosis may help to predict risk of future metastasis or risk of recurrence. The first quantitative evidence that intensity of angiogenesis correlated with future relapse was reported by Biberfeld.[259] Lymph nodes from patients with acquired immunodeficiency syndrome (AIDS) were stained with antibody to factor VIII–related antigen to highlight blood vessels. Overall high blood vessel counts correlated with increased future risk of mortality.

In a subsequent study of melanoma specimens, Srivastava et al. found a sharp breakpoint between a stage of relative absence of neovascularization in thin lesions

(<0.76 mm), which correlated with absence of metastasis, and a stage of increased neovascularization, which correlated with an increased metastatic rate.[62] In melanomas of 0.76 to 4.0 mm in thickness, the vascular area at the tumor base in patients developing metastases was twice that of patients without metastases.[63]

My colleagues and I found that histologic sections of invasive breast cancer stained with antibody to factor VIII–related antigen revealed abundant microvessels. These could be counted and expressed as the highest number of microvessels identified within any 200× field (i.e., 0.74 mm²).[37,64,260-262] Increasing microvessel count correlated significantly with risk of metastasis (Fig. 10–4). In this study we plotted the percentage of patients with metastatic disease in whom a vessel count was carried out within progressive 33-vessel increments. The incidence of metastatic disease increased with the number of vessels, reaching virtually 100 per cent for patients having invasive carcinomas containing microvessel counts greater than 100 per 200× field. Multivariate analysis showed that microvessel density in lymph node–negative patients was a better predictor of metastasis when compared to tumor grade, tumor size, or certain other prognostic markers, such as estrogen receptor positivity.[64] Subsequent confirmations that quantitation of microvessels within the area of most intense neovascularization of invasive breast cancer was associated with prognosis have been reported recently in several larger series of patients.[262-268] A five-year prospective study further confirms this correlation.[268] An antibody to CD31 appears to be a more sensitive endothelial marker than antibody to anti–factor VIII–related antigen for highlighting intratumoral vessels.

It is important to count vessels in the most dense area of neovascularization, rather than take an average over the whole section. It is also essential to count vessels with or without a lumen, because many new vessel tips are stained but have no lumen. The optimal field size is 0.74 mm² and the significance of microvessel density drops when

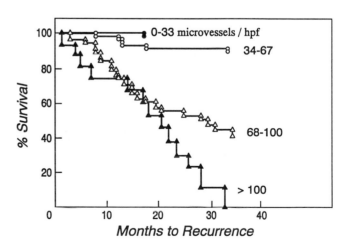

Figure 10–4. Correlation of microvessel count in breast cancer with recurrence-free survival for both node-negative and node-positive patients. hpf, high-power field. (From Weidner N, Folkman J, Pozza F, et al: Tumor angiogenesis: A new significant and independent prognostic indicator in early-stage breast carcinoma. J Natl Cancer Inst 84:1875, 1992, with permission.)

the field size is smaller than 0.19 mm^2.[37] It is also important to have adequate length of follow-up for either retrospective or prospective studies to determine those patients who will relapse. We have found that microvessel counts can be carried out by a pathologist in a few minutes per field and that automated image analysis has been unnecessary. In two reports of no association between microvessel density and relapse-free survival or overall survival of breast cancer patients, one investigator[269] used counting areas from 0.1225 to 0.476 mm^2 (i.e., 16 to 64 per cent of the optimal counting area reported by Weidner et al.[37]), and another[270] excluded vessels with single stained cells, believing that a lumen was necessary for classification as a vessel.[271]

A positive association between tumor angiogenesis and tumor aggressiveness also has been found for lung cancer,[272] prostate cancer,[273–275] and head and neck squamous cell carcinoma.[276,277] Additional data have been reported for melanoma neovascularization.[278–280]

These positive correlations between microvessel density and future risk of metastasis invite the speculation of a possible causal relationship. One clue to a mechanism is that tumor tissues contain focal areas of intense neovascularization, or "hot spots." This pattern suggests that subsets of tumor cells within a primary tumor are more highly angiogenic than other tumor cells. The presence of highly angiogenic and nonangiogenic tumor cells within the same tumor has been shown experimentally.[19,58] Areas of high microvessel density increase the opportunity for tumor cells to enter the circulation. In classic studies by Liotta et al., tumor cells began to enter the circulation only after the onset of neovascularization and then increased from 1.4×10^3 cells/day on day 5 after implantation to 1.5×10^5 cells/day on day 15.[40,281] The establishment of metastases also depends on the absolute number of cells shed into the circulation.[282] A tumor cell that is already angiogenic when it is shed from the primary tumor is more likely to generate a detectable metastasis when it arrives in a target organ than is a nonangiogenic cell, other conditions being similar. This is because the switch to the angiogenic phenotype in small populations of tumor cells takes time (weeks to months in transgenic animals, and possibly years in humans). In fact, tumor cells that are not angiogenic may become dormant micrometastases[72] (Fig. 10–5).

Intensity of tumor angiogenesis is also an indicator of risk of *local* recurrence of brain tumors. In a 2-year prospective study of brain tumors in childhood, we have found that microvessel counts (of tumor specimens stained with antibody to factor VIII–related antigen or CD34) were correlated significantly with tumor recurrence.[283]

A caveat about prognostic indicators for cancer should be considered. Various markers generally are used to analyze efficacy of therapy or to predict the course of disease, risk of future metastasis, and time to relapse. However, if there were a perfectly effective treatment for a given cancer (e.g., breast cancer) that could guarantee cure regardless of the severity of malignancy at initial diagnosis, prognostic markers would lose their value. Therefore, as cancer therapy improves in the future, it is possible that prognostic markers, including microvessel count, may appear to be less useful for certain tumors.

QUANTITATION OF ANGIOGENIC PEPTIDES IN SERUM AND URINE

A long-term goal of our laboratory has been to measure angiogenic peptides in cancer patients to determine if abnormally elevated levels could be used to guide therapy and to determine therapeutic efficacy. Chodak et al., working in our laboratory, measured endothelial chemokinetic activity in urine of patients with renal and bladder cancer in 1981,[284] (3 years before purification of the first known

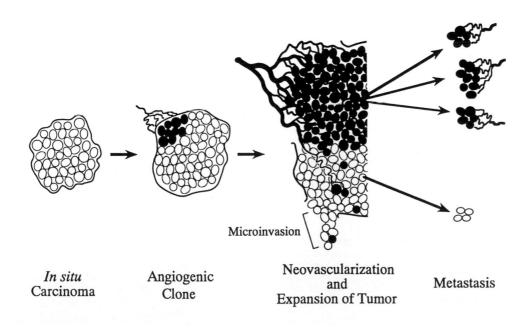

Figure 10–5. Model of the concept that subsets of tumor cells are angiogenic. (From Folkman J: Angiogenesis and breast cancer. J Clin Oncol 12:441, 1994, with permission.)

In situ Carcinoma   Angiogenic Clone   Neovascularization and Expansion of Tumor   Metastasis

Microinvasion

angiogenic peptide, bFGF.)[285] This activity subsequently was shown to be due to bFGF-like activity.[286] Urine from patients with nongenitourinary cancer was not analyzed in this study. An immunoassay for biologically active bFGF was reported by Watanabe et al. with a detection limit of 10 pg/mL.[287] The first clinical use of this method revealed that bFGF levels were elevated in the serum of patients with renal cell carcinoma.[288] We subsequently reported that bFGF was elevated abnormally in the serum of approximately 10 per cent of a wide variety of cancer patients, including those with breast cancer.[289] Normal levels of serum bFGF were less than 30 pg/mL; in contrast, bFGF levels in cancer patients were as high as 300 to 400 pg/mL. However, in urine, more than 37 per cent of patients had abnormally elevated levels of this angiogenic peptide (Fig. 10–6).[290] Of 950 patients having many different types of solid tumors, lymphoma or leukemia, the median level of bFGF was 312 pg/gm creatinine for those with local cancers and 479 pg/gm (with a 90th percentile level of 14,143 pg/gm) for those with metastatic disease. Thirty-one per cent of patients with local disease and 47 per cent of patients with metastatic disease had abnormally elevated bFGF levels (i.e., higher than the 90th percentile). By comparison, in control subjects (87 healthy volunteers and 198 patients with diseases unrelated to cancer, the median bFGF was 151 pg/gm for males, 237 pg/gm for females, and 619 pg/gm at the 90th percentile for both groups combined (Fig. 10–7).

In infants with hemangiomas, urine levels of bFGF also are elevated abnormally (e.g., from 20,000 to 150,000 pg/gm creatinine before therapy, compared to normal urine bFGF levels of less than 5000 pg/gm for newborns and infants up to 3 months of age and less than 1500 pg/gm after 3 months of age). These levels gradually return toward normal over a period extending to 2 to 4 years of age, as the lesions begin to undergo natural involution. When involution of life-threatening or vision-threatening hemangiomas is induced more rapidly by therapy, urine bFGF levels also fall toward normal as the hemangioma regresses (J. Folkman et al., unpublished data). In vascular malformations of children and adults, urinary bFGF levels have been uniformly normal. We are studying the value of urinary bFGF to help distinguish between hemangiomas and vascular malformations. Hemangiomas consist of rapidly proliferating capillary blood vessels. In contrast, vascular malformations contain mainly larger vessels (e.g., venous structures with deficiency of smooth muscle, arteriovenous malformations, or abnormal lymphatic vessels) that are not undergoing rapid proliferation. Hemangiomas respond to corticosteroid or α-IFN therapy; vascular malformations do not. It is sometimes difficult to distinguish correctly the diagnosis of hemangioma versus vascular malformation, especially because histologic names are confusing. Thus, a "cavernous hemangioma" is in fact a vascular malformation. To date, we have not seen an abnormally elevated urine bFGF level in more than 100 patients with vascular malformations (J. Folkman et al., unpublished data).

QUANTITATION OF bFGF IN CEREBROSPINAL FLUID OF PATIENTS WITH BRAIN TUMORS

Biologically active bFGF was detected in the cerebrospinal fluid of 62 per cent of 26 children with brain tumors (48 up to 1815 pg/mL), but in none of 18 control donors who had hydrocephalus or malignant disease outside of the central nervous system (down to the limit of detection of 30 pg/mL). Furthermore, the bFGF level in cerebrospinal fluid correlated significantly with microvessel density in histologic sections ($p \leq .005$).[283]

DETECTION OF OTHER ANGIOGENIC PEPTIDES

In cancer patients, we also have found abnormally elevated levels of VPF/VEGF in serum and of IL-8 in serum and urine, but these studies are incomplete and have not yet been reported. However, even these early results indicate that bFGF may not be the only angiogenic peptide

Figure 10–6. Distribution among patients with various types of cancer of abnormally elevated levels of the angiogenic peptide bFGF in urine. (From Nguyen M, Watanabe H, Budson AE, et al: Elevated levels of an angiogenic peptide, basic fibroblastic growth factor, in the urine of patients with a wide spectrum of cancers. J Natl Cancer Inst 86:356, 1994, with permission.)

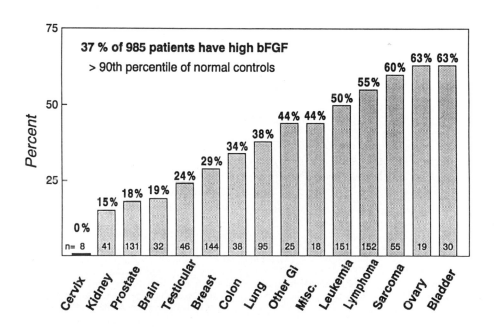

that can be quantitated in serum, urine, and cerebrospinal fluid of cancer patients. Perhaps it will be useful to obtain a "profile" of several angiogenic peptides at the time of initial diagnosis of cancer.

Therapeutic Inhibition of Angiogenesis

Antiangiogenic therapy began to be used in humans in 1988. There are currently seven angiogenesis inhibitors in phase I/II and III clinical trials, six for antitumor therapy and one for therapy of ocular angiogenesis. The angiogenesis inhibitors under study as antitumor agents include PF4, the fumagillin analogue AGM-1470 (TNP-470), α-IFN, CAI, the metalloproteinase inhibitor BB94, and the sulfated peptidoglycan DS4152. A complex of hydrocortisone and β-cyclodextrin tetradecasulfate is in a phase I clinical trial for topical treatment of refractory corneal neovascularization.

INTERFERON ALFA-2A FOR LIFE-THREATENING OR SIGHT-THREATENING HEMANGIOMAS

The discovery that IFN alfa-2a had antiangiogenic activity[140–142] led in 1988 to its successful use to treat a life-threatening pulmonary hemangioma in a child.[240,241] Subsequent experience[244,245,291,292] in treating other hemangiomas has led to some general principles that may be applied in clinical trials of antiangiogenic therapy of cancer.

Hemangiomas are benign vascular lesions that consist of rapidly proliferating capillary blood vessels. They are the most common tumor of infancy, appearing in 1 to 2 per cent of neonates,[293] in 12 per cent of children by age 1 year,[245,294] and in 22 per cent of premature infants with a birth weight below 1000 gm.[295] Their natural history is characterized by rapid postnatal growth for 8 to 12 months (the proliferating phase), followed by slowing of growth and then gradual regression over the next 1 to 5 years (the involuting phase).[296] Hemangiomas undergo complete regression in over 50 per cent of children by age 5 years and in over 70 per cent by age 7 years, with continued improvement in the remaining children up to 10 to 12 years (the involuted phase).[293,297] The majority of hemangiomas require no treatment. However, approximately 10 per cent cause serious tissue damage, interfere with a vital organ, or are life threatening (e.g., obstruct the airway, produce high-output heart failure, or cause platelet-trapping thrombocytopenic coagulopathy [Kasabach-Merritt syndrome]).[298] This coagulopathy has a mortality rate of 30 to 40 per cent from hemorrhage (intracranial, gastrointestinal, or pulmonary).[299] Hepatic hemangiomas have a mortality rate of 30 to 50 per cent.[300] These endangering or life-threatening hemangiomas are treated with corticosteroids (prednisone given orally at 2 to 3 mg/kg/day). Approximately 30 per cent of hemangiomas respond dramatically to corticosteroid therapy and show signs of regression within several days to 1 week, 40 per cent respond equivocally, and 30 per cent do not respond at all.[243] When there is a therapeutic response, prednisone is continued until involution is well underway, usually for 8 to 10 months, and then tapered gradually.[205] The side effects of corticosteroid therapy (e.g., anorexia, weight

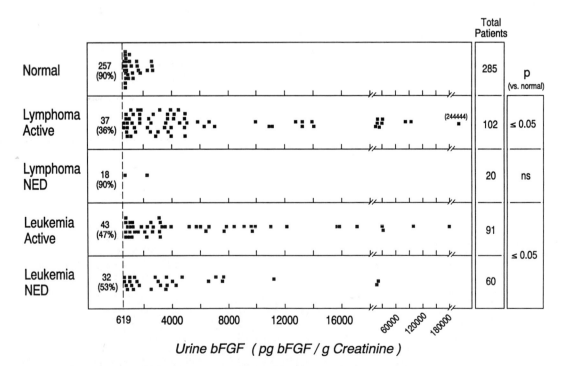

Figure 10–7. Urine bFGF levels in normal control subjects compared to patients with active local and active metastatic (NED) solid cancer (lymphoma or leukemia). Only those bFGF levels greater than the 90th percentile level of normal subjects were plotted individually. (From Nguyen M, Watanabe H, Budson AE, et al: Elevated levels of an angiogenic peptide, basic fibroblast growth factor, in the urine of patients with a wide spectrum of cancers. J Natl Cancer Inst 86:356, 1994, with permission.)

loss, growth retardation, Cushingoid facies, immunosuppression)[301] can be diminished by alternate-day therapy. When there is no effect, corticosteroid is discontinued in a rapid taper after a 2-week trial, because experience reveals that unresponsive hemangiomas will continue to grow despite corticosteroid for up to a year. Anecdotal evidence suggests that, occasionally, corticosteroid may accelerate hemangiomatous growth. When corticosteroids fail, there are no dependable, safe, and effective treatment alternatives for endangering hemangiomas, although there are anecdotal reports of favorable outcomes for radiation,[302] cyclophosphamide,[303,304] and embolization.[305,306]

There is now accumulating evidence that IFN alfa-2a is an effective treatment for life-threatening or sight-threatening hemangiomas even after failure of corticosteroid therapy. White et al. first observed regression of pulmonary hemangiomatosis in a 7-year-old boy after IFN alfa-2a therapy.[240] Orchard et al. reported two infants with hemangioma, one in the peritoneum and the other in the head and neck, both associated with thrombocytopenic coagulopathy. Both hemangiomas regressed and the coagulopathy was reversed with administration of α-IFN. White et al. also described two infants with life-threatening hemangiomas treated with α-IFN; one responded but the other died after less than 2 months of treatment.[343] At this writing, the empiric dose is 3 million units/m^2 given subcutaneously every day. There is a reported failure of IFN alfa-2a when given only three times per week.[307] IFN alfa-2b also has been used successfully,[308] although there is a report of failure with IFN alfa-2b.[309] We documented accelerated regression in 18 of 20 infants and children with life-threatening or sight-threatening hemangiomas treated with IFN alfa-2a.[244] Our ongoing experience in another 30 patients confirms this response. Others report similar experience.[246,291,292,310,311] IFN alfa-2a therapy must be continued for an average of 6 to 10 months. Accelerated regression is less dramatic with IFN than in hemangiomas that are highly responsive to corticosteroids. IFN alfa-2a appears to be particularly effective in the treatment of large cutaneous hemangiomas.

The toxicities associated with IFN alfa-2a in infants and children are less severe than in adults and are reversible. These are documented in detail in a recent review by Mulliken et al.[312] from our experience with 50 patients, and include fever for the first 1 to 2 weeks, transient neutropenia, anemia, and elevation of liver enzymes (up to fivefold). Most infants on IFN alfa-2a seem to gain weight and grow normally, in contrast to infants on prolonged corticosteroid therapy. A more problematic possible adverse reaction is spastic diplegia, reported in a child receiving IFN alfa-2a for nasopharyngeal papillomas.[313] We have observed one child with mild long-tract signs. Two other patients developed early signs of spastic diplegia but had confounding factors (e.g., prematurity in one child and spinal cord venous malformations in the other). We also are aware of two other children with similar neurologic signs at other centers. These signs improved after discontinuation of therapy. Thus, we currently advise neurologic/developmental evaluation before initiating IFN therapy and periodic assessments during and after therapy. We have not used corticosteroids and IFN alfa-2a together,

i.e., we taper corticosteroid therapy as soon as IFN alfa-2a therapy has begun. But, in a few patients in whom the two drugs have been used together at other centers, there has been no advantage of combination therapy and there is the possibility of increased toxicity.

At the Children's Hospital in Boston, we have an ongoing clinical study of the quantitation of urinary levels of bFGF in children with hemangiomas (J. Folkman et al., unpublished data). From the results to date, it appears that bFGF may be a good indicator of efficacy of therapy and may be useful in adjusting the dose of IFN alfa-2a in order to increase the regression rate, especially in cases of airway hemangiomas.

Our immunohistochemical studies of biopsies of hemangiomas show overexpression of bFGF and VEGF in endothelial cells and pericytes during the proliferating phase, and that bFGF overexpression persists into the involuting phase. Both angiogenic peptides return to normal levels in the involuted tissue.[245]

The recent finding by Fidler that mRNA and protein synthesis of bFGF in human renal and colon carcinoma cells is down-regulated by IFN-α and IFN-β, but not by IFN-γ suggests a possible mechanism for the antiangiogenic activity of IFN alfa-2a: that production of angiogenic peptides may be inhibited at their source.[138,314,342] This model is consistent with tissue levels and urinary levels of bFGF in patients with hemangiomas.

AGM-1470 (TNP-470)

This synthetic analogue of fumagillin currently is undergoing phase I clinical testing for AIDS-associated Kaposi's sarcoma at the National Cancer Institute. These Food and Drug Administration–approved dose escalation studies began in late 1992 and since have been extended to the treatment of metastatic carcinoma of the prostate and cervix (M.D. Anderson Hospital, Houston), and other solid tumors (Dana Farber Cancer Institute, Boston). Therapy is administered intravenously every other day.

In the preclinical animal studies, a wide variety of tumors in mice, rats, and rabbits (including human tumors in athymic mice) were inhibited significantly by AGM-1470 (TNP-470) so that T/C tumor volumes were suppressed to as low as 0.30. However, few were "cured," nor could "cures" be obtained with conventional cytotoxic therapy in these animals. However, combinations of AGM-1470 (or other angiogenesis inhibitors) with conventional cytotoxic agents produced durable "cures" in more than 50 per cent of animals.[46,315,316] This suggests that therapeutic attack against the tumor cell compartment as well as the endothelial cell compartment of a tumor may be more effective than treating either cell population alone. Therefore, although clinical trials of angiogenesis inhibitors such as AGM-1470 must be conducted as a single-drug study, after these inhibitors are approved for use, they could be most effective when used together with conventional therapy.

PLATELET FACTOR 4

This peptide is undergoing phase I/II clinical trials for Kaposi's sarcoma, melanoma, renal cell carcinoma, and colon cancer at four different centers in the United States. In Kaposi's sarcoma, it is being administered intralesionally in one study[317] and systemically in another. There have been few if any side effects to date.

CARBOXYAMINOIMIDAZOLE

This compound, which inhibits tumor growth and pulmonary metastases in in animals,[318] is undergoing phase I testing for solid tumors at the National Cancer Institute. It can be administered orally.[319]

METALLOPROTEINASE INHIBITOR BB94

BB94 (British Biotechnology 94) is a synthetic, low-molecular-weight inhibitor of matrix metalloproteinases. It has been shown to inhibit angiogenesis and tumor growth and metastasis in animals.[320] It is undergoing a phase I dose escalation trial for patients with malignant ascites at the ICRF Medical Oncology Unit (Western General Hospital) in Edinburgh, UK. The drug is administered intraperitoneally and efficacy is determined as the time to reaccumulation of ascites. In a recent report,[321] seven patients (five with ovarian carcinoma, one with endometrial carcinoma, and one with pancreatic carcinoma) tolerated the drug well and showed no significant toxicity, and only one patient reaccumulated ascites within the 28-day study period following administration of BB94.

THE PEPTIDOGLYCAN DS4152

DS4152 is a low-molecular-weight peptidoglycan extracted from the bacterial wall of the bacterium *Arthrobacter*. It is an angiogenesis inhibitor thought to operate by interfering with binding of bFGF to endothelial cells. It is undergoing phase I clinical trial for refractory malignancies, including breast, lung, and head and neck cancer and sarcoma. It is administered intravenously.[322] So far, toxicity mainly has been prolongation of the activated partial thromboplastin time, although this normalizes within

a few hours after termination of the infusion. No bleeding sequelae have been observed. Other side effects include fever and chills.

FUTURE DIRECTIONS

A new conceptual framework is beginning to emerge that outlines how certain principles of angiogenesis may be employed in the future management of patients with cancer. These ideas are based on preclinical studies taken together with the results of early clinical trials of antiangiogenic therapy, including IFN alfa-2a treatment of life-threatening hemangiomas.

At the time of diagnosis, it may be useful to ask how angiogenic is the the patient's tumor. A microvessel count could be obtained on the histologic section from the initial biopsy. For example, for patients with breast cancer, it is clear that, at the time of diagnosis, some tumors have a low intensity of neovascularization (i.e., 30 to 50 microvessels/200× field) and others are highly neovascularized (i.e., >100 microvessels/200× field).[260]

It also may be useful to determine if serum or urine contains elevated levels of an angiogenic peptide. Currently, we are accumulating experience with bFGF levels, but in the near future it may be feasible to determine a "profile" of angiogenic peptides, including VPF/VEGF and IL-8. The level of angiogenic peptide then could be measured periodically during therapy and follow-up, as a means of determining therapeutic efficacy and of detecting relapse. Thus, it may be informative to obtain urine levels of bFGF whenever IFN-α is used for anticancer therapy. For example, would urine bFGF levels predict which patients with AIDS-related Kaposi's sarcoma would respond to IFN?

At the start of conventional therapy, it may be useful to add antiangiogenic therapy as an adjunct to chemotherapy, radiotherapy, or surgery. The rationale for this approach is based on experimental studies by Teicher et

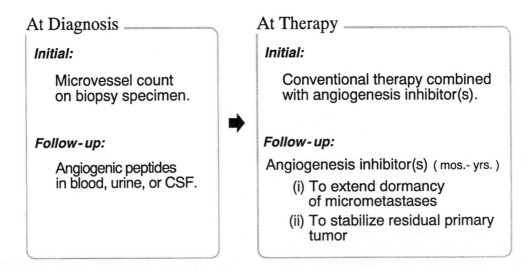

Figure 10–8. Proposed strategy for antiangiogenic therapy of neoplastic disease. CSF, cerebrospinal fluid.

al.[47,315,316] which show that combinations of cytotoxic therapy plus antiangiogenic therapy can produce durable "cures" in mice bearing Lewis lung carcinoma, but that either therapy alone cannot. Furthermore, an angiogenesis inhibitor such as AGM-1470 (TNP-470) can decrease DNA synthesis significantly in endothelial cells in a tumor bed, whereas cytotoxic agents such as Adriamycin and cisplatin do not decrease endothelial cell DNA synthesis.[323]

After conventional chemotherapy has been completed, it may be valuable to maintain antiangiogenic therapy for a prolonged period (months to years), with possibly short breaks. The rationale for this concept is based on our experience of treating life-threatening hemangiomas in infants by IFN alfa-2a. It was necessary to maintain therapy for at least 6 to 10 months, and at least 1 year in two children. Angiogenesis inhibitors generally down-regulate *neo*vascularization by inhibiting endothelial cell proliferation and migration, not by a cytotoxic effect on endothelial cells. Therefore, regression or involution of new capillary blood vessels is a slower process than lysis of tumor cells. The generally low level of toxicity of antiangiogenic therapy and the fact that drug resistance has not been a significant problem in long-term animal studies or in the use of IFN alfa-2a for hemangioma patients[244] or for tumor patients[324] offers the possibility that long-term antiangiogenic therapy may be well tolerated. A proposed strategy for antiangiogenic therapy in cancer is outlined in Figure 10–8.

Finally, the same angiogenesis inhibitors developed for anticancer therapy may turn out to be useful for non-neoplastic pathologic angiogenesis (e.g., diabetic retinopathy, macular degeneration, and arthritis).

REFERENCES

1. Folkman J, Long DM, Becker FF: Growth and metastasis of tumor in organ culture. Cancer 16:453, 1963
2. Coman DR, Sheldon WF: The significance of hyperemia around tumor implants. Am J Pathol 22:821, 1946
3. Warren BA: The vascular morphology of tumors. In Peterson H-I (ed): Tumor Blood Circulation: Angiogenesis, Vascular Morphology and Blood Flow of Experimental Human Tumors. Boca Raton, FL, CRC Press, 1979, pp 1–47
4. Ide AG, Baker N, Warren SL: Vascularization of the Brown-Pearce rabbit epithelioma transplant as seen in the transparent ear chamber. Am J Roentgenol 42:891, 1939
5. Algire G, Chalkely HW, Legallais FY, et al: Vascular reactions of normal and malignant tumors in vivo. I. Vascular reactions of mice to wounds and to normal and neoplastic transplants. J Natl Cancer Inst 6:73, 1945
6. Day ED: Vascular relationships of tumor and host. Prog Exp Tumor Res 4:57, 1964
7. Folkman J: Toward an understanding of angiogenesis: search and discovery. In Perspectives in Biology and Medicine. Chicago, The University of Chicago Press, 1985, pp 10–36
8. Folkman J: The intestine as an organ culture. In Burdette WJ (ed): Carcinoma of the Colon and Antecedent Epithelium. Springfield, IL, Charles C Thomas, 1970, pp 113–127
9. Folkman J, Cole P, Zimmerman S: Tumor behavior in isolated perfused organs: in vitro growth and metastasis of biopsy material in rabbit thyroid and canine intestinal segment. Ann Surg 164:491, 1966
10. Folkman J: Tumor angiogenesis: Therapeutic implications. N Engl J Med 285:1182, 1971
11. Folkman J: Angiogenesis. In Jaffe EA (ed): Biology of Endothelial Cells. Boston, Martinus Nijhoff Publishers, 1984, pp 412–428
12. Gimbrone MA Jr, Cotran RS, Leapman SB, et al: Tumor growth and neovascularization: An experimental model using rabbit cornea. J Natl Cancer Inst 52:413, 1974
13. Gimbrone MA Jr, Leapman SB, Cotran RS, et al: Tumor dormancy in vivo by prevention of neovascularization. J Exp Med 136:261, 1972
14. Brem S, Brem H, Folkman J, et al: Prolonged tumor dormancy by prevention of neovascularization in the vitreous. Cancer Res 36:2807, 1976
15. Folkman J: Tumor angiogenesis factor. Cancer Res 34:2109, 1974
16. Tannock IF: Population kinetics of carcinoma cells, capillary endothelial cells, and fibroblasts in a transplanted mouse mammary tumor. Cancer Res 30:2470, 1970
17. Knighton D, Ausprunk D, Tapper D, et al: Avascular and vascular phases of tumour growth in the chick embryo. Br J Cancer 35:347, 1977
18. Lien W, Ackerman NB: The blood supply of experimental liver metastases. II. A microcirculatory study of normal and tumor vessels of the liver with the use of perfused silicone rubber. Surgery 68:334, 1970
19. Folkman J, Watson K, Ingber D, et al: Induction of angiogenesis during the transition from hyperplasia to neoplasia. Nature 339:58, 1989
20. Thompson WD, Shiach KJ, Fraser RA, et al: Tumors acquire their vasculature by vessel incorporation, not vessel ingrowth. J Pathol 151:323, 1987
21. Skinner SA, Tutton PJ, O'Brien PE: Microvascular architecture of experimental colon tumors in the rat. Cancer Res 50:2411, 1990
22. Folkman J: What is the evidence that tumors are angiogenesis dependent? J Natl Cancer Inst 82:4, 1990
23. Ingber D, Fujita T, Kishimoto S, et al: Synthetic analogues of fumagillin that inhibit angiogenesis and suppress tumour growth. Nature 348:555, 1990
24. Gross JL, Herblin WF, Dusak BA, et al: Modulation of solid tumor growth in vivo by bFGF. Proc Am Assoc Cancer Res 31:79, 1990
25. Hori A, Sasada R, Matsutani E, et al: Suppression of solid tumor growth by immunoneutralizing monoclonal antibody against human basic fibroblast growth factor. Cancer Res 51:6180, 1991
26. Kim KJ, Li B, Winer J, et al: Inhibition of vascular endothelial growth factor-induced angiogenesis suppresses tumour growth in vivo. Nature 362:841, 1993
27. Plate KH, Breier G, Millauer B, et al: Up-regulation of vascular endothelial growth factor and its cognate receptors in a rat glioma model of tumor angiogenesis. Cancer Res 53:5822, 1993
28. Millauer B, Shawver LK, Plate KH, et al: Glioblastoma growth inhibited in vivo by a dominant-negative Flk-1 mutant. Nature 367:576, 1994
29. Ribatti D, Vacca A, Bertossi M, et al: Angiogenesis induced by B-cell non-Hodgkins lymphomas. Lack of correlation with tumor malignancy and immunological phenotype. Anticancer Res 10:401, 1990
30. Weiss L: Biophysical aspects of the metastatic cascade. In Weiss L (ed): Fundamental Aspects of Metastasis. Amsterdam, North-Holland Pub. Co. New York, American Elsevier, 1976, pp 51–70
31. Fidler IJ, Gersten DM, Hart IR: The biology of cancer invasion and metastasis. Adv Cancer Res 28:149, 1978
32. Nicolson GL: Cancer metastasis. Sci Am, 240:66, 1979
33. Zetter B: The cellular basis of site-specific tumor metastasis. N Engl J Med 322:605, 1990
34. Netland PA, Zetter BR: Organ-specific adhesion of metastatic tumor cells in vitro. Science 224:113, 1984
35. Nicolson GL: Organ specificity of tumor metastasis: Role of preferential adhesion, invasion and growth of malignant cells at specific secondary sites. Cancer Metastasis Rev 7:143, 1988
36. Boxberger HJ, Paweletz N, Spiess E, et al: An in vitro model

study of BSp73 rat tumour cell invasion into endothelial monolayer. Anticancer Res 9:1777, 1989

37. Weidner N, Semple JP, Welch WR: Tumor angiogenesis and metastasis—correlation in invasive breast carcinoma. N Engl J Med 324:1, 1991

38. Weinstat-Saslow D, Steeg PS: Angiogenesis and colonization in the tumor metastatic process: Basic and applied advances. FASEB J 8:401, 1994

39. Liotta LA, Tryggvason K, Garbisa S, et al: Metastatic potential correlates with enzymatic degradation of basement membrane collagen. Nature 284:67, 1980

40. Liotta LA, Saidel MG, Kleinerman J: The significance of hematogenous tumor cell clumps in the metastatic process. Cancer Res 36:889, 1976

41. Dvorak HF, Nagy JA, Dvorak JT, et al: Identification and characterization of the blood vessels of solid tumors that are leaky to circulating macromolecules. Am J Pathol 133:95, 1988

42. Nagy JA, Brown LF, Senger DR, et al: Pathogenesis of tumor stroma generation: A critical role for leaky blood vessels and fibrin deposition. Biochim Biophys Acta 948:305, 1989

43. Moscatelli D, Gross JL, Rifkin DB: Angiogenic factors stimulate plasminogen activator and collagenase production by capillary endothelial cells. J Cell Biol 91:201a, 1981

44. Kalebic T, Garbisa S, Glaser B, et al: Basement membrane collagen degradation by migrating endothelial cells. Science 221: 281, 1983

45. Smolin G, Hyndiuk RA: Lymphatic drainage from vascularized rabbit cornea. Am J Ophthalmol 72:147, 1971

46. Kerbel RS, Waghorne C, Korczak B, et al: Clonal dominance of primary tumors by metastatic cells: Genetic analysis and biological implications. Cancer Surv 7:597, 1988

47. Teicher BA, Sotomayor EA, Huang ZD: Antiangiogenic agents potentiate cytotoxic cancer therapies against primary and metastatic disease. Cancer Res 52:6702, 1992

48. Brem H, Gresser I, Grosfeld J, et al: The combination of antiangiogenic agents to inhibit primary tumor growth and metastasis. J Pediatr Surg 28:1253, 1993

49. Breslow A: Thickness cross-sectional areas and depth of invasion in the prognosis of cutaneous melanoma. Ann Surg 172:902, 1970

50. McGovern VJ, Murad TM: Pathology of melanoma: An overview. In Balch CM, Milton GW (eds): Cutaneous Melanoma: Clinical Management and Treatment Results Worldwide. Philadelphia, JB Lippincott Company, 1985, pp 29–53

51. Folkman J: What is the role of angiogenesis in metastasis from cutaneous melanoma? Eur J Cancer Clin Oncol 23:361, 1987

52. Jain RK: Delivery of novel therapeutic agents in tumors: Physiological barriers and strategies. J Natl Cancer Inst 81:570, 1989

53. Nicosia RF, Tchao R, Leighton J: Interactions between newly formed endothelial channels and carcinoma cells in plasma clot culture. Clin Exp Metastasis 4:91, 1986

54. Ziche M, Gullino PM: Angiogenesis and neoplastic progression in vitro. J Natl Cancer Inst 69:483, 1982

55. Brem SS, Gullino P, Medina D: Angiogenesis: A marker for neoplastic transformation of mammary papillary hyperplasia. Science 195:880, 1977

56. Brem SS, Jensen HM, Gullino PM: Angiogenesis as a marker of preneoplastic lesions of the human breast. Cancer 41:239, 1978

57. Chodak G, Haudenschild C, Gittes RF, et al: Angiogenic activity as a marker of neoplastic and preneoplastic lesions of the human bladder. Ann Surg 192:762, 1980

58. Kandell J, Bossy-Wetzel E, Radvanyi F, et al: Neovascularization is associated with a switch to the export of bFGF in the multistep development of fibrosarcoma. Cell 66:1095, 1991

59. Smith-McCune KK, Weidner N: Demonstration and characterization of the angiogenic properties of cervical dysplasia. Cancer Res 54:800, 1994

60. Sillman F, Boyce J, Fruchter R: The significance of atypical vessels and neovascularization in cervical neoplasia. Am J Obstet Gynecol 139:154, 1981

61. Hicks RM, Chowaniec J: Experimental induction, histology, and ultrastructure of hyperplasia and neoplasia of the urinary bladder epithelium. Int Rev Exp Pathol 18:199, 1978

62. Srivastava A, Laidler P, Hughes LE, et al: Neovascularization in human cutaneous melanoma: A quantitative morphological and Doppler ultrasound study. Eur J Cancer Clin Oncol 22: 1205, 1986

63. Srivastava A, Laidler P, Davies RP, et al: The prognostic significance of tumor vascularity in intermediate-thickness (0.76– 4.0 mm thick) skin melanoma. A quantitative histologic study. Am J Pathol 133:419, 1988

64. Weidner N, Folkman J, Pozza F, et al: Tumor angiogenesis: A new significant and independent prognostic indicator in early-stage breast carcinoma. J Natl Cancer Inst 84:1875, 1992

65. Weidner N, Carroll PR, Flax J, et al: Tumor angiogenesis correlates with metastasis in invasive prostate carcinoma. Am J Pathol 143:401, 1993

66. Hochberg MS, Folkman J: Mechanisms of size limitation of bacterial colonies. J Infect Dis 126:629, 1972

67. Folkman J: Tumor angiogenesis. Adv Cancer Res 43:175, 1985

68. Folkman J, Hochberg M: Self-regulation of growth in three dimensions. J Exp Med 138:745, 1973.

69. Folkman J: Tumor angiogenesis. In Becker FF (ed) Cancer: a comprehensive treatise, vol 3. New York, Plenum Press, 1975, pp 355–388

70. Rak JW, Hegmann EJ, Lu C, et al: Progressive loss of sensitivity to endothelium-derived growth inhibitors expressed by human melanoma cells during disease progression. J Cell Physiol 159: 245, 1994

71. Hamada J, Cavanaugh PG, Lotan O: Separable growth and migration factors for large-cell lymphoma cells secreted by microvascular endothelial cells derived from target organs for metastasis. Br J Cancer 66:349, 1992

72. Folkman J: Angiogenesis and breast cancer. J Clin Oncol 12: 441, 1994

73. Brown LF, Berse B, Jackman RW, et al: Increased expression of vascular permeability factor (vascular endothelial growth factor) and its receptors in kidney and bladder carcinoma. Am J Pathol 143:1255, 1993

74. Schweigerer L, Neufeld G, Friedman J, et al: Capillary endothelial cells express basic fibroblast growth factor, a mitogen that promotes their own growth. Nature 325:257, 1987

75. Motro B, Itin A, Sachs L, et al: Pattern of interleukin-6 gene expression in vivo suggests a role for this cytokine in angiogenesis. Proc Natl Acad Sci USA 87:3092, 1990

76. Podor TJ, Jirik FR, Loskutoff DJ, et al: Human endothelial cells produce IL-6: Lack of responses to exogenous IL-6. Ann N Y Acad Sci 557:374, 1989

77. Zsebo KM, Yuschenkoff VN, Schiffer S, et al: Vascular endothelial cells and granulopoiesis: Interleukin-1 stimulates release of G-CSF and GM-CSF. Blood 71:99, 1988

78. Shweiki D, Itin A, Soffer D, et al: Vascular endothelial growth factor induced by hypoxia may mediate hypoxia-initiated angiogenesis. Nature 359:843, 1992

79. Plate K, Breier G, Weich HA, et al: Vascular endothelial growth factor is a potential tumour angiogenesis factor in human gliomas in vivo. Nature 359:845, 1992

80. Long DM: Capillary ultrastructure in human metastatic brain tumors. J Neurosurg 51:53, 1979

81. Coomber BL, Steward PA, Hayakawa EM, et al: A quantitative assessment of microvessel ultrastructure in C6 astrocytoma spheroids transplanted to brain and to muscle. J Neuropathol Exp Neurol 47:29, 1988

82. Folkman J, Shing Y: Angiogenesis. J Biol Chem 267:10931, 1992

83. Senger DR, Galli SJ, Dvorak AM, et al: Tumor cells secrete a vascular permeability factor that promotes accumulation of ascites fluid. Science 219:983, 1983

84. Ferrara N, Henzel WJ: Pituitary follicular cells secrete a novel heparin-binding growth factor specific for vascular endothelial cells. Biochem Biophys Res Commun 161:851, 1989

85. Goldacre RJ, Sylvén B: On the access of blood-borne dyes to various tumour regions. Br J Cancer 16:306, 1962

86. Jain RK: Determinants of tumor blood flow. Cancer Res 48:2641, 1988

87. Kedar RP, Cosgrove DO, Smith IE, et al: Breast carcinoma: measurement of tumor response to primary medical therapy with color Doppler flow imaging. Radiology 190:825, 1994

88. Dobson DE, Kambe A, Block E, et al: 1-butyryl-glycerol: A novel angiogenesis factor secreted by differentiating adipocytes. Cell *61*:223, 1990

89. Form DM, Auerbach R: PGE$_2$ and angiogenesis. Proc Soc Exp Biol Med *172*:214, 1983

90. Ben Ezra D: Neovasculogenic ability of prostaglandins, growth factors and synthetic chemoattractants. Am J Ophthalmol *86*:455, 1978

91. Graeber JE, Glaser BM, Setty BNY, et al: 15-Hydroxyeicosatetraenoic acid stimulates migration of human retinal microvessel endothelium in vitro and neovascularization. Prostaglandins *39*:665, 1990

92. Kull FC Jr, Brent DA, Parikh I, et al: Chemical identification of a tumor-derived angiogenic factor. Science *236*:843, 1987

93. Dusseau J, Hutchins P, Malbasa D: Stimulation of angiogenesis by adenosine on the chick chorioallantoic membrane. Circulation *59*:164, 1986

94. West DC, Hampson IN, Arnold F, et al: Angiogenesis induced by degradation products of hyaluronic acid. Science *228*:1324, 1985

95. Raju KS, Alessandri G, Gullino PM: Characterization of a chemoattractant for endothelium induced by angiogenesis effectors. Cancer Res *44*:1579, 1984

96. Schulze-Osthoff K, Risau W, Vollmer E, et al: In situ detection of basic fibroblast growth factor by highly specific antibodies. Am J Pathol *137*:85, 1990

97. Paulus W, Grothe C, Sensenbrenner M, et al: Localization of basic fibroblast growth factor, a mitogen and angiogenic factor in human brain tumors. Acta Neuropathol (Berl) *79*:418, 1990

98. Folkman J, Klagsbrun M, Sasse J, et al: A heparin-binding angiogenic protein—basic fibroblast growth factor—is stored within basement membrane. Am J Pathol *130*:393, 1988

99. Gonzalez AM, Buscaglia M, Ong M, et al: Distribution of basic fibroblast growth factor in the 18-day rat fetus: localization in the basement-membranes of diverse tissues. J Cell Biol *110*:753, 1990

100. Soutter AD, Nguyen M, Watanabe H, et al: Basic fibroblast growth factor secreted by an animal tumor is detectable in urine. Cancer Res *53*:5297, 1993

101. Vlodavsky I, Bashkin P, Korner G, et al: Extracellular matrix-resident growth factors and enzymes: Relevance to angiogenesis and metastasis. Proc Am Assoc Cancer Res *31*:491, 1990

102. Polverini P, Leibovich S: Induction of neovascularization in vivo and endothelial proliferation in vitro by tumor-associated macrophages. Lab Invest *51*:635, 1984

103. Thompson RW, Whalen GF, Saunders KB, et al: Heparin-mediated release of fibroblast growth factor-like activity into the circulation of rabbits. Growth Factors *3*:221, 1990

104. Hondermarck H, Courty J, Boilly B, et al: Distribution of intravenously administered acidic and basic fibroblast growth factors in the mouse. Experientia *46*:973, 1990.

105. Li VW, Folkerth RD, Watanabe H, et al: Microvessel count and cerebrospinal fluid basic fibroblast growth factor in children with brain tumours. Lancet *344*:82, 1994

106. Connolly DT: Vascular permeability factor: A unique regulator of blood vessel function. J Cell Biochem *47*:219, 1991

107. Ferrara N, Houck K, Jakeman L, et al: Molecular and biological properties of the vascular endothelial growth factor family of proteins. Endocrinol Rev *13*:18, 1992

108. Dvorak HF, Sioussat TM, Brown LF, et al: Distribution of vascular permeability factor (vascular endothelial growth factor) in tumors: Concentration in tumor blood vessels. J Exp Med *174*:1275, 1991

109. Breier G, Albrecht U, Sterrer S, et al: Expression of vascular endothelial growth factor during embryonic angiogenesis and endothelial cell differentiation. Development *114*:521, 1992

110. Millauer B, Wizigmann-Voos S, Schnurch H, et al: High affinity VEGF binding and developmental expression suggest flk-1 as a major regulator of vasculogenesis and angiogenesis. Cell *72*:835, 1993

111. Jakeman LB, Armanini M, Phillips HS, et al: Developmental expression of binding sites and messenger ribonucleic acid for vascular endothelial growth factor suggests a role for this protein in vasculogenesis and angiogenesis. Endocrinology *133*:848, 1993

112. Peters KG, De Vries C, Williams LT: Vascular endothelial growth factor receptor expression during embryogenesis and tissue repair suggests a role in endothelial differentiation and blood vessel growth. Proc Natl Acad Sci USA *90*:8915, 1993

113. Shweiki D, Itin A, Neufeld G, et al: Patterns of expression of vascular endothelial growth factor (VEGF) and VEGF receptors in mice suggest a role in hormonally regulated angiogenesis. J Clin Invest *91*:2235, 1993

114. Houck KA, Leung DW, Rowland AM, et al: Dual regulation of vascular endothelial growth factor bioavailability by genetic and proteolytic mechanisms. J Biol Chem *267*:26031, 1992

115. Pertovaara L, Kaipainen A, Mustonen T, et al: Vascular endothelial growth factor is induced in response to transforming growth factor-beta in fibroblastic and epithelial cells. J Biol Chem *269*:6271, 1994

116. Pepper MS, Ferrara N, Orci L, et al: Potent synergism between vascular endothelial growth factor and basic fibroblast growth factor in the induction of angiogenesis in vitro. Biochem Biophys Res Commun *189*:824, 1992

117. Goto F, Goto K, Weindel K, et al: Synergistic effects of vascular endothelial growth factor and basic fibroblast growth factor on the proliferation and cord formation of bovine capillary endothelial cells within collagen gels. Lab Invest *69*:508, 1993

118. Takeshita S, Zheng LP, Brogi E, et al: Therapeutic angiogenesis. A single intra-arterial bolus of vascular endothelial growth factor augments revascularization in a rabbit ischemic hindlimb model. J Clin Invest *93*:662, 1994

119. Takeshita S, Pu LQ, Zheng L, et al: Vascular endothelial growth factor induces dose-dependent revascularization in a rabbit model of persistent limb ischemia. Circulation, in press, 1994

120. Shapiro R, Riordan JF, Vallee BL: Characteristic ribonucleolytic activity of human angiogenin. Biochemistry *25*:3527, 1986

121. St. Clair DK, Ryuak SM, Riordan JF, et al: Angiogenin abolishes cell-free protein synthesis by specific ribonucleolytic inactivation of ribosomes. Proc Natl Acad Sci USA *84*:8330, 1987

122. Bicknell R, Vallee BL: Angiogenin activates endothelial cell phospholipase C. Proc Natl Acad Sci USA *85*:5961, 1988

123. Bicknell R, Vallee BL: Angiogenin stimulates endothelial cell prostacyclin secretion by activation of phospholipase A2. Proc Natl Acad Sci USA *86*:1573, 1989

124. Miyazono K, Okabe T, Urabe A, et al: Purification and properties of an endothelial cell growth factor from human platelets. J Biol Chem *262*:4098, 1987

125. Furukawa T, Yoshimura A, Sumizawa T, et al: Angiogenic factor. Nature *356*:668, 1992

126. Haraguchi M, Miyadera K, Uemura K, et al: Angiogenic activity of enzymes. Nature *368*:198, 1994

127. Hobson D, Denekamp J: Endothelial proliferation in tumours and normal tissues: Continuous labelling studies. Br J Cancer *49*:405, 1984

128. Denekamp J: Review article: Angiogenesis, neovascular proliferation and vascular pathophysiology as targets for cancer therapy. Br J Radiol *66*:191, 1993

129. Sholley MM, Ferguson GP, Seibel HR, et al: Mechanisms of neovascularization: vascular sprouting can occur without proliferation of endothelial cells. *Lab. Invest. 51*:624, 1984

130. Hahnenberger R, Jakobson AM, Ansari A, et al: Low-sulphated oligosaccharides from heparan sulphate inhibit normal angiogenesis. Glycobiology *3*:567, 1993

131. Ingber DE: Fibronectin controls capillary endothelial cell growth by modulating cell shape. Proc Natl Acad Sci USA *87*:3579, 1990

132. Singhvi R, Kumar A, Lopez G, et al: Engineering cell shape and function. Science *264*:696, 1994

133. Ingber DE, Folkman J: How does the extracellular matrix control capillary morphogenesis? Cell *58*:803, 1989

134. Antonelli-Orlidge, Saunders KB, Smith SR, et al: An activated form of transforming growth factor-β is produced by cocultures of endothelial cells and pericytes. Proc Natl Acad Sci USA *86*:4544, 1989

135. Satoh Y, Rifkin DB: Inhibition of endothelial cell movement by pericytes and smooth muscle cells: Activation of key TGF-beta-like molecule by plasmin. J Cell Biol *109*:309, 1989

136. Satoh Y, Tsuboi R, Lyons R, et al: Characterization of the acti-

vation of latent TGF-beta by co-cultures of endothelial cells and pericytes or smooth muscle cells: A self-regulating system. J Cell Biol *111*:757, 1990

137. Schlingemann RO, Rietveld FJ, Kwaspen F, et al: Differential expression of markers for endothelial cells, pericytes, and basal lamina in the microvasculature of tumors and granulation tissue. Am J Pathol *138*:1335, 1991

138. Fidler IJ: Role of the organ environment in the pathogenesis of cancer metastasis. Proc Am Assoc Cancer Res *34*:570, 1993

139. Fabra A, Nakajima M, Bucana CD, et al: Modulation of the invasive phenotype of human colon carcinoma cells by organ specific fibroblasts of nude mice. Differentiation *52*:101, 1992

140. Brouty-Boye D, Zetter BR: Inhibition of cell motility by interferon. Science *208*:516, 1980

141. Dvorak HF, Gresser I: Microvascular injury in pathogenesis of interferon-induced necrosis of subcutaneous tumors in mice. J Natl Cancer Inst *81*:497, 1989

142. Sidky YA, Borden EC: Inhibition of angiogenesis by interferons: Effects on tumor- and lymphocyte-induced vascular responses. Cancer Res *47*:5155, 1987

143. Maione TE, Sharpe RJ: Development of angiogenesis inhibitors for clinical applications. Trends Pharmacol Sci *11*:457, 1990

144. Rastinejad F, Polverini P, Bouck NP: Regulation of the activity of a new inhibitor of angiogenesis by a cancer suppressor gene. Cell *56*:345, 1989

145. Good DJ, Polverini PJ, Rastinejad F, et al: A tumor suppressor-dependent inhibitor of angiogenesis is immunologically and functionally indistinguishable from a fragment of thrombospondin. Proc Natl Acad Sci USA *87*:6624, 1990

146. Sage EH, Bornstein P: Approaches for investigating matrix components produced by endothelial cells: Type VIII collagen, SPARC, and thrombospondin. *In* Haralson MA, Hassel J Jr (eds): Extracellular Matrix Molecules: A Practical Approach. New York, Oxford University Press, 1994, in press

147. Murphy-Ullrich JE, Schultz-Cherry S, Hook M: Transforming growth factor-beta complexes with thrombospondin. Mol Biol Cell *3*:181, 1992

148. Bagavandoss P, Kaytes P, Vogeli G, et al: Recombinant truncated thrombospondin-1 monomer modulates endothelial cell plasminogen activator inhibitor 1 accumulation and proliferation in vitro. Biochem Biophys Res Commun *192*:325, 1993

149. Tolsma SS, Volpert OV, Good DJ, et al: Peptides derived from two separate domains of the matrix protein thrombospondin-1 have antiangiogenic activity. J Cell Biol *122*:497, 1993

150. Moses MA, Sudhalter J, Langer R: Identification of an inhibitor of neovascularization from cartilage. Science *248*:1408, 1990

151. Liotta LA, Steeg PS, Stetler-Stevenson WG: Cancer metastasis and angiogenesis—an imbalance of positive and negative regulation. Cell *64*:327, 1991

152. Madri JA, Sankar S, Lu T: Matrix modulation of surface molecules during angiogenesis. J Cell Biochem Suppl *118A*:309, 1994

153. Ferrara N, Clapp C, Weiner R: The 16K fragment of prolactin specifically inhibits basal or fibroblast growth factor simulated growth of capillary endothelial cells. Endocrinology *129*:896, 1991

154. Crum R, Szabo S, Folkman J: A new class of steroids inhibits angiogenesis in the presence of heparin or a heparin fragment. Science *230*:1375, 1985

155. Folkman J, Szabo S, Stovroff M, et al: Duodenal ulcer: Discovery of a new mechanism and development of angiogenic therapy which accelerates healing. Ann Surg *214*:414, 1991

156. O'Reilly M, Rosenthal R, Sage EH, et al: The suppression of tumor metastases by a primary tumor. Surg Forum *XLIV*:474, 1993

157. Prehn RT: The inhibition of tumor growth by tumor mass. Cancer Res *51*:2, 1991

158. Prehn RT: Two competing influences that may explain concomitant tumor resistance. Cancer Res *53*:3266, 1993

159. Bouck NP: Tumor angiogenesis: The role of oncogenes and tumor suppressor genes. Cancer Cells *2*:179, 1990

160. Pientenpol JA, Vogelstein B: Tumour suppressor genes. No room at the p53 inn. Nature *365*:17, 1993

161. Bouck NP, Dameron KM, Volpert OV: Tumor suppressor gene

control of thrombospondin and angiogenesis. Presented at the Banbury Conference on Mechanisms of Developmental and Tumor Angiogenesis, Cold Spring Harbor Laboratory, Cold Spring Harbor, New York, November 11, 1993

162. Van Meir EG, Polverini PJ, Chazin VR, et al: Induction of wild type p53 expression in glioblastoma cells causes the release of an inhibitor of angiogenesis. Proc Am Assoc Cancer Res *35*:186, 1994

163. Stadler WM, Sherman J, Bohlander SK, et al: Homozygous deletions within chromosomal bands 9p21-22 in bladder cancer. Cancer Res *54*:2060, 1994

164. Diaz MO, Rubin CM, Harden A, et al: Deletions of interferon genes in acute lymphoblastic leukemia. N Engl J Med *322*:77, 1990

165. Folkman J: Anti-angiogenesis: New concept for therapy of solid tumors. Ann Surg *175*:409, 1972

166. Eisenstein R, Sorgente N, Soble L, et al: The resistance of certain tissues to invasion: Penetrability of explanted tissues by vascularized mesenchyme. Am J Pathol *73*:765, 1973

167. Brem H, Folkman J: Inhibition of tumor angiogenesis mediated by cartilage. J Exp Med *141*:427, 1975

168. Taylor S, Folkman J: Protamine is an inhibitor of angiogenesis. Nature *297*:307, 1982

169. Nguyen M, Shing T, Folkman J: Quantitation of angiogenesis and antiangiogenesis in the chick embryo chorioallantoic membrane. Microvasc Res *47*:31, 1994

170. Denekamp J: The current status of targeting tumour vasculature as a means of cancer therapy: An overview. Int J Radiat Biol *60*:401, 1991

171. Auerbach W, Auerbach R: Angiogenesis inhibition: A review. Pharmacol Ther, in press, 1994

172. Kerbel RS: Inhibition of tumor angiogenesis as a strategy to circumvent acquired resistance to anticancer therapeutic agents. BioEssays *13*:31, 1991

173. Maione T, Gray GS, Petro J, et al: Inhibition of angiogenesis by recombinant human platelet factor 4 and related peptides. Science *247*:77, 1990

174. Moore JV, West DC: Vasculature as a target for anti-cancer therapy. Cancer Cells *3*:100, 1991

175. Maragoudakis ME, Gullino P, Lelkes PI (eds): Angiogenesis in Health and Disease. New York, Plenum Press, NATO ASI Series A, Life Sciences, vol 227, 1992

176. Steiner R, Weisz PB, Langer R (eds): Angiogenesis: Key Principles—Science-Technology-Medicine. Boston, Birkauser Verlag, 1992

177. Denekamp J: Vascular attack as a therapeutic strategy for cancer. Cancer Metastasis Rev *3*:267, 1990

178. Brem S: The development of therapeutic angiosuppression: Problems and progress. *In* Maragoudakis M (ed): Angiogenesis in Health and Disease. NATO-ASI Series. Plenum, New York, 1882, pp 295–302

179. Folkman J, Ingber DE: Inhibition of angiogenesis. Semin Cancer Biol *3*:89, 1992

180. Langer R, Murray J: Angiogenesis inhibitors and their delivery systems. Appl Biochem Biotechnol *8*:9, 1983

181. Moses MA: The role of vascularization in tumor metastasis. *In* Orr FW, Buchanan MR, Weiss L (eds): Microcirculation in Cancer Metastasis. Boca Raton, FL, CRC Press, 1991, pp 257–276

182. Langer R, Folkman J: Polymers for the sustained release of proteins and other macromolecules. Nature *263*:797, 1976

183. Kuettner KE, Soble L, Croxen RL, et al: Tumor cell collagenase and its inhibition by a cartilage-derived inhibition. Science *196*:653, 1977

184. Langer R, Conn H, Vacanti J, et al: Control of tumor growth in animals by infusion of an angiogenesis inhibitor. Proc Natl Acad Sci USA *77*:4331, 1980

185. Kuettner K, Pauli B: Vascularity of cartilage. In Hall BK (ed): Cartilage: Structure Function and Biochemistry. New York, Academic Press, vol 1, 1983, pp 281–312

186. Sorgente N, Dorey CK: Inhibition of endothelial cell growth by a factor isolated from cartilage. Exp Cell Res *128*:63, 1980

187. Takigawa M, Shirai E, Enomoto M, et al: Cartilage-derived antitumor factor (CATF) inhibits the proliferation of endothelial cells in culture. Cell Biol Int Rep *9*:619, 1985

188. Takigawa M, Shirai E, Enomoto M, et al: A factor in conditioned medium of rabbit costal chondrocytes inhibits the proliferation of cultured endothelial cells and angiogenesis induced by B16 melanoma: Its relation with cartilage-derived anti-tumor factor (CATF). Biochem Int 14:357, 1987

189. Takigawa M, Pan H-O, Enomoto M, et al: A clonal human chondrosarcoma cell line produces an anti-angiogenic antitumor factor. Anticancer Res 10:311, 1990

190. Langer R, Brem H, Falterman K, et al: Isolation of a cartilage factor that inhibits tumor neovascularization. Science 193:70, 1976

191. Lee A, Langer R: Shark cartilage contains inhibitors of tumor angiogenesis. Science 221:1185, 1983

192. Oikawa T, Ashino-Fuse H, Shimamura M, et al: A novel angiogenic inhibitor derived from Japanese shark cartilage (I). Extraction and estimation of inhibitory activities toward tumor and embryonic angiogenesis. Cancer Lett 51:181, 1990

193. Greenwald RA, Golub LM, Lavietes B, et al: Tetracyclines inhibit human synovial collagenase in vivo and in vitro. J Rheumatol 14:28, 1987

194. Tamargo RJ, Bok RA, Brem H: Angiogenesis inhibition by minocycline. Cancer Res 51:672, 1991

195. Gross J, Azizkhan RG, Biswas C: Inhibition of tumor growth, vascularization, and collagenolysis in the rabbit cornea by medroxyprogesterone. Proc Natl Acad Sci USA 78:1176, 1981

196. Saksela O, Rifkin DB: Release of basic fibroblast growth factor-heparin sulfate complexes from endothelial cells by plasminogen activator-mediated proteolytic activity. J Cell Biol 110:767, 1990

197. Fujimoto J, Hosoda S, Fujita H, et al: Inhibition of tumor angiogenesis activity by medroxyprogesterone acetate in gynecologic malignant tumors. Invasion Metastasis 9:269, 1989

198. Yamamoto T, Terada N, Nishizawa Y, et al: Angiostatic activities of medroxyprogesterone acetate and its analogues. Int J Cancer 56:393, 1994

199. Saiki I, Murata J, Nakajima M, et al: Inhibition of sulfated chitin derivatives of invasion through extracellular matrix and enzymatic degradation by metastatic melanoma cells. Cancer Res 50:3631, 1990

200. Jakobsson A, Sorbo J, Norrby K: Protamine and mast-cell-mediated angiogenesis in the rat. J Exp Pathol 71:209, 1990

201. Folkman J, Langer R, Linhardt R, et al: Angiogenesis inhibition and tumor regression caused by heparin or a heparin fragment in the presence of cortisone. Science 221:719, 1983

202. Sharpe RJ, Byers HR, Scott CF, et al: Growth inhibition of murine melanoma and human colon carcinoma by recombinant human platelet factor 4. J Natl Cancer Inst 82:848, 1990

203. Maione TE, Gray GS, Hunt AJ, et al: Inhibition of tumor growth in mice by an analogue of platelet factor 4 that lacks affinity for heparin and retains potent angiostatic activity. Cancer Res 51:2077, 1991

204. Bagavandoss P, Wilks JW: Specific inhibition of endothelial cell proliferation by thrombospondin. Biochem Biophys Res Commun 170:867, 1990

205. Taraboletti G, Roberts D, Liotta LA, et al: Platelet thrombospondin modulates endothelial cell adhesion, motility, and growth: A potential angiogenesis regulatory factor. J Cell Biol 111:765, 1990

206. Iruela-Arispe ML, Bornstein P, Sage H: Thrombospondin exerts an antiangiogenic effect on cord formation by endothelial cells in vitro. Proc Natl Acad Sci USA 88:5026, 1991

207. Nickoloff BJ, Mitra RS, Varani J, et al: Aberrant production of interleukin-8 and thrombospondin-1 by psoriatic keratinocytes mediates angiogenesis. Am J Pathol 144:820, 1994

208. DiPietro LA, Polverini PJ: Angiogenic macrophages produce the angiogenic inhibitor thrombospondin 1. Am J Pathol 143:678, 1993

209. Sakamoto N, Tanaka N, Tohgo A, et al: Heparin plus cortisone acetate inhibits tumor growth by blocking endothelial cell proliferation. Cancer J 1:55, 1986

210. Sakamoto N, Tanaka NG, Tohgo A, et al: Inhibitory effects of heparin plus cortisone acetate on endothelial cell growth both in cultures and in tumor masses. J Natl Cancer Inst 78:581, 1987

211. Folkman J, Ingber DE: Angiostatic steroids. In Schleimer RP, Claman HN, Oronsky AL (eds): Anti-Inflammatory Steroid Action. New York, Academic Press, 1989, pp 330–350

212. Drago J: The evaluation of inhibitors of angiogenesis, platelet function and polyamine synthesis on metastasis in the NB rat prostatic carcinoma model. J Urology 135:337a, 1986

213. Benrezzak O, Madarnas P, Pageau R, et al: Evaluation of cortisone-heparin and cortisone-maltose tetrapalmitate therapies against rodent tumors. Anticancer Res 9:1883, 1989

214. Chen NT, Corey EJ, Folkman J: Potentiation of angiostatic steroids by a synthetic inhibitor of arylsulfatase. Lab Invest 59:453, 1988

215. Folkman J, Weisz PB, Joullié MM, et al: Control of angiogenesis with synthetic heparin substitutes. Science 243:1490, 1989

216. Pereles T, Ingber DE, Folkman J: Inhibition of capillary endothelial cell outgrowth: The role of complex formation between an angiostatic steroid and beta-cyclodextrin tetradecasulfate. J Cell Biol 109:311a, 1989

217. Sakamoto N, Tanaka NG: Mechanism of synergistic effect of heparin and cortisone against angiogenesis and tumor growth. Cancer J 2:9, 1988

218. Ingber DE, Madri JA, Folkman J: A possible mechanism for inhibition of angiogenesis by angiostatic steroids: Induction of capillary basement membrane dissolution. Endocrinology 119:1768, 1986

219. Blei F, Wilson EL, Mignatii P, et al: Mechanism of action of angiostatic steroids: Suppression of plasminogen activator activity via stimulation of plasminogen activator inhibitory synthesis. J Cell Physiol 155:568, 1993

220. Ingber DE, Folkman J: Inhibition of angiogenesis through modulation of collagen metabolism. Lab Invest 59:44, 1988

221. Nguyen NM, Lehr JE, Pienta KJ: Pentosan inhibits angiogenesis in vitro and suppresses prostate tumor growth in vivo. Anticancer Res 13:2143, 1993

222. Inoue K, Korenga H, Tanaka N, et al: The sulfated polysaccharide-peptidoglycan complex potently inhibits embryonic angiogenesis and tumor growth in the presence of cortisone acetate. Carbohydrate Res 181:135, 1988

223. Kusaka M, Sudo K, Fujita T, et al: Potent anti-angiogenic action of AGM-1470: Comparison to the fumagillin parent. Biochem Biophys Res Commun 174:1070, 1991

224. Oikawa T, Hirotani K, Shimamura M, et al: Powerful antiangiogenic activity of herbimycin A (named angiostatic antibiotic). J Antibiot 42:1202, 1989

225. Oikawa T, Hasegawa M, Shimamura M, et al: Eponemycin, a novel antibiotic, is a highly powerful angiogenesis inhibitor. Biochem Biophys Res Commun 181:1070, 1991

226. Oikawa T, Ashino H, Shimamura M: Inhibition of angiogenesis by erbstatin, an inhibitor of tyrosine kinase. J Antibiot 46:785, 1993

227. Oikawa T, Shimamura M, Ashino H: Inhibition of angiogenesis by staurosporine, a potent protein kinase inhibitor. J Antibiot 45:1155, 1992

228. Maragoudakis ME, Panoutsacopoulou M, Sarmonika M: Rate of basement membrane biosynthesis as an index to angiogenesis. Tissue Cell 20:531, 1988

229. Maragoudakis ME, Sarmonika M, Panoutsacopoulou M: Antiangiogenic action of heparin plus cortisone is associated with decreased collagenous protein synthesis in the CAM system. J Pharmacol Exp Ther 251:679, 1989

230. Missirilis E, Karakiulakis G, Maragoudakis ME: Antitumor effect of GPA1734 in rat walker 256 carcinoma. Invest New Drugs 8:145, 1990

231. Matsubara T, Saura R, Hirohata K, et al: Inhibition of human endothelial cell proliferation in vitro and neovascularization in vivo by D-penicillamine. J Clin Invest 83:158, 1989

232. Brem SS, Zagzag D, Tsanaclis AM, et al: Inhibition of angiogenesis and tumor growth in the brain. Am J Pathol 137:1121, 1990

233. Matsubara T, Ziff M: Inhibition of human endothelial cell proliferation by gold compounds. J Clin Invest 79:1440, 1987

234. Koch AE, Cho M, Burrows J, et al: Inhibition of production of macrophage-derived angiogenic activity by the anti-rheumatic agents gold sodium thiomalate and auranofin. Biochem Biophys Res Commun 154:205, 1988

235. Oikawa T, Hirotani K, Ogaswara H, et al: Inhibition of angiogenesis by vitamin D3 analogues. Eur J Pharmacol *178*:247–250, 1990

236. Strander H: Interferon treatment of human neoplasia. Adv Cancer Res *46*:1, 1986

237. Gutterman JU, Blumenschein GR, Alexanian R, et al: Leukocyte interferon-induced tumor regression in human metastatic breast cancer, multiple myeloma, and malignant lymphoma. Ann Intern Med *93*:399, 1980

238. Quesada JR, Reuben J, Manning JT, et al: Alpha interferon for induction of remission in hairy-cell leukemia. N Engl J Med *310*:15, 1984

239. Gutterman JU: Cytokine therapeutics: Lessons from interferon a. Proc Natl Acad Sci USA *91*:1198, 1994

240. White CW, Sondheimer HM, Crouch EC, et al: Treatment of pulmonary hemangiomatosis with recombinant interferon alfa-2a. N Engl J Med *320*:1197, 1989

241. Folkman J: Successful treatment of an angiogenic disease. N Engl J Med *320*:1211, 1989

242. Orchard PJ, Smith CM III, Woods WG, et al: Treatment of hemangioendotheliomas with alpha interferon. Lancet *2*:565, 1989

243. Enjroles O, Riche MC, Merland JJ, et al: Management of alarming hemangiomas in infancy: A review of 25 cases. Pediatrics *85*:491, 1990

244. Ezekowitz RA, Mulliken JB, Folkman J: Interferon alfa-2a therapy for life-threatening hemangiomas of infancy. N Engl J Med *326*:1456, 1992

245. Takahashi K, Mulliken JB, Kozakewich HPW, et al: Cellular markers that distinguish the phases of hemangioma during infancy and childhood. J Clin Invest *93*:2357, 1994

246. Ohlms LA, Jones DT, McGill TJ, et al: Interferon alfa-2a therapy for airway hemangiomas. Ann Otol Rhinol Laryngol *103*:1, 1994

247. Alesendro R, Spoonster J, Liotta LA, et al: Inhibition of angiogenesis by CAI, a novel inhibitor of signal transduction [abstr 1102]. Proc Am Assoc Cancer Res *35*:184, 1994

248. McBride WG: Thalidomide and congenital abnormalities. Lancet *2*:1358, 1961

249. Lenz W: Thalidomide and congenital abnormalities. Lancet *1*:45, 1962

250. Cahen R, Sautai M, Montagne J, et al: Evaluation of the teratogenicity of drugs. Med Exp *10*:201, 1964

251. Christie GA: Thalidomide and congenital abnormalities. Lancet *2*:249, 1962

252. Helm F: Tierexperimentelle untersuchungen und dysmeliesyndrom. Arzneim Forsch *16*:1232, 1966

253. Stertz H, Nothdurft H, Lexa P, et al: Teratologic studies on the Himalayan rabbit: New aspects of thalidomide-induced teratogenesis. Arch Toxicol *60*:376, 1987

254. Stephens TD: Proposed mechanisms of actions in thalidomide embryopathy. Teratology *38*:229, 1988

255. D'Amato RJ, Loughnan MS, Flynn E, et al: Thalidomide is an inhibitor of angiogenesis. Proc Natl Acad Sci USA *91*:4082, 1994

256. Cheresh DA: Human endothelial cells synthesize and express an Arg-Gly-Asp-directed adhesion receptor involved in attachment to fibrinogen and von Willebrand factor. Proc Natl Acad Sci USA *84*:6471, 1987

257. Leavesly DI, Schwartz MA, Rosenfeld M, et al: Integrin beta 1- and beta 3-mediated endothelial cell migration is triggered through distinct signaling mechanisms. J Cell Biol *121*:163, 1993

258. Brooks PC, Clark RAF, Cheresh DA: Requirement of vascular integrin avB3 for angiogenesis. Science *264*:569, 1994

259. Biberfeld P, Porwit-Ksiazek A, Bottiger B, et al: Immunohistopathology of lymph nodes in HTLV-III infected homosexuals with persistent adenopathy or AIDS. Cancer Res *45*:4665s, 1985

260. Weidner N: The relationship of tumor angiogenesis and metastasis with emphasis on invasive breast cancer. Adv Pathol Lab Med *5*:101, 1992

261. Gasparini G, Weidner N, Maluta S, et al: Intratumoral microvessel density and p53 protein: Correlation with metastasis in head-and-neck squamous-cell carcinoma. Int J Cancer *55*:739, 1993

262. Gasparini G, Harris AL: Does improved control of tumour growth require an anti-cancer therapy targeting both neoplastic and intratumoral endothelial cells? Int J Oncol *12*:454, 1994

263. Bosari S, Lee AK, DeLellis RA, et al: Microvessel quantitation and prognosis in invasive breast carcinoma. Hum Pathol *23*:755, 1992

264. Horak ER, Leek R, Klenk N, et al: Angiogenesis, assessed by platelet/endothelial cell adhesion molecule antibodies, as indicator of node metastases and survival in breast cancer. Lancet *340*:1120, 1992

265. Visscher DW, Smilanetz S, Drozdowicz S, et al: Prognostic significance of image morphometric microvessel enumeration in breast cancer. Anal Quant Cytol Histol *15*:88, 1993

266. Toi M, Kashitani J, Tominaga T: Tumor angiogenesis is a powerful prognostic indicator of primary breast carcinoma. Int J Cancer *55*:341, 1993

267. Fox SB, Leek RD, Smith K, et al: Tumor angiogenesis in node-negative breast carcinomas—relationship with epidermal growth factor receptor, estrogen receptor, and survival. Breast Cancer Res Treat *29*:109, 1994

268. Gasparini G, Weidner N, Bevilacqua P, et al: Tumor microvessel density, p53 expression, tumor size, and peritumoral lymphatic vessel invasion are relevant prognostic markers in node-negative breast carcinoma. J Clin Oncol *12*:441, 1994

269. Van Hoeff MEHM, Knox WF, Dhesi SS, et al: Assessment of tumor vascularity as a prognostic factor in lymph node negative invasive breast cancer. Eur J Cancer *29A*:1141, 1993

270. Hall NR, Fish DE, Hunt N, et al: Is the relationship between angiogenesis and metastasis in breast cancer real? Surg Oncol *1*:223, 1992

271. Weidner N: Tumor angiogenesis: Review of current applications in tumor prognostication. Semin Diagn Pathol, *10*:302, 1993

272. Macchiarini P, Fontani G, Hardin MJ, et al: Relation of neovascularisation to metastasis of non-small-cell lung cancer. Lancet *340*:145, 1993

273. Wakui S, Furusato M, Itoh T, et al: Tumour angiogenesis in prostatic carcinoma with and without bone marrow metastasis: A morphometric study. J Pathol *168*:257, 1992

274. Brawer MD, Keering RE, Brown M, et al: Predictors of pathologic stage in prostatic carcinoma. Cancer *73*:678, 1994

275. Brawer MK: The diagnosis of prostatic carcinoma. Cancer *71*:899, 1993

276. Makami, Y, Tsukunda M, Mochimatsu I, et al: Angiogenesis in head and neck tumor. Nippon Jibiinkoka Gakkai Kaiho *96*:645, 1991

277. Gasparini G: Quantitation of intratumoural vascularisation predicts metastasis in human invasive solid tumours. Oncol Rep *1*:7, 1994

278. Fallowfield ME, Cook MG: The vascularity of primary cutaneous melanoma. J Pathol *164*:241, 1991

279. Barnhill RL, Randrey K, Levy MA, et al: Angiogenesis and tumor progression of melanoma: Quantification of vascularity in melanocytic nevi and cutaneous malignant melanoma. Lab Invest *67*:332, 1992

280. Barnhill RL, Levy MA: Regressing thin cutaneous malignant melanomas (< or = 1.0 mm) are associated with angiogenesis. Am J Pathol *143*:99, 1993

281. Liotta L, Kleinerman J, Saidel G: Quantitative relationships of intravascular tumor cells, tumor vessels, and pulmonary metastases following tumor implantation. Cancer Res *34*:997, 1974

282. Blood CH, Zetter BR: Tumor interactions with the vasculature: Angiogenesis and tumor metastasis. Biochim Biophys Acta *1032*:89, 1990

283. Li V, Watanabe H, Yu C, et al: Cerebrospinal fluid from pediatric brain tumor patients contains a mitogen for capillary endothelial cells. Mol Biol Cell *3*:235a, 1992

284. Chodak G, Scheiner C, Zetter B: Urine from patients with transitional-cell carcinoma stimulates migration of capillary endothelial cells. N Engl J Med *305*:869, 1981

285. Shing Y, Folkman J, Sullivan R, et al: Heparin affinity: Purification of a tumor-derived capillary endothelial cell growth factor. Science *223*:1296, 1984

286. Chodak GW, Hospelhorn V, Judge SM, et al: Increased levels of fibroblast growth factor-like activity in urine from patients with bladder or kidney cancer. Cancer Res 48:2083, 1988

287. Watanabe H, Hori A, Seno M, et al: A sensitive enzyme immunoassay for human basic fibroblast growth factor. Biochem Biophys Res Commun 175:229, 1991

288. Fujimoto K, Ichimori Y, Kakizoe T, et al: Increased serum levels of basic fibroblast growth factor in patients with renal cell carcinoma. Biochem Biophys Res Commun 180:386, 1991

289. Watanabe H, Nguyen M, Schizer M, et al: Basic fibroblast growth factor in human serum—a prognostic test for breast cancer. Mol Biol Cell 3:324a, 1992

290. Nguyen M, Watanabe H, Budson AE, et al: Elevated levels of an angiogenic peptide, basic fibroblast growth factor, in the urine of patients with a wide spectrum of cancers. J Natl Cancer Inst 86:356, 1994

291. Blei F, Orlow SJ, Geronemus RG: Supraumbilical midabdominal raphe, sternal atresia, and hemangioma in an infant: Response of hemangioma to laser and interferon alfa-2a. Pediatr Dermatol 10:71, 1993

292. Blei F, Orlow SJ, Geronemus RG: Interferon alfa-2a therapy for extensive perianal and lower extremity hemangioma. J Am Acad Dermatol 23:98, 1993

293. Pratt GA: Birthmarks in infants. Arch Dermatol 67:302, 1953

294. Holmdahl K: Cutaneous hemangiomas in premature and mature infants. Acta Paediat 44:370, 1955

295. Amir J, Metzker A, Krikler R, et al: Strawberry hemangioma in preterm infants. Pediatr Dermatol 3:131, 1986

296. Mulliken JB, Young AE: Vascular Birthmarks: Hemangiomas and Malformations. Philadelphia, WB Saunders Company, 1988

297. Bowers RE, Graham EA, Tominson KM: The natural history of the strawberry nevus. Arch Dermatol 82:667, 1960

298. Kasabach HH, Merritt KK: Capillary hemangiomas with extensive purpura. Am J Dis Child 59:1063, 1940

299. El-Dessouky M, Azmy AF, Raine PAM, et al: Kasabach-Merritt syndrome. J Pediatr Surg 23:109, 1980

300. Cohen RC, Myers NA: Diagnosis and management of massive hepatic hemangiomas in childhood. J Pediatr Surg 21:6, 1986

301. Hyams JS, Carey DE: Corticosteroids and growth. J Pediatr 113:249, 1980

302. Schild SE, Buskirk SJ, Frick LM, et al: Radiotherapy for large symptomatic hemangiomas. Int J Radiat Oncol Biol Phys 21:729, 1991

303. Hurvitz CH, Alkalay AL, Sloninsky L, et al: Cyclophosphamide therapy in life-threatening vascular tumors. J Pediatr 109:360, 1986

304. al-Rashid RA: Cyclosphosphamide and radiation therapy in the treatment of hemangioendothelioma with disseminated intravascular clotting. Cancer 27:364, 1971

305. Argenta LC, Bishop E, Cho KJ, et al: Complete resolution of life-threatening hemangioma by embolization and corticosteroids. Plast Reconstr Surg 70:739, 1982

306. Stanley P, Gomperts E, Woolley MM: Kasabach-Merritt syndrome treated by therapeutic embolization with polyvinyl alcohol. Am J Pediatr Hematol Oncol 8:308, 1986

307. de Castelbajac D, Teillac D, Bodemer C, et al: Hemangiome cephalique tubereyx d'evolution fatale; inefficacite du traitment par inteferon alpha. Ann Dermatol Venereol 117:821, 1990

308. Loughnan MS, Elder J, Kemp A: Treatment of massive orbital capillary hemangioma with interferon alfa-2b: Short-term results. Arch Ophthalmol 110:1366, 1992

309. Teillac-Hamel D, De Prost Y, Bodemer C, et al: Serious childhood angiomas: Unsuccessful alpha-2b interferon treatment. A report of 4 cases. Br J Dermatol 129:473, 1993

310. Spiller JC, Sharma V, Woods GM, et al: Diffuse neonatal hemangiomatosis treated successfully with interferon alfa-2a. J Am Acad Dermatol 27:102, 1992

311. Dubois J, Leclerc JBM, Garel L, et al: Radiologic modifications induced by interferon alfa-2b in progressive hemangioma: Clinical and CT correlation. American Society of Pediatric Radiology abstract, Seattle, WA, May 12–15, 1993

312. Mulliken JB, Boon LM, Takahashi K, et al: An update on pharmacologic therapy for endangering hemangioma. Curr Opin Dermatol 2:109, 1995

313. Vesikari T, Nuutila A, Cantell K: Neurologic sequelae following interferon therapy of juvenile laryngeal papilloma. Acta Paediatr Scand 77:619, 1988

314. Fidler IJ: The biology of cancer metastasis and its implications [abstr 013]. Ann Oncol 5:71, 1994

315. Teicher BA, Holden SA, Ara G, et al: Response of the FSall fibrosarcoma to antiangiogenic modulators plus cytotoxic agents. Anticancer Res 13:2101, 1993

316. Teicher BA, Holden SA, Ara G, et al: Potentiation of cytotoxic cancer therapies by TNP-470 alone and with other antiangiogenic agents. Int J Cancer 57:1, 1994

317. Kahn J, Ruiz R, Kerschmann R, et al: A phase I/II study of recombinant platelet factor 4 (rPF4) in patients with AIDS related Kaposi's sarcoma (KS). Proc Am Soc Clin Oncol 12:50, 1993

318. Kohn E, Sandeen MA, Liotta LA: et al: In vivo efficacy of a novel inhibitor of selected signal transduction pathways including calcium, arachidonate, and inositol phosphates. Cancer Res 52:3208, 1992

319. Pluda J: Inhibitors of angiogenesis and metastasis: Preclinical and early clinical studies [abstr 014]. Ann Oncol 5:71, 1994

320. Davies B, Brown PD, East N, et al: A synthetic matrix metalloproteinase inhibitor decreases tumor burden and prolongs survival of mice bearing human ovarian carcinoma xenografts. Cancer Res 53:2087, 1993

321. Beattie GJ, Young HA, Smyth JF: Phase I study of intraperitoneal metallo-proteinase inhibitor BB94 in patients with malignant ascites [abstr 015]. Ann Oncol 5:72, 1994

322. Eckhardt G, Burris H III, Eckhardt J, et al: Initial phase I assessment of the novel angiogenesis inhibitor DS4152 [abstr 016]. Ann Oncol 5:72, 1994

323. Yamamoto T, Sudo K, Fujita T: Significant inhibition of endothelial cell growth in tumor vasculature by an angiogenesis inhibitor, TNP-470 (AGM-1470). Anticancer Res 14:1, 1994

324. Oberg KE: The role of interferons in neuroendocrine tumours and aspects of mechanisms of actions. In Crowther D (ed): Interferons: Mechanisms of Action and Role in Cancer Therapy. Berlin, Springer-Verlag, 1991, pp 43–52

325. Maciag T, Mehlman T, Friesel R, et al: Heparin binds endothelial cell growth factor, the principal endothelial cell mitogen in bovine brain. Science 225:932, 1984

326. Fett JW, Strydom DJ, Lob RR, et al: Isolation and characterization of angiogenin, an angiogenic protein from human carcinoma cells. Biochemistry 24:5480, 1985

327. Schreiber AB, Winkler ME, Derynck R: Transforming growth factor-alpha: A more potent angiogenic mediator than epidermal growth factor. Science 232:1250, 1986

328. Roberts AB, Sporn MB, Assoian RK, et al: Transforming growth factor type beta: Rapid induction of fibrosis and angiogenesis in vivo and stimulation of collagen formation in vitro. Proc Natl Acad Sci USA 83:4167, 1986

329. Lebovich SJ, Polverini PJ, Shepard HM, et al: Macrophage-induced angiogenesis is mediated by tumour necrosis factor-alpha. Nature 329:630, 1987

330. Connolly DT, Heuvelman DM, Nelson R, et al: Tumor vascular permeability factor stimulates endothelial cell growth and angiogenesis. J Clin Invest 84:1470, 1989

331. Leung DW, Cachianes G, Kuang WJ, et al: Vascular endothelial growth factor is a secreted angiogenic mitogen. Science 246:1306, 1989

332. Plouet J, Schilling J, Gospodarowicz D: Isolation and characterization of a newly identified endothelial cell mitogen produced by AtT-20 cells. EMBO J 8:3801, 1989

333. Ishikawa F, Miyazone K, Hellman U, et al: Identification of angiogenic activity and the cloning and expression of platelet-derived endothelial cell growth factor. Nature 338:557, 1989

334. Bussolino F, Ziche M, Wang JM, et al: In vitro and in vivo activation of endothelial cells by colony stimulating factors. J Clin Invest 87:986, 1991

335. Maglione D, Guerriero V, Viglietto G, et al: Isolation of a human placenta cDNA coding for a protein related to the vascular permeability factor. Proc Natl Acad Sci USA 88:9267, 1991

336. Koch A, Polverini PJ, Kunkel SL, et al: Interleukin-8 as a macrophage-derived mediator of angiogenesis. Science *258*: 1178, 1992

337. Rosen EM, Meromsky L, Setter E, et al: Purified scatter factor stimulated epithelial and vascular endothelial cell migration. Proc Soc Exp Biol Med *195*:34, 1990

338. Bussolino F, Di Renzo MF, Ziche M, et al: Hepatocyte growth factor is a potent angiogenic factor which stimulates endothelial cell motility and growth. J Cell Biol *119*:629, 1992

339. Folkman J: Oncology overview of antiangiogenesis. *In* Oncology Overview: Selected Abstracts on Antiangiogenesis: A Potential Therapeutic Strategy. Washington, DC, U.S. Government Printing Office, 1991, pp vii–xi

340. Ricketts RR, Hatley RM, Corden BJ, Sabio H, Howell CG. Interferon-Alpha-2a for the Treatment of Complex Hemangiomas of Infancy and Childhood. Annal Surg *219*:605, 1994

341. Dameron KM, Volpert OV, Tainsky MA, et al: Control of angiogenesis in fibroblasts by p53 regulation of thrombospondin-1. Science, in press, 1994

342. Singh RK, Gutman M, Bucana CD, et al. Interferons alpha and beta downregulate the expression of basic fibroblast growth factor in human carcinomas. Submitted to Proc Natl Acad Sci USA 1994

343. White CW, Wolf SJ, Korones DN, et al. Treatment of childhood angiomatous diseases with recombinant interferon alfa-2a. J Pediatr *118*:59, 1991

11

MOLECULAR MECHANISMS OF TUMOR CELL METASTASIS

MARY L. STRACKE
LANCE A. LIOTTA

Invasion and metastasis continue to present the greatest obstacles to successful cancer treatment. Despite advances made in conventional tumor therapies and surgical techniques, most cancer deaths still result from metastatic disease. Our lack of understanding of the molecular mechanisms involved in tumor cell invasion and metastasis has hindered the development of effective antimetastatic therapies; however, recent discoveries in this field are leading to novel therapeutic strategies.

The transition from in situ tumor growth to metastatic disease is defined by the ability of the tumor cells at the primary site to invade local tissues and to cross tissue barriers. To initiate the metastatic process, carcinoma cells first penetrate the epithelial basement membrane and then invade the interstitial stroma. This loss of epithelial basement membranes is a hallmark of invasion. Further basement membrane barriers are traversed by tumor cells when they enter or leave blood vessels as well as when they invade nerves and muscles. Once in the circulation, tumor cells must survive host immunologic assaults, arrest at a distant vascular bed, and subsequently extravasate. Ultimately, the cells must invade and proliferate in the tissue of the secondary site. Growth of the metastatic colony beyond 1 cu cm requires vascularization of the solid tumor.[1-3] Tumor-induced angiogenesis not only allows for expansion of the primary tumor, but also permits easy access to vascular compartment as a result of defects in the basement membranes of newly formed vessels.[4,5] Thus, angiogenesis may facilitate hematogenous spread of some tumors.

Metastasis is therefore a multistep process involving numerous tumor cell–host cell and cell–matrix associations[6-10] (Fig. 11–1). Interactions with the matrix, especially basement membranes, that characterize the process of invasion include attachment, proteolysis of matrix components, and migration through the matrix defect.[11] None of these functions is unique to tumor cell behavior. Attachment, proteolysis, and migration are steps of trophoblast implantation, mammary gland involution, embryonic morphogenesis, and tissue remodeling.[12,13] The difference between normal physiologic processes and the pathogenic process of tumor cell invasion therefore must be one of regulation. Thus, greater understanding of cellular adhesion, matrix proteolysis, and cell migration should provide new targets for therapeutic disruption of metastasis formation.

TUMOR CELL ADHESION

The capacity of tumor cells to adhere to other tumor cells, host cells, or components of the extracellular matrix could affect multiple components of the metastatic cascade. Several families of cell surface adhesion molecules have been identified, each with different functions and specificities (for review, see refs. 14,15). These include cadherins, the immunoglobulin superfamily, selectins, and integrins. Cadherins are calcium-dependent molecules that mediate homophilic (like-to-like) cell-cell adherence (for review, see refs. 16–18). Three subtypes (E-, N-, and P-cadherins) have been well characterized, distinguished primarily by tissue distribution. The immunoglobulin superfamily consists of divalent cation-independent receptors that have several repeats of immunoglobulin-like

233

folds characterized by β-pleated sheets held together by disulfide bonds (for review, see ref. 19). These molecules, which include neural cell adhesion molecule (NCAM), intercellular adhesion molecules (ICAM-1 and ICAM-2), vascular cell adhesion molecule (VCAM)-1, carcinoembryonic antigen (CEA), and "deleted in colorectal cancer" (DCC), mediate both homotypic and heterotypic (unlike) cell-cell adherence. Selectins, or LEC-CAMs, act through a terminal calcium-dependent lectin domain and are most prominently involved in heterotypic cell-cell adhesions between blood cells and endothelial cells. Integrins are a large class of αβ heterodimeric receptors that mediate primarily cellular adherence to the extracellular matrix (for review, see refs. 14,20). At least 14 α and 8 β subunits have been identified, which noncovalently associate to produce at least 20 different integrins. There is redundancy at the level of both receptor and ligand: Individual receptors can bind to more than one type of adhesion molecule, and ligands can be recognized by more than one integrin. Other adhesion receptors, not specifically characterized as members of these large superfamilies, also have been identified. These include the 65-kDa laminin receptor[21] and CD44, a homologue of cartilage link protein[22,23] that functions as a lymphocyte homing molecule and a cell surface receptor for hyaluronate.[24,25]

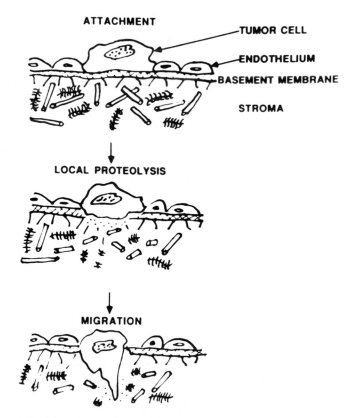

Figure 11–1. Three-step hypothesis of invasion. As depicted for a tumor cell exiting a capillary, the first step is attachment of the tumor cell to the subendothelial basement membrane. This is followed by secretion and activation of proteinases, including matrix metalloproteinases, which cleave extracellular matrix components. Proteolytic modification of the matrix barriers is followed by pseudopodial protrusion and locomotion. (From Stracke ML, Liotta LA: Multi-step cascade of tumor cell metastasis. In Vivo 6:309, 1992, with permission.)

In addition to their role as cell surface adhesion receptors, these molecules may activate and regulate various cellular functions. For example, integrins, cadherins, and CD44 may form structural links between the cell surface and components of the cytoskeleton.[17,20,26] Certain members of the immunoglobulin superfamily can anchor to the cell surface by covalent linkage to the membrane phospholipid phosphophatidylinositol, which can be hydrolyzed when the receptor is activated.[27] CD44 is a GTP-binding protein with intrinsic GTPase activity.[26] As a group, these molecules play major roles in determining such cellular characteristics as cell morphology, locomotor capacity, and state of differentiation (for review see refs. 14,17,19,28). It is therefore not surprising that the presence or absence of several of these adhesion molecules on the surface of tumor cells has been demonstrated to correlate with metastatic potential.

Tumor Adherence to the Extracellular Matrix

Tumor cells can attach to specific glycoproteins of the extracellular matrix, such as fibronectin, collagen, and laminin, through either integrin[29,30] or nonintegrin[31,32] cell surface receptors. Many studies have implicated this capacity of tumor cells to bind to the extracellular matrix as a crucial component of the metastatic process.[29,33–35] Evidence now suggests that tumor cells have altered adhesive properties involving changes in these matrix adhesion receptors.

A number of recent studies have examined the role of tumor cell attachment to fibronectin via the β_1 subclass of integrin receptors. The density of these integrins appears to be altered in transformed cells,[36] although no consistent pattern of change among different cell types has been defined.[36–39] However, on transformation some integrins become distributed in a more diffuse pattern on the cell membrane rather than being localized to sites of focal adhesion.[40,41] Transfection of Chinese hamster ovary cells with the cDNAs for the $\alpha_5\beta_1$ fibronectin receptor inhibits their ability to grow in soft agar, to establish tumors in nude mice, and to migrate.[42] In contrast, clonal sublines of erythroleukemia cells[43] or Chinese hamster ovary cells[44] expressing decreased levels of fibronectin receptor are characterized by increased tumorigenicity. These results suggest that enhancing the adhesive function of integrins may directly or indirectly modulate tumorigenesis.

Integrins appear to play a role in invasion and metastasis as well as tumorigenesis. For example, anti-β_1 monoclonal antibody inhibits both human tumor cell migration and in vitro (Matrigel assay) invasiveness at concentrations as low as 1 μg/mL.[45] In human melanomas, upregulation of the expression of certain integrins, including $\alpha_2\beta_1$, $\alpha_3\beta_1$, and $\alpha_6\beta_1$, have been shown to correlate with metastatic potential[45a] or progression of disease.[45b] For several integrin receptors whose functions can be competed by synthetic Arg-Gly-Asp (RGD) peptides, the addition of these peptides has been found to inhibit both in vitro and in vivo melanoma cell invasion.[29,34,35,46,47] However, these assays require a relatively high concentration of peptides (from 0.1 to 1 mg/mL for in vitro assays, 0.2 to 3 mg/injection with in vivo models) in order to achieve these effects.

Evidence also has been presented that expression of the vitronectin receptor ($\alpha_v\beta_3$ integrin) is elevated in malignant melanoma cells.[38,39] Most recently, experiments with the human melanoma cell line A375M have revealed that the enhanced ability of these cells to invade basement membranes results from increased expression of the matrix-degrading enzyme, 72-kDa type IV collagenase.[48] These data would indicate that signal transduction through the vitronectin receptor may modulate proteolytic enzyme production to enhance the invasive phenotype.

Cell surface receptors for laminin may play a role in adhesion of tumor cells to the basement membrane prior to invasion.[21,49] In the function of normal cell types, laminin is known to play a role in cell attachment, cell spreading, mitogenesis, neurite outgrowth, morphogenesis, and cell movement. Many types of neoplastic cells contain cell surface binding sites with affinity constants in the nanomolar range.[21] The isolated receptor is a 65-kDa protein[21] that binds to the "B" chain (short arm) region of the laminin molecule.[50] Laminin receptors may be altered in number or degree of occupancy in human carcinomas. This may be the indirect result of defective basement membrane organization in the carcinomas. Breast carcinoma and colon carcinoma tissue contains a higher number of unoccupied receptors compared with tissue of benign lesions. The laminin receptors of normal epithelium may be polarized at the basal surface and occupied with laminin in the basement membrane. In contrast, the laminin receptors on invading carcinoma cells are amplified and may be dispersed over the entire surface of the cell. The laminin receptor can be shown experimentally to play a role in hematogenous metastasis.[33] Treating tumor cells with the receptor-binding fragment of laminin at very low concentrations markedly inhibits or abolishes lung metastases from injected tumor cells.

CD44 has been shown to be elevated in highly metastatic human melanoma cell lines compared to poorly metastatic lines.[51] In rat pancreatic carcinoma cell lines, metastatic potential was found to correlate to the presence of a splice variant of *CD44* that has an expanded extracellular domain.[52,53] Transfection of the cDNA of this variant *CD44* gene into a nonmetastatic cell line conferred the metastatic phenotype. Recently, several human carcinoma cell lines have been shown to produce a homologous splice variant.[54] In addition, a cell surface chondroitin sulfate with a 110-kDa core protein immunologically related to CD44 was found to be important in murine melanoma motility and in vitro invasion in response to type I collagen.[55] Increased expression of CD44 thus appears to be important in a variety of tumor cell–matrix interactions.

Cell-Cell Adherence Molecules

Recent studies have indicated that cell-cell adhesion molecules may play a regulatory role in the development

of metastatic potential. For example, NCAMs exist as multiple splice variants with highly variable levels of *N*-glycosylation.[19] Highly metastatic glioma[56] and melanoma[57] cell lines have been found to have less total NCAM on their cell surface than poorly metastatic clones. However, neuroblastomas[58] and Wilms' tumors[59] were found to have elevated concentrations of highly sialylated isoforms of NCAM compared to normal cells. DCC is a member of the immunoglobulin superfamily with sequence homology to NCAM.[60] The *DCC* gene was cloned from the 18q chromosome region, which was found to have allelic deletions in more than 70 per cent of colorectal carcinomas. Mutations in this region appear to be an early event in the process of malignant transformation.[61] In contrast, the presence of MUC18, homologous to both NCAM and CEA, on the surface of melanoma cells has been found to correlate closely with the development of metastatic potential,[62] and ICAM-1 on melanoma cells has been shown to be an indicator of poor prognosis.[63] Thus, the immunoglobulin superfamily of adhesion molecules has a complex relationship to metastatic potential: Tumor cells can have down-regulation of these molecules on their cell surface, shifts in the level of glycosylation, or expression of new forms of adhesion molecules.[19] The result in all cases appears to be alterations in the adhesive properties of the tumor cells.

In contrast to the complex relationship between the metastatic phenotype and immunoglobulin-like adhesion molecules, cadherins appear to act as inhibitors of tumor invasion.[28] For example, in vitro assays with murine ovarian carcinoma cells,[64] epithelial Madin-Darby canine kidney (MDCK) cells,[65,66] rat Dunning prostatic cells,[67] and several human carcinoma cell lines[68,69] have demonstrated a negative correlation between E-cadherin (uvomorulin) levels and invasiveness. Cells that were treated with anti–E-cadherin monoclonal antibodies acquired in vitro invasive capability.[65] Transfection of plasmids containing the sense strand of E-cadherin mRNA into highly invasive clones resulted in overexpression of E-cadherin protein and loss of invasive capacity.[66] Partial down-regulation of E-cadherin by transfecting antisense mRNA into a noninvasive clone resulted in the acquisition of invasive behavior.[66] These data suggest that enhancing the capacity of tumor cells to bind to one another or to other host cells inhibits the ability of tumor cells to escape from their primary site to initiate invasion.

The current evidence regarding the involvement of cell-matrix and cell-cell interactions in the process of metastasis has pointed to the complexity of the malignant phenotype. Tumor cells that are more adherent either to substrata or to other cells appear to be generally less tumorigenic and less motile,[42–44] and may have reduced invasive capability.[16,65] However, studies of fibronectin, vitronectin, and laminin receptor function indicate that inhibition of tumor cell adhesion to extracellular matrix also results in less aggressive invasive behavior. Although these data seem to be somewhat contradictory, they might reflect the fact that tumor cell adherence is a regulated process with the capacity to change during different phases of the metastatic cascade.

PROTEOLYSIS OF THE EXTRACELLULAR MATRIX DURING INVASION

Although proteolysis and migration through tissue barriers are normal cell functions in specific physiologic circumstances, it is clear that a general aspect of malignant neoplasms includes a shift toward sustained invasive capacity. For invasion to take place, cyclic attachment to matrix components and subsequent release of proteolytic enzymes must occur in a directed and controlled manner. This implies that proteolysis, although enhanced in tumor cells, is still tightly regulated in a temporal and spatial fashion with respect to cell attachment. Proteolytic activity is the balance between the local concentration of activated enzymes and their endogenous inhibitors.

Positive correlation between tumor aggressiveness and protease levels has been documented for all four classes of proteases, including serine,[70–72] aspartyl,[73] cysteinyl,[74,75] and metal atom dependent.[76–79] In addition to proteolytic activity, augmented heparanase activity has been associated with malignancy.[80,81] Because inhibitors for the cysteinyl proteases, metalloproteinases, and serine proteases are all capable of blocking tumor cell invasion of native or reconstituted connective tissue barriers,[82–84] multiple enzymes appear to be involved in the metastatic process.

Matrix Metalloproteinases in Cancer

Significant evidence has accumulated to implicate directly members of the gene family of matrix metalloproteinases[85] in tumor invasion and metastasis formation. These enzymes, each of which is secreted as a proenzyme that requires activation, are divided into three general subclasses: interstitial collagenase, type IV collagenases (gelatinases), and stromelysins. Interstitial collagenase degrades type I collagen, as well as the fibrillar collagens II, III, and X.[86] The closely related enzyme neutrophil collagenase appears to have a similar substrate specificity.[87]

The stromelysins include two very similar enzymes, stromelysin-1 and stromelysin-2; matrilysin, which is a smaller truncated protein also referred to as PUMP-1[86]; and, most recently, stromelysin 3.[88] The stromelysins degrade proteoglycan core protein, laminin, fibronectin, gelatin, and the nonhelical portions of basement membrane collagens. The role of stromelysins in tumor progression has been reviewed recently.[89] Data on the most recently described member of the stromelysin gene family, stromelysin 3, suggest that its expression is associated with human breast cancer progression,[88] although its substrate specificity has yet to be defined. Matrilysin, but not stromelysin 1 or stromelysin 2, is prominent in human gastric and colonic carcinomas.[90] In epidermoid carcinomas of the head and neck, stromelysin-2 as well as interstitial collagenase mRNAs were detected in invasive cancer cells and associated stromal cells, whereas adjacent normal tissues were negative.[91] Furthermore, stromelysin-2 mRNA was localized in tumor cells arranged along disrupted basement membranes. These studies suggest that there may be organ or cell-type specificity associated with the up-regulation of proteolytic activity during malignant conversion.

Type IV Collagenases

The third group of enzymes of the matrix metalloproteinase gene family are the type IV collagenases. The 72- and 92-kDa enzymes are named for their ability to degrade pepsinized, triple-helical type IV collagens,[76,77,92] but it is important to note that the physiologic substrates of these enzymes have not been established. In addition to degrading the helical portion of type IV collagen, they also possess potent gelatinolytic activity, and can degrade collagen types V, VII, IX, and X, fibronectin, and elastin. The two enzymes arise from separate mRNA transcripts,[93,94] and are distinct from other members of the matrix metalloproteinases in that they possess a unique region immediately adjacent to the putative metal-binding domain that is homologous to the gelatin-binding domain of fibronectin. This sequence possibly provides an explanation for the enzyme affinity for denatured collagen. The 72- and 92-kDa type IV collagenases also differ from other members of the class by their ability to interact, as latent proenzymes, with the endogenous inhibitors of these enzymes, tissue inhibitors of metalloproteinases (TIMPs).[95–97] Both TIMP-1 and TIMP-2 have been isolated, cloned, and sequenced.[95–102] The 72-kDa proenzyme forms a complex with TIMP-2, and the 92-kDa proenzyme binds with TIMP-1.[94,96] TIMPs are not known to bind other latent matrix metalloproteinases, but will inhibit all matrix metalloproteinases once these enzymes are activated. TIMP-2 may preferentially inhibit the 72-kDa over the 92-kDa type IV collagenase.[103]

Correlative evidence for the involvement of type IV collagenase in the invasive phenotype is abundant.[77,80,104,105] Induction of the malignant phenotype using the *ras* oncogene has been shown to enhance expression of type IV collagenolytic activity.[106–109] In situ hybridization of human skin cancers detected message for 72- and 92-kDa type IV collagenase in most cases of infiltrating basal and squamous cell carcinomas, whereas the enzyme was absent from normal skin.[110] Most invasive colonic and gastric adenocarcinomas or the desmoplastic stroma are immunoreactive for 72-kDa type IV collagenase, whereas benign proliferative disorders of the breast and colon, and normal colorectal and gastric mucosa, show decreased or negative staining for this enzyme.[111–114] Similarly, recent immunohistochemical studies of serous tumors of the ovary were unable to detect 72-kDa type IV collagenase in benign cysts, yet invasive growths were positive.[115] Immunolocalization of the 72-kDa enzyme also has been found to correlate with tumor grade in neoplastic thyroid.[116] However, enzyme also was detected in benign disorders in which the tissue was undergoing remodeling and repair, such as in inflammation, fibrosis, and distortion of normal follicles. In contrast, normal thyroid, goiter, and Graves' disease tissue showed little or no immunoreactivity.[116]

In addition to correlative studies, recent direct evidence

has been provided establishing a causative role for these proteolytic activities in invasion. This has been accomplished primarily through the use of specific enzyme inhibitors. These studies have pointed to the potential role of endogenous enzyme inhibitors as tumor metastasis suppressors. TIMP-1, the first member of the TIMP family to be identified,[98] is a glycoprotein with an apparent molecular mass of 28.5 kDa. TIMP-1 forms a complex of 1:1 stoichiometry with activated interstitial collagenase, activated stromelysin, and the 92-kDa type IV collagenase. Native or recombinant TIMP-1 has been shown to inhibit in vitro invasion of human amniotic membranes[83,117] and in vivo metastasis in animal models.[117,118] Furthermore, transfection of antisense TIMP-1 RNA into mouse 3T3 cells, which down-regulates TIMP-1 expression, enhances their ability to invade human amnionic membranes and to form metastatic tumors in athymic mice.[117–119]

Similarly, TIMP-2 has been examined for its ability to inhibit tumor cell invasion. TIMP-2 is a 21-kDa nonglycosylated protein that shows 37 per cent identity and 65.6 per cent overall homology to TIMP-1, yet the proteins are immunologically distinct. TIMP-2 has been shown to successfully inhibit in vitro tumor cell invasion of extracellular matrices.[120,121] Antibodies to the 72-kDa type IV collagenase achieved a similar effect in experiments with HT-1080 fibrosarcoma cells.[121] This latter finding is important in specifying the proteolytic activity responsible for invasive behavior in this cell system, considering that TIMPs are capable of inhibiting multiple members of the metalloproteinase family and that the fibrosarcoma cells produce several species of matrix metalloproteinases. Most recently, overexpression of TIMP-2 in invasive and metastatic ras-transformed rat embryo fibroblasts suppressed the formation of lung metastases following intravenous injection in nude mice.[122] Moreover, the increased TIMP-2 levels significantly reduced the in vivo growth rate and invasive character of tumors following subcutaneous injection of these transfected cells.

Recent studies also have suggested that TIMPs are capable of inhibiting angiogenesis, which has many functional aspects similar to the process of tumor cell invasion. Mignatti et al. reported that TIMP-1 inhibited in vitro endothelial cell invasion of human amniotic membranes.[123] Moses et al. presented data that cartilage-derived inhibitor (CDI), a TIMP-related protein isolated from bovine articular cartilage, can block angiogenesis and also inhibits endothelial cell proliferation.[124,125] Additionally, both TIMP-1 and TIMP-2 have been shown to inhibit angiogenesis in the chick yolk sac.[126] Collectively, these data support a role for collagenolytic activity in at least two functional processes contributing to metastasis. That is, collagenases are involved in tumor cell invasion as well as neovascularization, on which solid tumor growth is dependent. These are important considerations in the design of proteolytic inhibitors for potential use as therapeutic agents.

Regulation of Type IV Collagenases

A greater understanding of the mechanisms of type IV collagenase inhibition by TIMPs is needed to estimate the potential for therapeutic use of these compounds. Currently, the significance of latent proenzyme-inhibitor complexes is not fully appreciated. Furthermore, little is known about the in vivo conversion of latent type IV procollagenases to their active forms. Histochemical and in situ hybridization studies have indicated that either tumor or stromal cells may contribute to tissue degradation during the transition from in situ to invasive carcinoma.[91,110,114] Regulation of type IV collagenolytic activities therefore may occur at many levels. Gaining insight into the transcriptional/translational regulation of type IV collagenase production, as well as its activation, may assist our understanding of the tissue localization of active proteases involved in the metastatic process.

Analysis of the transcriptional regulation of type IV collagenase expression has revealed that the 72-kDa type IV collagenase is regulated in a fundamentally unique manner when compared with other members of the collagenase family.[127] For example, exposure of cultured cells to phorbol ester has been shown to induce or enhance the expression of interstitial collagenase,[127,128] stromelysin-1,[129] and the 92-kDa type IV collagenase.[94] This regulation is mediated, at least in part, at the transcriptional level, and is consistent with the presence of a phorbol ester–responsive element (AP-1 site) in the promoter region of the interstitial collagenase[130] and stromelysin genes.[131] In contrast, no such element has been detected in the promoter region of the 72-kDa type IV collagenase gene,[132] and the expression of this enzyme is not induced or enhanced as a result of phorbol ester treatment of cells.[127] Similarly, treatment of cells with transforming growth factor (TGF)-β_1 decreases the expression of both interstitial collagenase[127,133] and stromelysin-1.[131] Again this effect appears to be mediated at the transcriptional level, as suggested by the discovery of a TGF-β_1 inhibitory element (TIE) in the promoter region of the stromelysin-1 gene.[134] A TIE consensus sequence also is present in the interstitial collagenase gene, as well as other genes that are negatively regulated by TGF-β_1.[134] Such an element is not found in the sequenced regions of the 72-kDa type IV collagenase upstream element,[132] and the expression of the 72-kDa type IV collagenase either unaffected or moderately up-regulated by TGF-β_1 treatment of human cell lines.[127,135]

Type IV collagenases, like other members of the collagenase family, are secreted by cells in culture as latent proenzymes. Unlike other members of the family, the 72-kDa and the 92-kDa type IV collagenases are complexed with TIMP-2 and TIMP-1, respectively.[94,95] The activation of these collagenases therefore constitutes an important level of regulation. Recently, in vitro studies of the mechanism of activation of these enzymes has yielded new insights into the molecular basis of proenzyme latency.[136–138] The collagenase proenzymes can be activated in vitro by a variety of agents, including organomercurials, chaotropic agents, and other proteases. Amino-terminal sequence analysis of the 72-kDa type IV collagenase following organomercurial treatment revealed the loss of an 80-residue amino-terminal domain.[139] Within this domain is a cysteine-containing sequence, PRCGXPDV, that is highly conserved among family members. Additionally, sequence comparison with other collagenases reveals that all proenzymes contain an odd number of cysteine residues.[93,94,136,137,139,140] The latency of the metalloproteinase now appears to be maintained by a specific metal atom–sulfhydryl side chain interaction.[136–138]

Recent studies have used synthetic peptides containing this highly conserved sequence from the matrix metalloproteinase enzyme profragment. These peptides have demonstrated protease inhibitory activity when present at less than 100-mM concentrations.[138] Control peptides in which the putative critical cysteinyl residue was replaced with serinyl residue did not show enzyme inhibitory activity. The same peptides were tested for their ability to block in vitro tumor cell invasion. The cysteinyl-containing peptide, at a concentration of 30 mmol/liter, was shown to inhibit by up to 80 per cent the invasion of reconstituted extracellular matrix by either human fibrosarcoma or melanoma cells, whereas the control peptide was not inhibitory.[141]

To date, the insights gained into the mechanism of activation by these agents in vitro has not led to an understanding of the cellular activation of the 72-kDa type IV collagenase in vivo. Proteases, specifically plasmin, have been shown to be responsible for the activation of both interstitial procollagenase and prostromelysin-1 in co-cultures of keratinocytes and dermal fibroblasts.[142] Furthermore, stromelysin-1 has been shown to activate interstitial collagenase and the 92-kDa gelatinase, suggesting a proteolytic cascade in the regulation of the activity of these enzymes.[143,144] However, plasmin and a variety of other proteases tested do not activate the 72-kDa type IV collagenase. More recently, treatment of HT-1080 fibrosarcoma cells with phorbol ester or treatment of fibroblasts with concanavalin A has been shown to induce processing of the 72-kDa IV collagenase to a 62-kDa activated form.[127,145] Analysis of the conditioned media from concanavalin A–treated gingival fibroblasts reveals a marked increase in type IV collagenase activity in the absence of organomercurial treatment.[145] The activation locus and amino-terminal sequence of the final cellular-activated species are identical to those of the organomercurially activated form. Treatment with phorbol ester or concanavalin A therefore induces cellular activation of 72-kDa type IV procollagenase.

The existence of a plasmin-independent cell surface mechanism for the specific activation of a single collagenase family enzyme has important physiologic implications. Such a mechanism would give a cell tight control over the degradation of matrix in its immediate vicinity. With respect to tumor invasion and metastasis, it might allow a cell that expresses the "activator," but not 72-kDa type IV collagenase, to activate and utilize exogenous type IV procollagenase in tissues such as brain and bone.[146,147] The identification of the molecular species responsible for the cellular activation of the 72-kDa type IV procollagenase, and other procollagenases, is likely to yield an important new series of target molecules in the development of treatments for invasive and degradative diseases.

Another critical level of regulation of type IV collagenase activity is the inhibition of active enzyme by the TIMP family of proteins. Although the purpose and fate of the TIMP molecules in the latent type IV collagenase complex is unclear, it is known that, once activated, both type IV collagenases are susceptible to inhibition by either TIMP-1 or TIMP-2.[93,94,127] TIMP-1 is secreted primarily in uncomplexed form, frequently by cells that secrete interstitial collagenase.[135] In contrast, TIMP-2 is secreted primarily as a complex with the latent 72-kDa type IV collagenase (Brown PD, Stetler-Stevenson WG, unpublished results).

ROLE OF TUMOR CELL MOTILITY IN METASTASIS

Active tumor cell motility, coupled with proteolysis, is required for the penetration of basement membranes and interstitial stroma during the transition from in situ to invasive carcinoma. Tumor cells also exhibit directional motility during intravasation and extravasation. The importance of tumor cell motility to invasion and metastasis has been appreciated for more than 40 years.[148,149] A pioneering study by Wood in 1958[150] used microcinematography to directly observe tumor cell movement in an in vivo system: V2 rabbit carcinoma cells were injected into the rabbit ear vasculature, and migration of the tumor cells out of the vasculature was detected. Later studies have focused on the relationship between the degree of tumor cell motility and metastatic potential[151–154] as well as on the loss of epithelial differentiation during tumor invasion.[154a] When parameters of motility such as pseudopod extension, chemotaxis, membrane ruffling, and vectorial translation were measured, the more highly invasive tumor cell lines exhibited a greater degree of motility than their less invasive counterparts.

Many agents have now been demonstrated to stimulate in vitro motility responses by tumor cells. These include both autocrine, or tumor-secreted, factors and paracrine, or host-derived, factors. The motility response stimulated by these factors in solution can be either random (chemokinesis) or directed toward a concentration gradient (chemotaxis). In addition, tumor cells can migrate in a directed manner toward substratum-bound, insoluble matrix proteins in the absence of soluble attractant (haptotaxis).[155] Thus, tumor cells are capable of responding to a variety of motility-promoting factors presented under a variety of conditions. This flexibility of response allows tumor cells to adapt to different microenvironments during the various stages of metastasis.

Autocrine Motility Factors

In early studies, Hayashi and colleagues described a 70-kDa chemotactic factor that was derived from extracts of solid rat hepatomas and was chemotactic for several tumor cell lines, including the cells of origin.[156] Later, it was observed that cultured human melanoma cells (the A2058 cell line) secreted an approximately 60-kDa attractant protein into serum-free media.[157] This factor stimulated both chemokinetic and chemotactic motility responses and appeared to have some degree of specificity for tumor cells, stimulating a wide variety of tumor cells[158] but failing to stimulate leukocytes.[157] Like autocrine growth factors that had been described earlier for tumor cells,[159,160] secretion of an autocrine motility factor (AMF) gave the tumor cells greater independence from their surroundings and allowed the cells to bypass the normal regulatory mechanisms that control physiologic processes of locomotion. Several tumor cell–derived motility-inducing cytokines have now been reported. These include a 53-kDa factor from rat mammary adenocarcinoma,[161] a 64-kDa protein from murine melanoma,[162] a greater than 10-kDa protein from rat and human malignant glioma cells,[163] a less than 30-kDa factor from rat prostatic adenocarcinoma cells,[164] and a 150- to 200-kDa protein from ras-transfected NIH 3T3 cells.[165] In addition, growth factors[166,166a] or glycosaminoglycans[167] may act as autocrine motility factors for certain tumor cells.

Recently, a potent new motility stimulant with higher molecular mass (120 kDa) was isolated from A2058 cell–conditioned medium and purified to homogeneity.[168] This new cytokine, termed autotaxin (ATX), is a basic glycoprotein with pI of approximately 7.7. ATX is active in the high picomolar range, stimulating both chemotactic and chemokinetic responses in A2058 cells. When cells are pretreated with pertussis toxin, this motile response is abolished. ATX thus is likely to stimulate the cell via a G protein–linked cell surface receptor. Sequence information, obtained on 19 purified tryptic peptides, confirmed that the protein is unique, with no significant homology to growth factors or previously described motility factors. ATX therefore appears to represent a new member of the AMF family.

Role of Extracellular Matrix Components in Tumor Cell Motility

Components of the extracellular matrix (ECM) are ubiquitous molecules that tumor cells encounter repeatedly during the process of metastasis, particularly in basement membranes and in tissue stroma. Several ECM glycoproteins have been found to stimulate locomotion in tumor cells. These include vitronectin,[169] fibronectin,[32,170–174] laminin,[32,50,170,175–178] type I collagen,[55,179,180] type IV collagen,[32,181] and thrombospondin.[182] Several fragments of these multidomain proteins have been shown to inhibit the formation of metastases when experimentally co-injected with tumor cells into mice.[29,183,184] A few of these ECM proteins have been demonstrated to induce a motility response in tumor cells through integrin receptors.[178,185] Others may act through cell surface proteoglycans.[55] However, for many ECM components, the motility receptors have not yet been defined.

The use of ECM proteins as attractants in motility assays has illustrated fundamental differences at the level of postreceptor signal transduction events between soluble and insoluble presentation of attractant. A2058 melanoma cells can respond chemotactically or haptotactically to laminin, fibronectin, type IV collagen,[32] and thrombospondin.[182] When cells were pretreated with pertussis toxin, the chemotactic response to laminin was diminished and the response to type IV collagen was abolished.[32] In contrast, haptotaxis to these same proteins was completely insensitive to pertussis toxin. Work done with thrombospondin[182] has provided a clue to the mechanism by which these multidomain proteins might stimulate different types of motility responses. The heparin-binding amino terminus of thrombospondin stimulated chemotaxis and was inhibited by the sulfatides heparin and fucoidan, as well as by a specific monoclonal antibody (A2.5). The carboxyl-terminus of thrombospondin stimulated haptotaxis and was inhibited by the synthetic peptide RGD, as well as by a different specific monoclonal antibody (C6.7). Taken together, these results suggested that soluble versus insoluble presentation of these ECM proteins might stimulate motility through different receptors that activate different signal transduction pathways. In contrast, for fibronectin, neither soluble nor insoluble presentation of attractant is sensitive to pertussis toxin. However, both types of motile responses are partially and specifically inhibited by RGD peptides. This suggests that, in A2058 melanoma cells, fibronectin may stimulate chemotactic and haptotactic responses at least partially through an integrin receptor.

Role of Growth Factors in Tumor Cell Motility

Formation of a successful metastatic nidus requires that the tumor cell find a microenvironment capable of supporting cell growth. Certain highly metastatic cell lines have been shown to produce their own necessary autocrine growth factors.[159,160,166,186–189] However, host-secreted growth supporting factors still may be advantageous to establishing colonies of metastatic cells. Several growth factors have now been demonstrated to stimulate chemotactic motility in tumor cells. These growth factors appear to be somewhat specific for cellular origin (Table 11–1). Many of these cytokines also appear to act as mitogens

TABLE 11–1. GROWTH FACTORS THAT AFFECT TUMOR CELL MOTILITY

FACTOR*	TUMOR CELL TYPES
Bombesin	Small-cell lung carcinoma[249]
acidic FGF	Bladder carcinoma[192]
basic FGF	Prostatic carcinoma,[193] teratocarcinoma[194]
HGF/SF	Carcinomas[250,251,251a]
Histamine	Melanoma/carcinoma[191]
IGF-I	Melanoma[195]
IGF-II	Rhabdomyosarcoma[166]
IL-6	Ductal breast carcinoma[252]
IL-8	Melanoma[253]
NGF	Embryonal carcinoma[254]
PDGF	Teratocarcinoma[190]
TGF-β₁	Adenocarcinoma of lung[180]

*Abbreviations: HGF/SF, hepatocyte growth factor/scatter factor; IL, interleukin, NGF, nerve growth factor; PDGF, platelet-derived growth factor; others as in the text.

for the same tumor cells that they stimulate to migrate.[166,190–194]

The insulin-like growth factors (IGFs) and insulin stimulate a pertussis toxin–insensitive chemotactic response in A2058 cells.[195] This response is strongest to IGF-I and appears to activate the cells through a type I IGF receptor, because a monoclonal antibody specific for the type I IGF receptor inhibited both ^{125}I-labeled IGF-I binding and IGF-I–induced motility in A2058 cells.[196] It might be noted that both insulin and IGF-I have been implicated as necessary growth factors for culture of primary human melanoma cells.[187] In similar experiments, IGF-II has been found to stimulate motility through a type II IGF/mannose-6-phosphate receptor in human rhabdomyosarcoma cells.[197] However, IGF-II stimulates mitogenesis in these same cells through a type I IGF receptor. Thus, these growth factors, acting through ''normal'' receptor mechanisms, may serve as homing factors for tumor cells that have reached the vasculature, directing the tumor cells to extravasate into a secondary site that provides a suitable microenvironment for growth.

Molecular Mechanisms of Tumor Cell Motility

The detailed molecular mechanisms by which motility stimuli cause a cell to migrate are incompletely understood. Morphologic studies have shown that tumor cells, like leukocytes, exhibit ameboid movement that is characterized by pseudopod extension.[151,154] It is generally agreed that the machinery for cell locomotion in eukaryotic cells resides in the peripheral cytoplasm, or cell cortex, which consists of a network of polymerized, cross-linked actin filaments.[198–200] For pseudopod protrusion and cell locomotion to occur, this network must be reversibly disassembled, then reassembled to stabilize the resulting extension. The precise manner in which this is accomplished, as well as its linkage to a localized, receptor-mediated chemotactic stimulus, is still not fully understood. Studies with neutrophils and with the lower eukaryote *Dictyostelium discoideum* have provided some insights that may be applicable to tumor cells. Models proposed by Condeelis et al.[200] and Stossel[198] both envision the localized polymerization and cross-linking of actin filaments at the site of a chemotactic stimulus, resulting in the directional protrusion of a pseudopod. Both models speculate that the signals generated by activated chemotactic receptors, and the resulting second messengers, regulate proteins that sever, cap, and cross-link actin filaments to generate pseudopods. The model based on studies with leukocytes links actin disassembly and reassembly with the activation of the phosphatidylinositol cycle,[201] which is mediated through a pertussis toxin–sensitive G protein.[202,203] In tumor cells, several lines of evidence also implicate the involvement of pertussis toxin–sensitive G proteins in motility and invasion.[32,168,195,204–206] However, migration of the A2058 human melanoma cell line is insensitive to pertussis toxin treatment when IGF-I[196] or fibronectin[32] is presented as a soluble attractant, and in haptotactic migration to laminin, fibronectin, and type IV collagen.[32] Thus, tumor cells appear to be capable of responding in a variety of ways to a diverse array of motility stimuli (Fig. 11–2).

REGULATION OF METASTASIS VERSUS TUMORIGENICITY

The process of metastasis is now believed to begin early in the growth of the primary tumor.[6–8] Although tumorigenesis is necessary for formation of a metastatic nidus, uncontrolled cellular proliferation alone will not produce a metastatic phenotype. The metastatic phenotype appears to require additional genetic and epigenetic changes, involving both the addition of positive modulators (oncogenes) and the loss of negative effectors (tumor growth suppressors; invasion and metastasis suppressors) in a multistep process of diversification and clonal selection (for review, see refs. 9,207).

Role of Oncogenes in Metastasis

Certain oncogenes, when transfected into appropriate recipient cells, result in a positive modulation or gain of function that can include the complete metastatic phenotype.[208] Although the search for specific metastasis-inducing genes continues, oncogene transfection has provided a model for activation of the effector processes that are required for tumor cells to develop a metastatic phenotype. These models also have revealed that some of the metastasis effector genes can be regulated independently from those that confer tumorigenicity.[209]

In 1985, several groups reported that activated (mutated) *ras* oncogene sequences, when transfected into mouse embryo–derived fibroblasts (NIH 3T3 cells), caused the transfected cells to produce numerous metastases.[210–212] Later studies showed that transfection of H-*ras* family oncogenes into fibroblasts and into epithelial cells of rodent and human origin also induced metastatic potential.[106,107,109,208,213–216] Several candidate effector proteins have been associated with metastasis in *ras* transfection models, including type IV collagenases,[93,107,109,210] cathepsin L,[217] and motility-associated cytokines.[157] Other oncogenes also induce a metastatic phenotype, although at lower efficiency. These include the serine-threonine kinase genes v-*mos* and v-*raf*,[208,218] tyrosine kinase genes v-*src*, v-*fes*, and v-*fms*,[208] and mutant *p53*.[219]

Although transfection of *ras* into appropriate cells can induce a metastatic phenotype, two observations indicate that there are differences in the downstream pathways for *ras* induction of tumorigenicity versus metastasis. First, certain recipient cells are capable of being transformed by *ras* without acquiring the capacity to metastasize.[106,220] Second, the adenovirus E1A gene has been demonstrated to suppress *ras* induction of metastatic potential with no inhibition of soft agar colony formation or tumorigenicity.[221] These data can be explained by assuming that invasion and metastasis require activation of a set of effector genes over and above those required for unrestrained growth. This observation provides a molecular basis for the slow, multistep development of tumorigenesis and metastatic capacity.

Suppressor Genes as Negative Regulators

Early evidence for the existence of tumor suppressor genes came from cell fusion experiments between normal and tumor cells.[105,122] In these experiments, the fused product reverted to a nontransformed phenotype, suggesting that tumor cells might fail to express certain recessive genes that down-regulate cell proliferation. Several such genes, encoding proteins that act at many levels of growth regulation, have now been identified and, in a few cases, cloned (for review, see refs. 223,224).

Analogous suppressor genes may play a role in conferring the metastatic phenotype. These suppressor genes could encode any protein that inhibits any portion of the metastatic cascade.[225] For example, protease inhibitors that affect invasive capacity of tumor cells, such as the TIMPs or plasminogen activation inhibitors (PAIs), could be considered to have suppressive properties. Similarly, E1A[221]

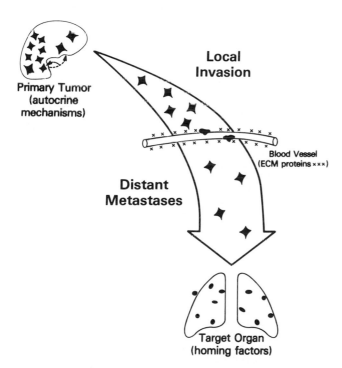

Figure 11–2. Tumor cell motility. Tumor cells are capable of responding to a variety of stimuli in a motile fashion. These different stimuli may take on greater or lesser significance during different stages of the metastatic cascade. The initial motile stimulus in or near the primary tumor may be an autocrine factor such as autotaxin. As the tumor cell moves into the stroma and invades local blood vessels and lymphatics, extracellular matrix (ECM) proteins, either insoluble within the matrix or in solution, may play a part in directing this motility. Once inside the vascular tree, the homing of the tumor cell to an appropriate metastatic site may depend on cytokines such as IGF-I that stimulate growth as well as a chemotactic response. (From Stracke ML, Liotta LA: Multi-step cascade of tumor cell metastasis. In Vivo 6:309, 1992, with permission.)

and the major histocompatibility complex H-2k^b gene[226,227] both inhibit metastasis formation in *ras*-transfected cells. The cell-cell adhesion molecule E-cadherin likewise appears to suppress the metastatic phenotype.[28,66] Other candidate suppressor genes have been identified by looking for differences in mRNA levels between metastatic and nonmetastatic cells. These include *nm23*,[228] *WDNM1*,[229] and *WDNM2*.[230]

Dear et al. used the technique of subtractive hybridization to select differentially expressed transcripts from nonmetastatic rat mammary adenocarcinoma cells, isolating the *WDNM1*[229] and *WDNM2*[230] genes. WDNM2 was later found to be completely homologous to DNA for rat NAD(P)H:menadione oxidoreductase, a flavoprotein that catalyzes the reduction of quinones.[231] WDNM1 has been found to be a member of the four-disulphide core family of proteins that include a number of protease inhibitors.[232] This tumor suppressor thus may function in a manner homologous to the TIMPs and PAI.

The *nm23* gene originally was identified on the basis of its reduced mRNA levels in five sublines of murine K1735 melanoma cells with high metastatic potential compared to two related lines with low metastatic potential using techniques of differential colony hybridization[228] (for review, see ref. 10). Transfection of murine melanoma cells with murine *nm23*-1 cDNA resulted in a reduced incidence of primary tumor formation and a significant reduction of metastatic potential.[233] The mRNA and protein levels of *nm23* have now been examined in a prospective series of human infiltrating ductal breast carcinomas. Reduced *nm23* expression was found to be associated with lymph node metastasis in two of the three reports,[234–236] as well as with disease recurrence of poor overall survival.[237–239] Additional human tumors have been found to be associated with low *nm23* expression, including hepatocellular carcinoma[240] and melanoma.[241] In other tumor types, structural alterations to *nm23*, and not reduced expression, have been associated with metastatic progression.[242] In still other tumor types, no correlation has been observed.

Clues to the function of the *nm23* gene have been found from divergent sources. The *nm23* amino acid sequence proved to be homologous to the *Drosophila awd* gene, which affects postembryonic development in the presumptive wing discs.[243–245] Mutations with reduced or abnormal *awd* expression result in altered morphology, aberrant differentiation, and cellular necrosis in multiple tissues. Loss of *nm23/awd* expression in tumors thus may lead to a disordered state, favoring aberrant development or progression to the metastatic state. The biochemical mechanism of nm23 suppression has not been established. Nm23 proteins possess nucleoside diphosphate (NDP) kinase activity, which transfers a terminal phosphate among nucleoside di- and triphosphates.[246] However, K1735 TK melanoma cell lines transfected with *nm23* failed to exhibit a significant increase in NDP kinase activity, thereby dissociating this enzymatic activity from *nm23* expression levels and metastatic potential.[247] Multiple other biochemical functions for nm23 protein have been proposed (for review, see ref. 248).

CONCLUSION

A group of coordinated cellular processes is responsible for metastasis. It is now clear that the loss or inactivation of negative regulatory processes may be just as important as acquisition of positive phenotypic effectors. Some genetic changes cause an imbalance of growth regulation, leading to uncontrolled proliferation. However, unrestrained growth does not, by itself, result in invasion and metastasis. Metastatic characteristics therefore require additional genetic alterations. Thus, tumorigenicity and metastatic potential have both overlapping and separate features. Invasion and metastasis can be facilitated by proteins that stimulate tumor cell attachment to host cellular or extracellular matrix determinants, tumor cell proteolysis of host barriers such as the basement membrane, tumor cell locomotion, and tumor cell colony formation in the target organ for metastasis. Facilitory proteins may act at many intracellular or extracellular levels, but are counterbalanced by factors that can block their production, regulation, or action. A common theme has emerged: In addition to loss of growth control, an imbalanced regulation of motility and proteolysis appears to be required for invasion and metastasis.

REFERENCES

1. Folkman J: Tumor angiogenesis: Therapeutic implications. N Engl J Med 285:1182, 1971
2. Folkman J, Klagsbrun M: Angiogenic factors. Science 235:442, 1987
3. Folkman J, Watson K, Ingber D, et al: Induction of angiogenesis during the transition from hyperplasia to neoplasia. Nature 339:58, 1989
4. Liotta L, Kleinerman J, Saidel G: Quantitative relationships of intravascular tumor cells, tumor vessels and pulmonary metastases following tumor implantation. Cancer Res 34:997, 1974
5. Furcht LT: Critical factors controlling angiogenesis: Cell products, cell matrix, and growth factors. Lab Invest 55:505, 1986
6. Fidler IJ, Hart IR: Biologic diversity in metastatic neoplasms—origins and implications. Science 217:998, 1982
7. Liotta LA, Rao CN, Barsky SH: Tumor invasion and the extracellular matrix. Lab Invest 49:636, 1983
8. Schirrmacher V: Experimental approaches, theoretical concepts, and impacts for treatment strategies. Cancer Res 43:1, 1985
9. Nicolson GL: Gene expression, cellular diversification and tumor progression to the metastatic phenotype. Bioessays 13:337, 1991
10. MacDonald NJ, Steeg PS: Molecular basis of tumor metastasis. Cancer Surv 16:175, 1993
11. Liotta LA, Stetler-Stevensen WG: Metalloproteinases and cancer invasion. Semin Cancer Biol 1:99, 1990
12. Lola PK, Graham CH: Mechanisms of trophoblast invasiveness and their control: The role of proteases and protease inhibitors. Cancer Metastasis Rev 9:369, 1990
13. Alexander CM, Werb Z: Extracellular matrix degradation. In Hay ED (ed): Cell Biology of the Extracellular Matrix, 2nd ed. New York, Plenum, 1991, p 255
14. McCarthy JB, Skubitz APN, Iida J, et al: Tumor cell adhesive mechanisms and their relationship to metastasis. Semin Cancer Biol 2:155, 1991
15. Hynes RO, Lander AD: Contact and adhesive specificities in the associations, migrations, and targeting of cells and axons. Cell 68:303, 1992
16. Takeichi M: Cadherins: A molecular family important in selective cell-cell adhesion. Annu Rev Biochem 59:237, 1990
17. Takeichi M: Cadherin cell adhesion receptors as a morphogenetic regulator. Science 251:1451, 1991
18. Magee AI, Buxton RS: Transmembrane molecular assemblies regulated by the greater cadherin family. Curr Opin Cell Biol 3:854, 1991
19. Johnson JP: Cell adhesion molecules of the immunoglobulin supergene family and their role in malignant transformation and progression to metastatic disease. Cancer Metastasis Rev 10:11, 1991
20. Hynes RO: Integrins: Versality, modulation, and signaling in cell adhesion. Cell 69:11, 1992
21. Wewer UM, Liotta LA, Jaye M, et al: Altered levels of laminin receptor mRNA in various human carcinoma cells that have different abilities to bind laminin. Proc Natl Acad Sci USA 83:7137, 1986
22. Stamenkovic I, Amiot M, Pesando JM, et al: A lymphocyte molecule implicated in lymph node homing is a member of the cartilage link protein family. Cell 56:1057, 1989
23. Goldstein LA, Zhou DFH, Picker LJ, et al: A human lymphocyte homing receptor, the hermes antigen, is related to cartilage proteoglycan core and link protein. Cell 56:1063, 1989
24. Miyake K, Underhill CB, Lesley J, et al: Hyaluronate can function as a cell adhesion molecule and CD44 participates in hyaluronate recognition. J Exp Med 172:69, 1990
25. Aruffo A, Stamenkovic I, Melnick M, et al: CD44 is the principal cell surface receptor for hyaluronate. Cell 61:1303, 1990
26. Lokeshwar VB, Bourguignon LYW: The lymphoma transmembrane glycoprotein GP85 (CD44) is a novel guanine nucleotide-binding protein which regulates GP85 (CD44)-ankyrin interaction. J Biol Chem 267:22073, 1992
27. Springer TA: Adhesion receptors of the immune system. Nature 346:425, 1990
28. Birchmeier W, Behrens J, Weidner KM, et al: Dominant and recessive genes involved in tumor cell invasion. Curr Opin Cell Biol 3:832, 1991
29. Humphries MJ, Olden K, Yamada KM: A synthetic peptide from fibronectin inhibits experimental metastasis of murine melanoma cells. Science 233:467, 1986
30. Hynes RO: Integrins: A family of cell surface receptors. Cell 48:549, 1987
31. Rao C, Castronovo V, Schmitt MC, et al: Evidence for a precursor of the high-affinity metastasis associated murine laminin receptor. Biochemistry 28:7476, 1989
32. Aznavoorian S, Stracke ML, Krutzsch HC, et al: Signal transduction for chemotaxis and haptotaxis by matrix molecules in tumor cells. J Cell Biol 110:1427, 1990
33. Barsky SH, Siegal GP, Jannotta F, et al: Loss of basement membrane components by invasive tumors but not by their benign counterparts. Lab Invest 49:140, 1983
34. Humphries MJ, Yamada KM, Olden K: Investigation of the biological effects of anticell adhesion synthetic peptides that inhibit experimental metastasis of B16-F10 murine melanoma cells. J Clin Invest 81:782, 1988
35. Saiki I, Murata J, Ida J, et al: The inhibition of murine lung metastasis by synthetic polypeptides [poly (arg-gly-asp) and poly (tyr-ile-gly-ser-arg)] with a core sequence of cell adhesion molecules. Br J Cancer 59:194, 1989
36. Plantefaber LC, Hynes RO: Changes in integrin receptors on oncogenically transformed cells. Cell 56:281, 1989
37. Dedhar S, Saulnier R: Alterations in integrin receptor on chemically transformed human cells: Specific enhancement of laminin and collagen receptor complexes. J Cell Biol 110:481, 1990
38. Abelda SM, Matte SA, Elder DE, et al: Integrin distribution in malignant melanoma: Association of the β_3 subunit with tumor progress. Cancer Res 50:6757, 1990
39. Gehlsen KR, Davis GE, Sriramarao P: Integrin expression in human melanoma cells with differing invasive and metastatic properties. Clin Exp Metastasis 10:111, 1992
40. Chen WT, Wang J, Hasegawa T, et al: Regulation of fibronectin receptor distribution by transformation, exogenous fibronectin, and synthetic peptides. J Cell Biol 103:1649, 1986
41. Roman J, LaChance RM, Brockelmann TJ, et al: The fibronec-

tin receptor is organized by extracellular matrix fibronectin: Implications for oncogenic transformation and for recognition of fibronectin matrices. J Cell Biol *108*:2529, 1989

42. Giancotti FG, Ruoslahti E: Elevated levels of the $\alpha_5\beta_1$ fibronectin receptor suppress the transformed phenotype of Chinese hamster ovary cells. Cell *60*:849, 1990

43. Symington BE: Fibronectin receptor overexpression and loss of transformed phenotype in a stable variant of the K562 cell line. Cell Regul *1*:637, 1990

44. Schreiner C, Fisher M, Hussein S, et al: Increased tumorigenicity of the fibronectin receptor deficient Chinese hamster ovary cell variants. Cancer Res *51*:1738, 1991

45. Yamada KM, Kennedy DW, Yamada SS, et al: Monoclonal antibody and synthetic peptide inhibitors of human tumor cell migration. Cancer Res *50*:4485, 1990

45a. Danen EHJ, van Muijen GNP, van de Wiel-van Klemenade E, et al: Regulation of integrin-mediated adhesion to laminin and collagen in human melanocytes and in non-metastatic and highly metastatic human melanoma cells. Int J Cancer *54*:315, 1993

45b. Natcli PG, Nicotra MR, Bartolazzi A, et al: Integrin expression in cutaneous malignant melanoma: Association of the α_3/β_1 heterodimer with tumor progression. Int J Cancer *54*:68, 1993

46. Yamada KM: Adhesive recognition sequences. J Biol Chem *266*:12809, 1991

47. Gehlsen KR, Argraves WS, Pierschbacher MD, et al: Inhibition of *in vitro* cell invasion by Arg-Gly-Asp-containing peptides. J Cell Biol *106*:925, 1988

48. Seftor REB, Seftor EA, Gehlsen KR, et al: Role of the $\alpha_v\beta_3$ integrin in human melanoma cell invasion. Proc Natl Acad Sci USA *89*:1557, 1992

49. Rao CN, Margulies I, Tralka TS, et al: Isolation of a subunit of laminin and its role in molecular structure and tumor cell attachment. J Biol Chem *257*:9740, 1982

50. Wewer UM, Taraboletti G, Sobel ME, et al: Role of laminin receptor in tumor cell migration. Cancer Res *47*:5691, 1987

51. Birch M, Mitchell S, Hart IR: Isolation and characterization of human melanoma cell variants expressing high and low levels of CD44. Cancer Res *51*:6660, 1991

52. Günthert U, Hofmann M, Rudy W, et al: A new variant of glycoprotein CD44 confers metastatic potential to rat carcinoma cells. Cell *65*:13, 1991

53. Sy MS, Guo Y-J, Stamenkovic I: Distinct effects of two CD44 isoforms on tumor growth *in vivo*. J Exp Med *174*:859, 1991

54. Hofmann M, Rudy W, Zöller M, et al: CD44 splice variants confer metastatic behavior in rats: Homologous sequences are expressed in human tumor cell lines. Cancer Res *51*:5292, 1991

55. Faassen AE, Schrager JA, Klein DJ, et al: A cell surface chrondroitin sulfate proteoglycan, immunologically related to CD44, is involved in Type I collagen-mediated melanoma cell motility and invasion. J Cell Biol *116*:521, 1992

56. Andersson AM, Moran N, Gaardsvoll H, et al: Characterization of NCAM expression and function in BT4C and BT4C$_n$ glioma cells. Int J Cancer *47*:124, 1991

57. Linnemann D, Raz A, Bock E: Differential expression of cell adhesion molecules in variants of K1735 melanoma cells differing in metastatic capacity. Int J Cancer *43*:709, 1989

58. Figarella-Branger DF, Durbec PL, Rougon GN: Differential spectrum of expression of neural cell adhesion molecule isoforms and L1 adhesion molecules on human neuroectodermal tumors. Cancer Res *50*:6364, 1990

59. Roth J, Zuber C, Wagner P, et al: Reexpression of poly(sialic acid) units of neural cell adhesion molecule in Wilms' tumor. Proc Natl Acad Sci USA *85*:2999, 1988

60. Fearon ER, Cho KR, Nigro JM, et al: Identification of chromosome 18q gene that is altered in colorectal cancers. Science *247*:49, 1990

61. Fearon ER, Vogelstein B: A genetic model for colorectal tumorigenesis. Cell *61*:759, 1990

62. Holzmann B, Bröcker EB, Lehmann JM, et al: Tumor progression in human malignant melanoma: Five stages defined by their antigenic phenotypes. Int J Cancer *39*:466, 1987

63. Johnson JP, Stade BG, Holzmann B, et al: *De novo* expression

of cell adhesion molecule ICAM-1 in melanoma and increased risk of metastasis. Proc Natl Acad Sci USA *86*:641, 1989

64. Hashimoto M, Niwa O, Nitta Y, et al: Unstable expression of E-cadherin molecules in metastatic ovarian tumor cells. Jpn J Cancer Res *80*:459, 1989

65. Behrens J, Marcell MM, Van Roy FM, et al: Dissecting tumor cell invasion: Epithelial cells acquire invasive properties after the loss of uvomorulin-mediated cell-cell adhesion. J Cell Biol *108*:2435, 1989

66. Vleminckx K, Vakaet L Jr, Mareel M, et al: Genetic manipulation of E-cadherin expression by epithelial tumor cells reveals an invasion suppressor role. Cell *66*:107, 1991

67. Bussemakers MJG, van Moorsclaar RJA, Giroldi LA, et al: Decreased expression of E-cadherin in the progression of rat prostatic cancer. Cancer Res *52*:2916, 1992

68. Frixen UH, Behrens J, Sachs M, et al: E-cadherin-mediated cell-cell adhesion prevents invasiveness of human colorectal carcinoma cells. J Cell Biol *113*:173, 1991

69. Sommers CL, Thompson EW, Torri JA, et al: Cell adhesion molecule uvomorulin expression in human breast cancer cell lines: Relationship to morphology and invasive capacities. Cell Growth Differ *2*:365, 1991

70. Wang BS, McLoughlin GA, Richie JP, et al: Correlation of the production of plasminogen activator with tumor metastasis in B16 mouse melanoma cell lines. Cancer Res *40*:288, 1980

71. Reich R, Thompson E, Iwamoto Y, et al: Effects of inhibitors of plasminogen activator, serine proteinases, and collagenase IV on the invasion of basement membranes by metastatic cells. Cancer Res *48*:3307, 1988

72. Axelrod JH, Reich R, Mishkin R: Expression of human recombinant plasminogen activators enhances invasion and experimental metastasis of H-ras-transformed NIH 3T3 cells. Mol Cell Biol *9*:2133, 1989

73. Rochefort H, Capony F, Garcia M, et al: A protease involved in breast cancer metastasis. Cancer Metastasis Rev *9*:321, 1990

74. Recklies AD, Poole AR, Mort JS: A cysteine proteinase secreted from human breast tumors is immunologically related to cathepsin B. Biochem J *207*:636, 1982

75. Sloane BR, Honn KV: Cysteine proteinases and metastasis. Cancer Metastasis Rev *3*:249, 1984

76. Liotta LA, Abe S, Robey P, et al: Preferential digestion of basement membrane collagen by an enzyme derived from a metastatic murine tumor. Proc Natl Acad Sci USA *76*:2268, 1979

77. Liotta LA, Tryggvason K, Garbisa S, et al: Metastatic potential correlates with enzymatic degradation of basement membrane collagen. Nature *284*:67, 1980

78. Ostrowski LE, Rinch J, Kreig P, et al: Expression pattern of a gene for a secreted metalloproteinase during late stages of tumor progression. Mol Carcinog *1*:13, 1988

79. Templeton NT, Brown PD, Levy AT, et al: Cloning and characterization of human tumor cell interstitial collagenase. Cancer Res *50*:5431, 1990

80. Nakajima M, Welch D, Belloni PN, et al: Degradation of basement membrane type IV collagen and lung subendothelial matrix by rat mammary adenocarcinoma cell clones of differing metastatic potentials. Cancer Res *47*:4869, 1987

81. Nakajima M, Morikawa K, Fabra A, et al: Influence of organ environment on extracellular matrix degradative activity and metastasis of human colon carcinoma cells. J Natl Cancer Inst *82*:1890, 1991

82. Thorgeirsson UP, Liotta LA, Kalebic T, et al: Effect of the natural protease inhibitors and a chemoattractant on tumor invasion in vitro. J Natl Cancer Inst *69*:1049, 1982

83. Mignatti P, Robbins E, Rifkin DB: Tumor invasion through the human amniotic membrane: Requirement for a proteinase cascade. Cell *47*:487, 1986

84. Wang M, Stearns ME: Blocking of collagenase secretion by estamustine during *in vitro* tumor cell invasion. Cancer Res *48*:6262, 1988

85. Liotta LA, Steeg PS, Stetler-Stevenson WG: Cancer metastasis and angiogenesis: An imbalance of positive and negative regulation. Cell *64*:327, 1991

86. Matrisian LM: Metalloproteinases and their inhibitors in matrix remodeling. Trends Genet 6:121, 1990

87. Hasty KA, Pourmotabbed TF, Goldberg GI, et al: Human neutrophil collagenase. J Biol Chem 265:11421, 1990

88. Basset P, Bellocq JP, Wolf C, et al: A novel metalloproteinase gene specifically expressed in stromal cells of breast carcinomas. Nature 348:699, 1990

89. Matrisian L, Bowden T: Stromelysin/transin and tumor progression. Semin Cancer Biol 1:107, 1990

90. McDonnell S, Naure M, Coffey RJ Jr, et al: Expression and localization of the matrix metalloproteinase Pump-1 (MMP-7) in human gastric and colon carcinomas. Mol Carcinog 4:527, 1991

91. Polette M, Clavel C, Muller D, et al: Detection of mRNA's encoding collagenase I and stromelysin 2 in carcinomas of the head and neck by in situ hybridization. Invasion Metastasis 11:76, 1991

92. Fessler L, Duncan K, Tryggvason K: Identification of the procollagen IV cleavage products produced by a specific tumor collagenase. J Biol Chem 259:9783, 1984

93. Collier IE, Wilhelm SM, Eisen AZ, et al: H-ras oncogene-transformed human bronchial epithelial cells (TBE-1) secrete a single metalloproteinase capable of degrading basement membrane collagen. J Biol Chem 263:6579, 1988

94. Wilhelm SM, Collier IE, Marmer BL, et al: SV40-transformed human lung fibroblasts secrete a 92-kDa type IV collagenase which is identical to that secreted by normal human macrophages. J Biol Chem 264:17213, 1989

95. Stetler-Stevenson WG, Krutzsch HC, Liotta LA: Tissue inhibitor of metalloproteinase (TIMP-2): A new member of the metalloproteinase inhibitor family. J Biol Chem 264:17374, 1989

96. Goldberg GI, Marmer BL, Grant GA, et al: Human 72-kilodalton type IV collagenase forms a complex with a tissue inhibitor of metalloproteinases designated TIMP-2. Proc Natl Acad Sci USA 86:8207, 1989

97. DeClerck YA, Yean TD, Ratzkin BJ, et al: Purification and characterization of two related but distinct metalloproteinase inhibitors secreted by bovine aortic endothelial cells. J Biol Chem 264:17445, 1989

98. Murphy G, Cawston T, Reynolds J: An inhibitor of collagenase from human amniotic fluid: Purification, characterization, and action on metalloproteinases. Biochem J 195:167, 1981

99. Stricklin GP, Welgus HC: Human skin fibroblast collagenase inhibitor: Purification and biochemical characterization. J Biol Chem 258:12252, 1983

100. Carmichael DF, Sommer A, Thompson RC, et al: Primary structure and cDNA cloning of human fibroblast collagenase inhibitor. Proc Natl Acad Sci USA 83:2407, 1986

101. Stetler-Stevenson WG, Brown PD, Onisto M, et al: Tissue inhibitor of metalloproteinase-2 (TIMP-2) mRNA expression in tumor cell lines and human tumor tissues. J Biol Chem 265:13933, 1990

102. Boone TC, Johnson MJ, DeClerck YA, et al: cDNA cloning and expression of a metalloproteinase inhibitor related to tissue inhibitor of metalloproteinase. Proc Natl Acad Sci USA 87:2800, 1990

103. Howard EW, Bullen EC, Banda MJ: Preferential inhibition of 72 kDa and 92 kDA gelatinases by TIMP-2. J Biol Chem 266:13070, 1991

104. Nakajima M, Lotan D, Baig MM, et al: Inhibition by retinoic acid of type IV collagenolysis and invasion through reconstituted basement membrane by metastatic rat mammary adenocarcinoma cells. Cancer Res 49:1698, 1989

105. Turpeenniemi-Hujanen T, Thorgeirsson UP, Hart IR, et al: Expression of collagenase IV (basement membrane collagenase) activity in murine tumor cell hybrids that differ in metastatic potential. J Natl Cancer Inst 75:99, 1985

106. Muschel RJ, Williams JE, Lowy DR, et al: Harvey ras induction of metastatic potential depends upon oncogene activation and the type of recipient cell. Am J Pathol 121:1, 1985

107. Garbisa S, Pozzati R, Muschel R, et al: Secretion of type IV collagenolytic protease and metastatic phenotype: Induction by transfection with c-Ha-ras but not c-Ha-ras plus Ad2-E1a. Cancer Res 47:1523, 1987

108. Bonfil RD, Reddel RR, Ura H, et al: Invasive and metastatic potential of a v-Ha-ras-transformed human bronchial epithelial cell line. J Natl Cancer Inst 81:587, 1989

109. Ura H, Bonfil RD, Reich R, et al: Expression of type IV collagenase and procollagen genes and its correlation with the tumorigenic, invasive and metastatic abilities of oncogene-transformed human bronchial epithelial cells. Cancer Res 49:4615, 1989

110. Pyke C, Ralfkiaer E, Huhtala P, et al: Localization of messenger RNA for M_r 72,000 and 92,000 type IV collagenases in human skin cancers by in situ hybridization. Cancer Res 52:1336, 1992

111. Monteagudo C, Merino M, San Juan J, et al: Immunohistologic distribution of type IV collagenase in normal, benign, and malignant breast tissue. Am J Pathol 136:585, 1990

112. D'Errico A, Garbisa S, Liotta A, et al: Augmentation of type IV collagenase, laminin receptor, and Ki67 proliferation antigen associated with human colon, gastric, and breast carcinoma. Mod Pathol 4:239, 1991

113. Levy A, Cioce V, Sobel ME, et al: Increased expression of the 72 kDa type IV collagenase in human colonic adenocarcinoma. Cancer Res 51:439, 1991

114. Poulsom R, Pignatelli M, Stetler-Stevenson WG, et al: Stromal expression of 72 kDa type IV collagenase (MMP-2) and TIMP-2 mRNA's in colorectal cancer. Am J Pathol 141:389, 1992

115. Campo E, Tavassoli FA, Charonis AS, et al: Evaluation of basement membrane components and the 72 kDa type IV collagenase in serous tumors of the ovary. Am J Pathol 16:500, 1992

116. Campo E, Merino MJ, Liotta LA, et al: Distribution of the 72 kDa type IV collagenase in non-neoplastic and neoplastic thyroid tissue. Hum Pathol 23:1395, 1992

117. Schultz RM, Silberman S, Persky B, et al: Inhibition by recombinant tissue inhibitor of metalloproteinase of human amnion invasion and lung colonization by murine B16-F10 melanoma cells. Cancer Res 48:5539, 1988

118. Alvarez OA, Carmichael DF, DeClerck YA: Inhibition of collagenolytic activity and metastasis of tumor cells by a recombinant human tissue inhibitor of metalloproteinases. J Natl Cancer Inst 82:589, 1990

119. Khokha R, Waterhouse P, Yagel S, et al: Antisense RNA-induced reduction in murine TIMP level confers oncogenicity on Swiss 3T3. Science 243:947, 1989

120. DeClerck YA, Yean TD, Chan D, et al: Inhibition of tumor invasion of smooth muscle cell layers by recombinant human metalloproteinase inhibitor. Cancer Res 51:2151, 1991

121. Albini A, Melchiori A, Santi L, et al: Tumor cell invasion inhibited by TIMP-2. J Natl Cancer Inst 83:775, 1991

122. DeClerck YA, Perez N, Shimada H, et al: Inhibition of invasion and metastasis in cells transfected with an inhibitor of metalloproteinases. Cancer Res 52:701, 1992

123. Mignatti P, Tsuboi R, Robbins E, et al: In vitro angiogenesis on the human amniotic membrane: Requirement for basic fibroblast growth factor-induced proteinases. J Cell Biol 108:671, 1989

124. Moses MA, Sudhalter J, Langer R: Identification of an inhibitor of neovascularization from cartilage. Science 248:1408, 1990

125. Moses MA, Langer R: A metalloproteinase inhibitor as an inhibitor of neovascularization. J Cell Biochem 47:230, 1991

126. Takigawa M, Nishida Y, Suzuki F, et al: Induction of angiogenesis in chick yolk-sac membrane by polyamines and its inhibition by tissue inhibitors or metalloproteinases (TIMP and TIMP-2). Biochem Biophys Res Commun 171:1264, 1990

127. Brown PD, Levy AT, Margulies I, et al: Independent expression and cellular processing of the 72-kDa type IV collagenase and interstitial collagenase in human tumorigenic cell lines. Cancer Res 50:6184, 1990

128. Brinckerhoff CE, Plucinska IM, Sheldon LA, et al: Half-life of synovial cell collagenase mRNA is modulated by phorbol myristate acetate but not by all-trans-retinoic acid or dexamethasone. Biochemistry 25:6378, 1986

129. Kreig P, Finch J, Furstenburger G, et al: Tumor promoters induce a transient expression of tumor-associated genes in both

basal and differentiated cells of the mouse epidermis. Carcinogenesis 9:95, 1988

130. Angel P, Baumann I, Stein B, et al: 12-O-tetradecanoyl-phorbol-13-acetate induction of the human collagenase gene is mediated by an inducible enhancer element located in the 5'-flanking region. Mol Cell Biol 7:2256, 1987

131. Matrisian LM, Leroy P, Ruhlmann C, et al: Isolation of the oncogene and epidermal growth factor-induced transin gene: Complex control in rat fibroblasts. Mol Cell Biol 6:1679, 1986

132. Huhlala P, Chow LT, Tryggvason K: Structure of the human type IV collagenase gene. J Biol Chem 265:11077, 1990

133. Edwards DR, Murphy G, Reynolds JJ, et al: Transforming growth factor beta modulates the expression of collagenase and metalloproteinase inhibitor. EMBO J 6:1899, 1987

134. Kerr LD, Miller DB, Matrisian LM: TGF-β_1 inhibition of transin/stromelysin gene expression is mediated through a fos binding sequence. Cell 61:267, 1990

135. Overall CM, Wrana JL, Sodek J: Independent regulation of collagenase, 72 kDa progelatinase, and metalloproteinase inhibitor expression in human fibroblasts by transforming growth factor-β. J Biol Chem 264:1860, 1989

136. Vallee BL, Auld DS: Zinc coordination, function, and structure of zinc enzymes and other proteins. Biochemistry 29:5647, 1990

137. Van Wart HE, Birkedal-Hansen H: The cysteine switch: A principal of regulation of metalloproteinase activity with potential applicability to the entire matrix metalloproteinase gene family. Proc Natl Acad Sci USA 87:5578, 1990

138. Stetler-Stevenson WG, Talano JA, Gallager ME, et al: Inhibition of human type IV collagenase by a highly conserved peptide sequence derived from its prosegment. Am J Med Sci 302:163, 1991

139. Stetler-Stevenson WG, Krutzsch HC, Wachter MP, et al: The activation of human type IV collagenase proenzyme. J Biol Chem 264:1353, 1989

140. Muller D, Quantin B, Gesnel MC, et al: The collagenase gene family in humans consists of at least four members. Biochem J 253:187, 1988

141. Melchiori A, Albini A, Ray JM, et al: Inhibition of tumor cell invasion by a highly conserved peptide sequence from the matrix metalloproteinase enzyme prosegment. Cancer Res 52:2353, 1992

142. Ho C, Wilhelm SM, Pentland AP, et al: Tissue cooperation in a proteolytic cascade activating human interstitial collagenase. Proc Natl Acad Sci USA 86:2632, 1989

143. Brinckerhoff CE, Suzuki K, Mitchell TI, et al: Rabbit procollagenase synthesized by a high-yield mammalian expression vector requires stromelysin (matrix metalloproteinase-3) for maximal activation. J Biol Chem 265:22262, 1990

144. Suzuki K, Enghild JJ, Morodomi T, et al: Mechanisms of activation of tissue procollagenase by matrix metalloproteinase 3 (stromelysin). Biochemistry 29:10261, 1990

145. Overall CM, Sodek J: Concanavalin A produces a matrix-degradative phenotype in human fibroblasts. J Biol Chem 265:22266, 1990

146. Apodaca G, Rutka JT, Bouhana K, et al: Expression of metalloproteinases and metalloproteinase inhibitors by fetal astrocytes and glioma cells. Cancer Res 50:2322, 1990

147. Rifas L, Halstead LR, Peck WA, et al: Human osteoblasts in vitro secrete tissue inhibitor of metalloproteinases and gelatinase but not interstitial collagenase as major cellular products. J Clin Invest 84:686, 1990

148. Enterline HT, Coman DR: The amoeboid motility of human and animal neoplastic cells. Cancer 3:1033, 1950

149. Coman DR: Mechanisms responsible for the origin and distribution of blood-borne tumor metastases: A review. Cancer Res 13:397, 1953

150. Wood S: Pathogenesis of metastasis formation observed in vivo in the rabbit ear chamber. Arch Pathol 66:550, 1958

151. Hosaka S, Suzuki M, Goto M, et al: Motility of rat ascites hepatoma cells with reference to malignant characteristics in cancer metastasis. Gann 69:273, 1978

152. Orr FW, Varani J, Delikatny J, et al: Comparison of the chemotactic responsiveness of two fibrosarcoma subpopulations of differing malignancy. Am J Pathol 102:160, 1981

153. Raz A, Ben-Ze'ev A: Cell-contact and -architecture of malignant cells and their relationship to metastasis. Cancer Metastasis Rev 6:3, 1987

154. Mohler JL, Partin AW, Coffey DS: Prediction of metastatic potential by a new grading system of cell motility: Validation in the Dunning R-3327 prostatic adenocarcinoma model. J Urol 138:168, 1987

154a. Birchmeier W, Weidner KM, Behrens J: Molecular mechanisms leading to loss of differentiation and gain of invasiveness in epithelial cells. J Cell Sci 17:159, 1993

155. McCarthy JB, Basara ML, Palm SL, et al: The role of cell adhesion proteins—laminin and fibronectin—in the movement of malignant and metastatic cells. Cancer Metastasis Rev 4:125, 1985

156. Hayashi H, Yoshida K, Ozaki T, et al: Chemotactic factor associated with invasion of cancer cells. Nature 226:174, 1990

157. Liotta LA, Mandler R, Murano G, et al: Tumor cell autocrine motility factor. Proc Natl Acad Sci USA 83:3302, 1986

158. Kohn EC, Francis EA, Liotta LA, et al: Heterogeneity of the motility response in malignant tumor cells: A biological basis for the diversity and homing of metastatic cells. Int J Cancer 46:287, 1990

159. Todaro GJ, Fryling C, DeLarco JE: Transforming growth factors produced by certain human tumor cells: Polypeptides that interact with epidermal growth factor receptors. Proc Natl Acad Sci USA 77:5258, 1980

160. Anzano MA, Roberts AB, Smith JM, et al: Sarcoma growth factor from conditioned medium of virally transformed cells is composed of both type α and type β transforming growth factors. Proc Natl Acad Sci USA 80:6264, 1983

161. Atnip KD, Carter LM, Nicolson GL, et al: Chemotactic response of rat mammary adenocarcinoma cell clones to tumor-derived cytokines. Biochem Biophys Res Commun 146:996, 1987

162. Siletti S, Watanabe H, Hogan V, et al: Purification of B16-F1 melanoma autocrine motility factor and its receptor. Cancer Res 51:3507, 1991

163. Ohnishi T, Arita N, Hayakawa T, et al: Motility factor produced by malignant glioma cells: Role in tumor invasion. J Neurosurg 73:881, 1990

164. Evans CP, Walsh DS, Kohn EC: An autocrine motility factor secreted by the Dunning R-3327 rat prostatic adenocarcinoma cell subtype AT2.1. Int J Cancer 49:109, 1991

165. Seiki M, Sato H, Liotta LA, et al: Comparison of autocrine mechanisms promoting motility in two metastatic cell lines: Human melanoma and ras-transfected NIH3T3 cells. Int J Cancer 49:171, 1991

166. El-Badry OM, Minniti C, Kohn EC, et al: Insulin-like growth factor II acts as an autocrine growth and motility factor in human rhabdomyosarcoma tumors. Cell Growth Differ 1:325, 1990

166a. Bellusci S, Moens G, Gaudino G, et al: Creation of an hepatocyte growth factor/scatter factor autocrine loop in carcinoma cells induces invasive properties associated with increased tumorigenicity. Oncogene 9:1091, 1994

167. Turley EA, Vandeligt K, Clary C: Hyaluronan and a cell-associated hyaluronan binding protein regulate the locomotion of ras-transformed cells. J Cell Biol 112:1041, 1991

168. Stracke ML, Krutzsch JC, Unsworth EJ, et al: Identification, purification, and partial sequence analysis of autotaxin, a novel motility-stimulating protein. J Biol Chem 267:2524, 1992

169. Basara ML, McCarthy JB, Barnes DW, et al: Stimulation of haptotaxis and migration of tumor cells by serum spreading factor. Cancer Res 45:2487, 1985

170. McCarthy JB, Furcht LT: Laminin and fibronectin promote the haptotactic migration of B16 melanoma cells in vitro. J Cell Biol 98:1474, 1984

171. Mensing H, Albini A, Krieg T, et al: Enhanced chemotaxis of tumor-derived and virus-transformed cells to fibronectin and fibroblast-conditioned medium. Int J Cancer 33:43, 1984

172. McCarthy JB, Hagen ST, Furcht LT: Human fibronectin con-

tains distinct adhesion- and motility-promoting domains for metastatic melanoma cells. J Cell Biol *102*:179, 1986

173. Aznavoorian S, Liotta LA, Kupchik HZ: Characteristics of invasive and noninvasive human colorectal adenocarcinoma cells. J Natl Cancer Inst *82*:1485, 1990

174. Makabe T, Saiki I, Murata J, et al: Modulation of haptotactic migration of metastatic melanoma cells by the interaction between heparin and heparin-binding domain of fibronectin. J Biol Chem *265*:14270, 1990

175. McCarthy JB, Palm SL, Furcht LT: Migration by haptotaxis of a Schwann cell tumor line to the basement membrane glycoprotein laminin. J Cell Biol *110*:1427, 1983

176. Situ R, Lee EC, McCoy JP Jr, et al: Stimulation of murine tumour cell motility by laminin. J Cell Sci *70*:167, 1984

177. Aresu O, Nicolò G, Allavena G, et al: Invasive activity, spreading on and chemotactic response to laminin are properties of high but not low metastatic mouse osteosarcoma cells. Invasion Metastasis *11*:2, 1991

178. Tashiro K-I, Sephel GC, Greatorex D, et al: The RGD containing site of the mouse laminin A chain is active for cell attachment, spreading, migration and neurite outgrowth. J Cell Physiol *146*:451, 1991

179. Tchao R: Novel forms of epithelial cell motility on collagen and on glass surfaces. Cell Motil *4*:333, 1982

180. Mooradian DL, McCarthy JB, Komanduri KV, et al: Effects of transforming growth factor-β_1 on human pulmonary adenocarcinoma cell adhesion, motility, and invasion *in vitro*. J Natl Cancer Inst *84*:523, 1992

181. Chelberg MK, Tsilibary EC, Hauser AR, et al: Type IV collagen-mediated melanoma cell adhesion and migration: Involvement of multiple, distinct domains of the collagen molecule. Cancer Res *49*:4796, 1989

182. Taraboletti G, Roberts DD, Liotta LA: Thrombospondin-induced tumor cell migration: Haptotaxis and chemotaxis are mediated by different domains. J Cell Biol *105*:2409, 1987

183. Iwamoto Y, Robey FA, Graf J, et al: YIGSR, a synthetic laminin pentapeptide, inhibits experimental metastasis formation. Science *238*:1132, 1987

184. McCarthy JB, Skubitz APN, Palm SL, et al: Metastasis inhibition of different tumor types of purified laminin fragments and a heparin-binding fragment of fibronectin. J Natl Cancer Inst *80*:108, 1988

185. Leavesly DI, Ferguson GD, Wayner EA, et al: Requirement of the integrin β_3 receptor for carcinoma cell spreading or migration on vitronectin and fibronectin. J Cell Biol *117*:1101, 1990

186. Huff KK, Kaufman D, Gabbay KH, et al: Secretion of an insulin-like growth factor-I-related protein by human breast cancer cells. Cancer Res *46*:4613, 1986

187. Rodeck U, Herlyn M, Menssen HD, et al: Metastatic but not primary melanoma cell lines grow *in vitro* independently of exogenous growth factors. Int J Cancer *40*:687, 1987

188. Halaban R, Kwon BS, Ghosh S, et al: bFGF as an autocrine growth factor for human melanomas. Oncogene Res *3*:177, 1988

189. Williams NN, Györfi T, Iliopoulos D, et al: Growth factor-independence and invasive properties of colorectal carcinoma cells. Int J Cancer *50*:274, 1992

190. Liapi C, Raynaud F, Anderson WB, et al: High chemotactic response to platelet-derived growth factor of a teratocarcinoma differentiated mesodermal cell line. In Vitro Cell Dev Biol *26*:388, 1990

191. Tilly BC, Tertoolen LGJ, Remorie R, et al: Histamine as a growth factor and chemoattractant for human carcinoma and melanoma cells: Action through Ca^{2+}-mobilizing H_1 receptors. J Cell Biol *110*:1211, 1990

192. Vallés AM, Boyer B, Badet J, et al: Acidic fibroblast growth factor is a modulator of epithelial plasticity in a rat bladder carcinoma cell line. Proc Natl Acad Sci USA *87*:1124, 1990

193. Pienta KJ, Murphy BC, Isaacs WB, et al: Effect of pentosan, a novel cancer chemotherapeutic agent, on prostate cell growth and motility. Prostate *20*:233, 1992

194. Schofield PN, Granerus M, Lee A, et al: Concentration-dependent modulation of basic fibroblast growth factor action on multiplication and locomotion of human teratocarcinoma cells. FEBS Lett *298*:154, 1992

195. Stracke ML, Kohn EC, Aznavoorian S, et al: Insulin-like growth factors stimulate chemotaxis in human melanoma cells. Biochem Biophys Res Commun *153*:1076, 1988

196. Stracke ML, Engel JD, Wilson LL, et al: The type I insulin-like growth factor receptor is a motility receptor in human melanoma cells. J Biol Chem *264*:21544, 1989

197. Minniti CP, Kohn EC, Grubb JH, et al: The insulin-like growth factor-II (IGF-II)/mannose 6-phosphate receptor mediates IGF-II-induced motility in human rhabdomyosarcoma cells. J Biol Chem *267*:9000, 1992

198. Stossel TP: How cells crawl: With the discovery that the cellular motor contains muscle proteins, we can begin to describe cell motility in molecular detail. Am Sci *78*:408, 1990

199. Cunningham CC: Actin structural proteins in cell motility. Cancer Metastasis Rev *11*:69, 1992

200. Condeelis J, Jones J, Segall JE: Chemotaxis of metastatic tumor cells: Clues to mechanisms from the *Dictyostelium* paradigm. Cancer Metastasis Rev *11*:55, 1992

201. Lester BR, McCarthy JB: Tumor cell adhesion to the extracellular matrix and signal transduction mechanisms implicated in tumor cell motility, invasion, and metastasis. Cancer Metastasis Rev *11*:31, 1992

202. Goldman DW, Chang FH, Gifford LA, et al: Pertussis toxin inhibition of chemotactic factor-induced calcium mobilization and function in human polymorphonuclear leukocytes. J Exp Med *162*:145, 1985

203. Spangrude GJ, Sacchi F, Hill HR, et al: Inhibition of lymphocyte and neutrophil chemotaxis by pertussis toxin. J Immunol *135*:4135, 1985

204. Lester BR, McCarthy JB, Sun Z, et al: G-protein involvement in matrix-mediated motility and invasion of high and low experimental metastatic B16 melanoma cells. Cancer Res *49*:5940, 1989

205. Lester BR, Winstein LS, McCarthy JB, et al: The role of G-protein in matrix-mediated motility of highly and poorly invasive melanoma cells. Int J Cancer *48*:113, 1991

206. Roos E, Van de Pavert IV: Inhibition of lymphoma invasion and liver metastasis formation by pertussis toxin. Cancer Res *47*:5439, 1987

207. Hunter T: Cooperation between oncogenes. Cell *64*:249, 1991

208. Greenberg AH, Egen SE, Wright JA: Oncogenes and metastatic progression. Invasion Metastasis *9*:360, 1989

209. Steeg PS: Genetic control of the metastatic phenotype. Cancer Biol *2*:105, 1991

210. Thorgeirsson UP, Turpeenniemi-Hujanen T, Williams JE, et al: NIH 3T3 cells transfected with human tumor DNA containing activated *ras* oncogenes express the metastatic phenotype in nude mice. Mol Cell Biol *5*:259, 1985

211. Bernstein SC, Weinberg RA: Expression of the metastatic phenotype in cells transfected with human metastatic tumor DNA. Proc Natl Acad Sci USA *82*:1726, 1985

212. Greig RG, Koestler TP, Trainer DL, et al: Tumorigenic and metastatic properties of "normal" and *ras*-transfected NIH-3T3 cells. Proc Natl Acad Sci USA *82*:3698, 1985

213. Bradley MO, Kraynak AR, Strorer RD, et al: Experimental metastasis in nude mice of NIH-3T3 cells containing various *ras* genes. Proc Natl Acad Sci USA *83*:5277, 1986

214. Nicolson GL: Tumor cell instability, diversification, and progression to the metastatic phenotype: From oncogene to oncofetal expression. Cancer Res *47*:1473, 1987

215. Hill SA, Wilson A, Chambers AF: Clonal heterogeneity, experimental metastatic ability, and p21 expression in H-ras-transformed NIH 3T3 cells. J Natl Cancer Inst *80*:484, 1988

216. Theodorescu D, Cornil I, Fernandez B, et al: Overexpression of normal and mutated forms of c-Ha-*ras* induce orthotopic bladder invasion in a human transitional cell carcinoma. Proc Natl Acad Sci USA *87*:9047, 1990

217. Mason RW, Gal S, Gottesman MM: The identification of the major excreted protein (MEP) from a transformed mouse fibroblast cell line as a catalytically active precursor form of cathepsin L. Biochem J *248*:449, 1987

218. Egan SE, Wright JA, Jarolim L, et al: Transformation by on-

cogenes encoding protein kinases induces the metastatic phyenotype. Science 238:202, 1987

219. Pohl J, Goldfnger N, Rader-Pohl A, et al: p53 increases experimental metastatic capacity of murine carcinoma cells. Mol Cell Biol 8:2078, 1988

220. Tuck AB, Wilson SM, Chambers AF: ras transfection and expression does not induce progression from tumorigenicity to metastatic ability in mouse LTA cells. Clin Exp Metastasis 8: 417, 1990

221. Pozzati R, Muschel R, Williams J, et al: Primary rat embryo cells transformed by one of two oncogenes show different metastatic potentials. Science 232:223, 1986

222. Sidebottom E, Clark SR: Cell fusion segregates progressive growth from metastasis. Br J Cancer 47:399, 1983

223. Marshall CJ: Tumor suppressor genes. Cell 64:313, 1991

224. Weinberg RA: Tumor suppressor genes. Science 254:1138, 1991

225. Sobel ME: Metastasis suppressor genes. J Natl Cancer Inst 82: 267, 1990

226. Gattoni-Celli S, Strauss RM, Willet CG, et al: Modulation of the transformed and neoplastic phenotype of rat fibroblasts by MHC-I expression. Cancer Res 49:3392, 1989

227. Gattoni-Celli S, Marazzi A, Timpale R, et al: Partial suppression of metastatic potential of malignant cells in immunodeficient mice caused by transfection of H-2K^b gene. J Natl Cancer Inst 243:947, 1990

228. Steeg PS, Bevilacqua G, Kopper L, et al: Evidence for a novel gene associated with low tumor metastatic potential. J Natl Cancer Inst 80:200, 1988

229. Dear TN, Ramshaw IA, Kefford RF: Differential expression of a novel gene, WDNM1, in nonmetastatic rat mammary adenocarcinoma cells. Cancer Res 48:5203, 1988

230. Dear TN, McDonald DA, Kefford RF: Transcriptional downregulation of a rat gene, WDNM2, in metastatic DMBA-8 cells. Cancer Res 49:5323, 1989

231. Dear TN: Note re: T. Neil Dear et al., Transcriptional downregulation of a rat gene, WDNM2, in metastatic DMBA-8 cells. Cancer Res 49:5323–5328, 1989. Cancer Res 50:1667, 1990

232. Dear TN, Kefford RF: The WDNM1 gene product is a novel member of the "four-disulphide core" family of proteins. Biochem Biophys Res Commun 176:247, 1991

233. Leone A, Flatow U, King CR, et al: Reduced tumor incidence, metastatic potential, and cytokine responsiveness of nm23-transfected melanoma cells. Cell 65:25, 1991

234. Bevilacqua G, Sobel ME, Liotta LA, et al: Association of low nm23 RNA levels in human primary infiltrating ductal breast carcinomas with lymph node involvement and other histopathological indicators of high metastatic potential. Cancer Res 49:5185, 1989

235. Sasre-Garau X, Lacombe M, Veron M, et al: Nucleoside diphosphate kinase/NM23 expression in breast cancer: Lack of correlation with lymph node metastasis. Cancer Res 50:533, 1992

236. Royds J, Stephenson T, Rees R, et al: nm23 product expression in ductal in situ and invasive human breast cancer. J Natl Cancer Inst 85:727, 1993

237. Barnes R, Masood S, Barker E, et al: Low nm23 protein expression in infiltrating ductal breast carcinomas correlates with reduced patient survival. Am J Pathol 139:245, 1991

238. Hennessy C, Henry JA, May FEB, et al: Expression of the anti-metastatic gene nm23 in human breast cancer, association with a good prognosis. J Natl Cancer Inst 83:281, 1991

239. Hirayama R, Sawai S, Takagi Y, et al: Positive relationship between expression of anti-metastatic factor (nm23 gene product or nucleoside diphosphate kinase) and good prognosis in human breast cancer. J Natl Cancer Inst 83:1249, 1991

240. Nakayama T, Ohtsuru A, Nakao K, et al: Expression in human hepatocellular carcinoma of nucleoside diphosphate kinase, a homologue of the nm23 gene product. J Natl Cancer Inst 84: 1349, 1992

241. Flørenes VA, Aamdal S, Myklebost O, et al: Levels of nm23 messenger RNA in metastatic malignant melanomas: Inverse correlation to disease progression. Cancer Res 52:6088, 1992

242. Leone A, Seeger R, Hong C, et al: Evidence for nm23 RNA overexpression, DNA amplication and mutation in aggressive childhood neuroblastomas. Oncogene 8:855, 1993

243. Dearolf CR, Hersperger E, Shearn A: Developmental consequences of awd^b3, a cell-autonomous lethal metation of Drosophila induced by hybrid dysgenesis. Dev Biol 129:159, 1988

244. Dearolf CR, Tripoulas N, Biggs J, et al: Molecular consequences of awd^b3, cell-autonomous lethal mutation of Drosophila induced by hybrid dysgenesis. Dev Biol 129:169, 1988

245. Rosengard AM, Krutzsch HC, Shearn A, et al: Reduced Nm23/Awd protein in tumor metastasis and aberrant Drosophila development. Nature 342:177, 1989

246. Gilles A, Presecan E, Vonica A, et al: Nucleoside diphosphate kinase from human crythrocytes. J Biol Chem 266:8784, 1991

247. Golden A, Benedict M, Shearn A, et al: Nucleoside diphosphate kinase, nm23 and tumor metastasis: Possible biochemical mechanisms. In Benz C, Liu E (eds): Oncogenes and Tumor Suppressor Genes in Human Malignancies. Boston, Klewer Academic Publishers, 1993

248. Steeg PS, De La Rosa A, Flatow U, et al: Nm23 and breast cancer metastasis. Breast Cancer Res Treat 25:175, 1993

249. Ruff M, Schiffmann E, Terranova V, et al: Neuropeptides are chemoattractants for human tumor cells and monocytes: A possible mechanism for metastasis. Clin Immunol Immunopathol 37:387, 1987

250. Stoker M, Gherardi E: Scatter factor and other regulators of cell motility. Br Med Bull 45:481, 1989

251. Weidner KM, Behrens J, Vandekerckhove J, et al: Scatter factor: Molecular characteristics and effect on the invasiveness of epithelial cells. J Cell Biol 111:2097, 1990

251a. Sunitha I, Meighen DL, Hartman D-P, et al: Hepatocyte growth factor stimulates invasion across reconstituted basement membranes by a new human small intestinal cell line. Clin Exp Metastasis 12:143, 1994

252. Tamm I, Cardinale I, Krueger J, et al: Interleukin 6 decreases cell-cell association and increases motility of ductal breast carcinoma cells. J Exp Med 170:1649, 1989

253. Wang JM, Taraboletti G, Matsushima K, et al: Induction of haptotactic migration of melanoma cells by neutrophil activating protein/interleukin-8. Biochem Biophys Res Commun 169:165, 1990

254. Kahan BW, Kramp DC: Nerve growth factor stimulation of mouse embryonal cell migration. Cancer Res 47:6324, 1987

SECTION
III

MOLECULAR ABNORMALITIES IN SPECIFIC MALIGNANCIES

MOLECULAR BIOLOGY OF LYMPHOID NEOPLASMS

MOLECULAR DIAGNOSIS AND THERAPY OF HEMATOPOIETIC NEOPLASMS

MOLECULAR BIOLOGY OF CHILDHOOD NEOPLASMS

MOLECULAR BIOLOGY OF LUNG CANCER

MOLECULAR ABNORMALITIES IN COLON AND RECTAL CANCER

MOLECULAR BASIS OF BREAST CANCER

12

MOLECULAR BIOLOGY OF LYMPHOID NEOPLASMS

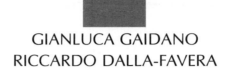

GIANLUCA GAIDANO
RICCARDO DALLA-FAVERA

CLASSIFICATION OF LYMPHOID NEOPLASIA

Biologic Basis of Lymphoid Neoplasia Heterogeneity

Lymphoid malignancies are neoplasms characterized by the proliferation of cells derived from the lymphoid tissue and its precursors. Despite this common tissue origin, these tumors exhibit a high degree of phenotypic heterogeneity, which reflects the diversity of their normal counterpart cells.[1,2] That lymphoid malignancies represent an extremely heterogeneous group of neoplastic diseases had been a common notion to clinicians and pathologists for many years; however, virtually no understanding of the biologic basis for this heterogeneity existed until the mid-1970s. The advent of cellular immunology first, and of molecular genetics in the following years, led to the discovery that normal lymphoid cells could be classified according to cell surface antigen expression and antigen receptor gene configuration, into distinct subsets populating discrete microenvironments and serving different functions.[3,4] It then became clear that, similarly to normal lymphoid cells, lymphoid malignancies can be distinguished on the basis of their immunophenotypic and immunogenotypic features, which closely mimic the normal lymphoid elements from which they originate.[1,2] Therefore, lymphoid malignancies are classified depending on (1) their derivation from either the B- or T-cell lineage, (2) the stage of differentiation of the involved cells, and (3) the acute or chronic clinical behavior.

B-Cell Lineage Lymphoid Malignancies

The physiologic B-cell differentiation pathways are schematically represented in Figure 12–1, together with the most common forms of B-cell neoplasms derived from each stage of B-cell maturation.

B-cell precursor stages, derived from a putative lymphoid stem cell and including *prepre* and *pre-B cells*, are characterized by the expression of terminal deoxynucleotidyltransferase (TdT), rearrangements of the immunoglobulin heavy-chain locus (Ig_H), and lack of surface immunoglobulins.[3,4] Prepre-B cells express the B lineage restricted antigens CD19 and CD20 and are characterized by the appearance of rearranged immunoglobulin light (Ig_L) chains.[3–5] The pre-B cell stage is characterized by cytoplasmic immunoglobulin expression.[3–5] Tumors derived from precursor B cells are classified as B-lineage acute lymphoblastic leukemia (ALL), because precursor cells arise in the bone marrow and tend to invade the bone marrow and, subsequently, a variety of other organs.

Mature B cells are characterized by completion of immunoglobulin gene rearrangement coupled to expression of cell surface immunoglobulins (sIgs). B-cell neoplasms arising from mature B cells include the large group of B-cell non-Hodgkin's lymphoma (B-NHL), B-cell chronic lymphocytic leukemia, and hairy-cell leukemia. These tumors arise in lymph nodes or extranodal sites, and for the most part are characterized by solid tumor burdens. Finally, the latest stages of B-cell neoplasms are represented by sIg^- cells, termed *plasma cells*, which secrete large amounts of monoclonal immunoglobulin, detectable in the cytoplasm (cIg).[3–5] B-cell tumors with the characteristics of terminally differentiated B cells are represented by multiple myeloma and plasma cell leukemia. These tumors arise in the bone marrow and, through early dissemination to the entire body axis, cause profound systemic bone erosion.

T-Cell Lineage Lymphoid Malignancies

Figure 12–2 illustrates the physiologic differentiation pathways of T cells and the most common forms of

251

T-cell tumors derived from each stage of differentiation. T-cell precursors reside in the thymus, where they undergo maturation and selection.[3-5] They usually are divided into three stages according to the sequential expression of differentiation antigens: *stage I* and *II* thymocytes reside in the thymus cortex, whereas *stage III* thymocytes are located in the medulla.[3-5] CD7, CD2, and CD5 are expressed throughout all stages, whereas CD4 and CD8 expression begins at stage II. Stage III thymocytes are characterized by the mutually exclusive expression of either CD4 or CD8, giving rise to the CD4+CD8− and CD8+CD4− *mature T cells (postthymic T cells)*. At the genetic level, T-cell maturation is accompanied by sequential rearrangement of the genes encoding the T-cell receptor (TCR) α, β, γ, and δ chains. TCR γ and β chain genes are the first to undergo rearrangement during T-cell maturation, followed by TCR δ rearrangements and, at a later stage, TCR α rearrangements.[2]

Tumors derived from T-lineage precursor cells (i.e., *thymocytes*) include ALL and lymphoblastic lymphoma and frequently present as a thymus mass. Clonal rearrangements of some, if not all, of the TCR genes commonly are detected in these tumors.[2] Mature T cells (i.e., postthymic T cells) give rise to a variety of T-cell tumors, including peripheral T-cell lymphomas (PTCLs), cutaneous T-cell lymphomas (CTCLs), T-cell chronic lymphocytic leukemia and prolymphocytic leukemia, and Tγ lymphoproliferative disorders. In western countries, mature T-cell neoplasms are relatively uncommon when compared to lymphoid malignancies arising from mature B cells; their incidence is higher in other specific geographic areas, namely Japan and the Caribbean.

GENERAL MECHANISMS OF PATHOGENESIS

The molecular lesions of lymphoid neoplasms can be grouped into broad categories according to the mechanisms of the lesion, which include activation of proto-oncogenes by chromosomal translocation or point mutation, proto-oncogene amplification, and tumor suppressor gene inactivation (Table 12–1).

Proto-oncogene activation by chromosomal translocation is the common result of a subset of molecular lesions that are typical of lymphoid neoplasms, are associated at high frequency with a specific subtype of lymphoproliferation, and can be found as the sole genomic alteration in a given tumor case. Chromosomal translocations of lymphoid tumors can have one of two effects. First, many translocations imply an antigen receptor locus (the immunoglobulin loci or the TCR loci in B- and T-cell malignancies, respectively) on one partner chromosome and a proto-oncogene on the other (Table 12–1). Once the proto-oncogene is juxtaposed to the antigen receptor locus, its expression becomes regulated by immunoglobulin or TCR promoters/enhancers, and deregulation occurs. Alternatively, chromosomal translocations may cause the formation of novel transcriptional units derived from the fusion of genes at the breakpoint sites (fusion transcripts). Proto-oncogene activation by fusion transcript formation leads to chimeric proteins displaying novel biochemical properties distinct from those of the wild-type proteins.

The proto-oncogenes involved in lymphoid neoplasm translocations belong to different classes of oncogenes. The overwhelming majority, particularly when considering acute lymphoproliferations of childhood, are represented by transcription factors directly involved in the

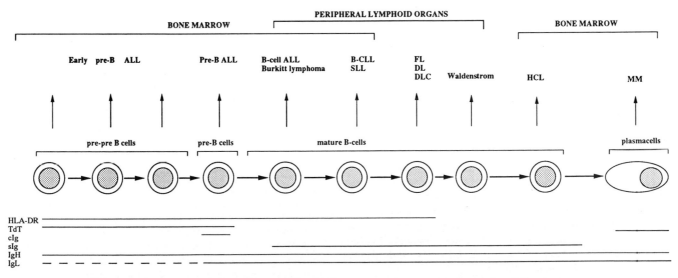

Figure 12–1. Scheme of B lymphocyte differentiation showing the normal stages of B-cell development, their anatomic compartmentalization, and their relationship to the major B-cell lineage lymphoproliferative disorders (indicated by arrows). ALL, acute lymphoblastic leukemia; B-CLL, B-cell chronic lymphocytic leukemia; SLL, small lymphocytic lymphoma; FL, follicular lymphoma; DL, diffuse lymphoma; DLCL, diffuse large-cell lymphoma; HCL, hairy-cell leukemia; MM, multiple myeloma; HLA-DR, human lymphocyte antigen; TdT, terminal deoxynucleodityltransferase; cIg, cytoplasmic immunoglobulins; sIg, surface immunoglobulins; IgH, immunoglobulin heavy-chain locus; IgL, immunoglobulin light-chain locus.

control of cell proliferation and differentiation. However, tyrosine kinases and growth factors also are implicated, although at a lower frequency. Conversely, the most frequent translocation in adult lymphoid tumors, which usually display a more chronic course, involves a novel type of proto-oncogene, *bcl-2*, that does not directly influence cell proliferation but rather prevents cell death.

Activation of proto-oncogenes by mutation in lymphoid neoplasms is restricted to the case of the *ras* family. These lesions are not specific to lymphoid tumors, and are found in a variety of human cancers. In lymphoid neoplasms, *ras* mutations usually accompany other molecular abnormalities typical of a given tumor type and frequently play a relevant role in tumor progression.

Gene amplification as a mechanism of proto-oncogene activation does not seem to play a major role in lymphoid

neoplasms, although it is a relatively common mechanism in the molecular pathogenesis of solid tumors.

Finally, *disruption of tumor suppressor genes* by chromosomal deletion of one allele and inactivation of the other allele, represents an additional general mechanism of pathogenesis in lymphoid tumors, best exemplified by the case of *p53*.

Overall, lymphoid malignancies are characterized by a relatively stable genome in comparison to solid tumors.[6] Indeed, many solid tumors carry random alterations that may involve more than 20 per cent of the total genome, whereas leukemias and lymphomas mostly carry nonrandom chromosomal breaks on a low background of random genomic disruption.[6] The biologic reason for the difference in genetic instability between solid and lymphoid tumors is presently not known.

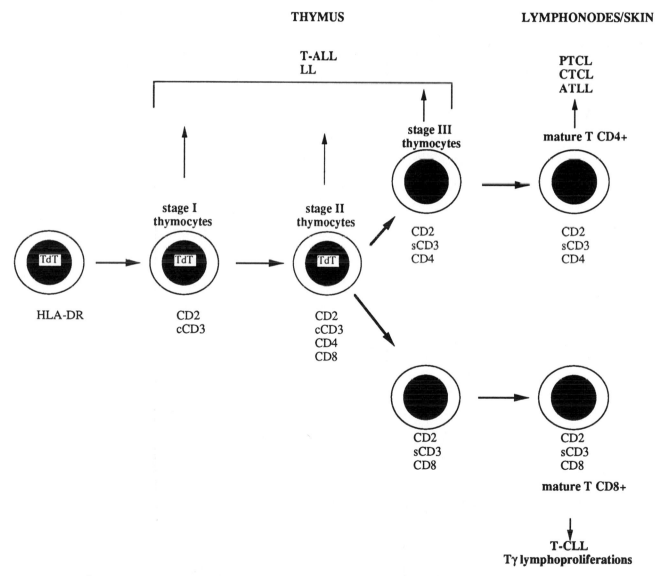

Figure 12–2. Scheme of T-lymphocyte differentiation showing cell phenotypes, their anatomic compartmentalization, and their relationship to the major T-cell lineage lymphoproliferative disorders. T-ALL, T-cell acute lymphoblastic leukemia; LL, lymphoblastic lymphoma; PTCL, peripheral T cell lymphoma; CTCL, cutaneous T cell lymphoma; ATLL, adult T cell leukemia/lymphoma; T-CLL, T-cell chronic lymphocytic leukemia; cCD3, cytoplasmic CD3; sCD3, cell surface CD3; HLA-DR, human lymphocyte antigen; TdT, terminal deoxynucleotidyltransferase.

ACUTE LYMPHOBLASTIC LEUKEMIA

General Overview

Acute lymphoblastic leukemia, a tumor of lymphocyte precursors, is the most frequent childhood cancer, accounting for up to one fourth of all malignancies and for 80 per cent of all leukemias occurring in children under 15.[7] In adults, ALL is more rare, representing 20 per cent of adult acute leukemias.[7] ALL is a malignant disorder resulting from unregulated clonal proliferation and impaired maturation of lymphocyte precursors, also called lymphoblasts.[7] The disease is highly heterogeneous, both clinically and biologically[1,8–12] (Table 12–2). More than 80 per cent of ALL cases arise from the B-cell lineage, whereas 10 to 20 per cent derive from T cells and are

TABLE 12–1. GENETIC LESIONS INVOLVED IN LYMPHOID MALIGNANCIES

	STRUCTURAL ABNORMALITY	MECHANISM OF LESION	TUMOR TYPE*	REFS.
Oncogenes				
Transcription factors				
E2A-PBX1	t(1;19)(q23;p13)	Fusion transcript	Early pre-B ALL, pre-B ALL	55,57,58
ALL-1/hrx–AF-4	t(4;11)(q21;q23)	Fusion transcript	Early pre-B ALL,	63–68
ALL-1/hrx–ENL	t(11;19)(q23;p23)		pre-B ALL, infant ALL	
E2A-Hlf	t(17;19)(q22;p13)	Fusion transcript	Early pre-B ALL	110,111
c-myc	t(8;14)(q24;q32), t(2;8)(p11;q24), t(8;22)(q24;q11)	Transcriptional deregulation	BL, B-cell ALL, diffuse B-NHL, immunoblastic B-NHL, AIDS-NHL	72–79, 169–174
	t(8;14)(q24;q11)		T-ALL	
tal-1	t(1;14)(p32;q11) Intragenic deletion	Transcriptional deregulation	T-ALL	80–91
HOX11	t(10;14)(q24;q11)	Transcriptional deregulation	T-ALL	92–94
rhom-1/ttg-1	t(11;14)(p15;q11)	Transcriptional deregulation	T-ALL	95–104
rhom-2/ttg-2	t(11;14)(p13;q11)	Transcriptional deregulation	T-ALL	95–104
tal-2	t(7;9)(q34;q32)	Transcriptional deregulation	T-ALL	113
lyl-1	t(7;19)(q35;p13)	Transcriptional deregulation	T-ALL	112
lyt-10	t(10;14)(q24;q11)	Removal of regulatory region	Low-grade B-NHL, CTCL	203–206
bcl-6	t(3;?)(q27)	Transcriptional deregulation	Diffuse B-NHL	200–202
Tyrosine Kinase				
bcr-abl	t(9;22)(q34;q11)	Fusion transcript	Early pre-B ALL, pre-B ALL	19–45
lck	t(1;7)(p34;q34)	Transcriptional deregulation	T-ALL	115
Other				
tan-1	t(7;9)(q34;q34.3)	?	T-ALL	114
IL-3	t(5;14)(q31;q32)	IL-3 overproduction	Pre-B ALL	108,109
bcl-1	t(11;14)(q13;q32)	*PRAD1* overexpression	Mantle zone B-NHL	190–197
bcl-2	t(14;18)(q32;q21)	*bcl-2* overexpression	Follicular B-NHL	146–168
ras	Point mutation	Constitutive activation	Early pre-B ALL, pre-B ALL, MM, AIDS-NHL	255–257
Tumor Suppressors				
p53	Point mutation	Loss of function	Early-pre B ALL, pre-B ALL, B-cell ALL, BL, MM, AIDS-NHL, B-CLL, ATLL	118,228, 262,269–271, 299,300
Viruses†				
EBV	—	—	BL	211–221
HTVL-I	—	—	ATLL	286–292

*ALL, acute lymphocytic leukemia; BL, Burkitt's lymphoma; B-NHL, B-cell non-Hodgkin's lymphoma; AIDS-NHL, AIDS-associated non-Hodgkin's lymphoma; T-ALL, T-cell acute lymphoblastic leukemia; CTCL, cutaneous T-cell lymphoma; MM, multile myeloma; B-CLL, B-cell chronic lymphocytic leukemia; ATLL, adult T-cell leukemia/lymphoma.

†EBV, Epstein-Barr virus; HTLV-I, human T-cell leukemia virus, type I.

known as T-ALL. Among B-cell–lineage ALL, three major subtypes are identified, known as *early pre-B, pre-B,* and *B-cell* ALL, according to the stage of differentiation. Finally, some ALLs express both lymphoid and myeloid markers; these cases, known as "biphenotypic" ALL, are most common in infants under 12 months.

Genetic Lesions

Several genetic lesions have been reported in ALL. A first subset of lesions, mainly involving genes located at the site of chromosomal translocation, is restricted to ALL or to its subtypes. In contrast, other molecular lesions, such as *p53* and *ras* mutations, are present throughout all the different subtypes of ALL at low frequency and also commonly are found in other human tumor types (the molecular mechanisms of alteration of this second subset of lesions are described in previous chapters of this book).

Almost half of ALL cases carry chromosomal translocations, and more than 15 distinct recurrent translocations have been described in ALL.[10,13–17] A number of these translocations involve the immunoglobulin or TCR loci, usually in B-lineage and T-lineage ALL, respectively, and are due to errors in the physiologic rearrangement process.[18] Chromosomal rearrangements in ALL can be grouped into two broad categories, according to the mechanism leading to oncogenic conversion of the proto-oncogene involved.[14–17] In the first category, the proto-oncogene involved is not normally expressed in the target tissue or is expressed at very low levels; the translocation or other structural abnormality causes its deregulated expression by juxtaposing it to an enhancer or promoter that is active in the cell type from which the tumor arises. In some cases, disruptions of the proto-oncogene regulatory regions add up to cause deregulation. Juxtaposition of a proto-oncogene to an antigen receptor locus, with or without truncation of regulatory elements, is the classic example of this mechanism; however, other structural abnormalities not involving antigen receptor loci (e.g., chromosome 1 interstitial deletions) might operate in the same way. This first type of mechanism is found in chromosomal rearrangements involving c-*myc*, *tal-1*, *HOX11*, *rhom-1/ttg-1*, *rhom-2/ttg-2*, *IL-3*, *tal-2*, and *lck*.[14–17] The second category of ALL chromosomal rearrangements is represented by translocations involving the *bcr-abl, E2A-*

PBX, E2A-hlf, and *HRX-ENL* or *ALL-1–AF-4* genes: Interchromosomal recombination occurs within an intron of the genes involved, leading to the formation of a fusion transcript. The resulting chimeric proteins display biochemical properties and/or expression patterns not associated with their normal counterparts.[14–17]

t(9;22)(q34;q11) AND *bcr-abl*

Because t(9;22)(q34;q11) represents the genetic hallmark of chronic myeloid leukemia (CML),[19] the general structure of this translocation, together with the physiopathologic functions of the loci involved, have been described in Chapter 2 of this book, to which the reader is referred. In almost 50 per cent of adult ALL cases showing a Ph[1] chromosome, the abnormality strictly resembles the one detected in CML both at the cytogenetic and at the molecular level.[20–24] The 5′ first four exons of the *bcr* gene at 22q11 are joined in the same transcriptional orientation to the second exon of the *abl* gene on chromosome 9q34 (Fig. 12–3). This novel transcriptional unit codes for a hybrid *bcr-abl* mRNA and protein called p210.[23,24] Experimental studies and analysis of p210 from patient samples both demonstrate that the *bcr* domain activates the tyrosine kinase activity of the *abl* protein[25] and converts it into a transforming protein for hematopoietic cells.[26–29]

In the remaining 50 per cent of ALL cases, the patients' cells exhibit a p190 *bcr-abl* fusion protein instead of the more common p210.[30–34] In these cases, the chromosome 22 breakpoints do not fall within the major breakpoint cluster region (MBCR) detected in p210-positive cases, but fall more 5′ in the *bcr* gene, and constitute the minor breakpoint cluster region (mbcr) located in the first intron of the *bcr* gene[30–38] (Fig. 12–3). Within the small percentage of childhood ALL cases carrying a *bcr-abl* translocation, p190 accounts for the majority,[38] whereas in adult ALL p190 and p210 are more equally distributed. In the face of the heterogeneity of *bcr-abl* rearrangements in Ph[1]-positive ALL, it has been proposed that ALL cases bearing a p210 protein represent the blast crisis arising from previous clinically silent CML, and that these cases should be considered as a disease distinct from de novo Ph[1] ALL harboring p190 *bcr-abl*.[38–40]

The p190 protein displays a more potent tyrosine kinase activity and transforming potential in vitro when com-

TABLE 12–2. IMMUNOLOGIC CLASSIFICATION OF ACUTE LYMPHOBLASTIC LEUKEMIA*

	TdT	CD19	CD10	I_{gH}	I_{gL}	cIg	sIg	CD7	TCR
B-Cell Lineage									
Early pre-B	+	+	+/−[†]	+	+ or −	−	−	−	−/+
Pre-B	+	+	+/−	+	+ or −	+	−	−	−/+
B cell	+	+	+/−	+	+ or −	−	+	−	−
T-Cell Lineage									
T-ALL	+	−	−/+[‡]	−/+	−	−	−	+	+

*TdT, terminal deoxynucleotidyl transferase; I_{gH}, immunoglobulin heavy-chain locus (+, rearranged, −, germline); I_{gL}, immunoglobulin light-chain locus (+, rearranged; −, germline); cIg, cytoplasmic immunoglobulins; sIg, surface immunoglobulins; TCR, T-cell receptor (+, rearranged; − germline).

[†] +/−, occasionally negative.

[‡] −/+, occasionally positive.

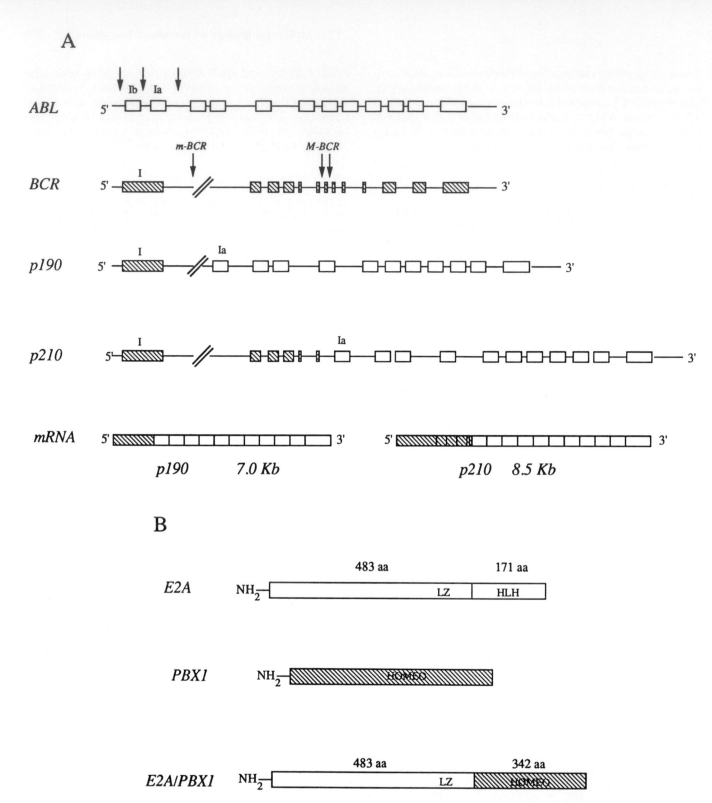

Figure 12–3. Schematic representation of the most common pathologic fusion transcripts generated by chromosomal rearrangement in ALL. *bcr-abl*, *E2A-PBX1*, *hrx-ENL*, and *SIL-tal-1* are included in panels A, B, C, and D, respectively. *A*, The configuration of normal genomic *abl* and *bcr*, together with the preferential breakpoint sites (indicated by arrows) are shown in the upper half of the panel. The lower half shows the result of the two *bcr-abl* types of translocation at the genomic and transcript level (p190, p210). *B*, The normal *E2A* and *PBX1* genes are shown, together with their functional domains (LZ, leucine zipper; HLH, helix-loop-helix; homeo, homeodomain) and the fusion transcript resulting from their reciprocal translocation. *C*, The normal *hrx* and *ENL* genes, involved in t(11;19)(q23;p23), are shown in the upper half of the panel, together with their functional domains. After the translocation, two distinct fusion transcripts are formed, represented in the lower half of the panel. *D*, The *SIL* and *tal-1* loci in the normal genomic configuration are shown in the upper half of the panel. The dotted lines indicate the portion of the *SIL* and *tal-1* loci that participate in giving the pathologic *tal*[d] fusion transcript, represented in the lower half of the panel. *Illustration continued on opposite page*

pared to p210.[41,42] In vivo models for Ph[1]-positive ALL have been developed to validate and elucidate the pathogenetic role of *bcr-abl*. These models involve the use of either p190 or p210. A high proportion of p190 transgenic animals developed ALL,[43] whereas irradiated mice whose bone marrow had been reconstituted with bone marrow cells infected with a p210 retroviral vector exhibited a wide variety of myeloid and lymphoid neoplastic disorders.[27–29] Clonal analysis of leukemic lymphoblasts from the p190 transgenes demonstrated that *bcr-abl*, in the absence of other chromosomal abnormalities, is sufficient to cause ALL.[44] In addition, *bcr-abl* confers growth factor independence in vitro to B cells and induces autocrine

release of interleukin 7.[45] Finally, recent studies have shown that, in t(9;22)(q34;q11) of both ALL and CML, the der(9) and the der(22) are consistently of paternal and maternal origin, respectively.[46] This phenomenon, known as parental bias, is found also in other tumor-associated chromosomal abnormalities and is considered to indicate that the chromosome regions involved in the translocation are subjected to parental imprinting.[47] It may be suggested that parental bias in *bcr-abl* translocations reflects differential expression of the parental versus maternal alleles of the normal genes, or, alternatively, that paternal and maternal copies of *bcr* and *abl* are characterized by differential predisposition to chromosomal rearrangement.

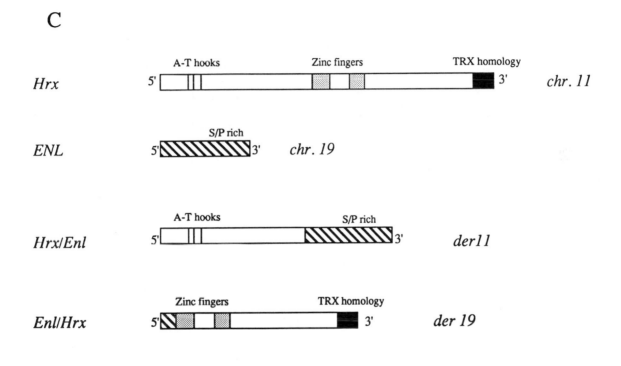

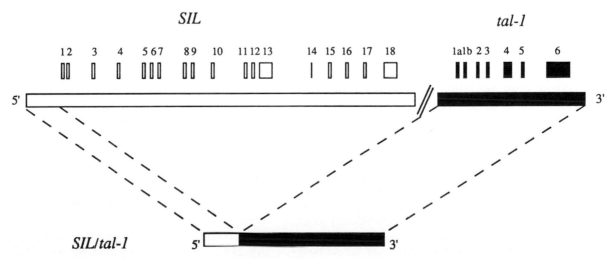

Figure 12–3. *Continued*

t(1;19)(q23;p13) AND *E2A-PBX1*

Twenty-five per cent of cases of pre-B ALL and 1 per cent of early pre-B ALL harbor a t(1;19)(q23;p13) translocation, making it the most common translocation of childhood ALL.[10,13,48–54] The *E2A* gene consistently is located at the breakpoint on chromosome 19.[55] It encodes for the E12 and E47 proteins, which contain DNA-binding domains, such as the basic helix-loop-helix (HLH) domain.[56] As a result of the translocation, *E2A* is juxtaposed with a homeobox gene, termed *PBX1*, normally located on chromosome 1 at q23[57,58] (Fig. 12–3) and a *5'E2A-3'PBX1* fusion transcript is expressed from the 19⁺ chromosome. The point of fusion for *E2A* and *PBX1* chimeric RNAs is highly consistent, occurring at precisely the same location in all cases of t(1;19)(q23;p13). *PBX1* is not normally expressed in lymphoid cells and, most notably, it is never detected in pre-B ALL cases lacking the translocation.[57,58] Conversely, *E2A* is expressed rather ubiquitously, including in lymphoid cells. In pre-B ALL cells carrying t(1;19)(q23;p13), *E2A-PBX1* fusion transcripts and proteins, consisting of the *E2A* transcriptional-activating motif and the *PBX1* DNA-binding homeodomain, are formed that are expressed at levels expected for *E2A*.[57,58] Among the various hypotheses proposed to explain the oncogenic conversion of *E2A-PBX1*, two are particularly attractive. On the one hand, it is possible that the fusion protein retains its ability to bind DNA sites recognized by *PBX1*, resulting in aberrant expression of *PBX1* target genes normally inactive in pre-B cells. On the other hand, it has been speculated that the translocated portion of *E2A* allows *PBX1* to interact with components of the transcription machinery with which it normally does not interact. Regardless of the mechanism of oncogenic conversion, the pathogenic action of *E2A-PBX1* is well documented because *E2A-PBX1* transfection causes malignant transformation in experimental models.[59]

LESIONS INVOLVING 11q23

Chromosomal breaks at 11q23 represent a frequent finding in ALL and in other hematopoietic tumors.[10,13,48] The t(4;11)(q21;q23), t(11;19)(q23;p23), and t(1;11)(p32;q23) translocations are detected in 10, 2 and less than 1 per cent of ALL cases, respectively.[60–62] Reciprocal translocations involving chromosomes 9 and 10, as well as interstitial deletions at 11q23, also are observed, although more rarely.

Recently, a gene on 11q23 was cloned from a t(4;11)(q21;q23) and a t(11;19)(q23;p23) translocation and was shown to undergo structural alterations in virtually all ALL cases harboring a break at 11q23.[63–68] This gene (named *ALL-1, hrx,* or *MLL*) codes for an unusually large protein that is a homologue of *Drosophila trithorax* and is involved in development through homeotic gene regulation.[66–68] The homology of *ALL-1/hrx/MLL* involves three domains within the coding sequence: Two regions in the middle of the protein contain DNA-binding motifs analogous to zinc finger domains in the *Drosophila* gene, and the third homologous region represents the carboxyl terminus of the protein[66–68] (Fig. 12–3). Unlike *trithorax*,

the amino terminus of *ALL-1/hrx/MLL* contains three small domains with significant homology to the AT hook motifs commonly observed in the DNA-binding high-mobility group I (HMG-I) proteins.[66–69] *ALL-1/hrx/MLL*, therefore, might bind to DNA in two independent ways: Its zinc fingers might bind DNA within the major groove, while the AT hooks would confer ability to bind DNA within the minor groove at AT-rich sites. Based on what is known for the *Drosophila* gene,[70] it is very likely that *ALL-1/hrx/MLL* is a transcription factor that might play a role in controlling genes involved in development and/or differentiation. Similarly to *trithorax, ALL-1/hrx/MLL* is expressed in a variety of tissues, including those of hematopoietic origin.[66–68]

In both t(4;11)(q21;q23) and t(11;19)(q23;p23), *ALL-1/hrx/MLL* is split between 11q23 and the partner chromosome and gives rise to fusion transcripts composed of either the 5' or the 3' portion of *ALL-1/hrx/MLL* and novel genes from chromosomes 4 or 19[66–68] (Fig. 12–3). *AF-4* on chromosome 4 and *ENL* on chromosome 19 are involved in the fusion transcripts; of the two, only *ENL* has been characterized in detail, and has been shown to be expressed in a variety of normal tissues, both lymphoid and nonlymphoid.[68] Sequence analysis of the ENL protein displayed no similarity to any previously reported protein; although none of the known DNA-binding motifs is recognizable in ENL, its high serine and proline contents are common features of activation domains found in transcription factors. Two chimeric transcripts are expressed as a consequence of t(411)(q21;q23) (i.e., *5'ALL-1/hrx/MLL–3'AF-4* and *5'AF-4–3'ALL/hrx/MLL*) and of t(11;19)(q23;p23) (i.e., *5'ALL-1/hrx/MLL–3'ENL* and *5'ENL–3'ALL-1/hrx/MLL*); in both translocations, the transcripts containing the 5' portion of *ALL-1/hrx/MLL* exhibit the AT hook motifs but lack the *trithorax*-homologous domains[66–68] (Fig. 12–3). Conversely, the *trithorax*-homologous domain is present in the transcripts containing the 3' portion of the gene.[66–68] As a consequence, both reciprocal proteins might bind DNA within either the major or the minor groove, supporting the hypothesis that the translocation products might function as a transcription factor. Although *ALL-1/hrx/MLL* seems to be the gene involved in all 11q23 translocations and deletions of ALL, the partner genes on the reciprocal chromosomes have not been identified yet.

The mechanism of t(4;11)(q21;q23) formation involves the V-D-J recombinase utilized for physiologic immunoglobulin gene rearrangement and is implicated in many chromosomal translocations involving antigen receptor loci.[71] This example, together with *tal-1* abnormalities in T-ALL (see later in this chapter), suggests that the recombinase enzymes might be active in mediating gene rearrangements in lymphoid neoplasms even if no antigen receptor locus is involved in the translocation.

TRANSLOCATIONS INVOLVING c-*myc*

Translocations between the c-*myc* proto-oncogene on chromosome 8 band q24 and an immunoglobulin locus [t(8;14)(q24;q32), t(2;8)(p11;q24), and t(8;22)(q24;q11)] are found in 100 per cent of B-cell ALL cases.[72–76] A preferential rearrangement of c-myc with the α heavy-chain locus on chromosome 14 has been reported in this form of leukemia, when compared to other lymphoid tumors carrying c-myc translocations.[75,76] A detailed description of the molecular mechanisms of c-myc translocations is presented in the section of this chapter regarding B-cell non-Hodgkin's lymphomas.

Rearrangements between c-myc and TCR α or δ in the form of t(8;14)(q24;q11) also have been described and are present in a small fraction of T-ALL cases.[77–79]

tal-1 TRANSLOCATIONS AND DELETIONS

Thirty per cent of T-ALL patients bear a rearranged tal-1 gene, making this abnormality the most frequent genetic lesion of T-ALL.[80,81] tal-1, also called SCL, codes for a protein containing an HLH DNA-binding and dimerization motif that is highly homologous to the ones found in other HLH proteins involved in lymphoid cell neoplasms, such as E2A, lyl-1, and c-myc.[82] The hypothesis that tal-1 functions as a transcription factor, initially based on its structural features, is confirmed by in vitro experiments showing that tal-1 indeed is capable of heterodimerizing with other proteins and of specific DNA binding.[83] The expression of tal-1 in lymphohematopoietic tissues is heterogeneous: It is present in cells with stem cell attributes but is consistently absent in thymocytes or other mature cells.[82]

Two mechanisms account for tal-1 disruption[80,81,84–90] (Fig. 12–3): In a small fraction of cases, the tal-1 locus at 1p32 is involved in translocations (designated tal[t]) with a TCR locus [t(1;14)(p32;q11) or t(1;7)(p32;q35)], whereas the most frequent type of lesion is represented by minute interstitial deletions (tal[d]) around the tal-1 locus that are not detectable at the level of cytogenetic resolution. In T-ALL cases showing the tal[t] abnormality, the translocation cleaves the tal-1 gene on chromosome 1 within a breakpoint cluster region of approximately 1 kb, separating the 5' end from the rest of the gene.[80,81,84–90] The truncated tal-1 is thus transposed from its normal location on chromosome 1 into the TCR α/δ chain locus on 14q11 or, more rarely, into the TCR β locus at 7q35.[84–90] In the most frequent tal[d] type of tal-1 rearrangement, a 90-kb deletion disrupts the tal-1 5' regulatory region.[80–90] In this case, the recombination event links tal-1 to another gene, called SIL, centromeric to tal-1 on chromosome 1p.[91] Despite the substantial size of the deletions, tal[d] abnormalities are indistinguishable in different T-ALL patients when probed by Southern blotting. The consistent site specificity of tal[d] rearrangements reflects the presence on both deletion ends of consensus heptamer sequences, which would function as substrates for illegitimate activity of the immunoglobulin-TCR recombinase, even in the absence of an associated nonamer element.[80–90]

Both tal[t] and tal[d] cause 5' truncation of tal-1 and lead to tal-1 ectopic expression as a result of juxtaposition with a heterologous promoter active in T cells, represented by TCR or SIL regulatory elements in tal[t] and tal[d], respectively.[80–91] Fusion transcripts, either between tal-1 and the δ locus or between tal-1 and SIL, arise in both situations and allow the coding of a full-length tal-1 protein.

tal-1 rearrangements are restricted to T-ALL and are never found in B-lineage ALL[81]; within T-ALL, patients with tal[d] or tal[t] do not differ significantly from T-ALL cases without tal-1 abnormalities in either clinical or immunophenotypic profile.[81]

t(10;14)(q24;q11) AND HOX11

The t(10;14)(q24;q11) translocation, found in approximately 7 per cent of T-ALL cases, involves the TCR δ chain locus on chromosome 14 and HOX11, a homeobox-containing gene, on chromosome 10.[92–94] The expression of this gene in normal adult tissues apparently is restricted to the liver, whereas it is highly transcribed in T-ALL cells carrying the translocation, but not in normal T cells or T-ALL cases lacking t(10;14)(q24;q11). The main effect of the translocation, therefore, seems to consist in redirecting the transcriptional control of HOX11 under the influence of the δ TCR promoter/enhancer, causing HOX11 ectopic expression in leukemic T cells.[92–94] In addition, because the breakpoints on chromosome 10 are tightly clustered and alter the 5' regulatory region of the gene, it is also possible that HOX11 overexpression results from loss of a silencer element or tissue-specific regulatory domain.[92–94]

LESIONS AT 11p15 AND 11p13

The short arm of chromosome 11 is involved in two distinct translocations found in T-ALL. Although the partner chromosome most commonly is represented by chromosome 14 at the TCR δ chain locus, resulting in t(11;14)(p15;q11) and t(11;14)(p13;q11),[10,13,48,60,61] variant translocations involving the TCR β chain gene on chromosome 7 also have been reported.[95] Breaks at 11p13 are detected in 10 per cent of T-ALL, whereas 11p15 is more rarely implicated. When compared to the bulk of T-ALL cases, patients harboring an 11p translocation display distinctive clinical features, as revealed by the common observation that these patients tend to co-express CD4 and CD8 on the leukemic blasts and are more prone to develop large mediastinal masses.[96]

The proto-oncogenes altered by these two translocations make up part of the family of transcription factors possessing LIM domains, and in particular of the rhombotin gene subfamily, and are called rhom-1/ttg-1 (11p15) and rhom-2/ttg-2 (11p13).[97–101] Both genes contain two highly conserved, cysteine-rich motifs (LIM domains) that show homology to zinc-binding proteins and iron-sulfur centers of ferridoxins. Although the exact function of the LIM domains is presently unknown, it has been proposed that LIM domain proteins might act, directly or through heterodimerization with other rhombotin-like proteins, by altering the expression of genes required for the determination of a specific cell fate. Consistent with this view is the proposed oncogenic mechanism of rhom-1/ttg-1 and rhom-2/ttg-2: Because expression of both genes is virtually absent in normal thymus, and in the case of rhom-1/ttg-1 is restricted to the neural lineage,[102,103] aberrant expression of rhom-1/ttg-1 and rhom-2/ttg-2 caused by the·

translocation would lead to ectopic activation of genes under the control of *rhom-1/ttg-1* and *rhom-2/ttg-2*.

Direct evidence of the oncogenicity of *rhom-1/ttg-1* has been gained recently using the transgenic mouse model: T-ALL developed at a high frequency in the transgenic animals, and displayed features similar to human leukemias with t(11;14)(p13;q11), including a high frequency of double-positive cases (i.e., cases expressing both CD4 and CD8) and marked thymus enlargement.[104]

OTHER STRUCTURAL ABNORMALITIES

Among B-cell–lineage ALL, t(5;14)(q31;32) and t(15;17)(q22;p13) have been associated with pre-B ALL with eosinophilia and early pre-B ALL with disseminated intravascular coagulation, respectively.[105–107] t(5;14)(q31;q32) causes the juxtaposition of the *IL-3* gene on chromosome 5 with the Ig_H locus on chromosome 14, resulting in *IL-3* deregulation.[108,109] t(17;19)(q22;p13) produces a chimeric transcription factor consisting of portions of the *E2A* gene [also involved in t(1;19)] fused to the basic DNA-binding and leucine zipper motifs of a new gene, called *hlf* (for hepatic leukemia factor).[110,111] Among translocations that are restricted to T-ALL, although at low frequency, t(7;19)(q35;p13), t(7;9)(q34;q32), t(7;9)(q34;q34.3), and t(1;7)(p34;q34) have been characterized in detail. Two transcription factors of the basic HLH family, *lyl-1* and *tal-2*, are involved in t(7;19)(q35;p13) and t(7;9)(q34;q32), respectively,[112,113] causing their deregulated expression. Although a common motif of T-ALL translocations is represented by activation of transcription factors, two different types of genes are involved in t(7;9)(q344.3) and t(1;7)(p34;q34): *tan-1*, a gene highly homologous to the *Drosophila* gene *notch*, is consistently altered in t(7;9)(q;34;q34.3) of T-ALL,[114] and t(1;7)(p34;q34) causes deregulated expression of the *lck* locus, which codes for a lymphocyte-specific tyrosine kinase.[115]

Point mutations in the *ras* family genes are restricted to a subset of ALL representing approximately 10 to 15 per cent of all cases, independent of the immunologic subtype.[116,117] Most commonly the N-*ras* gene at codons 12 or 13 is affected, in agreement with the mutational spectrum of *ras* genes in hematopoietic tumors. N-*ras* mutations are a potentially useful clinical marker because they correlate with a significantly high risk for hematologic relapse and a trend toward a lower rate of complete remission.[117]

Finally, the role of the *p53* tumor suppressor gene in ALL pathogenesis has been investigated widely. *p53* mutations are a rare event in early pre-B and pre-B ALL, whereas they are present in more than 50 per cent of B-cell ALL cases that also harbor a rearranged c-*myc*.[118] Other putative tumor suppressor genes are thought to map on the short arm of chromosome 9 and the long arm of chromosome 6, which are sites of frequent deletions in ALL.[60,61,119–121]

PLOIDY ABNORMALITIES

Variations in chromosomal numbers are a frequent event in ALL and are considered an important prognostic index. Cases with more than 50 chromosomes per leukemic cell represent one fourth of childhood ALL cases, and hyperdiploidy of more than 50 chromosomes has proved to be an index of durable responses to treatment.[10,122] Hyperdiploidy of more than 50 chromosomes is most frequently detected in early pre-B ALL and clusters with other favorable prognostic markers, such as CD10 expression, low leukocyte count, and age between 2 and 10.[123] Interestingly, within this group of ALL, cases with chromosomal structural abnormalities in addition to hyperdiploidy of more than 50 chromosomes have a less favorable prognosis.[124] Pseudiploidy, characterized by 46 chromosomes per cell in the presence of structural abnormalities, accounts for up to 40 per cent of childhood ALL cases and reflects a poor clinical outcome.[10] Finally, hyperdiploidy of 47 to 50 chromosomes, which is detectable in 15 per cent of children with ALL, implies an intermediate prognosis when compared to the previous two groups.[10]

Clinicopathologic Correlations

The genetic lesions previously described variously distribute in each ALL subtype. The frequency of association between a specific genetic lesion and a defined ALL subtype is reported in Table 12–3.

EARLY PRE-B ALL

Various genetic lesions are detected in early pre-B ALL, although only a few are specifically restricted to this type of leukemia (Table 12–3). *bcr-abl* rearrangements are detected in 5 per cent and 25 per cent of childhood and adult early pre-B ALL, respectively, representing the most common abnormality detected in ALL of adults.[10,13,125–128] Features closely associated with the presence of the Ph^1 chromosome in childhood ALL include an older age at presentation, high leukocyte counts, and a high incidence of central nervous system (CNS) disease.[125–128] Overall, children with Ph^1-positive ALL have a dismal prognosis, and are candidates for experimental therapy in the early phases of the disease.[126] *E2A-PBX* translocations, which characterize pre-B ALL, also are found in a small fraction of these cases (1 per cent), together with N-*ras* mutations and *p53* inactivation.[50–58,116–118] Like *bcr-abl* rearrangements, N-*ras* mutations in early pre-B ALL are well-established markers of a dismal prognosis when compared with cases lacking these lesions.[117] In contrast, hyperdiploidy of more than 50 chromosomes, which shows its highest incidence in early pre-B ALL, is considered a favorable prognostic marker.[122,123] A distinct subtype of early pre-B ALL is those cases harboring breaks at 11q23. The most common translocation, t(4;11)(q21;q23), characterizes more than two thirds of cases arising in infants; these cases frequently display a mixed lymphomonocytic phenotype and are characterized by a very poor prognosis.[63–71,129–136] Finally, *E2A-hlf* fusion transcripts identify those rare cases of early pre-B ALL that are accompanied by disseminated intravascular coagulation.[110,111] Uncharacterized molecular lesions in early pre-B ALL include deletions of 6q and 9p.[119-121]

PRE-B ALL

Twenty-five per cent of pre-B ALL cases bear a t(1;19)(q23;p13) translocation and form an *E2A-PBX1* fusion transcript.[55-58,137] These cases are associated with high-risk features, high leukocyte counts, and an adverse prognosis.[52-54] Recently, it has been shown that the prognosis improved significantly when patients were treated with an intensified chemotherapeutic protocol, emphasizing the clinical relevance of early detection of this gene rearrangement.[53,54,137] *bcr-abl* rearrangements also are present more frequently in adult (25 per cent) than in childhood (5 per cent) pre-B ALL.[125-128] The prognostic relevance of *bcr-abl* translocations is similar to that reported for early pre-B ALL. N-*ras* mutations are detected in 10 to 20 per cent of cases.[116,117] As in early pre-B ALL, both *bcr-abl* rearrangements and N-*ras* mutations signify a dismal prognosis.[117,126] *p53* inactivation, 6q⁻, and 9p⁻ also are found in variable proportions of patients.[119-121]

B-CELL ALL

B-cell ALL usually is considered as the leukemic counterpart of Burkitt's lymphoma (BL) and, like BL, is characterized by a very poor prognosis. The close clinical similarity between BL and B-cell ALL is further supported by molecular evidence showing an identical pattern of genetic lesions detected in the two types of tumors.[72-76] One hundred per cent of cases of B-cell ALL bear a translocated c-*myc*, accompanied in 50 to 60 per cent of cases by *p53* inactivation.[72-76,118] The frequent co-occurrence of these two lesions has suggested a putative synergic role of c-*myc* and *p53* in conferring tumorigenicity to B cells.

As in BL, c-*myc* translocations occur between chromosome 8 at q24, site of the c-*myc* gene, and an immunoglobulin locus[72-76]; B-cell ALL seems to display a preferential involvement of the immunoglobulin α chain locus on 14q32.[75,76] Other chromosomal translocations characteristic of B-lineage ALL are never detected in this type of leukemia.

ALL IN INFANTS

Altogether, breaks at 11q23, mainly represented by t(4;11)(q21;q23), comprise about two thirds of the chromosomal abnormalities in ALL in infants.[129-132,138] In clinical terms, patients with rearrangements at 11q23, in particular the t(4;11)(q21;q23) translocation, display distinct features, including prevalence in children under 1 year of age, hyperleukocytosis, organomegaly, early CNS disease, and a poor prognosis.[129-134,138] These cases are classified as early pre-B ALL, and many samples express the myeloid/monocytic CD15 and CD33 antigens in addition to B-cell markers, and are therefore considered as biphenotypic ALL.[135,136] The expression of mixed phenotypic character together with the potential of monocytic differentiation of 11q23-rearranged lymphoblasts would suggest that a gene involved in early lymphoid-myeloid differentiation might be altered in a stem or multipotent cell capable of either lymphoid or myelomonocytic differentiation.

T-CELL ALL

Whereas certain types of ALL are characterized by few or even unique chromosomal abnormalities that are found in a high proportion of the patient population [e.g., B-cell ALL and c-*myc* activation; infant ALL and t(4;11)], cytogenetic and molecular studies have not uncovered a

TABLE 12-3. MOLECULAR LESIONS ASSOCIATED WITH ALL

	EARLY PRE-B ALL	PRE-B ALL	B-CELL ALL	T-ALL
bcr-abl	5–25%*	5–25%*	—	—
E2A-PBX1	1%	25%	—	—
ALL-1/hrx/MLL	10–75%†	10%	—	—
IL-3	—	Rare	—	—
E2A-hlf	Rare	—	—	—
c-*myc*	—	—	100%	Rare
tal-1	—	—	—	30%
HOX11	—	—	—	7%
rhom-1/ttg-1	—	—	—	Rare
rhom-2/ttg-2	—	—	—	10%
TAN-1	—	—	—	Rare
lck	—	—	—	Rare
tal-2	—	—	—	Rare
lyl-1	—	—	—	Rare
ras	10–20%	10–20%	—	—
p53	10%	10%	60%	Rare§
9p⁻	30%	30%	NA‡	30%
6q⁻	10%	10%	NA	10%

* 5% in children and 25% in adults
† 75% in infants under 1 year.
‡ NA, not assessed.
§ More frequent cases at relapse.

major genetic lesion associated with T-ALL, but instead have defined a number of chromosomal abnormalities, each of which is found in a relatively small proportion of T-ALL cases (Table 12–3). The involvement of various members of different families of transcription factors in T-ALL pathogenesis is a frequent event; these factors include, in order of frequency, *tal-1*, *rhom-2/ttg-2*, *HOX11*, c-*myc*, and the more rarely implicated *tal-2*, *rhom-1/ttg-1*, and *lyl-1* proto-oncogenes.[77–103] With the exception of the rhombotin-like genes, the other transcription factors altered in T-ALL do not seem to be associated with specific features of T-ALL biologic and clinical behavior, nor to significantly influence prognosis.[10] It is possible that the different transcription factors altered in T-ALL may regulate expression of the same subordinate genes, leading to a common molecular pathway in T-ALL leukemogenesis. Besides transcription factors, other types of proto-oncogenes—such as *tan-1*, an integral membrane protein,[114] and *lck*, a tyrosine kinase[115]—participate in T-ALL leukemogenesis, although at lesser frequencies. 9p deletions are detected in 30 per cent of cases, and 6q$^-$ is present in around 10 per cent of T-ALL cases.[119–121]

DIAGNOSTIC RELEVANCE OF GENETIC LESIONS

From a diagnostic standpoint, the usefulness of genetic analysis of the described molecular lesions is twofold. On the one hand, at diagnosis, it is relevant to establish the presence of genetic markers carrying prognostic value: In this respect, the frequently poor diagnostic outcome of ALL metaphase preparations may be overcome by molecular methods, allowing the analysis of virtually all patients. On the other hand, specific genetic lesions in a patient can be used as markers for the evaluation of minimal residual disease after chemotherapy or bone marrow transplantation, which is best assessed by molecular assays with high sensitivity, such as polymerase chain reaction (PCR)–based assays.

Given the relevant prognostic value of t(9;22)(q34; q11), molecular assays aimed at establishing the presence of *bcr-abl* frequently are used in clinical practice to identify high-risk patients at diagnosis. Southern blotting allows the detection of rearrangements leading to p210, whereas a reverse PCR approach is needed to identify the p190 type of translocations, the breakpoints of which are highly heterogeneous.[139] In addition, PCR studies of *bcr-abl* rearrangements also have proved useful to monitor minimal residual disease after bone marrow transplantation or intensive chemotherapy.[38,139,140] t(1;19)(q23;p13) represents another marker that significantly influences therapeutic strategies[53,54,137]; recently, the consistency of the *E2A-PBX1* breakpoints in different cases has allowed researchers to design a PCR-based assay that detects the translocation in virtually all patients.[141,142] Finally, a PCR-based assay also has been proposed for the detection of *tal-1* rearrangements[143]; because *tal-1* lacks prognostic value at diagnosis, but it is present in a significant proportion of T-ALL cases, this assay will be useful mostly for minimal residual disease monitoring.

B-CELL NON-HODGKIN'S LYMPHOMA

General Overview

B-cell non-Hodgkin's lymphoma accounts for approximately 3 to 5 per cent of deaths from cancer in the western world.[144] B-NHL includes a group of neoplasms that share a target tissue, mature B cells, yet are characterized by a high degree of biologic and clinical heterogeneity. The frequency of B-NHL subtypes varies markedly with age: overall, low-grade B-NHL subtypes are most common in adult and elderly individuals, whereas high-grade B-NHL subtypes occur more frequently in children and young adults. The most widely used classification system for B-NHL is based on the degree of clinical aggressiveness correlated with the stage of differentiation and the pattern of growth (e.g., follicular or diffuse) of the tumor[145] (Fig. 12–1). B-NHL cells retain the characteristics of their normal counterpart cells to a greater or lesser extent, reproducing the same cytoarchitectonics (follicular versus diffuse), cell size (small or large), nuclear shape (cleaved or noncleaved), and immunologic features, all of which bear clinical and prognostic implications.[145] B-NHL may originate from primary B cells not yet exposed to antigens, as in the case of BL and small-cell lymphomas, or from germinal center cells, as in follicular and diffuse B-NHL. Although the etiopathogenesis of these neoplasms remains largely unclarified, it has become clear that the marked heterogeneity of B-NHL reflects distinct pathogenic mechanisms, characterized by the selective association of a genetic lesion with a specific type of B-NHL.

Genetic Lesions

Genetic lesions of B-NHL can be grouped into lesions that are present throughout all human cancers, although at different frequency (e.g., *p53* mutations), and lesions that are characteristic of B-NHL (Table 12–4). The following pages focus mainly on the latter group of genetic lesions, mostly represented by chromosomal translocations. A distinctive, although not constant, feature of B-NHL translocations is the involvement of an antigen receptor locus as one of the partner chromosomes (18): The immunoglobulin genes mainly are affected, most frequently at the Ig$_H$ locus on 14q32, but also in rarer cases at the Ig$_\kappa$ or Ig$_\lambda$ loci on 2p11 and 22q11, respectively. The molecular basis for the preferential involvement of antigen receptor loci in B-NHL translocations has been discussed in detail in a previous chapter of this book.

TRANSLOCATIONS INVOLVING *bcl-2*

The *bcl-2* gene was identified by molecular cloning of the t(14;18)(q32;q21) translocation, which is the most frequent chromosomal abnormality in B-NHL, being present in virtually all cases of follicular lymphomas as well as in a relatively small proportion of diffuse lymphomas.[146–149] The translocation joins the *bcl-2* gene at its 3' untranslated region to Ig$_H$ sequences, resulting in dereg-

TABLE 12–4. FREQUENCY OF GENETIC LESIONS IN B-NHL SUBTYPES

	bcl-2	c-myc	bcl-1	bcl-6	p53	6q−
Low Grade						
Small lymphocytic	—	—	—	—	—	20%
Mantle zone lymphoma	—	—	50%		—	NA
Follicular, small cell	70–90%	—	—	—	—	20%
Follicular, mixed	70–90%	—	—	—	—	20%
Intermediate Grade						
Follicular, large cell	70–90%	—	—	—	—	20%
Diffuse, small cell	—	5–20%	—	30%	—	20%
Diffuse, mixed	—	5–20%	—	30%	—	20%
Diffuse, large cell	—	5–20%	—	30%	—	20%
High Grade						
Immunoblastic	—	20%	—	—	—	20%
Lymphoblastic	—	NA†	—	—	NA	NA
Small noncleaved	—	100%	—	—	30%	20%
"Transformed"*	90%	10%	—	—	70%	NA

* B-NHLs that have undergone histologic progression from a follicular to a diffuse pattern.
† NA, not assessed.

ulation of the *bcl-2* gene expression because of the nearby presence of immunoglobulin transcriptional regulatory elements[146–152] (Fig. 12–4). Because *bcl-2* is placed in the same transcriptional orientation as Ig_H, a chimeric transcript is produced. However, the translocation does not interrupt the protein coding sequence of *bcl-2*, so that translocated alleles produce a normal protein. The consequence of the translocation is the presence within the cells of constitutively high levels of bcl-2 protein, as a result of both increased transcription and more efficient processing of the *bcl-2*-Ig fusion allele.[149–153] Approximately 70 per cent of the breakpoints on chromosome 18

are clustered within a MBCR, and the remaining cases usually break in the more distant mbcr.[146–148,154] Because neither of these two translocation hot spots possesses the typical heptamer-spacer-nonamer motif recognized by the immunoglobulin recombinase, the mechanism for localized *bcl-2* rearrangement remains elusive.[155,156]

Although it is still controversial, most data suggest that bcl-2 is a mitochondrial protein that makes up part of a distinct category of oncoproteins involved in programmed cell death regulation.[157] In contrast to most of the other oncoproteins involved in lymphoid neoplasia, which act as regulators of cell proliferation, bcl-2 has no obvious

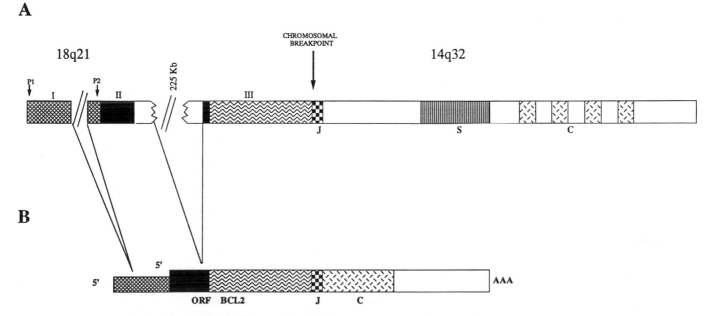

Figure 12–4. *bcl-2*–Ig fusion gene. The t(14;18) translocation introduces *bcl-2* into the immunoglobulin (Ig) locus, placing it in the same transcriptional orientation as Ig and generating a chimeric *bcl-2*–Ig mRNA. The genomic breakpoint of the der14 is shown in *A* and the fusion transcript in *B*. The *bcl-2* exons (I, II, III) and promoters (P1, P2) are shown, as well as the J, S, and C regions of the Ig locus.

proliferative effects, but instead it prevents programmed cell death or apoptosis. An example of this typically is represented by its ability to promote cell survival without simulating cell proliferation in growth factor–dependent cell lines deprived of cytokine.[158,159] Furthermore, the bcl-2 protein displays a topographic distribution restricted within mature tissues characterized by apoptotic cell death, such as the secondary germinal centers or proliferation zones of epithelia.[160] The location of bcl-2 within the cell coincides with the distribution of mitochondria, and the bcl-2 protein copurifies with mitochondrial enzymes such as succinate dehydrogenase[157,161,162]; however, the precise biochemical function through which bcl-2 exerts its antiapoptotic activity is not yet known.

In the normal settings, *bcl-2* plays a relevant role in normal generation of memory B cells, as suggested by the restriction of *bcl-2* expression to the zones of surviving B cells within germinal centers and as directly demonstrated by experiments in transgenic animals.[160,163] In contrast, the role of *bcl-2* in B cell neoplasia is complex. Although *bcl-2* as a single agent is not sufficient to confer tumorigenicity to B cells, it potentiates c-*myc*–transforming activity both in vitro and in vivo.[158,164,165] In addition, transgenic animals carrying an activated *bcl-2* gene develop a follicular lymphoproliferation involving the accumulation of long-lived resting B cells analogous to that seen in human follicular lymphoma.[166] Analogous to the human disease, over time some of these mice develop a more aggressive B cell lymphoma related to the occurrence of additional genetic alterations in a cell that already carries an activated *bcl-2* gene.[167] The fact that *bcl-2* activation per se is not fully tumorigenic is further supported by the puzzling finding of translocated *bcl-2* in 50 per cent of benign lymph nodes and tonsils displaying follicular hyperplasia.[168] Although it is difficult to assess the exact role of *bcl-2* translocations in normal tissues, these results impose the need for a certain caution when interpreting the results of PCR-based assays aimed at defining minimal residual disease (see later in this chapter).

TRANSLOCATIONS INVOLVING c-*myc*

Various types of lymphoid neoplasms are associated with chromosomal translocations involving the c-*myc* proto-oncogene and an antigen receptor locus[72] (Fig. 12–5). Indeed, the molecular analysis of c-*myc* translocations has provided the first example of the involvement of oncogenes in tumor-associated chromosomal abnormalities and has been the model for the study of other translocations involving antigen receptor loci.

Three types of reciprocal chromosomal translocations have been shown to involve the c-*myc* locus on chromosome 8q24 and one of the immunoglobulin loci, either Ig_H, Ig_κ, or Ig_λ[72–74,169–171] (Fig. 12–5). In 80 per cent of cases, a t(8;14)(q24;q32) translocation is detectable in which breakpoints located centromeric to c-*myc* lead to its translocation into the Ig_H locus on chromosome 14q32. In the less frequent variant t(2;8)(p11;q24) (15 per cent) and t(8;22)(q24;q11) (5 per cent) translocations, an Ig_L locus is translocated telomeric to the c-*myc* locus, which remains on chromosome 8.

These translocations have been found to be associated with a heterogeneous group of B-cell neoplasms that have as a common characteristic the involvement of mature B

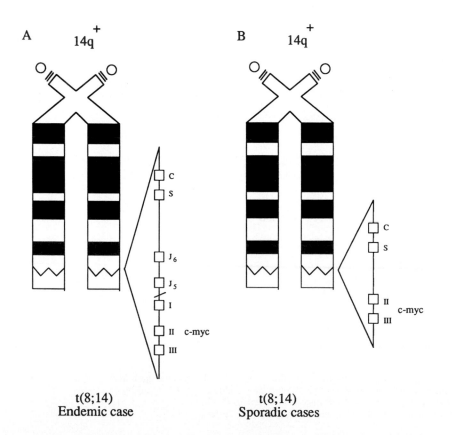

A 14q+   **B** 14q+

t(8;14)
Endemic case

t(8;14)
Sporadic cases

Figure 12–5. Schematic representation of the location of the chromosomal breakpoints within c-*myc* and Ig_H in t(8;14) of endemic BL (*A*) and of sporadic BL (*B*), t(8;22) (*C*), and t(2;8) (*D*). Boxes indicate functional regions of the Ig_H (J_H, S_μ, C_μ) and c-*myc* exons. *Illustration continued on opposite page*

cells expressing sIg. These neoplasms include: (1) B-NHL of both Burkitt and non-Burkitt type; (2) acquired immunodeficiency syndrome–associated NHL (AIDS-NHL; see also later in this chapter); and (3) B-cell ALL, as previously mentioned. Although fairly homogeneous at the microscopic level, these chromosomal recombinations are characterized by remarkable heterogeneity when dissected molecularly (Fig. 12–5). The first distinguishing feature is the position of the breakpoints, which are located 5' and centromeric to c-myc in the t(8;14) translocation, whereas they are located 3' to c-myc in the variant t(2;8) and t(8;22) translocations.[72–74,169–171] Further molecular heterogeneity can be found among t(8;14) translocations, which can be divided into two main types depending on the position of the chromosomal breakpoints on chromosomes 8 and 14.[172–174] One type, found more frequently in endemic-type BL, involves sequences on chromosome 8 at an undefined distance (>100 kb) 5' to the c-myc locus and sequences on chromosome 14 within or in proximity to the Ig_H J regions, which normally are involved in the first step (D-J) of the Ig_H gene rearrangements occurring early during B-cell differentiation. The second type, found in most B-NHL, AIDS-NHL, and B-cell ALL cases, involves sequences within or immediately 5' (<3 kb) to the c-myc gene on chromosome 8 and sequences on chromosome 14 within the Ig_H switch (S) regions, which normally are involved in heavy-chain constant region switching occurring relatively late during B-cell differentiation. Although recombinase-mediated rearrangement has been postulated as the mechanism of several translocations in lymphoid neoplasms,[18] this does not seem to be the case for translocations involving c-myc. In fact, the breakpoint sites can be outside S sequence motifs or typical J recognition signals in a proportion of cases, and, in addition, no homology is found between S sequences or D-J joining signals and breakpoint sites on chromosome 8.[174] Rather, the frequent finding of deletions and duplications at the chromosomal junctions suggests that the mechanism of c-myc translocation may rely on repair of staggered double-strand DNA breaks, leading to interchromosomal ligation of nonhomologous ends.[174]

C-myc expression is tightly regulated during normal cell proliferation and differentiation by transcriptional and posttranscriptional mechanisms.[175] Several experimental observations have indicated that this regulation is lost after chromosomal translocation and that translocated c-myc alleles may be expressed constitutively under the control immunoglobulin regulatory elements.[176–178] However, the precise mechanism by which the expression of translocated c-myc genes is deregulated and the precise role of immunoglobulin regulatory domains remain unclear. One additional feature of translocated c-myc genes that may be

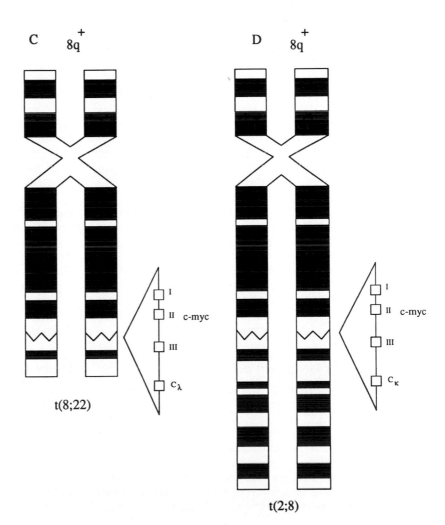

Figure 12–5. *Continued*

relevant to explain the mechanism involved in deregulation is the presence of structural alterations in the 5' regulatory domain of the gene. In a significant fraction of B-NHL, AIDS-NHL, and B-cell ALL cases, the t(8;14)(q24;q32) chromosomal breakpoint decapitates the c-*myc* gene at its first exon.[172] In all the remaining cases carrying either 5' or 3' breakpoints to the c-*myc* gene, an approximately 400-bp region spanning the first exon/first intron junction is selectively and consistently mutated in translocated c-*myc* alleles.[172,179,180] This region contains potentially important regulatory domains, and recent evidence suggests that at least one of these domains is consistently mutated, supporting a pathogenetic role of these alterations.[180]

Substantial experimental evidence documents that the constitutive expression of a normal c-*myc* protein can influence the growth and differentiation of B cells in vitro and in vivo, consistent with a role in B lymphomagenesis. In vitro, the expression of c-*myc* oncogenes transfected into Epstein-Barr virus (EBV)–immortalized human B cells, a potential natural target for c-*myc* activation in EBV-positive BL, leads to their malignant transformation.[181,182] In addition, antisense oligonucleotides directed against translocated c-*myc* mRNA are able to revert tumorigenicity of BL.[183] In vivo, the targeted expression of c-*myc* oncogenes in the B-cell lineage of transgenic mice leads to the development of B-cell malignancy at a relatively high frequency.[184]

Novel insights on the biologic role of c-*myc* in B lymphomagenesis have emerged with the identification of proteins that behave as a c-*myc* functional partner. The c-*myc* gene product is a nuclear DNA–binding phosphoprotein that contains a basic domain mediating specific DNA binding, as well as HLH and leucine zipper (LZ) domains that mediate homodimerization or heterodimerization with other specific HLH-LZ proteins.[185] A second basic-HLH-LZ protein called Max, has been identified based on its ability to form heterodimeric DNA-binding complexes with c-*myc*.[186] c-*myc* and Max together, but not c-*myc* alone, can directly regulate gene transcription; furthermore, differential target gene expression and growth phenotype can be obtained by varying the c-*myc*/Max ratio, with the heterodimeric c-*myc*/Max complex acting as a positive regulator of transcription and growth, while Max alone is a negative regulator.[187–189] Therefore, in BL or other lymphoid tumors carrying c-*myc* translocations, it may be postulated that constitutive expression of c-*myc* leads to increased formation of c-*myc*/Max complexes leading to positive growth stimulation.

TRANSLOCATIONS INVOLVING *bcl-1*

The *bcl-1* locus originally was identified as a breakpoint site on chromosome 11 in B-cell malignancies carrying the t(11;14)(q13;q32) translocation.[190–192] Translocations involving *bcl-1* characteristically are detected in 50 per cent of mantle zone lymphomas (also known as centrocytic or intermediate lymphocytic lymphomas).[193,194] Although this break initially was thought to be associated with B-cell chronic lymphocytic leukemia (B-CLL) and small-cell lymphocytic lymphoma (SCLL),[190–192] recent histologic reevaluation of *bcl-1*–positive B-CLL or SCLL cases has shown that they were in fact mantle zone lymphomas (i.e., lymphomas that derive from the mantle cells of the follicles).[193,194]

This translocation results in the juxtaposition of the Ig_H locus on chromosome 14 to sequences from chromosome 11.[190–192] Structurally, this translocation is reminiscent of the better characterized t(14;18) and t(8;14) translocations, in which a gene on chromosome 18 or 8 is transcriptionally deregulated as a result of its relocation in the vicinity of the immunoglobulin locus. By analogy, it was believed that the t(11;14) translocation would affect the transcription of a putative proto-oncogene near the *bcl-1* locus on chromosome 11. However, the predicted oncogene was not identified until recently, when the *PRAD1* gene was mapped 200 kb from the *bcl-1* locus.[195,196] The *PRAD1* gene has been shown to be identical to cyclin D1, a member of a family of proteins that regulate cell cycle progression, and seems to be consistently overexpressed in mantle zone lymphomas carrying a t(11;14)(q13;q32) translocation, but not in lymphomas with intact *bcl-1* loci.[197] The importance and mechanism of action of this putative oncogene in lymphomagenesis remains to be established through appropriate experimental studies aimed at testing the in vitro and in vivo pathogenic effect of this gene.

TRANSLOCATIONS INVOLVING *bcl-6*

Chromosomal translocations involving band 3q27 and various chromosomal sites, including the sites of the immunoglobulin loci, represent recurrent aberrations in B-NHL.[198,199] Overall, 3q27 breakpoints are detectable in 10 per cent of B-NHL cases by cytogenetic analysis. The clinicopathologic relevance of 3q27 breakpoints is underscored by their consistent association with diffuse-type B-NHL, a subtype for which no molecular lesion has yet been identified.[198,199] Recently, the 3q27 breakpoint has been cloned and a candidate proto-oncogene, termed *bcl-6*, has been identified.[200–202] The *bcl-6* gene belongs to the family of transcription factors containing zinc finger domains, and its 5' noncoding domain has been found to be rearranged in 30 per cent of diffuse large cell B-NHL cases; although the precise mechanism of activation is presently unknown, it seems that *bcl-6* transcriptional deregulation may play a role. The high frequency and selective association of *bcl-6* rearrangements with diffuse B-NHL render this genetic lesion a potentially important diagnostic marker.

OTHER STRUCTURAL ABNORMALITIES

A number of other structural abnormalities have been reported in B-NHL, although only a small fraction have been characterized at the molecular level. Breaks at 10q24 are a recurrent abnormality in 7 per cent of cases of low-grade B-NHL.[60,61] Recently, one of these breaks, represented by t(10;14)(q24;q32), has been cloned and the respective putative proto-oncogene identified.[203] As in other B-NHL–associated translocations, the recombination event involves the Ig_H locus on chromosome 14. On chromosome 10, the break occurs within the *lyt-10* gene (also called *NFKB-2*), a novel member of the NF-κB rel family of transcription factors.[204] The normal products of these genes have structural homologies within the DNA-binding rel domain and share the ability to bind to specific (κB) target sequences found in various inducible enhancer and promoter elements. In addition to the DNA-binding domain, the *lyt-10/NFKB-2* gene harbors an ankyrin motif, which is thought to regulate the physiologic nuclear/cytoplasm distribution of the *lyt-10/NFKB-2* protein.[203] The translocation breaks observed in B-NHL consistently disrupt the ankyrin domain, separating it from the DNA-binding domain. It is therefore conceivable that an intact DNA-binding domain, once separated from the regulatory ankyrin portion of the gene, might be constitutively activated and act as an oncogene to B cells. Curiously, the *lyt-10/NFKB-2* gene also seems to be involved in a small fraction (1 per cent) of mature lymphoid tumors, and slightly more frequently in T-cell malignancies[205,206] (Dalla-Favera et al., unpublished observations; see later in this chapter), whereas it is never involved in the t(10; 14)(q24;q32) translocation typically associated with T-ALL.[92–94]

Other chromosomal translocations may play a significant role in B-cell lymphomagenesis, based on their frequent association with a specific B-NHL subtype or their importance as prognostic markers. Chromosomal translocations involving 9p13 identify a subset of low-grade B-NHL cases with plasmacytoid features,[207] whereas breaks at 1p32-p36 and 1q21-q23 are associated with a shorter duration of complete remission and a shorter median survival.[208,209] The genes involved in these alterations have not been identified.

Tumor suppressor loci also seem to be involved in B-cell lymphomagenesis. Inactivation of the *p53* gene has been shown to be present in more than 30 per cent of BL cases in association with an activated *c-myc*.[118] Among B-NHL cases, this lesion typically is restricted to BL while it is consistently negative in other B-NHL cases.[118] Deletions of chromosome 6 have long since been recognized as a frequent genetic lesion of B-NHL.[60,61] Molecular mapping of chromosome 6 deletions in B-NHL has identified two discrete regions of minimal deletion, at 6q21-q23 and 6q25-q27 respectively, which are the sites of two distinct putative tumor suppressor loci.[208] Different histologic B-NHL types seem to associate preferentially with one or the other of the two regions of deletions, and the presence of a 6q⁻ abnormality is considered to correlate with a poor prognosis.[209,210]

EBV INFECTION

Infection with EBV, a DNA virus of the herpesvirus family, occurs asymptomatically in most individuals, and results in a lifelong immunity.[211] EBV initially was identified in cultured cells from an African BL case[212]; later studies have shown that EBV also is present in a fraction of other B-NHL types, including the sporadic form of BL, AIDS-NHL, and lymphomas arising in the posttransplant patient.[211]

The EBV viral genome has been cloned and entirely sequenced.[211] In the infectious virion, this DNA molecule is linear and flanked by terminal repeats at either end of the genome. On infection of a B lymphocyte, the viral genome is transported into the nucleus, where it exists predominantly as an extrachromosomal circular molecule (episome). The formation of circular episomes is mediated by the terminal repeats, which contain variable numbers of identical 500-bp sequences arranged as tandem repeats serving as cohesive sites for the circularization.[213] Because of this termini heterogeneity, the number of repetitive sequences enclosed in newly formed episomes may differ considerably, thus representing a constant clonal marker of the episome and, consequently, of the infected cell.[213] In EBV-infected lymphomas, usually a single form of fused EBV termini is detected, suggesting that the lymphoma cell population represents the clonally expanded progeny of a single infected cell.[214] Conversely, heterogeneous EBV termini are detected in polyclonal populations, as typically observed, for example, in cases of AIDS-associated persistent generalized lymphadenopathy (PGL).[215,216]

EBV is able to alter the growth of B-cells significantly. Among the EBV-encoded gene products, two are involved in B-cell growth regulation. The nuclear antigen EBNA-2 is thought to act as a *trans*-activator of cell and viral gene expression and is responsible for alterations in growth and morphology of the infected cells,[217] as demonstrated by the number of B-cell antigens that are modulated by EBNA-2, including CD23, CD21, LFA-1α/β, and LFA-3. In contrast, the latent membrane protein LMP1, representing a cell membrane protein associated with vimentin, is the only EBV-encoded protein with a proven transforming activity.[218,219] A certain heterogeneity exists, however, regarding EBNA-2 and LMP1 expression in EBV-infected B-cell tumors: For example, neither EBNA-2 nor LMP1 are expressed in BL, whereas their expression may be positive in AIDS-associated immunoblastic B-NHL and in lymphoproliferations occurring in posttransplant patients.[220,221] Recent studies suggest that EBV uses different cellular factors, depending on the differentiation stage of the host cell, to regulate the synthesis of its own growth transformation–associated proteins.[220,221]

Clinicopathologic Correlations

The molecular pathogenesis of B-NHL is a complex process involving multiple genetic lesions, which variously distribute into distinct B-NHL subtypes classified according to the Working Formulation.[145]

SMALL-CELL LYMPHOCYTIC LYMPHOMA

Small-cell lymphocytic lymphoma represents a tumor of mature B cells that usually is characterized by an indolent clinical course. It remains the least known among B-NHL types in terms of molecular pathogenesis. Despite the clinical and immunologic similarity between SCLL and B-CLL, *p53* mutations are restricted to the latter and never found in the former.[118] Recently, it has been shown that t(9;14)(p13;q32) specifically associates with a subgroup of SCLL showing signs of plasmacytoid differentiation.[207]

MANTLE ZONE LYMPHOMA

Mantle zone lymphoma is a relatively rare lymphoma of CD5+ B cells originating from the mantle zone surrounding reactive follicular centers. The t(11;14)(q13;q32) translocation and *bcl-1* rearrangement are the characteristic abnormalities of mantle zone lymphoma, being present in more than 50 per cent of cases.[193,194] Because mantle zone lymphoma might frequently simulate other low-grade lymphoproliferative diseases, the detection of *bcl-1* translocations is considered a relevant diagnostic marker for proper classification of this type of disorder.[193,194]

FOLLICULAR LYMPHOMA

Chromosomal translocations that involve *bcl-2* are the hallmark of follicular lymphoma, being detected in 80 to 90 per cent of cases, independently of the subtypes (small cleaved cell, mixed cell, large cell).[149,222,223] In contrast, cases of follicular lymphoma from specific geographic areas, namely Japan, display a surprisingly low frequency of *bcl-2* rearrangements when compared to those found in the western world.[224] Other oncogenes involved in lymphomagenesis, such as c-*myc* and *p53*, do not appear to be involved. Deletions of chromosome 6 are present in 20 per cent of cases.[210] Over time, follicular lymphomas tend to convert into an aggressive intermediate/high-grade lymphoma with a diffuse large cell architecture.[225] At present, a common genetic lesion responsible for transformation of follicular lymphoma has not been found; c-*myc* activation has been reported to occur in sporadic cases,[226] and recent evidence would suggest that *p53* inactivation also might play a role in a fraction of cases.[227,228]

DIFFUSE LYMPHOMA

The only genetic lesion known to be associated with and specific for de novo diffuse NHL is represented by activation of *bcl-6*.[200–202] Rearrangements of the *bcl-6* gene characterize over 30 per cent of cases of diffuse B-NHL and a very small minority of follicular NHL (<5 per cent), whereas they are not detected in other types of lymphoid malignancies.[200–202a] Most notably, rearrangements of the *bcl-6* gene identify a subset of diffuse NHL characterized by extra nodal presentation, lack of bone marrow involvement and significantly better prognosis.[202b] In addition to *bcl-6* activation, a certain number of diffuse NHL cases display c-*myc* translocation and lack of RB-1 protein expression.[72,229] *p53* inactivation does not appear to be involved in de novo diffuse lymphoma.[118] Although previous reports have shown *bcl-2* involvement in a small fraction of diffuse lymphomas,[223] recent evidence suggests that diffuse NHLs that carry a t(14;18)(q32;q21) translocation represent the transformation of follicular lymphoma into a more aggressive tumor, and *bcl-2* rearrangements are not detected in de novo diffuse lymphoma.[230] Breaks at 1p32-p36 or 1q21-q23, as well as deletions of the long arm of chromosome 6, are recurrent abnormalities in these tumors and are predictive of shortened duration of complete remission.[198,208–210] The genes implicated in these abnormalities have not been identified.

BURKITT'S LYMPHOMA

In virtually all cases of BL, c-*myc* deregulation occurs as an effect of chromosomal translocation or point mutations in regulatory regions of the gene.[72–74,169–174,179,180] With regard to the t(8;14) translocation, the endemic type of BL is associated predominantly with breakpoints at an undefined distance (>100 kb) 5' to the c-*myc* locus on chromosome 8 and within or in the proximity of the J_H region on chromosome 14[172,174]; conversely, in the sporadic type, as well as in AIDS-associated BL, the translocation involves sequences within or immediately 5' (<3 kb) to c-*myc* on chromosome 8 and sequences within the Ig_H switch regions on chromosome 14.[172,174] The differential involvement of distinct portions of the Ig_H locus in the two types of BL, together with some immunologic features, would suggest that endemic BL derives from a slightly more immature B cell than does sporadic BL.[72]

Another lesion that contributes to the development of this malignancy is EBV infection, present in virtually all cases of endemic BL and 30 per cent of cases of sporadic BL.[211] Finally, a role has been established for the loss/inactivation of *p53*, observed in more than 30 per cent of BL cases, and 6q deletions, present in 20 per cent of BL cases.[118,210]

IMMUNOBLASTIC LYMPHOMA

The pathogenesis of this highly aggressive lymphoma is still largely unclear. c-*myc* translocations are found in 20 per cent of the patients; in addition, EBV infection consistently is present in those cases associated with AIDS (see later in this chapter). A particularly high frequency of 6q deletions also has been reported in this B-NHL type.[231]

DIAGNOSTIC RELEVANCE OF GENETIC LESIONS

The general usefulness of genetic lesions as diagnostic markers has been outlined in the ALL section. Regarding B-NHL, the focused nature of the t(14;18) breakpoints has enabled the application of universal amplification procedures using PCR.[156,232,233] These assays can be used to detect residual lymphoma clones, to define the natural history of the disease, and to evaluate quickly the effects of therapy in removing pathologic cells.

B-CELL CHRONIC LYMPHOCYTIC LEUKEMIA

General Overview

B-cell chronic lymphocytic leukemia is the most common leukemia of adults in the western world, usually affecting individuals over 50 years of age.[234] Despite its rarity, however, well-characterized cases of B-CLL in children and young adults also have been reported, and appear to cluster with specific genetic abnormalities.[235,236] Genetic predisposition to B-CLL, suggested by the observation of familial aggregation in some cases, is a well-established notion, the molecular basis of which, however, remains elusive.[234]

B-CLL cells characteristically co-express B-cell antigens, such as sIg and CD19, and the pan-T marker CD5. It is thought that B-CLL originates from normal CD5+ B lymphocytes, which represent a rare B-cell subpopulation in adults.[234] Clinically, B-CLL is an indolent tumor, and a significant portion of patients remain stable for years. In a small proportion of cases, however, B-CLL may evolve into more aggressive forms, mainly by development of diffuse large cell lymphoma (Richter's syndrome).

Genetic Lesions

The molecular pathogenesis of B-CLL is still largely unknown. Mutations of the *p53* gene and loss of heterozygosity in 17p, the *p53* site, are found in a small fraction (10 to 15 per cent) of B-CLL cases.[118,237] A higher frequency of *p53* alterations is observed after transformation of B-CLL to Richter's syndrome, a highly aggressive lymphoma with a poor clinical outcome,[118] suggesting that *p53* may be involved in the genetic mechanisms underlying B-CLL progression.

A number of dominant oncogenes, including c-*myc*, *bcl-1*, *bcl-2*, and the *ras* family genes, have been widely investigated in B-CLL; however, none of these genes has shown clear associations with the disease.[116,190–192,237–240] Because high levels of *bcl-2* expression are seen consistently in B-CLL cells, it is conceivable that they result from mechanisms other than chromosomal translocation.[241] The rare cases of childhood B-CLL are associated with t(2;14)(p13;q32), involving the Ig_H locus on chromosome 14 and an as yet uncharacterized transcriptional unit on chromosome 2.[235,236,242,243]

Despite the paucity of information regarding the molecular lesions associated with B-CLL, cytogenetic studies point out several issues that need additional molecular clarification.[60,61,244] Trisomy 12 is found in approximately 10 to 20 per cent of B-CLL cases and correlates with poor survival.[244] Novel cytogenetic techniques (i.e., interphase fluorescent in situ hybridization) demonstrate that trisomy 12 is in fact present in a higher proportion of B-CLL (35 per cent) than that shown by conventional cytogenetic approaches.[245] Finally, breaks at 13q14 occur in more than 10 per cent of patients and represent the most frequent structural abnormality.[244] However, the *RB-1* gene, frequently disrupted in human tumors carrying breaks at 13q14, does not seem to be altered in B-CLL.[237,240]

MULTIPLE MYELOMA

General Overview

Multiple myeloma (MM) typically affects the elderly and represents the most common lymphoid malignancy in blacks and the second most common in whites.[246] MM makes up part of the group of B-cell malignancies known as plasma cell dyscrasias, representing the expansion of a single clone of plasma cell–like, immunoglobulin-secreting cells. The disease is characterized by osteolytic lesions, atypical marrow plasmacytoma, and a monoclonal gammopathy. A rare, terminal complication of MM is represented by plasma cell leukemia, consisting of massive invasion of peripheral blood by malignant plasma cells. Traditionally, the pathogenesis of MM has been ascribed to initial antigenic stimulation of B cells followed by a mutagenic event causing full malignant transformation.[246] Indeed, in individual cases, the putative initial antigenic stimulus has been identified on the basis of the antigenic specificity of the immunoglobulins secreted by the malignant plasma cells.

A role for autocrine and/or paracrine cytokine loops has emerged recently. Although initial investigation had suggested the presence of autocrine loops involving interleukins IL-4 and IL-6 in MM cells,[247,248] later studies have shown that MM growth more frequently is supported by paracrine mechanisms, whereby cytokines (IL-6, IL-3, IL-1β) produced by MM bone marrow stroma cells (fibroblasts, monocytes) and T lymphocytes provide a growth stimulus to the malignant plasma cells.[249–251] Conversely, MM plasma cells constitutively produce tumor necrosis factor β and IL-1, well-known osteoclast-activating factors (OAFs), which in turn would stimulate osteoclasts to cause the diffuse osteolysis consistently accompanying MM.[252–254] At present, however, it is not clear whether cytokine deregulation in MM is a primary event or instead is dependent on the genetic lesion of an as yet unidentified genetic locus.

Genetic Lesions

The molecular pathogenesis of MM is still largely obscure. Among dominantly acting oncogenes, *ras* is the only oncogene whose frequency of activation has been assessed conclusively. Mutations of the *ras* gene family have been reported in more than 30 per cent of cases of MM and have been found to associate with a partial or complete lack of response to therapy, suggesting that *ras* mutations in MM are a late event.[255–257] More recently, sequential analysis of cases at different stages of the disease has established that the frequency of *ras* mutations increases during the clinical course, strongly suggesting that *ras* mutations are associated with disease progression.[257] However, because patients in late MM stages usually have undergone intensive chemotherapy, it cannot be excluded that part of this increase might be due to a mutagenic effect of some chemotherapeutic agents on the *ras* genes. In addition, a correlation has been found between mutations of the *ras* oncogenes and a poor therapeutic response in cases examined at diagnosis.[255] As in other hematopoietic malignancies, the N-*ras* gene is involved preferentially in MM. The biologic relevance of *ras* activation in MM is suggested by in vitro models showing that the H-*ras* and N-*ras* genes are capable of causing terminal differentiation of B cells into plasma cells and of inducing their malignant transformation.[258]

No structural alteration has been detected in the c-myc locus in MM.[255,259] Because some authors have reported increased levels of c-myc in up to 25 per cent of MM cases,[260] it is likely that high c-myc levels in MM may represent a consequence of other genetic lesions present in the same cell.

Recently, rearrangements within the human homologue of the Moloney leukemia virus integration 4 locus (Mlvi-4) have been detected in 20 per cent of MM patients; because the Mlvi-4 locus maps 20 kb 3' to the c-myc locus, it has been proposed that changes in the region 3' to c-myc may contribute to MM pathogenesis by transcriptional deregulation of c-myc.[261]

Finally, the tumor suppressor gene p53 appears to play an important role in the mechanisms underlying MM tumor progression. Although the overall frequency of p53 inactivation is restricted to 15 per cent of MM cases, p53 mutations specifically cluster with the more advanced and clinically aggressive acute/leukemic forms of MM (45 per cent of cases) and are consistently absent in more indolent and chronic forms.[262] In particular, p53 mutations seem to carry an additional factor of dismal prognosis for MM patients in late stages, as indicated by a shorter survival of mutated versus nonmutated cases within the same clinical stage.[262]

LYMPHOPROLIFERATIVE DISEASES IN IMMUNOCOMPROMISED PATIENTS

General Overview

The association between an immunodeficiency state and the development of lymphoma has been long recognized in several clinical conditions, including congenital (e.g., Wiskott-Aldrich syndrome), iatrogenic (e.g., treatment with immunosuppressor agents) and viral-induced (e.g., AIDS) immunodeficiencies.[216,263,264] In recent years, the increasing frequency of two groups of immunodeficiencies, human immunodeficiency virus (HIV) infection and post-transplant iatrogenic immunosuppression, has emerged as a major risk factor for lymphomagenesis. The exact immune alterations that contribute to lymphoma development are not clear. In the instance of AIDS, at least three major components are thought to contribute to lymphomagenesis,[216] including (1) disturbed immunosurveillance; (2) chronic B-cell stimulation by antigens, viruses, and mitogens; and (3) EBV infection.

AIDS-NHL cases are almost invariably B-cell–derived NHL.[216,263,264] Systemic AIDS-NHLs are histologically heterogeneous, being represented by small noncleaved cell lymphoma (SNCCL), large-cell immunoblastic-plasmacytoid lymphoma (LC-IBPL), and diffuse large noncleaved cell lymphoma (LNCCL).[216,263,264] A distinct group of AIDS-NHLs is represented by NHLs arising in the CNS, the majority of which are LC-IBPLs. When compared to NHLs of similar histology in the immunocompetent patient, AIDS-NHLs are characterized by presentation in advanced stages, poor prognosis, and frequent involvement of extranodal sites.[216,263,264]

The definition of posttransplantation lymphoproliferative disorders (PT-LPDs) covers an entire spectrum of diseases, ranging from purely reactive to frankly neoplastic B-cell lymphoproliferations.[265] PT-LPDs display a high degree of immunophenotypic and immunogenotypic heterogeneity: Some are characteristically polyclonal or oligoclonal, whereas others express monoclonal surface immunoglobulins and show clonal immunoglobulin gene rearrangement. Finally, polyclonal and monoclonal lesions are commonly found at different sites in the same individual.[265]

Genetic Lesions

The molecular pathogenesis of AIDS-NHL has been clarified to a certain extent, whereas little is known about PT-LPD.

Among AIDS-NHL cases, EBV infection of the tumor clone is restricted to 30 to 40 per cent of SNCCL and LNCCL cases but is present in 100 per cent of cases of systemic LC-IBPL and AIDS-NHL arising in the CNS.[216,266–271] Activation of the c-myc oncogene is associated with 100 per cent of AIDS-associated SNCCL cases, whereas in LNCCL and LC-IBPL it is restricted to a minority of tumors.[215,266–271] The molecular mechanisms leading to c-myc activation in AIDS-NHL are similar to those in sporadic BL, as opposed to endemic BL. In addition, it has become evident that p53 inactivation through mutation and loss is found in 60 per cent of AIDS-associated SNCCL cases, whereas it is negative in the other AIDS-NHL types.[269–271] Furthermore, 6q deletions are found in 20 per cent of cases of AIDS-NHL, irrespective of the histologic type (G. Gaidano and R. Dalla-Favera, unpublished observation). Finally, mutations of the ras genes, which are never detected in B-NHL of the immunocompetent host, are present in AIDS-NHL, although at low frequency.[269,270]

It is now clear that the repertoire of genetic lesions differs substantially in different histologic types of AIDS-NHL, suggesting that AIDS-associated lymphomagenesis may be associated with distinct molecular pathways.[216,266–271] On the one hand, AIDS-NHLs displaying SNCCL histology are associated strictly with c-myc deregulation and p53 inactivation, whereas EBV infection is limited to the subset of these tumors. On the other hand, a monoclonal EBV infection is consistently associated with systemic LC-IBPL and CNS AIDS-NHLs in which additional genetic lesions (e.g., c-myc in a fraction of cases) may be necessary. It is of note that AIDS-associated lymphomagenesis is associated with multiple genetic lesions (c-myc activation, ras mutation, EBV infection, p53 inactivation, 6q deletions) accumulating in the relatively short time (4 to 6 years) corresponding to the development of these tumors[269–271] (Fig. 12–6). In this respect, the model of AIDS-NHL is in contrast to the general concept regarding multilesional tumorigenesis, which is derived mainly from solid tumors, in which a long time span (30 to 40 years) is necessary for the development of a fully transformed phenotype.[272]

The pathogenetic basis of PT-LPD is still unclear. The only genetic lesion consistently associated with PT-LPD is represented by EBV infection of the tumor cells, which is found in 90 per cent of PT-LPD cases.[273–278] Rearrangements of c-myc also have been detected in rare cases.[275] Recently, a classification of PT-LPDs on the basis of their genetic features has been proposed.[275] PT-LPDs are thus described as polymorphic (i.e., oligo- or polyclonal) and monomorphic (i.e., monoclonal), according to the clonality patterns of immunoglobulin gene rearrangements. The polymorphic group displays either a polyclonal or an oligoclonal immunoglobulin pattern, and frequently is associated with polyclonal EBV infection. Conversely, monomorphic PT-LPDs less frequently are associated with EBV, may exhibit c-myc rearrangements in some cases and, overall, mimic LC-IBPLs of HIV-infected individuals. The practical relevance of this classification is supported by the clinical observation that a high percentage of nonclonal or polyclonal PT-LPD patients regress when immunosuppression is reduced, whereas most oligoclonal and all the monoclonal cases progress despite the removal of the initial predisposing factor.[275]

MALIGNANCIES OF MATURE T CELLS

General Overview

Malignancies of mature T cells are a highly heterogeneous group of diseases, comprising four main groups: peripheral T-cell lymphoma (PTCL), cutaneous T-cell lymphoma (CTCL), adult T-cell leukemia/lymphoma (ATLL), and T-cell chronic lymphocytic leukemia (T-CLL). These malignancies greatly differ in clinical behavior, immunophenotypic features, and genetic lesions involved in their pathogenesis. In western countries, mature T-cell malignancies overall represent only 15 to 20 per cent of tumors derived from mature lymphocytes and are relatively uncommon when compared to mature B-cell malignancies.[279] A higher frequency of mature T-cell malignancies is reported in other parts of the world, namely Japan and the Caribbean. Most T-cell malignancies originate from CD4+ T cells, with the exception of T-CLL.[279]

PTCLs are diffuse proliferations arising in peripheral lymphoid organs and affecting most commonly the elderly. An exception is represented by Ki-1+ (CD30+) PTCL, also known as anaplastic large-cell lymphoma (ALCL), which tends to occur in children and young adults.[279] An intrinsic tropism for the skin is displayed by CTCLs, which include mycosis fungoides and its leukemic manifestation known as Sézary syndrome. The term ATLL encompasses a spectrum of lymphoproliferative diseases associated with the human retrovirus human T-cell leukemia virus, type I (HTLV-I) and characteristically expressing large amounts of IL-2 receptors (CD25). The geographical distribution of ATLL is mainly restricted to southwestern Japan and the Caribbean basin, although cases have been reported also in the United States and United Kingdom in long-term immigrants from the affected geographical areas.[279]

Genetic Lesions

The molecular pathogenesis of mature T-cell malignancies is poorly understood overall, and few genetic lesions have been found with significant frequency in these tumors.

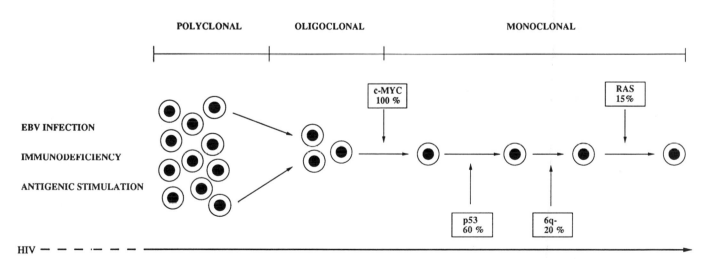

Figure 12–6. Multistep tumorigenesis in B-NHL. The example of AIDS-associated small noncleaved cell lymphoma is shown. In the case of small noncleaved cell lymphoma, c-myc activation is detected consistently in 100 per cent of cases, and p53 inactivation is found in 60 per cent of tumors; in addition, ras mutations and 6q deletions are associated with a fraction of samples. In the initial stages, host predisposing conditions (B-cell chronic stimulation, EBV infection, immunosurveillance alterations) favor the development of a polyclonal to oligoclonal B-cell hyperplasia known as persistent generalized lymphadenopathy. On this basis, multiple genetic lesions accumulate within one single clone, inducing its neoplastic transformation. Genetic lesions in AIDS-NHL accumulate in a relatively short period comprised between the HIV infection event and the clinical diagnosis of the tumor (4 to 5 years). The precise timing of the molecular events as depicted in the figure is derived arbitrarily from the frequency of each single genetic lesion in this type of tumor.

In PTCL, sporadic cases of c-*myc* rearrangements[280] and *p53* mutations[118] have been reported. A more frequent lesion is represented by t(2;5)(p23;q35), that is specifically associated with 50 per cent of Ki-1+ PTCL or ALCL cases.[281,282] The genetic loci implicated by this translocation are currently under investigation. Ki-1+ PTCLs also are associated consistently with high levels of *p53*, comparable to the ones detected in cases harboring *p53* mutations; however, genetic lesions in the *p53* gene have not been found in this group of PTCLs.[283] The role of autocrine loops involving a number of cytokines also has been proposed in PTCL pathogenesis.[284,285] CTCLs have not been associated with any known genetic lesions; recently, however, rearrangements of the *lyt-10/NFKB-2* gene at 10q24 have been demonstrated in a sizable fraction of these tumors[203-206] (Dalla-Favera et al., unpublished data). The detailed mechanism of activation of the *lyt-10/NFKB-2* proto-oncogene is described earlier in this chapter.

The molecular pathogenesis of ATLL has been elucidated to a wider extent in comparison to that of other mature T-cell tumors. ATLL is associated with HTLV-I infection of the tumor cells in 100 per cent of cases, although the rate of ATLL development among seropositive individuals is relatively low (<5 per cent lifetime risk).[286-291] The period between infection and onset of clinical disease is typically quite long, varying between 10 and 30 years.[292] Unlike acutely transforming animal retroviruses, the HTLV-I genome does not encode a known oncogene.[292] Furthermore, this retrovirus does not transform T cells by *cis*-activation of an adjacent proto-oncogene, because this provirus appears to integrate randomly within the host genome.[292] Rather, the pathogenic effect of HTLV-I in ATLL seems to be due to the viral production of a *trans*-regulatory protein (HTLV-I Tax) that markedly increases expression of all viral gene products and transcriptionally activates the expression of certain host genes, including *IL-2*, the α chain of the IL-2 receptor (CD25), c-*sis*, c-*fos*, and the granulocyte-macrophage colony-stimulating factor.[292-297] Indeed, a property of ATLL cells is the constitutive high-level expression of IL-2 receptors. The central role of these genes in normal T-cell activation and growth, together with the results of in vitro studies, support the notion that Tax-mediated activation of these host genes represents an important mechanism by which HTLV-I initiates T-cell transformation. In addition, recent studies have demonstrated that Tax represses the expression of β-polymerase, an enzyme involved in DNA repair.[298] Lack of β-polymerase could underlie the frequent karyotypic abnormalities seen in ATLL.

The long period of clinical latency that precedes the development of ATLL, the small percentage of infected patients that develop this malignancy, and the observation that leukemic cells from ATLL are monoclonal suggest that HTLV-I is not sufficient to cause the full malignant phenotype.[292] An attractive model for ATLL therefore would include an early period of Tax-induced polyclonal T-cell proliferation, mediated by the deregulated expression of IL-2 and its receptor, which in turn would facilitate the occurrence of additional genetic events leading to the monoclonal outgrowth of a fully transformed cell. This hypothesis is supported by the observation that the *p53* tumor suppressor gene is inactivated in 40 per cent of ATLL cases, representing the most frequent lesion of a cellular gene identified in ATLL.[299,300] Other tumor suppressor genes, specifically *RB-1*, and dominant-acting oncogenes, such as *ras* and c-*myc*, do not appear to play a role in ATLL pathogenesis.[300]

Finally, no genetic lesions have been found to be associated with T-CLL, although cytogenetic analysis has revealed inv(14;14)(q11;q32) in 65 per cent of cases.[60,61]

CONCLUSIONS

A number of general conclusions can be drawn from the extensive body of studies on genetic lesions in lymphoid neoplasms described in these pages.

First, the well-recognized clinical and histologic heterogeneity of lymphoid malignancies reflects, and possibly is due to an extreme degree of diversity among the molecular lesions associated with each type of lymphoid tumor. Distinct genetic lesions segregate the major categories of lymphoid tumors and, in addition, tumors of the same type, that are indistinguishable based on phenotype, may in fact be distinguishable based on pathogenic mechanisms. This is probably best exemplified by the case of ALL, the molecular pathogenesis of which has now been elucidated to a significant extent. Studies on the identification and distribution of genetic lesions in various leukemias and lymphomas therefore may provide the framework of potential clinical significance for a novel classification of these malignancies.

Second, lymphoid neoplasms result from the accumulation of multiple genetic lesions in the same clone (e.g., Fig. 12–6). In this respect, AIDS-NHLs are the best characterized example of multistep tumorigenesis in the immune system, wherein a number of genetic lesions variously interplay in the same cell. Even in lymphoid neoplasms consistently associated with a single genetic lesion with transforming potential per se (e.g., BL), other genetic accidents are likely to have occurred during the tumor's natural history. It is interesting that the pathogenesis of a number of lymphoid tumors (e.g., AIDS-NHL, PT-LPD, ATLL) is thought to consist of two phases, the first one represented by a polyclonal hyperplasia from which the second monoclonal phase arises at a later stage. In AIDS-NHL, for example, chronic antigen stimulation and diminished immunosurveillance may cause a persistent generalized lymphadenopathy, from which a neoplastic clone may emerge, conceivably on the occurrence of mutations in cellular genes.[216,301,302] Once the frank tumor is growing, progression through more aggressive stages also is accompanied by the emergence of novel genetic lesions.

Finally, because most genomic alterations in lymphoid neoplasms represent truly tumor-specific markers (*bcl-2* might be an exception to this rule) that are detectable at high sensitivity and high specificity by modern molecular genetic techniques, the identification of such lesions opens the way for improved early diagnosis and better monitoring of the clinical course.

ACKNOWLEDGMENTS: Work described in this chapter has been supported by grant CA-44029 to R.D.-F. G.G. has been supported by a Fellowship for AIDS Research from Istituto Superiore di Sanitá, Roma, Italy.

REFERENCES

1. Foon KA, Todd RF III: Immunologic classification of leukemia and lymphoma. Blood 68:1, 1986
2. Griesser H, Tkachuk D, Reis MD, et al: Gene rearrangements and translocations in lymphoproliferative diseases. Blood 73:1402, 1989
3. Chess L, Sclossman SF: Human lymphocyte subpopulations. Adv Immunol 25:213, 1977
4. Inghirami G, Knowles DM: The immune system: Structure and function. In Knowles DM (ed): Neoplastic Hematopathology. Baltimore, Williams & Wilkins, 1992, pp 27–72
5. Magrath I: Lymphocyte ontogeny: A conceptual basis for understanding neoplasia of the immune system. In Magrath I (ed): The Non-Hodgkin's Lymphomas. Baltimore, Williams & Wilkins, 1990, pp 29–48
6. Trent JM, Kaneko Y, Mitelman F: Report of the Committee on Structural Chromosome Changes in Neoplasia: Human gene mapping 10. Cytogenet Cell Genet 51:533, 1989
7. Mauer AM: Acute lymphocytic leukemia. In Williams WJ, Beutler E, Erslev AJ, Lichtman MA (eds): Hematology, 4th ed. New York, McGraw-Hill, 1990, pp 994–1005
8. Kamps WA, Humphrey GB: Heterogeneity of childhood acute lymphoblastic leukemia—impact on prognosis and therapy. Semin Oncol 12:268, 1985
9. Champlin R, Gale RP: Acute lymphoblastic leukemia: Recent advances in biology and therapy. Blood 73:2051, 1989
10. Pui C-H, Crist WM, Look AT: Biology and clinical significance of cytogenetic abnormalities in childhood acute lymphoblastic leukemia. Blood 76:1449, 1990
11. Greaves MF, Janossy G, Peto J, et al: Immunologically defined subclasses of acute lymphoblastic leukemia in children: Their relationship to presentation features and prognosis. Br J Haematol 48:179, 1981
12. Sobol RE, Royston I, LeBien TW, et al: Adult lymphoblastic leukemia phenotypes defined by monoclonal antibodies. Blood 65:730, 1985
13. Third International Workshop on Chromosomes in Leukemia: Chromosomal abnormalities and their clinical significance in acute lymphoblastic leukemia. Cancer Res 43:868, 1983
14. Sawyers CL, Denny CT, Witte ON: Leukemia and the disruption of hematopoiesis. Cell 64:337, 1991
15. Cleary ML: Oncogenic conversion of transcription factors by chromosomal translocations. Cell 66:619, 1991
16. Rabbits TH: Translocations, master genes, and differences between the origins of acute and chronic leukemias. Cell 67:641, 1991
17. Korsmeyer SJ: Chromosomal translocations in lymphoid malignancies reveal novel proto-oncogenes. Annu Rev Immunol 10:785, 1992
18. Tycko B, Sklar J: Chromosomal translocations in lymphoid neoplasia: A reappraisal of the recombinase model. Cancer Cells 2:1, 1990
19. Nowell PC, Hungerford DA: A minute chromosome in human granulocytic leukemia. Science 132:1497, 1960
20. Kurzrock R, Gutterman JU, Talpaz M: The molecular genetics of Philadelphia chromosome positive leukemias. N Engl J Med 319:990, 1988
21. Groffen J, Stephenson JR, Heisterkamp N, et al: Philadelphia chromosomal breakpoints are clustered within a limited region, bcr, on chromosome 22. Cell 36:93, 1984
22. Heisterkamp N, Stam K, Groffen J, et al: Structural organization of the bcr gene and its role in Ph¹ translocation. Nature 315:758, 1985
23. Shtivelman E, Lifshitz B, Gale RP, et al: Fusion transcript of abl and bcr in chronic myelogenous leukemia. Nature 315:550, 1985
24. Grosveld G, Verwoerd T, van Agthoven T, et al: The chronic myelocytic cell line K562 contains a breakpoint in bcr and produces a chimeric bcr/abl transcript. Mol Cell Biol 6:607, 1986
25. Konopka JB, Watanabe SM, Witte ON: An alteration of the human c-abl protein in K562 leukemia cells unmasks associated tyrosine kinase activity. Cell 37:1035, 1984
26. McLaughlin J, Chianese E, Witte ON: In vitro transformation of immature hematopoietic cells by the p210 bcr/abl oncogene product of the Philadelphia chromosome. Proc Natl Acad Sci USA 84:6558, 1987
27. Kelliher MA, McLaughlin J, Witte ON, et al: Induction of a chronic myelogenous leukemia-like syndrome in mice with v-abl and bcr/abl. Proc Natl Acad Sci USA 87:6649, 1990
28. Daley GQ, Van Etten RA, Baltimore D: Induction of chronic myelogenous leukemia in mice by the p210ᵇᶜʳ/ᵃᵇˡ gene of the Philadelphia chromosome. Science 247:824, 1990
29. Elefanty AG, Hariharan IK, Cory S: bcr-abl, the hallmark of chronic myeloid leukemia in man, induces multiple haematopoietic neoplasms in mice. EMBO J 9:1069, 1990
30. Chan LC, Karhi KK, Rayter SI, et al: A novel ABL protein expressed in Philadelphia-chromosome positive acute lymphoblastic leukemia. Nature 325:635, 1987
31. Clark SS, McLaughlin J, Champlin R, et al: Unique forms of the abl tyrosine kinase distinguish Ph¹-positive CML from Ph¹-positive ALL. Science 235:85, 1987
32. Feinstein E, Marcelle C, Rosner A, et al: A new fused transcript in Philadelphia chromosome positive acute lymphoblastic leukemia. Nature 330:386, 1987
33. Hermans A, Heisterkamp N, von Lindern M, et al: Unique fusion of bcr and c-abl genes in Philadelphia chromosome positive acute lymphoblastic leukemia. Cell 5:33, 1987
34. Kurzrock R, Shtalrid M, Romero P, et al: A novel c-abl protein product in Philadelphia-positive acute lymphoblastic leukemia. Nature 325:631, 1987
35. Rubin CM, Carrino JJ, Dickler MN, et al: Heterogeneity of genomic fusion of BCR and ABL in Philadelphia chromosome-positive acute lymphoblastic leukemia. Proc Natl Acad Sci USA 85:2795, 1988
36. Chen SJ, Chen Z, Hillion J, et al: Ph1-positive, bcr-negative acute leukemias: Clustering of breakpoints on chromosome 22 in the 3' end of the BCR gene first intron. Blood 73:1312, 1989
37. Heisterkamp N, Jenkins R, Thibodeau S, et al: The bcr gene in Philadelphia chromosome positive acute lymphoblastic leukemia. Blood 73:1307, 1989
38. Suryanarayan K, Hunger SP, Kohler S, et al: Consistent involvement of the BCR gene by 9;22 breakpoints in pediatric acute leukemias. Blood 77:324, 1991
39. de Klein A, Hagemeijer N, Bartram CR, et al: Bcr rearrangement and translocations of the c-abl oncogene in Philadelphia positive acute lymphoblastic leukemia. Blood 68:1369, 1986
40. Turhan AG, Eaves CJ, Kalousek DK, et al: Molecular analysis of clonality and bcr rearrangements in Philadelphia chromosome-positive acute lymphoblastic leukemia. Blood 71:1495, 1988
41. McLaughlin J, Chianese E, Witte ON: Alternative forms of the bcr/abl oncogene have quantitatively different potencies for stimulation of immature lymphoid cells. Mol Cell Biol 9:1866, 1989
42. Lugo TG, Pendergast AM, Muller A, et al: Tyrosine kinase activity and transformation potency of bcr-abl oncogene products. Science 247:1079, 1990
43. Heisterkamp N, Jenster G, ten Hoeve J, et al: Acute leukemia in BCR/ABL transgenic mice. Nature 344:251, 1990
44. Voncken JW, Morris C, Pattengale P, et al: Clonal development and karyotype evolution during leukemogenesis of BCR/ABL transgenic mice. Blood 79:1029, 1992
45. Griffiths SD, Healy LE, Ford AM: Clonal characteristics of

acute lymphoblastic cells derived from BCR/ABL p190 transgenic mice. Oncogene 7:1391, 1992

46. Haas OA, Argiryou-Tirita A, Lion T: Parental origin of chromosomes involved in the translocation t(9;22). Nature 359: 414, 1992

47. Ferguson Smith AC, Reik W, Surani MA: Genomic imprinting and cancer. Cancer Surv 9:487, 1990

48. Rowley JD: Recurring chromosome abnormalities in leukemia and lymphoma. Semin Hematol 27:122, 1990

49. Williams DL, Look AT, Melvin SL, et al: New chromosomal translocations correlate with specific immunophenotypes of childhood acute lymphoblastic leukemia. Cell 36:101, 1984

50. Carrol AJ, Crist WM, Parmley RT, et al: Pre-B cell leukemia associated with chromosome translocation 1;19. Blood 63: 721, 1984

51. Michael PM, Levin MD, Garson OM: Translocation 1;19—a new cytogenetic abnormality in acute lymphocytic leukemia. Cancer Genet Cytogenet 12:333, 1984

52. Pui C-H, Williams DL, Kalwinsky DK, et al: Cytogenetic features and serum lactic dehydrogenase level predict a poor treatment outcome for children with pre-B-cell leukemia. Blood 67:1688, 1986

53. Raimondi SC, Behm FG, Roberson PK, et al: Cytogenetics of pre-B acute lymphoblastic leukemia with emphasis on prognostic implications of the t(1;19). J Clin Oncol 8:1380, 1990

54. Crist WM, Carrol AJ, Shuster JJ, et al: Poor prognosis of children with pre-B acute lymphoblastic leukemia is associated with the t(1;19)(q23;p13). A Pediatric Oncology Group Study. Blood 63:407, 1984

55. Mellentin JD, Murre CM, Donlon TA, et al: The gene for enhancer binding proteins E12/E47 lies at the t(1;19) breakpoint in acute leukemias. Science 246:379, 1989

56. Murre C, McCaw PS, Baltimore D: A new DNA binding and dimerization motif in immunoglobulin enhancer binding, daughterless, MyoD, and c-myc proteins. Cell 56:777, 1989

57. Kamps MP, Murre C, Sun X-H, et al: A new homeobox gene contributes the DNA binding domain of the t(1;19) translocation protein in pre-B ALL. Cell 60:547, 1990

58. Nourse J, Mellentin JD, Galili N, et al: Chromosomal translocation t(1;19) results in synthesis of a homeobox fusion mRNA that codes for a potential chimeric transcription factor. Cell 60:535, 1990

59. Kamps MP, Look AT, Baltimore D: The human t(1;19) translocation in pre-B ALL produces multiple nuclear E2A/PBX1 fusion proteins with differing transforming potential. Genes Dev 5:528, 1991

60. Mitelman F: Catalog of Chromosome Aberrations in Cancer. New York, Wiley-Liss, 1991

61. Heim S, Mitelman F: Cancer Cytogenetics. New York, Liss, 1987

62. Raimondi SC, Peiper SC, Kitchingman GR, et al: Childhood acute lymphoblastic leukemia with chromosomal breakpoints at 11q23. Blood 73:1627, 1989

63. Cimino G, Moir DT, Canaani O, et al: Cloning of ALL-1, the locus involved in leukemias with the t(4;11)(q21;q23), t(9; 11)(p22;q23), and t(11;19)(q23;p13) chromosome translocations. Cancer Res 51:6712, 1991

64. Ziemin-Van der Poel S, McCabe NR, Gill HJ, et al: Identification of a gene, MLL, that spans the breakpoint in 11q23 translocations associated with human leukemias. Proc Natl Acad Sci USA 88:10735, 1991

65. Cimino G, Nakamura T, Gu Y, et al: An altered 11-Kb transcript in leukemic cell lines with the t(4;11)(q21;q23) chromosome translocation. Cancer Res 52:3911, 1992

66. Djabali M, Selleri L, Parry P, et al: A trithorax-like gene is interrupted by chromosome 11q23 translocations in acute leukemias. Nature Genet 2:113, 1992

67. Gu Y, Nakamura T, Alder H, et al: The t(4;11) chromosome translocation of human acute leukemias fuses the ALL-1 gene, related to Drosophila trithorax, to the AF-4 gene. Cell 71:701, 1992

68. Tkachuk DC, Kohler S, Cleary M: Involvement of a homolog of Drosophila trithorax by 11q23 chromosomal translocations in acute leukemias. Cell 71:691, 1992

69. Reeves R, Nissen MS: The AT-DNA-binding domain of mammalian high mobility group I chromosomal proteins: A novel peptide motif for recognizing DNA structure. J Biol Chem 265:8573, 1990

70. Mazo AM, Huang D-H, Mozer BA, et al: The trithorax gene, a trans-acting regulator of the bithorax complex in Drosophila, encodes a protein with zinc-binding domains. Proc Natl Acad Sci USA 87:2112, 1990

71. Gu Y, Cimino G, Alder H, et al: The t(4;11)(q21;q23) chromosome translocations in acute leukemias involve the VDJ recombinase. Proc Natl Acad Sci USA 89:10464, 1992

72. Dalla-Favera R: Chromosomal translocations involving the c-myc oncogene in lymphoid neoplasia. In Kirsch IR (ed): The Causes and Consequences of Chromosomal Aberrations. Boca Raton, FL, CRC Press, 1993, pp 313–332

73. Dalla-Favera R, Bregni M, Erickson J, et al: Human c-myc oncogene is located on the region of chromosome 8 that is translocated in Burkitt lymphoma cells. Proc Natl Acad Sci USA 79:7824, 1982

74. Dalla-Favera R, Martinotti S, Gallo RC, et al: Translocation and rearrangements of the c-myc oncogene locus in human undifferentiated B-cell lymphomas. Science 219:963, 1983

75. Peschle C, Mavilio F, Sposi NM, et al: Translocation and rearrangement of c-myc into immunoglobulin alpha heavy chain locus in primary cells from acute lymphocytic leukemia. Proc Natl Acad Sci USA 81:5514, 1984

76. Hibshoosh H, Neri A, Basso G, et al: Molecular analysis of the t(8;14) chromosomal translocation in L3-type acute lymphoblastic leukemia. Manuscript in preparation, 1994

77. Erikson J, Finger L, Sun L, et al: Deregulation of c-myc by translocation of the α-locus of T-cell receptor in T-cell leukemias. Science 232:884, 1986

78. Shima EA, Le Beau MM, McKeithan TW, et al: Gene encoding the α chain of the T-cell receptor is moved immediately downstream of c-myc in a chromosomal 8;14 translocation in a cell line from a human T-cell leukemia. Proc Natl Acad Sci USA 83:349, 1986

79. McKeithan TW, Shima EA, Le Beau MM, et al: Molecular cloning of the breakpoint junction of a human chromosomal 8;14 translocation involving the T-cell receptor α-chain gene and sequences on the 3' side of myc. Proc Natl Acad Sci USA 83:6636, 1986

80. Brown L, Cheng J-T, Chen Q, et al: Site-specific recombination of the tal-1 gene is a common occurrence in human T cell leukemia. EMBO J 9:3343, 1990

81. Aplan PD, Lombardi DP, Reaman GH, et al: Involvement of the putative haematopoietic transcription factor SCL in T-cell acute lymphoblastic leukemia. Blood 79:1327, 1992

82. Begley CG, Aplan PD, Denning SM, et al: The gene SCL is expressed during early hematopoiesis and encodes a differentiation-related DNA-binding motif. Proc Natl Acad Sci USA 86:10128, 1989

83. Hsu H-L, Cheng J-T, Chen Q, et al: Enhancer-binding activity of the tal-1 oncoprotein in association with the E47/E12 helix-loop-helix proteins. Mol Cell Biol 11:3037, 1991

84. Begley CG, Aplan PD, Davey MP, et al: Chromosomal translocation in human leukemic stem-cell line disrupts the T-cell antigen receptor δ-chain diversity region and results in a previously unreported fusion transcript. Proc Natl Acad Sci USA 86:2031, 1989

85. Finger LR, Kagan J, Cristopher G, et al: Involvement of the TCL5 gene on human chromosome 1 in T-cell leukemia and melanoma. Proc Natl Acad Sci USA 86:5039, 1989

86. Aplan PD, Lombardi DP, Ginsberg AM, et al: Disruption of the human SCL locus by "illegitimate" V-(D)-J recombinase activity. Science 250:1426, 1990

87. Chen Q, Cheng J-T, Tsai L-H, et al: The tal gene undergoes chromosomal translocation in T cell leukemia and potentially encodes a helix-loop-helix protein. EMBO J 9:415, 1990

88. Chen Q, Yang CY-C, Tsan JT, et al: Coding sequences of the tal-1 gene are disrupted by chromosome translocation in human T-cell leukemia. J Exp Med 172:1403, 1990

89. Bernard O, Lecointe N, Jonveaux P, et al: Two site-specific deletions and t(1;14) translocation restricted to human T-cell

acute leukemias disrupt the 5' part of the tal-1 gene. Oncogene 6:1477, 1991

90. Fitzgerald TJ, Neale GAM, Raimondi SC, et al: c-tal, a helix-loop-helix protein, is juxtaposed to the T-cell receptor-β chain gene by a reciprocal chromosomal translocation: t(1;7)(p32;q35). Blood 78:2686, 1991

91. Aplan PD, Lombardi DP, Kirsch IR: Structural characterization of SL, a gene frequently disrupted in T-cell acute lymphoblastic leukemia. Mol Cell Biol 11:5462, 1991

92. Dube ID, Kamel-Reid S, Yuan CC, et al: A novel human homeobox gene lies at the chromosome 10 breakpoint in lymphoid neoplasias with chromosomal translocation t(10;14). Blood 78:2996, 1991

93. Hatano M, Roberts CWM, Minden M, et al: Deregulation of a homeobox gene, HOX11, by the t(10;14) in T cell leukemia. Science 253:79, 1991

94. Kennedy MA, Gonzales-Sarmiento R, Kees UR, et al: HOX11, a homeobox-containing T-cell oncogene on human chromosome 10q24. Proc Natl Acad Sci USA 88:8900, 1991

95. Sanchez Garcia I, Kaneko Y, Gonzales-Sarmiento R, et al: A study of chromosome 11p13 translocations involving TCRβ and TCRδ in human T cell leukemia. Oncogene 6:577, 1991

96. Ribeiro RC, Raimondi SC, Behm FG, et al: Clinical and biologic features of childhood T-cell leukemia with the t(11;14). Blood 78:466, 1991

97. Boehm T, Baer R, Lavenir A, et al: The mechanism of chromosomal translocation t(11;14) involving the T-cell receptor $C_δ$ locus on human chromosome 14q11 and a translated region of chromosome 11p15. EMBO J 7:385, 1988

98. McGuire EA, Hockett RD, Pollock KM, et al: The t(11;14)(p15;q11) in a T-cell acute lymphoblastic leukemia cell line activates multiple transcripts, including Ttg-1, a gene encoding a potential zinc finger protein. Mol Cell Biol 9:2124, 1989

99. Boehm T, Greenberg JM, Buluwela M, et al: An unusual structure of a putative T-cell oncogene which allows production of similar proteins from distinct mRNAs. EMBO J 9:857, 1990

100. Boehm T, Foroni L, Kennedy M, et al: The rhombotin gene belongs to a class of transcriptional regulators with a potential novel protein dimerisation motif. Oncogene 5:1103, 1990

101. Boehm T, Foroni L, Yaneko Y, et al: The rhombotin family of cystein-rich LIM-domain oncogenes: Distinct members are involved in T-cell translocations to human chromosomes 11p15 and 11p13. Proc Natl Acad Sci USA 88:4367, 1991

102. Greenberg JM, Boehm T, Sofroniew MV, et al: Segmental and developmental regulation of a presumptive T-cell oncogene in the central nervous system. Nature 344:158, 1990

103. Boehm T, Spillantin M-G, Sofroniew MV, et al: Developmentally regulated and tissue specific expression of mRNAs encoding the two alternative forms of the LIM domain oncogene rhombotin: Evidence for thymus expression. Oncogene 6:695, 1991

104. McGuire EA, Rintoul CE, Sclar GM, et al: Thymic overexpression of Ttg-1 in transgenic mice results in T-cell acute lymphoblastic leukemia/lymphoma. Mol Cell Biol 12:4186, 1992

105. Hogan T, Koss W, Murgo A, et al: Acute lymphoblastic leukemia with chromosomal 5;14 translocation and hypereosinophilia: Case report and literature review. J Clin Oncol 5:382, 1987

106. Tono-oka T, Sato Y, Matsumoto T, et al: Hypereosinophilic syndrome in acute lymphoblastic leukemia with a chromosome translocation t(5q;14q). Med Pediatr Oncol 12:33, 1984

107. Raimondi SC, Privitera E, Williams DL, et al: New recurring chromosomal translocations in childhood acute lymphoblastic leukemia. Blood 77:2016, 1991

108. Grimaldi J, Meeker T: The t(5;14) chromosomal translocation in a case of acute lymphocytic leukemia joins the interleukin-3 gene to the immunoglobulin heavy chain gene. Blood 73:2081, 1989

109. Meeker TC, Hardy D, Willman C, et al: Activation of the interleukin-3 gene by chromosome translocation in acute lymphocytic leukemia with eosinophilia. Blood 76:285, 1990

110. Hunger SP, Ohyashiki K, Toyama K, et al: Hlf, a novel hepatic

111. Inaba T, Mark Roberts W, Shapiro LH, et al: Fusion of the leucine zipper gene HLF to the E2A gene in human acute B-lineage leukemia. Science 257:531, 1992

112. Mellentin JD, Smith SD, Cleary ML: lyl-1, a novel gene altered by chromosomal translocation in T cell leukemia, codes for a protein with a helix-loop-helix DNA binding motif. Cell 58:77, 1989

113. Xia Y, Brown L, Yang CY-C, et al: TAL2, a helix-loop-helix gene activated by the t(7;9)(q34;q32) translocation in human T-cell leukemia. Proc Natl Acad Sci USA 88:11416, 1991

114. Ellisen LW, Bird J, West DC, et al: TAN-1, the human homolog of the Drosophila notch gene, is broken by chromosomal translocations in T lymphoblastic neoplasms. Cell 66:649, 1991

115. Tycko B, Smith SD, Sklar J: Chromosomal translocations joining LCK and TCRB loci in human T cell leukemia. J Exp Med 174:867, 1991

116. Neri N, Knowles DM, Greco A, et al: Analysis of Ras oncogene mutations in human lymphoid malignancies. Proc Natl Acad Sci USA 85:9268, 1988

117. Lubbert M, Mirro J Jr, Miller CW, et al: N-Ras gene point mutations in childhood acute lymphocytic leukemia correlate with a poor prognosis. Blood 75:1163, 1990

118. Gaidano G, Ballerini P, Gong JZ, et al: p53 mutations in human lymphoid malignancies: Association with Burkitt lymphoma and chronic lymphocytic leukemia. Proc Natl Acad Sci USA 88:5413, 1991

119. Diaz MO, Ziemin S, Le Beau MM, et al: Homozygous deletion of the α- and β_1-interferon genes in human leukemia and derived cell lines. Proc Natl Acad Sci USA 85:5259, 1988

120. Diaz MO, Rubin CM, Harden A, et al: Deletions of interferon genes in acute lymphoblastic leukemia. N Engl J Med 322:77, 1990

121. Hayashi Y, Raimondi SC, Look AT, et al: Abnormalities of the long arm of chromosome 6 in childhood acute lymphoblastic leukemia. Blood 76:1626, 1990

122. Williams DL, Tsiatis A, Brodeur GM, et al: Prognostic importance of chromosome number in 136 untreated children with acute lymphoblastic leukemia. Blood 60:864, 1982

123. Pui C-H, Williams DL, Roberson PK, et al: Correlation of karyotype and immunophenotype in childhood acute lymphoblastic leukemia. J Clin Oncol 6:56, 1988

124. Pui C-H, Raimondi SC, Dodge RK, et al: Prognostic importance of structural chromosomal abnormalities in children with hyperdiploid (>50 chromosomes) acute lymphoblastic leukemia. Blood 73:1963, 1989

125. Ribeiro RC, Abromowitch M, Raimondi SC, et al: Clinical and biological hallmarks of the Philadelphia chromosome in childhood acute lymphoblastic leukemia. Blood 70:948, 1987

126. Crist W, Carrol A, Schuster J, et al: Philadelphia chromosome positive childhood acute lymphoblastic leukemia: Clinical and cytogenetic characteristics and treatment outcome. A Pediatric Oncology Group (POG) study. Blood 76:489, 1990

127. Berger R, Chen SJ, Chen Z: Philadelphia-positive acute leukemia: Cytogenetic and molecular aspects. Cancer Genet Cytogenet 44:143, 1990

128. Priest JR, Robison LL, McKenna RW, et al: Philadelphia chromosome positive childhood acute lymphoblastic leukemia. Blood 56:15, 1980

129. Pui C-H, Raimondi SC, Murphy SB, et al: An analysis of leukemic cell chromosomal features in infants. Blood 69:1289, 1987

130. Kaneko Y, Shikano T, Maseki N, et al: Clinical characteristics of infant acute leukemia with or without 11q23 translocations. Leukemia 2:672, 1988

131. Katz F, Malcolm S, Gibbons B, et al: Cellular and molecular studies on infant null acute lymphoblastic leukemia. Blood 71:1438, 1988

132. Gibbons B, Katz FE, Ganly P, et al: Infant acute leukemia with t(11;19). Br J Haematol 74:264, 1990

133. Arthur DC, Bloomfield CD, Lindquist LL, et al: Translocation

4;11 in acute leukemia: Clinical characteristics and prognostic significance. Blood 59:96, 1982

134. Pui C-H, Frankel LS, Carrol AJ, et al: Clinical characteristics and treatment outcome of childhood acute lymphoblastic leukemia with the t(4;11)(q21;q23): A collaborative study of 40 cases. Blood 77:440, 1991

135. Parkin JL, Arthur DC, Abramson CS, et al: Acute leukemia associated with the t(4;11) chromosome rearrangement: Ultrastructural and immunologic characteristics. Blood 60: 1321, 1982

136. Nagasaka M, Maeda S, Maeda H, et al: Four cases of t(4;11) acute leukemia and its myelomonocytic nature in infants. Blood 61:1174, 1983

137. Rivera GK, Raimondi SC, Hancock ML, et al: Improved outcome in childhood acute lymphoblastic leukemia with reinforced early treatment and rotational combination chemotherapy. Lancet 337:61, 1991

138. Abe R, Ryan D, Cecalupo A, et al: Cytogenetic findings in congenital leukemia: Case report and review of the literature. Cancer Genet Cytogenet 9:139, 1983

139. Kawasaki ES, Clark SS, Coyne MY, et al: Diagnosis of chronic myeloid leukemia and acute lymphocytic leukemias by detection of leukemia-specific mRNA sequences amplified in vitro. Proc Natl Acad Sci USA 85:5698, 1988

140. Kohler S, Galili N, Sklar JL, et al: Expression of BCR-ABL fusion transcripts following bone marrow transplantation for Philadelphia chromosome-positive leukemia. Leukemia 8: 541, 1990

141. Hunger SP, Galili N, Carrol AJ, et al: The t(1;19)(q23;p13) results in consistent fusion of E2A and PBX1 coding sequences in acute lymphoblastic leukemia. Blood 77:687, 1991

142. Izraeli S, Kovar H, Gadner H, et al: Unexpected heterogeneity in E2A/PBX1 fusion messenger RNA detected by the polymerase chain reaction in pediatric patients with acute lymphoblastic leukemia. Blood 80:1413, 1992

143. Jonsson OG, Kitchens RL, Baer R, et al: Rearrangements of the tal-1 locus as clonal markers for T cell acute lymphoblastic leukemia. J Clin Invest 87:2029, 1991

144. Magrath IT: The non-Hodgkin's lymphomas: An introduction. In Magrath IT (ed): The Non-Hodgkin's Lymphomas. Baltimore, Williams & Wilkins, 1991, pp 1–14

145. National Cancer Institute sponsored study of classification of non-Hodgkin lymphomas: Summary and description of a working formulation for clinical usage. Cancer 49:2112, 1982

146. Bakhshi A, Jensen JP, Goldman P, et al: Cloning the chromosomal breakpoint of t(14;18) human lymphomas: Clustering around J_H on chromosome 14 and near a transcriptional unit on 18. Cell 41:889, 1985

147. Tsujimoto Y, Finger LR, Yunis J, et al: Cloning of the chromosome breakpoint of neoplastic B cells with the t(14;18) chromosome translocation. Science 226:1097, 1984

148. Cleary ML, Sklar J: Nucleotide sequence of a t(14;18) chromosomal breakpoint cluster region near a transcriptionally active locus on chromosome 18. Proc Natl Acad Sci USA 82:7439, 1985

149. Korsmeyer SJ: Bcl-2 initiates a new category of oncogenes: Regulators of cell death. Blood 80:879, 1992

150. Cleary ML, Smith SD, Sklar J: Cloning and structural analysis of cDNAs for bcl-2 and a hybrid bcl-2/immunoglobulin transcript resulting from the t(14;18) translocation. Cell 47:19, 1986

151. Graninger WB, Seto M, Boutain B, et al: Expression of bcl-2 and bcl-2-Ig fusion transcripts in normal and neoplastic cells. J Clin Invest 80:1512, 1987

152. Seto M, Jaeger U, Hockett RD, et al: Alternative promoters and exons, somatic mutation and transcriptional deregulation of the Bcl-2-Ig fusion gene in lymphoma. EMBO J 7:123, 1988

153. Ngan B-Y, Chen-Levy Z, Weiss LM, et al: Expression in non-Hodgkin's lymphoma of the bcl-2 protein associated with the t(14;18) chromosomal translocation. N Engl J Med 318:1638, 1988

154. Cleary ML, Galili N, Sklar J: Detection of a second t(14;18)

breakpoint cluster region in human follicular lymphomas. J Exp Med 164:315, 1986

155. Bakhshi A, Wright JJ, Graninger W, et al: Mechanisms of the t(14;18) chromosomal translocation: Structural analysis of both derivative 14 and 18 reciprocal partners. Proc Natl Acad Sci USA 84:2396, 1987

156. Ngan B-Y, Nourse J, Cleary ML: Detection of chromosomal translocation t(14;18) within the minor cluster region of Bcl-2 by polymerase chain reaction and direct genomic sequencing of the enzymatically amplified DNA in follicular lymphomas. Blood 73:1759, 1989

157. Hockenberry D, Nunez G, Milliman C, et al: Bcl-2 is an inner mitochondrial membrane protein that blocks programmed cell death. Nature 348:334, 1990

158. Vaux DL, Cory S, Adams JM: Bcl-2 gene promotes hemopoietic cell survival and cooperates with c-myc to immortalize pre-B cells. Nature 335:440, 1988

159. Nunez G, London L, Hockenberry D, et al: Deregulated bcl-2 gene expression selectively prolongs survival of growth-factor-deprived hemopoietic cell lines. J Immunol 144:3602, 1990

160. Hockenberry D, Zutter M, Hickey W, et al: Bcl-2 protein is topographically restricted in tissues characterized by apoptotic cell death. Proc Natl Acad Sci USA 88:6961, 1991

161. Chen-Levy Z, Nourse J, Cleary ML: The bcl-2 candidate proto-oncogene product is a 24-kilodalton integral-membrane protein highly expressed in lymphoid cell lines and lymphomas carrying the t(14;18) translocation. Mol Cell Biol 9:701, 1989

162. de Jong D, Prins F, van Krieken HH, et al: Subcellular localization of bcl-2 protein. Curr Top Microbiol Immunol 182: 287, 1992

163. Nunez G, Hockenberry D, McDonnel TJ, et al: Bcl-2 maintains B-cell memory. Nature 353:71, 1991

164. Nunez G, Sato M, Seremetis S, et al: Growth and tumor promoting effects of deregulated bcl-2 in human B lymphoblastoid cells. Proc Natl Acad Sci USA 86:4589, 1989

165. Tsujimoto Y: Overexpression of the human bcl-2 gene product results in growth enhancement of Epstein-Barr virus-immortalized B cells. Proc Natl Acad Sci USA 86:1958, 1989

166. McDonnel TJ, Deane N, Platt FM, et al: bcl-2-immunoglobulin transgenic mice demonstrate extended B cell survival and follicular lymphoproliferation. Cell 57:79, 1989

167. McDonnel TJ, Korsmeyer SJ: Progression from lymphoid hyperplasia to high-grade malignant lymphoma in mice transgenic for the t(14;18). Nature 349:254, 1991

168. Limpens J, de Jong D, van Krieken JH, et al: Bcl-2/J_H rearrangements in benign lymphoid tissues with follicular hyperplasia. Oncogene 6:2271, 1991

169. Taub R, Kirsch I, Morton C, et al: Translocation of c-myc gene into the immunoglobulin heavy chain locus in human Burkitt lymphoma and murine plasmacytoma cells. Proc Natl Acad Sci USA 79:7837, 1982

170. Davis M, Malcolm S, Rabbits TH: Chromosome translocations can occur on either side of the c-myc oncogene in Burkitt lymphoma cells. Nature 308:286, 1984

171. Hollis GF, Mitchell KF, Battey J, et al: A variant translocation places the lambda immunoglobulin genes 3' to the c-myc oncogene in Burkitt's lymphoma. Nature 307:752, 1984

172. Pelicci PG, Knowles DK, Magrath I, et al: Chromosomal breakpoints and structural alterations of the c-myc locus differ in endemic and sporadic forms of Burkitt lymphoma. Proc Natl Acad Sci USA 83:2984, 1986

173. Haluska FG, Finger S, Tsujimoto Y, et al: The t(8;14) chromosomal translocation occurring in B-cell malignancies results from mistakes in V-D-J joining. Nature 324:158, 1986

174. Neri A, Barriga F, Knowles DM, et al: Different regions of the immunoglobulin heavy-chain locus are involved in chromosomal translocations in distinct pathogenetic forms of Burkitt lymphoma. Proc Natl Acad Sci USA 85:2748, 1988

175. Marcu KB, Bossone SA, Patel AS: Myc function and regulation. Annu Rev Biochem 61:809, 1992

176. Haluska FG, Tsujimoto Y, Croce CM: Oncogene activation by chromosomal translocation in human malignancy. Annu Rev Genet 21:321, 1987

177. Eick D, Bornkamm GW: Expression of normal and translocated c-myc alleles in Burkitt's lymphoma cells: Evidence for different regulation. EMBO J 8:1965, 1989
178. Grignani F, Lombardi L, Inghirami G, et al: Negative autoregulation of c-myc gene expression is inactivated in transformed cells. EMBO J 9:3913, 1990
179. Cesarman E, Dalla-Favera R, Bentley D, et al: Mutations in the first exon are associated with altered transcription of c-myc in Burkitt lymphoma. Science 238:1272, 1987
180. Murphy JP, Neri A, Richter R, et al: C-myc regulator sequences are consistently mutated in Burkitt's lymphoma. Manuscript in preparation, 1994
181. Lombardi L, Newcomb EW, Dalla-Favera R: Pathogenesis of Burkitt lymphoma: Expression of an activated c-myc oncogene causes the tumorigenic conversion of EBV-infected human B-lymphoblasts. Cell 49:161, 1987
182. Reed JC, Cuddy MP, Croce CM, et al: Deregulated bcl-2 expression enhances growth and tumorigenicity of a human B-cell line. Oncogene 4:1103, 1989
183. McManaway ME, Neckers LM, Loke SL, et al: Tumor-specific inhibition of lymphoma growth by an antisense oligodeoxynucleotide. Lancet 335:808, 1990
184. Adams JM, Harris AW, Pinkert CA, et al: The c-myc oncogene driven by immunoglobulin enhancers induces lymphoid malignancy in transgenic mice. Nature 318:533, 1985
185. Luscher B, Eisenman RN: New light on Myc and Myb. Part I: Myc. Genes Dev 4:2025, 1990
186. Blackwood EM, Eisenman RN: Max: A helix-loop-helix zipper protein that forms a sequence-specific DNA-binding complex with Myc. Science 251:1211, 1991
187. Gu W, Cechova K, Tassi V, et al: Differential regulation of target gene expression by Myc/Max ratio. Proc Natl Acad Sci USA 90:2935, 1993
188. Kretzner L, Blackwood EM, Eisenman RN: The Myc and Max proteins possess distinct transcriptional activities. Nature 359:426, 1992
189. Makela TP, Koskinen PJ, Vastrik I, et al: Alternative forms of Max as enhancers of suppressors of Myc-Ras cotransformation. Science 256:373, 1992
190. Tsujimoto Y, Yunis J, Onorato-Showe L, et al: Molecular cloning of the chromosomal breakpoint on chromosome 11 in human B-cell neoplasms with the t(11;14) chromosome translocation. Science 224:1403, 1984
191. Tsujimoto Y, Jaffe ES, Cossman J, et al: Clustering of breakpoints on chromosome 11 in human B-cell neoplasms with the t(11;14) chromosome translocation. Nature 315:340, 1985
192. Erikson J, Finan J, Tsujimoto Y, et al: The chromosome 11 breakpoint in neoplastic B cells with the t(11;14) translocation involves the immunoglobulin heavy chain locus. Proc Natl Acad Sci USA 81:4144, 1984
193. Raffeld M, Jaffe ES: bcl-1, t(11;14), and mantle zone lymphomas. Blood 78:259, 1991
194. Williams ME, Meeker TC, Swerdlow SH: Rearrangement of the chromosome 11 bcl-1 locus in centrocytic lymphoma: Analysis with multiple breakpoint probes. Blood 78:493, 1991
195. Motokura T, Bloom T, Goo KH, et al: A novel cyclin encoded by a bcl-1 linked candidate oncogene. Nature 350:512, 1991
196. Withers DA, Harvey RC, Faust JB, et al: Characterization of a candidate bcl-1 gene. Mol Cell Biol 11:4846, 1991
197. Rosenberg CL, Wong E, Petty EM, et al: PRAD1, a candidate BCL1 oncogene: Mapping and expression in centrocytic lymphoma. Proc Natl Acad Sci USA 88:9638, 1991
198. Offit K, Jhanwar S, Ebrahim SAD, et al: t(3;22)(q27;q11), a novel translocation associated with diffuse non-Hodgkin's lymphoma. Blood 74:1876, 1989
199. Bastard C, Tilly H, Lenormand B, et al: Translocations involving band 3q27 and Ig gene regions in non-Hodgkin's lymphoma. Blood 79:2527, 1992
200. Ye BH, Rao PH, Chaganti RSK, et al: Cloning of BCL-6, the locus involved in chromosome translocations affecting band 3q27 in B-cell lymphoma. Cancer Res 53:2732, 1993
201. Ye BH, Lista F, Lo Coco F, et al: Alterations of BCL-6, a novel zinc-finger encoding gene, in diffuse large cell lymphoma. Science 262:747, 1993
202. Baron BW, Nucifora G, McCabe N, et al: Identification of the gene associated with the recurring chromosomal translocations t(3;14)(q27;q32) and t(3;22)(q27;q11) in B-cell lymphomas. Proc Natl Acad Sci USA 90:5262, 1993
202a. Lo Coco F, Ye BH, Lista F, et al. Blood 83:1757, 1994
202b. Offit K, Lo Coco F, Louie DC, et al: Rearrangement of the BCL6 gene as a prognostic marker in diffuse large cell lymphoma. New Engl J Med, in press
203. Neri A, Chang C-C, Lombardi L, et al: B cell lymphoma-associated chromosomal translocation involves candidate oncogene lyt-10, homologous to NF-κB p50. Cell 67:1075, 1991
204. Lenardo MJ, Baltimore D: NF-κB: A pleiotropic mediator of inducible and tissue-specific gene control. Cell 58:227, 1989
205. Chang C-C, Zhang J, Lombardi L, et al: Mechanism of expression and role in transcriptional control of the proto-oncogene NFKB-2/LYT-10. Oncogene 9:923, 1994
206. Fracchiolla N, Lombardi L, Salina M, et al: Structure of the transcription factor NFKB-2/lyt-10 locus and its alterations in lymphoid malignancies. Oncogene 8:2839, 1993
207. Offit K, Parsa NZ, Jhanwar SC, et al: t(9;14)(p13;q32) denotes a subset of low grade non-Hodgkin's lymphoma with plasmacytoid differentiation. Blood 80:2594, 1992
208. Gaidano G, Hauptschein RS, Parsa NZ, et al: Deletions involving two distinct regions of 6q in B-cell non-Hodgkin lymphoma. Blood 80:1781, 1992
209. Offit K, Wong G, Filippa DA, et al: Cytogenetic analysis of 434 consecutively ascertained specimens of non-Hodgkin's lymphoma: Clinical correlations. Blood 77:1508, 1991
210. Offit K, Jhanwar SC, Ladanyi M, et al: Cytogenetic analysis of 434 consecutively ascertained specimens of non-Hodgkin's lymphoma: Correlations between recurrent aberrations, histology, and exposure to cytotoxic treatment. Genes Chromosome Cancer 3:189, 1991
211. Kieff E, Liebowitz D: Oncogenesis by herpesvirus. In Weinberg RA (ed): Oncogenes and the Molecular Origins of Cancer. Cold Spring Harbor, NY, Cold Spring Harbor Laboratory Press, 1989, pp 259–280
212. zur Hausen H, Schulte-Holthausen H, Klein G, et al: EBV DNA in biopsies of Burkitt tumors and anaplastic carcinomas of the nasopharynx. Nature 228:1056, 1970
213. Raab-Traub N, Flynn K: The structure of the termini of the Epstein-Barr virus as a marker of clonal cellular proliferation. Cell 47:883, 1986
214. Neri A, Barriga F, Inghirami G, et al: Epstein-Barr virus infection precedes clonal expansion in Burkitt's and acquired immunodeficiency-associated lymphoma. Blood 77:1092, 1991
215. Pelicci P-G, Knowles DM II, Arlin ZA, et al: Multiple monoclonal B cell expansions and c-myc oncogene rearrangements in acquired immunodeficiency syndrome-related lymphoproliferative disorders: Implications for lymphomagenesis. J Exp Med 164:2049, 1986
216. Gaidano G, Dalla-Favera R: Biologic aspects of human immunodeficiency virus-related lymphoma. Curr Opin Oncol 4:900, 1992
217. Wang F, Gregory CD, Rowe M, et al: Epstein-Barr virus nuclear antigen 2 specifically induces expression of the B-cell activation antigen CD23. Proc Natl Acad Sci USA 84:3452, 1987
218. Wang D, Liebowitz D, Kieff E: An EBV membrane protein expressed in immortalized lymphocytes transforms established rodent cells. Cell 43:831, 1985
219. Wang D, Liebowitz D, Wang F, et al: Epstein-Barr virus latent infection membrane protein alters the human B-lymphocyte phenotype: Deletion of the amino terminus abolishes activity. J Virol 62:2337, 1988
220. Klein G: Epstein-Barr virus-carrying cells in Hodgkin's disease. Blood 80:299, 1992
221. Contreras-Brodin BA, Anvret M, Imreh S, et al: B cell phenotype-dependent expression of the Epstein-Barr virus nuclear antigens EBNA-2 to EBNA-6: Studies with somatic cell hybrids. J Gen Virol 72:3025, 1991
222. Lipford L, Wright JJ, Urba W, et al: Refinement of lymphoma cytogenetics by the chromosome 18q21 major breakpoint region. Blood 70:1816, 1987

223. Lee M-S, Blick MB, Pathak S, et al: The gene located at chromosome 18 band q21 is rearranged in uncultured diffuse lymphomas as well as follicular lymphomas. Blood 70:90, 1987

224. Amakawa R, Fukuhara S, Ohno H, et al: Involvement of the bcl-2 gene in Japanese follicular lymphoma. Blood 73:787, 1989

225. Horning SJ, Rosenberg SA: The natural history of initially untreated low-grade non-Hodgkin's lymphomas. N Engl J Med 311:1471, 1984

226. Yano T, Jaffe ES, Longo DL, et al: MYC rearrangements in histologically progressed follicular lymphomas. Blood 80:758, 1992

227. Sander CA, Yano T, Karameris AM, et al: Association of p53 mutations with histologic transformation of follicular lymphoma and chronic lymphocytic leukemia. Blood 80(suppl 1):442a, 1992

228. Lo Coco, Gaidano G, Louie D, et al: p53 mutations are associated with histologic transformation of follicular lymphoma. Blood 82:2289, 1993

229. Inghirami G, Corradini P, Gu W, et al: Molecular analysis of the retinoblastoma gene in human lymphoid neoplasia. Manuscript in preparation, 1993

230. Athan E, Stefani S, Novero D, et al: BCL-2 rearrangements identify subgroup of diffuse non-Hodgkin lymphoma "transformed" from follicular form. Manuscript in preparation, 1993

231. Schouten HC, Sanger WG, Weisenburger DD, et al: Abnormalities involving chromosome 6 in newly diagnosed patients with non-Hodgkin lymphoma. Cancer Genet Cytogenet 47:73, 1990

232. Lee M-S, Chang K-S, Cabanillas F, et al: Detection of minimal residual cells carrying the t(14;18) by DNA sequence amplification. Science 237:175, 1987

233. Crescenzi M, Seto M, Herzig GP, et al: Thermostable polymerase chain amplification of t(14;18) breakpoints and the detection of minimal residual disease. Proc Natl Acad Sci USA 85:4869, 1988

234. Dighiero G, Travade P, Chevret S, et al: B-cell chronic lymphocytic leukemia: Present status and future directions. Blood 78:1901, 1991

235. Sonnier JA, Buchanan GR, Howard-Peebles PN, et al: Chromosomal translocation involving the immunoglobulin kappa-chain and heavy-chain loci in a child with chronic lymphocytic leukemia. N Engl J Med 309:590, 1983

236. Yoffe G, Howard-Peebles PN, Smith RG, et al: Childhood chronic lymphocytic leukemia with t(2;14) translocation. J Pediatr 116:114, 1990

237. Gaidano G, Gong JZ, Newcomb EW, et al: Genetic lesions in B-cell chronic lymphocytic leukemia. Am J Pathol 144:1312, 1994

238. Rechavi G, Katzir N, Brok-Simoni F, et al: A search for bcl1, bcl2, and c-myc oncogene rearrangements in chronic lymphocytic leukemia. Leukemia 3:57, 1989

239. Athan E, Foitl DR, Knowles DM: BCL-1 rearrangement: Frequency and clinical significance among B-cell chronic lymphocytic leukemias and non-Hodgkin's lymphomas. Am J Pathol 138:591, 1991

240. Raghoebier S, van Krieken JHJM, Kluin-Nelemans JC, et al: Oncogene rearrangements in chronic B-cell leukemia. Blood 77:1560, 1991

241. Schena M, Larsson L-G, Gottardi D, et al: Growth- and differentiation-associated expression of bcl-2 in B-chronic lymphocytic leukemia cells. Blood 79:2981, 1992

242. Fell HP, Graham Smith R, Tucker PW: Molecular analysis of the t(2;14) translocation of childhood chronic lymphocytic leukemia. Science 232:491, 1986

243. Richardson AR, Humphries CG, Tucker PW: Molecular cloning and characterization of the t(2;14) translocation associated with childhood chronic lymphocytic leukemia. Oncogene 7:961, 1992

244. Juliusson G, Oscier DG, Fitchett M, et al: Prognostic subgroups in B-cell chronic lymphocytic leukemia defined by specific chromosomal abnormalities. N Engl J Med 323:720, 1990

245. Anastasi J, Le Beau M, Vardiman JW, et al: Detection of trisomy 12 in chronic lymphocytic leukemia by fluorescent in situ hybridization to interphase cells: A simple and sensitive method. Blood 79:1796, 1992

246. Begsagel DE: Plasma cell myeloma. In Williams WJ, Beutler E, Erslev AJ, Lichtman MA (ed): Hematology, 4th ed. New York, McGraw-Hill, 1990, pp 1114–1141

247. Klein B, Jourdan M, Vasquez A, et al: Production of growth factors by human myeloma cells. Cancer Res 47:4856, 1987

248. Kawano M, Hirano T, Matsuda T, et al: Autocrine generation and requirement of BSF-2/IL-6 for human multiple myelomas. Nature 332:83, 1988

249. Bergui L, Schena M, Gaidano G, et al: Interleukin 3 and interleukin 6 synergistically promote the proliferation and differentiation of malignant plasma cell precursors in multiple myeloma. J Exp Med 170:613, 1989

250. Klein B, Zhang X-G, Jourdan M, et al: Paracrine rather than autocrine regulation of myeloma-cell growth and differentiation by interleukin-6. Blood 73:517, 1989

251. Caligaris-Cappio F, Bergui L, Gregoretti MG, et al: Role of bone-marrow stromal cells in the growth of human multiple myeloma. Blood 77:2688, 1991

252. Garret LR, Durie BGM, Nedwin GE, et al: Production of the bone resorbing cytokine lymphotoxin by cultured human myeloma cells. N Engl J Med 317:526, 1987

253. Kawano M, Yamamoto I, Iwato K, et al: Interleukin-1 beta rather than lymphotoxin is the major bone resorbing activity in human multiple myeloma. Blood 73:1646, 1989

254. Cozzolino F, Torcia M, Aldinucci D, et al: Production of interleukin-1 by bone marrow myeloma cells: Its role in the pathogenesis of lytic bone lesions. Blood 74:380, 1989

255. Neri A, Murphy JP, Cro L, et al: RAS oncogenes mutation in multiple myeloma. J Exp Med 170:1715, 1989

256. Paquette RL, Berenson J, Lichtenstein A, et al: Oncogenes in multiple myeloma: Point mutation of N-ras. Oncogene 5:1569, 1990

257. Corradini P, Ladetto M, Voena C, et al: Mutational activation of N- and K-Ras oncogenes in plasma cell dyscrasias. Blood 81:2708, 1993

258. Seremetis S, Inghirami G, Ferrero D, et al: Transformation and plasmacytoid differentiation of EBV-infected human B lymphoblasts by ras oncogenes, Science 243:660, 1989

259. Pegoraro L, Malavasi F, Bellone G, et al: The human myeloma cell line LP-1: A versatile model in which to study early plasma-cell differentiation and c-myc activation. Blood 73:1020, 1989

260. Selvanayagam P, Blick M, Marni F, et al: Alteration and abnormal expression of the c-myc oncogene in human multiple myeloma. Blood 71:30, 1988

261. Palumbo A, Boccadoro M, Battaglio S, et al: Human homologue of Moloney Leukemia Virus Integration-4 locus (MLVI-4), located 20 kilobases 3' of the c-myc gene, is rearranged in multiple myeloma. Cancer Res 50:6478, 1990

262. Neri A, Baldini L, Trecca D, et al: p53 gene mutations in multiple myeloma are associated with advanced forms of malignancy. Blood 81:128, 1993

263. Karp JE, Broder S: Acquired immunodeficiency syndrome and non-Hodgkin's lymphomas. Cancer Res 51:4743, 1991

264. Levine AM: Acquired immunodeficiency syndrome-related lymphoma. Blood 80:8, 1992

265. Frizzera G: Atypical lymphoproliferative disorders. In Knowles DM (ed): Neoplastic Hematopathology. Baltimore, Williams & Wilkins, 1992, pp 459–495

266. Subar M, Neri A, Inghirami G, et al: Frequent c-myc oncogene activation and infrequent presence of Epstein-Barr virus genome in AIDS-associated lymphoma. Blood 72:667, 1988

267. Hamilton-Dutoit SJ, Pallesen G, Franzmann MB, et al: AIDS-related lymphoma: Histopathology, immunophenotype, and association with Epstein-Barr virus as demonstrated by in situ nucleic acid hybridization. Am J Pathol 138:149, 1991

268. MacMahon EME, Glass JD, Hayward SD, et al: Epstein-Barr virus in AIDS-related primary central nervous system lymphoma. Lancet 338:969, 1991

269. Ballerini P, Gaidano G, Gong JZ, et al: Molecular pathogenesis of HIV-associated lymphoma. AIDS Res Hum Retroviruses 8:731, 1992

270. Ballerini P, Gaidano G, Gong JZ, et al: Multiple genetic lesions in acquired immunodeficiency syndrome-related non-Hodgkin's lymphoma. Blood 81:166, 1993

271. Gaidano G, Parsa NZ, Tassi V, et al: In vitro establishment of AIDS-related lymphoma cell lines: Phenotypic characterization, oncogene and tumor suppressor gene lesions, and heterogeneity in Epstein-Barr virus infection. Leukemia 7:1621, 1993

272. Fearon E, Vogelstein B: A genetic model for colorectal tumorigenesis. Cell 61:759, 1990

273. Ho M, Miller G, Atchison RW, et al: Epstein-Barr virus infections and DNA hybridization studies in posttransplantation lymphoma and lymphoproliferative lesions: The role of primary infection. J Infect Dis 152:876, 1985

274. Cleary ML, Nalesnik MA, Shearer WT, et al: Clonal analysis of transplant-associated lymphoproliferations based on the structure of the genomic termini of the Epstein-Barr virus. Blood 72:349, 1988

275. Locker J, Nalesnik M: Molecular genetic analysis of lymphoid tumors arising after organ transplantation. Am J Pathol 135:977, 1989

276. Weiss LM, Movahed LA: In situ demonstration of Epstein-Barr viral genomes in viral-associated B-cell lymphoproliferations. Am J Pathol 134:651, 1989

277. Patton DF, Wilkowski CW, Hanson CA, et al: Epstein-Barr virus-determined clonality in posttransplant lymphoproliferative disease. Transplantation 49:1080, 1990

278. Borisch-Chappuis B, Nezelof C, Muller H, et al: Different Epstein-Barr virus expression in lymphomas from immunocompromised and immunocompetent patients. Am J Pathol 136:751, 1990

279. Pinkus GS, Said JW: Peripheral T cell lymphomas. In Knowles DM (ed): Neoplastic Hematopathology. Baltimore, Williams & Wilkins, 1992, pp 837–867

280. Nagai M, Ikeda K, Tasaka T, et al: Genomic rearrangement of the c-myc proto-oncogene in non-AIDS-related lymphoma in Japan. Leukemia 5:462, 1991

281. Kaneko Y, Frizzera G, Edamura S, et al: A novel translocation, t(2;5)(p23;q35), in childhood phagocytic large T-cell lymphoma mimicking malignant hystiocytosis. Blood 73:806, 1989

282. Ebrahim SAD, Ladanyi M, Desai SB, et al: Immunohistochemical, molecular, and cytogenetic analysis of a consecutive series of 20 peripheral T-cell lymphomas and lymphomas of uncertain lineage, including 12 Ki-1 positive lymphomas. Genes Chromosome Cancer 2:27, 1990

283. Doglioni C, Pelosio P, Mombello A, et al: Immunohistochemical evidence of abnormal expression of the antioncogene-encoded p53 phosphoprotein in Hodgkin's disease and CD30⁺ anaplastic lymphomas. Hematol Pathol 5:67, 1991

284. Ohnishi K, Ichikawa A, Kagami Y, et al: Interleukin 4 and gamma-interpheron may play a role in the histopathogenesis of peripheral T-cell lymphoma. Cancer Res 50:8028, 1990

285. Merz H, Fliedner A, Orscheschek K, et al: Cytokine expression in T-cell lymphomas and Hodgkin's disease: Its possible implication in autocrine or paracrine production as a potential basis for neoplastic growth. Am J Pathol 139:1173, 1991

286. Poiesz BF, Ruscetti FW, Gazdar AF, et al: Detection and isolation of type C retrovirus particles from fresh cultured lymphocytes of a patient with cutaneous T-cell lymphoma. Proc Natl Acad Sci USA 77:7415, 1980

287. Catovsky D, Rose M, Goolden AWG, et al: Adult T-cell lymphoma-leukaemia in blacks from the West Indies. Lancet 1:639, 1982

288. Yoshida M, Miyoshi I, Hinuma Y: Isolation and characterization of retrovirus from cell lines of adult T-cell leukemia and its implication in the disease. Proc Natl Acad Sci USA 79:2031, 1982

289. Gallo RC, Kalyanaraman VS, Sarngadharan MG, et al: Association of the human type of C retrovirus with a subset of adult T-cell cancers. Cancer Res 43:3892, 1983

290. Wong-Staal F, Hahn B, Manzari V, et al: A survey of human leukemias for sequences of a human retrovirus. Nature 302:626, 1983

291. Yoshida M, Seiki M, Yamaguchi K, et al: Monoclonal integration of human T-cell leukemia provirus in all primary tumors of adult T-cell leukemia suggests causative role of human T-cell leukemia virus in the disease. Proc Natl Acad Sci USA 81:2534, 1984

292. Smith MR, Green W: Molecular biology of the type I human T-cell leukemia virus (HTLV-I) and adult T-cell leukemia. J Clin Invest 87:761, 1991

293. Inoue J, Seiki M, Taniguchi T, et al: Induction of interleukin-2 receptor gene expression by p40 encoded by human T-cell leukemia virus type I. EMBO J 5:2883, 1987

294. Cross SL, Feinberg MB, Wolf JB, et al: Regulation of the human interleukin-2 α chain promoter: Activation of a nonfunctional promoter by the transactivator gene of HTLV-I. Cell 49:47, 1987

295. Fujii M, Sassone-Corsi P, Verma IM: c-fos promoter transactivation by the tax1 protein of human T-cell leukemia virus type I. Proc Natl Acad Sci USA 85:8526, 1988

296. Wano Y, Feinberg M, Hosking JB, et al: Stable expression of the tax gene of type I human T-cell leukemia virus in human T-cells activates specific cellular genes involved in growth. Proc Natl Acad Sci USA 85:9733, 1988

297. Nimer SD, Gasson JC, Hu K, et al: Activation of the GM-CSF promoter by HTLV-I and -II tax proteins. Oncogene 4:671, 1989

298. Jeang KT, Widen SG, Semmes OJ, et al: HTLV-I transactivator protein, Tax, is a transrepressor of the human β-polymerase gene. Science 247:1082, 1990

299. Sakashita A, Hattori T, Miller CW, et al: Mutations of the p53 gene in adult T-cell leukemia. Blood 79:477, 1992

300. Cesarman E, Chadburn A, Inghirami G, et al: Structural and functional analysis of oncogenes and tumor suppressor genes in adult T-cell leukemia/lymphoma shows frequent p53 mutations. Blood 80:3205, 1992

301. Gaidano G, Dalla-Favera R: Biologic and molecular characterization of non-Hodgkin's lymphoma. Curr Opin Oncol, 5:555, 1993

302. Riboldi P, Gaidano G, Schettino EW, et al: Evidence for somatic selection by a self antigen in AIDS-associated Burkitt's lymphoma. Blood 83:2952, 1994

13

MOLECULAR DIAGNOSIS AND THERAPY OF HEMATOPOIETIC NEOPLASMS

ISSA KHOURI
HAGOP KANTARJIAN
MOSHE TALPAZ
DAVID CLAXTON
STEVEN KORNBLAU
ALBERT B. DEISSEROTH

Eighty per cent of cancers are thought to arise from exposure of somatic cells lining the epithelial surfaces to environmental carcinogens. This exposure often extends over years before sufficient numbers of somatic mutations are acquired to result in frankly invasive neoplasia. Consequently, the number of chromosomal changes as well as the number of changes at the nucleotide level are very large indeed. It is surprising, therefore, that only 20 to 30 per cent of individuals who are exposed to high levels of carcinogens develop cancer, suggesting that there are genetic factors that may determine susceptibility, such as tumor suppressor or DNA repair genes. The loss of such genes may increase the probability of developing cancer following carcinogen exposure.

In contrast to solid tumors, in which a very large number of genetic changes are acquired before frankly invasive cancer is generated, the development of hematopoietic neoplasms appears to involve the acquisition of a smaller number of genetic changes. In the early part of the 1970s, cytogenetic analysis of the leukemias resulted in the discovery of a number of balanced translocations [t(9;22), t(8;21), t(15;17)], monosomies (−7, −5), trisomies (+8), and other lineages (such as inversion 16 and inversion 3) that are associated with specific types of mye-

logenous leukemias. Each of these chromosomally defined subsets displays a unique clinical natural history and pattern of response to therapy.[1] A similar collection of changes already has been discovered in the lymphatic leukemias and, more recently, in the non-Hodgkin's lymphomas as well. The targets for these genetic changes may involve growth factor receptors, signal transduction molecules, tumor suppressor proteins, transcriptional regulatory genes, and the growth regulatory genes themselves, as shown in Figure 13–1.

CHRONIC MYELOGENOUS LEUKEMIA

Surprisingly, an even greater number of changes at the nucleotide level have been discovered in the subsets of leukemia, lymphoma, and solid tumors than are detectable at the cytogenetic level. Environmental exposures (such as radiation and chemical mutagens) are followed by the appearance of cytogenetic changes as well as the acquisition of point mutations in hematopoietic tissue. Changes such as the Philadelphia chromosome translocation of chronic myelogenous leukemia (CML) are induced re-

280

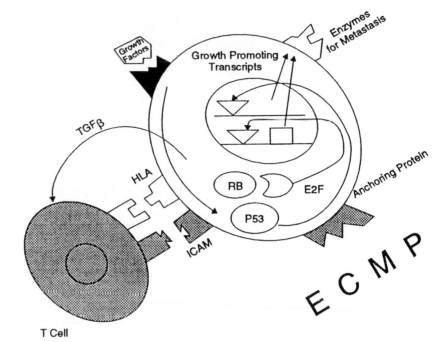

Figure 13–1. Recognition of the tumor antigens presented by the class I HLA by T cells. TGFβ indicates tumor growth factor-beta; ICAM, intercellular adhesion molecules; RB, retinoblastoma gene; p53, a tumor suppressor gene; E2F, a transcription factor involved in the activation of growth stimulatory genes; and ECMP, extracellular matrix protein.

producibly by exposure to radiation.[2] Moreover, there are also genetic elements that interact with transforming sequences at the junctions of the balanced chromosomal translocations such as *bcr-abl*. The reasons for believing that other changes must be present, in addition to those already discovered at the junctions of the chromosomal translocation breakpoints such as *bcr-abl*, in order for a decisive change in phenotype to occur are as follows.

First, not all individuals exposed to similar doses of irradiation therapy develop CML. Second, transduction of normal myeloid progenitor cells with viruses carrying *bcr-abl* cDNA in a transcription unit does not always result in phenotypic changes in the transduced cells that resemble CML. In fact, only a very small number of the animals transplanted with populations of cells transduced with *bcr-abl*–containing viruses develop CML. In contrast, the transduction of *bcr-abl* viruses into some very unique interleukin 3 (IL-3) growth-dependent cell lines makes the cells growth factor independent, suggesting that, in the correct regulatory and genetic environment, the *bcr-abl* virus can be transforming.[2]

Third, the results with animal model studies in transgenic mice and transplantation experiments in populations of marrow modified by the *bcr-abl* cDNA-containing viruses suggest that *bcr-abl* only very rarely alters the phenotype of the myeloid progenitor cells.

Fourth, the type of growth or "leukemia" that evolves following the transplantation of *bcr-abl*–modified populations of mice is very dependent on the genetic identity of the strain of mouse in which the *bcr-abl* mRNA sequences reside. For example, in certain strains of mice *bcr-abl* is associated with T-cell leukemias, whereas in others it causes B-cell leukemias, and, in still others, erythroleukemias or mast cell diseases. Only infrequently does one observe a phenotype that is suggestive of CML in animals transplanted with marrow cells transduced with

bcr-abl–expressing viruses. Clearly, the evolution of a population of cells that resemble CML following transfection with *bcr-abl* is a rare event, thus suggesting that, in both human and mouse, the evolution of the disease is dependent on both the presence of the *bcr-abl* translocation and the acquisition of changes in an unknown locus that complement the *bcr-abl* translocation. Animal model and in vitro cell data (*rat-1*) already have shown that *bcr-abl* can be transforming when complemented by known oncogenes, such as *myc* or *myb*. The cells that contain both *bcr-abl* and a dominant oncogene generate phenotypic changes consistent with tumor formation, anchorage-independent growth, and loss of contact inhibition.

Finally, CML is usually a disease that evolves in the fifth or sixth decade of life, suggesting that the t(9;22) translocation is occurring in the cells of normal individuals all the time, and that the alteration in a genetic locus of an as yet unknown identity must be acquired along with the Philadelphia chromosomal translocation to produce CML. It is further proposed that the acquisition of the altered second allele to generate the null genotype must be synchronous with the acquisition of the *bcr-abl* translocation breakpoint. The requirement for the loss of both normal alleles at the *bcr-abl* translocation explains the pattern of development of the disease late in life in the majority of patients and the observation that some of the patients (clearly the minority) develop the disease early in life. Presumably, these latter individuals are ones in whom the loss of the normal alleles at the unknown interacting genetic locus predisposes to the acquisition of CML early in life.

Natural History of CML

This leukemia starts in the chronic phase, which is an indolent disease characterized by leukocytosis (mature and immature myeloid cells), splenomegaly, thrombocytosis (at the beginning) or thrombocytopenia, mild anemia, and the presence of the Philadelphia chromosomal translocation, which is the cytogenetic hallmark of the disease. In addition, elevated vitamin B_{12}–binding protein levels and a low or absent leukocyte alkaline phosphatase level are encountered. Interestingly, CML is the one leukemia in which the incidence of *ras* mutations is very low at diagnosis, suggesting that the presence of the *bcr-abl* tyrosine-specific protein kinase makes the acquisition of the *ras* mutation irrelevant for the disease process. The biologic characteristic most commonly discussed is the relative independence of these cells of IL-3 and granulocyte-macrophage colony-stimulating factor (GM-CSF) for in vitro growth. In contrast to normal cells, the CML myeloid precursor cell does not stop proliferating when the white cell count rises above 10,000/cu mm, whereas the normal cell persists in shutting down proliferation when the white cell count rises to greater than normal levels. This results in a gradual reduction of the level of normal myeloid cells, and a continuing increase in the ratio of the leukemic to normal myeloid cells.

The prognosis in patients is thought to be related to the ratio of leukemic cells to the normal cells, because if the ratio of leukemic to normal cells is low, this indicates that the disease has not been present for very long, and that the possibility of achieving complete cytogenetic remission is very high with interferon therapy.

Following a variable period of time (a median of 4 years in older series but inexplicably increasing to 7 years in most recent series), the disease evolves from a chronic leukemia that does not affect the quality of life or survival of the patient, to a fulminant acute myelogenous leukemia, in which the patient dies of bleeding and infection, with only primitive leukemic blasts circulating in the patient's peripheral blood. The mechanism through which this transition takes place is the acquisition of somatic mutations, which is accompanied by the evolution of additional chromosomal abnormalities (additional Philadelphia chromosome, 17p deletion, isochromosome 17, trisomy 8, and a missing Y chromosome); severe anemia; severe thrombocytopenia; increasing blasts in the peripheral blood and bone marrow (15 per cent or more blasts); basophilia (15 per cent or more); and systemic symptoms such as fever, bone pain, and weight loss. This constellation of features is called the accelerated phase of CML. By the time the blast count reaches 30 per cent in the bone marrow, or the sum of the basophil count and the blast count rises above 30 per cent, the patient is described as being in blastic crisis. Patients apparently are subject to a 25 per cent risk of transformation into the blastic crisis every year of their life.

Therapy for CML

Patients seek therapy for CML, although the disease is indolent in the beginning, because they know that eventually the disease progresses to the blastic phase, and that the probability of controlling the disease, once it evolves into the blast crisis, is very low. All of the therapy for CML can be viewed as having as its purpose the reduction of the probability of entering blastic crisis, which, once it occurs, is associated with a survival of months.

The decision for therapy is becoming formalized for CML as a result of the wealth of systematic studies of this disease over the past 12 years, and the availability of several new approaches to therapy of CML. Most centers, following the diagnosis of CML, will advise a patient to attempt a short course of interferon, because 25 per cent of the patients who try this therapy enter complete cytogenetic remissions that are stable for years and are associated with a reduced (10 per cent) probability of entering into blast crisis.

At the time of the diagnosis, the family members, including siblings, parents, and children, are subjected to histocompatibility testing, in order to prepare for the eventuality that the patient will undergo an allogeneic bone marrow transplant. The success rate with matched related allogeneic bone marrow transplant is so good (60 to 80 per cent long-term disease-free survival, depending on the age and physiologic status of the patient) that the age of eligibility ranges up to 60 years in some centers. If a patient is 25 years of age or less, he or she may be referred directly to an allograft center, without a trial of interferon, but most centers will attempt a 6-month trial of interferon, providing the features of the disease are not those of a disease in evolution.

If there are no sibling donors, and if the patient is not sensitive to interferon, he or she will be referred to a center at which unrelated donor bone marrow transplantation is practiced. The best results are obtained with patients under the age of 30 years, because the lethal complications of graft-versus-host disease increase markedly above the age of 30 years.

If the patient is interferon resistant, has no allograft donor, or is ineligible for an allograft, he or she often is referred to an autologous bone marrow transplantation center. The results with this type of therapy are improving as the techniques for generating complete cytogenetic remissions improve. Moreover, better preparative regimens and improved methods for fractionation of the bone marrow afford further reduction of the level of leukemic cells in the autologous bone marrow infused after intensive systemic therapy.

The decision for therapy selection is determined by the age of the patient, the physiologic and performance status of the patient, the presence or absence of features of advanced disease, and the availability of a center in which all of the therapeutic options are available.

CHRONIC LYMPHOCYTIC LEUKEMIA

Chronic lymphocytic leukemia (CLL) is predominantly a disease of the elderly that starts to increase in incidence in the fifth decade and reaches a peak in the later part of the sixth decade. Interestingly, the natural history of the disease can be predicted by a staging system that measures the following parameters:

    I: lymphocytosis (Stage 0)
    II: lymphadenopathy (Stage I)

III: organomegaly (Stage II)

IV: severe anemia (Stage III)

V: severe thrombocytopenia (Stage IV)

The expectation of survival for these stages is 12 years for Stage 0 and 1 to 2 years for an individual in whom the features of Stage IV are present (lymphocytosis, lymphadenopathy, organomegaly, anemia, and thrombocytosis). Management plans must take account of these features of the disease and their implications for therapy, especially if the therapeutic intervention planned involves risk and is experimental. Thus, in an individual with Stage 0 CLL, one routinely does not treat, especially with a potentially toxic therapeutic intervention in a patient who is 60 years old, because the probability is that the presence of CLL will not alter survival. Conversely, the presence of the features of Stage IV in a patient who is 40 years old will mandate the implementation of an experimental intervention, even if it is potentially toxic, such as allogeneic or autologous bone marrow transplantation.

Clinical and Molecular Markers of the CLL

The clinical features of the disease are lymphocytosis, lymphadenopathy, splenomegaly, anemia, and thrombocytopenia. The molecular change that initiates this disease is unknown, but several molecular changes are associated with the disease, such as trisomy 12, clonal rearrangement of the immunoglobulin molecule, surface immunoglobulin, and decreased immunoglobulin levels. A deficiency of the CD4 helper T cell is also a frequent concomitant of the disease. In fact, although the disease always was thought to be an AB cell malignancy, because of the phenotype of the cell that dominates the clinical picture of the disease, many features of the disease, such as lowered immunoglobulin levels and susceptibility to opportunistic infections (i.e., *Cryptococcus neoformans* and gram positive bacteremias and pneumonias), can be explained by defective T-cell function.

The amount of disease that remains following chemotherapy or transplantation can be measured by a polymerase chain reaction (PCR) assay for the CDR3 domain of the V-D-J region of the immunoglobulin region, which generates during the somatic recombination event a unique molecular signature of nucleotides. In contrast to a population of immunoglobulin molecules in a normal person, which would generate a smear on a PCR or Southern blot analysis, the molecular signature of the population of the immunoglobulin in the CLL cells is clonality (i.e., a single molecular species).

Therapy of CLL

Decisions concerning treatment may range from close observation without any therapy to allogeneic bone marrow transplantation, depending on the age and physiologic condition of the individual, and the institutional availability of experimental or standard therapeutic interventions. Low-dose alkylating therapy has been the mainstay of the disease in former years. Although this therapy limits the level of the lymphocyte count, there is no effect on survival, the normal cells do not repopulate the marrow, and no complete remissions are achieved.

Although combination chemotherapy has been used in the past (i.e., combinations of chlorambucil with steroids, etc.), no complete remissions were achievable until the fludarabine-based regimens were developed. These regimens clearly generate complete remissions in 20 to 30 per cent of patients, but so far no survival advantage has been associated with this type of treatment. The combination chemotherapy regimens used for CLL have been useful, however, to prepare patients for allogeneic bone marrow transplantation, and especially to prepare patients for autologous bone marrow transplantation.

The decision to undertake a bone marrow transplantation in a patient with CLL usually is driven by the young age of the patient, as well as a good performance status and physiologic status. In allogeneic bone marrow transplantation, all other factors being equal, the availability of a donor and the age of the patient are the dominant factors in patient selection. For autologous bone marrow transplantation, the factors that drive the selection for a transplant include low chronologic age, excellent performance status and physiologic status, the attainment of a complete remission, the availability of a treatment center in which the bone marrow can be fractionated so as to remove the leukemic cells, and the availability of the PCR assay for the CDR3 region of the immunoglobulin region of the leukemic cell. Unfortunately, this PCR assay must be carried out with a set of primers that is tailor made for each patient, and therefore requires the cloning and characterization of the CDR3 region of the patient. However, with the advent of PCR cloning and the existence of sequencing cores in most institutions, this function is not beyond the reach of most academic medical centers.

TYPE OF CHROMOSOMAL TRANSLOCATION AND CLINICAL PHENOTYPE OF LEUKEMIAS

The characterization of cytogenetic changes in acute myelogenous leukemia (AML) has unveiled a significant degree of diversity of genetic change even at the chromosomal level. The major subsets of chromosomal change in AML are summarized in Table 13–1. We have summarized the most important changes in acute lymphocytic leukemia (ALL) and non-Hodgkin's lymphoma as well. There is evidence that the specific type of chromosomal translocations acquired in leukemias are relevant for defining the clinical phenotypes of leukemias.

As outlined by Keating et al.,[1] the occurrence of -7, -5, $7q-$, $5q-$, and $+8$ all confer an extremely poor prognosis on patients and predict a very low level of complete response to chemotherapy, whereas the occurrence of t(8;21), inv16, and t(15;17) are associated with a very high probability of remission induction. Similar changes at the chromosomal level have been identified in lym-

TABLE 13–1. CHROMOSOMAL TRANSLOCATIONS IN ACUTE AND CHRONIC LEUKEMIAS

DISEASE*	TRANSLOCATION CHROMOSOMES	GENE ASSOCIATED WITH TRANSLOCATION	PROGNOSIS
CML			
Chronic phase	(9;22)	*abl-bcr*	Poor
Blast crisis	Monosomy 7; isochromosome 17; trisomy 8, 18	?	Poor
ANLL			
M1	(q;22)	*abl-bcr*	Poor
M2	(8;21)	*ets*, "runt"	Good
M3	(15;17)	Retinoic acid receptor (myl-RARα)	Good
M4 with eosinophilia	Inversion 16		Good
M5	Translocations of 11q23	*ets-1*	Poor
M1, M2, M4, M5	Trisomy 8		Poor
M1, M2, M4	Monosomies 5, 7		Poor
M2 with basophilia	(6;9q)		
ANLL + thrombocytopenia (megakaryoblastic)	3 deletion or inversion		
M6	Monosomies 3, 5, 7; trisomy 8		
ALL	(9;22)	*abl-bcr*	Poor
ALL (hyperdiploidy)			Good
Burkitt's Lymphoma, Leukemia	(8;14); also (2;8), (8; 22)	*myc*	Poor
Nodular Non-Hodgkin's Lymphoma†	(14;18)	*bcl-2*, immunoglobulin	
T-Cell			
Lymphomas	Inversion 14	*tcl-1*, alpha chain of T-cell antigen receptor	
Leukemias and lymphomas	(11;14)	*tcl-2*, alpha chain of T-cell antigen receptor	
Neoplasms	7q34	Beta chain of T-cell receptor	
CLL			
CLL and other B-cell neoplasms (small-cell lymphocytic lymphoma, diffuse large-cell lymphoma)	(11;14), (p13;q13)	*bcl-1*	
CLL	Trisomy 12	?	Poor
Myelodysplasia	Monosomy 7, 5q- monosomy 5	*met*?	Poor Poor
Secondary ANLL following chemoradiotherapy	Monosomy 7, 5q- trisomy 8, monosomy 5	*met*?	Poor Poor
Myeloma	Trisomies 3, 5, 9, 15; monosomies 13, 16; t(11;14)(p13; q13)	?	Poor
Biphenotypic Leukemia (lymphoid/monocytoid)	(4;17), (11q;4)	?	Poor

*CML, chronic myelogenous leukemia; ANLL, acute nonlymphocytic leukemia; ALL, acute lympho-cytic leukemia; CLL, chronic lymphocytic leukemia.
†Follicular small cleaved cell, follicular mixed cell, and follicular large cell.

phatic leukemias. Thus, changes at the chromosomal level have been identified whose association with changes in prognosis and pattern of response suggest that they are very important biologically. Through the very persistent efforts that have been expended to identify the molecular origin of these rearrangements, the following genes have been identified at the breakpoints in AML: bcr-abl in CML[3] at the junction of the t(9;22) translocation; myl-rarα in acute promyelocytic leukemia[4] at the junction of the t(15;17) translocation; the "runt" Drosophila segmentation gene in AML[5] at the junction of the t(8;21) translocation; HLF in ALL[6] at the junction of the t(17;19) translocation; EVI-1 in AML[7] at the junction of the inv3 inversion; and altered expression and rearrangements in the bcl-2 gene at the junction of the t(14;18) translocation in non-Hodgkin's lymphoma.[8] Often, the clinical setting not only has been instrumental in providing the clues that are necessary to elucidate the molecular changes that have occurred at the chromosomal translocation junction, but also has resulted in the application and development of therapeutic interventions for other types of malignancy.

Acute Promyelocytic Leukemia

Acute promyelocytic leukemia (APML) is a distinct subset of acute leukemias (FAB M3) bearing the t(15;17)(q22;q12-21) translocation in most patient-derived cells. Its histopathology is characterized by a predominance of abnormal promyelocytes in the bone marrow that stain peroxidase positive and periodic acid–Schiff negative. Auer rods may be seen. It is associated clinically with disseminated intravascular coagulation and hemorrhagic complications. One of the best examples[4,9–13] of the importance of clues learned from the clinical phenotype and identifying the genes at a breakpoint is the molecular cloning of the reciprocal translocation of APML.[4,9–13] It is now known that the t(15;17) translocation rearranges a putative transcription factor on chromosome 15, PML (originally called myl) with RARα on chromosome 17, resulting in a fusion DNA, PML/RARα. Progress was made in the biology of APML when a group of clinicians working in the People's Republic of China, responding to sporadic reports of responses of APML patients to 13-cis retinoic acid, initiated a trial of all-trans retinoic acid (ATRA) in the treatment of APML.[12,13] The dramatic clinical remissions that were observed to be induced by ATRA from the experience of these investigators were confirmed by investigators in France.[11] These clinical responses to ATRA therapy are associated with in vivo maturation of leukemic cells.[10,11] Following the initial report, investigators at Memorial Sloan-Kettering Cancer Center[10] confirmed and extended these findings by showing that aberrant RARα mRNA expression resulting from the PML/RARα transcript was tightly linked to clinical response to ATRA in APML. This finding highlights a paradox in APML: The observed ATRA clinical responses are linked to expression of a rearranged RARα.

With the cloning of full-length PML/RARα cDNAs, it became possible to explore the function of the t(15;17) product. The function of PML/RARα was studied using transient transfection within several promoter and cellular contexts. Because the PML/RARα cDNAs retained the ligand and DNA-binding domains of RARα, the fusion cDNAs remain ligand-dependent transcription factors. However, as compared to the wild-type RARα, PML/RARα cDNAs exhibit altered transactivation profiles. Two attractive but not mutually exclusive hypotheses could explain the role of PML/RARα in APML biology: (1) the PML/RARα product antagonizes normal RARα function through a "dominant negative" mechanism; or (2) the fusion product antagonizes normal PML function.

The convergence of clinical and molecular genetic insights in APML led to improvements in its molecular diagnosis. As the presence of the bcr-abl product is diagnostically useful in CML, the appearance of the t(15;17) translocation clarifies the diagnosis of APML. This rearrangement can be diagnosed by routine cytogenics, Southern blot analysis, pulsed-field gel electrophoresis, or the reverse transcription polymerase chain reaction (RT-PCR) technique. The development of sensitive molecular assays to detect the APML rearrangement is diagnostically useful. These assays may be utilized to monitor patients during treatment and to tailor postremission therapy.

Several centers have undertaken clinical trials in APML combining ATRA with cytotoxic chemotherapy. Initial trials suggest more favorable outcomes following treatment with ATRA in combination with cytotoxic therapy than after cytotoxic chemotherapy or ATRA treatments alone. However, the optimal scheduling or sequencing of these combinations needs to be defined. Whether APML will become a paradigm for differentiation-based therapy of leukemia awaits future work.

Chromosomal Changes and Prediction of Therapeutic Outcome

This work in APML is an example of how important the patterns of response of leukemic cells are to the understanding of the biologic basis of the diseases that are associated with specific chromosomal translocations. Clearly, the clues developed in the course of clinical investigations may lead to discoveries as to how the genes involved in chromosomal rearrangements may contribute to the activation of oncogenes or to the loss of tumor suppression genes in leukemias and solid tumors.

A significant degree of genetic diversity may exist at the DNA level among patients who have an apparent homogeneity of the clinical phenotype of the disease. The degree of diversity becomes even more extensive when the analysis is extended to the nucleotide level. When one examines the rearrangements at the chromosomal level, an even greater degree of diversity exists in solid tumors. The challenge to the clinician, or to the biologist as well, is to identify the changes that are paramount in the evolution of a specific disease among the large number of chromosomal or molecular changes that involve almost every chromosome.

In order to identify those changes that are most important to the understanding of the disease and its therapy, many workers have tested for a correlation between the presence of a specific molecular change and response to therapy, the remission duration, and the survival. This allows for the identification of molecular changes that are important enough to affect survival or response. Those changes are the ones selected for use in developing chemotherapy or genetic therapy. Such an analysis in AML has determined that mutational changes in the *p53* antioncogene protein occur only at a very low frequency of 6 per cent.[14] In contrast, a substantially higher number of patients with solid tumors have point mutations in this gene, or exhibit deletion of the *p53* antioncogene.

Interestingly, AML cells in over 60 per cent of the patients contain p53 proteins in which altered conformal states can be detected.[15] Furthermore, the altered state of p53 conformation may equate to loss of the functional activity of the protein. Similarly, low levels of expression of the *Rb* gene result in a low level of the Rb protein in 30 per cent of AML patients.[16] In order to determine if either of these changes was relevant and important to the phenotype of AML cells, we tested for a correlation between the levels of Rb at diagnosis in over 110 patients with AML recently seen in our institution. As shown in Figure 13–2, the presence of low levels of Rb at diagnosis is associated with a very low probability of remission induction and a very short survival (40 days) as compared to the survival of individuals in whom high levels of Rb were present at diagnosis (survival was 400 days). We have thus identified a change within the AML patients in whom the loss of *Rb* expression is associated with a poor prognosis.[16]

These data have suggested that it is important first and foremost to follow very carefully the responses of leukemia cells in the clinical setting to identify clues as to those changes that may be the basis of the disease. It is important to test whether genetic, molecular, and chromosomal changes are predictive of response, survival, or remission duration in patients. These analyses serve to help identify changes that are important to the origin and evolution of disease. The identification of such changes may help identify targets for molecular and genetic therapy of these diseases. The targeting of therapy to the correction of genetic changes in leukemia cells may provide an opportunity to alter the unfavorable features of diseases through corrective molecular modifications of the cells contributing to these diseases.

ACUTE MYELOGENOUS LEUKEMIA

Acute myelogenous leukemia often presents with the symptoms of fatigue, bruising, and fever. At diagnosis, the patient often already is exhibiting a decrease in performance status, and the white cell count can be lower than normal, in the normal range, or between 10,000 and 50,000/cu mm. Rarely, the white cell count can reach above 100,000/cu mm, in which case emergency therapy or leukopheresis is necessary to avoid the complication of cerebral vascular accident, which occur at that level as a result of thrombosis and hemorrhage in the central nervous system caused by the aggregation of the blasts.

This disease is considered a medical emergency, because most of the patients will have a dangerously low absolute neutrophil count (less than 200/cu mm) despite there being a white cell count in the normal range. There is considerable variation in the precise mixture of normal residual cells and leukemic cells in any given patient, but all patients exhibit this mixture.

Therapy of AML

Combination chemotherapy is the mainstay of the initial approach to the therapy of this disorder. Regimens have been available for the past 20 years (TAD, daunomycin, continuous infusion ara-C) that are associated with a complete remission induction frequency of 75 per cent. The treatment death during induction therapy may range between 10 and 25 per cent. Unfortunately, the remission duration has been the major unsolved problem of therapy

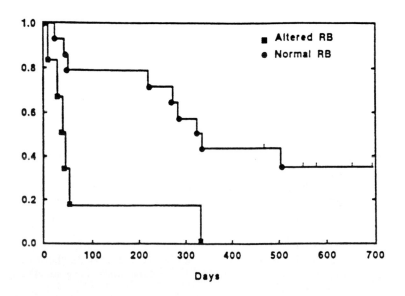

Figure 13–2. Rb protein gene expression and survival of patients with acute myelogenous leukemia.

in this disease. During the 1970s, two concepts were developed to attempt to increase the duration of remissions: intensive consolidation and cyclical reinduction therapy. The latter was associated with an increase in the remission duration to 24 months in a series that was dominated by younger individuals (below the age of 30 years). An 11-day regimen was developed by Vaughan that involved initial induction for 3 days, followed by an 8-day break, and then another intensive 3-day regimen; this also was associated with a 24-month remission duration frequency, but a 25 per cent treatment mortality as well.

Allogeneic bone marrow transplant in first remission has been successfully developed for AML. In addition, the use of autologous bone marrow transplantation has been widely recognized as having a role in the maintenance of remissions. Recently, the use of retroviral marking of autologous bone marrow cells, harvested for use in restoring hematopoietic function following intensive systemic preparative therapy, has demonstrated that there are sufficient leukemia cells in the marrow of some patients to contribute to the relapse. This discovery has focused attention on the need to develop fractionation procedures for remission AML marrows, but no standard way of accomplishing this has yet been established.

Again, the choice among these therapeutic options is dependent on the age and physiologic status of the patient, and the expertise of the center in which the patient is being treated. In addition, the cytogenetic subsets outlined in Table 13–1 contribute to therapy planning, because some subsets are associated with very good prognosis, such as inversion 16 and the balanced translocation between chromosomes 8 and 21. Among the most ominous chromosomal changes are monosomy 7 and 5, and trisomy 8.

New Directions of Therapy of AML

One of the challenges for chemotherapy is to increase the incidence of cells that are proliferating at the time of exposure to the chemotherapeutic agent. In the marrow of a leukemic patient at diagnosis, the higher-than-normal circulating myeloid cell mass suppresses the proliferative activity of the normal cells. Thus, there is a difference in the proliferative activity of normal and leukemic cells in AML patients at diagnosis. In order to increase the sensitivity of the leukemic cells, many workers have been testing schedules and doses of combination chemotherapy that can selectively induce the proliferation of leukemia cells and not stimulate the normal cells.

We recently have launched clinical protocols directed to the use of growth factors before initiation of chemotherapy to selectively sensitize the leukemic cells to therapy. As shown in Figures 13–3 and 13–4, stimulation of the leukemia cells with growth factors can result in proliferation induction of the leukemic population, but also can result in differentiation induction of the leukemic population if the exposure of cells is conducted for a sufficient period of time. This was confirmed in our studies of growth factors and chemotherapy in the therapy of AML. In the first growth factor trial, the cells were exposed to 4 to 7 days of GM-CSF before the initiation of chemotherapy.[17] In these trials, there was actually a reduction in the remission induction frequency, suggesting that differentiation induction had taken place following a 4- to 7-day exposure to the growth factor GM-CSF.

To increase the remission induction frequency, we exposed cells for a shorter time before initiation of chemotherapy. AML patients were given granulocyte colony-stimulating factor (G-CSF) for only 24 hours before chemotherapy was initiated. In this study, an actual increase in the remission induction frequency occurred in poor-prognosis patients when compared with a historic control group of poor-prognosis patients. The remission induction frequency was 75 per cent for patients who were treated with growth factor before initiation of chemotherapy, as compared with a 35 per cent remission induction frequency for patients treated without prior growth factor exposure. Thus, the schedule of growth factor administration is very important for the outcome of therapy.

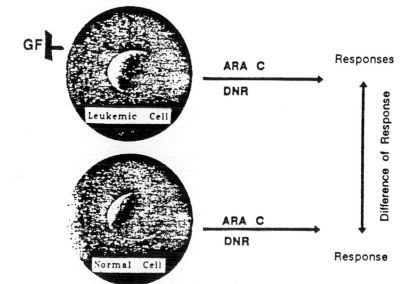

Figure 13–3. Induction of selective sensitization of leukemia cells to chemotherapy by growth factors.

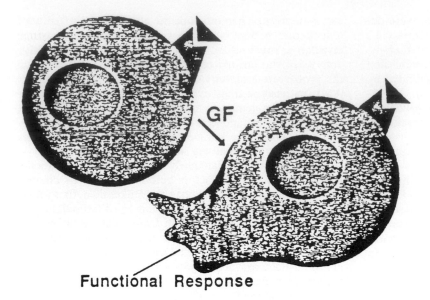

Figure 13–4. Induction of selective sensitization of leukemia cells to chemotherapy by growth factors.

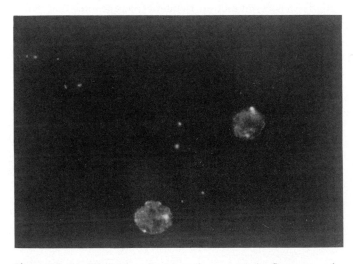

Figure 13–5. Monitoring of cytogenetic responses by fluorescence in situ hybridization (FISH).

Another factor, as mentioned earlier in this chapter and as shown in Table 13–1, is the heterogeneity of the cytogenetic change in AML. Actually, this heterogeneity of cytogenetic change at the chromosomal level can be used for identification of responses of normal versus leukemic cells. Fluorescence in situ hybridization (FISH) can be used for monitoring the response of the normal versus the leukemic cells, as shown in Figure 13–5. This figure shows that the use of fluorescent-conjugated probes can identify changes that are predictive for response outcomes and are important for identification of responses in the normal versus the leukemic cells following growth factor exposure or chemotherapy. Using multiparameter FISH, the genetic composition, the proliferative activity of the normal and abnormal cells (Fig. 13–6), the lineage distribution of cells, the stage of maturation, and the states of signal transduction molecules can be measured on the same slide. Thus, this method of analysis can be used to

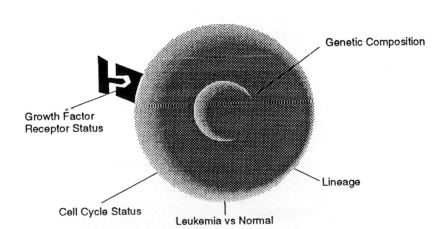

Figure 13–6. Multiparameter analysis relate leukemic cell to response.

establish conditions that are specific and optimal for proliferation induction of the leukemia cells.

Multiparameter FISH can be used not only to help identify the optimal condition for selective sensitization of the leukemic population, but also to characterize the phenotypic changes of the leukemic cells that may exist at every stage of the growth-regulatory signal induction pathway, as shown in Figure 13–6. Our group already has used this to show that the absence of the Rb tumor suppressor protein in AML cells at diagnosis is predictive of shortened remission duration and a decreased probability of entering into remission.

ACUTE LYMPHOCYTIC LEUKEMIA

Acute lymphocytic leukemia is associated with fatigue, fever, bleeding, and lymphocytosis. The cells that are circulating are lymphoblasts and are of three types: lymphoblasts without differentiation, lymphoblasts with some differentiation, and Burkitt's leukemia in which the blasts are large with blue, vacuolated cytoplasm. The cytogenetic changes of ALL include the Philadelphia chromosome translocation, which is found in 20 per cent of cases of adult ALL, and a host of other additional cytogenetic abnormalities, all of which are associated with a very grave prognosis. At the molecular level, the clonality of the T cell receptor in T-cell ALL, and of the immunoglobulin molecule in the majority of cases, which are pre–B-cell ALL, provides a tool for the estimation of minimal residual disease through the use of the PCR assay, and for diagnosis. The need to develop an individualized set of primers for each patient, based on the CDR3 region of the immunoglobulin molecule or the T cell receptor, has been facilitated by the advent of PCR cloning and automated sequencing methods. In addition, the pre–B-cell ALL cases also have clonality of the T-cell receptor in about 20 per cent of cases, the presence of terminal deoxynucleotidyltransferase, and the IL-2 growth factor receptor. In addition, myeloid growth factor receptors can be found on these cells, such as the receptor for IL-3, GM-CSF, G-CSF, and the c-KIT receptor, but the significance of these is not known.

Therapy of ALL

Very effective and relatively nontoxic combination chemotherapy regimens have been developed for this form of leukemia. The most nontoxic and simplest is the CVAD program, which consists of apoptosis-induction agents (discussed in detail later in this chapter). These drugs include cyclophosphamide, vincristine, daunomycin, and dexamethasone. The remission induction frequency reaches 80 to 90 per cent. Here again, the presence of additional cytogenetic abnormalities, such as the Philadelphia chromosome translocation, is predictive of a shortened remission duration.

For patients with mixed lineage or the presence of additional chromosomal abnormalities, the need for referral to a bone marrow transplant center arises from their shortened remission duration. This is done routinely following the achievement of a complete remission. The feasibility of this depends on the age of the patient (less than 55), the physiologic status of the patient, and the availability of donors. Autologous bone marrow transplant is an experimental therapeutic option that is still under development. There is great interest in this option at the present time because of the ease with which the normal myeloid cells can be separated from the lymphoid cells by CD34-positive selection and CD19-negative selection. The availability of PCR assays for documenting the presence of leukemia cells at a level of 1 leukemia cell in an excess of 100,000 to 1,000,000 nonmalignant cells further underscores the feasibility of this approach. Again, the choice among these options will be driven by the age of the patient, the prognostic category, the physiologic and performance status of the patient, and the availability of the therapeutic options at the center in which the patient is enrolled in therapy.

EX VIVO ANALYSIS OF LEUKEMIA CELLS IN PATIENTS UNDERGOING THERAPY

A large number of patients often is required to establish the optimal doses and schedules of administration of chemotherapeutic agents to evaluate whether changes in a program of therapy are having an impact on the therapeutic outcome. We have made use of a process called "ex vivo analysis" to increase the rate at which we can reach an interpretable result in a clinical trial. In this method, we administer a growth factor for a fixed period of time and, after a fixed interval, administer combination chemotherapy. If we sample the peripheral blood or marrow of patients at several intervals between the initiation of the growth factor and the initiation of chemotherapy, and then expose the cells to the drug combination used as well as a large number of alternative schedules of this combination or other combinations, we can develop data on a large number of schedules and drug combinations in the confines of a single clinical trial. With a few patients, a very large amount of data can be generated.

We also have applied this ex vivo analysis to the cells available following remission, using monoclonal antibodies specific for combinations of differentiation antigens that are not available on the hematopoietic cells of normal individuals. An example of such a combination is CD33 and CD19. Immature myeloid antigens such as CD33 are never found on a cell on which lymphoid antigens are found, such as CD19. Once such a combination has been identified, thereafter the marrow can be screened for persistence of leukemic cells that display that differentiation antigen combination. The persistence of such cells is predictive of a shortened remission duration, whereas the loss of such cells is associated with a prolonged remission duration. Thus, molecular endpoints that are predictive of the duration remission have been found. In addition, such a combination of differentiation antigens can be used to negatively select marrow so as to remove neoplastic hematopoietic cells from the marrow after therapy. The presence or absence of such cells can be used to evaluate the response to therapy. Finally, these molecular markers also can be used to help follow events in the normal versus the leukemic population in response to inductive events such as exposure to growth factor stimulation.

In addition, monoclonal antibody analysis and multiparameter FISH can be combined to follow the signal transduction pathways of growth factor stimulation from the extracellular membrane receptor through the cytoplasm, the nucleus, and the transcriptional activation of genes that are regulating proliferation. As stated earlier in this chapter, (see Fig. 13–2), we compared the survival of patients who have either normal levels or reduced levels of the Rb protein at diagnosis. There was a major statistically significant difference in the survival of patients who were shown to be positive for this negative regulatory protein (330 days) versus patients who lacked this protein (median survival of 45 days). Thus, the absence of this protein correlates with a shortened survival.[16] Further analysis has shown that this survival difference led to failure to enter into complete remission on exposure to chemotherapy. Thus, this change provides two markers: one for survival and one for chemotherapy response. We will use this protein: (1) to direct patients away from conventional dose chemotherapy to bone marrow transplantation when the levels of the protein are very low; and (2) as a target for corrective genetic therapy when viruses that can be targeted to the leukemic cell are developed.

GENETIC IMMUNOTHERAPY FOR AML

It is very clear from the studies with allogeneic bone marrow transplantation that T cells are an important factor in maintaining remissions after intensive therapy in myelogenous leukemias. The first indication of this was the fact that the relapse frequency among twins, in whom there is no T-cell reaction of the donor cells against the myelogenous cells of the recipient, is 60 per cent, whereas the relapse frequency of allografts among siblings, in which there is a graft-versus-leukemia effect mediated by T cells, is 30 per cent. This suggests that T cells of patients can mediate a graft-versus-leukemia effect providing there is antigen recognition. Also consistent with the idea that T cells are important in suppression of marrow cell growth is the fact that T-cell depletion invariably increases the relapse rate in patients following allogeneic bone marrow transplantation. Furthermore, among CML patients who have relapsed after an allograft, infusion of donor T cells at the time of relapse after allografting resulted in resolution of the relapse and a reinduction of complete remission. Thus, there is ample evidence among leukemic patients for the importance of T cells in suppressing the growth of neoplastic hematopoietic cells.

Emerson has shown that, even among normal myeloid cells, the autologous peripheral blood T cells can recognize and suppress cell growth.[18] He showed this by mixing the peripheral blood T cells with late myeloid progenitor cells in the autologous setting in vitro. He found that the

T cells undergo a mitogenic response when exposed to autologous myeloid cells, and that repetitive exposure of the T cells to the myeloid cells can result in a population of cells that are capable of recognizing and suppressing the growth of the normal myeloid hematopoietic tissue. Monoclonal antibodies have shown that this interaction is dependent on the presence of the CD2 antigen on the surface of the lymphoid cell, and the presence of the LFA-3 antigen on the surface of the myeloid cell. One can block the recognition event by monoclonal antibodies to LFA-3 or CD2. In addition, the loss of the LFA-1 surface cytoadhesion molecule from neoplastic B cells can result in the escape of Epstein-Barr virus–transformed B cells from T-cell depletion. This loss of LFA-1 expression accompanies unregulated *myc* expression generated by the 8;14 chromosomal translocation in these cells, which results in Burkitt's lymphoma. In CML as well as AML, the family of surface cytoadhesion molecules is expressed only at very low levels, as are the class I human lymphocyte antigens (HLAs). Both of these molecules are necessary for the type of recognition that is important in T-cell–dependent suppression of myeloid cell growth. In CML, interferon has been found to be an effective therapy for inducing cytogenetic remissions. Interferon increases the level of class I HLAs as well as the level of surface cytoadhesion molecules. If one looks at the ability of autologous T cells to recognize and suppress the growth of myeloid cells in CML patients, the T cells are usually ineffective and they do not exhibit a proliferative response to the presence of the myeloid cell in the patient before interferon exposure. However, after interferon exposure, the T cells once again recognize the presence of myeloid cells and suppress their growth. This is further evidence of the role of T cells in regulating myeloid cell growth. The changes that occur in leukemia cells sometimes result in a loss of expression of molecules necessary to this normal regulatory response of T cells in myeloid cell maturation and growth.

MOLECULAR VACCINES FOR LEUKEMIA

Several workers recently have developed data suggesting that molecular vaccines will be of importance for immune response.[19] Transduction of renal cells with retroviruses containing the cDNAs for γ-interferon or IL-2 resulted in changes within the cell that altered the responsiveness of T cells. Other workers have shown that com-

TABLE 13–2. IMMUNOENHANCEMENT MATERIALS

Lymphokines IL-2, IL-3, IL-4, IL-5, IL-6, IL-7, and IL-10
Viral proteins (E7)
Tumor-specific antigens
Human lymphocyte antigens
Monoclonal antibodies to tumor antigens
Mutant antigens
Transcriptional regulatory proteins
Viral particles (herpes simplex virus)

TABLE 13–3.   MECHANISMS OF IMMUNOENHANCEMENT

1.	IL-2: IL-2:	↑CTL + IFN: ↑CTL + NK
2.	IL-3:	↑PMN production and recruitment → IL-1β and TNF-α + CTL (LLCa)
3.	IL-4:	Dose effect Eosinophils ICAM in endothelium and eosinophils
4.	GM-CSF:	Presenting cells (M^0 + dendritic cells): ↑CD4 → ↑CD8 + HLA
5.	G-CSF:	↑PMN → fusion cell membranes
6.	IL-7:	↑T cells ↑ICAM Potentiates response to IL-2
7.	IL-10:	↑HLA class I

Abbreviations: CTL, cytotoxic T lymphocytes; IL, interleukin; IFN, interferon; NK, natural killer cells; PMN, polymorphonuclear leukocytes; TNF-α, tumor necrosis factor-α; ICAM, intercellular adhesion molecules, GM-CSF, granulocyte-macrophage colony-stimulating factor; G-CSF, granulocyte colony-stimulating factor; HLA, human lymphocyte antigen; ↑, increases; →, leads to.

binations of retroviruses containing IL-2 or GM-CSF actually can reduce regressions during the early stages of engraftment of tumor cells such as the B16 melanoma. This sensitization has been found to be durable and to be dependent on T cells and independent of natural killer (NK) cells. A large number of lymphokines have been studied in this way (Table 13–2) and have been found to be evolving by a variety of mechanisms (Table 13–3). Figure 13–7 shows an example of the types of mechanisms evolved in this response.

We are proposing the development of molecular vaccines for AML cells. As mentioned earlier in this chapter, our program of fludarabine plus Ara-C, preceded by G-CSF, is capable of inducing remissions at a frequency of 75 per cent in poor-prognosis subsets of AML patients in whom previous programs of therapy without growth factor stimulation induced only 35 to 40 per cent remissions. Twenty per cent of these patients are unable to continue with therapy because of physiologic status or sensitivity of major organ systems to the chemotherapy. We are proposing to use genetic vaccines as a form of therapy for these patients. We will take the IL-2 growth factor cDNA, insert it into the transcription unit of a safety-modified retrovirus, and use that retrovirus to transduce the AML cells. These AML cells will be administered weekly to patients subcutaneously and intravenously in an attempt to induce an expansion of a cohort of T cells that can recognize and suppress the growth function of the AML cells. The endpoint of the study will be to measure the ability of T cells in these patients to recognize and respond in a cytotoxic manner to the presence of the leukemia cells. We also will follow duration of remission and survival in these patients. The ability to immunoenhance the response of T cells to the autologous neoplastic myeloid cells will be tested in vitro. A comparison will be made of AML cells that contain the IL-2 retroviral transgenome and those that do not.

As shown in Figure 13–7, we are hypothesizing that the release of IL-2 from the neoplastic AML cell activates the release of lymphokines from accessory cells (other T cells and monocytes). One possible lymphokine is γ-interferon, which would up-regulate class I HLAs and surface cytoadhesion molecules that are necessary for the recognition and suppression of hematopoietic cells by T cells. Thus, this form of molecular therapy is an example of the treatment possibilities that arise when one is able to identify defects within leukemic populations that alter negative regulatory interaction among normal cells. The discovery that surface cytoadhesion molecules and class I HLAs were down-regulated in acute leukemia cells led to the elaboration of the strategy, which is designed to correct the altered immune response of the T cells to the leukemic progenitor cells. We will continue to elaborate mechanisms of immunomodulation for leukemic populations.

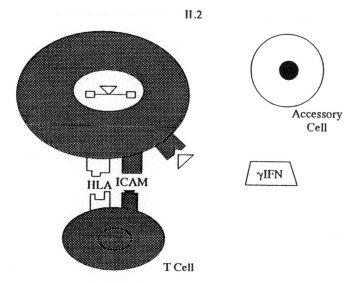

Figure 13–7. Recruitment of T-cell activation and cytotoxicity by the modified tumor cell. The interleukin-2 (IL-2)-modified tumor cell is lethally irradiated and injected and then locally releases IL-2, which activates the release of interferon-gamma (IFN-γ) and other lymphokines necessary for activation of the immune response by accessory cells.

CHEMOPROTECTION OF NORMAL HEMATOPOIETIC PROGENITOR CELLS BY RETROVIRUS-MEDIATED GENETIC MODIFICATION

If the hematopoietic cells of leukemic populations can be separated from the normal cells, then the normal hematopoietic progenitor cells of the marrow can be modified ex vivo so as to make them more resistant to chemotherapy. This will provide the opportunity of increasing the level of resistance in the hematopoietic progenitor cells above that which is present in the neoplastic myeloid cells. As shown in Figure 13–8, retroviruses will be armed with chemoprotection genes that can protect marrow cells against many therapeutic agents. Populations of normal hematopoietic progenitor cells from either CML or AML will be isolated by a two-step process: (1) positive selection of the normal early progenitor cells, and (2) negative selection of the neoplastic progenitor cells. The immunophenotype of the neoplastic progenitor cells can be identified and then monoclonal antibodies conjugated to beads can be used to negatively select these cells. This will be a much easier task in a lymphoid malignancy than in a myeloid malignancy. We have set up this type of separation in CLL as well as CML. If the neoplastic cells are removed, then chemotherapy resistance genes can be introduced into the normal hematopoietic progenitor cells and they can be reconstituted following intensive systemic preparative therapy. The presence of chemotherapy resistance genes in the normal myeloid progenitor cells that reconstitute marrow function following intensive therapy will provide the opportunity of continuing and extending the patient's therapy over time through cyclical reexposure of the genetically modified normal hematopoietic progenitor cells to intensive combination chemotherapy. Usually, chemotherapy is difficult to administer following transplant because of the sensitivity of the graft. Under this method of chemoprotection, it will be possible to extend chemotherapy-induced maintenance at an intensive level without endangering the normal progenitor cells. Instead of being consumed in terms of stem cell reserve, the normal progenitor cells will become stronger and more resistant to chemotherapy with each succeeding cycle as a result of the selective enrichment of the genetically modified progenitor cells in this population.

SUMMARY

The field of leukemia therapy and research is a rapidly evolving one, in which the accumulation of information about the molecular changes responsible for the disease process was driven in the beginning by the clues arising from the presence of balanced chromosomal translocations, and is now driven by a much more systematic study of the genetic changes in leukemia using the newer techniques of comparative chromosomal hybridization, fluorescent in situ hybridization, and interphase fluorescent in situ hybridization.

The advent of effective remission induction regimens for virtually all of the leukemias has improved the prospect for control in the short term. The development of allogeneic bone marrow transplantation and the improvement of support technologies have improved the outlook for a greater number of patients for whom donors are available. The development of unrelated donor registries for allogeneic bone marrow transplantation has not yet had an impact on this disease. Increasingly, many centers are investing effort in the development of autologous bone marrow transplantation programs in an attempt to provide a therapeutic option that can prolong the duration of the complete remissions that are achievable in the majority of patients.

The molecular diagnostic techniques, such as PCR and especially FISH on interphase and metaphase cells, are producing an opportunity to optimize the schedules and the doses of therapy, because these techniques enable the investigator to maximize the differential toxicity of these regimens between the normal and leukemic cells. The explosion of information as to the mechanism of chemotherapy-induced cell death, especially the information on apoptosis induction of chemotherapy, and the per-

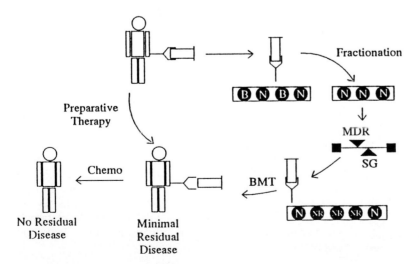

Figure 13–8. Use of multidrug resistant (MDR) retroviruses. SG, selection gene; BMT, bone marrow transplantation.

sistence of this therapy-induced cell death, such as loss or mutational inactivation of *p53*, the loss of other tumor suppressor genes such as the Rb protein, and the accumulation of other somatic changes such as mutations in the *ras* family of genes, is providing hope that, through optimization of the differential toxicity to normal and leukemic cells, the remission duration can be maximized. Finally, the availability of PCR techniques to measure and track the level of residual disease and the direction of changes of the level of leukemia cells with maintenance therapy promises to accelerate the rate at which more effective, less toxic, and individualized programs of therapy can be developed for each patient's disease, depending on the specific combination of genetic changes present in each leukemic population. The availability of molecular diagnostic information, as well as the emerging technology of molecular approaches to therapy, increases the likelihood that decisive approaches to induction and remission duration therapy will be available for all patients with leukemia. Over the next few years, the ability to couple specific laboratory tests, which provide information as to the precise defects within each patient's disease, and the outcome of therapy will likely play a major role in the drive to translate this information into new, more decisive, less toxic, and more effective therapy for all of these patients.

ACKNOWLEDGMENTS: The authors recognize the support from the Anderson Chair for Cancer Treatment and Research, the NCI (PO1 CA49639, The Therapy of CML; P01 CA 55164, The Therapy of AML; AND R01 CA 58655), ACS grant IM 66559, the Bush Fund for Leukemia Research, and the Wiley Fund, and support from Genta, Inc., Aastrom Biosciences, Inc., and Ingenex, Inc. Technological contributions from CellPro are also recognized, as are the editorial activities of Rosemarie Lauzon.

REFERENCES

1. Keating M, Cork MA, Broach Y, et al: Toward a clinically relevant cytogenetic classification of acute myelogenous leukemia. Leukemia Res *11*:119, 1987
2. Clarkson B, Strife A: Discordant maturation in chronic myelogenous leukemia. *In* Deisseroth AB, Arlinghaus R (eds): Chronic Myelogenous Leukemia: Molecular Approaches to Research and Therapy. New York, Marcel Dekker, 1990, pp 3–90
3. Groffen J, Stephenson JR, Heisterkamp N, et al: Philadelphia chromosomal breakpoints are clustered within a limited region, bcr, on chromosome 22. Cell *36*:93, 1984
4. de Thé H, Chromienne C, Lanotte M, et al: The t(15;17) translocation of acute promyelocytic leukaemia fuses the retinoic acid receptor α gene to a novel transcribed locus. Nature *347*: 558, 1990
5. Erickson P, Gao J, Chang KS, et al: Identification of breakpoints in t(8;21) acute myelogenous leukemia and isolation of a fusion transcript, AML 1/ETO, with similarity to drosophilia segmentation gene, runt. Blood *80*:1825, 1992
6. Inaba T, Roberts M, Shapiro L, et al: Fusion of the leucine zipper gene HLF to E2A gene in human acute b-lineage leukemia. Science *257*:531, 1992
7. Morishita K, Parganas E, Willman C, et al: Activation of EVI1 gene expression in human acute myelogenous leukemias by translocations spanning 300–400 kilobases on chromosome band 3q26. Proc Natl Acad Sci USA *89*:3937, 1992
8. Limpens J, De Jong D, Van Kri=sen JH, et al: Bcl-2/J_H rearrangements in benign lymphoid tissues with follicular hyperplasia. Oncogene *6*:2271, 1991
9. Claxton DF, Plunkett W Jr, Andreeff M, et al: Retinoids and cancer therapy. J Natl Cancer Inst *84*:1306, 1992
10. Warrell R, Frankel S, Miller W, et al: Differentiation therapy of acute promyelocytic leukemia with tretinoin (all-trans-retinoic acid). N Engl J Med *324*:1385, 1991
11. Castaigne S, Chomuenne C, Daniel M, et al: All-trans retinoic acid as a differentiation therapy for acute promyelocytic leukemia. I. Clinical results. Blood *76*:1704, 1990
12. Chen Z, Xue X, Zhang R, et al: A clinical and experimental study on all-trans retinoic acid-treated acute promyelocytic leukemia patients. Blood *78*:1413, 1991
13. Huang M, Ye Y, Chen S, et al: Use of all-trans retinoic acid in the treatment of acute promyelocytic leukemia. Blood *72*:567, 1988
14. Hu G, Zhang W, Deisseroth AB: P 53 gene mutations in acute myelogenous leukaemia. Br J Haematol *81*:489, 1992
15. Zhang W, Hu G, Estey E, et al: Altered conformation of the p53 protein in myeloid leukemia cells and mitogen-stimulated normal blood cells. Oncogene *7*:1645, 1992
16. Kornblau SM, Xu H-J, del Giglio A, et al: Clinical implications of decreased retinoblastoma protein expression in acute myelogenous leukemia. Cancer Res *52*:4587, 1992
17. Estey E, Thall P, Kantarjian H, et al: Treatment of newly diagnosed acute myelogenous leukemia with granulocyte-macrophage colony-stimulating factor (GM-CSF) before and during continuous-infusion high-dose ara-c + daunorubicin: comparison to patients treated without GM CSF. Blood *79*: 2246, 1992
18. Guba S, Emerson S: Hematopoietic regulation of stem cell dynamics in chronic myelogenous leukemia. *In* Deisseroth A, Arlinghaus R (eds): Chronic Myelogenous Leukemia: Molecular Approaches to Research and Therapy. New York, Marcel Dekker, Inc, 1990, pp 337–348
19. Gastl G, Finstad C, Guarini A, et al: Retroviral vector-mediated lymphokine gene transfer into human renal cancer cells. Cancer Res *52*:6229, 1992

14

MOLECULAR BIOLOGY OF CHILDHOOD NEOPLASMS

MARK A. ISRAEL

Tumors that arise during childhood are biologically distinct from tumors occurring in adults (Table 14–1). Tumors of childhood frequently resemble the embryonic precursor of the cell type in which they arise, and they have short latency periods. Oftentimes these tumors are highly invasive, metastasizing early in their course. Perhaps of more importance, pediatric tumors as a group are very responsive to currently available modalities of therapy, especially chemotherapy. It is appealing to think that the differential responsiveness of these tumors to therapy may be associated with biological differences that distinguish them from carcinomas, the most common tumors in adults. To date, however, the molecular and cellular basis for either these apparent biologic differences or differing responses to therapy remain enigmatic.

Rarely, it has been possible to identify an association between the incidence of a particular childhood tumor and an environmental carcinogen. Tumors occurring early in life have distinctly different histologies and occur in distinctly different tissues from those tumors that occur in adults. Sometimes childhood tumors apparently arise even before birth, suggesting that environmental influences play less of a role in the pathogenesis of childhood tumors than they do in tumors of adults. Childhood tumors occur prominently in association with a variety of different hereditary syndromes (Table 14–2). Disorders such as xeroderma pigmentosum, which renders children at increased risk for the development of skin cancers, and ataxia–telangiectasia, which oftentimes is complicated by the development of lymphoid malignancies, are examples of inherited disorders that put children at increased risk for the development of cancer.

Some cancer predisposition syndromes are not recognized to be associated with prominent nonmalignant stigmata. Hereditary retinoblastoma,[1] the Li-Fraumeni syndrome,[2,3] and familial polyposis[4] are among the best characterized of these syndromes. Interestingly, each syndrome is associated with a recognizably increased predisposition to a number of different tumors. We can anticipate that the enhanced sensitivity of molecular analysis over clinical observation to study cancer epidemiology will lead to the identification of additional inherited syndromes that increase the risk of childhood cancer. The likelihood of this occurring, and our ability to detect genetic changes in patients at risk for known cancer predisposition syndromes, enhance the importance of genetic counseling in the care of children with cancer.[5]

Current evidence suggests that many of the tumors occurring during childhood are associated with a rather limited number of recurring cytogenetic changes. This findings stands in contrast to tumors of adults, in which the frequency of any particular rearrangement in any specific tumor type varies considerably. Because the cell types recognizable in childhood tumors closely resemble undifferentiated cells seen during normal embryologic development, it seems likely these genetic changes alter the ability of such cells to achieve a fully differentiated phenotype. For the majority of tumors, it has not been possible to determine whether the lack of differentiated features in tumor cells reflects arrested differentiation or dedifferentiation. Regardless of which is accurate, it is possible that the many different biologic characteristics of tumor cells, including their ability to proliferate, invade normal tissues, migrate to neighboring locations and reestablish their growth, and exhibit differential sensitivities to relatively nonspecific cytotoxic agents, reflect normal cellular activities present in the cell types from which a specific cancer arises. Because of these biologic and genetic features of childhood tumors, and the contrast they provide in tumors of adults, pediatric malignancies may provide particularly important opportunities to better understand both normal cellular processes and alterations of these processes that contribute to the development of malignancy.

TABLE 14–1. COMMON TUMORS OF CHILDHOOD

Leukemia
Brain tumors
Lymphoma
Peripheral nervous system tumors, including neuroblastoma
Soft tissue sarcomas, including rhabdomyosarcoma
Wilms' tumor
Bone tumors, including osteosarcoma
Retinoblastoma

BRAIN TUMORS

Clinical Description and Pathology

Tumors of the central nervous system (CNS) constitute approximately 20 per cent of all childhood tumors, and they are responsible for a considerably higher proportion of all deaths from pediatric cancer. The incidence of these tumors is second only to that of hematopoietic malignancies; they occur with an annual incidence of approximately 25 per 1 million children per year, approximately 85 per cent of the incidence of acute lymphoblastic leukemia, the most common of childhood malignancies.[6] Childhood brain tumors include a very heterogeneous group of malignancies that have proved to be therapeutic challenges because of their intimate proximity to critical structures and their apparent resistance to available chemotherapeutic agents. These tumors are therefore a particularly important problem in pediatric oncology, although less is known of their pathogenesis than that of most other childhood tumors.

Childhood CNS tumors are most commonly sporadic, and their clinical presentation is highly unpredictable, reflecting both the child's developmental status and the tumor's location and growth rate. Rapidly growing tumors tend to present in a more precipitous manner than that observed in children with slower growing tumors. Typically, the onset of symptoms in children with CNS tumors is slow and not easily localized to an intracranial mass at a precise anatomic location. Prominent features of such presentations include morning headaches, vomiting, and lethargy, attributable to increased intracranial pressure. Tumor infiltration of vital structures also can contribute significantly to the development of symptoms, and these are rarely localizing.

CNS tumors occurring during childhood are most commonly infratentorial.[7] These tumors include medulloblastomas, cerebellar astrocytomas, and brain stem gliomas. The localizing signs associated with infratentorial tumors include diminished coordination, altered gait, and cranial nerve palsies. Brain stem invasion by these tumors often is marked by deficits of cranial nerves V, VII, or IX. Supratentorial tumors are usually gliomas or primitive neuroectodermal tumors (PNETs). These tumors most commonly present with headaches, seizures, and other nonlocalizing symptoms sometimes associated with increased intracranial pressure. Evidence of upper motor neuron disease or disturbances of vision occasionally can direct attention to specific tumor sites; however, the cornerstone of current diagnosis and evaluation of such tumors is radiographic imaging, especially magnetic resonance imaging.

The evaluation of most pediatric CNS tumors includes a pretreatment biopsy. Tumors of the brain stem and optic tract occasionally are treated without histologic examination because of the morbidity associated with such procedures. Although tumors that are highly infiltrative and present with diffuse involvement of normal structures are invariably malignant, the pathologic grade of more circumscribed masses presenting as localized masses on imaging studies is less predictable.[8] The pathologic classification of pediatric CNS tumors is an area of continuing controversy and revision. As is the case for nervous system tumors of adults, tumors that occur in astrocytes are classified primarily based on their degree of anaplasia and cellularity.[8,9] In addition to astrocytomas, there are a num-

TABLE 14–2. HEREDITARY SYNDROMES ASSOCIATED WITH CHILDHOOD TUMORS

HEREDITARY DISORDER	PROMINENTLY ASSOCIATED MALIGNANCIES
Neurofibromatosis type 1	Multiple tumor types, including sarcomas and gliomas
Neurofibromatosis type 2	Meningioma, acoustic neuroma
Hereditary retinoblastoma	Retinoblastoma
Multiple endocrine neoplasia, types I and II	Adenomas and carcinomas of endocrine tissues
Familial polyposis coli	Intestinal polyps, colon carcinomas
Peutz-Jeghers syndrome	Intestinal polyps
Familial Wilms' tumor	Wilms' tumor
Ataxia-telangiectasia	Lymphomas, brain tumors
Bloom syndrome	Leukemia
Beckwith-Wiedemann syndrome	Wilms' tumor, rhabdomyosarcoma, hepatoma, adrenocortical carcinoma
Li-Fraumeni syndrome	Sarcomas, brain tumors, leukemia

ber of distinctive embryonal tumors of the CNS seen almost invariably during childhood. These include medulloblastomas, PNETs (primitive neuroectodermal tissue), and pineal cell tumors.[10] Although the cellular origins of these tumors have been a controversial aspect of pediatric neuropathology for several decades,[11] only recently have data emerged on which to base an informed opinion as to the precise cell types in which they arise.[12] It is possible that medulloblastomas and PNETs are ontologically very closely related.

The term PNET was first used by Hart and Earle in 1973 to describe poorly differentiated childhood CNS tumors that did not seem to correspond to any of the recognized groups of poorly differentiated tumors, such as medulloblastoma, central neuroblastoma, and ependymoblastoma[13] (Fig. 14–1). This concept has been broadened by a proposed comprehensive nomenclature for such tumors.[10] A number of cogent critiques of this system have been offered,[11,14] although no more comprehensive or practical schema has emerged. This classification contrasts most sharply with the earlier, but largely untested, histogenetic classification originally suggested by Bailey and Cushing[15] and expanded on in considerable detail by Russell and Rubinstein.[11] Ongoing genetic and cell biologic studies strongly suggest that there might soon be a substantive data base on which to either develop novel nosologies or pursue an evaluation of these histologically based, but divergent approaches to tumor classification.

Genetics

A considerable number of childhood CNS tumors are associated with hereditary syndromes, including Gorlin syndrome, tuberous sclerosis,[16] neurofibromatosis,[17] and the Li-Fraumeni syndrome.[2,3] The recent description of genes involved in the development of von Recklinghausen's disease (neurofibromatosis type 1; NF-1)[18] and neurofibromatosis type 2 (NF-2)[19] suggests the direct involvement of these genes in the development of different CNS malignancies. The *NF-1* gene encodes a protein structurally related to regulators of *ras* proteins, the *ras* GTPase-activating proteins, and has the expected GTPase-stimulating activity.[18,20,21] The homozygous inactivation of this gene has been identified in glial malignancies that occur in association with NF-1,[22,23] and it can be expected that this gene will contribute to sporadically occurring tumors of glial origin as well.[23]

The *NF-2* gene encodes a protein that is structurally related to the ezrin/moesin/talin family of genes, whose products localize to the internal surface of the plasma membrane and may interact with the cytoskeleton.[19] Mutations in this gene occur in patients with NF-2. Tumors from NF-2 patients have lost both copies of the *NF-2* gene, suggesting that these tumors arise by a process that includes the inactivation of the *NF-2* gene. Schwannomas and meningiomas are the most common tumors occurring in patients with NF-2; ependymomas are encountered less frequently. The *NF-2* gene also has been observed to be inactivated in these tumors when they occur in individuals not affected by NF-2.[19]

It now seems likely that tumor suppressor genes important for the pathogenesis of adult glioblastoma multiforme may reside on chromosomes 7, 9, 10, 13, 17, and 22.[24-28] Also, mutation of the *p53* gene[29] and amplification of the epidermal growth factor (EGF) receptor[30] occur in a significant number of high-grade gliomas. Deletions of the short arm of chromosome 9, involving several members of the interferon gene family, also have been described.[31] Glial tumors arising in childhood may be characterized by some of these same alterations, but there is little evidence to support this hypothesis. Cytogenetic studies of childhood glial tumors have not yet confirmed the alterations described above, and few molecular studies have been reported. Indeed, the studies reported to date do not provide either a comprehensive or a clear picture of frequently encountered cytogenetic changes in pediatric glial tumors.

In childhood PNETs, loss of heterozygosity on chromosomes 6q, 16q, 22, and 17p has been detected,[32] although the incidence of these changes may be infrequent. Medulloblastoma is an important and common CNS tumor of childhood. In this and closely related PNETs, i(17q) seems to occur quite frequently.[32,33] The loss of ge-

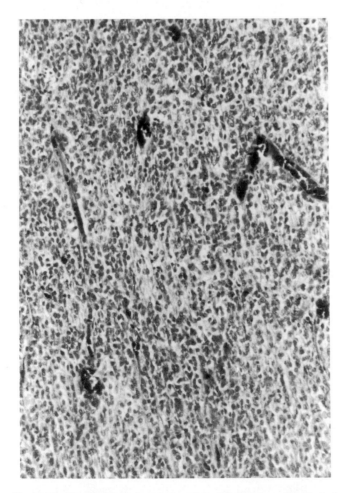

Figure 14–1. Histologic appearance of medulloblastoma. The typical cytology of medulloblastoma tumor cells includes undifferentiated, basophilic round nuclei with a high nuclear-to-cytoplasmic ratio. The minimal cytoplasm that can be detected has few if any distinguishing features. (Prepared by Dr. A. Bollen.)

netic material from 17p is now well documented,[34-36] although alterations in the *p53* tumor suppressor gene, which is located on 17p, seem to be very rare.[37] Also, c-*myc*, N-*myc*, and EGF receptors each have been found to be amplified in at least a single medulloblastoma cell line,[38,39] although the incidence of such amplification is unclear.[38-41] Cytogenic evidence of gene amplification, such as double minute chromosomes, is common in medulloblastoma.[42,43] Point mutations of various *ras* genes also have been detected occasionally in medulloblastoma tumor specimens, a finding that distinguishes medulloblastoma from most other embryonal tumors, in which *ras* gene alterations have been found only very rarely.[44] These findings are consistent with the likelihood that multiple genetic alterations are involved in the pathogenesis of medulloblastoma.

Cell Biology

In contrast to what is known about embryonal tumors of the childhood peripheral nervous system (see later in this chapter), little is known about the cellular characteristics of childhood CNS tumors that might identify biologically distinctive subgroups among them. Similarly, there is little molecular evidence relating these tumors to CNS precursors, although recently reported data suggest strongly that it will be possible to relate PNETs to such cell types.[12] A novel intermediate filament protein, nestin, may be of use in neuropathology as a marker of early CNS precursors.[45] This intermediate filament is expressed in medulloblastomas, other PNETs, and some gliomas.[46,47] There is an extensive body of literature that documents the differentiation of PNETs along different morphologically recognizable pathways, such as those corresponding to neuronal, glial, muscle, ependymal, and pineal cells. The finding that nestin is expressed in an embryonal CNS tumor cell line with the potential to differentiate in vitro along several of the multiple different cellular lineages often seen in medulloblastomas suggests that this tumor arises in a multipotential CNS precursor. The usefulness of nestin as a marker of tumor cell origin is speculative, because work from other laboratories has documented that the expression of intermediate filaments in PNETs of the CNS is promiscuous.[48] Nonetheless, nestin expression in childhood CNS tumors suggests that it may be possible to identify other markers of primitive CNS precursors in these tumors as well.

Treatment

CNS tumors of childhood usually are treated initially with a craniotomy to debulk the tumor as completely as possible without increasing the patient's neurologic deficit.[17] Following surgery, irradiation is utilized for the control of residual disease, especially if the tumor being treated is either anaplastic or has evidence of a rapid growth rate. As opposed to embryonal tumors of the CNS such as medulloblastoma and ependymoma, the glial tumors that occur during childhood are often of low histologic grade and often are treated with surgery alone. Che-

motherapy has an important role in the treatment of medulloblastoma and also is used for the treatment of childhood PNETs and glioblastoma multiforme. In an effort to minimize and delay the use of irradiation, which can have very significant toxic effects on the CNS of young patients, there has been an effort to increase the use of adjuvant chemotherapy.[49]

TUMORS OF THE PERIPHERAL NERVOUS SYSTEM

Neuroblastoma

CLINICAL DESCRIPTION AND PATHOLOGY

Neuroblastoma (NB) is the best known of the childhood tumors arising in the peripheral nervous system (PNS). Other tumor types that occur less frequently include neuroepitheliomas, schwannomas, and neurofibrosarcomas. The embryonic neural crest gives rise to the PNS, including the cranial and spinal sensory ganglia, the autonomic ganglia, the adrenal medulla, and a variety of paraendocrine cells found throughout the body. Tumors of the human PNS occur in the various cellular lineages that make up these structures, including neuronal, fibroblastic, and glial cells. For example, Schwann cell tumors can arise in the nerve sheath of peripheral neurons. Of these tumor cell types, only those arising in the neuronal lineage have been studied extensively, and these are the focus of this section. Because nervous system maturation is completed at an early age, most neuronal tumors including NBs and neuroepitheliomas arise during early childhood.

NB most commonly occurs in the abdominal retroperitoneum, arising in cells of the adrenal medulla and at other sites of known sympathetic nervous system tissue. NB originating in the thoracic cavity, usually in close association with a dorsal root ganglion, represents about 15 per cent of cases.[50] Overall, metastatic disease is present when patients first are seen in 60 to 70 per cent of cases.[50] Children with disseminated NB are often cachexic, pale, and in substantial pain from marrow and bony metastases at the time they present in the clinic.

A particularly interesting presentation of NB, Stage IV-S (IV-special),[51] frequently is associated with spontaneous remission. Stage IV-S NB is diagnosed in infants less than 1 year of age with primary tumors of limited size and evidence of remote disease that does not involve the bone, a common site of metastases in older children with advanced-stage disease. It is not known for certain whether IV-S NB represents metastatic disease or if it might be a multifocal, nonclonal disorder of neuroblast development. Such a possibility would be compatible with the finding that, during remission, Stage IV-S can be associated with evidence of differentiation, although other potential mechanisms of remission, including immunologically mediated ones, are possible. A considerable proportion of children initially thought to have Stage IV-S NB, and who do not receive cytotoxic therapy, go on to develop more aggressive disease. At present, there is no definitive way to distinguish Stage IV-S disease from advanced-stage metastatic (Stage IV) disease, and the precise relationship of these tumors to one another is not known. Analysis of survival in patients with NB has resulted in the identification of numerous prognostic factors.[50] NB was the first tumor in which an oncogenetic alteration, N-*myc* amplification, was identified to be of prognostic importance.[52] More recently, other prognostic variables of potential biologic importance—for example, expression of the nerve growth factor[53] and evidence of neuronal differentiation[54]—have been identified.

Histologic examination of NB specimens usually reveals small, round cells with hyperchromatic nuclei and stippled chromatin.[55] A hallmark of its light-microscopic appearance is the presence of Homer-Wright rosettes characterized by tumor cells clustered around a central mesh of cell processes (neuropil). Although sheets of monomorphic tumor cells interrupted by these abortive attempts at histologic differentiation usually dominate the light-microscopic appearance of NB, necrosis and calcification sometimes are seen. Undifferentiated NB occasionally can be a diagnostic dilemma, mimicking other small round-cell tumors of childhood. Ultrastructural examination of tumor tissue by electron microscopy always demonstrates the presence of cytoplasmic, neurosecretory, dense-core granules and neural processes, providing important diagnostic information in tumors without other evidence of neuroblastic differentiation.[55]

Various enzymes and proteins of neural origin are expressed in NB and aid in its diagnosis. These include neuron-specific enolase,[55] neuropeptide Y,[56,57] and sympathomimetic catecholamines, which along with their precursors and metabolites can be measured in blood or urine. These measurements frequently corroborate the histopathologic diagnosis and may be useful adjuncts with which to follow tumor response during therapy.[50]

GENETICS

With modern cytogenetic banding techniques, nearly 80 per cent of NBs studied to date have shown some chromosomal abnormality.[58] The cytogenetic characteristics of NB tumors have been studied extensively,[58,59] and many of the observed changes have been documented in NB-derived cell lines as well.[60] The most common cytogenetic abnormality is a deletion or rearrangement of the short arm of chromosome 1.[61,62] Other chromosomal alterations found in NB include chromosomal loss, gain, and rearrangements of chromosomes 10, 14, 17, and 19.

The chromosomal rearrangements in NB of greatest recent interest have been homogeneous staining regions (HSRs) and double minute chromosomes (DMs), which first were detected in human NB cell lines[59,61] (Fig. 14–2). These cytogenetic structures are now widely recognized to contain regions of gene amplification and frequently can be identified in tissue from NB tumors. It has been shown that the N-*myc* gene, a gene with considerable homology to the cellular proto-oncogene c-*myc*, is amplified within HSRs and DMs found in NB-derived cell lines and tumor specimens.[63–65] It is now believed that N-*myc* amplification in NB, as well as other cytogenetic alterations, is associated with a shorter time to tumor relapse.[66] These genetic changes can be detected in the tumors of approximately one third of patients with advanced-stage disease.[66,67]

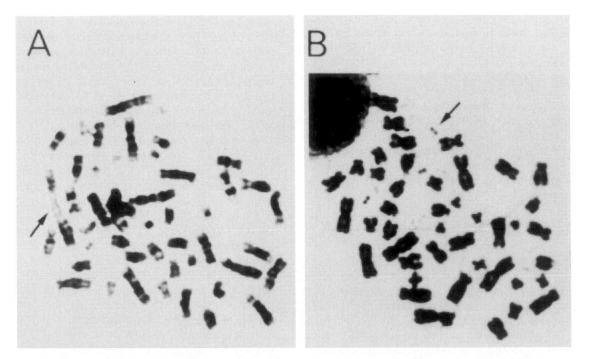

Figure 14–2. Cytogenetic evidence of gene amplification. *A*, G-banded metaphase chromosomal spread from a tumor cell in which the arrow marks a homogeneously staining region. *B*, Conventionally stained tumor cell metaphase chromosomal spread in which double minute chromosomes are marked by an arrow.

Several different proto-oncogenes, including N-*myc*, c-*myc*, c-*myb*, ets-1, src, and rdc-1, have been recognized to be highly expressed in NB cell lines.[64,68–72] With the exception of N-*myc*, none of these genes has yet been implicated in the pathogenesis of this tumor. Many NB tumor cell lines have been identified as having amplified N-*myc*, although several NB cell lines without evidence for amplification of the N-*myc* gene have been described as well.[73]

CELL BIOLOGY

Study of ganglionic differentiation has provided insight into the cellular mechanisms that contribute to the regulation of NB maturation and may be important for the pathogenesis of NB. When NB tumor cell lines are induced to differentiate, the expression of several different proto-oncogenes has been documented to change.[69,74] Following the treatment of NB tumor cell lines with retinoic acid, there is a sharp decline in the steady-state levels—of N-*myc* mRNA, although the enhanced expression of genes marking the neuronal lineage and the morphologic changes associated with neuronal differentiation become evident only much later.[74] When expressed at high levels, N-*myc* can block retinoic acid–induced NB differentiation.[75]

These findings suggest that the arrested differentiation of developing neuroblasts may be an important feature of NB pathogenesis. Compatible with this possibility is the observation that NB cell lines and tumors seem to correspond to recognizable neural crest precursors that appear during the maturation of the developing adrenal medulla, the most common site at which NBs arise[54,76] (Fig. 14–3). The identification of genes that are developmentally regulated during neural crest differentiation has made it possible to determine both the specific tissue lineage and the degree of maturation to which a particular tumor corresponds.[76,77] In tumor specimens, evidence for differentiation along multiple neural crest lineages, including the ganglionic, chromaffin, and glial lineages, can be detected.[54] NBs are thought to be clonal tumors, and this lineage infidelity may represent plasticity of the tumor to express multiple different genetic programs. Because tumors demonstrating the ability to differentiate along a ganglionic lineage may have a distinctly better response to therapy,[54] it is of importance to understand the molecular mechanisms that underlie the regulation of differentiation in these tissues.[75]

NB cells expressing the high-affinity nerve growth factor (NGF) receptor trk A[78] may be terminally differentiated by NGF and often may demonstrate morphologic evidence of ganglionic differentiation. The observation that evidence of ganglionic differentiation[54] and trk gene activation[53] has a favorable prognosis suggests that cellular properties of neurons may facilitate their therapeutic responsiveness. Remarkably, NBs never appear as mature chromaffin tissues, such as is seen in pheochromocytoma.

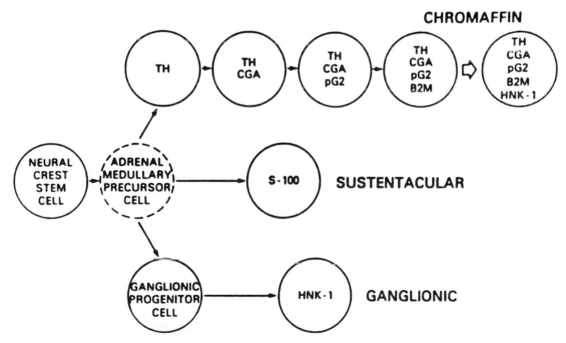

Figure 14–3. Model of adrenal medullary histogenesis. Neuroblastoma consists of cell types seen during the normal histogenesis of the adrenal medulla, which is depicted here. Specific stages in differentiation are marked by developmentally regulated expression of tissue-specific markers, including tyrosine hydroxylase (TH), chromogranin A (CGA), an anonymous marker (pG2), and β2-microglobulin (B2M). HNK-1 immunoreactivity marks an additional stage in chromaffin maturation that is reached in normal tissues after 5 years of age.[76,244] S-100 marks the sustentacular lineage and HNK-1 marks the ganglionic lineage, when chromaffin markers are not detected. All of these cell types can be found in neuroblastoma tumors. (From Cooper MJ, Hutchins GM, Israel MA: Histogenesis of the human adrenal medulla: An evaluation of the ontogeny of chromaffin and nonchromaffin lineages. Am J Pathol *137*:613, 1990, with permission.) See also ref. 54.

This is an unexpected finding, because most NBs arise in the adrenal medulla, where cells of the chromaffin lineage greatly outnumber cells of the ganglionic lineage after early fetal development. The lack of evidence for chromaffin cell differentiation in most NBs contrasts to the finding that these tumors express high levels of the *mdr* gene, a cytoplasmic pump that can confer antineoplastic drug resistance on tumor cells when it is highly expressed.[79] Chromaffin cells of the adrenal medulla express high levels of the *mdr* gene, perhaps related to their secretory functions. It is not known if the high levels of *mdr* expression in NB tumors reflect this ontologic relationship, but it is of interest that NBs have long been recognized to be particularly resistant to chemotherapeutic agents.

Insulin-like growth factor II (IGF-II) is another developmentally regulated gene that may contribute to the pathogenesis of NB. IGF-II is an important stimulatory ligand for the in vivo and in vitro growth of NB tumor cells.[80,81] IGF-II expression is found in the adrenal cortex during embryonic life and in the adrenal medulla of adult tissue. In tumor cell lines that express a pattern of developmentally regulated genes found late in the chromaffin lineage, IGF-II is highly expressed, compatible with the suggestion that these cell lines correspond to mature cells of this lineage.[76] In such cell lines IGF-II functions in an autocrine growth pathway.[80] Other NB cell lines that express markers suggesting they correspond to more immature cells[76] respond to IGF-II but do not produce the mitogen themselves. These in vitro findings may have in vivo correlates. Occasional NB tumors can be identified in which the tumor cells themselves have evidence of *IGF-II* gene expression.[81] More commonly IGF-II seems to function in vivo as a paracrine growth mediator in NB. In such tumor tissue specimens, IGF-II expression can be detected in infiltrating tumor and adjacent normal tissues.

TREATMENT

Treatment for NB reflects primarily the patient's age and clinical stage of the tumor at presentation. Lower stage disease (Stages I and II) is limited in its localization, whereas Stages III and IV represent more extensive local and regional or metastatic disease. The mainstay of therapy for young children with Stage I and II tumors is surgical excision. Chemotherapy does not improve the outcome of these patients.[82] Multimodality therapy including high-dose chemotherapy is the mainstay of therapy for Stage III and IV disease, and is effective in inducing complete, although usually transient, remissions in 30 to 40 per cent of patients.[50,83,84] Currently the efficacy of very intensive therapy requiring bone marrow transplantation and other extensive supportive approaches is being examined.[85]

Neuroepithelioma

CLINICAL DESCRIPTION AND PATHOLOGY

Peripheral neuroepithelioma (PN) first was recognized as a distinctive pathologic entity in 1918 by Stout when he characterized a tumor with neuronal characteristics arising in a peripheral nerve.[86] PN occurs in patients ranging in age from infants to adults; it most commonly presents in the second decade of life.[87,88] When metastases occur, they most commonly are found in lung and bone.[87] Bone marrow involvement, both at diagnosis and in relapse, appears to be more frequent than previously recognized. PN probably occurs more commonly than is generally appreciated. It has been described by many different names, including adult NB, peripheral NB, and PNET of the chest wall (Askin's tumor).[89–91] Recent studies have determined, however, that tumors such as these carry an easily recognized and almost invariant chromosomal translocation, t(11;22)(q24;q12)[60,92,93] (Fig. 14–4). This finding, along with a variety of recently recognized biologic differences,[72,94,95] strongly suggests that PN originates in a cell of the PNS that is different from that in which the histologically indistinguishable tumor undifferentiated NB arises.[72] Ewing's sarcoma (ES), a round-cell tumor of unknown histogenesis, also is characterized by a t(11;22)(q24;q12) translocation[96] and a number of other characteristics suggesting it is closely related or identical to PN[97] (Table 14–3), although this has been questioned by some investigators.[98] Current data suggest that PN, like ES, tends to recur locally, although it can be metastatic either at presentation or on recurrence.

Histologically, PN appears as an undifferentiated, small, blue, round-cell tumor with varying degrees of neuronal differentiation. PN can be periodic acid–Schiff positive, another common feature of ES. Although not always present, an important feature of the light-microscopic appearance of this tumor is the presence of rare rosettes. Ultrastructural analysis invariably reveals evidence of neuronal differentiation, including neurites, neurofilaments, neurotubules, and neurosecretory granules.[99]

PN expresses neuron-specific enolase and is usually negative for S-100 protein. Biochemical evaluation of PN cells has demonstrated high levels of choline acetyltransferase, an enzyme important for the synthesis of acetylcholine.[97] Outside the CNS, this neurotransmitter is largely confined to postganglionic parasympathetic neurons, which suggest that these are the cells of origin of PN. This finding contrasts to high levels of catecholamine biosynthetic enzymes in NB.[72] Urine catecholamine excretion is therefore absent in patients with PN, further distinguishing this disease from NB. Cholecystokinin also may be a marker capable of distinguishing ES and PN from NB.[95] Although the immunocytochemical profile of ES may be different from that characterizing PN,[94] it seems likely that evidence of commitment to a neuronal differentiation pathway will be typical of ES tissues as well as those tumors currently designated as neuroepithelioma.

GENETICS

The identification of a t(11;22)(q24;q12) chromosomal rearrangement in PN was an important observation in helping to clarify the relationship of this tumor to other neuroblastic malignancies, especially childhood NB.[92,93] It also was the first evidence suggesting a close relationship

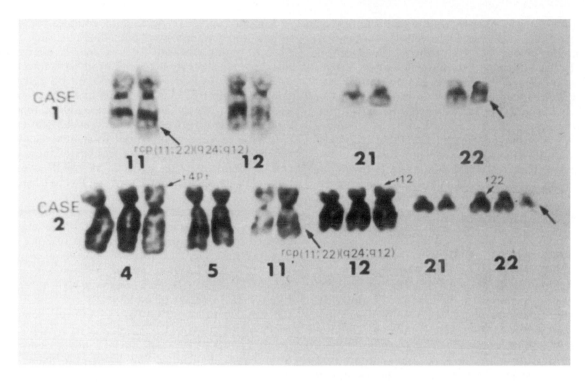

Figure 14–4. Cytogenetic appearance of the t(11;22)(q23;q12) translocation found in Ewing's sarcoma and peripheral neuroepithelioma. These karyotypes are from patients with neuroepithelioma. (From Whang -PJ, Triche JJ, Knutsen T, et al: Chromosome translocation in peripheral neuroepithelioma. N Engl J Med *311*:584, 1984, with permission.)

between this tumor and ES. t(11;22)(q24;q12) has now been reported in several other malignancies, such as Askin's tumor.[91] Interestingly, many PNs that have been examined for cytogenetic rearrangements also contain more than the expected two copies of chromosome 8.[93] The significance of this is unknown, although the tumors do express high steady-state levels of mRNA encoded by the c-*myc* gene, which is located on chromosome 8.[72]

Both PN- and ES-derived cell lines typically carry a

t(11;22)(q24;q12) chromosomal rearrangement, although variations of this rearrangement have been observed.[60,93,100,101] Recently this translocation breakpoint has been molecularly cloned, and most tumors that have been examined have translocations lying within an approximately 7-kb region on chromosome 22 and a 40-kb region on chromosome 11.[101] This translocation results in a chimeric mRNA involving a previously unknown gene on chromosome 22 termed *esw* and the human homologue of

TABLE 14–3. COMPARISON OF NEUROEPITHELIOMA AND EWING'S SARCOMA

	NEUROEPITHELIOMA	EWING'S SARCOMA
Morphology	Small round cells; primitive neuronal features	Small round cells; undifferentiated cytology
Enzyme Expression		
Neuron-specific enolase	+	
Dopamine β-hydroxylase	−	−
Choline acetyltransferase	+	+
Cholecystokinin Expression	+	+
Cytogenetics	t(11;22)(q24;q12);8	t(11;22)(q24;q12);8
Proto-oncogene Expression		
N-*myc*	+	+
c-*myc*	++	++
c-*myb*	+	+
ets-1	+	+
c-*sis*	−	−
rdc-1	+	+
dbl	−	+

fli-1, a member of the *ets-1* transcription factor family on chromosome 11. The *ews* gene encodes a protein that has limited homology with a portion of the large subunit of eukaryotic RNA polymerase II protein, and it has an RNA-binding domain. The *ews* gene is constitutively expressed in a wide variety of tissues, in sharp contrast to *fli-1*, which has a more restricted pattern of expression. The resultant chimeric protein replaces the RNA-binding domain of *ews* with the *ets*-like DNA-binding domain of *fli-1*.

The patterns of expression of a number of different oncogenes have been characterized in PN cell lines and tumor tissues[72,97] and are distinguishable from that observed in NB tumor cell lines[72] (Table 14–3). Of particular interest is the high level of c-*myc* expression. In contrast, the pattern of oncogene expression in PN cell lines is virtually indistinguishable from that observed in cell lines derived from ES,[97] providing additional evidence for the close relationship between these tumors. One putative oncogene that has an apparently limited range of expression, but is expressed in all PN- and ES-derived cell lines that have been examined, is *rdc-1*.[71] *rdc-1* maps to chromosome 13 and seems to have a *myc*-like transforming activity when assayed in vitro. *rdc-1* is expressed in a limited set of normal tissues, most prominently in developing human retina but also in brain and spinal cord. The only significant difference in oncogene expression by PN and ES cell lines to date is the expression of *dbl* in ES but in neither NB nor PN.[102]

CELL BIOLOGY

The biochemical features of PN-derived cell lines are indistinguishable from those of ES-derived cell lines and constitute strong evidence for the origin of both tumors in cells of the PNS. In all cell lines from these tumors that have been examined to date, evidence for the expression of choline acetyltransferase[97] and cholecystokinin[95] has been detected. Other markers of neuronal differentiation in addition to the neurotransmitters mentioned above also have been examined in PN tumor cell lines.[94] Although these cell lines are invariably reactive with antibodies against neuron-specific enolase, the expression of other genes that are typically detectable in ganglionic cells is somewhat less predictable. Recently, a newly derived monoclonal antibody recognizing a cell surface glycoprotein encoded by the *mic*-2 gene has been characterized and found to be reactive with PN and ES cell lines but not NB-derived tumor cell lines.[103,104] PN and ES cell lines also can be distinguished from most NB tumor cell lines in that they express high levels of human lymphocyte antigens (HLAs) and β_2-microglobulin.[94] PN cells also express fibronectin.[94]

It has been difficult to induce the differentiation of PN cells lines in culture, although there has not yet been a systematic effort in this regard.[105] It is possible to induce neural differentiation of ES-derived cell lines.[106] Treatment with either cyclic AMP (cAMP) or 12-*O*-tetradecanoylphorbol-13-acetate (TPA) results in cells developing elongated processes with varicosities that are visible by phase-contrast microscopy. Neurofilaments, microtubules,

and uraniffin-positive dense-core granules are detectable by electron microscopy. Neural markers such as neurofilament protein also are detected readily after treatment. Increased neurite extension and synthesis of acetylcholinesterase have been detected in PN and ES cell lines cultured in serum-free medium in the presence of cAMP and TPA. Nerve growth factor does not induce morphologic differentiation of PN cell lines and apparently cannot enhance the expression of neuronal characteristics in these cell lines.[105] The growth of a number of these cell lines can be inhibited by agents such as cAMP, cytosine arabinoside, tumor necrosis factor α (TNF-α), and γ-interferon without evidence of differentiation.[107]

There have been few studies examining the biochemical pathways over which the growth of PN is mediated. In contrast to the role of IGF-II in promoting the proliferation of NB-derived cell lines, there is some evidence that IGF-I may be of importance in the growth of PN tumor cells.[108] Most PN cell lines express mRNA encoding IGF-I, and their secretion of biologically active IGF-I and an IGF-binding protein (IGFBP-2) has been demonstrated. Blockade of the type I IGF receptor by a monoclonal antibody known to interrupt ligand binding inhibits serum-free growth, indicating that IGF-I can be an autocrine growth factor for PN.[108]

TREATMENT

Because this rare tumor has been identified as a separate entity from "adult NB" only in the last decade, there is limited information available about its optimal treatment. The average survival of patients presenting with metastatic is less than 1 year even with a multimodality approach to therapy consisting of surgery, radiation, and chemotherapy.[87] Most often, a combination of vincristine, actinomycin D, doxorubicin, and cyclophosphamide has been used.[87,88] Other agents known to be active in PN are VM-26, cisplatin, and VP-16. Local radiation at doses of 45 to 60 Gy generally is given to primary unresectable tumors. Given the poor prognosis of this tumor and the presence of a genetic alteration indistinguishable from that seen in ES, treatment of these patients in a manner reflective of the experience gathered in the management of ES patients holds hope for the identification of more efficacious treatments.

WILMS' TUMOR

Clinical Description and Pathology

Several distinct kidney tumors occur during the course of childhood. These originally all were thought to be variants of Wilms' tumor (WT), but further study has led to the recognition of clear-cell sarcoma of the kidney, rhabdoid tumor of the kidney, and anaplastic nephroblastoma as distinctive pathologic entities. WT is among the more common tumors of childhood, occurring approximately once in 7 million children under the age of 16.[109] Other kidney tumors occur infrequently compared to WT. The age distribution of children afflicted with these tumors is similar to that of WT, primarily under 3 years of age. Most childhood kidney tumors are highly malignant, although their degree of aneuploidy and the proliferative indices that characterize them vary greatly.[110]

WT most commonly occurs in very young children and typically presents as an asymptomatic abdominal mass. A minority of children will have symptoms such as hematuria[111] or hypertension,[112] which are directly referable to the primary tumor. Approximately 20 per cent of children present with distant metastatic disease[113–115] and, like other pediatric tumors, the patterns of spread are highly predictable. Beyond regional lymph nodes, metastatic WT at diagnosis most commonly involves the lung and occasionally the liver.

Of all childhood embryonal tumors, the relationship of WT to aberrations in normal development seems most evident. Early in development, the embryonal mesonephros emerges from a complex interaction between epithelial-derived ureteric bud tissue and mesenchymally derived metanephric blastema through a series of reciprocal, inductive differentiation events. Mature nephrons that develop from the mesonephros consist of nephroblasts, tubules, and stromal tissues, which together ultimately will form the adult kidney. These different tissues, in turn, contribute to the most distinctive characteristic of WT, which is its histopathologic diversity.

WT is characterized pathologically by a remarkable histologic diversity of cell types. The triphasic presentation in which blastemal, epithelial, and stromal elements each are easily detectable is the most frequent. These elements typically appear to reflect normal developmental stages, and the arrested differentiation of embryonal cells may play an important role in the pathogenesis of this tumor. Consistent with this possibility is the observation that nephrogenic rests have been observed in a high percentage of normal kidney biopsies obtained from WT patients, although the occurrence of such structures in tissues examined at autopsy of age-related individuals dying of non–cancer-related events is less than 1 per cent.[116] WT arising in younger individuals seems to occur more commonly in an intralobar distribution than in the perilobar distribution observed in older individuals.[116] It is possible that inappropriately proliferating nephroblasts, perhaps a reflection of either a clonal or nonclonal disorder of differentiation, may be the target in which subsequent pathologic events such as sequential mutations lead directly to the development of WT.

Tumors arising in the intralobar area are typically triphasic in their histology and also may contain such heterotopic elements as muscle and bone. Tumors arising in the perilobar area tend to be biphasic or monomorphic,

typically epithelial. This pattern is consistent with the concept that they arise from a cell that is prevalent later in development and has a more limited potential to differentiate along multiple lineages.

Genetics

Data collected in association with the National Wilms' Tumor Studies suggest that as many as 1 per cent of cases of WT occur in individuals who have at least one other affected family member.[117] The observation that familial cases have an increased incidence of bilateral tumors and a younger age at diagnosis suggests that the mode of inheritance of WT is autosomal dominant.[114,118] Few reports have observed the occurrence of WT in the offspring of affected parents or in parents of affected children; however, the apparently autosomal dominant mode of inheritance of WT is thought to be of highly variable penetrance.

Children with WT typically have a normal constitutional karyotype.[119] The rare occurrence of aniridia and WT in association with a constitutional deletion at 11p13 called attention to the possibility of a gene at this locus that might be related to the development of WT.[120,121] Aniridia is a rare condition, although it has been estimated that approximately 30 per cent of children with aniridia go on to develop WT. The occurrence of WT and aniridia with anomalies of the genitourinary tract and mental retardation has been called the WAGR syndrome. Individuals with this syndrome frequently have deletions of chromosome 11 and these typically include 11p13.[120] Further evidence suggesting the role of 11p13 in WT comes from the observation that a deletion in this region could be identified by molecular biological techniques in tumors appearing karyotypically normal.[122] Most patients who exhibit evidence of a deletion of 11p13 in tumor tissue do not have constitutional deletions at this location.

Identification of 11p13 as a location in which a WT gene might be located led several investigators to pursue the isolation of candidate genes in this region[123,124] from individuals with the WAGR syndrome. WT-1 was identified as a candidate gene responsible for WT on the basis of its differentially high level of expression in embryonic compared to adult kidney and its highly conserved sequence homology across species[123] (Fig. 14–5). The 3.0-kb cDNA now recognized to encode the WT-1 gene maps to a 50-kb region of 11p13. In most WT specimens examined to date, it has not been possible to identify alterations in the WT-1 gene. However WT specimens with tumor-specific deletions of this locus have been identified and provide evidence that this allele is specifically inac-

Figure 14–5. Structural characteristics of the WT-1 gene product. The WT-1 gene encodes a protein of 429 amino acids. The carboxy-terminal 122 amino acids consist of four zinc fingers of the C_2H_2 class[127] that are required for DNA binding. The amino-terminal region is required for the transcriptional repression mediated by WT-1.[130]

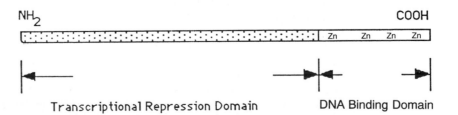

NH$_2$ COOH

| | Zn | Zn | Zn | Zn |

Transcriptional Repression Domain   DNA Binding Domain

tivated during the pathogenesis of some WT.[124,125] In one well-described case, it has been possible to demonstrate the homozygous deletion of this locus in a bilateral WT patient who carried on one chromosome a constitutional deletion of 11p13, including the WT-1 locus.[126]

The highest levels of expression in WT tissues are in blastemal components corresponding to cells arrested during the formation of tubular structures. WT-1 expression during the course of normal development also seems to be highest in tubular structures and lower in the stromal elements. This theme of tumor cells expressing a pattern of genes reflective of the embryonal cell type in which the tumor arises is consistent with the pattern of gene expression seen in other embryonal tumors as well.[76] It is not yet known which precise function of the WT-1–encoded protein inactivated during oncogenesis is of pathologic importance. The WT-1 protein is approximately 53 kDa and contains four zinc fingers in the carboxy-terminal region.[127] The zinc fingers of the WT-1 gene fall into a class of genes related to the Kruppel gene of Drosophila. WT-1 shares approximately a 65 per cent homology with the zinc finger regions of the human early response genes, EGR-1 and EGR-2 (Krox-24 and -20 in the mouse).[128] The EGR genes are thought to regulate the expression of genes that mediate the G_0-to-G_1 transition of the cell cycle, a cellular activity of obvious importance for malignant transformation. These genes and WT-1 recognize the DNA sequence element 5'-GCGGGGGCG-3',[129] although EGR-family transcription factors seem to activate genes whose regulatory regions contain this binding motif, whereas WT-1 functions to repress transcription.[130] Mutations in WT-1 found in WT inactivate its DNA-binding activity.[129] Expression of the genes for IGF-II and the A chain of platelet-derived growth factor (PDGF) can be regulated by WT-1 and are candidate targets suggesting a possible mechanism by which WT-1 might contribute to both the normal and neoplastic proliferation of kidney cells.[131–134]

An important hint regarding the functions of the WT-1 gene that are of oncologic significance may be the observation that WT-1 seems to be important for the proper development of the urogenital system.[135] The adult male genital organs share with the kidney a common embryologic anlage in the metanephros, and the developing genitalia express high levels of WT-1. Patients with bilateral WT frequently have urogenital abnormalities, and among patients with the WAGR syndrome there is approximately a 25-fold increase in the frequency of such abnormalities compared to that in the general population. Such observations may reflect inductive interactions between these two distinct organ systems during development or a pleiotrophic effect of WT-1 reflecting contributions to the development of each of these systems. Patients with the Denys-Drash syndrome,[135] in which the occurrence of pseudohermaphroditism is associated with WT, have heterozygous germline alterations of the WT-1 gene, suggesting that the latter of these hypotheses is correct. Also consistent with this possibility is the observation of WT-1 alterations in individuals with hypospadias and other developmental anomalies of the male genitalia.[135]

The occurrence of multiple genetic alterations in individual tumors is now recognized as commonplace in most if not all tumors. Following the characterization of 11p13 in WT patients, it was recognized that some tumors have alterations restricted to 11p15. Some WAGR patients with a loss of genetic material at 11p15 who were heterozygous at 11p13 could be identified. Subsequently, several rare instances of familial Beckwith-Wiedemann syndrome (BWS) exhibiting linkage at 11p15 were observed. BWS is characterized by hemihypertrophy and the development of embryonal solid tumors, the most common of which are WT and soft tissue sarcomas. These findings and the observation that 11p15 deletions can occur in sporadic cases of WT in which mutations of WT-1 cannot be identified strongly suggest that a second WT predisposition locus is located at this site.[136] Consistent with this possibility is the observation that WT in BWS patients is associated with perilobar nephrogenic rests and occurs outside the infancy period. These characteristics contrast sharply to those of WT occurring in association with germline lesions at 11p13. Clearly 11p13 and 11p15 both contain genetic loci important for the pathogenesis of WT. Other sites at which other tumor suppressor genes important for the pathogenesis of WT may be present include 1p, 16q, and 17p.[119]

In addition to the important role of recessive oncogenes in the development of WT, a role for several dominantly acting oncogenes has been hypothesized. Among these, the possible role of N-myc seems most convincing. Although N-myc is expressed in a limited number of tissues early in development, it is expressed at high levels in developing renal tissues and in WT tissues. Interestingly, c-myc is expressed at low levels in these tissues.[137]

Patients with BWS can exhibit paternal uniparental disomy (both alleles derived from the father) for 11p15.[138] Germline duplication of the paternal allele also has been observed in BWS patients.[138] The gene for IGF-II, an important embryonic mitogen that is highly expressed in WT, maps to this region and is imprinted in humans.[139,140] Imprinting is a gamete-specific modification causing differential expression of the two alleles of a gene in somatic cells. In human tissues, only the paternally derived allele of IGF-II is expressed.[141] In contrast, WTs that have not lost heterozygosity at 11p15 frequently show biallelic expression.[141] These findings suggest that the overexpression of IGF-II, through either gene amplification or inappropriate loss of maternal allelic repression, may contribute to the malignant growth of WT tissue.[138,142] Methylation is thought to be a mechanism by which such imprinting might occur,[143] and it has been suggested that chromosome 11 may carry an imprinting locus. Mutations in such a locus could explain the pattern of WT inheritance that is characterized by the occurrence of the disease in cousins and siblings rather than in the offspring of affected individuals.

Cell Biology

As indicated earlier in this chapter, IGF-II is a potent growth stimulator that is widely expressed during fetal development. High levels of IGF-II are detectable in cells of the metanephric blastema, and these decrease over the course of development.[144] In WT specimens, high levels of IGF-II mRNA are detectable in cells that appear to exhibit evidence of epithelial or rhabdoid maturation.[145,146] These observations and the finding that the type I IGF receptor also is expressed in WT tissue specimens[147] suggest the possibility that IGF-II may serve as an autocrine growth factor for this tumor. A particularly interesting observation in this regard has been the finding that the product of the *WT-1* gene can act as a transcriptional repressor of the *IGF-II* gene.[148] This finding suggests that *WT-1* alterations modify the ability of this factor to repress *IGF-II* expression, which in turn leads to the inappropriate proliferation of WT. Other growth factor–related genes, including acidic growth factor–like activity[149] and PDGF,[150] also might contribute to the growth regulation of WT, but their characterization remains incomplete.

Treatment

WT was the first of the solid tumors recognized as being curable even when metastases were present. The sequential studies carried out by the National Wilms' Tumor Study Group[114] have led to the development of effective treatment approaches.[111,112] The cornerstone of therapy is surgery, and key to its success is the lack of tumor spread into the abdominal cavity at the time of tumor removal. Chemotherapy with a variety of agents is the mainstay of treatment for minimal residual disease that may remain following surgical removal of the tumor and for metastatic disease that cannot be removed at surgery. Actinomycin D and vincristine are used routinely, and Adriamycin is added for the treatment of patients with more extensive disease.[111] More aggressive therapy is used for tumors of poor prognosis, the key prognostic factors being the size of the tumor and the clinical stage of the patient at presentation.[151] WT is also sensitive to radiation therapy. The focus of recent studies has been to tailor therapy in a manner to limit toxicity without compromising the excellent treatment results currently achieved in experienced treatment centers.

CHILDHOOD SARCOMAS

Rhabdomyosarcoma

CLINICAL DESCRIPTION AND PATHOLOGY

Sarcomas arise in supportive tissues that have their origin in embryonic mesenchyme. These tissues include fibrous tissue, muscle, cartilage, and bone. Each of the different sarcomas that have been recognized exhibits evidence of differentiation along one or more of these cellular lineages and, like other childhood tumors, their rather undifferentiated appearance is their most characteristic feature.

Among the soft tissue sarcomas, the best characterized to date has been rhabdomyosarcoma, a tumor exhibiting evidence of skeletal muscle differentiation, although it occasionally occurs in sites such as the bladder where skeletal muscle does not exist. Like other pediatric solid tumors, tumors classified as rhabdomyosarcoma long have been recognized to be a morphologically and biologically heterogeneous group, the genetic basis of which is only now emerging. The relationship of these tumors to the undifferentiated sarcomas of adulthood is poorly understood, and the designation of malignant fibrous histiocytoma has been adopted to describe this group of tumors when it occurs in adults.[152]

Rhabdomyosarcoma is the most common of the soft tissue sarcomas of childhood, accounting for approximately 50 per cent of these tumors, which together account for between 5 and 10 per cent of all childhood malignancies.[109,153] Rhabdomyosarcoma is therefore somewhat less frequent than NB or WT. Undifferentiated sarcomas, which account for the largest portion of soft tissue sarcomas with evidence of skeletal muscle differentiation, are a very heterogeneous group of tumors defined largely by the lack of any recognizable histologic evidence of differentiation along a specific tissue lineage. In many cases, this diagnosis is made to indicate the apparent origin of a primitive, undifferentiated tumor of mesenchymally derived tissue.

Rhabdomyosarcoma is pathologically characterized by the presence of cytologic evidence for skeletal muscle differentiation. Light-microscopic identification of cross striations mimicking those seen in normal skeletal muscle commonly are absent from tumors in which rhabdomyoblasts are recognized by immunocytochemical detection of muscle-specific gene proteins such as myoglobin[154] and creatinine kinase,[155] and by electron microscopic evidence of muscle-specific differentiation such as sarcomeric structures.[156] These features unambiguously identify tumors as belonging to this group.

Rhabdomyosarcomas, despite evidence of skeletal muscle differentiation, remain a morphologically and biologically heterogeneous group of tumors that continue to resist optimal classification. Despite the lack of a strong prognostic impact, the most widely recognized histologic designations used to distinguish these tumors include embryonal rhabdomyosarcoma, which is characterized by a round or slightly spindle-shaped tumor cell embedded in a meshwork of abundant myxomatous stroma, and alveolar rhabdomyosarcoma, which is a highly cellular tumor of small round cells appearing in monotonous sheets delimited histologically by apparent spaces in the tissue resembling lung alveoli. These spaces in the tissue arise during the preparation of the histologic sections and presumably reflect the distinctive intercellular components of this tumor tissue. Other histologic schemas for characterizing rhabdomyosarcoma have been suggested, although no comprehensive classification system based on either histology or etiology has yet emerged.

The sites at which rhabdomyosarcomas arise have implications for treatment and outcome. Rhabdomyosarcomas arising in the head and neck tend to be smaller at the time of diagnosis than sarcomas at other sites. They also are infrequently metastatic at the time of presentation. Sarcomas arising at other sites invade tissues adjacent to their site of origin and metastasize throughout the body following invasion into either the lymphatic or vascular systems.

Most commonly, early metastatic foci are found in the lung, bone marrow, and bone. These findings suggest that the improved prognosis of head and neck rhabdomyosarcomas compared to rhabdomyosarcomas occurring at other locations may reflect earlier detection, although it is also noteworthy that these tumors almost invariably have an embryonal histology. Similarly, rhabdomyosarcomas of the genitourinary tract, with the exception of those arising in the prostate, tend to be of the embryonal variant and also have a good prognosis. This is especially true of those tumors arising in subepithelial tissues and presenting as protruding, grape-like (botryoid) structures.

GENETICS

Several different cytogenetic alterations have been recognized to occur repeatedly in childhood sarcomas, although recognition that a t(2;13)(q35;q14) translocation is typical of alveolar rhabdomyosarcoma has been a particularly important observation because it provides a genetic correlation for this widely recognized clinicopathologic variant of rhabdomyosarcoma.[157] This translocation results in a rearrangement of chromosome 2 within the *pax-3* gene, which includes homeodomain and paired box elements. The translocation juxtaposes *pax-3* DNA-binding elements to chromosome 13 sequences, perhaps resulting in the formation of a novel, hybrid transcription factor.[158] This translocation is not found in embryonal rhabdomyosarcoma, but these tumors frequently do have a loss of heterozygosity at 11p15, which is detectable by the evaluation of restriction fragment length polymorphisms known to map to this region.[159] Attention was first drawn to 11p15 in studies of sarcomas because of the occurrence of rhabdomyosarcomas in patients with BWS.[142] This sort of correlation between histology and genetics has largely eluded the field of solid tumors, with a few exceptions such as the t(11;22) translocation that distinguishes neuroepithelioma from NB. In contrast, such correlations have become routine in oncologic hematopathology.

The early observation in 1969 by Li and Fraumeni that there was an association between the occurrence of soft tissue sarcomas in children and breast cancer in the mothers of these children[2] has led to an extensive and fruitful search to define a cancer syndrome characterized by the familial inheritance of a predisposition for the development of a number of different tumors, but especially sarcomas.[2,3] The recognition that this syndrome was associated with the germline transmission of a mutated *p53* tumor suppressor gene[160,161] has provided considerable insight into the possible genetic basis for inherited cancer predisposition.[162,163] For example, *p53* functions to mediate the genetic stability of cells in tissue culture.[164,165] It is possible that, when *p53* mutation occurs early in the pathogenesis of tumors, the cellular genome is predisposed to developing additional genetic alterations. *p53* mutations also have been described in apparently sporadically occurring childhood sarcoma.[166]

Constitutional alterations in *p53* now are thought generally to be null mutations that inactivate the allele. When this occurs, inactivation of the second allele by subsequent mutation leads to tumor development.[167,168] A large body of studies has now detailed the mechanisms by which the *p53* gene can be inactivated in a variety of tumors.[167] In sporadically occurring tumors, including sarcomas, it appears that mutations that inactivate the first *p53* allele most commonly are point mutations. The second allele can be lost through one of a number of different mechanisms that all functionally result in a conversion of the first mutated allele to homozygosity.

p53 acts to arrest cell growth. Inactivation of this locus either through the loss of both functional alleles or as the result of a dominant negative mutation in one allele can contribute to the unregulated growth of tumor cells. The involvement of other tumor suppressor genes in soft tissue sarcomas is being investigated. To date, it appears that mutations of the retinoblastoma gene (*Rb*) locus frequently occur in sarcomas, including tumors that also carry a mutated *p53* locus.[169] Because such tumors presumably arise from the selection of a subpopulation of cells in which both loci are inactivated, the activity of *p53* and *Rb* may not be totally redundant, although both genes are involved in the regulation of cells during the transition from G_1 into S phase.

Only a few dominantly acting oncogenes have been examined to determine if they may contribute to the pathogenesis of childhood rhabdomyosarcoma. Of these, the ones most commonly recognized to be involved have been the *ras* genes, which may be mutated in approximately one third of these tumors.[170] More rarely, amplifications of *myc* family genes, including both c-*myc* and N-*myc*, have been recognized.[171] Another gene whose expression pattern has not been examined extensively in rhabdomyosarcoma but that may be expected to contribute to the pathogenesis of this tumor is c-*raf*, because its expression is regulated in association with the differentiation of muscle cell precursors.[172,173]

CELL BIOLOGY

As has been the case in other solid tumors of childhood, rhabdomyosarcoma has been recognized to be a tumor tissue in which the dichotomy of differentiation and cell growth is sharply contrasted. In the adult, cells corresponding to those in which rhabdomyosarcoma arises are unlikely to be present, and several lines of investigation suggest that rhabdomyosarcoma is a tumor of a cell that has been arrested during its ontogenic maturation.[171] Treatment of rhabdomyosarcoma cells with retinoic acid or other "differentiating agents" can induce evidence of muscle differentiation[173] and also decreases the growth potential of such cells.[174]

Extensive studies of the molecular mechanisms mediating the differentiation of normal muscle tissue have provided considerable insight, which can be expected to contribute to the understanding of rhabdomyosarcoma. Muscle cell development begins with the expression of one or more genes important for the commitment of multipotential stem cells to the myogenic lineage. The most studied of these genes are myogenin,[175] *myoD*,[176] and *myf-5*.[177] Expression of these genes, which encode transcription factors belonging to the basic helix-loop-helix family of DNA-binding proteins, initiates a cascade of gene expression that activates several known muscle-specific genes such as creatine kinase and the myosin heavy-chain locus. Although *myoD* expression is sufficient to induce myogenic differentiation in a wide variety of different cell types, overexpression apparently does not lead to the differentiation of rhabdomyosarcoma cells.[178,179] This suggests that the block to differentiation in these tumor cells is either in some co-factor that is required for the action of *myoD* or in a step distal to *myoD*-mediated commitment.[179]

Although the role of extracellular factors in the initiation of the process that leads precursor cells to commitment along a specific differentiation pathway is poorly understood, it is clear that maturation along the myogenic lineage can be influenced by the exposure of precursor cells to a number of different cytokines. Among these, IGF-II may be of particular importance because it is highly expressed both in developing mesodermal tissues and in rhabdomyosarcoma. Furthermore, at different doses IGF-II can have different effects on the induction of muscle differentiation. Low doses of IGF-II stimulate the expression of muscle differentiation, whereas at higher doses the proliferative effects seem to predominate.[180] In some cases IGF-II may act as an autocrine growth factor, stimulating the proliferation of rhabdomyosarcoma cells.[181] Both basic fibroblast growth factor (bFGF)[182] and transforming growth factor β (TGF-β)[183] have been shown to be capable of blocking myogenic differentiation. This may be of importance for the pathogenesis of rhabdomyosarcoma, because FGF is produced by these tumor cells.[184] The mechanism by which bFGF and TGF-β mediate the inhibition of muscle cell differentiation is unknown, although this seems to be independent of their mitogenic activity.[183]

TREATMENT

Most soft tissue sarcomas, including rhabdomyosarcoma, initially are responsive to radiation and chemotherapy. Therefore, the management of patients with these tumors typically includes control of the local tumor by surgery and irradiation and treatment of both known and micrometastatic disease with chemotherapy.[185] Current approaches to the management of patients with localized rhabdomyosarcoma are highly efficacious, although the treatment of disease that is metastatic at presentation or that has recurred following an initial attempt at therapy is still very inadequate; the majority of these patients still die of their disease. Molecular approaches to studying metastases and relapse of sarcomas have been rather limited, although recognition of the role of IGF-II in stimulating the motility of rhabdomyosarcoma cells suggests that it eventually may be possible to develop an integrated approach to therapy based on interrupting the IGF-II—mediated growth and motility pathways in these tumor cells.[181,186] Interestingly, an antibody against the type I IGF receptor can block the growth of rhabdomyosarcoma cells but it does not interrupt the IGF-II—induced increase in cell motility, suggesting that these two different effects may be mediated by different cell surface receptors.[181,187]

Osteosarcoma

CLINICAL DESCRIPTION AND PATHOLOGY

Sarcomas of bone are considerably less common than sarcomas of soft tissues in children. Among the sarcomas of bone, osteosarcoma has been studied most extensively. Osteosarcoma occurs most frequently during adolescence, when bone growth is rapid,[188] and among children of this age group it is the most common tumor other than those of the hematopoietic tissues.[153] The sites at which osteosarcoma most commonly occur are the metaphyseal growth plates. These findings and the occurrence of this tumor earlier in girls than in boys[189] and in taller children[190] strongly suggest an important role for cellular proliferation in the oncogenic conversion of immature bone precursors in which these tumors are thought to arise.

The histologic diagnosis of osteosarcoma is made when tumor osteoid and disorganized bone can be identified within malignant stromal tissues. As is the case with other pediatric solid tumors, a wide range of different histologic patterns are seen in osteosarcoma specimens. The natural histories of these histologic variants are not yet clinically distinguishable. At least one widely recognized classification system for bone tumors is based on the degree of tissue-specific differentiation of tumor cells.[191] In this schema, tumors are classified as osteoblastic, chondroblastic, or fibroblastic osteosarcoma depending on whether the predominant differentiation is along bone, cartilage, or stromal tissue pathways, respectively. Although none of the available histologic classification systems for osteosarcoma have been of importance for either optimizing treatment or prognostication, the use of a system that provides insight into the biologic potential of individual tumors may offer a basis on which to initiate laboratory studies of these tumors.

GENETICS

Several conditions are known to predispose patients to the development of osteosarcoma, although the genetic basis for this tendency is not yet known. Osteosarcoma invariably is associated with Paget's disease when it develops in the adult,[192] and other benign growth disorders of bone such as Ollier's disease (endochondromatosis) can be associated with this malignancy when it develops during adolescence.[192]

Constitutional genetic rearrangements that predispose specifically to the development of osteosarcoma are not known, although patients who carry constitutional alterations of the *Rb* gene[193] or the *p53* gene[2] are at increased risk for the development of osteosarcoma. These patients, who belong to families with either hereditary retinoblastoma or the Li-Fraumeni syndrome, respectively, also may develop other tumor types, although in each case osteosarcoma is among the most frequent. This finding is compatible with the observation that alterations in both copies of the *Rb* and *p53* genes often are found in sporadically occurring osteosarcomas.[169,194] Also of interest in this regard is the finding that there are rare patients presenting with apparently multifocal osteogenic sarcoma who carry a constitutional mutation in *p53*[195] (Fig. 14–6). Transgenic mice expressing high levels of a mutant *p53* gene also develop osteosarcomas, suggesting a key role for the *p53* gene product in the regulation of bone growth.[196]

A role for other oncogenes in the development of osteosarcoma also has been sought, including c-*fos*.[197] The viral homologue of c-*fos*, v-*fos*, was identified as the transforming gene of the FBJ murine osteosarcoma virus, which induces bone tumors in mice. Transgenic mice constitutively expressing c-*fos* also develop bone tumors.[198] v-*fos* differs from c-*fos* at the carboxy-terminal region of the protein, which is deleted in the viral-transforming gene. c-*fos* protein levels have been observed to be significantly elevated in human osteosarcoma and may contribute to the development of these tumors.[197] Other oncogenes, including c-*sis*, *myc*, and c-*raf*, also have been found to be infrequently amplified in osteosarcoma as well.[199]

CELL BIOLOGY

There is an extensive literature on bone growth and remodeling, although the implications of these data for the pathogenesis of tumors arising in precursors of bone have not been fully exploited. Bone repair involves mesenchymally derived precursor cell proliferation that is mediated by PDGF, EGF, IGFs, γ-interferon, and other peptide mitogens.[200–202] The B chain of PDGF is a homologue of the transforming protein of simian sarcoma virus. The PDGF receptor encodes a tyrosine kinase activity, and when PDGF binds the expression of *fos*, *myc* and a cascade of cellular genes important for initiating proliferation is induced. Several tumor cell lines isolated from osteogenic sarcomas have been found to produce PDGF that may stimulate growth through an autocrine mechanism.[201] Such autocrine pathways mediated by PDGF include intracellular growth stimulatory pathways. This indicates that there may be several different sites along the PDGF-mediated mitogenic pathway at which inappropriate expression or activation can trigger oncogenesis.[203] EGF also may contribute to the pathogenesis of osteosarcoma. Some cell lines derived from osteosarcoma express the EGF receptor on their surface, and these receptors can proliferate in response to treatment with EGF.[204] Interestingly, the mitogenic response of osteosarcoma cells to both EGF and PDGF may be blocked by TGF-β,[205] although at low doses TGF-β may stimulate proliferation of the cells.[206] IGF-I also contributes to the regulation of childhood bone sarcoma proliferation.[207] Both IGF-I–stimulated osteogenic tumor cell proliferation and proliferation caused by EGF and PDGF can be blocked by suramin when these pathways have an extracellular component.[208,209]

TREATMENT

Surgery is the key therapeutic modality in the management of osteosarcoma, whereas chemotherapy is used to control micrometastases even when only local disease is identifiable. If surgery other than amputation—for example, "limb-sparing surgery" or subtotal tumor removal—is performed, chemotherapy also is used to control the primary tumor. Osteosarcoma is generally thought to be relatively resistant to conventional doses of γ-irradiation. To date, biologic response modifiers, monoclonal antibodies, and other agents developed by the use of modern molecular technologies have not impacted on the treatment of osteosarcoma, although there is considerable research activity in this area. Therapeutic trials using various forms of immunologic augmentation also have

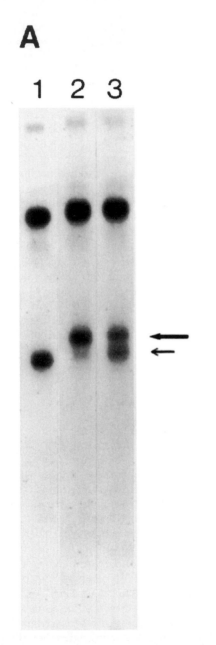

A

1 2 3

Figure 14–6. Single-strand conformation analysis of exon 8 of the *p53* gene from a patient with multifocal osteogenic sarcoma. DNA from peripheral blood lymphocytes of a normal individual (lane 1), from the patient's tumor tissue (lane 2), and from peripheral blood lymphocytes (lane 3) are shown. The normal alleles are identified by the slowest migrating gel band and the band marked by the thin arrow. The thick arrow indicates the mutated allele. (From Iavarone A, Matthay KK, Steinkirchner TM, et al: Germ-line and somatic p53 gene mutations in multifocal osteogenic sarcoma. Proc Natl Acad Sci USA 89:4207, 1992, with permission.)

been undertaken for the treatment of this tumor, but opportunities to improve outcome of patients with bone sarcomas have not yet emerged. Most recently, liposome-encapsulated muramyl tripeptide–phosphatidylethanolamine, a molecule present in the bacille Calmette-Guerin vaccine, has been administered intravenously because of its potential for activating monocytes to become cytotoxic.[210,211] The initial evaluation of this approach has been promising, and further evaluation is in progress.

RETINOBLASTOMA

Clinical Description and Pathology

Retinoblastoma (Rb) is a rare childhood tumor thought to arise in embryonic retinal epithelium.[212] It occurs with an incidence of approximately 1 in 20,000 new births[213] or approximately 200 new cases per year in the United States. Despite the infrequency with which this tumor occurs, it has been the target of intense research interest. This interest has been spurred by recognition that Rb can be an inherited disorder and that patients with Rb have an enhanced predisposition to develop other tumors, such as osteosarcoma.[214,215] The discovery of the gene that encodes the predisposition to Rb,[216] and recognition that this gene is important in cell cycle regulation,[217] provided important research opportunities in several areas of molecular biology.

Rb occurs almost invariably in early childhood, and can be congenital. Less than 10 per cent of Rb occurs in children with a positive family history for the disease.[218] An additional 10 per cent of Rb patients have acquired the disease as the result of a new germline mutation, and therefore have the heritable form of the disease as well. Patients with heritable Rb have a significantly enhanced predisposition to developing a second tumor,[214,215] and by 30 years after their first tumors such patients may have an extraordinarily high chance of having a second tumor.[214] For these patients, the use of radiation or chemotherapy may contribute to this increased tumor incidence, although it cannot explain the increased incidence of tumors outside the radiation field in patients who have not received chemotherapy.[214] The most common second tumors are sarcomas, especially osteosarcomas, a tumor in which the Rb gene is known to be mutated frequently even when the tumor presents in a sporadic form.[219]

Rb is characterized by the rapid growth of undifferentiated neuroblastic precursors derived from various layers of retinal ganglion cells.[212] Histologically, Rb resembles other embryonal, solid tumors of childhood. The cells are small and round with a high nuclear-to-cytoplasmic ratio, with numerous mitoses reflecting their rapid growth rate. Typically Rb tumor cells appear very undifferentiated, with evidence of ganglionic differentiation, such as the presence of Flexner-Wintersteiner rosettes. Electron microscopy oftentimes reveals structural features found only in retinal cells.[220]

Tumors that are limited to the globe at the time of di-

agnosis are staged according to the schema of Reese and Ellsworth, which is based on the number and size of tumors.[221] This classification predicts the likelihood of obtaining local tumor control and the preservation of vision. Each eye is staged individually. Rb can spread beyond the orbit by both direct invasion of adjacent tissue and hematogenous spread.[222] Rb typically invades along blood vessels or along the optic nerve itself. Spread along the optic nerve oftentimes leads to invasion of the brain parenchyma itself or to seeding of the cerebral spinal fluid and neuraxis. Hematogenous spread can lead to wide dissemination with metastases to bone, bone marrow, and brain, although this is rare in developed countries, where definitive treatment is undertaken early in the course of the disease.

Genetics and Cell Biology

Rb is the prototype tumor for the study of inherited cancer predispositions for the development of any specific tumor[1] (Fig. 14–7). The occurrence of bilateral disease is strong evidence for a germline mutation in the Rb gene. In about 50 per cent of individuals with bilateral disease this mutation is inherited from an affected parent. Other patients who present with bilateral Rb now are recognized to have newly occurring germline mutations. This finding is consistent with the observation that hereditary Rb is expressed with a very high penetrance, although occasionally a generation is spared in a pedigree in which the gene seems to be highly penetrant.[1]

Based on the occurrence rates of bilateral and unilateral disease, Knudson proposed a model of carcinogenesis that predicted these tumors arising as the result of two independent genetic events.[169,223] In patients with the heritable (bilateral) form of the disease, the first of these two mutations would have been inherited from an affected parent by germline transmission. Such mutations would be present in every cell of the offspring. A second mutation in the remaining Rb allele of such a cell would lead to complete inactivation of the gene and the development of Rb. Sporadically occurring cases of Rb arise when these two mutations occurred stochastically in a single cell. The obviously increased chance that patients carrying a germline alteration will inactivate both Rb alleles provides an explanation for the observation that patients with hereditary Rb typically have bilateral disease, have multiple tumors by the time a diagnosis is made, and present with tumors at an earlier age than patients with tumors that occur sporadically.

The Rb gene initially was isolated based on its position at 13q14.[216] The product of the Rb gene, a 105-kDa phosphoprotein,[224] is encoded in 27 exons that span approximately 200 kb of DNA.[225] Virtually all normal tissues that have been examined express Rb,[226] and mice lacking the Rb gene are viable only through day 16 of gestation.[227] The finding that the Rb gene is expressed in all tissues is consistent with its role as a critical mediator of cellular growth, but contrasts sharply with the observation that there are no obvious growth defects in embryonic mice lacking Rb. Indeed, the finding that these mice only have defects in the development of their hematopoietic and nervous systems has led to speculation that the critical role of *Rb* may be in the differentiation of these affected tissues rather than in the control of growth.[227]

Tumors in which the *Rb* gene has been homozygously inactivated typically do not contain detectable Rb RNA or protein, although occasionally a truncated form of the protein is found. This may be due to the actual deletion of the gene, destabilization of the protein, or premature termination of the protein. Mutations have been identified throughout the *Rb* gene in tissue from both Rb and a wide variety of other tumors. The most common of these are osteosarcoma,[216] breast cancer,[228] and small-cell lung cancer.[229] Interestingly, the incidence of breast cancer and small-cell lung cancer has not been reported to be increased in patients who survive bilateral Rb.

Studies to elucidate the function of the *Rb* gene have focused primarily on its role as a suppressor of cell proliferation. Transfection of *Rb* into cells from which it has been lost as a result of mutation leads to a variable response, but in some cell types this results in a diminished proliferative capacity and a loss of tumorigenicity.[230,231] It is currently thought that *Rb* functions to suppress growth by sequestering the E2F family of transcription factors during the G_1 phase of the cell cycle. E2F transcription factors contribute to the activation of several different genes encoding S-phase functions related to the synthesis of DNA, including dihydrofolate reductase, thymidine kinase, and DNA polymerase.[232] When complexed to Rb, E2F gene–mediated transcriptional activation does not occur. E2F is only bound to the underphosphorylated (active) forms of Rb and is present in an active form only when Rb is inactivated by phosphorylation. As the cell cycle progresses through G_1 and into S phase, Rb becomes phosphorylated and is no longer able to bind E2F, releasing these mediators of cellular proliferation.[232]

Cell lines of human Rb are available for study. Little is known of the growth-regulatory molecules that mediate their proliferation, although the type I IGF receptor is expressed on the surface of these cells.[233] These cell lines differentiate in vitro in response to such agents as nerve growth factor and cAMP.[234] Rb cell lines express markers of both the glial and neuronal lineages[235–237] consistent with the origin of these tumors in immature, multipotential epithelium.[212] Rb cells also respond to a wide variety of different cytokines, including interferons and TNF, although the therapeutic potential of such biologicals in this disease has not yet been pursued.[237]

Treatment

The identification and characterization of the gene responsible for the dominant transmission of Rb[216,238] and an extensive data base documenting the incidence of Rb have provided a sound basis for genetic counseling. Accurate mapping of *Rb* mutations and their detection in the germline of patients greatly enhances the precision of genetic counseling regarding both transmissibility of the trait and the likelihood of secondary tumors. Detection of *Rb* mutations in new Rb cases is complicated by the large size and complex organization of exons in the *Rb* gene.[225,239] Once a particular mutation in a proband is identified, the evaluation of other family members is frequently facilitated by the identification of restriction fragment length polymorphisms that co-segregate with the mutant allele.

The management of patients with Rb depends on the size of the tumor and the extent of tumor invasion at the time of diagnosis. Children with sporadic disease typically have larger tumors when they are first diagnosed than children with familial histories and bilateral disease, because these children are usually under close observation from the time of birth. Surgery and irradiation are the mainstays of treatment for patients with Rb. More than 90 per cent of children with local disease can be cured of Rb.[240] Rare patients who present with metastatic disease or disease that has spread locally beyond the orbit are treated with varying chemotherapeutic regimens, but less than 10 per cent of these patients survive beyond 2 years.[241] Expres-

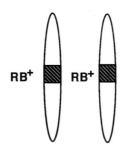

All somatic cells of a normal individual contain two wild-type alleles

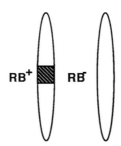

All somatic cells of an individual with hereditary retinoblastoma contain 1 wild-type and 1 mutated allele

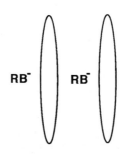

Tumor cells contain two mutated alleles

Figure 14–7. Knudson model of inherited cancer predisposition. (From Knudson AG: Retinoblastoma: A prototypic hereditary neoplasm. Semin Oncol 5:57, 1978, with permission.)

sion of P-glycoprotein encoded by the *mdr-1* gene has been implicated in the resistance of Rb to several different chemotherapeutic agents.[242]

The excellent treatment outcome for children with localized disease has enhanced the importance of attempting to preserve vision in planning for the treatment of this tumor. For this reason, radiation has taken a prominent role in the management of Rb patients.[243] For small tumors (<3 mm), cryotherapy and photocoagulation frequently are used, whereas enucleation of the eye is reserved for cases in which there is no prospect for preserving vision. Patients with bilateral Rb do not have as high a survival rate as patients with unilateral disease because of the frequent occurrence of second tumors in these patients.[214]

ACKNOWLEDGMENTS: I wish to thank Dr. David Eisenstat for his critical reading of this manuscript and Ms. L. de la Calzada for her assistance in its preparation.

REFERENCES

1. Knudson AG: Retinoblastoma: A prototypic hereditary neoplasm. Semin Oncol 5:57, 1978
2. Li FP, Fraumeni JF Jr: Rhabdomyosarcoma in children: Epidemiologic study and identification of a familial cancer syndrome. J Natl Cancer Inst 43:1365, 1969
3. Li FP, Fraumeni JF Jr: Prospective study of a family cancer syndrome. JAMA 247:2692, 1982
4. Leppert M, Burt R, Hughes JP, et al: Genetic analysis of an inherited predisposition to colon cancer in a family with a variable number of adenomatous polyps. N Engl J Med 322: 9048, 1990
5. Mulvihill JJ, Byrne J: Genetic counseling of the cancer survivor. Semin Oncol Nurs 5:29, 1989
6. Cancer Statistics Review 1973–1986. Publication No. 89-2789. Bethesda, MD, National Institutes of Health, 1989
7. Rorke LB, Schut L: Introductory survey of pediatric brain tumors. In McLaurin RL, et al (eds): Pediatric Neurosurgery, 2nd ed. Philadelphia, WB Saunders Company, 1989, pp 335–337
8. Daumas-Duport C, Scheithauer B, O'Fallon J, et al: Grading of astrocytomas: A simple and reproducible method. Cancer 62: 2152, 1988
9. Burger PC, Vogel FS, Green SB, et al: Glioblastoma multiforme and anaplastic astrocytoma: Pathologic criteria and prognostic implications. Cancer 56:1106, 1985
10. Rorke LB, Gilles FH, Davis RL: Revision of the World Health Organization classification of brain tumors for childhood brain tumors. Cancer 56:1869, 1985
11. Russell DS, Rubinstein LJ: Pathology of Tumours of the Nervous System, 5th ed. Baltimore, Williams & Wilkins, 1989
12. Trojanowski JQ, Tohyama T, Lee VM: Medulloblastomas and related primitive neuroectodermal brain tumors of childhood recapitulate molecular milestones in the maturation of neuroblasts. Mol Chem Neuropathol 17:121, 1992
13. Hart MN, Earle KM: Primitive neuroectodermal tumors of the brain in children. Cancer 32:890, 1973
14. Becker L: Primitive neuroectodermal tumors: Views on a working classification. In Fields WS (ed): Primary Brain Tumors: A Review of Histologic Classification. New York, Springer-Verlag, 1989, pp 59–69
15. Bailey P, Cushing H: A Classification of the Tumors of the Glioma Group on a Histogenetic Basis with a Correlated Study of Prognosis. Philadelphia, JB Lippincott Company, 1926
16. Schoenberg B: Multiple primary neoplasms and the nervous system. Cancer 40:1961, 1977
17. Heideman RL, Packer RJ, Albright LA, et al: Tumors of the central nervous system. In Pizzo PA, Poplack DG (eds): Principles and Practice of Pediatric Oncology, 2nd ed. Philadelphia, JB Lippincott Company, 1993, pp 633–681
18. Marchuk DA, Saulino AM, Tavakkol R, et al: cDNA cloning of the type 1 neurofibromatosis gene: Complete sequence of the NF1 gene product. Genomics 11:931, 1991
19. Rouleau GA, Merel P, Lutchman M, et al: Alteration in a new gene encoding a putative membrane-organizing protein causes neuro-fibromatosis type 2. Nature 363:515, 1993
20. DeClue JE, Cohen BD, Lowy DR: Identification and characterization of the neurofibromatosis type 1 protein product. Proc Natl Acad Sci USA 88:9914, 1991
21. Gutmann DH, Boguski M, Marchuk D, et al: Analysis of the neurofibromatosis type 1 (NF1) GAP-related domain by site-directed mutagenesis. Oncogene 8:761, 1993
22. Viskochil D, Buchberg AM, Xu G, et al: Deletions and a translocation interrupt a cloned gene at the neurofibromatosis type 1 locus. Cell 62:187, 1990
23. Steck PA, Saya H: Pathways of oncogenesis in primary brain tumors. Curr Opin Oncol 3:476, 1991
24. Bigner SH, Mark J, Mahaley MS, et al: Pattern of the early, gross chromosomal changes in malignant human glioma. Hereditas 101:103, 1984
25. James CD, Carlbom E, Dumanski JP, et al: Clonal genomic alterations in glioma malignancy stages. Cancer Res 48:5546, 1988
26. Jenkins RB, Kimmel DWV, Moertel CA, et al: A cytogenetic study of 53 human gliomas. Cancer Genet Cytogenet 39:253, 1989
27. Bigner SH, Mark J, Burger PC, et al: Specific chromosomal abnormalities in malignant human gliomas. Cancer Res 48:405, 1988
28. Yamada K, Kondo T, Yoshioka M, et al: Cytogenetic studies in twenty human brain tumors: Association of no. 22 chromosome abnormalities with tumors of the brain. Cancer Genet Cytogenet 2:293, 1980
29. Frankel RH, Bayona W, Koslow M, et al: p53 mutations in human malignant gliomas: Comparison of loss of heterozygosity with mutation frequency. Cancer Res 52:1427, 1992
30. Libermann TA, Nusbaum HR, Razon N, et al: Amplification, enhanced expression and possible rearrangement of EGF receptor gene in primary human brain tumors of glial origin. Nature 313:144, 1985
31. James CD, He J, Carlbom E, et al: Chromosome 9 deletion mapping reveals interferon alpha and interferon beta-1 gene deletions in human glial tumors. Cancer Res 51:1684, 1991
32. James CD, He J, Carlbom E, et al: Loss of genetic information in central nervous system tumors common to children and young adults. Genes Chromosom Cancer 2:94, 1990
33. Bigner SH, Mark J, Friedman HS, et al: Structural chromosomal abnormalities in human medulloblastoma. Cancer Genet Cytogenet 30:91, 1988
34. Thomas GA, Raffel C: Loss of heterozygosity on 6q, 16q, and 17p in human central nervous system primitive neuroectodermal tumors. Cancer Res 51:639, 1991
35. Biegel JA, Burk CD, Barr FG, et al: Evidence for a 17p tumor related locus distinct from p53 in pediatric primitive neuroectodermal tumors. Cancer Res 52:3391, 1992
36. Cogen PH, Daneshvar L, Metzger AK, et al: Involvement of multiple chromosome 17p loci in medulloblastoma tumorigenesis. Am J Hum Genet 50:584, 1992
37. Saylors RL, Sidransky D III, Friedman HS, et al: Infrequent p53 gene mutations in medulloblastomas. Cancer Res 51:4721, 1991
38. Bigner SH, Friedman HS, Vogelstein B: Amplification of the c-myc gene in human medulloblastoma cell lines and xenografts. Cancer Res 50:2347, 1990
39. Garson JA, Pemberton LF, Sheppard PW, et al: N-myc gene expression and oncoprotein characterisation in medulloblastoma. Br J Cancer 59:889, 1989
40. Fuller GN, Bigner SH: Amplified cellular oncogenes in neoplasms of the human central nervous system. Mutat Res 276: 299, 1992
41. MacGregor DN, Ziff EB: Elevated c-myc expression in childhood medulloblastomas. Pediatr Res 28:63, 1990

42. Sawyer JR, Swanson CM, Roloson GJ, et al: Molecular cytogenetic analysis of a medulloblastoma with isochromosome 17 and double minutes. Cancer Genet Cytogenet 57:181, 1991

43. Badiali M, Pession A, Basso G: N-myc and c-myc oncogenes amplification in medulloblastomas: Evidence of particularly aggressive behavior of a tumor with c-myc amplification. Tumori 77:118, 1991

44. Iolascon A, Lania A, Badiali M, et al: Analysis of N-ras gene mutations in medulloblastomas by polymerase chain reaction and oligonucleotide probes in formalin-fixed, paraffin-embedded tissues. Med Pediatr Oncol 19:24, 1991

45. Lendahl U, Zimmerman LB, McKay RD: CNS stem cells express a new class of intermediate filament protein. Cell 60:585, 1990

46. Tohyama T, Lee VM, Rorke LB, et al: Monoclonal antibodies to a rat nestin fusion protein recognize a 220-kDa polypeptide in subsets of fetal and adult human central nervous system neurons and in primitive neuroectodermal tumor cells. Am J Pathol 143:258, 1993

47. Dahlstrand J, Collins VP, Lendahl U: Expression of the class VI intermediate filament nestin in human central nervous system tumors. Cancer Res 52:5334, 1992

48. Molenaar WM, Jansson DS, Gould VE, et al: Molecular markers of primitive neuroectodermal tumors and other pediatric central nervous system tumors: Monoclonal antibodies to neuronal and glial antigens distinguish subsets of primitive neuroectodermal tumors. Lab Invest 61:635, 1989

49. Duffner PK, Horowitz ME, Krischer JP, et al: Postoperative chemotherapy and delayed radiation in children less than three years of age with malignant brain tumors. N Engl J Med 328:1725, 1993

50. Brodeur GM, Castleberry RP: Neuroblastoma. In Pizzo PA, Poplack DG (eds): Principles and Practice of Pediatric Oncology, 2nd ed. Philadelphia, JB Lippincott Company, 1993, pp 739–769

51. Evans A, D'Angio G, Randolph J: A proposed staging system for children with neuroblastoma. Cancer 27:374, 1971

52. Brodeur GM: Neuroblastoma: Clinical significance of genetic abnormalities. Cancer Surv 9:673, 1990

53. Nakagawara A, Nakagawa MA, Scavarda NJ, et al: Association between high levels of expression of the TRK gene and favorable outcome in human neuroblastoma. N Engl J Med 328:847, 1993

54. Cooper MJ, Steinberg SM, Chatten J, et al: Plasticity of neuroblastoma tumor cells to differentiate along a fetal adrenal ganglionic lineage predicts for improved patient survival. J Clin Invest 90:2402, 1992

55. Triche T, Askin F: Neuroblastoma and the differential diagnosis of small, round, blue cell tumors. Hum Pathol 14:569, 1983

56. Cohen PS, Cooper MJ, Helman LJ, et al: Neuropeptide Y expression in the developing adrenal gland and in childhood neuroblastoma tumors. Cancer Res 50:6055, 1990

57. Kogner P, Bjork O, Theodorsson E: Neuropeptide Y as a marker in pediatric neuroblastoma. Pediatr Pathol 10:207, 1990

58. Brodeur G, Sekhon G, Goldstein M: Chromosomal aberrations in human neuroblastoma. Cancer 40:2256, 1977

59. Biedler J, Ross R, Sharske S, et al: Human neuroblastoma cytogenetics: Search for significance of homogeneously staining regions in double minute chromosomes. In Evans A (ed): Advances in Neuroblastoma Research. New York, Raven Press, 1980, pp 81–96

60. Potluri VR, Gilbert F, Helsen C, et al: Primitive neuroectodermal tumor cell lines: Chromosomal analysis of five cases. Cancer Genet Cytogenet 24:75, 1987

61. Biedler JL, Spengler BA: A novel chromosome abnormality on human neuroblastoma and anti-folate resistant Chinese hamster cell lines in culture. J Natl Cancer Inst 57:683, 1976

62. Brodeur GM, Green AA, Hayes FA, et al: Cytogenetic features of human neuroblastomas and cell lines. Cancer Res 41:4678, 1981

63. Montgomery K, Biedler JL, Spengler BA, et al: Specific DNA sequence amplification in human neuroblastoma cells. Proc Natl Acad Sci USA 80:5724, 1983

64. Schwab M, Alitalo K, Lempnauer K, et al: Amplified DNA with limited homology to myc cellular oncogene is shared by human neuroblastoma cell lines and a neuroblastoma tumor. Nature 305:245, 1983

65. Kohl NE, Gee CE, Alt FW: Activated expression of the N-myc gene in human neuroblastomas and related tumors. Science 226:1335, 1984

66. Seeger R, Brodeur GS, et al: Association of multiple copies of the N-myc oncogene with rapid progression of neuroblastomas. N Engl J Med 313:1111, 1985

67. Brodeur G, Seeger R, Schwab M, et al: Amplification of N-myc in untreated human neuroblastomas correlates with advanced disease stage. Science 224:1121, 1984

68. Sacchi N, Wendtner CM, Thiele CJ: Single-cell detection of ETS-1 transcripts in human neuroectodermal cells. Oncogene 6:2149, 1991

69. Thiele CJ, Deutsch LA, Israel MA: The expression of multiple proto-oncogenes is differentially regulated during retinoic acid induced maturation of human neuroblastoma cell lines. Oncogene 3:281, 1988

70. Bolen JB, Rosen N, Israel MA: Increased pp60^{c-src} tyrosylkinase activity in human neuroblastomas is associated with amino-terminal tyrosine phosphorylation of the src gene product. Proc Natl Acad Sci USA 82:7275, 1985

71. Collum RG, DePinho R, Mellis S, et al: A novel gene expressed specifically in neuroepitheliomas and related tumors. Cancer Cells 113:6, 1989

72. Thiele CJ, McKeon C, Triche TJ, et al: Differential protooncogene expression characterizes histopathologically indistinguishable tumors of the peripheral nervous system. J Clin Invest 80:804, 1987

73. Cohn SL, Salwen H, Quasney MW, et al: High levels of N-myc protein in a neuroblastoma cell line lacking N-myc amplification. Prog Clin Biol Res 366:21, 1991

74. Thiele CJ, Reynolds PC, Israel MA: Decreased expression of N-myc precedes retinoic acid induced phenotypic differentiation of human neuroblastoma. Nature 313:404, 1985

75. Thiele CJ, Israel MA: Regulation of N-myc expression is a critical event controlling the ability of human neuroblasts to differentiate. Exp Cell Biol 56:321, 1988

76. Cooper MJ, Hutchins GM, Cohen PS, et al: Human neuroblastoma tumor cell lines correspond to the arrested differentiation of chromaffin adrenal medullary neuroblasts. Cell Growth Differ 2:149, 1990

77. Helman LJ, Thiele CJ, Linehan WM, et al: Molecular markers of neuroendocrine development and evidence of environmental regulation. Proc Natl Acad Sci USA 84:2336, 1987

78. Marchetti D, Perez PJR: Nerve growth factor receptors in human neuroblastoma cells. J Neurochem 49:475, 1987

79. Chan HS, Thorner PS, Haddad G, et al: Multidrug resistance in cancers of childhood: Clinical relevance and circumvention. Adv Pharmacol 24:157, 1993

80. El-Badry OM, Romanus JA, Helman LJ, et al: Autonomous growth of a human neuroblastoma cell line is mediated by insulin-like growth factor II. J Clin Invest 84:829, 1989

81. El-Badry OM, Israel MA: Growth regulation of human neuroblastoma. Cancer Treat Res 63:105, 1992

82. Matthay KK, Sather HN, Seeger RC, et al: Excellent outcome of stage II neuroblastoma is independent of residual disease and radiation therapy. J Clin Oncol 17:236, 1989

83. Finkelstein J, Kemperer M, Evans A, et al: Multiagent chemotherapy for children with metastatic neuroblastoma: A report from the Children's Cancer Study Group. Med Pediatr Oncol 6:179, 1979

84. Shafford E, Rogers D, Pritchard J: Advanced neuroblastoma: Improved response rate using a multiagent regimen (OPEC) including sequential cisplatin and VM26. J Clin Oncol 2:742, 1984

85. Yaniv I, Bouffet E, Irle C, et al: Autologous bone marrow transplantation in pediatric solid tumors. Pediatr Hematol Oncol 7:35, 1990

86. Stout AP: A tumor of the ulnar nerve. Proc NY Pathol Soc 18:2, 1918

87. Miser J, Steis R, Longo D, et al: Treatment of newly diagnosed high risk sarcoma and primitive neuroectodermal tumors (PNET) in children and young adults. Proc Am Soc Clin Oncol 4:240, 1985

88. Marina NM, Etcubanas E, Parham DM, et al: Peripheral primitive neuroectodermal tumor (peripheral neuroepithelioma) in children: A review of the St. Jude experience and controversies in diagnosis and management. Cancer 64:1952, 1989

89. Askin KF, Rosai J, Sibley R, et al: Malignant small cell tumor of the thoracopulmonary region in childhood: A distinctive clinicopathologic entity of uncertain histogenesis. Cancer 43:2438, 1979

90. Llombart-Bosch A, Lacombe MJ, Peydro-Olaya A, et al: Malignant peripheral neuroectodermal tumours of bone other than Askin's neoplasm: Characterization of 14 new cases with immunohistochemistry and electron microscopy. Virchows Arch A Pathol Anat Histopathol 412:421, 1988

91. Gonzalez-Crussi F, Wolfson S, Misugi K, et al: Peripheral neuroectodermal tumors of the chest wall in childhood. Cancer 54:2519, 1984

92. Whang PJ, Triche JJ, Knutsen T, et al: Chromosome translocation in peripheral neuroepithelioma. N Engl J Med 311:584, 1984

93. Whang PJ, Triche TJ, Knutsen T, et al: Cytogenetic characterization of selected small round cell tumors of childhood. Cancer Genet Cytogenet 21:185, 1986

94. Donner L, Triche TJ, Israel MA, et al: A panel of monoclonal antibodies which discriminate neuroblastoma from Ewing's sarcoma, rhabdomyosarcoma, neuroepithelioma, and hematopoietic malignancies. Prog Clin Biol Res 175:347, 1985

95. Friedman JM, Vitale M, Maimon J, et al: Expression of the cholecystokinin gene in pediatric tumors. Proc Natl Acad Sci USA 89:5819, 1992

96. Turc-Carel C, Philip I, Berger M, et al: Chromosomal translocations in Ewing's sarcoma. N Engl J Med 309:497, 1983

97. McKeon C, Thiele CJ, Ross RA, et al: Indistinguishable patterns of protooncogene expression in two distinct but closely related tumors: Ewing's sarcoma and neuroepithelioma. Cancer Res 48:4307, 1988

98. Rettig WJ, Garin CP, Huvos AG: Ewing's sarcoma: New approaches to histogenesis and molecular plasticity. Lab Invest 66:133, 1992

99. Triche T, Carazzana AO: Principles in pediatric pathology. In Pizzo PA, Poplack DE (eds): Principles and Practice of Pediatric Oncology. Philadelphia, JB Lippincott Company, 1989, pp 93–125

100. Miozzo M, Sozzi G, Calderone C: t(11;22) in three cases of peripheral neuroepithelioma. Genes Chromsom Cancer 2:163, 1990

101. Zucman J, Delattre O, Desmaze C, et al: Cloning and characterization of the Ewing's sarcoma and peripheral neuroepithelioma t(11;22) translocation breakpoints. Genes Chromosom Cancer 5:271, 1992

102. Vecchio G, Cavazzana AO, Triche TJ, et al: Expression of the dbl proto-oncogene in Ewing's sarcomas. Oncogene 4:897, 1989

103. Fellinger EJ, Garin CP, Su SL, et al: Biochemical and genetic characterization of the HBA71 Ewing's sarcoma cell surface antigen. Cancer Res 51:336, 1991

104. Fellinger EJ, Garin CP, Glasser DB, et al: Comparison of cell surface antigen HBA71 (p30/32MIC2), neuron-specific enolase, and vimentin in the immunohistochemical analysis of Ewing's sarcoma of bone. Am J Surg Pathol 16:746, 1992

105. Chen J, Chattopadhyay B, Venkatakrishnan G, et al: Nerve growth factor-induced differentiation of human neuroblastoma and neuroepithelioma cell lines. Cell Growth Differ 1:79–85, 1990

106. Cavazzana AO, Miser JS, Jefferson J, et al: Experimental evidence for a neural origin of Ewing's sarcoma of bone. Am J Pathol 127:507, 1987

107. Noguera R, Triche TJ, Navarro S, et al: Dynamic model of differentiation in Ewing's sarcoma cells: Comparative analysis of morphologic, immunocytochemical, and oncogene expression parameters. Lab Invest 66:143, 1992

108. Yee D, Favoni RE, Lebovic GS, et al: Insulin-like growth factor I expression by tumors of neuroectodermal origin with the t(11;22) chromosomal translocation: A potential autocrine growth factor. J Clin Invest 86:1806, 1990

109. Young JL Jr, Ries LG, Silverberg E, et al: Cancer incidence, survival and mortality for children less than 15 years of age. Cancer 58:598, 1986

110. Arnold HH, Gerharz CD, Gabbert HE, et al: Retinoic acid induces myogenin synthesis and myogenic differentiation in the rat rhabdomyosarcoma cell line BA-Han-1C. J Cell Biol 118:877, 1992

111. Green DM: Diagnosis and Management of Malignant Solid Tumors in Infants and Children. Boston, Martinus Nijhoff, 1985, p 522

112. Ganguly A, Gribble J, Tune B, et al: Renin-secreting Wilms' tumor with severe hypertension; report of a case and brief review of renin-secreting tumors. Ann Intern Med 79:835, 1973

113. D'Angio GJ, Breslow N, Beckwith JB, et al: Treatment of Wilms' tumor: Results of the Third National Wilms' Tumor Study. Cancer 64:349, 1989

114. D'Angio GJ, Evans AE, Breslow N, et al: The treatment of Wilms' tumor: Results of the National Wilms' Tumor Study. Cancer 38:633, 1976

115. D'Angio GJ, Evans A, Breslow N, et al: The treatment of Wilms' tumor: Results of the Second National Wilms' Tumor Study. Cancer 47:2302, 1981

116. Beckwith JB, Kivat NB, Bonadio JF: Nephrogenic rests, nephroblastomatosis, and the pathogenesis of Wilms' tumor. Pediatr Pathol 10:1, 1990

117. Breslow NE, Beckwith JB: Epidemiological features of Wilms' tumor: Results of the National Wilms' Tumor Study. J Natl Cancer Inst 68:429, 1982

118. Knudson AG, Strong LC: Mutation and cancer: A model for Wilms' tumor of the kidney. J Natl Cancer Inst 48:313, 1978

119. Ferrell RE, Strong LC, Riccardi VM, et al: A clinical cytogenetic and gene marker survey of 106 patients with Wilms' tumor (WT) and/or aniridia (AN). Am J Hum Genet 32:104, 1980

120. Francke U, Holmes LB, Atkins L, et al: Aniridia-Wilms' tumor association: Evidence for specific deletion of 11p13. Cytogenet Cell Genet 24:185, 1979

121. Junien C, Turleau C, de Grouchy J, et al: Regional assignment of catalase (CAT) gene to band 11p13: Association with the aniridia-Wilms' tumor gonadoblastoma (WAGR) complex. Ann Genet 23:165, 1980

122. Koufos A, Hansen MF, Lamplin BC, et al: Loss of alleles at loci on human chromosome 11 during genesis of Wilms' tumor. Nature 309:170, 1984

123. Call K, Glaser T, Ito CY, et al: Isolation and characterization of a zinc finger polypeptide gene at the human chromosome 11 Wilms' tumor locus. Cell 60:509, 1990

124. Gessler M, et al: Homozygous deletion in Wilms' tumours of a zinc-finger gene identified by chromosome jumping. Nature 343:774, 1990

125. Haber DA, Buckler AJ, Glaser T, et al: An internal deletion within an 11p13 zinc finger gene contributes to the development of Wilms' tumor. Cell 61:1257, 1990

126. Brown KW, Watson JE, Poirier V, et al: Inactivation of the remaining allele of the WT1 gene in a Wilms' tumour from a WAGR patient. Oncogene 7:763, 1992

127. Morris JF, Madden SL, Tournay OE, et al: Characterization of the zinc finger protein encoded by the WT1 Wilms' tumor locus. Oncogene 6:2339, 1991

128. Sukhatme VP: Early transcriptional events in cell growth: The Egr family. J Am Soc Nephrol 1:859, 1990

129. Rauscher FJ, Morris JF III, Tournay OE, et al: Binding of the Wilms' tumor locus zinc finger protein to the EGR-1 consensus sequence. Science 250:1259, 1990

130. Madden SL, Cook DM, Morris JF, et al: Transcriptional regression mediated by the WT1 Wilms' tumor gene product. Science 253:1550, 1991

131. Wang ZY, Madden SL, Deuel TF, et al: The Wilms' tumor gene product, WT1, represses transcription of the platelet-derived growth factor A-chain gene. J Biol Chem 267:2199, 1992

132. Drummond IA, Madden SL, Rohwer NP, et al: Repression of the insulin-like growth factor II gene by the Wilms' tumor suppressor WT1. Science 257:674, 1992

133. Gashler AL, Bonthron DT, Madden SL, et al: Human platelet-

derived growth factor A chain is transcriptionally repressed by the Wilms' tumor suppressor WT1. Proc Natl Acad Sci USA 89:10984, 1992

134. Fraizer GE, Bowen-Pope DF, Vogel AM: Production of platelet-derived growth factor by cultured Wilms' tumor cells and fetal kidney cells. J Cell Physiol 133:169, 1987

135. Pelletier J, Bruening W, Kashtan CE, et al: Germline mutations in the Wilms' tumor suppressor gene are associated with abnormal urogenital development in Denys-Drash syndrome. Cell 67:437, 1991

136. Reeve AE, Sih SA, Raizis AM, et al: Loss of allelic heterozygosity at a second locus on chromosome 11 in sporadic Wilms' tumor cells. Mol Cell Biol 9:1799, 1989

137. Nisen PD, Zimmerman KA, Cotter SV, et al: Enhanced expression of the N-myc gene in Wilms' tumors. Cancer Res 46: 6217, 1986

138. Henry I, Bonaiti-Pellie C, Chehensse V, et al: Uniparental paternal disomy in a genetic cancer-predisposing syndrome. Nature 351:665, 1991

139. Ohlsson R, Nystrom A, Pfeifer OS, et al: IGF2 is parentally imprinted during human embryogenesis and in the Beckwith-Wiedemann syndrome. Nat Genet 4:94, 1993

140. Giannoukakis N, Deal C, Paquette J, et al: Parental genomic imprinting of the human IGF2 gene. Nat Genet 4:98, 1993

141. Ogawa O, Eccles MR, Szeto J, et al: Relaxation of insulin-like growth factor II gene imprinting implicated in Wilms' tumor. Nature 362:749, 1993

142. Brown KW, Gardner A, Williams JC, et al: Paternal origin of 11p15 duplications in the Beckwith-Wiedemann syndrome: A new case and review of the literature. Cancer Genet Cytogenet 58:66, 1992

143. Reik W, Surani MA: Genomic imprinting and embryonal tumours. Nature 338:112, 1989

144. Brice AL, Cheetham JE, Bolton VN, et al: Temporal changes in the expression of the insulin-like growth factor II gene associated with tissue maturation in the human fetus. Development 106:543, 1989

145. Haselbacher GK, Irminger JC, Zapf J, et al: Insulin-like growth factor II in human adrenal pheochromocytomas and Wilms' tumors: Expression at the mRNA and protein level. Proc Natl Acad Sci USA 84:1104, 1987

146. Paik S, Rosen N, Jung W, et al: Expression of insulin-like growth factor-II mRNA in fetal kidney and Wilms' tumor: An in situ hybridization study. Lab Invest 61:522, 1989

147. Gansler T, Allen KD, Burant CF, et al: Detection of type 1 insulin-like growth factor (IGF) receptors in Wilms' tumors. Am J Pathol 130:431, 1988

148. Drummond IA, Madden SL, Rohwer NP, et al: Repression of the insulin-like growth factor II gene by the Wilms' tumor suppressor WT1. Science 257:674, 1992

149. Witte DP, Nagasaki T, Stambrook P, et al: Identification of an acidic fibroblast growth factor-like activity in a mesoblastic nephroma. Lab Invest 60:353, 1989

150. Fraizer GE, Bowen PDF, Vogel AM: Production of platelet-derived growth factor by cultured Wilms' tumor cells and fetal kidney cells. J Cell Physiol 133:169, 1987

151. Breslow N, Sharples K, Beckwith JB, et al: Prognosis in non-metastatic, favorable histology Wilms' tumor: Results of the Third National Wilms' Tumor Study. Cancer 68:2345, 1991

152. Fletcher CD: Pleomorphic malignant fibrous histiocytoma: Fact or fiction? A critical reappraisal based on 159 tumors diagnosed as pleomorphic sarcoma. Am J Surg Pathol 16:213, 1992

153. Kramer S, Meadows AT, Jarrett P, et al: Incidence of childhood cancer: Experience of a decade in a population-based registry. J Natl Cancer Inst 70:49, 1983

154. Corson JM, Pinkus GS: Intracellular myoglobin—a specific marker for skeletal muscle differentiation in soft tissue sarcomas: An immunoperoxidase study. Am J Pathol 103:384, 1981

155. Tsokos M, Howard R, Costa J: Immunohistochemical study of alveolar and embryonal rhabdomyosarcoma. Lab Invest 48: 148, 1983

156. Kahn HJ, Yeger H, Kassim O, et al: Immunohistochemical and electron microscopic assessment of childhood rhabdomyosarcoma: Increased frequency of diagnosis over routine histologic methods. Cancer 51:1897, 1983

157. Barr FG, Biegel JA, Sellinger B, et al: Molecular and cytogenetic analysis of chromosomal arms 2q and 13q in alveolar rhabdomyosarcoma. Genes Chromosom Cancer 3:153, 1991

158. Barr FG, Galili N, Holick J, et al: Rearrangement of the PAX3 paired box gene in the paediatric solid tumour alveolar rhabdomyosarcoma. Nat Genet 3:113, 1993

159. Scrable HJ, Johnson DK, Rinchik EM, et al: Rhabdomyosarcoma-associated locus and MYOD1 are syntenic but separate loci on the short arm of human chromosome 11. Proc Natl Acad Sci USA 87:2182, 1990

160. Malkin D, Li FP, Strong LC, et al: Germ line p53 mutations in a familial syndrome of breast cancer, sarcomas, and other neoplasms. [see comments] Science 250:1233, 1990

161. Srivastava S, Zou ZQ, Pirollo K, et al: Germ-line transmission of a mutated p53 gene in a cancer-prone family with Li-Fraumeni syndrome. [see comments] Nature 348:747, 1990

162. Kuerbitz SJ, Plunkett BS, Walsh WV, et al: Wild-type p53 is a cell cycle checkpoint determinant following irradiation. Proc Natl Acad Sci USA 89:7491, 1992

163. Kastan MB, Zhan Q, El Deiry WS, et al: A mammalian cell cycle checkpoint pathway utilizing p53 and GADD45 is defective in ataxia-telangiectasia. Cell 71:587, 1992

164. Yin Y, Tainsky MA, Bischoff FZ, et al: Wild-type p53 restores cell cycle control and inhibits gene amplification in cells with mutant p53 alleles. Cell 70:937, 1992

165. Livingstone LR, White A, Sprouse J, et al: Altered cell cycle arrest and gene amplification potential accompany loss of wild-type p53. Cell 70:923, 1992

166. Miller CW, Aslo A, Tsay C, et al: Frequency and structure of p53 rearrangements in human osteosarcoma. Cancer Res 50: 7950, 1990

167. Mulligan LM, Matlashewski GJ, Scrable HJ, et al: Mechanisms of p53 loss in human sarcomas. Proc Natl Acad Sci USA 87: 5863, 1990

168. Knudson A: Mutation and cancer: Statistical study of retinoblastoma. Proc Natl Acad Sci USA 68:620, 1971

169. Reissmann PT, Simon MA, Lee WH, et al: Studies of the retinoblastoma gene in human sarcomas. Oncogene 4:839, 1989

170. Stratton MR, Fisher C, Gusterson BA, et al: Detection of point mutations in N-ras and K-ras genes of human embryonal rhabdomyosarcomas using oligonucleotide probes and the polymerase chain reaction. Cancer Res 49:6324, 1989

171. Hayashi Y, Sugimoto T, Horii Y, et al: Characterization of an embryonal rhabdomyosarcoma cell line showing amplification and over-expression of the N-myc oncogene. Int J Cancer 45: 705, 1990

172. Ramp U, Gerharz CD, Doehmer J, et al: Increase in proto-oncogene raf expression precedes differentiation induction in different clonal rhabdomyosarcoma subpopulations. Anticancer Res 12:537, 1992

173. Gabbert HE, Gerharz CD, Ramp U, et al: Enhanced expression of the proto-oncogenes fos and raf in the rhabdomyosarcoma cell line BA-HAN-1C after differentiation induction with retinoic acid and N-methylformamide. Int J Cancer 45:724, 1990

174. Crouch GD, Helman LJ: All-trans-retinoic acid inhibits the growth of human rhabdomyosarcoma cell lines. Cancer Res 51:4882, 1991

175. Wright WE, Sassoon DA, Lin VK: Myogenin, a factor regulating myogenesis, has a domain homologous to MyoD. Cell 56:607, 1989

176. Li L, Olson EN: Regulation of muscle cell growth and differentiation by the MyoD family of helix-loop-helix proteins. Adv Cancer Res 58:95, 1992

177. Braun T, Winter B, Bober E, et al: Transcriptional activation domain of the muscle-specific gene-regulatory protein myf5. Nature 346:663, 1990

178. Tapscott SJ, Thayer MJ, Weintraub H, et al: Deficiency in rhabdomyosarcomas of a factor required for MyoD activity and myogenesis. Science 259:1450, 1993

179. Hosoi H, Sugimoto T, Hayashi Y, et al: Differential expression of myogenic regulatory genes, MyoD1 and myogenin, in human rhabdomyosarcoma sublines. Int J Cancer 50:977, 1992

180. Magri KA, Ewton DZ, Florini JR: The role of the IGFs in myogenic differentiation. Adv Exp Med Biol 293:57, 1991

181. El-Badry OM, Minniti C, Kohn EC, et al: Insulin-like growth factor II acts as an autocrine growth and motility factor in human rhabdomyosarcoma tumors. Cell Growth Differ 1:325, 1990

182. Schweigerer L, Neufeld G, Mergia A, et al: Basic fibroblast growth factor in human rhabdomyosarcoma cells: Implications for the proliferation and neovascularization of myoblast-derived tumors. Proc Natl Acad Sci USA 84:842, 1987

183. Johnson SE, Allen RE: The effects of bFGF, IGF-I, and TGF-beta on RMO skeletal muscle cell proliferation and differentiation. Exp Cell Res 187:250, 1990

184. McCune BK, Patterson K, Chandra RS, et al: Expression of transforming growth factor-beta isoforms in small round cell tumors of childhood: An immunohistochemical study. Am J Pathol 142:49, 1993

185. Rancy RB, Hays DM, Tefft M, et al: Rhabdomyosarcoma and the undifferentiated sarcomas. In Pizzo PA, Poplack DG (eds): Principles and Practice of Pediatric Oncology, 2nd ed. Philadelphia, JB Lippincott Company, 1993, p 769

186. Minniti CP, Maggi M, Helman LJ: Suramin inhibits the growth of human rhabdomyosarcoma by interrupting the insulin-like growth factor II autocrine growth loop. Cancer Res 52:1830, 1992

187. Minniti CP, Kohn EC, Grubb JH, et al: The insulin-like growth factor II (IGF-II)/mannose 6-phosphate receptor mediates IGF-II-induced motility in human rhabdomyosarcoma cells. J Biol Chem 267:9000, 1992

188. Dahlin DC, Unni KK: Bone Tumors: General Aspects and Data on 8542 Cases, 4th edition. Springfield, IL, Charles C Thomas, 1986

189. Price C: Primary bone-forming tumours and their relationship to skeletal growth. J Bone Joint Surg (Br) 40:574, 1958

190. Fraumeni J: Stature and malignant tumors of bone in childhood and adolescence. Cancer 20:967, 1967

191. Dahlin D, Unni K: Osteosarcoma of bone and its important recognizable varieties. Am J Surg Pathol 1:61, 1977

192. Huvos A: Bone Tumors: Diagnosis, Treatment and Prognosis, 2nd ed. Philadelphia, WB Saunders Company, 1991

193. Schimke R, Lowman J, Cowan G: Retinoblastoma and osteogenic sarcoma in siblings. Cancer 34:2077, 1974

194. Araki N, Uchida A, Kimura T, et al: Involvement of the retinoblastoma gene in primary osteosarcomas and other bone and soft-tissue tumors. Clin Orthop 270:271, 1991

195. Iavarone A, Matthay KK, Steinkirchner TM, et al: Germ-line and somatic p53 gene mutations in multifocal osteogenic sarcoma. Proc Natl Acad Sci USA 89:4207, 1992

196. Donehower LA, Harvey M, Slagle BL, et al: Mice deficient for p53 are developmentally normal but susceptible to spontaneous tumours. Nature 356:215, 1992

197. Wu JX, Carpenter PM, Gresens C, et al: The proto-oncogene C-fos is over-expressed in the majority of human osteosarcomas. Oncogene 5:989, 1990

198. Ruther U, Komitowski D, Schubert FR, et al: c-fos expression induces bone tumors in transgenic mice. Oncogene 4:861, 1989

199. Ikeda S, Sumii H, Akiyama K, et al: Amplification of both c-myc and c-raf-1 oncogenes in a human osteosarcoma. Jpn J Cancer Res 80:6, 1989

200. Bolander ME: Regulation of fracture repair by growth factors. Proc Soc Exp Biol Med 200:165, 1992

201. Graves DT, Valentin OA, Delgado R, et al: The potential role of platelet-derived growth factor as an autocrine or paracrine factor for human bone cells. Connect Tissue Res 23:209, 1989

202. Hauschka PV, Chen TL, Mavrakos AE: Polypeptide growth factors in bone matrix. Ciba Found Symp 136:207, 1988

203. Westermark B, Heldin CH: Platelet-derived growth factor: Structure, function and implications in normal and malignant cell growth. Acta Oncol 32:101, 1993

204. Yamada K, Yoshitake Y, Norimatsu H, et al: Roles of various growth factors in growth of human osteosarcoma cells which can grow in protein-free medium. Cell Struct Funct 17:9, 1992

205. Mioh H, Chen JK: Differential inhibitory effects of TGF-beta on EGF-, PDGF-, and HBGF-1-stimulated MG63 human osteosarcoma cell growth: Possible involvement of growth factor

206. Datta HK, Zaidi M, Champaneri JB, et al: Transforming growth factor-beta-induced mitogenesis of human bone cancer cells. Biochem Biophys Res Commun 161:672, 1989

207. Pollak MN, Polychronakos C, Richard M: Insulinlike growth factor I: A potent mitogen for human osteogenic sarcoma. J Natl Cancer Inst 82:301, 1990

208. Olivier S, Formento P, Fischel JL, et al: Epidermal growth factor receptor expression and suramin cytotoxicity in vitro. Eur J Cancer 26:867, 1990

209. Pollak M, Richard M: Suramin blockade of insulinlike growth factor I-stimulated proliferation of human osteosarcoma cells. J Natl Cancer Inst 82:1349, 1990

210. Kleinerman ES, Snyder JS, Jaffe N: Influence of chemotherapy administration on monocyte activation by liposomal muramyl tripeptide phosphatidylethanolamine in children with osteosarcoma. J Clin Oncol 9:259, 1991

211. Murray JL, Kleinerman ES, Cunningham JE, et al: Phase I trial of liposomal muramyl tripeptide phosphatidylethanolamine in cancer patients. J Clin Oncol 7:1915, 1989

212. Gonzalez FF, Lopes MB, Garcia FJM, et al: Expression of developmentally defined retinal phenotypes in the histogenesis of retinoblastoma. Am J Pathol 141:363, 1992

213. Devesa SS: The incidence of retinoblastoma. Am J Ophthalmol 80:263, 1975

214. Abramson DH, Ellsworth RM, Kitchin FD, et al: Second nonocular tumors in retinoblastoma survivors: Are they radiation induced? Ophthalmology 91:1351, 1984

215. Smith LM, Donaldson SS, Egbert PR, et al: Aggressive management of second primary tumors in survivors of hereditary retinoblastoma. Int J Radiat Oncol Biol Phys 17:499, 1989

216. Friend S, Bernards R, Rogelj S, et al: A human DNA segment with properties of the gene that predisposes to retinoblastoma and osteosarcoma. Nature 323:643, 1986

217. Goodrich DW, Wang NP, Qian YW, et al: The retinoblastoma gene product regulates progression through the G1 phase of the cell cycle. Cell 67:293, 1991

218. Francois J, Matton MTh, deBie S, et al: Genesis and genetics of retinoblastoma. Ophthalmologica 170:405, 1975

219. Hansen MF, Koufos A, Gallie BL, et al: Osteosarcoma and retinoblastoma: A shared chromosomal mechanism revealing recessive predisposition. Proc Natl Acad Sci USA 82:6216, 1985

220. Tso MOM, Zimmerman LE, Fine BS: The nature of retinoblastoma II: Photoreceptor differentiation: An electron microscopic study. Am J Ophthalmol 69:350, 1970

221. Ellsworth RM: The practical management of retinoblastoma. Trans Am Ophthalmol Soc 67:462, 1969

222. Zimmerman LE: Retinoblastoma and retinocytoma. In Spencer WH (ed): Ophthalmic Pathology: An Atlas and Textbook, 3rd edition. Philadelphia, WB Saunders Company, 1985, p 1292

223. Knudson AG, Hethcote HW, Brown BW: Mutation and childhood cancer: A probabilistic model for the incidence of retinoblastoma. Proc Natl Acad Sci USA 72:5116, 1975

224. Lee WH, Shew JY, Hong FD, et al: The retinoblastoma susceptibility gene encodes a nuclear phosphoprotein associated with DNA binding activity. Nature 329:642, 1987

225. Yandell DW, Campbell TA, Dayton SH, et al: Oncogenic point mutations in the human retinoblastoma gene: Their application to genetic counseling. N Engl J Med 321:1689, 1989

226. Goddard AD, Balakier H, Canton M, et al: Infrequent genomic rearrangement and normal expression of the putative RB1 gene in retinoblastoma tumors. Mol Cell Biol 8:2082, 1988

227. Lee EY, Chang CY, Hu N, et al: Mice deficient for Rb are nonviable and show defects in neurogenesis and haematopoiesis. Nature 359:288, 1992

228. Fung YK, Tang A: The role of the retinoblastoma gene in breast cancer development. Cancer Treat Res 61:59, 1992

229. Harbour JW, Lai SL, Whang-Peng J, et al: Abnormalities in structure and expression of the human retinoblastoma gene in SCLC. Science 241:353, 1988

230. Huang HJS, Yee JK, Shew JY: Suppression of the neoplastic

phenotype by replacement of the retinoblastoma gene product in human cancer cells. Science 242:1563, 1988

231. Bookstein R, Shew JY, Chen PL, et al: Suppression of tumorigenicity of human prostate carcinoma cells by replacing a mutated RB gene. Science 247:712, 1990

232. Nevis JR: E2F: A link between the Rb tumor suppressor protein and viral oncoproteins. Science 258:424, 1992

233. Yorek MA, Dunlap LA, Ginsberg BH: Amino acid and putative neurotransmitter transport in human Y79 retinoblastoma cells: Effect of insulin and insulin-like growth factor. J Biol Chem 262:10986, 1987

234. Pineda R, Chan DD, Ni M, et al: Human retinoblastoma cells express alpha B-crystallin in vivo and in vitro. Curr Eye Res 12:239, 1993

235. Herman MM, Perentes E, Katsetos CD, et al: Neuroblastic differentiation potential of the human retinoblastoma cell lines Y-79 and WERI-Rb1 maintained in an organ culture system. An immunohistochemical, electron microscopic, and biochemical study. Am J Pathol 134:115, 1989

236. Campbell M, Chader GJ: Retinoblastoma cells in tissue culture. Ophthalmic Paediatr Genet 9:171, 1988

237. Detrick B, Evans CH, Chader G, et al: Cytokine-induced modulation of cellular proteins in retinoblastoma: Analysis by flow cytometry. Ophthalmol Vis Sci 32:1714, 1991

238. Lee WH, Bookstein R, Hong F, et al: Human retinoblastoma susceptibility gene: Cloning, identification and sequence. Science 235:1394, 1987

239. Dunn JM, Phillips RA, Zhu X, et al: Mutations in the RB1 gene and their effects on transcription. Mol Cell Biol 9:4594, 1989

240. Stannard C, Lipper S, Sealy R, et al: Retinoblastoma: Correlation of invasion of the optic nerve and choroid with prognosis and metastasis. Br J Ophthalmol 63:560, 1979

241. Rootman J, Ellsworth RM, Hofbauer J, et al: Orbital extension of retinoblastoma: A clinicopathological study. Can J Ophthalmol 13:72, 1978

242. Chan HS, Thorner PS, Haddad G, et al: Multidrug-resistant phenotype in retinoblastoma correlates with P-glycoprotein expression. Ophthalmology 98:1425, 1991

243. Bagshaw MA, Kaplan HS: Supervoltage linear accelerator radiation therapy VIII: Retinoblastoma. Radiology 86:242, 1966

244. Cooper MJ, Hutchins GM, Israel MA: Histogenesis of the human adrenal medulla: An evaluation of gene expression in chromaffin and non-chromaffin lineages. Am J Pathol 137:605, 1990

15

MOLECULAR BIOLOGY OF LUNG CANCER

BRUCE E. JOHNSON

There will be an estimated 172,000 new cases of lung cancer in the United States in 1994 and 85 per cent of these patients will die from their cancer, comprising one fourth of cancer deaths in the United States.[1] Lung cancer is the fourth most common cancer after skin, prostate, and breast cancer and is the most common cause of cancer deaths in the United States.

The World Health Organization histologic classification of lung cancer is the most commonly used in the United States.[2] The four major histologies, which represent 95 per cent of the lung cancers, include epidermoid or squamous cell carcinoma in 30 to 40 per cent of patients, adenocarcinomas in 30 to 40 per cent, small-cell carcinoma in 20 per cent, and large-cell carcinoma in 5 per cent[2-4] (Fig. 15-1). The most important clinical distinction is recognizing small-cell carcinoma versus the other three histologies, because small-cell carcinoma is managed principally by systemic chemotherapy, whereas patients with non–small-cell lung cancer are managed primarily by local measures, including surgery and/or radiation therapy.[5] The squamous cell cancers tend to present with exophytic endobronchial lesions that are clinically localized within the chest at presentation.[6] In contrast, small-cell lung cancers are most commonly infiltrating submucosal lesions and have the greatest tendency to develop clinically evident systemic metastases very early in their clinical course.[5,7,8] Adenocarcinomas and large-cell carcinomas tend to present with peripheral lesions and commonly are not visualized using fiberoptic bronchoscopy.[6] The identification of adenocarcinoma of the lung by pathologists is rising in most series of patients with lung cancer in the United States.[1,3,9]

The availability of hundreds of tumor cell lines and tumor specimens comprising the major histologic types have allowed characterization of the major molecular changes of established human lung cancer (see Tables 15–1 through 15–5 later in this chapter). However, the initial molecular changes that give rise to cancer have been difficult to study because of the paucity of identifiable early lesions in lung cancer and lack of appropriate animal models of lung cancer caused by cigarette smoke, the most common etiology of lung cancer in humans. Therefore, many of the data on early molecular changes in the lung come from studies of the human lung exposed to cigarette smoke and data on cell culture systems of tracheobronchial cells. The data presented in this chapter concentrate on the molecular changes caused by cigarette smoking in the lung and in lung cancer. Animal data are used when data on humans are not available or the information is pertinent to the understanding of the disease process. This chapter covers the molecular and cellular response to injury of the lung, gene activation of peptide hormones, their interaction with receptors, dominant oncogenes, and tumor suppressor genes in lung cancer. The focus is on the molecular changes that are associated with changes in growth patterns, specific histologies, and patient outcome.

NORMAL RESPIRATORY EPITHELIUM

The proximal normal respiratory epithelium (first 16 of the 23 generations) is composed of pseudostratified columnar epithelium with cilia at the luminal surface with interspersed goblet cells (Fig. 15–2). As the airway continues out distally, the epithelium becomes cuboidal and then squamous in the alveolus.[10] Lung cancers most commonly arise in the proximal airways of the lung, so the

The opinions and assertions contained herein are the expressed views of the authors and are not to be construed as official or as reflecting the views of the Department of the Navy or the Department of Defense.

All material in this chapter is in the public domain, with the exception of any borrowed figures or tables.

most common site of origin is in the pseudostratified epithelium (Fig. 15–2).

In addition, neuroendocrine and neuroepithelial bodies are scattered throughout the respiratory epithelium and are recognized histologically by groups of large polyhedral cells in the basal layer of the epithelium with clear cytoplasm and numerous dark granules.[11,12] These granules have been identified as neurosecretory granules by electron microscopy and contain the structural protein chromogranin[13] (Fig. 15–3). These cells produce biogenic amines such as serotonin or different peptide hormones that can include calcitonin and gastrin-releasing peptide.[13,14]

ETIOLOGIC AGENTS OF LUNG CANCER

Lung cancer is an unusual human solid tumor because the cause is known in the vast majority of patients. Eighty-five to 90 per cent of lung cancer is caused by cigarette smoking.[15] In addition to cigarette smoking, environmental agents have been implicated in the development of lung cancer in the minority of cases. Environmental exposures to radon and passive smoke can increase the risk of lung cancer. The molecular changes caused by cigarette smoking, and the different molecular

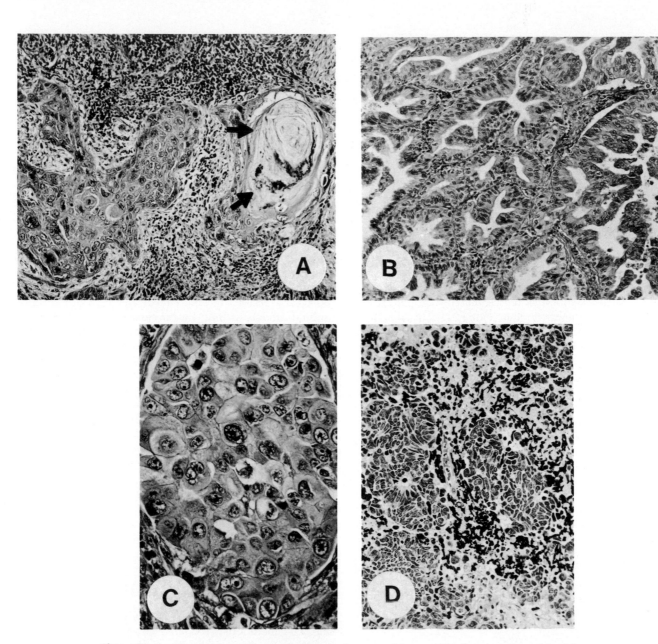

Figure 15–1. Photomicrographs of major histologic types of lung cancer (hematoxylin-eosin stain). *A*, Squamous cell carcinoma with a well-differentiated focus of keratinization (arrows; ×130). *B*, Adenocarcinoma with papillary features (×130). *C*, Large-cell carcinoma; note lack of any features of differentiation (×330). *D*, Small-cell carcinoma of the lung with well-preserved fusiform cells with nuclear molding and fine chromatin pattern mixed with dark hyperchromatic crushed and necrotic cells (×200). (Courtesy of RI Linnoila, MD.)

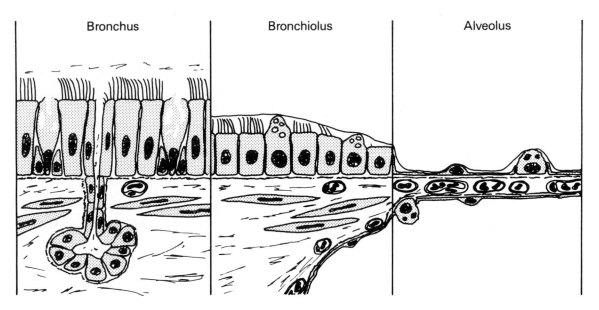

| Bronchus | Bronchiolus | Alveolus |

Figure 15–2. Airway wall structure at three principal levels. The epithelium is located at the top of the figure, the basement membrane just below the epithelium, and the smooth muscle and fibrous coat below that. The epithelium in the bronchi is a pseudostratified layer with columnar cells, with the cilia located at the luminal surface and normal proliferation going on in the basal layer of cells. The epithelium also contains goblet cells that produce mucus interspersed among the columnar cells. The epithelium becomes progressively thinner as the airway proceeds distally, changing to cuboidal and then to squamous in the alveolus. The smooth muscle and fibrous coat also decreases in size and thickness. (Modified from Wiebel ER, Taylor CR: Design and structure of the human lung. *In* Fishman AP [ed]: Pulmonary Diseases and Disorders. ed. 2. New York, McGraw-Hill, 1988, p 14, with permission.)

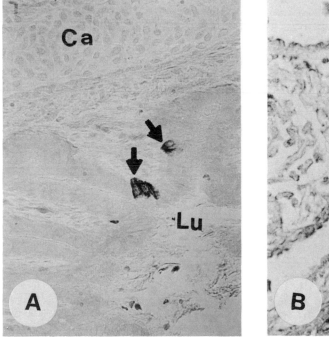

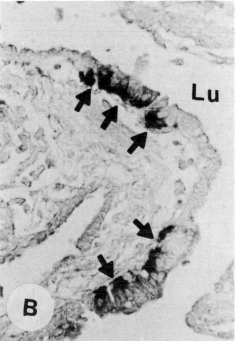

Figure 15–3. Photomicrographs of pulmonary neuroendocrine cells in human lung. *A*, Scattered neuroendocrine cells (arrows) in a fetal bronchus (note cartilage on the top) with chromogranin-like immunoreactivity (immunoperoxidase stain; ×360). Ca, cartilage; Lu, bronchial lumen. *B*, Linear hyperplasia of adult pulmonary neuroendocrine cells (arrows) with chromogranin-like immunoreactivity in a terminal bronchiolus (immunoperoxidase stain; ×360). Lu, bronchial lumen. (Courtesy of RI Linnoila, MD.)

changes in nonsmokers and associated with radon exposure, are pointed out here.

Smoking

Cigarette smoking causes a 15-fold increased risk of developing lung cancer in smokers compared to non-smokers.[15] In addition, the risk increases with increased number of cigarettes smoked per day as well as the duration of smoking.[16,17] Lung cancer mortality closely parallels the smoking habits of both men and women, with a lag of approximately 20 years. The age-adjusted death rate from lung cancer in the United States is increasing in women, relatively stable in men, and increasing overall.[15] The risk of lung cancer declines from an increased risk of approximately 15-fold for current smokers to a 1.5- to 4-fold risk for lung cancer 15 years after stopping smoking compared to a nonsmoker.[15] The exposure of a nonsmoker to smoking by a spouse or parent in the household causes an increased risk of 1.2- to 1.5-fold compared to that of a nonsmoker who is not exposed to a spouse or parent smoking.[18,19] Different histologies of lung cancer have varying associations with smoking. More than 95 per cent of patients with small-cell lung cancer are current or ex-smokers, compared to 80 per cent of patients with adenocarcinoma.[17,20,21] Adenocarcinoma is the most common histologic type identified in nonsmokers.[17,20–22]

Radon

The interest in radon as a potential cause of lung cancer has increased because of the identification of high levels of radon gas in some homes that can approach levels associated with an increased risk of lung cancer in underground miners.[23–25] Radon is a chemically inert gas that decays to radon daughters that release radioactive α particles and interact with the respiratory epithelium. There is an increase in the relative risk of 1.5- to 4.0-fold for each 100 working level–month exposure in underground miners. This increased risk of lung cancer caused by radon decay products in the mining industry adds to the risk caused by cigarette smoking. Extrapolation of the data from underground miners and information from a case control study show residential radon is associated with development of lung cancer.[25]

RESPONSE TO RESPIRATORY INJURY

The most common cause of lung cancer is cigarette smoking, so the studies of early lesions in smokers have focused on the early proliferative responses observed in patients' airways. The initial studies of smokers characterized the histologic changes in the epithelium of smokers who had pulmonary resection and in postmortem examinations of patients who died from lung cancer and other causes. Later studies have investigated the abnor-malities observed in the neuroendocrine cell population found in the airways.

The histologic changes observed with cigarette smoking include the loss of cilia, cellular atypia, and proliferation of the bronchial epithelium.[26,27] The changes were more pronounced in the proximal than distal airways and were more common with increased cigarette usage, reaching their maximum in the airways uninvolved with lung cancer in patients who died of lung cancer.[26,27] In addition, the number of patients with carcinoma in situ increased with the number of cigarettes smoked per day, and was most common in patients who died of lung cancer.

In addition to these histologic changes associated with smoking, the dispersed neuroendocrine cells and neuroepithelial bodies can increase in number.[28] This system is important in the lung because these cells may play a role in growth regulation and differentiation and may be the cells of origin of small-cell lung cancer. Approximately 70 per cent of these neuroendocrine cells are located proximally in the bronchi, 25 per cent in the bronchioles, and only 4 per cent in the alveolar ducts.[13]

These neuroendocrine cells can be recognized by antibodies directed against biogenic amines (serotonin) and peptide hormones (gastrin-releasing peptide, calcitonin, and chromogrannin),[13] which are discussed individually in detail later in this chapter (Fig. 15–3). The numbers of these neuroendocrine cells and neuroendocrine bodies are increased in the bronchial epithelium of patients with chronic bronchitis, emphysema,[29] bronchiectasis and in airways uninvolved with cancer from patients with lung cancer.[28] There is an increase in the number of neuroendocrine cells in lungs exposed to lower partial tensions of oxygen in Bolivian natives living at altitudes of 3500 to 4300 meters, suggesting that hypoxia stimulates the proliferation of neuroendocrine cells as well.[13]

Animal model systems have shown that rodents exposed to nitrosamines found in cigarette smoke and hyperoxia also show proliferation of neuroendocrine cells, production of bombesin-like immunoreactivity in the lungs, and development of lung cancer with neuroendocrine features.[30,31]

Growth Factor Production in Lung Cancer and Smokers

The peptide hormones that are produced by the neuroendocrine cells may function to stimulate their own growth or the growth of surrounding cells (Fig. 15–4).[32] Understanding of these systems has been facilitated greatly by the advances in molecular biology and immunology for characterizing individual peptides in the normal lung and in lung cancer tumors and tumor cell lines and their receptors. These systems typically have multiple related peptides and related peptide hormone receptors, making the investigation of each system more complex. Therefore, the cloning of genes and development of specific immunologic reagents are important for determining individual genes and gene products and their roles in growth, differentiation, and malignant transformation. The best characterized has been gastrin-releasing peptide and

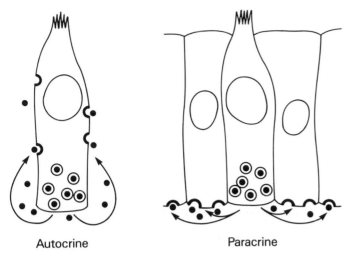

Autocrine   Paracrine

Figure 15–4. Autocrine and paracrine growth stimulation of cells. The figure on the left diagrammatically represents autocrine growth. The cell produces a peptide hormone that is released from the cell, binds to receptors on its surface, and stimulates growth. The figure on the right depicts paracrine growth. The cell produces a peptide hormone that is released by the cell and diffuses to a neighboring cell that has receptors for the peptide hormone. The peptide hormone binds to the neighboring cell and stimulates the growth of the neighboring cell. (Adapted from Sporn MB, Todaro GJ: Autocrine secretion and malignant transformation of cells. Reprinted from N Engl J Med 303:878, 1980, with permission.)

its role in growth regulation of normal and neoplastic lung. The other peptides and their receptors covered here include neuromedin B, epidermal growth factor, transforming growth factor α, insulin-like growth factor I, and arginine vasopressin. These peptides have been well characterized, and there is evidence to demonstrate a role for growth regulation of the normal lung and/or lung cancer cells.

GASTRIN-RELEASING PEPTIDE AND NEUROMEDIN B

The tetradecapeptide bombesin was first discovered in the frog skin,[33] and a bombesin-like immunoreactivity was detected in fetal and neonatal lungs by immunohistochemistry and radioimmunoassay.[34] Bombesin-like immuno-

reactivity subsequently was discovered in small-cell lung cancer cell lines[35,36] and an athymic nude mouse tumor established from a tumor specimen from a patient with small-cell lung cancer.[37]

Bombesin-like immunoreactivity subsequently was determined to be caused by the production of gastrin-releasing peptide, a mammalian peptide in which 9 of the 10 carboxy-terminal amino acids are identical to those of bombesin (Fig. 15–5). The cDNA has been cloned and sequenced from both a human pulmonary carcinoid tumor[38] and small-cell lung cancer cell lines.[39] The gene codes for a preprohormone of 145 amino acids that processes to the smaller gastrin-releasing peptide[38–40] (Fig. 15–6). The carboxy-terminal portion of the prohormone can vary because of alternative splicing of the mRNA, and the different forms of the carboxy-terminal portion of the protein have unknown biologic function.[39,40]

Gastrin-releasing peptide production in lung cancer has been demonstrated by gastrin-releasing peptide mRNA expression using Northern blotting, S1 nuclease analyses,[39,41,42] and in situ hybridization.[42,43] Gastrin-releasing peptide has been identified in lung cancer and lung cancer cell lines by radioimmunoassay of lung cancer tumors and tumor cell lines.[35–37,41] It also has been detected by immunohistochemical analyses of tumors and tumor specimens from patients with small-cell lung cancer.[44,45] Gel filtration and high-performance liquid chromatography of cell pellet extracts in conditioned media demonstrate that the major immunoreactive form of gastrin-releasing peptide elutes similarly to the 14–amino acid form of bombesin.[35–37,45,46] The exact form of the peptide has not been determined because the amino acid sequence has not been determined from a lung cancer tumor or tumor cell line. Bombesin-like immunoreactivity is present in the minority of lung cancers, approximately 30 per cent of small-cell lung cancer and 5 per cent of non–small-cell lung cancer tumors and tumor cell lines.

A related peptide, neuromedin B, has been cloned and sequenced from a human hypothalamic cDNA library.[47] The preprohormone is 76 amino acids long, and gives rise to a 32–amino acid peptide (Fig. 15–6). The carboxy-terminal portions of gastrin-releasing peptide and neuromedin B share close homology (Fig. 15–5). Small-cell

Bombesin

Gastrin Releasing Peptide

Neuromedin B

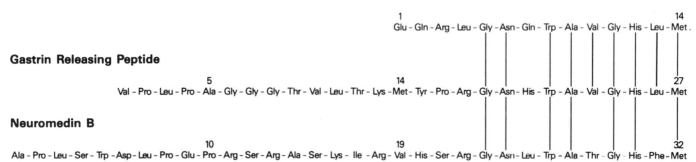

Figure 15–5. Peptide hormone sequences of bombesin, gastrin-releasing peptide, and neuromedin B. The vertical lines represent amino acid homology among the three peptides. The numbers represent the sequence of amino acids from the amino-terminal end of the peptide to the carboxy-terminal end.[33,38,152]

Gastrin Releasing Peptide

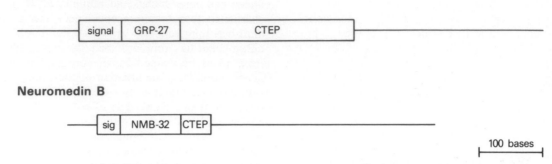

Neuromedin B

Figure 15–6. Gastrin-releasing peptide and neuromedin B. The gastrin-releasing peptide mRNA gives rise to a 145–amino acid preprohormone that has a 23–amino acid signal peptide, a 27–amino acid gastrin-releasing peptide (GRP-27), and a carboxy-terminal extension peptide (CTEP) that can be different lengths because of alternate splicing of the three exons of the gene. The neuromedin B mRNA gives rise to a 74–amino acid preprohormone with a 24–amino acid signal peptide, a 32–amino acid neuromedin B peptide (NMB-32), and a carboxy-terminal peptide that is 18 amino acids long.[40]

lung cancer cells have been observed to express neuromedin B mRNA by Northern blotting, S1 nuclease analyses, and polymerase chain reactions.[41,48] The protein has been identified by radioimmunoassays of lung cancer cell lines and media. Neuromedin B immunoreactivity has similar characteristics in a gel filtration profile and high-performance liquid chromatography column as synthetic 32–amino acid neuromedin B.[48]

GASTRIN-RELEASING PEPTIDE, NEUROMEDIN B, AND BRS-3 RECEPTORS

The receptors for gastrin-releasing peptide and neuromedin B have been cloned and sequenced from the human small-cell lung cancer cell line NCI-H345[49] and bombesin receptor subtype 3 (BRS-3) from N417.[49b] The nucleotide sequences predict receptors to have 384, 390, and 399 amino acids, respectively, with seven transmembrane domains and a 45 to 55 per cent amino acid homology between the three receptors.[49] mRNA expression of gastrin-releasing peptide, neuromedin B, and BRS-3 receptors has been demonstrated by RNase protection assay or reverse transcriptase/polymerase chain reaction (RT/PCR) in both small-cell and non–small-cell lung cancer cell lines.[49,49a] The receptors also have been shown to be present by binding studies of small-cell lung cancer cell lines.[50–53] The antibodies to the receptors have not been developed to allow further immunologic characterization of the receptors.

The mechanism for intracellular activation following binding of the agonists gastrin-releasing peptide, bombesin, and neuromedin B to their receptors has been well worked out in lung cancer. The agonists bind to their receptors, activate phospholipase C,[54] generate inositol triphosphates,[52,55] and mobilize intracellular calcium.[56–60]

Gastrin-releasing peptide and bombesin can function as mitogens in vitro in the soft agarose cloning assay with some small-cell lung cancer cell lines[52,61–63] and in vivo in athymic nude mouse models.[61] A monoclonal antibody directed against gastrin-releasing peptide or bombesin, 2A11 (Fig. 15–7), functions to inhibit the growth of small-cell lung cancer cells in vitro in a clonogenic assay

and in vivo in athymic nude mouse models.[61] In addition, bombesin or gastrin-releasing antagonists that block the binding of bombesin to their receptors inhibit the growth of small-cell lung cancer cells in vitro as measured by clonogenic assay and thymidine incorporation.[53,64,65] The antagonists, when injected around the tumors in athymic nude mice bearing small-cell lung cancer, also inhibited the growth of two of four tumor cell lines tested.[64] The

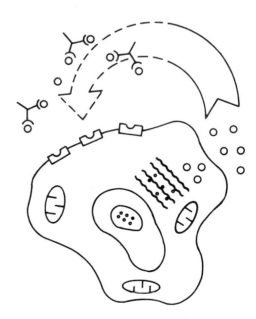

INHIBITION

Figure 15–7. Monoclonal antibody 2A11 blocks the autocrine stimulation of small-cell lung cancer cells. This figure diagrammatically depicts gastrin-releasing peptide (circles) being produced by small-cell lung cancer cells and secreted into the extracellular media. Normally this peptide binds to the receptors, represented by the half circles on the surface of the cell. The monoclonal antibody, represented by the branched figures, binds to the gastrin-releasing peptide, making it unavailable to the receptors, and thus inhibits the growth of the small-cell lung cancer cells.

monoclonal antibody 2A11 has reached clinical trials and has shown evidence of antitumor activity.

The studies of gastrin-releasing peptide are of considerable interest because of its potential role in growth stimulation of the fetal and neonatal lung and of the bronchial epithelium's response to respiratory injury. Bombesin and gastrin-releasing peptide have been shown to be growth factors in normal human bronchial epithelial cells in a clonogenic assay[66] and stimulate growth of murine lung cells as assayed by tritiated thymidine incorporation.[67] Fetal and neonatal lungs produce gastrin-releasing peptide mRNA, with both Northern blotting analysis and in situ hybridization showing expression in the neuroendocrine cells of the lung.[68,69] Immunoreactive gastrin-releasing peptide also is localized to the neuroendocrine cells of the fetal and neonatal lung.[68,69] Immunoreactive gastrin-releasing peptide also is localized to the neuroendocrine cells of the fetal and neonatal lung.[68,69] Immunoreactive gastrin-releasing peptide is present in the hyperplastic neuroendocrine cells of the lungs in patients with bronchiectasis and chronic obstructive pulmonary disease.[14] The level of bombesin-like immunoreactivity is elevated in the bronchoalveolar lavage fluid and urine of patients who smoke.[70,71] Therefore, the increased production of gastrin-releasing peptide can take place both in lung cancer and during development of the respiratory epithelium and when the respiratory epithelium is responding to injury.

Thus, the molecular components of the gastrin-releasing peptide system have been well worked out, and existing experimental evidence supports gastrin-releasing peptide's important role in the growth and differentiation of normal epithelium as well as in established small-cell lung cancer tumor cell lines. Therapeutic interventions have been designed using this system and have achieved success in vivo in animal model systems and in humans.

EPIDERMAL GROWTH FACTOR AND TRANSFORMING GROWTH FACTOR α

The nucleotide sequence of the normal human epidermal growth factor cDNA predicts a 53–amino acid peptide sequence.[72] Human transforming growth factor α, a related peptide, also has been sequenced.[73] The gene codes for a 160–amino acid precursor that gives rise to the 50–amino acid transforming growth factor α, which shares a 42 per cent amino acid homology with epidermal growth factor.

The production of epidermal growth factor by human lung cancer has been demonstrated by immunohistochemical studies in approximately 60 per cent of tumors from patients with squamous cell and adenocarcinoma of the lung.[74,75] The production of transforming growth factor α has been demonstrated in lung cancer tumors and tumor cell lines by mRNA production[75a–78] and in approximately 60 per cent of adenocarcinomas and squamous cell carcinomas of the lung by immunohistochemical studies.[74,75]

EPIDERMAL GROWTH FACTOR RECEPTORS c-erbB-1 AND c-erbB-2

The epidermal growth factor receptor (also referred to as c-erbB-1 because of its sequence homology to the tyrosine kinase domain of the avian erythroblastosis retrovirus) has been cloned and sequenced.[79] The human epidermal growth factor receptor gene codes for a 1210–amino acid protein with an extracellular epidermal growth factor–binding domain, a transmembrane domain, and an intracellular tyrosine kinase domain. A related human gene, c-erbB-2, also has been cloned and sequenced.[80,81] The c-erbB-2 gene gives rise to a 1255–amino acid protein with a structure similar to that produced by the c-erbB-1 gene. The intracellular tyrosine kinase domain shares a 70 per cent nucleotide sequence and an 80 per cent amino acid sequence homology with the epidermal growth factor receptor (c-erbB-1) and v-erbB product.

The presence of epidermal growth factor receptors in lung cancer has been demonstrated by epidermal growth factor receptor mRNA expression,[77,82,83] detection of the epidermal growth factor receptor protein by immunoprecipitation or affinity labeling,[83–86] and binding studies.[83–85,87–90] The epidermal growth factor receptor has been found to be amplified in some non–small-cell lung cancer cell lines and tumors that have high levels of mRNA expression and epidermal growth factor receptor protein.[82,86,90] Immunohistochemical analyses of surgically resected non–small-cell lung cancers show that approximately 70 per cent of squamous cell lung cancers and 40 per cent of adenocarcinomas of the lung, have detectable epidermal growth factor receptors; they are undetectable in small-cell lung cancer.[74,75,86,91]

The presence of c-erbB-2 receptors in lung cancer has been demonstrated by c-erbB-2 receptor mRNA expression in tumors and tumor cell lines from patients with small-cell and non–small-cell lung cancer[92,93] and by detection of the c-erbB-2 protein by immunoprecipitation or Western blotting analysis.[93,94] The receptor has been detected by immunohistochemical analyses in 40 to 50 per cent of adenocarcinomas and squamous cell carcinomas but was not detected in three small-cell lung cancers tested.[93,94]

The exogenous addition of transforming growth factor α can stimulate the growth of lung cancer cells in a clonogenic assay at concentrations up to 0.1 ng/ml,[95] and inhibited their growth at higher concentrations (1.0 ng/ml or higher) in a clonogenic assay system and in a cell growth assay system.[78,95] A monoclonal antibody directed against transforming growth factor α has been shown to inhibit the growth of two different adenocarcinoma cell lines by MTT (3-[4,5-dimethyl-2-thiazolyl]-2,5-diphenyltetrazolium bromide) assay.[96]

Two different monoclonal antibodies directed against the epidermal growth factor receptor have been shown to inhibit the growth of non–small-cell lung cancer cell lines in vitro and in vivo.[97,98] The antibodies are in clinical trials as antitumor agents for patients with lung cancer, but no clinical responses have yet been reported.[98,98a] A clinical study that did immunohistochemical analyses of patients with adenocarcinoma of the lung showed that patients who had either epidermal growth factor or transforming growth factor α and the c-erbB-1 receptor lived a shorter period of time than patients who did not have both molecules needed for the autocrine loop.[74]

INSULIN-LIKE GROWTH FACTOR I

The human insulin-like growth factor I gene has been cloned and sequenced.[99] Human insulin-like growth factor I contains 70 amino acids, and 50 of these amino acids share homology with human insulin.[100] Insulin-like growth factor I mRNA has been detected in lung cancer cell lines by polymerase chain reactions,[101] and insulin-like growth factor I protein in lung cancer tumors by radioimmunoassay[102] and immunohistochemistry[103] and in tumor cell lines by Western blot analyses.[104] Insulin-like growth factor I immunoreactivity has been detected in the media of both small-cell and non–small-cell lung cancer cell lines.[105–107]

The receptors for insulin-like growth factors I and II have been cloned and the nucleotide sequence determined.[108,109] Insulin-like growth factor I receptor mRNA has been detected by Northern blot analysis,[110] cross linking of the receptor protein to radiolabeled insulin-like growth factor I,[110] binding studies of iodinated insulin-like growth factor I,[103,104,106] and detection with antibodies directed against the insulin-like growth factor in lung cancer tumors and tumor cell lines.[103,106]

The addition of exogenous insulin-like growth factor I can stimulate the growth of small-cell and non–small-cell lung cancer tumors and tumor cell lines measured by cell counting,[111] clonogenic assay,[95,110,112] tritiated thymidine uptake,[105,106] and MTT assay.[104] Monoclonal antibody against either insulin-like growth factor I or the insulin-like growth factor I receptor can block the growth stimulation of insulin-like growth factor I and inhibit the growth of lung cancer cells.[104–106] The percentages of lung cancers and lung cancer cell lines that make insulin-like growth factor have not been well established. In addition, the growth effects of insulin and insulin-like growth factor II have not been extensively studied in lung cancer.

ARGININE VASOPRESSIN

Human arginine vasopressin has been cloned and sequenced.[113] The preprohormone is processed to a biologically active 9–amino acid peptide (Fig. 15–8). Arginine vasopressin mRNA has been detected by Northern blotting, S1 nuclease analysis, and RNase protection assay in tumors and tumor cell lines from patients with small-cell lung cancer and hyponatremia.[113–115] The peptide has been detected in tumors and tumor cell lines by radioimmunoassay,[114,115] secretion by small-cell lung cancer cell lines into media has been verified,[116] and synthesis in a small-cell lung cancer tumor has been verified by incorporation of radioactive amino acids into arginine vasopressin.[117]

Exogenously added arginine vasopressin elevates cytosolic calcium,[56,118,119] increases tritiated thymidine uptake, and increases the clonogenicity of selected cell lines in soft agarose assays.[119,120] In addition, there is a close relationship between elevated arginine vasopressin production in small-cell lung cancer and hyponatremia.[115] Hyponatremia in patients with small-cell lung cancer is associated with shortened survival.[115,121–123] Therefore, there is in vitro evidence that arginine vasopressin can stimulate the growth of lung cancer cells and clinical evidence that the peptide hormone that causes hyponatremia in small-cell lung cancer is associated with shortened survival. Further studies of this peptide in lung cancer await the cloning of the human arginine vasopressin receptor. Arginine vasopressin mRNA expression and immunoreactive peptide have not been detected in tumor cell lines established from patients with non–small-cell lung cancer.[115]

SURFACE EPITOPES

Cancer cells can have alteration of the carbohydrates on the surface of their cells involving the ABO system. Two different studies of surface epitopes on tumors from patients with lung cancer show that the presence or absence of a surface marker can be associated with differences in patient survival. A retrospective study of patients with surgically resectable non–small-cell lung cancer (surgical stages I through IIIb) showed that 43 patients with blood type A or AB whose tumors stained with an antibody directed against the blood group A antigen lived longer than 28 patients with blood type A or AB whose tumor did not have blood group A antigen.[124] Another retrospective study of patients with surgically resectable

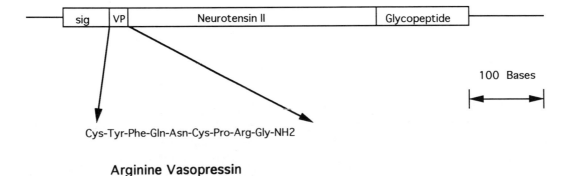

Arginine Vasopressin

Figure 15–8. Arginine vasopressin. The 700-base arginine vasopressin mRNA is translated into a 103–amino acid preprohormone with an amino-terminal signal peptide (sig); the arginine vasopressin nonapeptide (VP), with its amino acid sequence shown below; and a carboxy-terminal neurotensin II and glycopeptide.[113]

non–small-cell lung cancer (surgical stages I through IIIa) showed that 91 patients whose tumors stained with a migration-inhibiting antibody (MIA) directed against the precursors to the ABO blood group antigens (H/Le^y/Le^b) survived a shorter period of time than patients whose tumor did not stain with MIA.[125] The presence of the precursors to the ABO blood group antigens are associated with the loss of ABO blood group antigens, so the two studies have similar findings. These observations of surface epitopes in lung cancer currently are being examined in prospective trials.

DOMINANT ONCOGENES

myc Family DNA Amplification in Lung Cancer

SMALL-CELL LUNG CANCER CELL LINES

The myc family is comprised of c-myc, N-myc, and L-myc. DNA amplification of c-myc initially was discovered in a human leukemia cell line because of sequence homology between the c-myc gene and the avian retrovirus gene v-myc.[126] N-myc, a gene with sequence homology with v-myc and c-myc, was discovered because it was found to be amplified in a neuroblastoma and neuroblastoma cell lines.[127] L-myc, a gene with sequence homology with c-myc and N-myc, was discovered because it was found to be amplified in small-cell lung cancer cell lines and tumors.[128]

myc family DNA amplification commonly is detected in tumor and tumor cell lines from patients with small-cell lung cancer (Table 15–1). c-myc DNA amplification and expression is associated with the variant phenotype of small-cell lung cancer cell lines.[129,130] The variant cell lines have an altered morphology in cell culture (growth in loose chains), altered athymic nude mouse xenotrans-

plant histology (large cells with abundant cytoplasm and prominent nucleoli), and different biochemical properties compared to classic small-cell lung cancer cell lines. The variant small-cell lung cancer cell lines produce low or undetectable levels of L-dopa decarboxylase and bombesin-like immunoreactivity, markers of neuroendocrine differentiation. The variant cell lines also have a more rapid doubling time, have a higher cloning efficiency in soft agarose, and are less sensitive to radiation than the classic cell lines.[130,131]

The transfection of the normal human c-myc gene into a small-cell lung cancer cell line that did not express detectable c-myc mRNA caused c-myc mRNA expression.[132] This was associated with a more rapid growth rate, increased cloning efficiency, altered morphology in cell culture (Fig. 15–9), and altered histology in athymic nude mouse xenotransplants. There were no significant changes in the biochemical properties. Therefore, the expression of c-myc appears to correlate with the growth and morphologic phenotypic properties associated with the variant small-cell lung cancer cell lines.

myc family DNA amplification also has been associated with shortened survival.[133–135] c-myc DNA amplification in tumor cell lines established from patients with small-cell lung cancer who had been treated previously with chemotherapy have been associated with shortened survival.[133,134] In addition, greater than tenfold myc family DNA amplification in tumor samples has been associated with shortened survival as well.[135] myc family DNA amplification also has been found more commonly in tumor cell lines established from patients who have previously received chemotherapy than those who have not.[133,136]

myc family DNA amplification is present in approximately one third of tumor cell lines from patients with small-cell lung cancer (Table 15–1). Only 1 of more than 100 small-cell lung cancer cell lines studied has DNA amplification of more than two myc family genes, L-myc, and c-myc.[137] Studies of myc family DNA amplification in 11 tumor cell lines established from patients with small-

TABLE 15–1. myc FAMILY DNA AMPLIFICATION OF SMALL-CELL LUNG CANCER

STUDY	c-myc		N-myc		L-myc	
Small-Cell Lung Cancer Cell Lines						
Little et al.[129]	2/4	(50%)	0/4	(0%)		
Morstyn et al.[197]	0/6	(0%)	0/6	(0%)		
Kiefer et al.[138]	4/5	(80%)	0/5	(0%)		
Waters et al.[160]	0/9	(0%)	3/9	(33%)	3/9	(33%)
Takahashi et al.[139]	3/15	(20%)	0/15	(0%)	4/15	(27%)
Brennan et al.[133]	7/69	(10%)	4/69	(6%)	5/69	(7%)
Total	16/108	(15%)	7/108	(6%)	12/93	(13%)
Small-Cell Lung Cancer Tumors						
Wong et al.[141]	2/45	(4%)	3/45	(7%)		
Johnson et al.[134]	0/38	(0%)	4/38	(10%)	2/38	(5%)
Gemma et al.[142]	0/5	(5%)	0/5	(0%)	3/5	(60%)
Yokota et al.[137]	0/17	(0%)	1/17	(6%)	3/17	(18%)
Takahashi et al.[139]	2/23	(9%)	0/23	(0%)	3/23	(13%)
Shiraishi et al.[143]	1/8	(13%)	0/8	(0%)	2/6	(33%)
Noguchi et al.[135]	1/47	(2%)	5/47	(11%)	5/47	(11%)
Total	6/183	(3%)	13/183	(7%)	18/136	(13%)

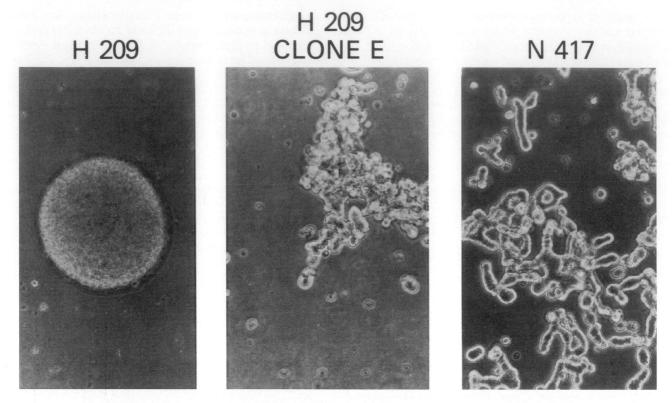

H 209   H 209 CLONE E   N 417

Figure 15–9. Cellular morphology of small-cell lung cancer cell lines and a transfected clone. From left to right, photomicrographs of small-cell lung cancer cell lines NCI-H209, NCI-H209 transfected with multiple copies of the normal c-*myc* gene, and NCI-N417 growing in log phase. The cells have been photographed using a phase-contrast Nikon photomicroscope (×100). (From Johnson BE, Battey JF, Linnoila I, et al: Changes in the phenotype of human small cell lung cancer lines after transfection and expression of the c-myc. J Clin Invest 78:525, 1986, with permission.)

cell lung cancer at different times during their clinical course showed similar *myc* family DNA amplification status in different tumor cell lines from five patients.[138,139] One patient with small-cell lung cancer had N-*myc* DNA amplification in a tumor cell line established prior to the initiation of therapy, whereas two cell lines established after the patients' tumors recurred had c-*myc* DNA amplification.[140]

SMALL-CELL LUNG CANCER TUMORS

Seven different studies have evaluated *myc* family DNA amplification of tumors from 5 to 47 patients with small-cell lung cancer (Table 15–1). *myc* family DNA amplification is present in approximately 20 per cent of tumors from patients with small-cell lung cancer (Table 15–1).

Three studies showed that *myc* family DNA copy number was similar in multiple sites of metastatic disease from 35 different patients with small-cell lung cancer[135,139,141] (Table 15–1). Two other reports have described three small-cell lung cancer patients with different *myc* family DNA copy numbers in different metastatic sites from the same patient. Yokota et al. reported on a patient with small-cell lung cancer in whom the primary tumor and two metastatic sites had about 100-fold amplification of N-*myc* while two other metastases did not.[137] Noguchi et al. reported that one of two patients had N-*myc* DNA am-

plification in part of the primary tumor and three metastatic sites while a different part of the primary tumor and three other metastatic sites did not have N-*myc* DNA amplification.[135] The other patient had L-*myc* DNA amplification in metastatic lymph nodes present at postmortem examination, but this was not present in the primary lesion, which had been resected prior to the patient's death. No investigators found DNA amplification of multiple members of the *myc* family DNA in the same tumor sample.

TUMORS AND TUMOR CELL LINES FROM THE SAME PATIENT WITH SMALL-CELL LUNG CANCER

The *myc* family DNA copy number is similar in tumors and tumor cell lines from 21 of 23 evaluable patients with small-cell lung cancer.[133,137,139,140] Figure 15–10 shows results in two patients who have similar degrees of N-*myc* DNA amplification in the tumor and the derived tumor cell line, whereas a single copy is present in the normal tissue from the same patients. The exceptions were Lu-135 and Lu-139. Lu-135 was amplified for both c-*myc* and L-*myc*, whereas the tumor from which Lu-135 was established had L-*myc* DNA amplification but did not have c-*myc* DNA amplification.[137] The second tumor cell line, Lu-139, had c-*myc* DNA amplification while the original tumor did not.[137]

NON–SMALL-CELL LUNG CANCER

myc family DNA amplification was detected in only 10 per cent of 200 tumors from patients with non–small-cell lung cancer.[137,142,143] c-*myc* DNA amplification was detected in 10 per cent, L-*myc* in 2 per cent, and N-*myc* DNA in none. Fewer than 20 non–small-cell lung cancer cell lines have been studied. Although the c-*myc* gene may

play an important role in the biology of some lung cancers and lung cancer cell lines, *myc* family DNA amplification is uncommon in lung cancer and appears to be a relatively late event in the genesis of lung cancer.

ras Family Gene Mutations in Lung Cancer

MUTATIONS IN TUMORS AND TUMOR CELL LINES FROM PATIENTS WITH LUNG CANCER

The *ras* family of genes is composed of H-*ras*, K-*ras*, and N-*ras*, which code for membrane-associated proteins with 189 amino acids.[144,145] These genes normally bind guanine nucleotides (GTP and GDP), have GTPase activity, and are thought to play a role in the transduction of signals across cellular membranes, thereby regulating cellular proliferation. These *ras* genes can be activated to play a role in the development of cancer by a point mutation that most commonly occurs at the 12th, 13th, or 61st amino acid of the 189 amino acids in the protein.[144,145] The *ras* family of genes are mutated in approximately 19 per cent of non–small-cell lung cancer tumors and tumor cell lines (Table 15–2), whereas none of 51 small-cell lung cancer tumors and tumor cell lines studied have these mutations.[146–149,154a] The mutations most commonly are found in adenocarcinomas of the lung (23 per cent), in contrast to a 10 per cent incidence in squamous cell carcinomas, large-cell carcinomas of the lung, and carcinoid tumors.[146–150] In addition, the K-*ras* gene is the most commonly mutated of the *ras* family of genes in tumors from patients with non–small-cell lung cancer, representing approximately 90 per cent of the mutations identified in adenocarcinomas of the lung. Mutations of the H-*ras* and N-*ras* gene are found in less than 2 per cent of non–small-cell lung cancer tumors and tumor cell lines.

Mutations of the 12th amino acid in the K-*ras* gene represent 85 per cent of the mutations identified in the K-*ras* gene in adenocarcinomas of the lung.[146–154e] The mutation of the normal codon (GGT), the 3–base pair sequence that codes for glycine, is most commonly a G→T transversion (change from a purine to a pyrimidine) in the first two bases. These mutations to TGT and GTT represent approximately 70 per cent of the mutations identified at the 12th amino acid in the K-*ras* protein and code for cysteine and valine, respectively (Fig. 15–11).[152]

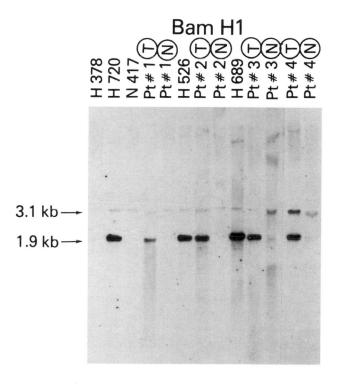

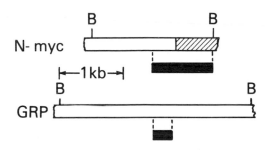

Figure 15–10. N-*myc* DNA amplification in patients' tumors and tumor cell lines. Southern blot of 10 μg of DNA digested with the Bam H1 restriction endonuclease from small-cell lung cancer tumors, normal tissues, and tumor cell lines hybridized to N-*myc* and a gastrin-releasing peptide (GRP) fragment. The tumor for each patient is designated T and the normal tissue is designated N. Small-cell lung cancer cell line NCI-H526 was derived from a tumor from patient 2 and NCI-H689 was derived from a tumor from patient 3. The signals that appear at 1.9 kb represent the signal from the N-*myc* fragment, whereas the signals that appear at 3.1 kb represent the (GRP) single copy control. The intense signals from NCI-H720, patients' tumors 1 through 4, and NCI-H526 and NCI-H689 show that the N-*myc* gene is amplified while the normal tissue has a single copy. (From Johnson BE, Makuch RW, Simmons AD, et al: myc family DNA amplification in small cell lung cancer patients' tumors and corresponding cell lines. Cancer Res 48:5163, 1988, with permission.)

K-RAS MUTATIONS IN LUNG CANCERS FROM SMOKERS, NONSMOKERS, AND PATIENTS WITH OCCUPATIONAL EXPOSURE TO RADON

The K-*ras* gene mutations found in lung cancers of smokers are different from those found in lung cancers of nonsmokers and patients who have had occupational exposure to radon. Three studies of adenocarcinomas of the lung showed that tumors from 85 patients who smoked had K-*ras* mutation in 31 per cent of tumors compared to 10 per cent in the tumors from 59 patients who did not smoke.[152,154,154a] In addition, one of the two K-*ras* mutations in adenocarcinomas of the lung from the patients who did not smoke did not have the typical G:C→T:A

TABLE 15–2. *ras* FAMILY MUTATIONS IN NON–SMALL CELL LUNG CANCER

STUDY	SAMPLE SIZE	ADENOCARCINOMAS		OTHER HISTOLOGIES	
		K-*ras*	H-*ras*	K-*ras*	H-*ras*
Rodenhuis et al.[148]	36	5/10	0/10	0/26	0/26
Rodenhuis et al.[149]	43	10/35	1/35	0/8	0/8
Slebos et al.[151]	69*	19/69			
Suzuki et al.[146]	121	14/66	1/66	2/55	2/55
Slebos et al.[152]	27	8/27			
Mitudomi et al.[147]	61†	9/32	0/32	11/29	1/29
Kobayashi et al.[153]	67*	10/67			
Sugio et al.[154]	115	17/115	0/115		
Lung et al.[150]	130	6/63	0/63	1/67	0/67
Husgafvel-Pursiainen et al.[154a]	44	12/21	0/21	2/23	0/23
Rosell et al.[154b]	66	3/22		10/44	
Bongiorno et al.[154c]	29*	7/29			
Li et al.[154d]	41	8/41			
Kern et al.[154e]	42	16/42			
Total	891	144/639 (23%)	2/342 (1%)	26/252 (10%)	3/206 (1%)

*Studied only codon 12 of the K-*ras* gene.
†Tumor cell lines.

transversion seen in the tumors from patients who did smoke.[152] The mutation was from GGT to CGT and GAT. The *ras* family of genes has been studied in lung cancer patients who have been exposed to radon, another environmental agent associated with the development of lung cancer, while working underground as uranium miners.[156] Eighteen of these 19 patients also were cigarette smokers. In contrast to patients who were exposed only to cigarette smoke, none of the 19 lung cancers had mutations of the K-*ras* gene in codons 12 or 13.

The K-*ras* gene appears to mutate early in the development of lung cancer. The K-*ras* gene mutations were present in 18 of 57 (32 per cent) adenocarcinomas resected from patients who had discontinued smoking one to 10 or more years before their resection,[156a] similar to adenocarcinomas in current smokers (Table 15–2). In addition, K-*ras* mutations have been studied in the sputum collected from adult smokers participating in a lung cancer screening trial.[156b] The smokers who eventually developed an adenocarcinoma or large carcinoma had their tumor studied for K-*ras* mutations. The 10 patients who had K-*ras* mutations identified in their lung cancers had detectable K-*ras* mutations in their sputum before the clinical detection of lung cancer. Therefore, it appears the K-*ras* mutation associated with smoking appears years before the clinical detection of adenocarcinoma of the lung.

In contrast to lung cancer, the mutations of the K-*ras* gene in gastrointestinal malignancies and colon and pancreatic cancer do not typically have G→T transversions in the first position of the 12th codon.[155] These adenocarcinomas are not as closely associated with smoking compared to adenocarcinomas of the lung. Despite a similar histologic appearance (adenocarcinoma) and a similar mutated oncogene (K-*ras*), the mutagenic effects of smoking may lead to different patterns of K-*ras* mutations in adenocarcinomas of the lung than in gastrointestinal malignancies.[155]

CLINICAL OUTCOMES OF PATIENTS WITH NON–SMALL-CELL LUNG CANCER AND MUTATIONS OF THE K-RAS GENE

The identification of K-*ras* gene mutations in non–small-cell lung cancer tumors and tumor cell lines has been associated with shortened survival in five retrospective studies. Four studies reported on 236 patients with early-stage adenocarcinoma of the lung (stages I through IIIa) treated with curative intent by surgical resection.[154,154b,154e,157] The patients whose tumors had K-*ras* mutations lived a shorter period of time than those who did not in all four studies.

In addition, one of these studies examined the K-*ras* oncogene in tumor cell lines from 66 patients with non–small-cell lung cancer. These patients had predominantly advanced-stage disease, 21 with stages I through IIIa treated with surgical resection or chest radiotherapy and 45 with stage IIIb or IV treated with chemotherapy, palliative radiotherapy, or supportive treatment.[157] The patients whose tumor cell lines had mutations of the 12th codon of the K-*ras* gene lived a shorter time than the patients whose tumor cell lines did not. A subset analysis of the 21 patients with stages I, II, and IIIa non–small-cell lung cancer also showed that the patients who had K-*ras* mutations in their tumor cell lines lived a shorter period of time than those who did not. Therefore, in these three studies of patients with early and late stages of non–small-cell lung cancer, mutation of the K-*ras* gene was associated with shortened survival. Additional prospective studies will need to be performed to confirm this observation.

TUMOR SUPPRESSOR GENES

Studies of nonrandom cytogenetic changes and loss of alleles from specific portions of the chromosome in lung

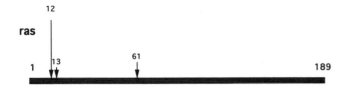

Figure 15–11. Location of *ras* family gene mutations. The bar diagrammatically represents the K-*ras*, H-*ras*, and N-*ras* genes, which are 189 amino acids in length. The vertical arrows represent the sites of the common amino acid mutations.

cancer cell lines and tumors have identified potentially important chromosomal regions and have helped identify chromosomal regions where tumor suppressor genes may reside.[158,159]

3p Chromosome Deletions in Lung Cancer

The loss of a portion of one of the two short arms of chromosome 3 is the most common abnormality identified in tumor cell lines and tumors from patients with small-cell lung cancer. Chromosomal analyses first identified the loss of one of two short arms of chromosome 3 in small-cell lung cancer cell lines and tumors, but there was not universal agreement about its incidence, ranging from 20 to 100 per cent.[160–166] The loss of the short arm of chromosome 3 appears to be an early event in carcinogenesis because 3p deletions are detectable in dysplastic lesions of the bronchus in smokers with or without evidence of lung cancer.[166a]

The development of molecular tools for evaluation of chromosomal deletions aided in resolving the controversy about the incidence of deletions of chromosome 3 and allowed studies of tumor tissues without having to do karyotypic analyses. Figure 15–12 gives an example of normal and small-cell lung cancer DNA studied using a DNA fragment that detects a restriction fragment length polymorphism. These restriction fragment length polymorphism studies show that a portion of the short arm of chromosome 3 is lost in nearly 100 per cent of tumors and tumor cell lines from patients with small-cell lung cancer[158,159,162,167–170] and 50 per cent of tumor cell lines and tumor from patients with non–small-cell lung cancer.[159,162,168,169,171–173]

This has prompted the search for a specific gene that, when lost, can give rise to lung cancer. The strategies used for identifying this gene include searching for homozygous deletions (loss of both copies of the gene), mapping the area most consistently deleted in lung cancers with large numbers of probes that identify loci on the short arm of chromosome 3, and studying genes that have been cloned and are found to map to the short arm of chromosome 3.

Homozygous deletions in the region of chromosome 3p12–3p22 have been identified in six small-cell lung cancer cell lines and one non-small cell lung cancer cell line.[174,174a,174b] The cell line, U2020, has a homozygous deletion of approximately 4 to 7 megabases (4 to 7 million base pairs) and maps to chromosome 3p12–14.[174,175,175a] The homozygous deletions in the other six cell lines (five

small-cell lung cancer and one non-small cell lung cancer) involve chromosomal regions 3p21–3p22 but have not yet been studied as thoroughly as U2020.[174a,174b]

The mapping of the most consistently deleted region of 3p in lung cancer tumors and tumor cell lines has been facilitated by the development of more than 800 probes that detect sequences on the short arm of chromosome 3.[175a,178,179] The large number of fragments that detect sequences on the short arm of chromosome 3 allow more precise localization of the region of the chromosome that is consistently lost in lung cancer. The identification of chromosomal region 18q, which was consistently deleted in colorectal cancer, was the successful strategy for identifying the *DCC* gene, a gene frequently altered in colorectal cancer.[180] The region that most often is deleted in lung cancer samples detected by restriction fragment length polymorphisms appears to be in the area of 3p21 and 3p25.[158,162,166a,169–171,173,174a,181,182]

Multiple candidate tumor suppressor genes that map to the consistently deleted segment of chromosome 3p include aminoacylase,[183] a thyroid hormone receptor,[169] B receptor for retinoic acid,[184] protein-tyrosine phosphatase γ,[185] the von Hippel-Lindau disease tumor suppressor gene,[185a] and DNA fragments from 3p21 with reduced mRNA expression in small-cell lung cancer cell lines.[186,186a] Two other loci have been identified at 3p14 by cloning the regions of chromosomal translocations in the germline DNA in families with hereditary renal cancer[186b] and hematologic malignancies.[186c] Candidate genes near these two chromosomal breakpoints on chromosome 3 have been identified and are undergoing study.

The introduction of chromosome 3 into the cell line derived from an adenocarcinoma of the lung[186d] or the short arm of chromosome 3 into a murine fibrosarcoma cell line[186e] reduces the tumorigenicity of the cells when injected into athymic nude mice. There is compelling evidence that the short arm of chromosome 3 has one or more tumor suppressor genes and intensive efforts are underway to identify the gene or genes in this area.

Retinoblastoma Gene Abnormalities in Lung Cancer

The retinoblastoma (*Rb*) gene was the initial tumor suppressor gene discovered in childhood retinoblastoma.[176,177] The *Rb* gene normally codes for a nuclear phosphoprotein, and both copies of the gene are inactivated in retinoblastomas.[176,177] The *Rb* gene can be inactivated in lung cancer cell lines or tumors by DNA mutations, deletions, undetectable or reduced mRNA expression, or undetectable or aberrant protein production. The DNA in the *Rb* locus shows a deletion or rearrangement of the locus in 21 per cent, absent or barely detectable mRNA expression in 55 per cent, and undetectable protein in 70 per cent of the small-cell lung cancer tumors and tumor cell lines studied (Table 15–3). In addition to these abnormalities, studies of one of the tumor cell lines showed that a point mutation within exon 21 prevented phosphorylation that caused a loss of function of the *Rb* protein.[187,187a]

In contrast to these findings in small-cell lung cancer,

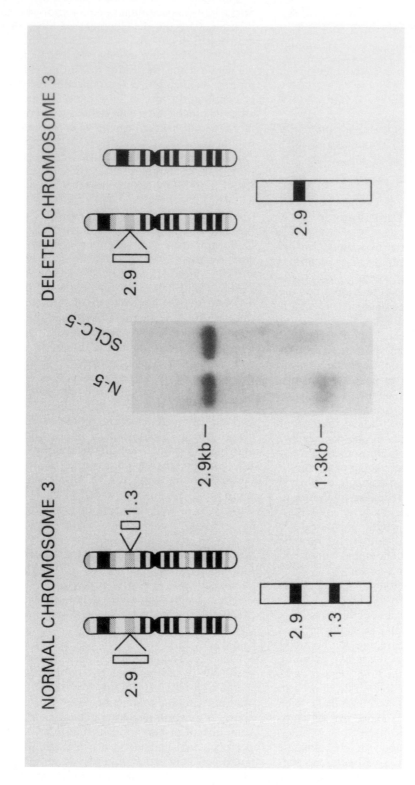

Figure 15–12. Restriction fragment length polymorphism studies in small-cell lung cancer. This figure diagrammatically represents the results of a Southern blot of normal DNA compared to small-cell lung cancer DNA with an interstitial deletion of the short arm of chromosome 3 when hybridized to a DNA fragment that recognizes a restriction fragment length polymorphism on the short arm of chromosome 3. The DNA fragment D3S2 recognizes a restriction fragment length polymorphism that localizes to the chromosomal band 3p14–21.[167,173] The copy of the gene on one chromosome gives rise to a band at 2.9 kb on a Southern blot of DNA digested with the restriction endonuclease MSP I. The copy of the gene on the other chromosome gives rise to a band of 1.3 kb on the same Southern blot, giving two bands. This is recognized by the two bands under N-5, the normal tissue from patient 5. An interstitial deletion of one of the two arms of chromosome 3 causes the loss of one of the two bands (1.3 kb), so the small-cell lung cancer tissue (SCLC-5) from the same patients has a single band. This is referred to as the loss of heterozygosity. In this way, the study of tumor and normal tissue can document the loss of loci on specific parts of a chromosome.

abnormalities of the *Rb* gene, mRNA, and protein are less common in tumor cell lines from patients with non–small-cell lung cancer. The retinoblastoma gene has a mutation, deletion, or rearrangement in 3 per cent, absent or barely detectable mRNA expression in 11 per cent, and undetectable protein in 29 per cent of tumors and tumor cell lines from patients with non-small cell lung cancer (Table 15–3). Two series of 101 and 163 patients with non-small cell lung cancer have shown that 24 and 33 per cent have undetectable protein by immunohistochemistry.[200a,200c] One study showed that patients with undetectable *Rb* protein in their Stage I and II non-small cell lung cancer lived a shorter time than patients who did not.[200c] In contrast, the other study showed no difference in survival between patients with non-small cell lung cancer who did and did not have undetectable protein.[200a] We await additional prospective studies of tumors from patients with non-small cell lung cancer to resolve this issue.

Two studies have shown that transfection of a normal retinoblastoma gene into four cell lines derived from small cell lung cancer reduced their efficiency, slowed their rate of growth, decreased their cloning efficiency, and reduced the tumorigenicity of the cells when injected into athymic nude mice.[187b,197c] Therefore, there is a high incidence of retinoblastoma gene inactivation in small cell lung cancer, and replacement of the gene product by transfection can decrease the growth and suppress the tumorigenicity of these lung cancer cells. The impact of absent retinoblastoma protein on survival of patients with non-small cell lung cancer will be assessed by currently ongoing prospective studies.

p53 Mutations in Lung Cancer

Mutations of the *p53* tumor suppressor gene are currently the most common genetic alteration identified in human cancers.[188–190] The *p53* gene is a tumor suppressor gene that normally codes for a nuclear phosphoprotein and was identified because it bound to the large T antigen of the DNA tumor virus simian virus 40 (SV40) to form an oligomeric complex.

The abnormalities in the region of the *p53* gene in human lung cancer were first identified by frequent loss of heterozygosity of probes that detect restriction fragment length polymorphisms on the short arm of chromosome 17.[159] Southern blots of DNA from lung cancer cell lines showed homozygous deletions and rearrangements of the *p53* gene in 3 of 30 lines examined.[191] RNase protection assays of mRNA and cDNA sequencing from these lung cancer cell lines showed reduced expression of *p53* and/or mutations in the protein coding portion of the gene in 22 of 30 lines examined.[191]

More than 550 lung cancer tumors and tumor cell lines have been characterized for their *p53* mutations (Table 15–4). In contrast to the K-*ras* gene, in which the mutations tend to occur in specific portions of the gene, the mutations of the *p53* gene occur throughout the length of the entire gene (Fig. 15–13). The mutations can be missense mutations, nonsense mutations, deletions, insertions, or mutations within the splicing region of the gene giving rise to an abnormal mRNA and thus an abnormal protein (Table 15–4). Mutations of the *p53* gene have been found in 74 per cent of the tumors and tumor cell lines from patients with small-cell lung cancer and 49 per cent of the tumors and tumor cell lines from patients with non–small-cell lung cancer. Despite the difference in the incidence of *p53* mutations, the mechanisms of mutation are similar. Missense mutations make up approximately 72 per cent of the mutations, with nonsense mutations, deletions and insertions, and splicing mutations making up the rest (Table 15–4).

The *p53* gene mutations appear relatively early in the course of carcinogenesis. Three studies of preneoplastic lesions have demonstrated cytogenetic abnormalities of chromosome 17p, loss of heterozygosity of 17p, and mutations in the *p53* gene.[191a–191c] In addition, two additional studies have shown antibodies directed against the *p53* protein stain areas of preneoplastic lesions located near squamous cell cancers.[191d,191e] Therefore, genetic lesions of the *p53* gene and increased *p53* protein are detectable in the bronchial mucosa before the appearance of lung cancer.

The relationship of smoking and *p53* mutations or increased *p53* protein have been examined in patients with lung cancer. Two studies of 138 patients with lung cancer showed an association between cigarette smoking and *p53* mutations,[192,192a] while another study of 51 patients did not.[193] In addition, two studies of 129 patients with lung cancer showed an association between cigarette smoking and increased *p53* protein detected by immunostaining in the lung cancer,[193a,193b] while another study of 88 patients

TABLE 15–3. RETINOBLASTOMA GENE ABNORMALITIES IN LUNG CANCER

STUDY	DNA	mRNA	PROTEIN
Small-Cell Lung Cancer Portion Unchanged			
Non-Small Cell Lung Cancer			
Harbour et al.[198]	0/20	4/19	
Yakota et al.[199]	1/9	2/9	2/9
Horowitz et al.[200]			0/3
Reissmann et al.[200a]	2/219	22/219	53/163
Sachse et al.[200b]	5/44		
Xu et al.[200c]			24/101
Total	8/300 (3%)	28/247 (11%)	79/276 (29%)

TABLE 15-4. INCIDENCE OF *p53* MUTATIONS IN LUNG CANCER

Study	# mut/Total	Missense	Nonsense	Deletion or Insertion	Splicing
Small Cell Lung Cancer and Carcinoid Tumors					
Hensel et al.[203]	7/16	2	1		1
Takahashi et al.[204]	11/15	10	1		
Lehman et al.[205]	1/1*	1			
D'Amico et al.[206]	21/21*	12	4		5
D'Amico et al.[206]	16/20†				
Miller et al.[207]	20/27	15	3	1	2
Sameshima et al.[208]	23/27	6		1	1
Lohmann et al.[213]	15/28	12	2		1
Total	114/155 (74%)	58 (72%)	11 (14%)	2 (2%)	10 (12%)
Non-Small Cell Lung Cancer					
Chiba et al.[193]	23/51	21		2	
Lehman et al.[205]	4/8*	2	2		
Suzuki et al.[192]	14/30	11		3	
Miller et al.[207]	3/13	2	1		
Mitsudomi et al.[209]	57/77	34	8	6	4
Kishimoto et al.[210]	60/115	43	4	11	2
Ryberg et al.[192a]	34/108	26	4	4	
Total	195/402 (49%)	139 (73%)	19 (10%)	26 (14%)	6 (3%)

*Lung cancer cell lines.
†Not sequenced.

with lung cancer did not.[193c] Smoking in patients who develop lung cancer appears to increase the chance of developing a *p53* mutation or detecting *p53* protein by immunostaining, but the final conclusions await additional studies.

The nucleotide mutations in the *p53* gene in cancers from the lung tend to differ from the *p53* mutations identified in other cancers that are not as tightly linked to cigarette smoking. The mutations of the *p53* gene in both non–small-cell lung cancer and small-cell lung cancer are most commonly a G:C→T:A transversion (Table 15–5), whereas the most common mutation in cancers other than lung cancer is a G:C→A:T transition.[188]

Two studies of 191 patients with surgically resected non-small cell lung cancer studied the impact of *p53* mutations on survival. Both showed patients with *p53* mutations in their lung cancer lived a shorter period of time than patients who did not.[192,193d] A study of patients with non-small cell lung cancer who had 77 tumor cell lines established showed no difference in survival between patients who did and did not have *p53* mutations.[209] These cell lines were established from patients with more advanced non-small cell lung cancer than the patients in the two studies of surgically resected non-small cell lung cancer, perhaps explaining why there was no difference in survival.

The mechanism for increased staining of lung cancer specimens with antibodies that detect epitopes of the *p53*

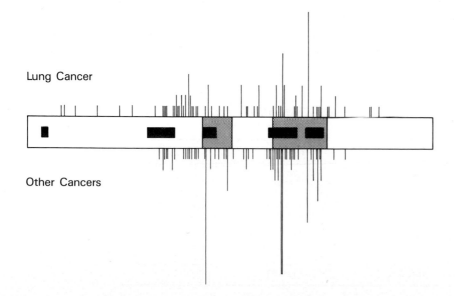

Lung Cancer

Other Cancers

Figure 15–13. Distribution of *p53* gene mutations in lung cancer. The five black boxes indicate the evolutionary conserved regions of the *p53* gene, and the shaded gray areas represent the simian virus 40 large T antigen–binding domains. The vertical lines represent the location of mutations and the taller lines represent multiple mutations in the same amino acid. The vertical lines above the bar represent the mutations found in 97 lung cancers (75 non–small-cell lung cancer specimens and 22 small-cell lung cancers). The vertical lines below the bar represent mutations in 121 cancers of the breast, colon, esophagus, liver, bladder, brain, and stomach, as well as leukemia and sarcoma. (Adapted from Mitsudomi T, Steinberg SM, Nau MM, et al: p53 gene mutations in non–small-cell cancer cell lines and their correlation with the presence of ras mutations and clinical features. Oncogene 7:171, 1992, with permission.)

TABLE 15-5. NUCLEOTIDE SUBSTITUTION PATTERN OF p53 MUTATIONS IN LUNG CANCER

Nucleotide Substitution	Number (percentage)
Small-Cell Lung Cancer, n = 70	
G:C → T:A	32 (46)
G:C → A:T	14 (20)
G:C → C:G	9 (13)
A:T → G:C	8 (11)
T:A → G:C	5 (7)
T:A → A:T	2 (3)
Non-Small Cell Lung Cancer, n = 162	
G:C → T:A	62 (38)
G:C → A:T	51 (32)
G:C → C:G	21 (13)
A:T → G:C	15 (9)
A:T → T:A	8 (5)
T:A → G:C	5 (3)

*Data from refs. 192, 193, 203–208, 211–213.

molecule have been reported recently.[194] Lung cancer cell lines with missense mutations in exons 5 through 8 had increased staining with antibodies that detect p53 in 16 of 17 tumor cell lines studied. The p53 mutations that give rise to mRNA splicing abnormalities, nonsense, deletions, or mutations outside exons 5 through 8 were unlikely to have high levels of p53 detected by p53 antibodies. This provides information about the molecular findings or tumor specimens with increased amounts of staining.

Three different studies of 279 patients with adenocarcinoma or squamous cell carcinoma of the lung compared the survival of patients who did and did not have immunoreactivity detectable by 1–5 antibodies directed against p53 in their lung cancer. One study showed shortened survival in patients whose tumor had detectable p53 immunoreactivity,[194a] while the other two did not.[194b,194c] The study which showed a difference in survival used a single antibody which stained 43 percent of the lung cancers compared to the other studies using 4 or 5 antibodies which stained 56 per cent of the lung cancers, potentially explaining the difference in the findings of the different studies.

Three different studies have evaluated p53 mutations in patients exposed to radiation. Two studies of 71 patients exposed to radon while working as uranium miners report very different findings. All but 6 of these miners also smoked cigarettes. One study of 19 uranium miners showed 7 (37 per cent) had mutations of the p53 gene.[156] None of these 7 had G:C to T:A mutations typical of smoking related malignancies (Table 15–5). In contrast, the other study showed 29 of the 52 (56 per cent) had mutations of the p53 gene including 19 who had G:C to T:A (37 per cent or 66 per cent of those with p53 mutations).[194d] Seventeen of these 29 G:C to T:A mutations were in codon 249. A potential explanation for the difference in these findings is that the exposure to radon of the 52 patients in the group with the G:C to T:A mutations was 5-fold greater than the other 19 patients.[194d] The third study evaluated p53 mutations in lung cancers from 9 non-smoking patients exposed to radiation following the

atomic-bomb detonation in Hiroshima.[194e] Four of the nine had mutations in the p53 gene and one had the typical G:C to T:A transversion (Table 15–5).

Therefore, the genetic lesions in these tumors, which were associated with a different environmental pathogen (radon), were different from the lesions typically found in patients who developed lung cancer after chronic cigarette smoking. In addition, the studies of p53 mutations in different histologies suggest smoking may play a role in the type of mutation that occurs. The G:C→A:T mutations of the p53 gene made up 20 per cent of the mutations in small-cell lung cancers (Table 15–5), the histology most closely linked with cigarette smoking. The G:C→A:T mutations are found more commonly in non–small-cell lung cancers (32 per cent), which include adenocarcinomas, the histology most commonly found in patients with lung cancer who did not smoke and the histology least linked to cigarette smoking.

The potential biologic role of p53 in lung cancer has been recently reported. The insertion of wild type p53 into four different non-small cell lung cancer cell lines suppressed the number of colonies generated by transfection or growth rate compared to an antisense construct or mutant p53.[195–195c] In addition, the cells were not tumorigenic when injected into athymic nude mice or mice with severe combined immunodeficiency. In contrast, the same cells transfected with mutated p53 had no effect on the number of colonies following transfection and the cells were tumorigenic in severe combined immunodeficiency or athymic nude mice. This provides evidence of p53 suppressing tumor growth in lung cancer cells.

Patients with lung cancer have detectable antibody directed against p53 in only about 10 per cent of cases.[196] Again, all of the patients who developed antibody were those who had p53 missense mutations. Therefore, the immunologic reaction may be increased in these patients because of the large amounts of protein produced by the missense mutations, which can be recognized by immunohistochemistry and give rise to an antibody response in patients with lung cancer.[195,196]

REFERENCES

1. Boring CC, Squires TS, Tong T, et al: Cancer statistics, 1994. CA Cancer J Clin 44:7, 1994
2. World Health Organization: The World Health Organization histologic typing of lung tumors: Second edition. Am J Clin Pathol 77:123, 1982
3. Humphrey EW, Smart CR, Winchester DP, et al: National survey of the pattern of care for carcinoma of the lung. Thorac Cardiovasc Surg 100:837, 1990
4. El-Torky M, El-Zeky F, Hall JC: Significant changes in the distribution of histologic types of lung cancer. Cancer 65:2361, 1990
5. Ihde DC: Drug therapy: Chemotherapy of lung cancer. N Engl J Med 327:1434, 1992
6. Rosenow EC, III, Carr DT: Bronchogenic carcinoma. CA Cancer J Clin 29:233, 1979
7. Ihde DC, Cohen MH, Bernath AM, et al: Serial fiberoptic bronchoscopy during chemotherapy for small cell carcinoma of lung. Chest 74:531, 1978
8. Tondini M, Rizzi A: Small-cell lung cancer: Importance of fi-

beroptic bronchoscopy in the evaluation of complete remission. Tumori 75:266, 1989

9. Reyes CV, Chua D, Aranha GV: Changing incidence of adenocarcinoma of the lung: A brief review. J Surg Oncol 35: 50, 1987

10. Weibel ER, Taylor CR: Design and structure of the human lung. In Fishman AP (ed): Pulmonary Diseases and Disorders. New York, McGraw-Hill, 1988, p 11

11. Gmelich JT, Bensch KG, Liebow AA: Cells of Kultschitzky type in bronchioles and their relation to the origin of peripheral carcinoid tumor. Lab Invest 17:88, 1967

12. Bensch KG, Gordon GB, Miller LR: Studies on the bronchial counterpart of the Kultschitzky (argentaffin) cell and innervation of bronchial glands. J Ultrastruc Res 12:668, 1965

13. Gould VE, Linnoila RI, Memoli VA, et al: Neuroendocrine components of the bronchopulmonary tract: Hyperplasia, dysplasias, and neoplasms. Lab Invest 49:519, 1983

14. Sunday ME, Kaplan LM, Motoyama E, et al: Gastrin-releasing peptide (mammalian bombesin) gene expression in health and disease. Lab Invest 59:5, 1988

15. Garfinkel L, Silverberg E: Lung cancer and smoking trends in the United States over the past 25 years. CA Cancer J Clin 41:137, 1991

16. Jedrychowski W, Becher H, Wahrendorf J, et al: Effect of tobacco smoking on various histologic types of lung cancer. J Cancer Res Clin Oncol 118:276, 1992

17. Morabia A, Wynder EL: Cigarette smoking and lung cancer cell types. Cancer 68:2074, 1991

18. Fielding JE, Phenow KJ: Health effects of involuntary smoking. N Engl J Med 319:1452, 1988

19. Janerich DT, Thompson WD, Varela LR, et al: Lung cancer and exposure to tobacco smoke in the household. N Engl J Med 323:632, 1990

20. Brownson RC, Chang JC, Davis JR: Gender and histologic type variations in smoking-related risk of lung cancer. Epidemiology 3:61, 1992

21. McDuffie HH, Klassen DJ, Dosman JA: Determinants of cell type in patients with cancer of the lungs. Chest 98:1187, 1990

22. Capewell S, Sankaran R, Lamb D, et al: Lung cancer in lifelong non-smokers. Thorax 46:565, 1991

23. American Medical Association Council on Scientific Affairs: Health effects of radon exposure: Report of the Council on Scientific Affairs, American Medical Association. Arch Intern Med 151:674, 1991

24. Samet JM: Indoor radon and lung cancer: Estimating the risks. West J Med 156:25, 1992

25. Pershagen G, Akerblom G, Axelson O, et al: Residential radon exposure and lung cancer in Sweden. N Engl J Med 330:159, 1994

26. Auerbach O, Stout AP, Hammond EC, et al: Changes in bronchial epithelium in relation to cigarette smoking and in relation to lung cancer. N Engl J Med 265:253, 1961

27. Auerbach O, Gere JB, Forman JB, et al: Changes in bronchial epithelium in relation to smoking and cancer of the lung: A report of progress. N Engl J Med 256:97, 1957

28. Gosney JR, Sissons MCJ, Allibone RO: Neuroendocrine cell populations in normal human lungs: A quantitative study. Thorax 43:878, 1988

29. Gosney JR, Sissons MCJ, Allibone RO, et al: Pulmonary endocrine cells in chronic bronchitis and emphysema. J Pathol 157:127, 1989

30. Nylen ES, Becker KL, Joshi PA, et al: Pulmonary bombesin and calcitonin in hamsters during exposure to hyperoxia and diethylnitrosamine. Am J Respir Cell Mol Biol 2:25, 1990

31. Schuller HM, Becker KL, Witschi HP: An animal model for neuroendocrine lung cancer. Carcinogenesis 9:293, 1988

32. Sporn MB, Todaro GJ: Autocrine secretion and malignant transformation of cells. N Engl J Med 303:878, 1980

33. Erspamer V, Espamer GF, Inselvini M: Some pharmacological actions of alytesin and bombesin. J Pharm Pharmacol 22:875, 1970

34. Wharton J, Polak JM, Bloom SR, et al: Bombesin-like immunoreactivity in the lung. Nature 273:769, 1978

35. Sorenson GD, Bloom SR, Ghatei MA, et al: Bombesin production by human small cell carcinoma of the lung. Reg Peptides 4:59, 1982

36. Moody TW, Pert CB, Gazdar AF, et al: High levels of intracellular bombesin characterize human small-cell lung carcinoma. Science 214:1246, 1981

37. Erisman MD, Linnoila RI, Hernandez O, et al: Human lung small-cell carcinoma contains bombesin. Proc Natl Acad Sci USA 79:2379, 1982

38. Spindel ER, Chin WW, Price J, et al: Cloning and characterization of cDNAs encoding human gastrin-releasing peptide. Proc Natl Acad Sci USA 81:5699, 1984

39. Sausville EA, Lebacq-Verheyden AM, Spindel ER, et al: Expression of the gastrin-releasing peptide gene in human small cell lung cancer: Evidence for alternative processing in three distinct mRNAs. J Biol Chem 261:2451, 1986

40. Spindel ER, Krane IM: Molecular biology of bombesin-like peptides: Comparison of cDNAs encoding gastrin-releasing peptide, human neuromedin B, and amphibian ranatensin. Ann NY Acad Sci 456:10, 1988

41. Cardona C, Rabbits PH, Spindel ER, et al: Production of neuromedin B and neuromedin B gene expression in human lung tumor cell lines. Cancer Res 51:5205, 1991

42. Hamid QA, Corrin B, Dewar A, et al: Expression of gastrin-releasing peptide (human bombesin) gene in large cell undifferentiated carcinoma of the lung. J Pathol 161:145, 1990

43. Hamid QA, Bishop AE, Springall DR, et al: Detection of human probombesin mRNA in neuroendocrine (small cell) carcinoma of the lung: In situ hybridization with cRNA probe. Cancer 63:266, 1989

44. Tsutsumi Y: Immunohistochemical localization of gastrin-releasing peptide in normal and diseased human lung. Ann N Y Acad Sci 456:336, 1988

45. Polak JM, Hamid Q, Springall DR, et al: Localization of bombesin-like peptides in tumors. Ann N Y Acad Sci 456: 322, 1988

46. Vangsted AJ, Schwartz TW: Production of gastrin-releasing peptide (18–27) and a stable fragment of its precursor in small cell lung carcinoma cells. J Clin Endocrinol Metab 70: 1586, 1990

47. Krane IM, Naylor SL, Helin-Davis D, et al: Molecular cloning of cDNAs encoding bombesin-like peptide neuromedin B. J Biol Chem 263:13317, 1988

48. Giaconne G, Battey J, Gazdar AF, et al: Neuromedin B is present in lung cancer cell lines. Cancer Res 52:2732s, 1992

49. Corjay MH, Dobrzanski DJ, Way JM, et al: Two distinct bombesin receptor subtypes are expressed and functional in human lung carcinoma cells. J Biol Chem 266:18771, 1991

49a. Fathi Z, Corjay MH, Shapira H, et al: BRS-3: A novel bombesin receptor subtype selectively expressed in testis and lung carcinoma cells. J Biol Chem 268:5979, 1993

50. Kane MA, Aguayo SM, Portanova LB, et al: Isolation of the bombesin/gastrin releasing peptide receptor from human small cell lung carcinoma NCI-H345. J Biol Chem 266:9486, 1991

51. Cardona C, Bleehen NM, Reeve JG: Characterization of ligand binding and processing by gastrin-releasing peptide receptors in a small-cell lung cancer cell line. Biochem J 281:115, 1992

52. Kado-Fong H, Malfroy B: Effects of bombesin on human small cell lung cancer cells: Evidence for a subset of bombesin non-responsive cell lines. J Cell Biochem 40:431, 1989

53. Layton JE, Scanlon DB, Soveny C, et al: Effects of bombesin antagonists on the growth of small cell lung cancer cells in vitro. Cancer Res 48:4783, 1988

54. Sharoni Y, Viallet J, Trepel JB, et al: Effect of guanine and adenine nucleotides on bombesin-stimulated phopholipase C activity in membranes from Swiss 3T3 and small cell carcinoma cells. Cancer Res 50:5257, 1990

55. Trepel JB, Moyer JD, Heikkila R, et al: Modulation of bombesin-induced phosphatidylinositol hydrolysis in a small-cell lung-cancer cell line. Biochem J 255:403, 1988

56. Bunn PA Jr, Chan D, Dienhart DG, et al: Neuropeptide signal transduction in lung cancer: Clinical implications of bradykinin sensitivity and overall heterogeneity. Cancer Res 52: 24, 1992

57. Woll PJ, Rozengurt E: Multiple neuropeptides mobilise calcium in small cell lung cancer: Effects of vasopressin, bradykinin, cholecystokinin, galanin, and neurotensin. Biochem Biophys Res Commun 164:66, 1989

58. Takuwa N, Takuwa Y, Ohue Y, et al: Stimulation of calcium mobilization but not proliferation by bombesin and tachykinin neuropeptides in small cell lung cancer cells. Cancer Res 50:240, 1990

59. Bunn PA Jr, Dienhart DG, Chan D, et al: Neuropeptide stimulation of calcium flux in human lung cancer cells: Delineation of alternative pathways. Proc Natl Acad Sci USA 87:2162, 1990

60. Heikkila R, Trepel JB, Cuttitta F, et al: Bombesin-related peptides induce calcium mobilization in a subset of human small cell lung cancer cell lines. J Biol Chem 262:16456, 1987

61. Cuttitta F, Carney DN, Mulshine J, et al: Bombesin-like peptides can function as autocrine growth factors in human small-cell lung cancer. Nature 316:123, 1985

62. Carney DN, Cuttitta F, Moody TW, et al: Selective stimulation of small cell lung cancer clonal growth by bombesin and gastrin-releasing peptide. Cancer Res 47:821, 1987

63. Weber S, Zuckerman JE, Bostwick DG, et al: Gastrin releasing peptide is a selective mitogen for small cell lung cancer in vitro. J Clin Invest 75:306, 1985

64. Thomas F, Arvelo F, Antoine E, et al: Antitumoral activity of bombesin analogues on small cell lung cancer xenografts: Relationship with bombesin receptor expression. Cancer Res 52:4872, 1992

65. Mahmoud S, Staley J, Taylor J, et al: [Psi13,14] bombesin analogues inhibit the growth of small cell lung cancer in vitro and in vivo. Cancer Res 51:1798, 1991

66. Willey JC, Lechner JF, Harris CC: Bombesin and the C-terminal tetradecapeptide of gastrin-releasing peptide are growth factors for normal human bronchial epithelial cells. Exp Cell Res 153:245, 1984

67. Sunday ME, Hua J, Dai IIB, et al: Bombesin increases fetal lung growth and maturation in utero and in organ culture. Am J Respir Cell Mol Biol 3:199, 1990

68. Spindel ER, Sunday ME, Hofler H, et al: Transient elevation of messenger RNA encoding gastrin-releasing peptide, a putative growth factor in human fetal lung. J Clin Invest 80:1172, 1987

69. Sunday ME: Tissue-specific expression of the mammalian bombesin gene. Ann N Y Acad Sci 456:95, 1988

70. Aguayo SM, Kane MA, King TE Jr, et al: Increased levels of bombesin-like peptide in the lower respiratory tract of asymptomatic cigarette smokers. J Clin Invest 84:1105, 1989

71. Aguayo SM, King TE Jr, Kane MA, et al: Urinary levels of bombesin-like peptides in asymptomatic cigarette smokers: A potential risk marker for smoking-related diseases. Cancer Res 52:2727s, 1992

72. Bell GI, Fong NM, Stempien MM, et al: Human epidermal growth factor precursor: cDNA sequence, expression in vitro and gene organization. Nucleic Acids Res 14:8427, 1986

73. Derynck R, Roberts AB, Winkler ME, et al: Human transforming growth factor-alpha: Precursor structure and expression in E. coli. Cell 38:287, 1984

74. Tateishi M, Ishida T, Mitsudomi T, et al: Immunohistochemical evidence of autocrine growth factors in adenocarcinoma of the human lung. Cancer Res 50:7077, 1990

75. Gorgoulis V, Aninos D, Mikou P, et al: Expression of EGF, TGF-alpha, and EGFR in squamous cell lung carcinomas. Anticancer Res 12:1183, 1992

75a. Rusch V, Baselga J, Cordon-Cardo C, et al: Differential expression of the epidermal growth factor receptor and its ligands in primary non-small cell lung cancers and adjacent benign lung. Cancer Res 53:2379, 1993

76. Falco JP, Baylin SB, Lupu R, et al: v-rasH induces non-small cell phenotype, with associated growth factors and receptors, in a small cell lung cancer cell line. J Clin Invest 85:1740, 1990

77. Derynck R, Goeddel DV, Ullrich A, et al: Synthesis of messenger RNAs for transforming growth factor alpha and beta and the epidermal growth factor receptor by human tumors. Cancer Res 47:707, 1987

78. Rabiasz GJ, Langdon SP, Bartlett JMS, et al: Growth control by epidermal growth factor and transforming growth factor-alpha in human lung squamous carcinoma cells. Br J Cancer 66:254, 1992

79. Ullrich A, Coussens L, Hayflick JS, et al: Human epidermal growth factor receptor cDNA sequence and aberrant expression of the amplified gene in A431 epidermoid carcinoma cells. Nature 309:418, 1984

80. Semba K, Kamata N, Toyoshima K, et al: A v-erbB-related protooncogene, c-erbB-2, is distinct from the c-erbB-1/epidermal growth factor-receptor gene and is amplified in a human salivary gland adenocarcinoma. Proc Natl Acad Sci USA 82:6497, 1985

81. Coussens L, Yang-Feng TL, Liao YC, et al: Tyrosine kinase receptor with extensive homology to the EGF receptor shares chromosomal location with neu oncogene. Science 230:1132, 1985

82. Ozanne B, Richards CS, Hendler F, et al: Over-expression of the EGF receptor is a hallmark of squamous cell carcinomas. J Pathol 149:9, 1986

83. Damstrup L, Rygaard K, Spang-Thomsen M, et al: Expression of the epidermal growth factor receptor in human small cell lung cancer cell lines. Cancer Res 52:3089, 1992

84. Haeder M, Rotsch M, Bepler G, et al: Epidermal growth factor receptor expression in human lung cancer cell lines. Cancer Res 48:1132, 1988

85. Moody TW, Lee M, Kris RM, et al: Lung carcinoid cell lines have bombesin-like peptides and EGF receptors. J Cell Biochem 43:139, 1990

86. Berger MS, Gullick WJ, Greenfield C, et al: Epidermal growth factor receptors in lung tumours. J Pathol 152:297, 1987

87. Sherwin SA, Minna JD, Gazdar AF, et al: Expression of epidermal and nerve growth factor receptors and soft agar growth factor production by human lung cancer cells. Cancer Res 41:3538, 1991

88. Hwang DL, Tay YC, Lin SS, et al: Expression of epidermal growth factor receptors in human lung tumors. Cancer 58:2260, 1986

89. Veale D, Kerr N, Gibson GJ, et al: Characterization of epidermal growth factor receptor in primary human non-small cell lung cancer. Cancer Res 49:1313, 1989

90. Kaseda S, Ueda M, Ozawa S, et al: Expression of epidermal growth factor receptors in four histologic cell types of lung cancer. J Surg Oncol 42:16, 1989

91. Cerny T, Barnes DM, Haselton P, et al: Expression of epidermal growth factor receptor (EGF-R) in human lung tumours. Br J Cancer 54:265, 1986

92. Schneider PM, Hung MC, Chiocca SM, et al: Differential expression of the c-erbB-2 gene in human small cell and non-small cell lung cancer. Cancer Res 49:4968, 1989

93. Kern JA, Schwartz DA, Nordberg JE, et al: p185neu expression in human lung adenocarcinomas predicts shortened survival. Cancer Res 50:5184, 1990

94. Weiner DB, Nordberg J, Robinson R, et al: Expression of the neu gene-encoded protein (P185neu) in human non-small cell carcinomas of the lung. Cancer Res 50:421, 1990

95. Siegfried JM, Owens SE: Response of primary human lung adenocarcinomas to autocrine growth factors produced by a lung carcinoma cell line. Cancer Res 43:4976, 1988

96. Imanishi K, Yamaguchi K, Kuranami M, et al: Inhibition of human lung adenocarcinoma cell lines by anti-transforming growth factor alpha monoclonal antibody. J Natl Cancer Inst 81:220, 1989

97. Lee M, Draoui M, Zia F, et al: Epidermal growth factor receptor monoclonal antibodies inhibit the growth of lung cancer cell lines. J Natl Cancer Inst Monogr 13:117, 1992

98. Mendelsohn J: Epidermal growth factor receptor as a target for therapy with antireceptor monoclonal antibodies. J Natl Cancer Inst Monogr 13:125, 1992

98a. Perez-Soler R, Donato NJ, Shin DM, et al: Tumor epidermal growth factor receptor studies in patients with non-small cell lung cancer or head and neck cancer treated with monoclonal antibody RG 83852. J Clin Oncol 12:730, 1994

99. Steenbergh PH, Koonen-Reemst A, Cleutjens C, et al: Complete

nucleotide sequence of the high molecular weight human IGF-I mRNA. Biochem Biophys Res Commun 175:507, 1991

100. Rinderknecht E, Humbel RE: The amino acid sequence of human insulin-like growth factor I and its structural homology with proinsulin. J Biol Chem 253:2769, 1978

101. Reeve JG, Brinkman A, Hughes S, et al: Expression of insulin-like growth factor (IGF) and IGF-binding protein genes in human lung tumor cell lines. J Natl Cancer Inst 84:628, 1992

102. Minuto F, Del Monte P, Barreca A, et al: Evidence for an increased somatomedin-C/insulin-like growth factor I content in primary human lung tumors. Cancer Res 46:985, 1986

103. Shigematsu K, Kataoka Y, Kamio T, et al: Partial characterization of insulin-like growth factor I in primary human lung cancers using immunohistochemical and receptor autoradiographic techniques. Cancer Res 50:2481, 1990

104. Nakanishi Y, Mulshine JL, Kasprzyk PG, et al: Insulin-like growth factor-I can mediate autocrine proliferation of human small cell lung cancer cell lines in vitro. J Clin Invest 82:354, 1988

105. Minuto F, Del Monte P, Barreca A, et al: Evidence for autocrine mitogenic stimulation by somatomedin-C/insulin-like growth factor I on an established human lung cancer cell line. Cancer Res 48:3716, 1988

106. Macaulay VM, Everard MJ, Teale JD, et al: Autocrine function for insulin-like growth factor I in human small cell lung cancer cell lines and fresh tumor cells. Cancer Res 50:2511, 1990

107. Reeve JG, Payne JA, Bleehen NM: Production of immunoreactive insulin-like growth factor-I (IGF-I) and IGF-I binding proteins by human lung tumors. Br J Cancer 61:727, 1990

108. Ullrich A, Gray A, Tam AW, et al: Insulin-like growth factor I receptor primary structure: Comparison with insulin receptor suggests structural determinants that define functional specificity. EMBO J 5:2503, 1986

109. Morgan DO, Edman JC, Standring DN, et al: Insulin-like growth factor II receptor as a multifunctional binding protein. Nature 329:301, 1987

110. Rotsch M, Maasberg M, Erbil C, et al: Characterization of insulin-like growth factor I receptors and growth effects in human lung cancer cell lines. J Cancer Res Clin Oncol 118:502, 1992

111. Ankrapp DP, Devan DR: Insulin-like growth factor-I and human lung fibroblast-derived insulin-like growth factor-I stimulate the proliferation of human lung carcinoma cells in vitro. Cancer Res 53:3399, 1993

112. Siegfried JM: Culture of primary lung tumors using medium conditioned by a lung carcinoma cell line. J Cell Biochem 41:91, 1989

113. Sausville E, Carney D, Battey J: The human vasopressin gene is linked to the oxytocin gene and is selectively expressed in a cultured lung cancer cell line. J Biol Chem 260:10236, 1985

114. Bliss DP, Battey JF, Linnoila RL, et al: Expression of the atrial natriuretic factor gene in small cell lung cancer tumors and tumor cell lines. J Natl Cancer Inst 82:305, 1990

115. Gross AJ, Steinberg SM, Reilley JG, et al: Atrial natriuretic factor and arginine vasopressin production in tumor cell lines from patients with lung cancer and their relationship to serum sodium. Cancer Res 53:67, 1993

116. Pettengill OS, Faulkner CS, Hurster-Hill DH, et al: Isolation and characterization of a hormone-producing cell line from human small cell anaplastic carcinoma of the lung. J Natl Cancer Inst 58:511, 1977

117. George JM, Capen CC, Phillips AS: Biosynthesis of vasopressin in vitro and ultrastructure of a bronchogenic carcinoma. J Clin Invest 51:141, 1972

118. Hong M, Moody TW: Vasopressin elevates cytosolic calcium in small cell lung cancer cells. Peptides 12:1315, 1991

119. Sethi T, Rozengurt E: Multiple neuropeptides stimulate clonal growth of small cell lung cancer: Effects of bradykinin, vasopressin, cholecystokinin, galanin, and neurotensin. Cancer Res 51:3621, 1991

120. Sethi T, Langdon S, Smyth J, et al: Growth of small cell lung

121. Osterlind K, Andersen PK: Prognostic factors in small cell lung cancer: Multivariate model based on 778 patients treated with chemotherapy with or without irradiation. Cancer Res 46:4189, 1986

122. Rawson NSB, Peto J: An overview of prognostic factors in small cell lung cancer: A report from the Subcommittee for the Management of Lung Cancer of the United Kingdom Coordinating Committee on Cancer Research. Br J Cancer 61:597, 1990

123. Sagman U, Maki E, Evans WK, et al: Small-cell carcinoma of the lung: Derivation of a prognostic staging system. J Clin Oncol 9:1639, 1991

124. Lee JS, Ro JY, Sahin AA, et al: Expression of blood-group antigen A—a favorable prognostic factor in non-small cell lung cancer. N Engl J Med 324:1084, 1991

125. Miyake M, Taki T, Hitomi S, et al: Correlation of expression of $H/L^{ey}/L^{eb}$ antigens with survival in patients with carcinoma of the lung. N Engl J Med 327:14, 1992

126. Collins S, Groudine M: Amplification of endogenous myc-related DNA sequences in a human myeloid leukaemia cell line. Nature 298:679, 1982

127. Schwab M, Alitalo K, Klempnauer KH, et al: Amplified DNA with limited homology to myc cellular oncogene is shared by human neuroblastoma cell lines and a neuroblastoma tumour. Nature 305:245, 1983

128. Nau MM, Brooks BJ, Battey J, et al: L-myc, a new myc-related gene amplified and expressed in human small cell lung cancer. Nature 318:69, 1985

129. Little CD, Nau MM, Carney DN, et al: Amplification and expression of the c-myc oncogene in human lung cancer cell lines. Nature 306:194, 1983

130. Gazdar AF, Carney DN, Nau MM, et al: Characterization of variant subclasses of small cell lung cancer cell lines having classic and variant features. Cancer Res 45:2924, 1985

131. Carney DN, Mitchell JB, Kinsella TJ: In vitro radiation and chemosensitivity of established human small cell lung cancer and its large cell morphologic variants. Cancer Res 43:2806, 1983

132. Johnson BE, Battey JF, Linnoila I, et al: Changes in the phenotype of human small cell lung cancer cell lines after transfection and expression of the c-myc. J Clin Invest 78:525, 1986

133. Brennan J, O'Connor T, Makuch RW, et al: myc family DNA amplification in 107 tumor cell lines from patients with small cell lung cancer treated with different combination chemotherapy regimens. Cancer Res 51:1708, 1991

134. Johnson BE, Makuch RW, Simmons AD, et al: myc family DNA amplification in small cell lung cancer patients' tumors and corresponding cell lines. Cancer Res 48:5163, 1988

135. Noguchi M, Hirohashi S, Hara F, et al: Heterogenous amplification of myc family oncogenes in small cell lung carcinoma. Cancer 66:2053, 1990

136. Johnson BE, Ihde DC, Makuch RW, et al: myc family oncogene amplification in tumor cell lines established from small cell lung cancer patients and its relationship to clinical status and course. J Clin Invest 79:1629, 1987

137. Yokota J, Wada M, Yoshida T, et al: Heterogeneity of lung cancer cells with respect to the amplification and rearrangement of myc family oncogenes. Oncogene 2:607, 1988

138. Kiefer PE, Bepler G, Kubasch M, et al: Amplification and expression of protooncogenes in human small cell lung cancer cell lines. Cancer Res 47:6236, 1987

139. Takahashi T, Obata Y, Sekido Y, et al: Expression and amplification of myc gene family in small cell lung cancer and its relation to biological characteristics. Cancer Res 49:2683, 1989

140. Kok K, Osinga J, Schotanus DC, et al: Amplification and expression of different myc-family genes in a tumor specimen and 3 cell lines derived from one small-cell lung cancer patient during longitudinal follow-up. Int J Cancer 44:75, 1989

141. Wong AJ, Ruppert JM, Eggleston J, et al: Gene amplification

of c-myc and N-myc in small cell carcinoma of the lung. Science 233:461, 1986

142. Gemma A, Nakajima T, Shiraishi M, et al: myc family gene abnormality in lung cancers and its relation to xenotranplantability. Cancer Res 48:6025, 1988

143. Shiraishi M, Noguchi M, Shimosato Y, et al: Amplification of protooncogenes in surgical specimens of human lung carcinomas. Cancer Res 49:6474, 1989

144. Barbacid M: ras genes. Annu Rev Biochem 56:779, 1987

145. Slebos RJC, Rodenhuis S: The ras gene family in human non-small cell lung cancer. J Natl Cancer Inst Monogr 13:23, 1992

146. Suzuki Y, Orita M, Shiraishi M, et al: Detection of ras gene mutations in human lung cancers by single-strand conformation polymorphism analysis of polymerase chain reaction products. Oncogene 5:1037, 1990

147. Mitsudomi T, Viallet J, Mulshine JL, et al: Mutations of ras genes distinguish a subset of non-small cell lung cancer cell lines from small-cell cancer cell lines. Oncogene 6:1353, 1991

148. Rodenhuis S, Van De Wetering ML, Mooi WJ, et al: Mutational activation of the K-ras oncogene: A possible pathogenetic factor in adenocarcinoma of the lung. N Engl J Med 317:929, 1987

149. Rodenhuis S, Slebos RJC, Boot AJM, et al: Incidence and possible clinical significance of K-ras oncogene activation in adenocarcinoma of the lung. Cancer Res 48:5738, 1988

150. Lung ML, Wong M, Lam WK, et al: Incidence of ras oncogene activation in lung carcinomas in Hong Kong. Cancer 70:760, 1992

151. Slebos RJC, Kibbelaar RE, Dalesio O, et al: K-ras oncogene activation as a prognostic marker in adenocarcinoma of the lung. N Engl J Med 323:561, 1990

152. Slebos RJC, Hruban RH, Dalesio O, et al: Relationship between K-ras oncogene activation and smoking in adenocarcinoma of the human lung. J Natl Cancer Inst 83:1024, 1991

153. Kobayashi T, Tsuda H, Noguchi M, et al: Association of point mutation in c-K-ras oncogene in lung adenocarcinoma with particular reference to cytologic subtypes. Cancer 66:289, 1990

154. Sugio K, Ishida T, Yokoyama H, et al: ras gene mutations as a prognostic marker in adenocarcinoma of the human lung without lymph node metastases. Cancer Res 52:2903, 1992

154a. Husgafvel-Pursiainen K, Hackman P, Ridanpaa M, et al: K-ras mutations in human adenocarcinoma of the lung: Association with smoking and occupational exposure to asbestos. Int J Cancer 53:250, 1993

154b. Rosell R, Li S, Skacel Z, et al: Prognostic impact of mutated k-ras gene in surgically resected non-small cell lung cancer patients. Oncogene 8:2407, 1993

154c. Bongiorno PF, Whyte RI, Lesser EJ, et al: Alteration of K-ras, p53, and erbB-2/neu in human lung adenocarcinomas. J Thorac Cardiovasc Surg 107:590, 1994

154d. Li ZH, Zheng J, Weiss LM, Shibata D: c-K-ras and p53 mutations occur very early in adenocarcinoma of the lung. Am J Pathol 144:303, 1994

154e. Kern JA, Slebos RJC, Top B, et al: C-erbB-2 expression and codon 12 K-ras mutations both predict shortened survival for patients with pulmonary adenocarcinomas. J Clin Invest 93:516, 1994

155. Capella G, Mitra-Cronauer S, Peinado MA, et al: Frequency and spectrum of mutations at codons 12 and 13 of the c-K-ras gene in human tumors. Environ Health Perspect 93:149, 1991

156. Vahakangas KH, Samet JM, Metcalf RA, et al: Mutations of p53 and ras gene in radon-associated lung cancer from uranium miners. Lancet 336:576, 1992

156a. Westra WH, Slebos RJC, Offerhaus GJA, et al: K-ras oncogene activation in lung adenocarcinomas from former smokers. Cancer 72:432, 1993

156b. Mao L, Hruban RH, Boyle JO, et al: Detection of oncogene mutations in sputum precedes diagnosis of lung cancer. Cancer Res 54:1634, 1994

157. Mitsudomi T, Steinberg SM, Oie HK, et al: ras gene mutations in non-small cell lung cancers are associated with shortened survival irrespective of treatment intent. Cancer Res 51:4999, 1991

158. Johnson BE, Sakaguchi AY, Gazdar AF, et al: Restriction fragment length polymorphism studies show loss of chromosome 3p alleles in small cell lung cancer patients' tumors. J Clin Invest 88:502, 1988

159. Yokota J, Wada M, Shimosato Y, et al: Loss of heterozygosity of chromosomes 3, 13, 17 in small-cell carcinoma and on chromosome 3 in adenocarcinoma of the lung. Proc Natl Acad Sci USA 84:9252, 1987

160. Waters JJ, Ibson JM, Twentyman PR, et al: Cytogenetic abnormalities in human small cell lung carcinoma: Cell lines characterized for myc gene amplification. Cancer Genet Cytogenet 30:213, 1988

161. Whang-Peng J, Kao-Shan CS, Lee EC, et al: Specific chromosome defect associated with human small-cell lung cancer: Deletion 3p(14–23). Science 215:181, 1982

162. Kok K, Osinga J, Carritt B, et al: Deletion of a DNA sequence at the chromosomal region 3p21 in all major types of lung cancer. Nature 330:578, 1987

163. DeFusco PA, Frytak S, Dahl RJ, et al: Cytogenetic studies in 11 patients with small cell carcinoma of the lung. Mayo Clin Proc 64:168, 1989

164. Wurster-Hill DH, Cannizzaro LA, Pettengill OS, et al: Cytogenetics of small cell carcinoma of the lung. Cancer Genet Cyto-genet 13:303, 1984

165. Falor WH, Ward-Skinner R, Wegryn S: A 3p deletion in small cell lung carcinoma. Cancer Genet Cytogenet 16:175, 1985

166. Ibson JW, Waters JJ, Twentyman PR, et al: Oncogene amplification and chromosomal abnormalities in small cell lung cancer. J Cell Biochem 33:267, 1987

166a. Sundaresan V, Ganly P, Hasleton P, et al: p53 and chromosome 3 abnormalities, characteristic of malignant lung tumors, are detectable in preinvasive lesions of the bronchus. Oncogene 7:1989, 1992

167. Naylor SL, Johnson BE, Minna JD, et al: Loss of heterozygosity of chromosome 3p markers in small cell lung cancer. Nature 329:451, 1987

168. Brauch H, Johnson BE, Hovis J, et al: Molecular analysis of the short arm of chromosome 3 in small cell and non-small cell carcinoma of the lung. N Engl J Med 317:1109, 1987

169. Leduc F, Brauch H, Haij C, et al: Loss of heterozygosity in a gene coding for a thyroid hormone receptor in lung cancers. Am J Hum Genet 44:282, 1989

170. Mori N, Yokota J, Oshimura M, et al: Concordant deletions of chromosome 3p and loss of heterozygosity of chromosomes 13 and 17 in small cell lung cancer. Cancer Res 49:5130, 1989

171. Brauch H, Tory K, Kotler F, et al: Molecular mapping of deletion sites in the short arm of chromosome 3 in human lung cancer. Genes Chromosom Cancer 1:240, 1990

172. Weston A, Willey JC, Modali R, et al: Differential DNA sequence deletions from chromosomes 3, 11, 13 and 17 in squamous-cell carcinoma, large-cell carcinoma and adenocarcinoma of the human lung. Proc Natl Acad Sci USA 86:5009, 1989

173. Rabbitts P, Douglas J, Daly M, et al: Frequency and extent of allelic loss in the short arm of chromosome 3 in nonsmall-cell lung cancer. Genes Chromosom Cancer 1:95, 1989

174. Rabbitts P, Bergh J, Douglas J, et al: A submicroscopic homozygous deletion at the D3S3 locus in a cell line isolated from a small cell lung carcinoma. Genes Chromosom Cancer 2:231, 1990

174a. Daly MC, Xiang RH, Buchhagen D, et al: A homozygous deletion on chromosome 3 in a small cell lung cancer cell line correlates with a region of tumor suppressor activity. Oncogene 8:1721, 1993

174b. Yamakawa K, Takahashi T, Horio Y, et al: Frequent homozygous deletions in lung cancer cell lines detected by a DNA marker located at 3p21.3-p22. Oncogene 8:327, 1993

175. Latif F, Tory K, Modi WS, et al: Molecular characterization of a large homozygous deletion in the small cell lung cancer cell line U2020: A strategy for cloning the putative tumor suppressor gene. Genes Chromosom Cancer 5:119, 1992

175a. Drabkin HA, Mendez MJ, Rabbitts PH, et al: Characterization of the submicroscopic deletion in the small-cell lung carcinoma (SCLC) cell line U2020. Genes Chromosom Cancer 5: 67, 1992

176. Friend SH, Bernards R, Rogelj S, et al: A human DNA segment with properties of the gene that predisposes to retinoblastoma and osteosarcoma. Nature 323:643, 1986

177. Lee WH, Bookstein R, Hong F, et al: Human retinoblastoma susceptibility gene: Cloning, identification and sequence. Science 235:1394, 1987

178. Drabkin H, Wright M, Jonsen M, et al: Development of a somatic cell hybrid mapping panel and molecular probes for human chromosome 3. Genomics 8:435, 1990

179. Lerman MI, Latif F, Glenn GM, et al: Isolation and regional localization of a large collection (2,000) of single-copy DNA fragments on chromosome 3 for mapping and cloning tumor suppressor genes. Hum Genet 86:567, 1991

180. Fearon ER, Cho KR, Nigro JM, et al: Identification of a chromosome 18q gene that is altered in colorectal cancers. Science 247:49, 1990

181. Ganly PS, Jarad N, Rudd RM, et al: PCR-based RFLP analysis allows genotyping of the short arm of chromosome 3 in small biopsies from patients with lung cancer. Genomics 12:221, 1992

182. Hibi K, Takahashi T, Yamakawa K, et al: Three distinct regions involved in 3p deletion in human lung cancer. Oncogene 71: 445, 1992

183. Cook RM, Burke BJ, Buchhagen DL, et al: Human aminoacylase-1: Cloning, sequence, and expression analysis of a chromosome 3p21 gene inactivated in small cell lung cancer. J Biol Chem 268:17010, 1993

184. Houle B, Leduc F, Bradley WEC: Implication of RARB in epidermoid (squamous) lung cancer. Genes Chromosom Cancer 3:358, 1991

185. LaForgia S, Morse B, Levy J, et al: Receptor protein-tyrosine phosphatase gamma is a candidate tumor suppressor gene at human chromosome 3p21. Proc Natl Acad Sci USA 88:5036, 1992

185a. Latif F, Tory K, Gnarra J, et al: Identification of the von Hippel-Lindau Disease tumor suppressor gene. Science 260:1317, 1993

186. Carritt B, Kok K, van den Berg A, et al: A gene from human chromosome 3p21 with reduced expression in small cell lung cancer. Cancer Res 52:1536, 1992

186a. Kok K, Hofstra R, Pilz A, et al: A gene in the chromosomal region 3p21 with greatly reduced expression in lung cancer is similar to the gene for ubiquitin-activating enzyme. Proc Natl Acad Sci USA 90:6071, 1993

186b. Boldog FL, Gemmill RM, Wilke CM, et al: Positional cloning of the hereditary renal cell carcinoma 3;8 chromosome translocation breakpoint. Proc Natl Acad Sci USA 90:8509, 1993

186c. Smith SE, Joseph A, Nadeau S, et al: Cloning and characterization of the human t(3;6) (p14;p11) translocation breakpoint associated with hematologic malignancies. Cancer Genet Cytogenet 71:15, 1993

186d. Satoh H, Lamb PW, Dong JT, et al: Suppression of tumorigenicity of A529 lung adenocarcinoma cells by human chromosomes 3 and 11 introduced via microcell-mediated chromosome transfer. Mol Carcinog 7:157, 1993

186e. Killary AM, Wolf ME, Giambernardi TA, et al: Definition of a tumor suppressor locus within human chromosome 3p21–p22. Proc Natl Acad Sci USA 89:10877, 1992

187. Kaye FJ, Kratzke RA, Gerster JL, et al: A single amino acid substitution results in a retinoblastoma protein defective in phosphorylation and oncoprotein binding. Proc Natl Acad Sci USA 87:6922, 1990

187a. Kratzke RA, Otterson GA, Lin AY, et al: Functional analysis of the Cys706 residue of the retinoblastoma protein. J Biol Chem 267:25998, 1992

187b. Kratzke RA, Shimizu E, Geradts J, et al: RB-mediated tumor suppression of a lung cancer cell line is abrogated by an extract enriched in extracellular matrix. Cell Growth & Diff 4:629, 1993

187c. Ookawa K, Shiseki M, Takahashi R, et al: Reconstitution of the

RB gene suppresses the growth of small-cell lung carcinoma cells carrying multiple genetic alterations. Oncogene 8:2175, 1993

188. Harris CC, Hollstein M: Clinical implications of the p53 tumor-suppressor gene. N Engl J Med 329:1318, 1993

189. Levine AJ, Momand J, Finlay CA: The p53 tumor suppressor gene. Nature 351:453, 1991

190. Hollstein M, Sidransky D, Vogelstein B, et al: p53 mutations in human cancers. Science 253:49, 1991

191. Takahasi T, Nau MM, Chiba I, et al: p53: A frequent target for genetic abnormalities in lung cancer. Science 246:491, 1989

191a. Sundaresan V, Ganly P, Hasleton P, et al: p53 and chromosome 3 abnormalities, characteristic of malignant lung tumors, are detectable in preinvasive lesions of the bronchus. Oncogene 7:1989, 1992

191b. Sozzi G, Miozzo M, Donghi R, et al: Deletions of 17p and p53 mutations in preneoplastic lesions of the lung. Cancer Res 52:6079, 1992

191c. Mitsudomi T, Lam S, Shirakusa T, Gazdar AF: Detection and sequencing of p53 gene mutations in bronchial biopsy samples in patients with lung cancer. Chest 104:362, 1993

191d. Klein N, Vignaud JM, Sadmi M, et al: Squamous metaplasia expression of protooncogenes and p53 in lung cancer patients. Lab Invest 68:26, 1993

191e. Hirano T, Franzen B, Kato H, et al: Genesis of squamous cell lung carcinoma: Sequential changes of proliferation, DNA ploidy, p53 expression. Am J Pathol 144:296, 1994

192. Suzuki H, Takahashi T, Kuroishi T, et al: p53 mutations in non-small cell lung cancer in Japan: Association between mutations and smoking. Cancer Res 52:734, 1992

192a. Ryberg D, Kure E, Lystad S, et al: p53 mutations in lung tumors: Relationship to putative susceptibility markers for cancer. Cancer Res 54:1551, 1994

193. Chiba I, Takahashi T, Nau MM, et al: Mutations in the p53 gene are frequent in primary, resected non-small cell lung cancer. Oncogene 5:1603, 1990

193a. Westra WH, Offerhaus GJ, Goodman SN, et al: Overexpression of the p53 tumor suppressor gene product in primary lung adenocarcinomas is associated with cigarette smoking. Am J Surg Pathol 17:213, 1993

193b. Gosney JR, Butt SA, Gosney MA, et al: Exposure to cigarette smoke and expression of the protein enclolded by the p53 gene in bronchial carcinoma. Ann NY Acad Sci 686:243, 1993

193c. Hiyoshi H, Matsuno Y, Kato H, et al: Clinicopathological significance of nuclear accumulation of tumor suppressor gene p53 product in primary lung cancer. Jpn J Cancer Res 83: 101, 1992

193d. Mitsudomi T, Oyama T, Kusano T, et al: Mutations of the p53 gene as a predictor of poor prognosis in patients with non-small-cell lung cancer. J Natl Cancer Inst 85:2018, 1993

194. Bodner SM, Minna JD, Jensen SM, et al: Expression of mutant p53 proteins in lung cancer correlates with the class of p53 gene mutation. Oncogene 7:743, 1992

194a. Quinlan DC, Davidson AG, Summers CL, et al: Accumulation of p53 protein correlates with a poor prognosis in human lung cancer. Cancer Res 52:4828, 1992

194b. Brambilla E, Gazzeri S, Moro D, et al: Immunohistochemical study of p53 in human lung carcinomas. Am J Pathol 143: 199, 1993

194c. McLaren R, Kuzu I, Dunnill M, et al: The relationship of p53 immunostaining to survival in carcinoma of the lung. Br J Cancer 66:735, 1992

194d. Taylor JA, Watson MA, Devereux TR, et al: p53 mutation hot-spot in radon-associated lung cancer. Lancet 343:86, 1994

194e. Takesima Y, Seyama T, Bennett WP, et al: p53 mutations in lung cancer from non-smoking atomic-bomb survivors. Lancet 342:1520, 1993

195. Takahashi T, Carbone D, Takahashi T, et al: Wild-type but not mutant p53 suppresses the growth of human lung cancer cells bearing multiple genetic lesions. Cancer Res 52:2340, 1992

195a. Fujiwara T, Grimm EA, Mukhopadhyay T, et al: A retroviral wild-type p53 expression vector penetrates human lung cancer spheroids and inhibits growth by inducing apoptosis. Cancer Res 53:4129, 1993

195b. Cajot JF, Anderson MJ, Lehman TA, et al: Growth suppression mediated by transfection of p53 in Hut292DM human lung cancer cells expressing endogenous wild-type p53 protein. Cancer Res 52:6956, 1992

195c. Cai EW, Mukhopadhyay T, Liu Y, et al: Stable expression of the wild-type p53 gene in human lung cancer cells after retrovirus-mediated gene transfer. Hum Gene Ther 4:617, 1993

196. Winter SF, Minna JD, Johnson BE, et al: Development of antibodies against p53 in lung cancer patients appears to be dependent on the type of p53 mutation. Cancer Res 52:4168, 1992

197. Morstyn G, Brown J, Novak U, et al: Heterogeneous cytogenetic abnormalities in small cell lung cancer cell lines. Cancer Res 47:3322, 1987

198. Harbour JW, Lai SL, Whang-Peng J, et al: Abnormalities in structure and expression of the human retinoblastoma gene in SCLC. Science 241:353, 1988

199. Yokota J, Akiyama T, Fung YKT, et al: Altered expression of the retinoblastoma (RB) gene in small-cell carcinoma of the lung. Oncogene 3:471, 1988

200. Horowitz JM, Park SH, Bogenmann E, et al: Frequent inactivation of the retinoblastoma anti-oncogene is restricted to a subset of human tumor cells. Proc Natl Acad Sci USA 87:2774, 1990

200a. Reissmann PT, Koga H, Takahashi R, et al: Inactivation of the retinoblastoma susceptibility gene in non-small-cell lung cancer. Oncogene 8:1913, 1993

200b. Sachse R, Murakami Y, Shiraishi M, et al: DNA aberrations at the retinoblastoma gene locus in human squamous cell carcinomas of the lung. Oncogene 9:39, 1994

200c. Xu HJ, Quinlan DC, Davidson AG, et al: Altered retinoblastoma protein expression and prognosis in early-stage non-small-cell lung carcinoma. J Natl Cancer Inst 86:695, 1994

201. Rygaard K, Sorenson GD, Pettengill OS, et al: Abnormalities in structure and expression of the retinoblastoma gene in small cell lung cancer cell lines and xenografts in nude mice. Cancer Res 50:5312, 1990

202. Hensel CH, Hsieh CL, Gazdar AF, et al: Altered structure and expression of the human retinoblastoma susceptibility gene in small cell lung cancer. Cancer Res 50:3067, 1990

203. Hensel CH, Xiang RH, Sakaguchi AY, et al: Use of the single strand conformation polymorphism technique and PCR to detect p53 gene mutations in small cell lung cancer. Oncogene 6:1067, 1991

204. Takahashi T, Suzuki H, Hida T, et al: The p53 gene is frequently mutated in small-cell lung cancer with a distinct nucleotide substitution pattern. Oncogene 6:1775, 1991

205. Lehman TA, Bennett WP, Metcalf RA, et al: p53 mutations, ras mutations, and p53-heat shock protein complexes in human lung carcinoma cell lines. Cancer Res 51:4090, 1991

206. D'Amico D, Carbone D, Mitsudomi T, et al: High frequency of somatically acquired p53 mutations in small-cell cancer cell lines and tumors. Oncogene 7:339, 1992

207. Miller CW, Simon K, Aslo A, et al: p53 mutations in human lung tumors. Cancer Res 52:1695, 1992

208. Sameshima Y, Matsuno Y, Hirohashi S, et al: Alterations of the p53 gene are common and critical events for the maintenance of malignant phenotypes in small-cell lung carcinoma. Oncogene 7:451, 1992

209. Mitsudomi T, Steinberg SM, Nau MM, et al: p53 gene mutations in non-small-cell cancer cell lines and their correlation with the presence of ras mutations and clinical features. Oncogene 7:171, 1992

210. Kishimoto Y, Murakami Y, Shiraishi M, et al: Aberrations of the p53 tumor suppressor gene in human non-small cell carcinomas of the lung. Cancer Res 52:4799, 1992

211. Takahashi T, D'Amico D, Chiba I, et al: Identifications of intronic point mutations as an alternative mechanism for p53 inactivation in lung cancer. J Clin Invest 86:363, 1990

212. Sameshima Y, Akiyama T, Mori N, et al: Point mutation of the p53 gene resulting in splicing inhibition in small cell lung carcinoma. Biochem Biophys Res Commun 173:697, 1990

213. Lohmann D, Putz B, Reich U, et al: Mutational spectrum of the p53 gene in human small-cell lung cancer and relationship to clinicopathological data. Am J Pathol 142:907, 1993

16
MOLECULAR ABNORMALITIES IN COLON AND RECTAL CANCER

ERIC R. FEARON

The development of colon and rectal cancer is undoubtedly a complex process. Among the possible causal agents and mechanisms are environmental and dietary factors and both inherited and somatic mutations. Although rather limited progress has been made over the past decade in the treatment and clinical management of patients with colorectal cancer, and particularly those with advanced disease, a great deal of progress has been made toward characterizing some of the molecular alterations that underlie the development and progression of colorectal tumors. Indeed, recombinant DNA–based studies have demonstrated quite convincingly that colorectal cancer is a genetic disease at the cellular level.[1–5] Specific alterations in both oncogenes and tumor suppressor genes have been identified in tumors of various stages. As reviewed previously in this text, activation of alleles of cellular oncogenes can result from specific mutations that alter gene function or from alterations, such as chromosomal rearrangements, that deregulate the normal controls on expression of the oncogene. In somewhat similar fashion, tumor suppressor gene function can be inactivated by specific mutations or by complete loss of the gene.[1,2] At present, only somatic (arising in nongerm cells during the patient's lifetime) genetic alterations have been detected in oncogenes. Although the majority of alterations detected in tumor suppressor genes are somatic mutations, in some cases inherited mutations also can inactivate tumor suppressor genes.[3,6,7]

The primary focus of this chapter is to review the molecular alterations present in colorectal tumors of various stages, the means by which these alterations can be identified in primary tumors, and the possible role(s) for these alterations in the biology and clinical behavior of colorectal cancer. It should be noted that a large number of clinical and histopathologic studies have provided ample documentation that many colorectal cancers do not arise de novo; rather, the majority of carcinomas are believed to arise from preexisting adenomas. Therefore, it is important to relate the molecular alterations identified with the multistep process—the natural history—of colorectal cancer. The clinical and pathologic features of colorectal tumors that are relevant to the molecular genetic studies therefore are addressed first. Then the molecular alterations, both inherited and somatic, that have been detected in adenomas and carcinomas are discussed. Finally, based on the data obtained thus far from the studies of molecular alterations in colorectal tumorigenesis, it seems reasonable to predict that molecular genetics studies will have a number of future clinical applications for improving the diagnosis and clinical management of patients with colorectal cancer. Some of these possible clinical applications are illustrated.

CLINICAL AND HISTOPATHOLOGIC STUDIES

Nearly 160,000 cases of colorectal cancer were diagnosed in the United States in 1992; about 70 per cent of those were colon cancers, and 40 to 45 per cent of the patients diagnosed with colorectal cancer will die from

340

their disease.[8] As is reviewed later in this chapter, the adenomatous polyp or adenoma is believed to be the precursor lesion to cancer in the vast majority of cases, and the number of patients with adenomatous polyps may be tenfold or greater the number with colorectal cancers. By some estimates, the prevalence of adenomas in asymptomatic individuals in the United States who are over 40 years of age is 10 to 20 per cent.[9] Thus, colorectal tumors not only represent a significant fraction of the cancer cases diagnosed annually, but may affect between 1 in 10 and 1 in 5 individuals in their lifetime.

The proposal that the majority of colorectal cancers arise from adenomatous polyps is supported by at least three independent lines of evidence. First, a small number of longitudinal studies have assessed the risk of subsequent cancer development in individuals with adenomas. A large study by Gilbertsen was perhaps the first to suggest that polypectomy resulted in a reduction in cancer incidence.[10] Perhaps a more direct demonstration has been provided in a recent study by Murakami et al.[11] These investigators either treated a sizeable cohort of patients with polyps with primary excision of their polyps or biopsied the polyps and left the polyps in situ for the duration of the study. All patients with polyps and a similar cohort of patients without polyps then were followed. Those patients who had their adenomatous polyps excised at the initiation of the study had no increased risk of cancer compared to the control group, whereas those patients whose polyps were not excised had an approximately eight-fold increase in their risk of cancer. Recent findings from the National Polypectomy Study also support the proposal that removal of adenomatous polyps significantly reduces the incidence of cancer development.[12] Second, histopathologic studies have shown that foci of carcinoma often can be detected in adenomatous polyps, particularly those of increased size, dysplasia, and villous histopathology. In addition, residual regions of adenomatous cells often are noted in cancer specimens.[13–15] Finally, individuals affected by syndromes that strongly predispose them to the development of hundreds of adenomas, such as familial adenomatous polyposis (discussed later in this chapter), invariably develop colorectal cancers by the third to fifth decades of life if their colons are not removed.[16,17] Thus, there is ample clinical and histopathologic support for the relevance of the adenoma-carcinoma sequence in the development of colorectal cancer.[13–15]

Adenomatous polyps arise from glandular epithelium, and their primary common features are the unrestricted division of the cells in the lesion and the failure of these cells to differentiate appropriately. Both gross and histopathologic features can be used to distinguish the tumors. Grossly, the lesions can be described as pedunculated (with a stalk), sessile (flat), or semi-sessile. Histopathologic features, including size, dysplasia, and glandular architecture, are used to distinguish tumors and may be useful for predicting the likelihood that a lesion contains a focus of cancer or that it will progress to cancer. Although the normal configuration of intestinal glands is maintained in adenomatous lesions with tubular architecture, the crypts are elongated and the cells in the glands are incompletely differentiated (Fig. 16–1). In villous architecture,

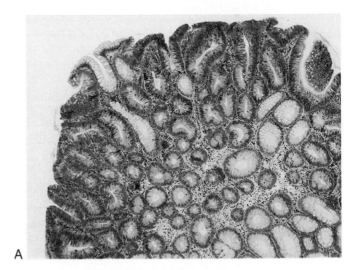

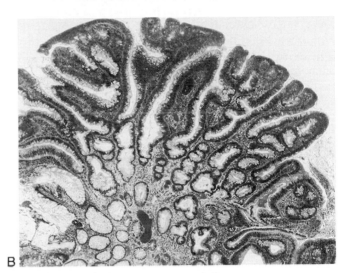

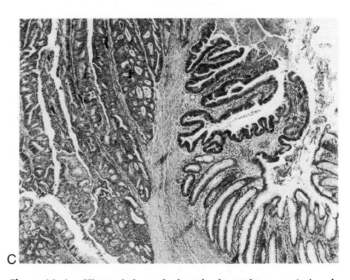

Figure 16–1. Histopathology of selected colorectal tumors. *A*, An adenoma containing glands predominantly of tubular architecture. *B*, An adenoma containing glands of predominantly villous architecture. *C*, A carcinoma that displays an adjacent region of adenomatous cells. The carcinoma glands are present at the left and a region of adenoma glands (presumably residual) is present at the right. At the extreme right is a region of normal epithelium.

the glands consist of finger-like processes extending outward from the surface of the adenoma. In many adenomas, regions of both tubular and villous architecture often can be observed.[13–15] Although exceptions to the following generalizations are common, adenomas composed predominantly of regions with tubular architecture often are smaller and have cells that are more well differentiated and less dysplastic than do adenomas that are composed predominantly of regions of tubulovillous and villous architecture.[18,19]

In addition to adenomatous polyps, other polyps, such as hyperplastic polyps, can be seen in the colon and rectum. Although some studies have suggested that the development of hyperplastic polyps may be associated with an increased risk of adenomatous polyps, most data suggest that only adenomatous polyps are capable of progressing to cancer.[13–15] At the present time, although it is presumed that only stem cells are susceptible to transformation and that one to five stem cells are present in each crypt, little is known about the precise cell population(s) within the colon that give rise to adenomatous polyps on transformation. A number of studies have suggested that adenomatous polyps arise from areas of mucosa with hyperproliferative features or abnormal tissue architecture (aberrant crypt foci).[18,19] Some of these small adenomas progress, with increases in size and cellular atypia, to larger adenomas with increased malignant potential, or even to intraepithelial neoplasia or carcinoma in situ. Finally, a subset of these lesions may progress to invasive and metastatic cancer. This multistep process of tumor initiation and progression probably occurs over a period measured in years or even decades.

At least one other clinical situation besides adenomatous polyp development provides a very marked increase in the risk of colorectal cancer—ulcerative colitis (UC). UC is a chronic inflammatory bowel disease of unknown etiology. Patients with longstanding and severe UC have a 20- to 40-fold increase in their risk of colorectal cancer compared to the general population.[14] It is generally believed that carcinomas arise in these patients as a combined result of the chronic cycles of injury to the mucosa

and its subsequent renewal and regrowth. The possible precursor lesions to cancer in patients with UC include dysplasia and flat adenomatous plaques. However, these precursor lesions, their relationship to one another and to the villous regeneration seen in UC patients, and the relative risks of progression of the various lesions are much less well defined than the adenoma-carcinoma sequence reviewed earlier.

GENETICS OF INHERITED COLORECTAL CANCER

By some estimates, more than 10 per cent of colorectal cancer cases may result, at least in part, from an inherited predisposition to the disease.[20] Clinical criteria can be used to distinguish a number of the predisposition syndromes from one another. Familial adenomatous polyposis (FAP) is an autosomal dominant syndrome that has been estimated to affect about 1 in 10,000 individuals in the United States.[16,17,20] Hundreds, and in some cases even a thousand or more, of adenomas can be seen in the large bowel and rectum of affected individuals by the third to fourth decades of life (Fig. 16–2). Although only a fraction of these adenomas progress to cancer, some inevitably do so, necessitating the prophylactic removal of the patient's colon. A number of variants of FAP have been described in which there is marked variability in the number of adenomas seen in affected individuals or in which tumors in tissues other than the colon and rectum also are seen (Table 16–1). Among these variant syndromes are Gardner syndrome, in which affected individuals have extensive polyposis, epidermoid cysts, desmoid tumors, and osteomas; and Turcot's syndrome, in which polyposis and brain tumors can be seen.[16,17,20] The gene that, when mutated, is responsible for FAP and Gardner syndrome (and perhaps other variants of adenomatous polyposis) initially was localized to chromosome 5q. Recent studies have led to the molecular cloning of this gene, termed the adenomatous polyposis coli (APC) gene (discussed in more detail

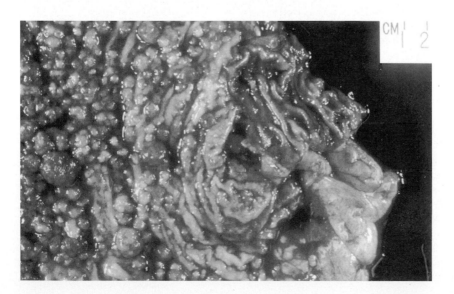

Figure 16–2. Surgical resection specimen from a patient with familial adenomatous polyposis (FAP) In the specimen, there are perhaps a hundred or more adenomatous polyps present. Some of these polyps inevitably will progress to cancer if the patient's colon is not removed prophylactically. (Photograph courtesy of Dr. David Rimm, Yale University School of Medicine.)

TABLE 16-1. GENETICS OF INHERITED COLORECTAL TUMOR SYNDROMES

SYNDROME	FEATURES SEEN IN AFFECTED INDIVIDUALS	GENE/CHROMOSOME
Familial adenomatous polyposis (FAP)	Multiple adenomatous polyps (> 100) of the large intestine; occasionally gastric polyps	*APC* gene; chromosome 5q
Gardner syndrome	Same as FAP; also, desmoid tumors, osteomas, retinal pigmentation changes	*APC* gene; chromosome 5q
Turcot's syndrome	Same as FAP; in addition, brain tumors	?*APC* gene; chromosome 5q?
Attenuated adenomatous polyposis coli	Same as FAP, except marked variation in polyp number (from 10 to >100)	*APC* gene; chromosome 5q (at least some kindreds)
Hereditary nonpolyposis colorectal cancer		Unknown
Lynch Type I	Colorectal cancer without extensive polyposis	hMSH2 gene; chromosome 2p
Lynch Type II	Colorectal cancer, stomach cancer, endometrial cancer, urothelial cancer	hMLH1 gene; chromosome 3p
Peutz-Jeghers syndrome	Hamartomatous polyps throughout the gastrointestinal (GI) tract; mucocutaneous pigmentation; estimated 9- to 13-fold increased risk of GI and non-GI cancers	Unknown
Juvenile polyposis	Multiple hamartomatous/juvenile polyps; increase in GI cancer risk is poorly defined	Unknown
Cowden's syndrome	Hamartomas of all three embryonal layers; thyroid disease—adenomas, goiter, and cancer; breast cancer; increase in GI cancer risk is poorly defined	Unknown

later in this chapter).[21-24] Other intestinal polyposis syndromes in which patients manifest nonadenomatous polyps have been described, and patients with some of these syndromes may have an increased risk of both gastrointestinal and nongastrointestinal tumors (Table 16-1). The inherited genetic alterations predisposing to these syndromes have not been identified, but they are thought to be distinct from those involved in FAP and its related variants.[20]

In addition to the inherited polyposis syndromes, several forms of inherited colorectal cancer that are not associated with extensive polyposis have been described by Lynch and others[20] (Table 16-1). Presumably, cancers in affected individuals with these hereditary nonpolyposis colorectal cancer (HNPCC) syndromes arise from adenomas through a multistep process; however, more rapid progression from a small adenoma to invasive cancer may be a feature of these syndromes. In some kindreds with the HNPCC syndromes, only colorectal cancers are seen (Lynch type I); in others, epithelial cancers other than colorectal cancer also are seen (Lynch type II).[20] The genetics of the HNPCC syndromes are described in more detail later in this chapter.

In the majority of patients with colorectal cancer, no obvious genetic component can be identified, and thus these cases are termed sporadic. Nevertheless, even some of these apparently sporadic cases may have an inherited genetic basis. Studies by Burt, Cannon-Albright, and their colleagues have suggested that a large number of the colorectal cancer cases in the general population may be due, in part, to a dominantly inherited predisposition to the development of adenomas.[25] In fact, these studies suggest the alleles predisposing to increased rates of adenoma formation may have a frequency in North American Caucasian populations of nearly 20 per cent. The variation in the number of adenomas that develop in predisposed individuals, as well as the rate at which these polyps progress to cancer, might be due to environmental or dietary agents or even other inherited genetic factors. Given the proposed frequency of the adenoma predisposition alleles in the U.S. population (approximately 20 per cent) and the frequency of colorectal cancer in the U.S. population (<4 per cent), it would be predicted that, as in FAP, only a small subset of the adenomas that arise progress to cancer.

FAMILIAL POLYPOSIS AND THE *APC* GENE

The initial observation that led to the mapping of the *APC* gene was the demonstration in 1986 by Herrera and Sandberg of an interstitial deletion on chromosome 5q, affecting band 5q21, in a unique patient with mental retardation, colorectal cancer, and extensive polyposis of the colon.[26] Subsequent linkage analyses confirmed that, in multiple kindreds with FAP or Gardner syndrome, the disease phenotype segregated with DNA markers near 5q21.[27,28] Additional molecular genetics studies eventually led to the identification and molecular cloning of the *APC* gene in 1991.[21-24] The *APC* gene is a relatively large gene, with at least 15 exons encoding a protein of 2843 amino acids. Analysis of the predicted amino acid sequence of the *APC* gene reveals no strong similarity to previously characterized proteins. Based on the absence of a number of key sequence features, the protein is predicted to be localized in the cytoplasm, although experimental studies have not yet substantiated this proposal.[21,23] The predicted coiled-coil secondary structure of the APC protein suggests that it may oligomerize with itself and/or other cellular proteins. Among the cellular proteins which complex with the APC protein are α- and β-cartenin.[28a,28b] At present, although the *APC* gene appears to be expressed in most tissues, little is known about its expression pattern in development. Similarly, the role of the *APC* gene product in the regulation of normal cell growth in the colon or other tissues is unknown.

Germline mutations have been identified thus far in one of the two *APC* alleles of affected individuals in more than two thirds of the families affected by FAP or Gardner syndrome who have been studied.[29,30] All germline *APC* mutations identified appear to inactivate the function of the gene; they include gross deletions of the gene in a few cases, and more often localized mutations that cause frameshifts or create stop codons or missense mutations in the gene product (Table 16–2). Mutations that inactivate the gene therefore are consistent with the proposed function of the *APC* gene as a tumor suppressor gene. Thus far, comparison of the nature and location of the germline mutations identified in FAP and Gardner syndrome patients (who also manifest extracolonic tumors) has yielded few, if any, insights into the variation in phenotype between these two syndromes.[24] In fact, in at least some patients, the mutations identified are identical at the DNA level in patients with Gardner syndrome to those who have only colonic polyposis. However, preliminary findings from some studies suggest that a reasonable correlation between genotype and phenotype may exist for the mutations present in the *APC* gene and the extent of polyposis seen. In one study, it was observed that the relative location of a mutation within the *APC* gene was well correlated with the severity of the disease phenotype.[30] In addition, several kindreds have been described that are remarkable in that marked variation in disease phenotype, with regard to the number of polyps that occur, can be noted between the affected family members of a single kindred. For example, in a kindred with attenuated adenomatous polyposis coli (AAPC), as this polyposis variant is termed, some affected individuals may have hundreds of polyps by their early 30s, whereas others may have only 10 to 20 polyps by 50 years of age. In at least some of these AAPC kindreds, it has been established that mutations in the *APC* gene are responsible for polyposis, although the genetic basis for the variation in phenotype between individuals who have inherited the same mutant APC allele is unclear.[31] Nevertheless, it will be of interest in future studies to ascertain if the relative location of a mutation within the *APC* gene is responsible for determining the severity and expressivity of the disease phenotype, as well as to determine the molecular basis for these relationships. Of note, preliminary studies suggest mutations in more amino-terminal APC sequences are associated with the attenuated phenotype.[31a]

Recently, in a somewhat remarkable fashion, a murine model for colorectal tumorigenesis known as the Min (for multiple intestinal neoplasia) mouse has been described.[32] The Min mouse has been found to have a germline mutation in the murine homologue of the *APC* gene.[33] Data from DNA sequence analysis of the mutant Min allele has shown that it harbors a mutation that would be predicted to result in a prematurely truncated APC protein. Presumably, this is the basis for the multiple intestinal tumors that develop in these mice. It should be noted that the intestinal tumor phenotype of Min mice is not identical to that seen in FAP patients. In particular, whereas large benign tumors of the small intestine develop in Min mice, adenomatous polyps usually are restricted to the colon and rectum in FAP and Gardner syndrome patients (although some gastric and duodenal polyps can be seen). In addition, the Min mice usually die as a result of blood loss from their large, benign tumors, rather than from invasive and metastatic colorectal cancer. Nevertheless, the Min mouse may prove to be an interesting and useful model for colorectal tumor development. It also has been shown that other cellular genes can influence significantly the number of polyps that arise in mice harboring the mutant Min allele.[34] Specifically, when the Min mutation was transferred to various genetic backgrounds, variations in the number of intestinal tumors that arose were observed. This variation in the expression and severity of the disease phenotype bears some similarity to the AAPC syndrome and to other findings reviewed earlier in this chapter, where it was suggested that an inherited genetic component for adenoma predisposition might be present in upward of 20 per cent of the North American Caucasian population.[25] Perhaps other cellular genes might modify the phenotype produced by the adenoma predisposition gene(s), such that colorectal cancers would arise only in a small subset of the individuals who inherit a predisposition allele. Recent studies have demonstrated that a gene that modifies the number of tumors arising in mice harboring that mutant Min allele maps to mouse chromosome 4.[34a] Interestingly, the modifier gene lies in a region of synteny conservation with human chromosome 1p35-36, a region frequently affected by chromosome loss events in a variety of human tumors, including those of the colon.

GENETICS OF HEREDITARY NONPOLYPOSIS COLORECTAL CANCER

For more than 25 years, HNPCC has been recognized as a distinct clinical entity. A number of investigators, including Lynch, Utsonyimama, and their colleagues, have described kindreds with apparently autosomal dominant patterns of colorectal cancer not accompanied by extensive intestinal polyposis.[20] Some studies have suggested that perhaps 5 to 10 per cent of colorectal cancer cases may be attributed to the HNPCC syndromes. As noted in Table 16–1, two different variations of the HNPCC syndrome have been described. In kindreds with the Lynch type I pattern, colorectal cancer is the sole tumor type seen. In kindreds with Lynch type II syndrome,

TABLE 16–2. NATURE OF GERMLINE MUTATIONS (*n* = 63) IN THE *APC* GENE.*

Point mutations
    Nonsense—33%
    Missense—8%

Frameshift
    Deletion (1–5 bp)—56%
    Insertion (1–2 bp)—3%

*Data on germline mutations are abstracted from refs. 29 and 30.

endometrial, stomach, hepatobiliary, and urinary tract cancers may be seen in addition to colorectal cancers (Fig. 16–3). Preliminary findings from Lynch and his colleagues suggested that, in kindreds with the Lynch type II syndrome, the predisposition gene was linked to the Kidd blood group.[35] Subsequently, the Kidd blood group was assigned to chromosome 18q.[36] In recent studies of five unrelated Finnish kindreds with features of the Lynch type II syndrome, no evidence for linkage of the disease predisposition gene to chromosome 18q has been obtained.[37] Furthermore, no evidence for linkage of chromosome 5q sequences or the *APC* gene to the HNPCC disease predisposition has been obtained.[38] Thus, a search of the entire genome for the HNPCC gene(s) was carried out. After much work, great progress has recently been made in localizing and identifying at least two of the genes responsible for HNPCC.[38a–d] Both of the genes encode proteins involved in the recognition and repair of DNA mismatches. One gene is termed hMSH2. It maps to chromosome 2p and is the homolog of the mutS bacterial mismatch repair gene. The other gene is termed hMLH1. It maps to chromosome 3p and is the homolog of the mutL bacterial mismatch repair gene. A sizeable fraction of those with the HNPCC syndrome harbor germline mutations in one allele of either the hMSH2 gene or the hMLH1 gene. In cells with one mutant and one normal allele, DNA repair is not impaired. However, inactivation of the remaining allele can occur during tumor development (e.g., in an adenoma) and thousands of errors/mutations arise as the tumor progresses. While many of these mutations may be detrimental to cell growth, a subset of the mutations are likely to activate oncogenes or inactivate tumor suppressor genes. Thus, inactivation of hMSH2 or hMLH1 gene leads to a "mutator" phenotype in tumor cells and presumably allows the small adenomas that arise in HNPCC individuals to progress rapidly to cancer.

The molecular genetic studies to date of the HNPCC syndromes are perhaps illustrative of the difficulties that can be encountered in attempting to identify genes that predispose to common adult cancers. The HNPCC syndromes are heterogeneous at the level of the disease phenotype, and perhaps this may reflect genotypic heterogeneity. Indeed, other inherited genetic diseases in humans have provided evidence that inherited mutations in several different genes can produce similar or overlapping disease phenotypes. In addition, given the possible variability in the expression of the disease phenotype and age of onset in kindreds with HNPCC, reliable identification of affected and unaffected individuals within a kindred is difficult. Indeed, the mean age of cancer onset in the Finnish HNPCC kindreds studied was 62 years.[37,38] Moreover, the lack of any clear-cut precursor lesion, such as the abundant adenomas seen in FAP patients, makes it difficult to ascertain patients affected by the disease until they may have developed and died from metastatic cancer. Nevertheless, it seems reasonable to predict that the recent progress in the molecular genetics of HNPCC should yield powerful tests for presymptomatic detection of those individuals in HNPCC kindreds who are at risk for the development of colorectal cancer.

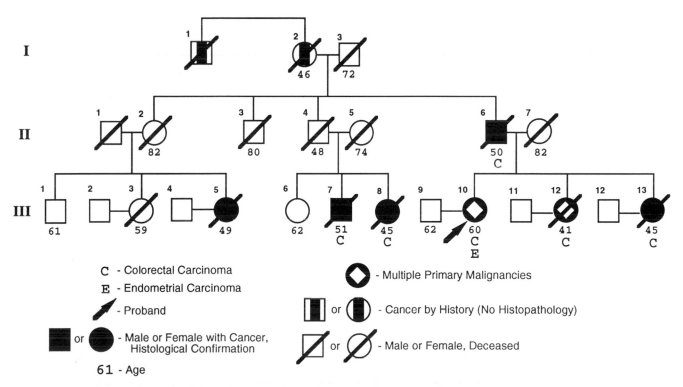

Figure 16–3. Partial pedigree of a kindred with inherited nonpolyposis colorectal cancer and other cancers (Lynch type II syndrome). The explanations for the symbols are indicated below the pedigree.

SOMATIC MUTATIONS UNDERLIE TUMOR INITIATION AND PROGRESSION

Although the specific genetic events that are responsible for the initiation of colorectal tumors are rather poorly understood, evidence suggests that both colorectal adenomas and carcinomas arise as the result of somatic mutations.[1,2] Studies of the clonal composition of carcinomas and adenomas have been carried out using recombinant DNA–based techniques to determine the pattern of X-chromosome inactivation in tumors from females.[39] The rationale for this approach is based on the observation that inactivation of one X chromosome occurs in all cells of a female at an early stage of embryonic development. The pattern of X-chromosome inactivation is maintained stably in all daughter cells, and therefore can be used to determine whether a particular cell population (such as the neoplastic cells in a tumor) arose from either one cell or a number of precursor cells (Fig. 16–4). In general, normal tissues (even very small tissue specimens) and hyperplastic and reactive lesions have been shown to have a polyclonal pattern of X inactivation, and therefore are presumed to have arisen from multiple independent cells. In contrast, leukemias and a number of advanced solid tumors each have been found to have a clonal pattern of X inactivation.

Using this X-chromosome inactivation strategy, adenomas and carcinomas from female patients with either inherited or sporadic tumors have been examined. The results of the analysis demonstrated that all colorectal tumors examined, including very small adenomas of 3 to 4 mm maximal diameter, had a clonal composition.[39] The lesions are presumed, therefore, to have had a clonal

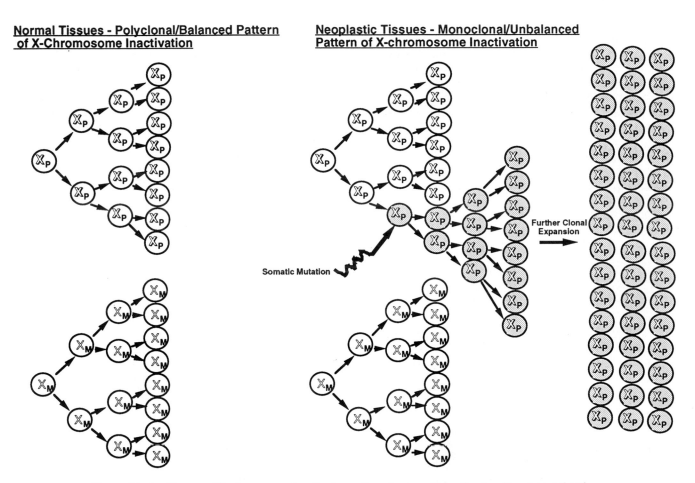

Figure 16–4. The use of X-chromosome inactivation patterns to characterize the clonality of normal and neoplastic cell populations in females. During embryogenesis, one of the two X chromosomes in the somatic cells of every female is randomly inactivated. Thus, each cell from a female has either the maternal (X_M) or paternal (X_P) X chromosome active. In normal female somatic tissues, polyclonal or balanced patterns of X-chromosome inactivation are seen. The precise ratio of active to inactive maternal X chromosomes (and similarly, paternal X chromosomes) is determined early in the development of each female; this ratio normally is distributed around the mean ratio of 50 per cent active maternal X chromosomes and 50 per cent active paternal X chromosomes. If neoplastic transformation is initiated by a rare somatic genetic event, such as a somatic mutation, and subsequent clonal expansion occurs, a tumor comprised of neoplastic cells that harbor a monoclonal or unbalanced pattern of X-chromosome inactivation can be observed. The pattern of X-chromosome inactivation in normal and tumor cell populations can be studied using recombinant DNA techniques that allow the maternal and paternal X chromosomes to be distinguished by DNA polymorphisms, and the activity of the X chromosomes can be determined by the methylation status of the DNA sequences. The results obtained in studies of the clonality of colorectal adenomas and carcinomas are reviewed in the text.

origin. In addition, examination of multiple independent adenomas from individual patients with FAP demonstrated that each tumor was a unique clone and apparently arose independently. Similar studies of the clonality of early-stage colorectal tumors also have been carried out using chimeric mice.[40] Following treatment of these mice with dietary carcinogens, mucosal lesions and tumors were studied. Analysis of small adenomas and even early dysplastic lesions from these mice demonstrated that colorectal adenomas and carcinomas, and even microscopic foci of neoplastic cells, were clonal. Normal colonic mucosa from the mice and from patients with colorectal tumors has been found to have a polyclonal composition. Therefore, the clonality data suggest that the process of clonal selection is an early event in colorectal tumorigenesis. Moreover, the observations obtained in both the human and the murine systems are consistent with the proposal that a somatic mutational event caused one or a small number of cells from a single crypt to initiate the tumorigenic process in the colon.[4]

It is generally believed that additional somatic mutations are responsible for tumor progression, and some of the alterations in oncogenes and tumor suppressor genes that are thought to be crucial to colorectal tumor progression are described later in this chapter. However, it is useful to review the rationale for inferring that the genetic alterations that have been identified are not merely associated with, but are *causal* in, tumor progression. It has been proposed that the progression of initiated, but not fully tumorigenic, cells is driven by additional somatic mutations, through cycles of somatic mutation and subsequent clonal expansion and evolution.[41,42] The genetic alterations that are of greatest interest, therefore, are those that are clonal in tumors (i.e., present in all, or nearly all, neoplastic cells of a primary tumor at any given stage but not present in the normal cells of the patient). It is inferred that such clonal genetic alterations are causal in promoting further tumor outgrowth/progression, because somatic mutations can become clonal only by a limited number of mechanisms.[42] The genetic alteration itself could have been selected for because it provided the tumor cell with a growth advantage over other tumor cell progeny, allowing it to become the predominant cell type in the tumor (clonal expansion). Alternatively, the specific alteration detected might have arisen coincident with another, perhaps undetected, alteration that was the crucial change underlying clonal outgrowth. If the specific genetic alteration can be shown to promote tumorigenesis or transformation in in vitro or animal experiments, or if the same gene or chromosomal region is affected in a particular tumor type from many different patients, it seems reasonable to suggest that the genetic alteration might indeed be causal in tumor progression.

ALTERATIONS IN ONCOGENES IN COLORECTAL TUMORS

As reviewed previously in this text, a large number of cellular oncogenes have been identified. These genes have varied but critical roles in the proper regulation of cell growth and differentiation. The normal function of oncogenes can be subverted by somatic mutations that alter either the normal activity of the oncogene product or the proper regulation of its expression.[1,2,43] Alleles of the three members of the *ras* gene family—K-*ras*, H-*ras*, and N-*ras*—frequently are altered by somatic mutations in multiple different human and animal tumor types.[44,45] In addition, multiple lines of evidence have established that these mutated *ras* alleles are critically involved in tumorigenesis.[2] Mutations in one of the three *ras* genes can be identified in approximately 50 per cent of colorectal carcinomas and in about 50 per cent of colorectal adenomas greater than 1 cm in diameter.[46] In contrast, the frequency of *ras* mutations in adenomas less than 1 cm in diameter is approximately 10 per cent or less. In studies in which the adenomas have been distinguished from one another on the basis of the degree of dysplasia, *ras* mutations are more frequently detected in tumors with increased dysplasia.[47] Thus, *ras* mutations are associated with at least two histopathologic features—increased size and dysplasia—that are predictive of progression of the lesion to cancer. Perhaps *ras* mutations have a direct role in increasing the likelihood of tumor progression.

Nevertheless, at the present time, the precise role and timing of *ras* mutations in colorectal tumor development has not been determined. Based on the increased prevalence of *ras* mutations in later-stage adenomas and carcinomas as compared to small, early adenomas, at least two possible proposed roles for *ras* mutations in colorectal tumor initiation and progression can be suggested. First, *ras* mutations may arise in one cell of a small, preexisting adenoma and may cause it to progress to a larger and more dysplastic adenoma, with a greater risk of subsequent progression to cancer. Alternatively, in a subset of adenomas, mutations in the *ras* gene may occur very early and may even be an initiating event. Perhaps the subset of adenomas with *ras* mutations increase in size and dysplasia more rapidly than adenomas without *ras* mutations. It seems likely that further studies of adenomas of various sizes and histopathologies, as well as studies of *ras* mutations in animal models of colorectal cancer, will be necessary to establish more precisely the role of *ras* mutations in the adenoma-carcinoma sequence.

The spectrum of *ras* mutations observed in colorectal tumors is also of some interest. Mutations have been detected in both the K-*ras* and N-*ras* genes in colorectal tumors, but have not been observed in the H-*ras* gene in any cases. The vast majority of the mutations detected are present at codons 12 and 13 of K-*ras* (in about 70 per cent and 18 per cent of cases, respectively, in some studies). N-*ras* mutations at codons 12, 13, and 61 are present in only a small percentage of cases. All three *ras* genes are believed to be expressed at relatively equivalent levels in colonic mucosa. In addition, specific mutations (codons 12, 13, and 61) in any of the three *ras* genes will activate those mutant alleles for in vitro transformation of rodent fibroblasts.[44,45] Therefore, the biologic basis for the spectrum of *ras* mutations observed in colorectal tumors (and several other human epithelial cancers as well) is unclear. Future studies may identify the particular cells in the mucosa that express each of the various *ras* genes at high levels, as well as the growth regulatory pathways controlled by each *ras* gene. Perhaps then it will be clear why K-*ras* mutations, but not N-*ras* and H-*ras* mutations, are observed frequently in colorectal tumors.

Although mutations in the *ras* genes are prevalent in colorectal tumors, specific alterations in the alleles of other cellular oncogenes have not been detected in a significant percentage of colorectal tumors of any stage. A number of oncogenes have been found to be amplified or rearranged in a small percentage of the cases studied. Among the oncogenes found to be affected by gene amplification are *neu* (also known as *HER-2* or *erbB-2*), c-*myc*, and *myb*[48–52] (Table 16–3); only the *trk* oncogene (encoding the nerve growth factor receptor) has been found to be activated by gene rearrangement.[53] Although specific genetic alterations affecting oncogenes other than *ras* appear to be infrequent in tumors, alterations in oncogene expression or activity have been observed to be prevalent in colorectal carcinomas. The kinase activity of c-*src* has been demonstrated to be increased in colorectal adenomas and carcinomas, without a demonstrable genetic alteration in the c-*src* locus or a concomitant increase in the level of c-Src protein present in the cells.[54] Presumably, the increased kinase activity reflects an alteration in the proteins or pathways that regulate c-*src*. In addition to alterations in oncogene activity, it has been proposed that c-*myc* gene and protein expression is increased in the majority of colorectal cancers, without accompanying alterations in the c-*myc* locus.[52,55] Astrin and co-workers have suggested that the deregulation of c-*myc* expression might be attributable to defects in trans-acting factors of regulatory pathway.[56] In particular, preliminary studies in which chromosome 5q sequences have been returned to colorectal cancer cell lines with increased c-*myc* expression suggest that a locus on chromosome 5q (perhaps the *APC* gene) might be involved in the appropriate regulation of c-*myc*. Inactivation of the function of these *trans*-acting factors and pathways results in in-

creased levels of c-*myc* in colorectal tumor cells. If the *APC* gene is involved in regulation of c-*myc* expression, it would seem likely that this regulation would not occur through direct protein-protein interactions, given the apparent localization of the APC product to the cytoplasm and the c-*myc* protein to the nucleus. The observations of increased oncogene expression and/or activity are of great interest; however, further studies are necessary to determine the functional significance of these alterations in oncogene expression or activity, in the absence of specific genetic alterations that affect the sequence, structure, or copy number of an oncogene. The alterations of c-*src* activity and c-*myc* expression may be of causal importance or may simply reflect the altered tumor phenotype.

It also should be noted that one of the major difficulties in the identification of novel oncogenes with critical roles in colorectal cancer specifically, and human tumors in general, is that only a small number of strategies for the identification of activated oncogene alleles exist. If oncogenes other than the *ras* genes play a key role in colorectal tumor development, they may fail to be identified in DNA transfection assays because they are unable to transform NIH 3T3 cells or other rodent fibroblasts in vitro. The further development of additional strategies for identification of oncogenic alleles from colorectal tumors will be necessary if a more complete picture of the role of oncogene alterations in colorectal tumors is to be obtained.

ALTERATIONS IN TUMOR SUPPRESSOR GENES IN COLORECTAL TUMORS

Alterations in Chromosome 5q and the *APC* Gene

As reviewed previously, familial polyposis, with germline mutation of the *APC* gene, is a relatively uncommon

TABLE 16–3. SOMATIC MUTATIONS IN ONCOGENES AND TUMOR SUPPRESSOR GENES IN COLORECTAL CANCER

GENE	TYPE OF MUTATION*	% OF CANCERS WITH ALTERATION
Oncogenes		
K-*ras*	Point mutation	48
N-*ras*	Point mutation	< 2
neu (HER-2/erbB-2)	Amplification	< 5
c-*myc*	Amplification	< 5
myb	Amplification	< 5
Tumor Suppressor Genes		
p53	Point mutation, LOH†	75–85
APC	Point mutation, small deletion/ insertion, LOH	> 65
DCC	LOH, insertion, deletion, point mutation	70–75
MCC	Point mutation (also 5q LOH)	10–15 (5q LOH has frequency of 40–50%)
NF-1‡	Point mutation	Unknown

*Manuscripts describing the data on the frequencies of the various mutations are referenced in the text.
†LOH, loss of heterozygosity (see text).
‡NF-1, neurofibromatosis type I gene. Only one case with a somatic mutation in the gene has been described.[83]

cause of colorectal cancer in the general population. However, recent findings suggest that mutations that inactivate the *APC* gene are of critical importance in the majority of colorectal adenomas and carcinomas. The preliminary observation that suggested inactivation of the *APC* gene might be common in colorectal tumors was that the chromosome 5q region containing the gene frequently was affected by loss-of-heterozygosity (LOH) events in colorectal adenomas and carcinomas from patients without polyposis.[46,57,58] LOH is so termed because, at a gross chromosomal level, only one of the two parental chromosome sets present in each normal cell appears to be affected in the tumor cells. However, in accord with a hypothesis originally proposed by Knudson and supported by more recent molecular studies, the remaining copy of a tumor suppressor gene within the chromosomal region affected by LOH often is found to be inactivated by more localized mutations, such as a point mutation or a small insertion or deletion.[3,6,59] Studies of LOH (also termed allelic loss) events in retinoblastoma, Wilms' tumor, and several other pediatric tumors had demonstrated previously that LOH was a common mechanism for the inactivation of one copy of the retinoblastoma and Wilms' tumor suppressor genes. Therefore, it was suspected that LOH would be a possible mechanism for the inactivation of novel tumor suppressor genes in adult tumors. The initial findings obtained from studies of sporadic adenomas and carcinomas, demonstrating LOH for 5q in approximately 40 to 50 per cent of cases, were consistent with this proposal.

Since the identification of the *APC* gene in 1991, more detailed analyses of the somatic mutations that inactivate the gene in sporadic colorectal tumors have been carried out. In general, the frequency of mutations, the nature of the mutations, and their distribution appear to be relatively similar in both adenomas and carcinomas.[60,61] Moreover, the somatic mutations identified in sporadic tumors are similar to those observed in the germline of patients with familial polyposis or Gardner syndrome (Fig. 16–5). Currently, it is believed that at least 60 to 70 per cent of colorectal tumors, regardless of their size or histopathologic status, have somatic mutations in the *APC* gene. *APC* mutations even have been found in adenomas of only 0.5 cm in maximal dimension.[61] With regard to the timing of *APC* mutations in the adenoma-carcinoma sequence, of five sporadic adenomas studied that were less than 1 cm in maximal dimension and that had *APC* mutations, only one of the lesions had a *ras* mutation.[61] Thus, based on comparison of the prevalence of *APC* mutations in small early adenomas to that of *ras* mutations, it seems reasonable to suggest that *APC* mutations may precede the development of *ras* mutations. Furthermore, somatic mutations in the *APC* gene may even be the initiating genetic event in a sizeable proportion of tumors.

In some of the sporadic colorectal tumors studied, only one copy of the *APC* gene was found to be affected by mutation,[60,61] rather than both, as might be predicted based on the Knudson hypothesis or as has been demonstrated for the retinoblastoma gene in a number of different tumor types. The following picture has emerged thus far: In some cases, the mutant APC allele may encode a protein that can function in a dominant negative fashion to inactivate the function of the wild-type protein (e.g., by oligomerization with wild-type APC and/or other cellular proteins, such as the catenins). In other cases, the change in *APC* gene dosage caused by inactivation of one allele is sufficient to alter normal APC function and may alter cell growth regulation. In support of this proposal, studies of

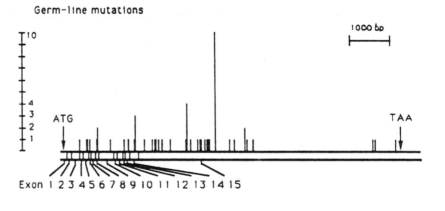

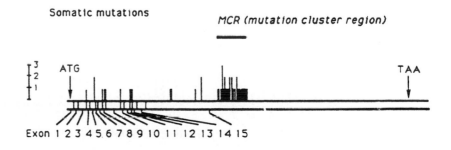

Figure 16–5. A comparison of the distribution of germline mutations and somatic mutations in the adenomatous polyposis coli (*APC*) gene. The length of the bar indicates the number of FAP patients or colorectal tumors for which germline or somatic mutations were detected at the indicated position. The relative positions of the *APC* exons are numbered, and the translation initiation (ATG) and termination (TAA) codons are marked with arrows. (From Miyoshi Y, Nagase H, Ando H, et al: Somatic mutations of the APC gene in colorectal tumors: Mutation cluster region in the APC gene. Hum Mol Genet *1*:229, 1992, with the permission of Oxford University Press.)

adenomas from patients with polyposis (and germline mutation in one *APC* allele) suggest that inactivation of the remaining wild-type *APC* allele, at least by 5q LOH, does not occur commonly in early-stage adenomas. In addition, in some studies, approximately 50 per cent or more of the *APC* somatic mutations detected were heterozygous in the tumor tissues of sporadic colorectal adenomas and carcinomas. Thus, chromosome 5q LOH is seen in combination with a specific mutation in the remaining *APC* allele in only a subset of colorectal tumors.[62] Inactivation of the remaining wild-type *APC* allele may not be a necessary event to provide a growth advantage to tumor cells; rather, it may be a progression event in some tumors from patients with or without polyposis.

In addition to the *APC* gene, another gene on chromosome 5q that is affected by somatic mutations in colorectal tumors has been identified. This gene, termed *MCC* (for "mutated in colorectal cancer"), is a candidate tumor suppressor gene.[63] The *MCC* gene maps very close to the *APC* gene in chromosome band 5q21, and is predicted to encode a protein product of 829 amino acids. The MCC protein shares little similarity with any known proteins, and virtually nothing is known about the pattern of expression of the protein or its function. Somatic mutations have been identified in the *MCC* gene in about 10 to 15 per cent of colorectal cancers; however, no germline genetic alterations have yet been identified in patients with familial polyposis or other inherited colorectal cancer syndromes. It is of interest to note that the *MCC* gene product does, however, share some similarity with the *APC* gene product.[23] Both protein products are predicted to contain heptad repeat motifs that might be capable of mediating protein-protein interactions. Perhaps the *APC* and *MCC* gene products might oligomerize with each other or an overlapping subset of proteins. Furthermore, it might be possible that the *APC* and *MCC* gene products have crucial roles in similar or overlapping growth regulatory pathways in colonic cells.

Using cytogenetic or molecular genetic techniques, the loss of chromosomal sequences other than 5q can be detected in colorectal adenomas and carcinomas.[64] It has been presumed that these LOH events also arise and are selected for during tumor development because they result in the inactivation of a tumor suppressor gene in the affected chromosomal region. Among the chromosomal regions (besides chromosome 5q) most frequently affected by LOH events in colorectal cancers are chromosomes 8p, 17p, and 18q (Fig. 16–6). Although a candidate tumor suppressor gene on chromosome 8p that might be inactivated by the allelic losses has not been identified, candidate tumor suppressor genes have been identified for chromosomes 17p and 18q, and they are discussed next.

Alterations in Chromosome 18q and the *DCC* Gene

LOH involving chromosome 18q can be identified in about 70 per cent of colorectal carcinomas, in approximately 50 per cent of large, late-stage adenomas, and in only about 10 per cent of early-stage adenomas.[46] A common region of LOH on 18q has been identified for which LOH was observed when any allelic loss involving a contiguous segment of 18q was noted. From this common region of LOH, the *DCC* (for "deleted in colorectal cancer") gene was identified on the basis of specific genetic alterations that affected the *DCC* locus in several colorectal cancer specimens, but that were not present in the normal tissues of the patients.[65] The *DCC* gene is extremely large, spanning greater than 1.35 million base pairs, and it contains 29 or more exons.[66] The predicted protein product, based on the cDNA sequences characterized thus far, contains 1447 amino acids, with a signal peptide of approximately 30 amino acids, an extracellular domain of about 1050 amino acids, a transmembrane domain of 24 amino acids, and a cytoplasmic domain of about 324 amino acids. The extracellular domain is predicted to encode a protein with similarity to the neural cell adhesion

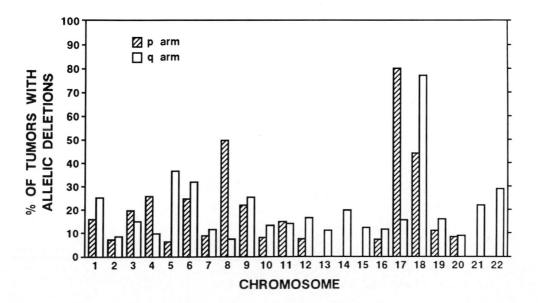

Figure 16–6. Allelotype of colorectal carcinomas. The results of loss-of-heterozygosity (LOH) studies in a group of 60 colorectal cancers are shown. DNA markers from all nonacrocentric, autosomal chromosomes were used to determine the frequency of allelic losses affecting the indicated chromosomal arms. The percentage of tumors in which allelic losses were detected is shown; chromosomes 17p, 18q, 8p, and 5q were affected most frequently. (Modified from Vogelstein B, Fearon ER, Kern SE, et al: Allelotype of colorectal carcinomas. Science *244*:207, 1989. Copyright 1989 by the AAAS, with permission.)

molecule (NCAM) family, with four immunoglobulin-like domains and six fibronectin type III domains. The cytoplasmic domain sequence of *DCC* shares little similarity with any other characterized sequences.

Several lines of evidence support the proposal that the *DCC* gene may be inactivated frequently by genetic alterations during colorectal tumor development, and thus should be considered to be a candidate tumor suppressor gene.[65,66] First, the *DCC* gene is affected by allelic losses in greater than 70 per cent of colorectal cancers. Second, although the *DCC* gene appears to be expressed in most normal tissues, including colonic mucosa, *DCC* gene expression was found to be absent or greatly reduced in over 85 per cent of the colorectal tumor cell lines studied. Finally, somatic mutations in the *DCC* gene have been observed in about 15 per cent of colorectal carcinomas. The somatic alterations detected include complete (homozygous) deletion of the 5′ region of the gene in one case, point mutations affecting intron sequences in another case, and multiple cases in which insertions were present in a specific DNA sequence immediately downstream of one of the exons. In addition, the search for mutations within either coding regions of the gene or intronic sequences immediately flanking its exons has identified several somatic point mutations that might be expected to inactivate the function of the *DCC* gene.

Nevertheless, the identification of somatic mutations affecting the *DCC* gene in colorectal tumors does not establish that the *DCC* gene functions as a tumor suppressor gene. Support for this hypothesis might be obtained by demonstrating that some aspect of the tumorigenic phenotype can be suppressed in colorectal tumor cell lines following the transfer of a normal copy of the *DCC* gene. Indeed, preliminary studies suggest that transfer of a normal copy of chromosome 18q to colorectal cancer cells, by microcell-mediated chromosome transfer, resulted in increased *DCC* gene expression in the cells and the suppression of their tumorigenic phenotype in vitro and in immunocompromised mice.[67,68] Given the similarity of the *DCC* gene product to the NCAM family, the DCC protein may be involved in the negative regulation of cell growth through recognition of extracellular signals from either cell-cell or cell–extracellular matrix interactions. Perhaps inactivation of *DCC* may be responsible, in part, for some of the alterations in cell adhesion, invasion, motility, and metastasis seen in cells from later stage colorectal lesions. However, the specific function of the *DCC* gene in normal cell growth and in the suppression of neoplastic cell growth has yet to be identified. In addition, although present data support the proposal that the *DCC* gene is inactivated in colorectal cancers, further studies are necessary to determine more precisely the prevalence of *DCC* gene inactivation in colorectal cancers, as well as the specific alterations that underlie *DCC* gene inactivation in the majority of cases.

Alterations in Chromosome 17p and the *p53* Gene

The chromosomal region most frequently affected by LOH in colorectal cancers is chromosome 17p.[64] Allelic losses affecting 17p are observed in about 75 per cent of colorectal cancers, but are seen infrequently in any stage of adenoma, including large, late-stage adenomas.[46] In some individual tumor specimens containing regions of both adenoma and carcinoma, LOH for 17p has been found to be present only in the regions that have progressed to cancer. The common region of LOH on 17p includes the *p53* gene, and multiple independent lines of evidence have provided support for the hypothesis that the wild-type *p53* gene functions as a tumor suppressor gene[69,70] (see Chapter 5). Sequence analysis of the remaining *p53* allele from a large number of colorectal carcinomas that had suffered allelic losses for 17p revealed that missense mutations were present in the overwhelming majority of cases.[71] In contrast, studies of adenomas without 17p LOH have shown that they infrequently contain mutations. Most adenomas with 17p allelic losses have been found to have *p53* mutations. Thus, point mutation of one *p53* allele coupled with loss of the remaining wild-type allele occurs frequently only in later stages of colorectal tumorigenesis (i.e., colorectal cancers). Mutations in the *p53* gene rarely are seen in adenomas, but can be seen with some frequency in the small subset of adenomas with 17p LOH. It is inferred, based on data from a limited number of colorectal primary tumor cases, that mutant *p53* alleles can exert a phenotype effect in the tumor cell, despite the presence of a wild-type *p53* allele. Presumably, with further cell divisions and tumor progression, the remaining wild-type allele is selectively lost by 17p LOH in the majority of cases. It is unknown whether 17p LOH in colorectal cancers also inactivates other tumor suppressor genes besides the *p53* gene.

The *p53* mutations observed in colorectal tumors have been found predominantly in the most conserved regions of the gene, similar to the findings obtained in studies of other human cancers. However, the spectrum of mutations differs from that seen in several other human tumor types, such as lung cancers. In particular, codons 175, 284, and 273 have been found to be mutated at a high frequency in colorectal tumors.[5,71] Based on the sequence of the codons affected and the base pair substitutions seen, the data suggest that many of the mutations in colorectal tumors may arise as the result of deamination of 5-methylcytosine bases—an endogenous process in both humans and prokaryotes—with the resultant change of a G:C base pair to an A:T base pair.[5]

There are a number of unexplained observations with regard to the role of *p53* mutations in colorectal tumorigenesis. Many of the individuals with Li-Fraumeni syndrome have been found to harbor one *p53* allele with a missense mutation. Although these individuals are at increased risk for soft tissue sarcomas, osteosarcomas, breast cancer, and leukemia, they do not appear to be at a greatly increased risk of colorectal cancer, as compared to the general population.[70] In addition, as reviewed earlier in this section, mutational inactivation of *p53* is seen frequently at later stages of colorectal tumorigenesis, but is infrequent in earlier stage tumors. Presumably, the combination of a missense mutation in one *p53* allele and loss of the wild-type *p53* allele could arise in earlier stage lesions, but there is selection for *p53* inactivation only in later stage lesions. The biologic basis for inactivation of *p53* preferentially in later stage lesions is unknown. There are at least two possible explanations for this phenomenon, which are not necessarily mutually exclusive:

1. Inactivation of the *p53* gene may provide a growth advantage in a colorectal tumor cell only when genetic alterations in oncogenes and/or other tumor suppressor genes already have occurred (i.e., the wild-type alleles of other cellular genes may modify or abrogate completely the effect of a mutated *p53* gene in a colonic cell).

2. Inactivation of the *p53* gene may be selected for at later stages of tumorigenesis because of the role of *p53* in arresting the cell cycle progression in response to DNA damage.[72] Specifically, other genetic or epigenetic alterations in the tumor cell may continually promote some degree of genetic instability and DNA damage. Following detection of this DNA damage, wild-type *p53* might be induced and cell cycle progression would be arrested. Inactivation of wild-type *p53* function at later stages of colorectal tumorigenesis would become necessary to escape this control on cell growth, and thus would allow the tumor cells to progress and develop further genetic alterations.

A GENETIC MODEL FOR COLORECTAL TUMORIGENESIS AND ITS RELEVANCE IN OTHER GASTROINTESTINAL CANCERS

Based on the data on oncogene and tumor suppressor gene alterations in colorectal tumors that has been reviewed thus far, a present view is that multiple genetic alterations are present, and presumed critical, in colorectal cancer development. These alterations have a relative temporal preference with regard to their occurrence/presence in the various stages of tumor development (Fig. 16–7). The model is based on the assumption that most carcinomas arise from preexisting adenomas through a series of stages. Each genetic alteration shown in the scheme in Figure 16–7 is seen at high frequency only at particular stages of tumor development, and this is the basis for assigning a relative order to the alterations in the multistep pathway. However, this order is not invariant, because early adenomas with *p53* mutations have been identified and K-*ras* mutations can be associated with progression to cancer in some late-stage adenomas. Furthermore, although the majority of colorectal cancers can be demonstrated to have several of the genetic alterations described in the scheme (K-*ras* oncogene activation and *APC*, *p53*, and *DCC* gene inactivations), most cases do not have all of these genetic alterations present. It seems most likely, therefore, that the accumulation and interaction of the multiple genetic alterations in the tumor cell may determine its phenotype, and may be responsible in part for the biologic and clinical heterogeneity seen in colorectal cancer. In addition, novel oncogenes and tumor suppressor genes that are critical to colorectal tumorigenesis, such as the tumor suppressor gene on chromosome 8p, remain to be identified. Therefore, although the genetic model shown in Figure 16–7 accurately reflects much of the data obtained thus far in studies of colorectal tumors, it is

likely to be incomplete and overly simplistic. Indeed, the model does not take into account alterations in the HNPCC genes, oncogene expression or activity (e.g., the c-*myc* and c-*src* genes), growth factor responsiveness, angiogenesis, cell motility, or other properties that distinguish colorectal cancer cells from normal colonic mucosal cells.

Studies of a number of other gastrointestinal tumors, including gastric, pancreatic, and biliary tract cancers, suggest that they may have present many of the genetic alterations seen in colorectal cancer. Indeed, K-*ras* gene mutations can be seen in more than 75 per cent of pancreatic adenocarcinomas, as well as in about 50 per cent of biliary tract cancers.[73,74] Missense mutations in the *p53* gene and 17p LOH have been found to be prevalent in pancreatic and gastric cancers, as well as esophageal and hepatocellular carcinomas.[75] Somatic mutations that inactivate the *APC* gene are common in gastric carcinomas.[76] Inactivation of the *DCC* gene in gastrointestinal cancers has been suggested by the presence of frequent LOH events affecting 18q in gastric and pancreatic cancers.[77,78] Thus, although the relationship of the genetic alterations observed in these other tumors to the various stages of tumor development is not yet as well elucidated as it is for colorectal tumorigenesis, it seems that there may be some common themes shared between the genetic alterations present in colorectal cancer and those present in other gastrointestinal cancers.

APPLICATIONS OF GENETIC ALTERATIONS TO CLINICAL MEDICINE

The identification of inherited and somatic genetic alterations in colorectal cancers has made possible several clinical applications that should improve the diagnosis and care of patients and families affected by colorectal cancer (Table 16–4). The identification of inherited genetic alterations that predispose to the development of adenomatous polyps or carcinomas should prove useful for determining the risk of colorectal cancer development in kindreds affected by inherited forms of colorectal tumor development. For example, the identification of the *APC* gene on chromosome 5q and the demonstration of germline alterations in the gene in more than 60 per cent of families with FAP and Gardner syndrome provide the basis for genetic counseling of families at risk for polyposis. Individuals from polyposis kindreds who are not found to have inherited a disease-causing allele will be spared anxiety and frequent colonoscopic examinations in their adolescent and early adult years. In turn, those who have inherited a mutant allele can be closely monitored, and perhaps can be treated with chemopreventive regimens to delay the onset or perhaps even prevent the development of adenomas and carcinomas. Preliminary studies by Waddell and colleagues suggest that the nonsteroidal anti-inflammatory agent Sulindac can cause regression of polyps in FAP patients.[79] Further studies will be necessary to substantiate these results and to identify additional agents, as well as to determine the basis for the effects seen.

Presently, it is possible to use either direct or indirect

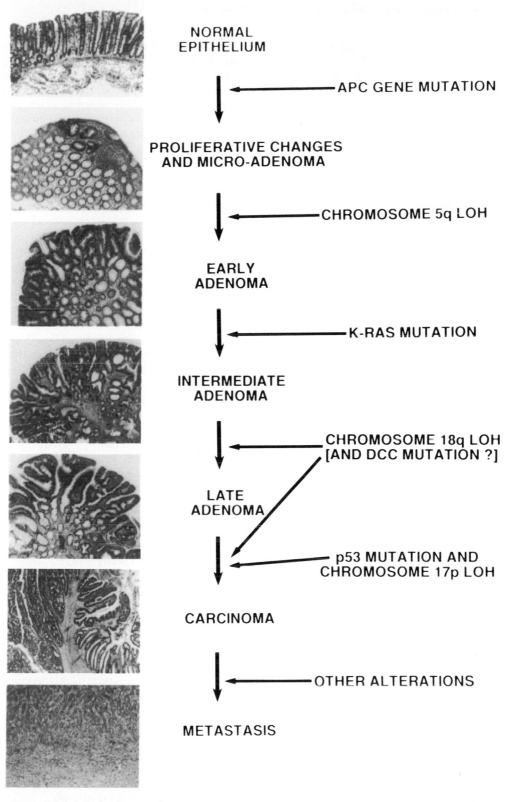

NORMAL
EPITHELIUM

⟵ APC GENE MUTATION

PROLIFERATIVE CHANGES
AND MICRO-ADENOMA

⟵ CHROMOSOME 5q LOH

EARLY
ADENOMA

⟵ K-RAS MUTATION

INTERMEDIATE
ADENOMA

⟵ CHROMOSOME 18q LOH
[AND DCC MUTATION ?]

LATE
ADENOMA

⟵ p53 MUTATION AND
CHROMOSOME 17p LOH

CARCINOMA

⟵ OTHER ALTERATIONS

METASTASIS

Figure 16–7. A genetic model for colorectal tumorigenesis. As reviewed in the text, it is proposed that, in the majority of cases, carcinomas arise from preexisting adenomas. In addition, several studies have suggested that proliferative changes in the mucosa and microscopic lesions may precede the formation of visible adenomas, both in patients with polyposis and in those without. Although multiple stages of adenomas may exist, only three are shown; in general, they represent tumors of increasing size, dysplasia, and villous content. The relative timing of the genetic events is indicated. Although a preferred order for the genetic alterations appears to exist, the order of the changes is not invariant. Thus, it seems most likely that the accumulation of multiple genetic alterations both in oncogenes and in tumor suppressor genes is most important in promoting tumor progression, not the order of the alterations per se. (From Fearon ER, Jones PA: Progressing toward a molecular description of colorectal cancer development. FASEB J 6:2783, 1992, with permission.)

detection strategies to identify which individuals within a kindred with polyposis carry mutant *APC* alleles. Prior to the identification of a specific mutation within an *APC* allele of an affected individual, linkage analysis methods can be used to determine whether a particular member of a polyposis kindred has inherited the disease-causing *APC* allele. By using polymorphic DNA markers from the *APC* locus (normal variations in the DNA sequence, not mutations in the *APC* gene that result in polyposis), the inheritance of the disease-causing *APC* allele can be traced in some kindreds with polyposis, and individuals who have inherited the mutant *APC* allele can be identified presymptomatically or even prenatally (Fig. 16–8). However, in some kindreds with few affected and/or unaffected members, using this linkage analysis method, it may not be possible to determine unambiguously whether an asymptomatic individual has inherited the disease predisposition allele or not.

For direct detection of mutant *APC* alleles in members of a polyposis kindred, the first step is to identify the specific mutant *APC* allele in any affected member. The identification of a mutation often requires detailed DNA sequencing studies of both copies of the *APC* gene. However, a rapid technique for the identification of mutations in the APC gene has recently been described.[79a] Although many of the mutant *APC* alleles that have been studied in polyposis patients have mutations that are somewhat similar to one another (see Fig. 16–5), given the large size of the *APC* gene and the multitude of different mutations that can inactivate the function of the gene, very few unrelated kindreds have been found to have identical mutations.[29,30] However, once the specific *APC* mutation in a kindred is identified, subsequent affected family members (who must carry the same mutated *APC* allele) can be identified presymptomatically by strategies such as the direct allele-specific oligonucleotide hybridization strategy illustrated in Figure 16–8. As noted previously, in about two thirds of the kindreds with FAP or Gardner syndrome, a germline mutation in the *APC* gene has been identified either in exons or in nearby flanking intron sequences.

Although FAP and Gardner syndrome are rare causes of colorectal cancer, it seems reasonable to predict that similar recombinant DNA–based strategies could be used in a more general fashion in the future to determine presymptomatically an individual's risk of colorectal cancer. Such strategies would be useful for identification of affected individuals in kindreds who have inherited genetic alterations that predispose to HNPCC, as well as to identify affected individuals in kindreds with mildly elevated rates of adenoma formation.

Molecular genetics studies also may prove useful for the specific detection of colorectal tumors at an earlier stage than is currently possible using fecal occult blood testing or through colonoscopy or radiographic studies for a patient's symptomatic complaints. It may be possible to screen for colorectal carcinomas and adenomas by identifying the mutated oncogene or tumor suppressor gene DNA sequences in tumor cells shed into the stool or blood. Similarly, some patients may produce antibodies against mutated oncogene or tumor suppressor gene products, and these antibodies could be identified in the blood. In fact, preliminary findings from studies of DNA isolated from stool samples of patients who were known to have carcinomas or large, advanced adenomas support this proposal.[80] If a K-*ras* gene mutation was present in the primary tumor specimen and the tumor specimen was of sufficient size, the mutant *ras* gene sequences could be detected readily in the DNA of cells shed into the stool. The sensitivity and specificity of the present detection system for identifying *ras* gene mutations in the stool of normal individuals and patients with various types of colorectal tumors have not been determined, nor have the preliminary results been confirmed yet in a larger study. Nevertheless, the results are encouraging given that about 50 per cent of colorectal cancers and advanced adenomas contain *ras* gene mutations. Furthermore, the results suggest that it might be possible to design similar screening strategies to detect mutations in other oncogenes and tumor suppressor genes and to detect tumors in other anatomic locations. Perhaps patients at increased risk for other gastrointestinal cancers also could be followed using molecular genetics techniques to examine epithelial cells obtained by biopsy or scraping.

In addition to presymptomatic diagnosis (risk assessment) and early detection of tumors, several studies suggest that characterization of the genetic alterations present in cancers may provide improved/increased prognostic information about the likelihood of local and distant tumor recurrence.[81,82] In the future, if differences are noted in the response rates between patients whose tumors have differing constellations of genetic alterations, it may prove useful to characterize some of the genetic alterations present in a tumor, so that a patient might receive the particular chemotherapeutic regimen that has been shown to have greatest efficacy on tumors of that specific genotype.

TABLE 16–4. CLINICAL APPLICATIONS OF GENETIC ALTERATIONS IN COLORECTAL CANCERS

INHERITED SUSCEPTIBILITY/ RISK ASSESSMENT	EARLY DETECTION OF TUMORS	PROGNOSTIC SIGNIFICANCE
APC gene/chromosome 5q markers	K-*ras* mutation	Chromosome 18q loss/*DCC* alterations
HNPCC gene(s)	N-*ras* mutation	Chromosome 17p loss/*p53* mutations
Other predisposition genes	*APC* mutation	
	p53 mutation	Multiple chromosome losses
	Other genetic alterations	K-*ras* mutations

Furthermore, some of the oncogene and tumor suppressor gene alterations in colorectal tumors may provide specific targets for novel chemotherapeutic agents. Some of these agents might antagonize or act selectively on the mutated oncogene products or the growth pathways in which they function; other agents might mimic or restore some of the normal tumor suppressor gene function in affected cells.

SUMMARY AND FUTURE DIRECTIONS

During the past decade, molecular genetics studies of colorectal tumorigenesis have yielded a number of insights into the pathogenesis of colorectal cancer. It is now evident that mutations in both oncogenes and tumor sup-

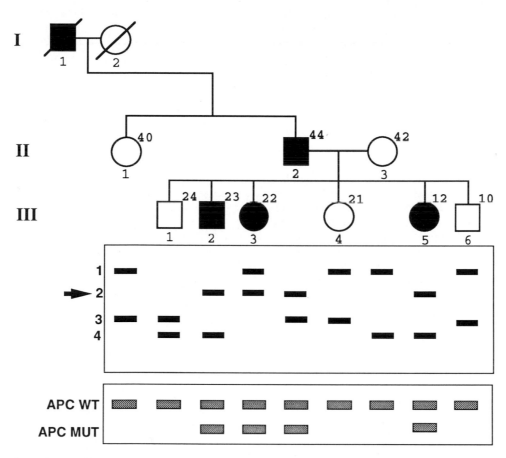

Figure 16–8. Determination of the inheritance of the familial adenomatous polyposis (FAP) syndrome by DNA analysis. A three-generation kindred with polyposis is shown. Individuals in the kindred are denoted by generation (I, II, III) and number (1, 2, 3, etc.) shown below their symbol. The age of each individual is indicated at the right above the symbol. Affected individuals, according to either clinical criteria or genetic diagnosis (individual III-5; see below), are indicated by solid symbols. Deceased individuals are denoted by symbols with slashes. In the upper panel, the patterns of DNA fragments detected by a region of the adenomatous polyposis coli (*APC*) gene exhibit polymorphism or normal variation among the population (*note*: this type of variation is *not* a mutation within the *APC* gene that alters the function of the gene). Each individual has two differently sized DNA fragments detected, corresponding to the two parental copies of chromosome 5 (and the specific *APC* gene) inherited—one from each parent. The father in the second generation (individual II-2) is affected by polyposis and has alleles 2 and 3. His wife (II-3), who is not affected, has alleles 1 and 4. Two children (III-2 and III-3) have polyposis, and two children (III-1 and III-4) have reached an age where they would be expected to have polyps but they have none. The affected children have inherited allele 2 from the father, and the unaffected children have inherited allele 3 from him. The other two children (III-5 and III-6) have not exhibited the polyposis phenotype, but are rather young. Thus, no firm diagnosis can be reached based on clinical criteria. Based on the observation that the affected individuals have inherited *APC* allele 2 from the father, the prediction would be that individual III-5 will develop polyposis because she has inherited the mutant *APC* allele from the father. Similarly, individual III-6 has inherited a normal *APC* allele from the father and he is predicted to be unaffected from polyposis. Thus, the polyposis disease phenotype can be predicted presymptomatically. In the bottom panel, if the specific mutation that causes polyposis in this kindred is identified, the mutant *APC* allele can be detected in affected individuals using a specific DNA oligonucleotide in an allele-specific oligonucleotide hybridization analysis (see Fig. 16–4). Affected individuals have both normal (APC WT) and mutant (APC MUT) *APC* alleles; unaffected individuals have only normal *APC* alleles. (Modified from Fearon ER: The genetics of colorectal tumor development: The emerging picture and clinical implications. Semin Colon Rectal Surg 2:253, 1991, with permission of WB Saunders Company.)

pressor genes are critical to tumor development. A relatively small number of oncogenes and tumor suppressor genes—the K-*ras*, *APC*, *p53*, and *DCC* genes—have been found to be altered frequently in colorectal tumors, and studies are underway to address the function and regulation of these genes in normal and neoplastic cell growth. However, much work lies ahead before a more complete understanding of the pathogenesis of colorectal cancer will be obtained. First, the relative significance to the cancer cell phenotype of each of the various inherited and somatic mutations has not yet been defined. Second, it is likely that additional oncogenes and tumor suppressor genes with important roles in colorectal cancer remain to be identified. Characterization of the function of these novel cancer-causing genes, as well as those genes already identified, will be an important but difficult task. Third, at present, there is little understanding of the relationship between dietary and environmental agents associated with increased risk of colorectal cancer and the mutation rate and nature of the mutations seen in normal and tumor cells from the colon. Finally, although some preliminary studies have suggested possible clinical applications of the molecular genetics studies to improved diagnosis and management of patients at risk for and harboring colorectal tumors, the significance and generality of the observations obtained thus far are limited. Nevertheless, an optimistic outlook is that further molecular genetic studies of colorectal tumorigenesis not only will yield insights into the molecular basis of colorectal cancer, but also will improve the diagnosis and treatment of patients with colorectal tumors.

REFERENCES

1. Bishop JM: The molecular genetics of cancer. Science 235:305, 1987
2. Weinberg RA: Oncogenes, antioncogenes, and the molecular bases of multistep carcinogenesis. Cancer Res 49:3717, 1989
3. Weinberg RA: Tumor suppressor genes. Science 254:1138, 1991
4. Fearon ER, Vogelstein B: A genetic model for colorectal tumorigenesis. Cell 61:759, 1990
5. Fearon ER, Jones PA: Progressing toward a molecular description of colorectal cancer development. FASEB J 6:2783, 1992
6. Stanbridge EJ, Cavenee WK: Heritable cancer and tumor suppressor genes: a tentative connection. *In* Weinberg RA (ed): Oncogenes and the Molecular Origins of Cancer. Cold Spring Harbor, NY, Cold Spring Harbor Laboratory Press, 1989, pp 281 306
7. Marshall CJ: Tumor suppressor genes. Cell 64:313, 1991
8. Boring CC, Squires TS, Ting T: Cancer statistics. CA Cancer J Clin 41:19, 1991
9. Eddy TM: Screening for colorectal cancer. Ann Intern Med 113:377, 1990
10. Gilbertson VA: Proctosigmoidoscopy and polypectomy in reducing the incidence of rectal cancer. Cancer 34:936, 1974
11. Murakanni R, Tsukuma H, Kanamori S, et al: Natural history of colorectal polyps and the effect of polypectomy on occurrence of subsequent cancer. Int J Cancer 46:159, 1990
12. Winawer SJ, Zauber AG, O'Brien MJ, et al: The National Polyp Study: Design, methods and characteristics of patients with newly diagnosed polyps. Cancer 70:1236, 1992
13. Muto T, Bussey HJR, Morson BC: The evolution of cancer of the colon and rectum. Cancer 36:2251, 1975
14. Cohen AM, Shenk B, Friedman MA: Colorectal cancer. *In* DeVita VT, Hellman S, Rosenberg SA (eds): Cancer: Principles and Practices of Oncology. Philadelphia, JB Lippincott Company, 1989, pp 895–964
15. Fenoglio CM, Lane N: The anatomical precursors of colorectal carcinoma. Cancer 34:819, 1974
16. Burt RW, Samowitz WS: The adenomatous polyp and the hereditary polyposis syndromes. Gastroenterol Clin North Am 17:657, 1988
17. Bussey HJR: Familial Polyposis Coli: Family Studies, Histopathology, Differential Diagnosis, and Results of Treatment. Baltimore, Johns Hopkins University Press, 1975
18. Lipkin M: Biomarkers of increased susceptibility of gastrointestinal cancer: New application to studies of cancer prevention in human subjects. Cancer Res 48:235, 1988
19. Tudek WR, Bird RP, Bruce WR: Foci of aberrant crypts in the colon of mice and rats exposed to carcinogens associated with foods. Cancer Res 49:1236, 1989
20. Utsunomiya J, Lynch HT (eds): Hereditary Colorectal Cancer. New York, Springer-Verlag, 1990
21. Groden J, Thlivers A, Samowitz W, et al: Identification and characterization of the familial adenomatous polyposis coli gene. Cell 66:589, 1991
22. Joslyn G, Carlson M, Thlivers A, et al: Identification of deletion mutations and three new genes at the familial polyposis locus. Cell 66:601, 1991
23. Kinzler KW, Nilbert MC, Su L-K, et al: Identification of FAP locus genes from chromosome 5q21. Science 253:661, 1991
24. Nishisho I, Nakamura Y, Miyoshi Y, et al: Mutations of chromosome 5q21 genes in FAP and colorectal cancer patients. Science 253:665, 1991
25. Cannon-Albright LA, Skolnick MH, Bishop DT, et al: Common inheritance of susceptibility to colonic adenomatous polyps and associated colorectal cancers. N Engl J Med 319:533, 1988
26. Herrera L, Kakati S, Gibas L, et al: Brief clinical report: Gardner syndrome in a man with an interstitial deletion of 5q. Am J Med Genet 25:473, 1986
27. Bodmer WF, Bailey C, Bodmer J, et al: Localization of the gene for familial polyposis on chromosome 5. Nature 328:614, 1987
28. Leppert M, Dobbs M, Scambler P, et al: The gene for familial polyposis coli maps to the long arm of chromosome 5. Science 238:1411, 1987
28a. Rubinfeld B, Souza B, Albert I, et al: Association of the APC gene product with β-catenin. Science 262:1731, 1993
28b. Su L-K, Vogelstein B, Kinzler KW: Association of the APC tumor suppressor protein with catenins. Science 262:1734, 1993
29. Miyoshi Y, Ando H, Nagase H, et al: Germ-line mutations of the APC gene in 53 adenomatous polyposis patients. Proc Natl Acad Sci USA 89:4452, 1992
30. Nagase H, Miyoski, Horii A, et al: Correlation between the location of germ-line mutations in the APC gene and the number of colorectal polyps in familial adenomatous polyposis patients. Cancer Res 52:4055, 1992
31. Leppert M, Burt R, Hughes JP, et al: Genetic analysis of an inherited predisposition to colon cancer in a family with a variable number of adenomatous polyps. N Engl J Med 322:904, 1990
31a. Spirio L, Olschwang S, Groden J, et al: Allelas of the APC gene: An attenuated form of familial polyposis. Cell 75:951, 1993
32. Moser AR, Pitot HC, Dove WF: A dominant mutation that predisposes to multiple intestinal neoplasm in the mouse. Science 247:322, 1990
33. Su L-K, Kinzler KW, Vogelstein B, et al: Multiple intestinal neoplasia caused by a mutation in the murine homolog of the APC gene. Science 256:668, 1992
34. Moser A, Dove W, Drinkwater W, et al: Genetic models and multistage carcinogensis in the gastrointestinal system of the mouse and rat. *In* Brugge J, Curran T, Harlow E, et al (eds): Origins of Human Cancer: A Comprehensive Review. Cold Spring Harbor, NY, Cold Spring Harbor Laboratory Press, 1991, pp 601–608
34a. Dietrich WF, Lander ES, Smith JS, et al: Genetic identification of Mom-1, a major modifier locus affecting Min-induced intestinal neoplasia in the mouse. Cell 75:631, 1993
35. Lynch HT, Scheulke GS, Kimberling WJ, et al: Hereditary non-

polyposis colorectal cancer (Lynch syndromes I and II) biomarker studies. Cancer 56:939, 1985

36. Geitvik GA, Hoyheim B, Gedde-Dahl T, et al: The Kidd (JK) blood group assigned to chromosome 18 by close linkage to a DNA-RFLP. Hum Genet 77:205, 1987

37. Peltomaki P, Sistonen P, Mecklin J-P, et al: Evidence supporting exclusion of the DCC gene and a portion of chromosome 18q as the locus for susceptibility to hereditary non-polyposis colorectal cancer in 5 kindreds. Cancer Res 51:4135, 1991

38. Peltomaki P, Sistonen P, Mecklin J-P, et al: Evidence that the MCC-APC gene region in 5q21 is not the site for susceptibility to hereditary non-polyposis colorectal carcinoma. Cancer Res 52:4530, 1992

38a. Fishel R, Lecoe K, Rao MRS, et al: The human mutator gene homolog MSH2 and its association with hereditary nonpolyposis colon cancer. Cell 75:1027, 1993

38b. Leach FS, Nicolaides NC, Papadopoulos N, et al: Mutations of a mutS homolog in hereditary nonpolyposis colorectal cancer. Cell 75:1215, 1993

38c. Bronner CE, Baker SM, Morrison PT, et al: Mutation in the DNA mismatch repair gene homologue hMLH1 is associated with hereditary nonpolyposis colon cancer. Nature 368:258, 1994

38d. Papadopoulos N, Nicolaides NC, Wei Y-F, et al: Mutation of a mutL homolog in hereditary colon cancer. Science 263:1625, 1994

39. Fearon ER, Hamilton SR, Vogelstein B: Clonal analysis of human colorectal tumors. Science 238:193, 1987

40. Ponder BAJ, Wilkinson MM: Direct examination of the clonality of carcinogen-induced colonic epithelial dysplasia in chimeric mice. J Natl Cancer Inst 77:967, 1986

41. Foulds L: The natural history of cancer. J Chron Dis 8:2, 1958

42. Nowell P: The clonal evolution of tumor cell populations. Science 194:23, 1976

43. Bishop JM: Viral oncogenes. Cell 42:23, 1985

44. Barbacid M: ras genes. Annu Rev Biochem 56:779, 1987

45. Bos JL: ras oncogene in human cancer: A review. Cancer Res 49:4682, 1989

46. Vogelstein B, Fearon ER, Hamilton SR, et al: Genetic alterations during colorectal tumor development. N Engl J Med 319:525, 1988

47. Miyaki M, Seki M, Okamoto M, et al: Genetic changes and histopathological types in colorectal tumors from patients with adenomatous polyposis. Cancer Res 50:7166, 1990

48. Alitalo K, Schwab M, Linn CC, et al: Homogeneously staining chromosomal regions contain amplified copies of an abundantly expressed cellular oncogene (c-myc) in malignant neuroendocrine cells from a human colon carcinoma. Proc Natl Acad Sci USA 80:1707, 1983

49. Alitalo K, Winquist R, Linn CC, et al: Aberrant expression of an amplified c-myb oncogene in two cell lines from a colon carcinoma. Proc Natl Acad Sci USA 81:4535, 1984

50. D'Emilia J, Bulovas K, D'Erole D, et al: Expression of the c-erbB-2 gene product (P-185) at different stages of neoplastic progression in the colon. Oncogene 4:1233, 1989

51. Ramsay RG, Thompson MA, Hayman JA, et al: Myb expression is higher in malignant human colonic carcinoma and premalignant adenomatous polyps than in normal mucosa. Cell Growth Differ 3:723, 1992

52. Melhem MF, Meisler AI, Finley GG, et al: Distribution of cells expressing myc proteins in human colorectal epithelium, polyps, and malignant tumors. Cancer Res 52:5853, 1992

53. Martin-Zanca D, Hughes SH, Barbacid M: A human oncogene formed by the fusion of truncated tropomyosin and protein tyrosine kinase sequences. Nature 319:743, 1986

54. Bolen JB, Veillette A, Schwartz AM, et al: Activation of pp60[c-src] protein kinase activity in human colon carcinoma. Proc Natl Acad Sci USA 84:2251, 1987

55. Stewart J, Evan G, Watson J, et al: Detection of the c-myc oncogene product in colonic polyps and carcinomas. Br J Cancer 53:1, 1986

56. Erisman MD, Scott JK, Astrin SM: Evidence that the FAP gene is involved in a subset of colon cancers with a complementable defect in c-myc regulation. Proc Natl Acad Sci USA 86:4264, 1989

57. Solomon E, Voss R, Hall V, et al: Chromosome 5 allele loss in human colorectal carcinomas. Nature 328:616, 1987

58. Ashton-Rickardt PG, Dunlop MG, et al: High frequency of APC loss in sporadic colorectal carcinoma due to breaks clustered in 5q21-22. Oncogene 4:1169, 1989

59. Knudson AG Jr: Hereditary cancer, oncogenes, and anti-oncogenes. Cancer Res 45:1437, 1985

60. Miyoshi Y, Nagase H, Ando H, et al: Somatic mutations of the APC gene in colorectal tumors: Mutation cluster region in the APC gene. Hum Mol Genet 1:229, 1992

61. Powell SM, Zilz N, Beazer-Barclay Y, et al: APC mutations occur early during colorectal tumorigenesis. Nature 359:235, 1992

62. Ichii S, Horii A, Nakatsuru S, et al: Inactivation of both APC alleles in an early stage of colon adenomas in a patient with familial adenomatous polyposis (FAP). Hum Mol Genet 6:387, 1992

63. Kinzler KW, Nilbert MC, Vogelstein B, et al: Identification of a gene located at chromosome 5q21 that is mutated in colorectal cancers. Science 251:1366, 1991

64. Vogelstein B, Fearon ER, Kern SE, et al: Allelotype of colorectal carcinomas. Science 244:207, 1989

65. Fearon ER, Cho KR, Nigro JM, et al: Identification of a chromosome 18q gene which is altered in colorectal cancers. Science 247:9, 1990

66. Hedrick L, Cho K, Fearon ER, et al: The role of the DCC gene in colorectal tumorigenesis. Cancer Res Clin 1:90, 1992

67. Tanaka D, Oshimura M, Kikuchi R, et al: Suppression of tumorigenicity in human colon carcinoma cells by introduction of normal chromosomes 5 or 18. Nature 349:340, 1991

68. Goyette MC, Cho K, Fasching CL, et al: Progression of colorectal cancer is associated with multiple tumor suppressor gene defects but inhibition of tumorigenicity is accomplished by correction of any single defect via chromosome transfer. Mol Cell Biol 12:1387, 1992

69. Baker SJ, Fearon ER, Nigro JM, et al: Chromosome 17 deletions and p53 gene mutations in colorectal carcinomas. Science 24:207, 1989

70. Levine AJ, Momand J, Finlay CA: The p53 tumor suppressor gene. Nature 351:453, 1991

71. Baker SJ, Preisinger AC, Jessup JM, et al: p53 gene mutations occur in combination with 17p allelic deletions as late events in colorectal tumorigenesis. Cancer Res 50:7717, 1990

72. Kastan MB, Zhan Q, El-Deiry WS, et al: A mammalian cell cycle checkpoint pathway utilizing p53 and GADD45 is defective in ataxia-telangiectasia. Cell 71:587, 1992

73. Almoguera C, Shibata D, Forrester K, et al: Most human carcinomas of the exocrine pancreas contain mutant c-k-ras genes. Cell 53:549, 1988

74. Tada M, Yokosuka O, Omata M, et al: Analysis of ras gene mutations in biliary and pancreatic tumors by polymerase chain reaction and direct sequencing. Cancer 66:930, 1990

75. Hollstein M, Sidransky D, Vogelstein B, et al: p53 mutations in human cancers. Science 253:49, 1991

76. Nakatsuru S, Yanagisawa A, Ichii S, et al: Somatic mutation of the APC gene in gastric cancer: Frequent mutations in very well differentiated adenocarcinoma and signet-ring carcinoma. Hum Mol Genet 1:559, 1992

77. Uchino S, Tsuda H, Noguchi M, et al: Frequent loss of heterozygosity at the DCC locus in gastric cancer. Cancer Res 52:3099, 1992

78. Hohne MW, Halatsch M-E, Kahl GF, et al: Frequent loss of expression of the potential tumor suppressor gene DCC in ductal pancreatic adenocarcinoma. Cancer Res 52:2616, 1992

79. Waddell WR, Gansen GF, Cerice EJ, et al: Sulindac for polyposis of the colon. Am J Surg 157:175, 1989

79a. Powell SM, Petersen GM, Krush AJ, et al: Molecular diagnosis of familial adenomatous polyposis. N Engl J Med 329:1982, 1993

80. Sidransky D, Tokino T, Hamilton SR, et al: Identification of ras oncogene mutations in the stool of patients with curable colorectal tumors. Science 256:102, 1992

81. Kern SE, Fearon ER, Tersmette KWF, et al: Allelic loss in colorectal carcinoma. JAMA 261:3099, 1989

82. Bell SM, Scott N, Cross D, et al: Prognostic value of p53 overexpression and c-Ki-ras gene mutations in colorectal cancer. Gastroenterology 104:57, 1993

83. Li Y, Bollay G, Clark R, et al: Somatic mutations in the neurofibromatosis 1 gene in human tumors. Cell 69:275, 1992

17

MOLECULAR BASIS OF BREAST CANCER

■

ROBERT B. DICKSON
MARC E. LIPPMAN

■

OVERVIEW

Description of the Disease

Breast cancer is the most prevalent malignancy in women of western industrialized nations (Europe and North America). In striking contrast, it appears to be of much lower incidence in Oriental and in developing nations. Although it is generally thought of as a disease of women, men do contract breast cancer with a frequency of 1 per cent of that observed in the opposite sex. These demographics are thought to be the result of a profound influence of the female sex hormones, diet, and other undefined environmental factors on the disease.[1]

Although breast cancer cases were described in the literature of ancient Egypt, perhaps the Greeks were the first to suspect the systemic influence of blood-borne substances (later shown to include hormones) on the disease. Hippocrates proposed that disease represented an imbalance of body humors (fluids) with universal elements. Galen pioneered the use of experimental animals and proposed that a "congestion of black bile" was the cause of cancer (which he termed *scirrhus*, a hard, heavy, malignant cancer with a tendency toward ulceration). Galen described breast cancer as a swelling with distended veins resembling a crab's legs. Thus the universal symbol for cancer initially was derived from early Greek descriptions of breast cancer.[2]

The tendency of breast and other cancers to metastasize was first clearly appreciated by the Frenchman Henri Francois le Dran in the late 17th century. He proposed that cancer was a local disease in early stages but that its later spread to the lymphatic system signaled a poorer prognosis. Probably the most important theoretical insights into breast cancer as a unique tumor type were provided by observations in the late 19th century on the con-

nection of the ovaries to the disease. In 1889, Albert Schinzer of Germany proposed the use of premenopausal oophorectomy prior to mastectomy based on his belief that the postmenopausal disease was of better prognosis than the premenopausal form. In his widely quoted papers of 1896 and 1901, George Thomas Beatson of Scotland reported the use of oophorectomy to obtain favorable responses with several breast cancer patients. The rationale for his study was based on observations that removal of the ovaries in cows prolonged lactation. He thus reasoned that interference with ovarian function in breast cancer also might have some favorable effect. In these and other early surgical experiences, it was observed that approximately one third of patients responded to this form of what eventually would be recognized as antihormonal therapy. These early insights into ovarian-breast interactions still pervade nearly all aspects of breast cancer diagnosis, treatment, prevention, and basic mechanistic research.[2]

Characteristics of Clinical Presentation

Breast cancer usually presents as a postmenopausal disease. However, as previously mentioned, it can be of particularly poor prognosis when premenopausal. The disease usually is detected as a mass by self-examination or mammography sometimes with skin involvement and nipple retraction. As mammography and biopsy methods are being increasingly applied toward early detection, smaller and smaller malignant lesions are characterized based on the appearance of microcalcifications in the tumor area and on histopathologic characteristics of frozen tissue sections.

It has been estimated that, from the time of earliest possible detection, a 1-cm tumor mass requires up to 8

358

years to grow. During this "preclinical" period, the tumor may widely metastasize to distant sites. A single metastatic site may contain 10^9 cells. Metastases seem to be detected initially in regional lymph nodes prior to more distant spread to bone, brain, lung, and other sites. The disease is staged I through IV, depending on primary tumor size, lymph node involvement, and combined histologic grading. Stages I and II are intraductal, III is locally invasive, and IV is more widely metastatic disease.[3,4]

Pathology

The first case of pathologic analysis in breast cancer diagnosis was reported in 1822 when James Elliott carried out a study of a lymph node biopsy that contained metastatic tumor cells. A major advance occurred in 1891 when William Welch, a pathologist at Johns Hopkins, reported the first use of frozen sections of tissue in breast cancer diagnosis. Current biopsy techniques also include fine-needle aspirates and nipple aspirates.[2]

Pathologic analysis of such specimens allows description of the tumor as intraductal, locally invasive, or metastatic. Furthermore, it allows appreciation of the degree of dedifferentiation of epithelial structure that has occurred (nuclear morphology and glandular characteristics) or identification of a mesenchymal-appearing tumor type. Frozen or paraffin sections and other biopsy methodologies also allow detection of specific antigens, gene expression, or gene amplifications in tumor or surrounding stromal cells by the current techniques of immunohistochemistry, flow cytometry, and in situ hybridization. Pathologic analysis of biopsy specimens has begun to allow a distinction to be drawn between benign and malignant early breast lesions. A complicated complex of fibrocystic diseases is considered to be relatively nonmalignant. Conditions termed hyperplasia, papilloma, and sclerosing adenosis are considered to have a 1.5- to 2-fold increased risk of cancer, and the condition of atypical hyperplasia is considered to have a four- to fivefold increased risk. Carcinoma in situ, a disease either of mammary secretory lobules or ductules is considered to carry an eight- to tenfold increased risk of breast cancer.[5]

Disease Syndromes

The risk of breast cancer seems to depend on a complex of familial, hormonal, and environmental factors. Epidemiologic analysis has shown that early puberty and late menopause are risk factors, whereas loss of ovarian function early in life is protective. Pregnancy is protective early in life, but becomes a risk factor after approximately 30 to 40 years of age. The possible risk associated with use of oral contraceptives or postmenopausal replacement hormones represents an area of current controversy, although they do not appear to be major risk factors. Prepubertal and pubertal exposure to ionizing radiation is also a risk factor. Much current study surrounds dietary influences, with high dietary intake of fat considered to be possibly a major risk factor. Age is clearly a strong risk factor; breast cancer is predominantly postmenopausal in onset.[1]

Finally, an especially interesting, emergent area is the study of breast cancer as an inherited tendency. Although most breast cancers are considered to be "sporadic," approximately 10 per cent are "familial," with perhaps 1 per cent considered to be "hereditary." Hereditary breast cancer is characterized by a very high incidence of the disease in association with other cancers and consistent with an autosomal dominant factor, premenopausal onset, excess bilateral disease, and multiple primary tumors. Among the hereditary syndromes that have been described are the breast-ovarian cancer syndrome, Li-Fraumeni disease (also called SBLA complex disease, for sarcoma, breast cancer, brain, lung, laryngeal, leukemia, and adrenal cortical). Cowden's disease (breast cancer plus a cutaneous condition marked by trichilemmomas), and an "extraordinary early onset" breast cancer syndrome.[6] Current studies, described later in this chapter, are beginning to unravel the molecular details of familial and hereditary breast cancer and to draw interesting parallels with mutations later in the progression of sporadic disease.

Treatment and Prevention

The first description of breast cancer treatment was that of the Greek physician Leonides, who in the 1st century A.D. described repeated incision and cautery. As previously mentioned, in the 19th century Beatson pioneered oophorectomy and in the 20th century Huggins succeeded in applying adrenalectomy in surgical-endocrine approaches to the disease. In the early 20th century, Halstead and Mager systematized radical mastectomy and theorized its importance in removing metastatic cells embedded in the regional lymph nodes. Local treatment with radiotherapy then was added to mastectomy by McWhirter of Scotland. More recently, the mastectomy has been refined to be less mutilating and the subcutaneous bilateral mastectomy has been utilized in a prevention sense for hereditary breast cancer. Also, the antiestrogenic drug tamoxifen has become a mainstay of therapy of hormone-dependent disease. In addition, cytotoxic chemotherapeutic drugs such as Adriamycin (doxorubicin) are used in both hormone-dependent and -independent breast cancer. In contrast, immunotherapy of breast cancer has not been a particularly promising avenue of investigation to the present time.[2,7,8]

Although the local therapies of surgery and radiation are highly successful in stages I and II of breast cancer, metastatic disease has required procedures combining antihormonal and chemotherapeutic drugs. Success of such combined regimens critically depends on tumor size, timing of surgery, and dosage and timing of the drugs. The use of antihormonal and cytotoxic drugs after surgery is termed adjuvant therapy, whereas preoperative drug therapy to shrink the tumor is called neoadjuvant therapy. Also, clinical trials currently are underway in the United States and United Kingdom using tamoxifen prophylactically in an attempt to decrease incidence of the disease in high-risk women.[7-9]

Prognosis

The prognosis of breast cancer and its response to therapy strongly depend on characteristics of the disease discernible by pathologic analysis. As previously mentioned, a major distinction in disease classification is whether or not lymph nodes are involved. Metastatic dissemination is a hallmark of poor prognosis. Current studies also are focused on establishing characteristics of a subset(s) of lymph node–negative disease that are of poor prognosis. Some of the most important indicators of poor prognosis are poor nuclear grade, large tumor size, and increasing numbers of lymph nodes involved. Other useful indicators of poor prognosis are a high DNA content (ploidy), a high proliferative index, and the presence of an amplified oncogene known as c-erbB_2 (described later in this chapter). Of particular interest in prognosis is the presence of the estrogen receptor (ER, pioneered by William McGuire) and the presence of the estrogen-inducible progesterone receptor (PR, pioneered by Kathryn Horowitz). These markers not only are of good prognostic value but also predict good response to antihormonal therapy.[2,4,10,11]

MOLECULAR AND CELLULAR PATHOPHYSIOLOGY OF BREAST CANCER

Hormonal Control of Mammary Development, Proliferation, and Differentiation

The regulation of normal breast development, breast carcinogenesis, and growth and progression of breast cancer is dependent on hormonal factors. The most well defined of these hormonal factors are the endocrine steroids, peptides, and other molecular molecules produced by the glandular epithelium of the ovaries, pituitary, endocrine pancreas, thyroid, and adrenal cortex (Table 17–1). These hormones act through either nuclear or cell surface receptors. In addition, normal and malignant mammary tissues themselves are able to synthesize locally acting hormone-like substances. One general class is that of the paracrine hormones, factors released by one cell type that then modulate the function of neighboring cells of the same or different mammary cell type. A second general class is that of the autocrine hormones, factors released by one cell type that act back on the same cell type through surface receptors. The polypeptide growth factors are the most widely studied of these local factors at present, but pros-

taglandins, fatty acids, and other molecular classes may serve such functions as well. Polypeptide growth factors appear to act usually through cell surface receptors, many of which function to add phosphate groups to protein substrates (protein kinases). In the mammary gland, it appears likely that the three main differential cell types (stromal, myoepithelial, and epithelial) communicate by paracrine factors and that additional autocrine mechanisms also may exist, particularly for epithelial cells[12] (Fig. 17–1).

The mammary gland develops from a prepubertal interaction between an epithelial rudiment at the nipple and underlying fatty stroma. The initial ductal penetration into the fat seems to depend only on poorly defined, local inductive factors. During puberty, ductal elongation and branching occurs. This is under positive regulation by ovarian estrogen and pituitary growth hormone (or its local mediator, the growth factor termed insulin-like growth factor I [IGF-I]. During pregnancy, the final stage in differentiation—lobuloalveolar development—occurs. This process is under the influence of many endocrine hormones: prolactin, growth hormone, insulin, glucocorticoids, estrogen, and progesterone (Table 17–1). This terminal epithelial differentiation process results in epithelial cells characterized by the ability to produce milk proteins (such as casein) and lipids.[13,14] Milk is also a very rich source of growth factors, which may be important in mammary growth and differentiation as well as in neonatal development.[15] Following weaning, withdrawal of the lactating gland from hormones of pregnancy is characterized by the programmed death process (termed apoptosis) in the differentiated luminal cells.[16,17] The cells degrade their own DNA and the tissue undergoes autoproteolytic destruction as differentiated function is lost. A somewhat similar cyclicity occurs in the proliferation and development of the gland in the normal woman undergoing cyclicity of reproductive hormones. Proliferation of the epithelium is maximal in the luteal phase as progesterone (in the presence of estrogen) peaks.[16,17] A wave of apoptosis then follows cessation of proliferation. It is particularly notable that the cyclicity of proliferation in the mammary gland is 180 degrees out of phase with that in the endometrium (where mitoses are primarily follicular). Thus, the concept of progesterone as a hormone that opposes the actions of estrogen on proliferation is without a firm basis in the breast.

It is considered probable that two different types of ovarian-controlled, hormonally dependent proliferative processes occur in the mammary gland, depending on the stage of development. During puberty, an estrogen-dependent growth may depend on expansion of the stem cell population within the invading, terminal ramifications of the ductal network. During normal cyclic proliferation and the proliferation of pregnancy-lactation, an estrogen- and progesterone-dependent growth process may depend on expansion of a different or more evoked "stem cell" population within the ducts and their terminal alveoli.[18] It is likely that each of these two distinct hormone-dependent proliferative processes also depends on poorly defined local influences from stromal cells. Such influences appear to be important throughout mammary development. Most studies of breast development, proliferation, differentia-

TABLE 17–1. ENDOCRINE HORMONES REGULATING GROWTH OF THE BREAST

Prepubertal	?
Pubertal	Estrogen, growth hormone (IGF-I)
Pregnancy/lactation	Estrogen, progesterone, insulin, thyroid hormone, growth hormone (IGF-I), prolactin, hydrocortisone
Cancer	Estrogen, progesterone (insulin, IGF-I?)

IGF-I, insulin-like growth factor type I.

tion, and carcinogenesis have focused on the epithelium. However, a rapidly developing undercurrent has become the characterization of different mammary stromal cell types and the study of their role in the aforementioned processes.[19]

An additional feature of mammary differentiation is the organizing influence exerted by the basement membrane[20] (Fig. 17–1). The basement membrane is synthesized and assembled at the interface of epithelium and its underlying stroma. Its primary constituents are collagen IV, laminin, fibronectin, and heparin sulfate proteoglycans. Regulatory influences governing its synthesis, assembly, and degradation (or remodeling) are not certain at present. However, the basally located, scattered myoepithelial cells seem to possess high levels of collagenase IV[21] and may be critical in basement membrane turnover and gland remodeling.

Hormonal Control of Breast Cancer

Breast cancer is characterized by dysregulated proliferation, sometimes by loss of certain epithelial character-

istics ("epithelial-mesenchymal transition"), by genomic instability (mutations, deletions, amplifications, and chromosomal rearrangements), and by a loss of normal organization and compartmentalization (metastasis). The classic observations by Beatson in the 1890s established the fact that endocrine influences are of primary importance in growth control of metastatic breast cancer.[22] More recent studies have implicated ovarian estrogens as primary among these endocrine influences. In rodent models of carcinogen-induced mammary cancer, it has been shown that both progesterone and estrogens are able to support initial tumor formation and early tumor growth.[23–25] It also has been shown that administration of sustained, high doses of a synthetic progestin (medroxyprogesterone acetate; MPA) to adult BALB/c mice with intact ovaries leads to development of malignant mammary tumors.[26] Presumably, the mechanism of interaction of estrogens and progestins in both normal and malignant rodent and human breast is based on the requirement of estrogen to induce expression of PR. However, other mechanisms of interaction may exist as well.[27] Current controversy continues

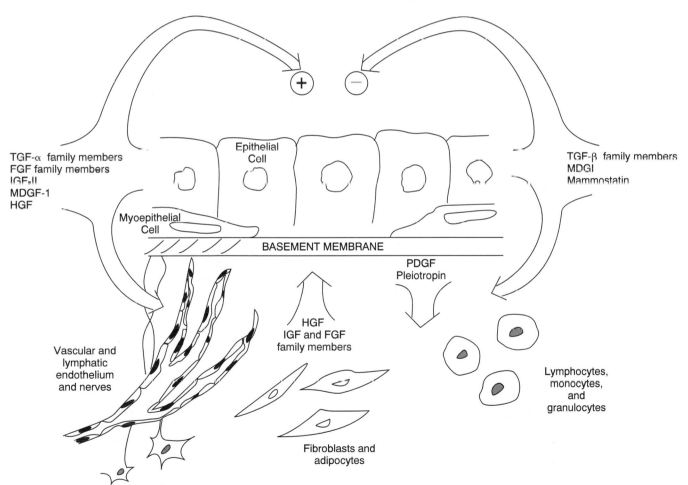

Figure 17–1. Known principal endocrine, autocrine, and paracrine regulators of breast cancer.[12] Growth factors are released by stromal and epithelial cells in the mammary gland. Both autocrine and paracrine positive and negative growth-regulatory functions have been described. Some growth factors, such as heregulin and amphiregulin, may have either positive or negative effects on the epithelium. TGF-β seems to act positively on the stroma and negatively on the epithelium. FGF, fibroblast growth factor; IGF, insulinlike growth factor; MDGF, mammary-derived growth factor; MDGI, mammary-derived growth inhibitor; PDGF, platelet-derived growth factor; TGF, transforming growth factor; HGF, hepatocyte growth factor.

to surround both estrogenic and progestational components of oral contraceptives as risk factors in developing breast cancer,[16,28,29] although it now appears that the majority of women taking these drugs do not have an increased risk of breast cancer.[29] Established risk factors in breast cancer are a family history, prior patient history, a prolonged reproductive phase of life, a late pregnancy, and a high-fat diet (although the latter is still controversial). An early pregnancy is protective.[1]

Estrogen and progesterone receptors have been localized to a luminal subpopulation of ductal and lobular epithelial cells in women and rodents. Paradoxically, receptors appear to be absent from terminal end bud epithelial cells in rodents, the most proliferative region of the gland. Thus, ER and PR appear to be present in at least partially differentiated epithelium. It is not yet clear whether these steroid receptor–positive cells are precursors to breast cancer, although circumstantial evidence would appear to suggest the possibility.[30,31] Hormonal responsiveness is evident in about one third of breast cancers by the time they are metastatic. In human breast cancer treatment, a variety of antihormonal therapies such as ovariectomy, hypophysectomy, luteinizing hormone–releasing hormone (LHRH) agonists, antiestrogen, and antiprogestin, as well as high-dose estrogen or progestin, have been used successfully to control metastatic disease.[7,8]

As a class, hormone unresponsive, ER- and PR-negative breast cancers seem to differ in many respects from their steroid receptor–positive counterparts. These differences encompass proliferative and invasive rates in vivo and in vitro, expression of certain growth factor receptors, enzymes of drug metabolism, morphology, and other loosely defined indicators of differentiation. These differences do not appear to be random but would seem to indicate at least two distinct stages of differentiation or biologic types of breast cancer.[5,11,32] It is not yet clear whether this comes about because of different cell types of tumor origin or because of different stages of malignant progression from a single cancer precursor. It is of note that essentially all breast cancers possess a ductal luminal keratin signature.[33] Furthermore, ER-positive cell lines have been observed in vitro (but not yet in the patient) to acquire multiple characteristics of ER-negative lines during acquisition of resistance to stepwise increasing concentration of the chemotherapeutic drug Adriamycin or during prolonged withdrawal from estrogen.[32] These observations would tend to argue that breast cancers may be derived from a luminal stage of differentiation and that malignant progression could encompass wholesale phenotypic modulations within this luminal lineage.

Estrogen and Progesterone Receptors

ROLE OF ESTROGEN AND PROGESTINS IN HUMAN BREAST CANCER

Because breast cancer is characterized by hormonal control of its growth, measurements of levels of the ER currently are used to predict which patients have a good prognosis and may benefit from antihormonal therapy. Although qualitative or quantitative measurements of the ER are employed to predict the responsivity of a tumor to antihormonal therapy, the response to such endocrine therapy is not absolute. Significant levels of ER have been detected in more than 60 per cent of human breast cancers. However, at best, only two thirds of these ER-positive tumors respond to endocrine therapy.[34–37] In addition, 5 to 10 per cent of those patients identified as ER-negative respond to endocrine therapy.[38,39] To increase the prognostic value of the ER, the presence of an estrogen-regulated protein such as the PR also has been measured. In normal endometrial tissue as well as in breast cancer cell lines, PR expression is positively regulated by estrogen.[40,41] It is not yet known if ER regulates PR in normal human mammary epithelium or if ER and PR coexist in the same luminal cells. Although the presence of PR improves the predictability of hormone dependency of a tumor, this relationship is not perfect. Retrospective studies show that only 70 per cent of PR-positive and 25 to 30 per cent of PR-negative tumors respond to hormone therapy. The reasons for the discrepancies among the levels of receptors and their predictive values are not completely clear but may be attributed to laboratory error, to differential metabolism of tamoxifen, to the ability of defective ER to regulate gene expression in the absence of ligand, to the ability of defective ER to bind ligand but not regulate gene expression, or to the constitutive synthesis of estrogen-regulated proteins independent of a functional ER pathway. Of particular interest are recent studies[42–44] establishing that mutant ERs with the potential to be constitutively activated appear to be common in breast cancer. Additional ER assays, such as binding of the ER to an estrogen-responsive DNA element (ERE) or mutational analysis of ER by the polymerase chain reaction or other techniques, may be necessary to predict more accurately tumor response to endocrine therapy.

Some uncertainty underlies the function of ER as expressed endogenously versus heterotypically by expression vector in formerly ER-negative breast cancer cell lines. Several groups have shown that, in contrast to its function in ER-positive cell lines, ER expressed in ER-negative cell lines functions to suppress cell growth while functioning normally in other respects to regulate expression of certain responsive genes.[45,46] It is not yet known whether the lack of expression of ER in ER-negative breast cancer is due to dominant or recessive mechanisms at the level of the endogenous gene. A recent study with an antiestrogen-resistant, ER-positive but PR-negative subline of MCF-7 suggests that loss of PR expression is a recessive phenotype.[47] Other studies have begun to implicate the cellular enzyme protein kinase C (PKC) in down-modulation of ER, inactivation of ER function, and independently inducing some estrogen-responsive genes during malignant progression. PKC is an intracellular enzyme with serine-threonine specificity for phosphate addition to other cellular proteins. It has been observed that PKC is expressed to an elevated extent in ER-negative and drug-resistant breast cancer relative to ER-positive breast cancer. Stimulation of ER-positive breast cancer with an activator of PKC, the phorbol ester 12-O-tetradeanoylphorbol-13-acetate (TPA or PMA), leads to down-

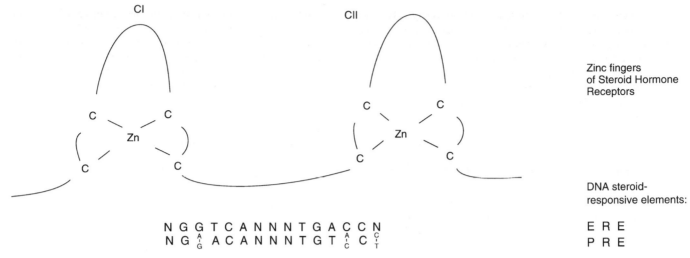

Figure 17–2. DNA-binding zinc finger structures of steroid receptors and the consensus elements for DNA binding of receptors for estrogen and progesterone.[315] CI, first zinc finger (C is cysteine, coordinately bonded to zinc); CII, second zinc finger; ERE, estrogen-responsive element (binds to zinc fingers of estrogen receptor); PRE, progestin-responsive element (binds to zinc fingers of progesterone, glucocorticoid, or androgen receptor); A, T, C, and G, specific nucleotides; N, any of the four nucleotides.

regulation of ER and destabilization of its mRNA, and phosphorylation of residual ER coincident with loss of its function.[48,49] Other current investigations suggest that other sites of phosphorylation of ER and PR induced by growth factors, dopamine agonists, and cAMP and that other hormones may constitutively activate the steroid receptors.[50,51]

MECHANISMS OF STEROID HORMONE ACTION

Receptors for steroid hormone are members of a class of *trans*-acting factors that stimulate gene transcription by binding to specific DNA elements termed hormone responsive elements (HREs) (Fig. 17–2). These genetic elements generally are located in the promoter regions of responsive genes (for review, see ref. 52). It has been demonstrated that these HREs have a palindromic sequence and exhibit the properties of "enhancers" of transcription. Enhancers exert their action in an orientation-independent manner when situated at variable distances upstream from gene promoters.[53] It also has become evident that nonclassic ERE may exist. For example, it was shown recently that ER can modulate transcription after binding to AP-1 sites, previously thought to be specific for *fos/jun* transcription factors.[54] Because the stimulation of transcription of steroid-responsive genes is dependent on binding of steroids to their cognate receptors, these receptors represent inducible enhancers. It has become increasingly evident that, in addition to regulation of transcription, steroid hormone action involves posttranscriptional regulation of mRNA stability[53] and regulation of translation of mRNA to protein.[55] However, the biochemical mechanisms of the effects are not fully understood at present.

Steroid receptors are encoded by a family of closely related genes that include the glucocorticoid, progesterone, androgen, mineralocorticoid, estrogen, thyroid, retinoic acid, and vitamin D receptors and a collection of "orphan" receptor-like genes (for review, see ref. 56). All known receptors in this family of genes appear to be structured in a similar way. There are two forms of the PR, termed A and B; they are closely related proteins derived from the same gene. In contrast, only a single form of the ER is known to exist. The ER, a 66-kDa protein originally was divided into domains termed A through F based on regions of sequence homology comparing the human and chicken forms (Fig. 17–3). Region A/B is the variable amino-terminal region of the receptor; it has a modulatory effect on the *trans*-activation of transcription.[42] The conserved central domain, region C, is a short, cysteine-rich region that corresponds to a DNA-binding domain. Two DNA-binding "fingers" are formed when the cysteines

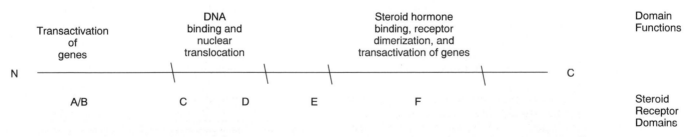

Figure 17–3. Domain structure of receptors for estrogen and progesterone and other steroid hormones.[54]

tetrahedrally coordinate a zinc ion; the intervening amino acids form regions that interact with specific DNA sequences. The amino-terminal zinc finger contacts the major groove of one half of the palindrome of the ERE, whereas the carboxy-terminal zinc finger contacts the sugar phosphate backbone of the flanking sequences. In addition to a role in DNA binding, the amino-terminal zinc finger appears to play a role in *trans*-activation of genes. Structurally and functionally, the most complex region of the receptor is the carboxy-terminal domain (regions D, E, and F). Region E is the hydrophobic hormone-binding domain; it forms a hydrophobic pocket for estradiol. Region E also appears to contain an estradiol-inducible transcription activation function (TAF) and a heat shock protein-binding domain.[57] Region D is believed to function as a hinge between the hormone- and DNA-binding domains.[57] In the absence of steroid, the DNA-binding domain is masked by the hormone-binding domain; binding of hormone appears to relieve this masking effect. Recently it has been suggested that region D also mediates certain inhibitory effects of the ER on gene transcription. The carboxy-terminal regions also play a role in the hormone-induced dimerization of the receptor[58]; a weak, constitutive dimerization domain also is found in the DNA-binding domain. The importance of receptor dimerization for action of ER has been underscored recently by the characterization of a dominant-negative variant of the ER.[59] Also, it has been proposed that the most potent, pharmacologically pure antiestrogens and antiprogestins prevent dimerization of their cognate receptors.[60]

REGULATION OF ESTROGEN AND PROGESTERONE RECEPTOR EXPRESSION

Expression of the ER in human breast cancer appears to be a complex process involving multiple steps, many of which themselves are subject to regulation by estrogen. Previously it had been shown that treatment of MCF-7 breast cancer cells with estrogen results in a down-regulation of estrogen-binding sites.[61–64] Recent studies indicate that transcriptional as well as posttranscriptional events contribute to the estrogen-induced decrease in ER expression.[65] Treatment of MCF-7 cells with estrogen results in the decline in the steady-state level of ER protein. The level of ER binding also decreases in a manner similar to the decline in receptor protein. The decline in receptor protein to a new steady-state level accompanies a parallel decrease in the level of receptor mRNA.[66–68] In contrast to the effect on protein and mRNA, estrogen treatment results in a transiently decreased transcription of the ER gene followed by an enhanced transcriptional level. The regulation by ER by its own mRNA has been observed to depend on cellular protein synthesis,[69] tissue culture conditions, and individual characteristics of cell lines[66–71] or tissues.[72–74] These findings suggest that estrogen may function at transcriptional, translational, and perhaps posttranslational levels.

In addition to ER receptor, autoregulation has been demonstrated for other steroid hormones, such as progestins,[75,76] glucocorticoids,[77–80] and thyroid hormones.[81] Autoregulation of the PR by progestins also has been demonstrated in the breast cancer cell lines MCF-7[76] and T47D.[75–78] Treatment of breast cancer cells with progestins results in a suppression of PR expression. The decline in receptor protein accompanies a parallel decrease in the steady-state level of PR mRNA and a decrease in the level of PR gene transcription. In contrast to the effects of estrogen on ER expression, progestins have no effect on PR mRNA half-life but mediate a decrease in PR protein half-life.[77] It appears that the predominant mechanisms regulating PR expression are transcriptional and posttranslational events.

Growth Factors

LOCAL REGULATION OF PROLIFERATION AND INTERACTION WITH ESTROGEN AND PROGESTERONE

Recent studies have begun to address the local tissue mechanisms of action of estrogen and progesterone in the promotion and growth of malignancy. A poorly understood serum requirement has been characterized as necessary for estrogen- or progesterone-regulated, anchorage-independent proliferation of steroid receptor–positive breast cancer.[82,83] Many investigators also are examining defective or overexpressed growth-regulatory genes (oncogenes or proto-oncogenes) and locally acting polypeptide hormones (growth factors) as mediators and modulators of steroid action (Table 17–2). Early studies identified the transforming growth factors (TGFs) in breast cancer. TGFs derive their name from their ability to reversibly induce the transformed phenotype (initially defined as the capacity for anchorage-independent growth) in certain rodent fibroblasts. They are a diverse group of polypeptides that initially were found to be synthesized and secreted by a variety of retrovirally, chemically, or oncogene-transformed human and rodent cell lines.[84–87]

Two major classes of structurally and functionally distinct TGF families are the TGF-α and TGF-β families. TGF-α and TGF-α–like peptides are members of a mul-

TABLE 17–2. PROTEINS KNOWN TO BE DIFFERENTIALLY REGULATED BY ESTROGEN AND PROGESTERONE IN BREAST CANCER

	ESTROGEN	PROGESTERONE
Induced	TGF-α	TGF-α
	EGF	EGF
	Amphiregulin	
	EGF receptor	EGF receptor
	pS2	pS2
	IGF-II	IGF-II
	c-*myc*	c-*myc*
	c-*fos*	c-*fos*
	c-*jun*	c-*jun*
	Cathepsin D	Cathepsin D
	Progesterone receptor	Fatty acid synthetase
Inhibited	c-*erbB*₂	c-*erbB*₂
	TGF-β₁	TGF-β₁
	TGF-β₂	

TGF, transforming growth factor; EGF, epidermal growth factor; IGF-II, insulin-like growth factor type II.

TABLE 17–3. TYROSINE KINASE–ASSOCIATED RECEPTORS IN BREAST CANCER

EPITHELIAL*	STROMAL
EGF	EGF
FGF*	FGF†
c-*erbB₂*	PDGF
c-*erbB₃*	Insulin
c-*erbB₄*	IGF-I
Insulin	
c-met	
IGF-I	

*Tyrosine kinase–associated receptor for the mammary-derived growth factor MDGF-1 also has been detected in mammary epithelium and stroma but has not been fully characterized in either cell type.[109]

FGF, fibroblast growth factor; PDGF, platelet-derived growth factor; IGF-I, insulin-like growth factor type I.

†The FGF receptor actually consists of a family of at least 4 gene products and multiple splice variants.

tiple-species family with apparent molecular masses ranging from 6 to 44 kDa. Most compete with epidermal growth factor (EGF) for binding to the same receptor, activate receptor tyrosine-specific kinase activity, and are generally growth stimulatory[88–91] (Table 17–3; Fig. 17–4). The TGF-α–related growth factors are all single-chain species with a consensus pattern of three intrachain disulfide bonds; the most well-characterized members include TGF-α, EGF, vaccinia growth factor (VGF), amphiregulin, heparin-binding EGF, and a factor termed cripto. Most recently, a separate heparin-binding subfamily with members called heregulin (human) and NDF (*neu* differentiating factor, rat) has been cloned.[92–94] The rat and human homologues are virtually identical in sequence and do not appear to bind to the EGF receptor

(EGFR), unlike the aforementioned species. Instead, NDF and herregulin were initially reported to bind to *erbB₂(neu)*, an EGFR-related protein. EGFR, c-*erbB₂*, c-*erbB₃*, and c-*erbB₄* make up a closely related family of tyrosine kinase–linked receptors.[95] After the description of *erbB₃* and *erbB₄* it was shown that NDF/heregulin directly binds *erbB₄* and, to a lesser extent, *erbB₃*. Due to cross dimerization of both gene products with *erbB₂*, there may be an indirect action with *erbB₂*.[95a] A recently discovered additional factor appears to bind *erbB₂* directly.[95b] All four receptors and all of the EGF-related growth factors except VGF have been detected in breast cancer.

The TGF-β family consists of at least three related gene products, each forming 25-kDa homodimeric species[96] and all of which are found in breast cancer. There appears to be a complex pattern of interaction of these species with the TGF-β receptors, which have been described as three different molecular-weight species. Two of these receptors have been cloned and sequenced. While one appears to be a nonsignaling binding protein, the other appears to mediate its signal via a serine-threonine–specific kinase activity.[96–99] TGF-β, and more recently TGF-α, have been found in the urine and pleural and peritoneal effusions of cancer patients.[100–102] These growth factors also have been observed in some normal tissues.[85–87,89] Treatment of both normal and malignant epithelial tissue with TGF-β of all subtypes generally has a growth-inhibitory and sometimes differentiating effect. Three other inhibitory factors may be relevant to breast cancer: mammary-derived growth inhibitor (MDGI),[103] mammostatin,[104] and α lactalbumin.[105]

At least six other classes of growth factors are also relevant. Insulin-like growth factors (IGF-I and IGF-II, and their binding proteins), platelet-derived growth factor

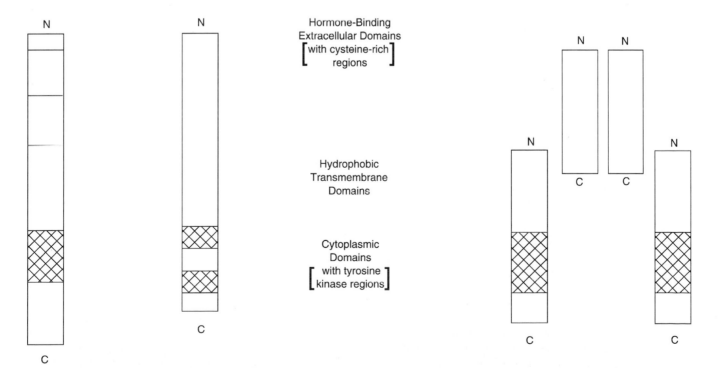

Figure 17–4. Domain structures of principal families of tyrosine kinase receptors in human breast cancer.[85]

(PDGF), and fibroblast growth factors (FGFs, a family of at least seven members) have been studied for several years.[85-87] Each of these factors binds to its own multi-member class of tyrosine kinase–encoding receptors. Another tyrosine kinase, c-met is bound and activated on breast cancer cells by its ligand, hepatocyte growth factor (HGF, or scatter factor). This factor may regulate both cell motility and cell growth. A more recently described growth factor, mammary-derived growth factor type 1 (MDGF-1), has been found in human milk and in conditioned medium from human breast cancer cell lines.[106-109] This glycosylated, monomeric, and non–disulfide-linked 62-kDa growth factor stimulates stromal collagen production and also may play a role in growth regulation of normal and malignant human mammary epithelium. Its receptor is a 130-kDa protein that also stimulates tyrosine phosphorylation of a 180-kDa cellular protein.[106,109]

It has been hypothesized that transformation of cells from normal to malignant may indirectly associate with or directly result from increased production of growth-stimulatory factors or decreased production of growth-inhibitory substances. Alternative hypotheses invoke altered responsiveness to either or both transforming groups of growth factors.[87] To evaluate these hypotheses, it is important to understand pathways of growth control in neoplastic cells, the normal cells from which the cancer derived. To date, this area of investigation has advanced rather slowly for normal epithelial cells because of the difficulties involved in their culture. However, the recent development of specialized serum-free culture conditions has facilitated the study of growth regulation in normal human keratinocytes,[110] normal human bronchial epithelial cells,[111] and normal human mammary epithelial cells.[112,113] Although human mammary epithelial cells may now be cultured in vitro, it is not yet clear that the cultured subtype is of the lineage or differentiation type(s) that would give rise to breast cancer in a woman. For example, receptors for estrogen and progesterone have not been demonstrated in these cells, and they appear to have a basal epithelial "stem cell" character.[112,113]

Studies on steroid–growth factor interactions in human mammary tissue have been restricted to the malignant epithelium. In hormone-responsive human breast cancer cells, growth stimulation by estrogen is accompanied by an increase in growth-stimulatory TGF-α amphiregulin and IGF-II production,[88,114,115,115a] whereas growth inhibition of hormone-responsive breast cancer cell lines in vitro and primary tumors in vivo by an antiestrogen is paralleled by inhibition of TGF-α and augmented secretion of growth-inhibitory TGF-β.[116-118,118a] Similar effects have been observed with progestins: TGF-α, EGF, and the EGFR were induced, whereas TGF-β was inhibited (antiprogestins had the opposite effect).[119-122] Steroids and growth factors also have been observed to cooperate in induction of certain other indicator genes, such as pS2 and cathepsin D.[123] In hormone-independent breast cancer cell lines, growth factors are constitutively produced.[124-126] These results are consistent with, but do not prove, a role for growth factors in the expression of a more malignant phenotype and escape from normal hormonal control in vivo.

Recent studies have begun to evaluate the mechanisms and consequences of induction of TGF-α and TGF-β family members. TGF-α and TGF-β₂ are both under transcriptional control by estrogen and antiestrogen; effects of progestins and antiprogestins have been less well characterized. The transcriptional regulation of TGF-α depends on a palindromic, imperfect consensus ERE in the region of the gene 5′ to the coding region.[127,128] Under typical cell culture conditions in plastic dishes, estrogen stimulates while progestins inhibit proliferation of hormone-responsive breast cancer cell lines. In contrast, in anchorage-independent colony formation in soft agar culture, both estrogen and progesterone are growth stimulatory. Under such anchorage-independent conditions, it has been shown, using anti–growth factor antibodies and antisense nucleotide sequences, that estrogen- and progesterone-induced TGF-α and estrogen- and progesterone-inhibited TGF-β play at least a modulatory role in steroid control of growth.[124,129,130,130a] One study[131] has shown that, under anchorage-dependent conditions, the novel synthetic progestin gestodine inhibits hormone-dependent breast cancer cells at least partially via TGF-β induction.

Other studies have utilized growth factor and receptor gene transfection into hormone-responsive breast cancer cell lines to assess possible effects on malignant progression. Although transfection of TGF-α or EGFR had very little effect, slightly growth-enhancing effects have been reported for the *IGF-II* gene and for the *erbB₂* proto-oncogene.[132-134] In striking contrast, very strong enhancement of hormone-independent tumor growth and metastases was observed after transfection of FGF-4 into MCF-7 cells. Whether the mechanism of enhancement is direct or indirect (depending on tumor-host interactions) is not yet known.[135,136]

Finally, studies in vivo in the nude mouse are providing additional perspectives on the roles of growth factors in breast cancer proliferation. Infusion of EGF or IGF-I is capable of limited stimulation of tumor growth of MCF-7 implanted in the athymic nude mouse. Tumors were nonprogressing in either case.[137] Other studies infused TGF-β in the nude mouse to attempt to block proliferation of the highly responsive MDA-MB-231 cell line. Unexpectedly, the tumor growth was unaffected in vivo and the animals exhibited cachexia, multiple organ fibrosis, and splenic regression.[138] A subsequent study[139] further characterized the effects of release of endogenous TGF-β from hormone-independent breast tumors in vivo, observing that neutralizing anti–TGF-β antibodies suppressed tumor growth and enhanced natural killer (NK) cell immune function. Thus, a new picture of growth factor function is emerging from in vivo studies. Local functions of growth factors in normal breast tissue may include stimulation of epithelial proliferation by TGF-α, IGF, and FGF family members and inhibition of epithelial proliferation by TGF-β and other inhibitory factors. However, in cancer, growth factor overproduction, perturbation of signal transduction mechanisms, and loss of tissue compartmentalization may lead to aberrant action of growth factors. These actions may contribute to tumor growth and metastases and include angiogenesis or blood vessel infiltration (TGF-β, FGF), desmoplasia and collagen deposition (MDGF-1, TGF-β, TGF-α), and immune suppression (TGF-β). Some of these tumor-host interactions are described in greater detail in later sections of this chapter.

MULTIPLE ROLES FOR BREAST-DERIVED TGF-α AND EGF IN NEONATAL DEVELOPMENT, MAMMARY PROLIFERATION, CARCINOGENESIS, AND TUMOR GROWTH

The natural secretory product of the mammary epithelial cell, milk, is an extraordinarily rich source of growth factors.[140] It seems possible that milk-derived growth factors play multiple roles in newborn development, mammary growth, and mammary carcinogenesis. EGF, a milk-derived growth factor, appears to be an important regulator both of the proliferation and differentiation of the mouse mammary gland in vivo and of mouse mammary explants in vitro.[140–142] EGF is also a required supplement for the clonal anchorage-dependent growth, in vitro, of normal human mammary epithelial cells.[143] It is of interest, therefore, that human breast cancer cells in culture do not require exogenous EGF for continuous growth. However, many breast cancer cell lines retain receptors and growth-stimulatory responses to EGF.[144,145] It would appear plausible that growth factors might be critical during mammary carcinogenesis processes. In this regard, it has been observed that circulating mouse salivary gland–derived EGF appears to be necessary for spontaneous mammary tumor formation in the mouse model as well as for growth of the tumors once they are formed.[146]

TGF-α and amphiregulin, structural and functional homologues of EGF, can produce essentially the same biologic effects in mouse mammary explants and cultured human and mouse mammary epithelial cell lines as EGF.[141,147,149a] Their role in normal and malignant mammary development has been emerging in the past few years. It is of interest that TGF-α mRNA has been detected in mammary epithelium by in situ hybridization during the proliferative, lobuloalveolar development stage of rodent and human pregnancy.[148] A detailed immuno-histochemical study in the mouse gland revealed that TGF-α expression predominates in the basal epithelial, proliferative, and bud cap cells, whereas EGF expression is in scattered ductal luminal secretory cells.[149] TGF-α and amphiregulin[149a] mRNA and protein and EGFR are detected in vitro in proliferating human mammary epithelial cells, but are very low in resting organoids.[150,151] TGF-α and amphiregulin both appear to act as autocrine growth factors in normal human mammary epithelial cells in mass culture; an anti-EGFR antibody (or heparin, to block amphiregulin) reversibly inhibits proliferation.[151,152] As mentioned previously, newer members of this growth factor family, such as cripto-1,[115a] amphiregulin,[152] and heparin-binding EGF,[153] have been discovered in breast cancer cell lines, but their exact physiologic role in normal and malignant proliferation remains to be determined. For example, amphiregulin appears to inhibit breast tumor cells, but not some normal cell types, in vitro.[154]

TGF-α has been implicated directly as a modulator of cellular transformation in a number of studies. Overex-

pression of TGF-α following transfection of a human TGF-α cDNA expression vector into the immortal, but nontumorigenic, mouse mammary epithelial cell line NOG-8 led to its capacity for anchorage-independent growth (but not full tumorigenicity).[155] Another study utilized MCF-10, a newly described, spontaneously immortalized human breast ductal epithelial cell line, as recipient for the TGF-α gene. This cell line, which is negative for ER and PR but contains a high level of EGFR also was phenotypically transformed in vitro by TGF-α transfection.[156] In contrast, TGF-α transfection into fully malignant MCF-7 cells, which have low levels of EGFR, does not confer a significant growth advantage in vitro or in vivo.[157] In some studies using immortalized rodent fibroblasts as recipients for human or rat TGF-α cDNA, transformation to full tumorigenicity also was achieved.[158] In contrast, in other studies, TGF-α transfection induced increased proliferation but not full malignant progression to tumorigenicity.[159] EGF also can act as an oncogene when transfected and overexpressed in immortalized rodent fibroblasts.[160] There is also evidence to suggest that the level of secretion of TGF-α in breast cancer and rodent fibroblasts is associated with expression of other oncogenes. A direct correlation among TGF-α production, ras oncogene expression, and malignant transformation has been demonstrated in vitro.[156] The relationships among expression of oncogenes, TGF-α expression, and TGF-α function probably are dependent on the cell type in question.

In studies of human breast cancer biopsies, TGF-α mRNA and protein were detected in 70 per cent or more of the specimens[88,161] and in approximately 30 per cent of benign breast lesions.[162] Immunoreactive TGF-α has been found in fibroadenomas and 20 to 25 per cent of primary human mammary carcinomas,[114,163] and an EGF-related protein of 43 kDa has been isolated recently from breast cancer patient urine.[164] The relevance of expression of these mitogenic growth factors is not yet certain for primary human breast cancer. Perhaps detection of TGF-α/EGF in tumor biopsies, serum, or urine eventually will be found useful in determining prognosis or tumor burden.

A very recent group of studies has addressed the effect of TGF-α overexpression (with MMTV or metallothionine promoters) in the mammary glands of transgenic mice. These studies suggest the possibility that TGF-α expression may be important in early stages of onset of mammary cancer. In one study using outbred mice, the mammary gland was hyperproliferative and exhibited delayed penetration of the epithelial ducts into the stromal fat pad.[165] Such a delayed penetration also has been observed with local mammary implants of EGF.[166] Two other TGF-α transgenic mouse studies using inbred strains also have shown the mammary glands to be hyperproliferative, often resulting in mammary cancer after multiple pregnancies.[167,168] The significance of the different results with outbred versus inbred strains and different gene promoters is not yet clear.

In human breast cancer cell lines in vitro, clear evidence of significant autocrine growth control by the TGF-α/EGFR system has been seen only in the hormone-independent MDA-MB-468 cell line. This line has a high expression of TGF-α and an amplified EGFR.[169] Such studies would appear to have clear implications for developing novel therapeutic strategies. However, it seems likely that, excepting the few per cent of breast cancers overexpressing EGFR by such a gene amplification, this growth factor receptor system will not be of primary importance in autocrine growth regulation of malignant and metastatic disease. It seems more likely that the EGFR/TGF-α system may be much more critical in normal gland growth and early stages of breast tumorigenesis. Therapeutic strategies employing EGFR ligands or antibodies coupled to toxins or therapeutic drugs could conceivably find future utility, because a large portion of hormone-independent breast cancers express significant levels of this receptor even though a direct function of this receptor has not been proven.[126,145] TGF-α also may contribute to aberrant tumor-host interactions in breast cancer.

EGFR/Proto-oncogene

In comparing hormone-dependent and hormone-independent breast cancer cell lines and primary tumors, the absence of ER in conjunction with expression of high levels of EGFR often is noted.[170–172] The EGFR is a 170,000-Da transmembrane glycoprotein with tyrosine kinase activity[173] (Fig. 17–4). Binding of EGF to its receptor results in the intracellular internalization and down-regulation of the receptor,[174] and also leads to autophosphorylation of EGFR in addition to phosphorylation of other substrates.[175,176] Overexpression of EGFR has been shown to result in EGF-dependent transformation of rodent fibroblasts,[177,178] implicating the receptor in the process of cellular transformation. The extensive homology between EGFR and the avian erythroblastosis v-erbB oncogene also strongly suggests that EGFR is the cellular homologue of v-erbB.[179–182]

Clinically, high EGFR levels in breast tumors have been shown to correlate strongly with a poor prognosis, independent of ER status.[170–172] Most studies with clinical specimens have utilized a membrane-binding assay for EGFR. There is a great need to develop a standardized immunohistochemical approach to quantify EGFR in paraffin-fixed clinical material. High expression of EGFR often is accompanied by a low-level expression of ER, suggesting a mechanistic link between up-regulation of EGFR and hormone independence.[170–172] This inverse correlation also holds true in many breast cancer cell lines, with EGFR expression varying by more than two orders of magnitude from ER+ to ER− cells.[145] Additionally, substances that alter EGFR and ER expression, such as estrogen and phorbol esters (TPA, for example), generally have opposite effects on these two receptors.[65,183–186]

The usefulness of EGFR as a prognostic indicator and its inverse relationship with ER in both tumors and cell lines point out our need to understand the mechanisms that control EGFR in breast cancer. To date, there are few data on the molecular basis of EGFR gene expression in this disease. In general, human tumor cell lines exhibit substantial variation in their level of EGFR,[187,188] and the mechanisms responsible for elevated EGFR also can dif-

fer. Cell lines have been identified with EGFR gene amplification accompanied by gene rearrangements that produce altered transcripts, gene amplification without rearrangement, and overexpression of EGFR in the absence of gene amplification[188] (Table 17–4). Human cell lines with a nonrearranged EGFR gene contain two major species of EGFR mRNA (10 kb and 5.6 kb), and the level of these transcripts generally correlates with the amount of EGFR protein.[187] It has been shown that messenger RNA levels correlate with the amount of protein, and that these differences in expression are controlled at least in part at the transcriptional level; EGFR gene amplification appears to be a rare event (less than 5 per cent) in breast cancer.[145]

A variety of substances, such as EGF, phorbol esters, and estrogen, can utilize different mechanisms to alter the level of EGFR. EGF stimulates both protein and message levels of its receptor in hormone-independent MDA-MB-468 breast cancer cells,[189,190] WB rat hepatic cells,[191] and KB cells (a line derived from HeLa cervical carcinoma cells).[192] However, it has been shown by nuclear transcription run-on assays that EGF does not affect EGFR transcription in KB cells, suggesting that EGF regulates the level of its receptor through a posttranscriptional mechanism.[193] The phorbol ester TPA also causes an increase in EGFR levels in MDA-MB-468 and MCF-7 breast cancer cells[186,190]; however, there appears to be both a transcriptional and a posttranscriptional component to this regulation as seen by nuclear run-on and RNase protection assays in MCF-7 cells.[186] In the rat uterus, estrogen has been shown to transiently increase both EGFR message and protein; the effect on message is completely blocked by the transcription-blocking drug actinomycin D, suggesting a strong transcriptional component to estrogen regulation of EGFR.[183,184] Treatment with nonestrogenic steroids produces no effect on EGFR mRNA, and the protein synthesis–blocking drug puromycin fails to modulate the estrogen-induced increase in message.[183] These results imply a specific estrogenic effect on EGFR transcription mediated by direct action of the estrogen receptor on the EGFR gene. To date, no ERE has been identified in the promoter of the EGFR gene.

Studies on the molecular mechanisms of EGFR tran-

TABLE 17–4. PRINCIPLE GENETIC ALTERATIONS IN HUMAN BREAST CANCER

TUMOR SUPPRESSORS (MUTATED OR ELIMINATED)	ONCOGENES (AMPLIFIED OR OVEREXPRESSED)
p53	c-myc
RB-1	c-erbB₂
BRCA-1(?)*	EGFR‡
nm23†	cyclin D₁
CDK 4 inhibitor	cyclin E

*Breast and ovarian cancer familial cancer locus; not yet isolated or proven to be a tumor suppressor.

†Known to be down-regulated in metastases; mutations not yet commonly demonstrated.

‡Amplified in only a few per cent of tumors but frequently overexpressed.

scriptional regulation have for the most part been carried out using A431 epidermoid carcinoma cells and HeLa cells. In these studies, several binding sites for proteins, including SP1, were found in the promoter region and exon 1[192,194–196] (Fig. 17–5). The EGFR gene promoter is typical of many "housekeeping" genes in that it is extremely GC rich and contains no TATA or CAAT box.[197] Among the regulatory factors that are present in A431 cells and interact with the 5' flanking region of the EGFR gene is one known as ETF1, which appears to specifically stimulate in vitro transcription of genes whose promoters lack a TATA box.[192] Another factor with positive transcriptional activity in vitro, known as TCF, binds to a region that contains four repeats, each 10 to 15 bp in length, of the sequence "TCC." However, numerous other factors have been found to bind to the EGFR promoter; some showing the strongest sequence-specific binding have little or no effect on transcription either in vitro or in vivo.[196] Transient transfection assays with EGFR promoter/reporter chloramphenicol acetyltransferase (CAT) constructs in HeLa cells also have identified regions of the promoter and intron I that show enhancer activity, and several binding sites for HeLa cell nuclear factors were found in the intron I enhancer.[198] However, this sequence did not appear to have enhancer activity in MCF-7 breast cancer cells, an estrogen-dependent line.

Additional studies of EGFR promoter function, using transient transfection assays in HeLa cells with EGFR promoter/reporter luciferase constructs, have shown that sequences from -485 to -19 (relative to the start of translation) produce the same level of luciferase activity as does 1100 bp of the promoter.[185] Luciferase activity is decreased fivefold when the EGFR promoter is shortened to -153 (a position downstream of the major in vivo transcriptional start site). However, in HeLa cells, all three of these constructs are capable of responding to stimulation by EGF, TPA, retinoic acid, (Bu)$_2$-cAMP, and dexamethasone. This is in contrast to the studies described previously,[193] wherein EGF did not affect transcription of the endogenous EGFR gene in KB cells, and to a report[184] that dexamethasone did not affect EGFR transcript levels. These differences raise the possibility that regulation of the EGFR gene involves complex interactions, requiring additional sequences either upstream or downstream of the proximal promoter region to correctly modulate its expression.

c-*erbB*$_2$ Receptor/Oncogene

AN EGF RECEPTOR-LIKE SYSTEM?

c-*erbB*$_2$ protein (also called p185, p185^{erbB-2}, p185^{neu}, and p185^{HER-2}) is a transmembrane protein with substantial homology to EGFR (Table 17–3; Fig. 17–4). It also was initially reported to be a receptor for a human TGF-α–related ligand termed herregulin[92] and its rat homologue NDF.[93,94] However, recent studies suggest a different li-

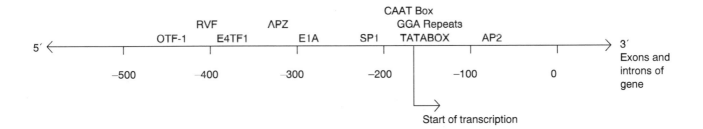

EGF Receptor Gene Promoter

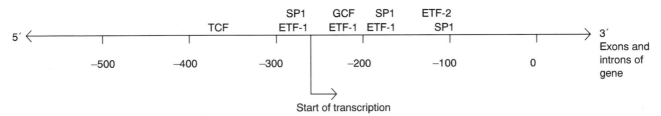

Figure 17–5. Promoter features of the genes for epidermal growth factor receptor (EGFR) and c-*erbB*$_2$ receptor tyrosine kinases. The regulation of these two tyrosine kinases in breast cancer is very different. Overexpression of EGFR, likely the result of increased transcription, is associated with lack of estrogen receptor and other aspects of poorly differentiated breast cancer. In contrast, the c-*erbB*$_2$ gene is commonly amplified, driving its overexpression in a class of poor-prognosis breast cancers.[316,317]

gand interaction with $erbB_2$.[95a] Herregulin/NDF actually represents a highly complex family of alternately spliced ligands interaction, primarily with other receptors in the $erbB_2$ family.[199–202] Herregulin/NDF, like ligands for the EGF receptor are thought to indirectly phosphor and activate $erbB_2$ through heterodimerization.[95b] About 10 to 30 per cent of breast, gastric, and ovarian cancers over-express c-$erbB_2$ protein at a sufficiently high level that the protein can be detected by immunohistochemical staining of formalin-fixed and paraffin-embedded sections. This characteristic has facilitated rapid development of c-$erbB_2$ as a tumor prognostic marker. Overexpression in cancers from other organ systems, including adenocarcinoma of the lung, ovaries, stomach,[203] and pancreas[204] and endometrial carcinoma,[205] have been reported.

There has been some confusion in the literature because of the terminology used by different groups who independently identified the c-$erbB_2$ gene. c-$erbB_2$[206] and HER-2[207] both refer to an identical human homologue of the *neu* oncogene in rat.[208] In this review, we will use the term c-$erbB_2$ protein. The normal function of the c-$erbB_2$ protein is not known; however in cancers overexpressing c-$erbB_2$, the growth factor NDF slightly stimulates (low concentrations) and inhibits (higher concentrations) proliferation in association with promotion of differentiation. Thus, the exact role of c-$erbB_2$ as either an oncogene or as a differentiation-inducing factor remains problematic. It is also of interest that c-$erbB_2$ and EGFR seem to form heterodimers when co-expressed at high levels.[209,210]

c-$erbB_2$ AS A PROGNOSTIC FACTOR IN BREAST AND OTHER CANCERS

Many studies have been published utilizing various methods to quantitate c-$erbB_2$, ranging from measurement of gene copy number (Southern blot), to transcript amount (Northern blot), to protein amount (Western blot), to immunohistochemistry with or without image analysis. In general, overexpression of c-erb_2 protein is due to amplification of its gene rather than other mechanisms of disregulated expression (Table 17–4). However, because of the occasional overexpression of c-$erbB_2$ protein without gene amplification, in some tumors an assay for the protein products appears to be the method of choice. In this respect, immunohistochemistry gives a reasonable threshold when used on formalin-fixed and paraffin-embedded sections, so that a simple all-or-nothing scoring can be applied with excellent clinical correlation and reproducibility. It has been shown that there is a good agreement between immunohistochemistry and Western blot assay.[211] Although some investigators are concerned about a decrease in sensitivity when performing immunohistochemistry with paraffin-embedded sections,[212] this seems to be due to poorer affinity/specificity of the reagents used in these studies. With cocktail monoclonal antibody preparation, we have reported excellent reproducibility of staining.[213]

There exists a confusing body of literature about the prognostic role of c-$erbB_2$ in breast cancer. Most of the negative studies generally have utilized specimens from heterogeneous treatment groups. In at least two large studies that examined relatively homogeneous treatment groups,[214,215] the prognostic role of c-$erbB_2$ in node-positive breast cancer was evident. Data from gastric cancer as well as findings in vitro suggest that this discrepancy may be due to the fact that c-$erbB_2$ may affect response to chemotherapy. It has been reported that c-$erbB_2$ is of prognostic value even in good-nuclear-grade breast tumors[214] and ovarian carcinoma.[216] Although several groups have shown amplification and overexpression of c-$erbB_2$ in gastric cancer, only one study actually examined its prognostic role.[217]

ROLE OF c-$erbB_2$ IN PATHOGENESIS OF BREAST CANCER

Data including cell line transfections in vitro and transgenic mouse experiments in vivo have suggested a role of oncogenically mutated c-$erbB_2$ in the onset of breast cancer.[218–220] Immunostaining of primary human tumors revealed that, when a tumor is positive, it usually shows a very homogeneous staining of all tumor cells, including preinvasive components (intraductal cancer or ductal carcinoma in situ). Indeed, a number of groups now have reported higher incidence of c-$erbB_2$ overexpression in ductal cancer in situ than in infiltrating ductal carcinoma.[221] This raises the question as to the role of c-$erbB_2$ in carcinogenesis and tumor progression in vivo. It is possible that c-$erbB_2$ gene amplification is an early event in the pathogenesis of these tumors. To become invasive cancer, activation or deletion of at least one other gene may be necessary. Candidate genes are EGFR, c-$erbB_2$ ligand, or a suppressor gene. An interesting body of literature is accumulating that shows that there may be a functional relationship between overexpression of EGF receptor and simultaneous overexpression of c-$erbB_2$. Several clinical studies have noted that an especially poor patient prognosis is associated with such co-overexpression.[222] On a molecular level, this interaction apparently is manifested as receptor heterodimerization and cross phosphorylation.[209,210] Presumably, such complex formation and cross phosphorylation contribute to increased affinity for ligands and/or increased activation of tyrosine kinases. An additional active area of investigation is the function of retrodimerization of $erbB_2$ with the $erbB_3$ and $erbB_4$ family members.[95b] Study of c-$erbB_2$ and its ligands by radioligand binding assay is likely to be complicated by shedding of the extracellular domain of c-$erbB_2$ by some breast cancer cell lines.[223] Although the function of this shedding is unknown, it may be of use in monitoring patient sera.

Relevance of $erbB_2$ and EGFR to Treatment

Prognostic factors and factors that can influence or associate with therapeutic response should be recognized separately. For example, as previously noted, ER is an indicator for good prognosis. However, ER is not the best prognostic indicator in comparison to other indicators (e.g., lymph node status or tumor size). Despite this caveat, ER is important in therapeutic decision making because it predicts response to antiestrogen. Likewise, poor nuclear grade is an indicator of a poor prognosis, but its effect on response to adjuvant therapy is greater. c-erbB₂ and EGFR-positive tumors impose a difficult problem because the prognostic value of each receptor generally has been determined in groups of patients who were treated with adjuvant therapy. Thus it is possible, for example, that c-erbB₂ is not only an indicator for poor prognosis but also an indicator for poor response to adjuvant therapy. Future studies are required to fully evaluate this hypothesis.

Two major types of treatments may be explored for c-erbB₂-positive or EGFR-positive patients: (1) receptor-directed experimental therapeutics, including monoclonal antibodies, antisense oligodeoxynucleotides, blocking peptides, high-dose inhibitory ligands, or extracellular domain of c-erbB₂; and (2) known chemotherapeutic regimens to which these receptor-overexpressing tumors might better respond. The second approach may turn out to be more practical and rapidly achievable.

Although there are studies that have shown inhibition of tumor growth by monoclonal antireceptor antibodies,[224–226] such approaches may not be useful when employed in the absence of other agents because they may be only relatively weak cytostatic agents. However, monoclonal antibodies may unexpectedly change other aspects of tumor biology. For example, in an ovarian cancer cell line, a noninhibitory dose of anti–c-erbB₂ monoclonal antibody sensitizes the cells to killing by cisplatin.[219] Thus, it may be possible to use such an approach with antireceptor reagents as biologic response modifiers to sensitize the tumor cells to conventional, less toxic regimens, which alone are not effective. Antibody or toxin conjugation is an additional, exciting approach for the future[226] and eventually may contribute to response to treatment as single agents or in combination with other agents.[227,228]

Signal Transduction–Associated Nuclear Oncogenes

A common link between the actions of growth-promoting steroids and growth factors in diverse tissues are the nuclear proto-oncogenes. These may represent convergent pathways of growth-regulatory stimuli. The proto-oncogenes c-fos, c-myc, c-myb, and c-jun commonly are observed to be induced shortly after mitogenic treatment of cells. Considerable evidence supports a causal link between their induction and proliferation processes. At least three nuclear proto-oncogene products—c-myc, c-fos, and c-jun—appear to be induced by both estrogen and progesterone in breast cancer.[229] Tamoxifen down-regulates c-myc expression during treatment-induced tumor regression in patient tumors.[230] It is not yet known if any of these nuclear proto-oncogenes are involved in induction of growth of the normal mammary gland, but c-myc, c-fos, and c-jun induction has been shown to occur in the rat uterus in response to estrogen treatment.[231,232] Protein products of the c-fos and c-jun genes function through heterodimerization and subsequent interaction with gene promoter consensus sequences termed AP-1. Similarly,

the c-myc product dimerizes with another protein termed Max (or Myn in the mouse) to modulate genes through a different consensus sequence. It is also thought that the Myc protein binds and inactivates the retinoblastoma tumor suppressor gene product[233] (discussed later in this chapter). Using antisense oligonucleotides complimentary to c-myc mRNA, it has been shown recently that Myc is necessary for estrogen induction of proliferation of breast cancer.[234]

Amplification of the c-myc gene is one of the most common genetic alterations in breast cancer (Table 17–4). Probably about one third of breast cancers express this genetic change. Study of c-myc gene expression in breast cancer has been hampered by difficulties in measuring the protein in tumor biopsies. These difficulties include the exceedingly short half-life to the protein and the lack of a wide range of monoclonal antibodies capable of staining paraffin sections. In spite of these difficulties, several studies have shown amplification of the c-myc gene to be associated with poor prognosis[234,235] and postmenopausal diseases,[236] but independently of c-erbB₂ gene amplification. An interesting literature is developing in the study of various epithelial malignancies, including those of the ovary and liver,[237,238] which shows that c-myc amplification is associated with TGF-α overexpression. The potential functional significance of this observation is discussed in a later section. A very active area of current investigation is study of the ultimate cell cycle regulators, cyclins and their associated cyclin dependent kinases and inhibitors. For example, it is now known that cyclin D is very commonly amplified in breast cancer (as is cyclin E) and the cyclin dependent kinase inhibitor-4 (CDKI-4) is very commonly deleted or mutated in breast cancer.[238a,238b] Amplified cyclins may act as oncogenes and cyclin inhibitors may be tumor suppressors.

An additional signal transduction–associated proto-oncogene is the c-ras family. This oncogene is intimately associated with signal transduction from tyrosine kinase-encoding receptors. Mutations in this family are common in experimental rodent mammary tumors, but seldom seen in human breast cancer. The ras family is not discussed further here.

Tumor Suppressor Genes in Sporadic, Hereditary, and Familial Breast Cancer

Cancer is being viewed increasingly as a process involving not only proliferative factors and activations of oncogenes but also loss of suppressor gene function. In breast cancer, recent studies have underscored the role of germline deletion or mutation of suppressor genes in familial breast cancer and somatic mutation or deletion during breast tumor progression. It is likely that the identification of breast tumor suppressor genes is only in its infancy at present (Table 17–4).

It has been estimated that approximately 10 per cent of breast cancers show a strongly familial pattern. These cancers tend to appear in a younger subset of women than the majority of breast cancers (which are postmenopausal). Of great interest are the observations that a short region on chromosome 17 is consistently rearranged or deleted in tumor and nontumor tissue of these patients. This region (17q21) contains the cancer-associated *BRCA-1* locus; the individual mutated gene(s) are not yet identified. This locus is thought to contain a new candidate tumor suppressor gene for breast (and possibly ovarian) cancers.[230–232] Other studies have characterized loss of the previously characterized tumor suppressor genes retinoblastoma (*Rb-1*; on 17p) and *p53* (on chromosome 11) in breast cancer. However, germline alterations in these genes probably only account for a small fraction of familial breast cancer. It has long been appreciated that the few patients carrying deletions at the *Rb-1* locus who live long enough express susceptibility to multiple organ neoplasia. Also, it has been shown recently that women carrying mutated *p53* seem to define the multiple organ neoplasia (frequently including breast and ovary) syndrome termed Li-Fraumeni.[239–241] An additional hypothesis for familial breast cancer is that women who are heterozygous for a defective DNA repair gene on chromosome 11 (ataxia-telangiectasia) are susceptible to the disease.[242]

Mutation and/or loss of suppressor genes is thought to play a role in tumor progression as well as familial predisposition. These mutations may interact. For example, hereditary *BRCA-1* alterations often appear to be associated with amplification of c-*erbB₂* (also on 17q) in breast tumors.[243] Both *Rb-1* and *p53* seem to be lost with relatively high frequency as breast tissue progresses through various stages of malignancy.[244–246] *p53* alterations also are associated in some cases with inherited *BRCA-1* alterations.[243] However, a tremendous number of mutations occur during tumor progression either spontaneously or in response to cytotoxic chemotherapy.[243,247] Loss of heterozygosity, an indicator of the presence of suppressor genes, appears to be common at the following chromosomal sites: 1p, 1q, 3p, 7, 11p, 13q, 17p, 17q, and 18q.[243,248] It seems likely, therefore, that multiple tumor suppressors may be mutated in cancer and that their collective presence may be required to suppress the disease. In agreement with such a proposal, a recent study has reported failure of transfection of the *Rb-1* gene to reverse malignancy of tumor cell lines carrying this deletion.[249] A very recent discovery is the *nm23* gene, whose loss seems to parallel metastatic progression of breast cancer.[250] This gene product seems to have the ability to attenuate metastases in melanoma and in breast cancer in model systems.[251] Finally, much effort is being expended currently on study of protein tyrosine phosphatases as candidate tumor suppressor genes. Loss of expression of such genes would be expected to enhance dramatically the growth-promoting and oncogenic activities of tyrosine kinases such as EGFR and c-*erbB₂*.[252,253]

Genetic Changes during Tumor Progression: Interaction of Oncogenes and Suppressor Genes

The malignant progression of breast cancer is likely to involve a transition from normal mechanisms of prolif-

eration in its early stages to highly abnormal regulation of metastatic disease.[254,255] Early proliferation probably depends on systemic hormones (estrogen and progesterone) and local growth factors (such as TGF-α). Some critical damage or repair error event(s) then may occur (or were already present, in the case of familial breast cancer). An early manifestation of such events must be to allow gene amplification,[256] because amplification of c-*erbB₂* and c-*myc* in breast cancer seems to occur in all stages of the disease. In addition, mutations of *p53* and *Rb-1* suppressors and down-modulation of *nm23* appear to be frequent and associated with poorer prognosis.[244–246,250] However, it is not yet certain at what stage in progression these genes become mutated or dysregulated. As additional amplifications and mutations occur, the cancer cells with the greatest growth, invasive, apoptosis suppression, or survival advantage will undergo positive selection.[257] Several studies both in vitro and in vivo have begun to address potential synergistic mechanisms whereby mutations may interact in breast cancer to the advantage of the tumor. A large array of suspected prognostic variables for breast cancer begins to indicate the scope of molecular lesions whose interactions may be significant (Table 17–5).

Some studies utilizing cell lines in vitro are attempting to sort out potentially significant factors and their interactions. As previously noted, EGFR and c-*erbB₂* seem to

TABLE 17–5. PROGNOSTIC FACTORS IN BREAST CANCER

TUMOR AGGRESSIVENESS/DIFFERENTIATION INDICATORS
Tumor size
Nuclear grade
Histologic subtype
DNA ploidy
c-*erbB₂*, c-myc, cyclin D, amplification
Overexpression of EGFR
Expression of other growth factors/receptors
Loss of *Rb-1*, *nm23* CDKI-4 expression
Overexpression of mutated *p53*
ER, PR expression
Vimentin-keratin co-expression

PROLIFERATION INDICES
Mitotic rate
Thymidine labeling
S-phase fraction
Ki67 antigen
PCNA/cyclin expression
c-myc amplification

METASTASIS-RELATED INDICES
Nodal status
Distant metastases
Local invasion
Degree of neoangiogenesis
Laminin receptor
Gelatinase expression
Plasminogen activator (UPA) expression

OTHER MARKERS OF INTEREST
Heat shock proteins
Haptoglobin-related protein
pS2 protein
Cathepsin D
p170 glycoprotein

interact in the small percentage of breast tumors in which both are co-overexpressed.[209,210,222] The mechanism seems to be the formation of an interactive heterodimeric receptor species of high affinity that cross phosphorylates itself. A recent in vitro study with the MCF-10A mammary epithelial cell line also has observed that c-*erbB₂* and TGF-α co-transfection is capable of additive action to promote anchorage-independent growth. However, this additive interaction was not sufficient to promote tumorigenesis fully.[258] A second type of interaction apparently occurs with c-*myc* amplification. c-*myc* is known to bind and inactivate the *Rb-1* gene product;[233] thus Myc may simultaneously stimulate proliferation and decrease tumor suppression. An additional effect of c-*myc* amplification seems to be sensitization of mammary (and other) cell types to anchorage-independent growth-promoting effects of EGF and FGF receptor stimulus.[259] Additionally, as previously mentioned, the hereditary *BRCA-1* locus may interact with *p53*, c-*erbB₂*, and possibly other loci in an unknown fashion during malignant progression.[243,248] Finally, c-*erbB₂* and *p53* loci themselves may interact in an unknown manner.[243]

A separate approach to the study of interactive mechanisms in tumorigenesis has utilized the transgenic mouse. Exogenous genes are expressed under strong, sometimes tissue-specific promoters in the mouse. At present, the effects of interactions of growth factors and oncogenes have only begun to be evaluated in such a system. In the transgenic mouse model system, it has been observed that c-*myc* and c-*ras*[H] oncogenes strongly interact in tumorigenesis.[260] However, few studies have yet focused on combinations of oncogenes, growth factors, and loss of suppressor genes thought to be important in the human disease. A recent line of investigation has demonstrated that TGFα and myc strongly synergise to induce mammary tumors in a bitransgenic system.[260a]

CELL AND TISSUE BIOLOGY OF BREAST CANCER

Dedifferentiation, Stromal-Epithelial Interactions, and Metastases

Two separate, but apparently interactive, cellular processes seem to occur during malignant progression of breast cancer: loss of differentiated properties and loss of proper tissue compartmentalization (metastases) (Fig. 17–6). Several molecular determinants have been proposed to relate to each process. In the case of dedifferentiation, it appears that loss of cell-cell attachment, altered cell substratum attachment, and altered cytoskeletal organization seem to play a role. In metastases, the same three influences are thought to prevail but, in addition, cell locomotion, proteolysis, and the ability to survive and proliferate at distant sites[261,262] are considered to be essential.

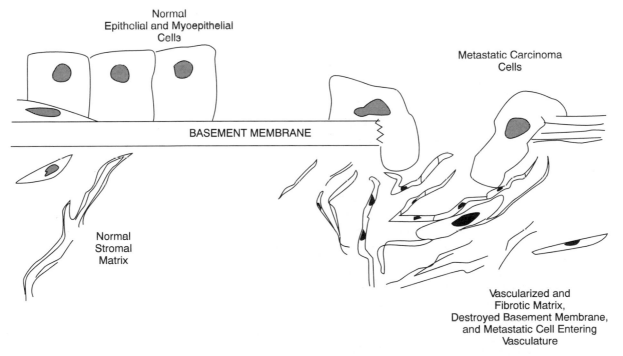

Figure 17–6. Epithelial cell-cell and cell-substratum and epithelial-endothelial interactions in the mammary epithelium. Transitions that may be important in dedifferentiation and metastasis of breast cancer include increased attachment of epithelial cells to basement membrane and matrix through integrin and nonintegrin molecules, decreased cell-cell attachment through cadherins (such as E-cadherin/uvomorulin), increased motility and matrix proteolysis, disruptions in intermediate filament regulation (co-expression of vimentin and keratin), and increased neoangiogenesis (blood vessel infiltration).[266,275]

A principle cell-cell adhesion molecule thought to be involved in mammary epithelial differentiation is uvomorulin (also called E-cadherin or LCAM). Cell-cell adhesion through these molecules is thought to restrict motility[261] and to promote differentiation.[263] Loss of expression of E-cadherin is associated with acquisition of a more motile, fibroblastic morphology in breast cancer and with increased invasiveness.[264] A subset of E-cadherin–negative breast cancer cells exist that express the mesenchymal intermediate filament vimentin (along with epithelial keratins) and that express a strongly motile, invasive phenotype.[264,265] This progression to phenotype has been observed by other investigators in bladder cancer epidermal carcinogenesis and melanoma cancer, wherein it has been termed an epithelial-mesenchymal transition (EMT). In addition, the EMT process is known to occur frequently during embryogenesis.[261,266–268]

Metastases initially are marked by local invasion of the cancer across the basement membrane to the stromal area. This transition is thought to depend on local proteolysis and tumor cell motility. Several proteolytic enzymes are thought to be critical. The two collagen IV–selective degrading enzymes termed 92-kDa and 72-kDa gelatinases are currently under intense scrutiny in this respect.[269] Other investigators have focused on plasmin production (caused by tumor cell–secreted plasminogen activator termed UPA[269a]), cathepsin D, and a novel 80-kDa, broad-substrate, matrix-degrading metalloproteinase as potentially important.[270,271] Although cathepsin D is a marker of poor prognosis as measured in breast tumor homogenates and is under hormonal regulation in breast cancer, it is considered unlikely to be a critical mediator of metastasis. First, its pH optimum is extremely acidic (as opposed to the other enzymes mentioned); second, it is apparently present in tumor homogenates primarily as a result of inflammatory cell infiltration and release; and, finally, its levels do not correlate with invasive potential of breast cancer cells in vitro. Proteolysis may depend on a balance between enzymes and their inhibitors. For example, the gelatinases are secreted with endogenous tissue inhibitors of metalloproteinase (TIMP-1 and TIMP-2).[269] It appears that loss of expression of the estrogen and progesterone receptors may be associated with an EMT process in breast cancer.[255] The exact mechanism of EMT remains unknown, but it seems to be associated with primary defects in arrangement of desmosomal and cytoskeletal proteins.[258] Because PKC expression seems to increase during malignant progression, and because a primary substrate of PKC is an actin filament cross-linking protein thought to be involved in motility,[272–274] it is possible that PKC plays a role in EMT regulation.

Cell-substratum attachment also seems critical both in differentiation[20] and in metastases.[275] Expression of high levels of a nonintegrin, 67-kDa receptor for laminin have been reported to be correlated with progression of breast and colon cancer.[275] This laminin receptor is strongly induced by estrogen and progesterone in breast cancer cell lines.[276] Other studies have implicated the heterodimeric integrin class of attachment molecules as necessary for attachment, particularly the $\alpha_5\beta_1$ integrin, also known as the fibronectin receptor.[277]

Growth Factors, Proteases, Angiogenesis, and Metastases

It is not yet known what cellular events trigger the cascade of processes in local invasion and metastases. c-erbB₂ is an oncogene whose amplification is known to be associated with poor prognosis, node-negative breast cancer, and it may be involved in this process at the cellular level.[278] Increased cellular motility almost certainly is involved as well. Several motility-promoting molecules have been proposed to act in this transition: the FGF family members,[261,279] a molecule termed autocrine motility factor, and a growth factor termed hepatocyte growth factor (or scatter factor), which acts through the c-met tyrosine kinase oncogene.[280] Several model systems have been established for in vitro study of invasion. In particular, the repolymerized basement membrane extract matrigel has been utilized extensively. Using this system, it has been observed that ER-negative cells are generally more invasive than ER-positive cells and that estrogen enhances invasiveness of ER-positive cell lines. Interestingly, tamoxifen is sufficiently estrogenic also to induce invasion of breast cancer cell lines; the pure antiestrogen ICI-164384 is suppressive.[281]

Invasive breast cancer is, by definition, marked by abnormal stromal-epithelial interaction. This was noted several years ago in the context of increased motility of tumor fibroblasts.[282] More recently, this type of study has been extended to include characterization of FGF secretions. Interestingly, the growth factor IGF-II is expressed by breast tumor–derived fibroblasts, whereas IGF-I is expressed by normal breast fibroblasts.[283] Many other growth factors, including acidic FGF, basic FGF, and FGF-5, also are secreted by breast fibroblasts, regardless of source.[283] A recent study also has implicated stromal production of the protease stromelysin III as an early marker of invasive breast cancer.[284] Finally, the matrix component tenacein appears to be synthesized in areas of local invasion, including invasion into metastatic sites.[285]

An important final event leading to full metastatic dissemination of breast cancer is the process of angiogenesis (blood vessel invasion into the tumor area).[3] Angiogenesis has for many years been appreciated as necessary for tumor growth beyond a few millimeters in size as a result of tumor tissue requirements for a proper metabolic environment. Necrosis is thought to be the result of an improperly vascularized tissue, such as the lumen of a large tumor. It appears from recent studies that the degree of tumor metastasis is also directly proportional to the number of capillaries infiltrating the tumor (neoangiogenesis). It would appear that at least two mechanisms for this effect are possible. First, it has been suggested for many years that simple tumor size is a poor prognostic indicator. The ability of a tumor to induce a high degree of local microvasculature will lead to large size. Large tumors may allow a greater diversity of mutational events and a greater likelihood of highly aggressive, metastatic cells. A second mechanism could directly involve the vasculature as a necessary escape route for tumor cells. Tumor cells preferentially accumulate in local lymph nodes, perhaps prior to organ capillary beds. It is not completely clear why the local lymph nodes appear to be such good pathologic indicators of tumor metastases. Perhaps there is also lymphatic infiltration of tumors.[286] It is of great interest that a recent study has observed a close, perhaps causal relationship between breast tumor neoangiogenesis and metastases in patients.[287]

Several in vivo model systems of human breast cancer metastases have been developed recently. In general, hormone-independent breast cancer cells are more likely to be locally invasive in the nude mouse than are hormone-dependent cells.[265] One hormone-independent line, in particular, has been developed into a hematogenesis-metastasis model in the nude mouse: the MDA-MB-435 cell line. This line can be widely metastatic in 6 to 9 months, yielding some macrometastases.[288] In addition, the inoculation site and dietary fat content strongly modulate tumor growth and metastatic spread in experimental models of breast cancer.[289,290]

Studies in a variety of systems suggest that release of heparin-binding growth factors such as the members of the FGF family can contribute significantly to angiogenesis and metastases. For example, in multistep development of human fibrosarcoma, basic FGF release is associated closely with angiogenesis.[291] Also, FGF-4 expression is associated closely with metastases in spontaneous mouse mammary carcinoma.[292] Amplification of the gene for FGF-3 (int-2) and FGF-4 occurs with a 15 per cent frequency in human breast cancer; both genes are located at 11q13. However, expression of these two genes at the mRNA and protein levels is not common, and it is now suspected that a more important gene also exists on the amplicon. A likely candidate is cyclin D1—a cell cycle–related gene.[293] A recent study also has shown that FGF-4 transfection into human MCF-7 breast cancer cells strongly promotes tumor growth and lymphatic/hematogenous metastases. In this study, a gene encoding an enzyme (lacZ, which renders cells easily stainable) was utilized in preparing the model. LacZ gene co-transfection with FGF-4 afforded clear indication of metastatic cells. By 3 weeks ipsilateral lymph nodes were 100 per cent positive; by 6 weeks other more distant lymph nodes, lung, and kidney were positive; and by 12 weeks multiple organs showed evidence of metastases.[135,136] The nature of the most important heparin-binding growth factors in human breast cancer is still under investigation. For example, a recent report identified the heparin-binding, growth-associated neurotropic molecule known as pleiotropin in breast cancer cell lines.[294]

THERAPY

Surgery, Radiation, Antihormonal Therapy, and Chemotherapy

Surgery has remained the centerpiece of breast cancer therapy for millennia. However, the propensity for the disease to metastasize has led to the use of radiation therapy, hormonal therapy, chemotherapy, and immunotherapy as additional measures. All but immunotherapy have had

some limited success. It now appears clear that the failure to achieve a cure in approximately 70 per cent of patients is due to primary lack of therapeutic effect on undetected or detected metastases and to acquired drug and hormonal resistance during therapy.[3,295]

Systemic adjuvant therapy was designed to combat undetected metastases after surgery. Although ovariectomy and adrenalectomy have met with some success, they largely have been replaced by hormonal and antihormonal drugs. Initial studies achieved success with high-dose estrogens, androgens, and progestins, but now these hormonal treatments usually are reserved as second-line therapy after the tumor becomes unresponsive to the antiestrogen tamoxifen. Although ovariectomy, adrenalectomy, and tamoxifen clearly appear to function by diminishing systemic estrogen levels or by preventing estrogen attachment to its receptor in the tumor, the mechanism of action of high-dose steroids is less clear. Newer approaches for antihormonal therapy include LHRH analogues, which seem to act both at the level of the pituitary and directly on the tumor; aromatase inhibitors, which act on adrenals and other sites of peripheral conversion of androgens to estrogens; and antiprogestational drugs, which seem to have a direct effect on receptor-containing tumors.[296,297]

Cytotoxic chemotherapeutic drugs include the following: methotrexate, 5-fluorouracil, Adriamycin (doxorubicin), melphalan (L-PAM), cyclophosphamide, vincristine, chlorambucil, mitoxantrone, mitomycin C, thiotepa, and cisplatin. Adriamycin is one of the newest and most effective of these when given as a single agent. A very new arrival that may show promise is taxol. Usually, two or three of these drugs are combined, sometimes with the glucocorticoid prednisone. Although initially rationalized as an antiadrenal therapy, it now appears that prednisone has useful immunomodulatory and antiangiogenic properties and is helpful in combatting the later tumor sequelae of intracranial pressure, spinal compression, and hypercalcemia. Current clinical trials involve attempts to optimally order and dose antihormonal and chemotherapeutic drugs, sometimes giving them prior to surgery in protocols termed neoadjuvant. Current emphasis is also on maximal-dose intensification and rescue of nontumor tissue with leucovorin (folinic acid). Other attempts to utilize autologous bone marrow transplantation after aggressive chemotherapy are underway. The terminal cancer patient requires additional supportive care because of lymphoedema, anorexia, nausea and vomiting, respiratory problems, and bone pain and bone resorption.[296,298]

Resistance to Therapy by Antihormones and Chemotherapeutic Drugs

In the malignant progression of breast cancer, it is all too often observed that the patient ultimately will fail to respond to treatments. This usually is associated with widely metastatic disease. There is no obvious relationship between initial tumor resistance to chemotherapy, resistance to antiestrogens, and metastatic capacity either clinically or in model systems in vitro.[299,300] It would appear, however, that resistance that develops during clinical application of therapeutic agents clinically is associated either directly or indirectly with malignant progression.

Resistance to antiestrogens occurs rapidly in vitro but is associated with no obvious changes in estrogen, progesterone, or growth factor levels. However, one relatively stable, resistant cell line exists—the LY2 clone of MCF-7, which has lost expression of the progesterone receptor.[301] In this cell line, loss of antigestrogen sensitivity appears to be a recessive characteristic.[47] A peculiarity of in vitro selection for antiestrogen resistance in anchorage-dependent growth is that resistant cell lines usually appear to have lost their tumorigenic characteristics. Tamoxifen resistance also has been proposed to be associated with abnormal tumor drug metabolism, producing high levels of estrogenic metabolites.[302] Several studies in the nude mouse have established that resistance to tamoxifen proceeds more slowly in vivo than in vitro. After approximately 6 months of treatment, MCF-7 cells are observed to switch from growth inhibition to growth stimulation by tamoxifen. This appears to be a receptor-mediated phenomenon that depends on the slight estrogenic character of tamoxifen, because the pharmacologically pure antiestrogen ICI-164384 is capable of blockade of this growth stimulation.[303] An in vitro study[304] also has noted the phenomenon of the evolution of another hormone-dependent cell line (T47D), certain clones of which are tamoxifen stimulated after prolonged treatment. There seems to be little association of resistance to antiprogesterone or other hormonal treatments with resistance to antiestrogen in vivo in patients. It remains to be seen whether clinical trials of a new steroid pure antiestrogen with favorable pharmacokinetics will show it to be effective in patients with tumors who have relapsed on tamoxifen.[305]

Resistance to chemotherapeutic drugs has become a topic of much recent interest, with identification of the p170 glycoprotein pump (the *mdr-1* gene product) as an important mechanism.[306] Many, but not all, studies have shown this protein to be slightly but significantly elevated in relapsing patient breast tumors.[307] Much energy has been expended to find inhibitors of this drug efflux pump to clinically enhance chemotherapy effectiveness. Of interest is the recent suggestion that both antiestrogens[308] and progestins[309] may have some potential in this respect, at least in vitro. An interesting consequence of selection of MCF-7 human breast cancer cells in vitro for stepwise resistance to Adriamycin is that expression of the receptors for estrogen and progesterone are greatly diminished or lost and the receptor for EGF is strongly increased. Phenotypically, the MCF-7 Adr[R] cell line is hormone independent and tumorigenic in vivo, quite invasive, and cross resistant to antiestrogens.[310] These phenotypic changes are not due to the presence of the amplified *mdr-1* gene.[311] It remains to be seen whether these interesting observations in vitro have clinical relevance for the scheduling of hormonal and chemotherapy.

Potential Novel Therapies

There is now the hope that identification of molecular determinants of growth, apoptosis, angiogenesis-metasta-

sis, and drug resistance can lead to new breast cancer therapies. In particular, strategies for coupling bacterial toxins to growth factors and antibodies directed toward receptors and tumor antigens on the cancer surface seem to be a real possibility. A second pont of vulnerability may be the induction of programmed cell death with the appropriate treatment. Antihormones, chemotherapeutic drugs, and differentiation agents may contribute to this process. A third point of tumor vulnerability seems to be processes of angiogenesis-metastasis. The literature would suggest that prevention of endothelial invasion of the tumor with antiprotease antigrowth factor or antiadhesion strategies would inhibit metastases. Likewise, similar strategies also might have direct effects on the invasive ability of tumor cells themselves. There is also much current enthusiasm concerning the potential for gene therapy. Ideal candidates for this would be the attempted reexpression of *Rb-1*, *p53*, or *nm23* tumor suppressor genes in breast tumors that either have lost expression entirely or express mutant proteins. Theoretically, this could be achieved by a retroviral vector strategy. Obvious hurdles in such approaches, however, would be development of systemic routes and target cell specificities and efficient incorporation techniques for such therapy, and the probability that multiple tumor suppressors become mutated. Finally, novel inhibitors for the p170 glycoprotein resistance pump are on the horizon and could be used to increase effectiveness of current chemotherapeutic agents. However, many other mechanisms of resistance might exist for antihormonal and cytotoxic drugs.

PREVENTION

Prevention of breast cancer seems to be a realistic hope. At present, there are ongoing trials to use tamoxifen for prevention in high-risk women with the rationale of inhibition of proliferation and progression of early lesions. Other potentially viable prevention strategies have been proposed using retinoids, vitamin D, progestins, antiprogestins, or contraceptive measures utilizing LHRH analogues. Other prevention strategies have diet as their focus. Lowered fat and increased vegetable consumption coupled with adequate exercise have been proposed. Finally, better application of mammography and biopsy techniques is almost certain to make a positive impact on the disease.[9,312–314]

Perhaps one of the most exciting long-term hopes is a better understanding of the role of mammary differentiation, such as that which occurs in early pregnancy and protects against the disease. Knowledge of how to interrupt proliferative processes pharmacologically or dietarily and how to induce differentiation likely will lead to new effective future strategies in breast cancer prevention and treatment.[314]

REFERENCES

1. Mant DM, Vessey MP: Epidemiology of breast cancer. *In* Bland KI, Copeland EM (eds): The Breast. Philadelphia, WB Saunders Company, 1991, pp 235–245

2. Coagner FB: History of breast disease and its treatment. *In* Bland KI, Copeland EM (eds): The Breast. Philadelphia, WB Saunders Company, 1991, pp 1–16

3. Fidler IJ, Nicolson GL: Concepts and mechanisms of breast cancer metastases. *In* Bland KI, Copeland EM (eds): The Breast. Philadelphia, WB Saunders Company, 1991, pp 395–408

4. Yeatman TJ, Bland KI: Staging of breast cancer. *In* Bland KI, Copeland EM (eds): The Breast. Philadelphia, WB Saunders Company, 1991, pp 313–330

5. Simpson JF, Page DL: Prognostic value of histopathology of the breast. Semin Oncol *19*:254, 1992

6. Lynch HT, Marcus JN, Watson P, Lynch J: Familial breast cancer, family cancer syndromes, and predisposition to breast neoplasia. *In* Bland KI, Copeland EM (eds): The Breast. Philadelphia, WB Saunders Company, 1991, pp 262–291

7. Early Breast Cancer Trialists' Collaborative Group: Systemic treatment of early breast cancer by hormonal, cytotoxic, or immune therapy. Lancet *339*:1, 1992

8. Early Breast Cancer Trialists' Collaborative Group: Systemic treatment of early breast cancer by hormonal, cytotoxic, or immune therapy. Lancet *339*:71, 1992

9. Powles TJ, Jones AL: Chemoprevention of breast cancer. *In* Powles TJ, Smith IE (eds): Medical Management of Breast Cancer. London, Martin Dunitz, 1991, pp 289–298

10. Leis HP: Prognostic parameters for breast carcinoma. *In* Bland KI, Copeland EM (eds): The Breast. Philadelphia, WB Saunders Company, 1991, pp 331–350

11. Elledge RM, McGuire WL, Osborne CK: Prognostic factors in breast cancer. Semin Oncol *19*:244, 1992

12. Dickson RB, Lippman ME: Growth regulation of normal and malignant breast epithelium. *In* Bland KI, Copeland EM (eds): The Breast. Philadelphia, WB Saunders Company, 1991, pp 363–394

13. Sakakura T: Mammary embryogenesis. *In* Neville MC, Daniel CW (eds): The Mammary Gland. New York, Plenum, 1987, pp 37–66

14. Russo J, Russo I: Development of the human mammary gland. *In* Neville MC, Daniel CW (eds): The Mammary Gland. New York, Plenum, 1987, pp 67–96

15. Salomon DS, Kidwell WR: Tumor associated growth factors in malignant rodent and human mammary epithelial cells. *In* Lippman ME, Dickson RB (eds): Breast Cancer: Cellular and Molecular Biology. Boston, Kluwer, 1988, pp 363–390

16. Anderson TJ, Battersby S, Macintyre CCA: Proliferative and secretory activity in human breast during natural and artificial menstrual cycles. Am J Pathol *130*:193, 1988

17. Longacre TA, Bartow SA: A correlative morphologic study of human breast and endometrium in the menstrual cycle. Am J Surg Pathol *10*:382, 1986

18. Daniel CW, Silberstein GB: Developmental biology of the mammary gland. *In* Neville MC, Daniel CW (eds): The Mammary Gland. New York, Plenum, 1987, pp 3–36

19. Haslam SZ: Stromal-epithelial interactions in normal and neoplastic mammary gland. *In* Lippman ME, Dickson RB (eds): Regulatory Mechanisms in Breast Cancer. Boston, Kluwer, 1990, pp 401–420

20. Streuli CH, Bailey N, Bissell MJ: Control of mammary epithelial differentiation: Basement membrane induces tissue-specific gene expression in the absence of cell-cell interaction and morphological polarity. J Cell Biol *115*:1383, 1991

21. Monteagudo C, Merino MJ, San-Juan J, et al: Immunohistochemical distribution of type IV collagenase in normal, benign, and malignant breast tissue. Am J Pathol *136*:585, 1990

22. Beatson GT: On the treatment of inoperable cases of carcinoma of the mamma: Suggestion for a new method of treatment, with illustrative cases. Lancet *2*:104, 1896

23. Welsch CW: Host factors affecting the growth of carcinogen-induced rat mammary carcinomas: A review and tribute to Charles Brenton Huggins. Cancer Res *45*:3415, 1985

24. Jabara AG, Toyne PH, Harcourt AG: Effects of time and duration of progesterone administration on mammary tumors induced by DMBA in Sprague Dawley rats. Br J Cancer *27*:63, 1973

25. Robinson SP, Jordan VC: Reversal of the antitumor effects of tamoxifen by progesterone in the DMBA-induced rat mammary carcinoma model. Cancer Res *47*:5386, 1987

26. Molinolo AA, Lanari C, Charreau EH, et al: Mouse mammary tumors induced by medroxy progesterone acetate: Immunohistochemistry and hormonal receptors. J Natl Cancer Inst *79*:1341, 1987

27. Clarke CL, Sutherland RL: Progestin regulation of cellular proliferation. Endocr Rev *11*:266, 1990

28. McCarty KS: Proliferative stimuli in the normal breast: Estrogens or progestins. Hum Pathol *20*:1137, 1989

29. Committee on the Relationship between Oral Contraceptives and Breast Cancer, IOM, DHPDP: Oral Contraceptives and Breast Cancer. Washington, DC, National Academy Press, 1991, pp 1–185

30. Daniel CW, Silberstein GA, Strickland P: Direct action of 17β estradiol in mouse mammary ducts analyzed by sustained release implants and steroid autoradiography. Cancer Res *47*:6052, 1987

31. Dulbecco R: Experimental studies in mammary development and cancer: Relevance to human cancer. Adv Oncol *5*:3, 1990

32. Vickers PJ, Dickson RB, Cowan KH: Multidrug-resistance in human breast cancer. Trends Pharmacol Sci *9*:443, 1988

33. Taylor-Papadimitriou J, Lane EB: Keratin expression in the mammary gland. *In* Neville MC, Daniel CW (eds): The Mammary Gland. New York, Plenum, 1987, pp 181–216

34. Osborne CK, Yochmowitz MG, Knight WA III, et al: The value of estrogen and progesterone receptors in the treatment of breast cancer. Cancer *46*:2884, 1980

35. Allegra JC, Lippman ME: Estrogen receptor status and the disease-free interval in breast cancer. Recent Results Cancer Res *71*:20, 1980

36. DeSombre ER, Jensen EV: Estrophilin assays in breast cancer: Quantitative features and application to the mastectomy specimens. Cancer *46*:2783, 1980

37. Paridaens R, Sylvester RJ, Ferrazzi E, et al: Clinical significance of the quantitative assessment of estrogen receptors in advanced breast cancer. Cancer *46*:2889, 1980

38. Edwards DP, Chamness GC, McGuire WL: Estrogen and progesterone receptor proteins in breast cancer. Biochim Biophys Acta *560*:457, 1979

39. DeSombre ER, Green GL, Jensen EV: Estrophilin and endocrine responsiveness of breast cancer. *In* McGuire WL (ed): Hormones, Receptors and Breast Cancer. New York, Raven Press, 1978, pp 1–25

40. Kassis JA, Sakai D, Walent JH, Gorski J: Primary cultures of estrogen-responsive cells from rat uteri: Induction of progesterone receptors and a secreted protein. Endocrinology *114*:1558, 1984

41. Eckert RL, Katzenellenbogen BS: Human endometrial cells in primary tissue culture: Modulation of the progesterone receptor level by natural and synthetic estrogens in vitro. J Clin Endocrinol Metab *52*:699, 1981

42. Kumar V, Green S, Stack G, et al: Functional domains of the human estrogen receptor. Cell *51*:941, 1987

43. McGuire WL, Chamness GC, Fuqua SAW: Estrogen receptor variants in clinical breast cancer. Mol Endocrinol *5*:1571, 1991

44. Dotzlaw H, Alkhalaf M, Murphy LC: Characterization of estrogen receptor variant mRNA's from human breast cancers. Mol Endocrinol *5*:773, 1992

45. Jiang SY, Jordan VC: Growth regulation of estrogen receptor-negative breast cancer cells transfected with complementary DNAs for estrogen receptor. J Natl Cancer Inst *84*:580, 1992

46. Touitou I, Vignon F, Cavailles V, et al: Hormonal regulation of cathepsin D following transfection of the estrogen or progesterone receptor into three sex hormone resistant cancer cell lines. J Steroid Biochem Mol Biol *40*:231, 1991

47. Paik S, Blair O, Lippman ME: Dominance of tamoxifen sensitive phenotype in MCF-7/LY-2 somatic cell hybrids [abstract]. Proc Annu Meeting Am Assoc Cancer Res *33*:1645, 1992

48. Tzukerman M, Zhang XK, Pfahl M: Inhibition of estrogen receptor activity by the tumor promoter 12-O-tetradecanyl-

phorbol-13-acetate: A molecular analysis. Mol Endocrinol 5: 1983, 1991

49. Saceda M, Knabbe C, Dickson RB, et al: Post transcriptional destabilization of estrogen receptor mRNA in MCF-7 cells by 12-O-tetradecanoylphorbol-13-acetate. J Biol Chem 266: 17809, 1991

50. Power RF, Mani SK, Codina J, et al: Dopaminergic and ligand-independent activation of steroid hormone receptors. Science 254:1636, 1991

51. Power RF, Conneely OM, O'Malley BW: New insights into activation of the steroid hormone receptor superfamily. Trends Pharmacol Sci 13:318, 1991

52. Yamamoto KR: Steroid receptor regulated transcription of specific genes and gene networks. Annu Rev Genet 19:209, 1985

53. Brock ML, Shapiro DJ: Estrogen stabilizes vitellogenin mRNA against cytoplasmic degradation. Cell 34:207, 1983

54. Kushner PJ, Webb P: A novel mechanism of transcriptional stimulation by the antiestrogens tamoxifen and ICI 164,384 [abstract]. In Proceedings of the Cold Spring Harbor Meeting on Genetics and Molecular Biology of Breast Cancer. Cold Spring Harbor, NY, Cold Spring Harbor Laboratory Press, 1992

55. Martin MB, Lindsey R, Saceda M: Anti-estrogen regulation of estrogen receptor expression in MCF-7 cells [abstract 932]. In Proceedings of the Endocrine Society 70th Annual Meeting, 1988

56. Beato M: Gene regulation by steroid hormones. Cell 56:335, 1989

57. Kumar V, Green S, Staub A, et al: Localisation of the oestradiol-binding and putative DNA-binding domains of the human oestrogen receptor. EMBO J 5:2231, 1986

58. Kumar V, Chambon P: The estrogen receptor binds tightly to its responsive element as a ligand-induced homodimer. Cell 55:145, 1988

59. Wang Y, Miksicek RJ: Identification of a dominant negative form of the human estrogen receptor. Mol Endocrinol 5:1707, 1991

60. Fawell SE, White R, Hoare S, et al: Inhibition of estrogen receptor DNA binding by the pure antiestrogen ICI 164,384 appears to be mediated by impaired receptor dimerization. Proc Natl Acad Sci USA 87:6883, 1990

61. Horwitz KB, McGuire WL: Actinomycin D prevents nuclear processing of estrogen receptor. J Biol Chem 253:6319, 1978

62. Horwitz KB, McGuire WL: Nuclear estrogen receptors. J Biol Chem 255:9699, 1980

63. Kasid A, Strobl JS, Huff K, et al: A novel nuclear form of estradiol receptor in MCF-7 human breast cancer cells. Science 225:1162, 1984

64. Monsa FJ Jr, Katzenellenbogen BS, Miller MA, et al: Characterization of the estrogen receptor and its dynamics in MCF-7 human breast cancer cells using a covalently attaching antiestrogen. Endocrinology 115:143, 1984

65. Saceda M, Lippman ME, Chambon P, et al: Regulation of the estrogen receptor in MCF-7 cells by estradiol. Mol Endocrinol 2:1157, 1988

66. Berkenstam A, Glaumann H, Martin M, et al: Hormonal regulation of estrogen receptor messenger ribonucleic acid in T47Dco and MCF-7 breast cancer cells. Mol Endocrinol 3: 22, 1989

67. Read LD, Greene GL, Katzenellenbogen BS: Regulation of estrogen receptor messenger ribonucleic acid and protein levels in human breast cancer cell lines by sex steroid hormones, their antagonists and growth factors. Mol Endocrinol 3:295, 1989

68. Ree AH, Landmark BF, Eskild W, et al: Autologous down-regulation of messenger ribonucleic acid and protein levels for estrogen receptors in MCF-7 cells: An inverse correlation to progesterone receptor levels. Endocrinology 124:2577, 1989

69. Saceda M, Lippman ME, Lindsey RK, et al: Role of an estrogen receptor-dependent mechanism in the regulation of estrogen receptor mRNA in MCF-7 cells. Mol Endocrinol 3:1782, 1989

70. Westley BR, May FEB: Oestrogen regulates oestrogen receptor

71. Piva R, Bianchini E, Kumar VL, et al: Estrogen induced increase of estrogen receptor RNA in human breast cancer cells. Biochem Biophys Res Commun 155:943, 1988

72. Dickson RB, Eisenfeld AJ: Estrogen receptor in liver of male and female rats: Endocrine regulation and molecular properties. Biol Reprod 21:1105, 1979

73. Beers PC, Rosener W: The binding of estrogens in the liver of the rat: Demonstration and endocrine influences. J Steroid Biochem 8:251, 1977

74. Shupnik MA, Gordon MS, Chin WW: Tissue-specific regulation of rat estrogen receptor mRNAs. Mol Endocrinol 3:660, 1989

75. Wei L, Krett NL, Francis MD, et al: Multiple human progesterone receptor messenger ribonucleic acids and their auto-regulation by progestin agonists and antagonists in breast cancer cells. Mol Endocrinol 2:62, 1988

76. Read LD, Snider CE, Miller JS, et al: Ligand-modulated regulation of progesterone receptor messenger ribonucleic acid and protein in human breast cancer cell lines. Mol Endocrinol 2:263, 1988

77. Kalinyak JA, Dorin RI, Hoffman AR, et al: Tissue-specific regulation of glucocorticoid receptor mRNA by dexamethasone. J Biol Chem 262:10441, 1987

78. Alexander IE, Clarke CL, Shine J, et al: Progestin inhibition of progesterone receptor gene expression in human breast cancer cells. Mol Endocrinol 3:1377, 1989

79. Okert S, Poellinger L, Dong Y, et al: Down-regulation of glucocorticoid receptor mRNA by glucocorticoid hormones and recognition by the receptor of a specific binding sequence within a receptor cDNA clone. Proc Natl Acad Sci USA 83: 5899, 1986

80. Dong Y, Poellinger L, Gustafsson J-A, et al: Regulation of glucocorticoid receptor expression: Evidence for transcriptional and posttranslational mechanisms. Mol Endocrinol 2:1256, 1988

81. Lazar MA, Chin WW: Regulation of two c-erbA messenger ribonucleic acids in rat GH3 cells by thyroid hormone. Mol Endocrinol 2:479, 1988

82. Zugmaier G, Knabbe C, Fritsch C, et al: Tissue culture conditions determine the effects of estrogen and growth factors on the anchorage independent growth of human breast cancer cell lines. J Steroid Biochem Mol Biol 39:684, 1991

83. Van Der Burg B, Kulkhoven E, Isbruecken L, et al: Effects of progestins on the proliferation of estrogen-dependent human breast cancer cells under growth factor-defined conditions. J Steroid Biochem Mol Biol 42:457, 1992

84. Paul D, Schmidt GH: Immortalization and malignant transformation of differentiated cells by oncogenes in vitro and in transgenic mice. Crit Rev Oncog 1:307, 1989

85. Heldin CH, Westermark B: Growth factors: Mechanism of action and relations to oncogenes. Cell 37:9, 1984

86. Goustin AS, Leof EB, Shipley GD, et al: Growth factors and cancer. Cancer Res 46:1015, 1986

87. Sporn MB, Roberts AB: Peptide growth factors and inflammation, tissue repair, and cancer. J Clin Invest 78:329, 1986

88. Bates SE, Davidson NE, Valverius EM, et al: Expression of transforming growth factor alpha and its mRNA in human breast cancer: Its regulation by estrogen and its possible functional significance. Mol Endocrinol 2:543, 1988

89. Massague J: Epidermal growth factor-like transforming growth factor. J Biol Chem 258:13606, 1983

90. Derynck R: Transforming growth factor α. Cell 54:593, 1988

91. Eckert K, Granetzny A, Fischer J, et al: Relationship between 43 kDa epidermal growth factor-related activity, clonogenic activity and clinical parameters for breast cancer. Anticancer Res 11:2125, 1991

92. Holmes WE, Sliwkowski MX, Akita RW, et al: Identification of heregulin, a specific activator of p185^{erbB2}. Science 256: 1205, 1992

93. Wen D, Peles E, Cupples R, et al: Neu differentiation factor: A transmembrane glycoprotein containing an EGF domain and an immunoglobulin homology unit. Cell 69:559, 1992

94. Peles E, Bacus SS, Koski RA, et al: Isolation of the neu/HER-

2 stimulatory ligand: A 44 kd glycoprotein that induces differentiation of mammary tumor cells. Cell 69:205, 1992

95. Cadena DL, Gill GN: Receptor tyrosine kinases. FASEB J 6:2332, 1992

95a. Plowman GD, Green JM, Couscou JM, et al: Herregulin induces tyrosine phosphorylation of Her4/p180 (erbB₄). Nature 366:473, 1993

95b. Samanta A, LeVea CM, Dougall WC, et al: Ligand and p185^{c-neu} destiny govern receptor interactions and tyrosine kinase activation. Proc Natl Acad Sci USA 91:1711, 1994

96. Cheifetz S, Bassols A, Stanley K, et al: Heterodimeric transforming growth factor β. J Biol Chem 263:10783, 1988

97. Ohtsuki M, Massague J: Evidence for the involvement of protein kinase activity in transforming growth factor-β signal transduction. Mol Cell Biol 12:261, 1992

98. Shibanuma M, Kuroki T, Nose K: Release of H₂O₂ and phosphorylation of 30 kilodalton proteins as early responses of cell cycle-dependent inhibition of DNA synthesis by transforming growth factor β₁. Cell Growth Differ 2:583, 1991

99. Massague J: Receptors for the TGFβ family. Cell 69:1067, 1992

100. Stromberg K, Hudgins R, Orth DN: Urinary TGFs in neoplasia: Immunoreactive TGF-α in the urine of patients with disseminated breast carcinoma. Biochem Biophys Res Commun 144:1059, 1987

101. Artega CL, Hanauske AR, Clark GM, et al: Immunoreactive alpha transforming growth factor (IrαTGF) activity in effusions from cancer patients: A marker of tumor burden and patient prognosis. Cancer Res 48:5023, 1988

102. Sairenji M, Suzuki K, Murakami K, et al: Transforming growth factor activity in pleural and peritoneal effusions from cancer and non-cancer patients. Jpn J Cancer Res 78:814, 1987

103. Grosse R, Bohmer FD, Binas B, et al: Mammary-derived growth inhibitor. In Dickson RB, Lippman ME (eds): Genes, Oncogenes and Hormones. Boston, Kluwer, 1992, pp 69–96

104. Ervin PR, Kaminski M, Cody RL, et al: Production of mammostatin, a tissue-specific growth inhibitor, by normal human mammary cells. Science 244:1585, 1989

105. Thompson MP, Farrell HM, Mohanam S, et al: Identification of human milk α-lactalbumin as a cell growth inhibitor. Protoplasma 167:134, 1992

106. Bano M, Kidwell WR, Lippman ME, et al: Characterization of MDGF-1 receptor in human mammary epithelial cell liver. J Biol Chem 265:1874, 1990

107. Bano M, Solomon DS, Kidwell WR: Purification of mammary derived growth factor 1 (MDGF 1) from human milk and mammary tumors. J Biol Chem 260:5745, 1985

108. Bano M, Lupu R, Kidwell WR, et al: Production and characterization of mammary-derived growth factor 1 in mammary epithelial cells. Biochemistry 31:610, 1992

109. Bano M, Worland P, Kidwell WR, et al: Receptor-induced phosphorylation by mammary derived growth factor 1 in mammary epithelial cells. J Biol Chem 267:10389, 1992

110. Coffey RJ, Derynck R, Wilcox JN, et al: Production and auto-induction of transforming growth factor-α in human keratinocytes. Nature 328:817, 1987

111. Masui T, Wakefield LM, Lechner JF, et al: Type β transforming growth factor is the primary differentiation-inducing serum factor for normal human bronchial epithelial cells. Proc Natl Acad Sci USA 83:2438, 1986

112. Stampfer MR, Bartley JC: Induction of transformation and continuous cell lines from normal human mammary epithelial cells after exposure to benzo-a-pyrene. Proc Natl Acad Sci USA 82:2394, 1985

113. Hammond SL, Ham RG, Stampfer MR: Serum-free growth of human mammary epithelial cells: Rapid clonal growth in defined medium and extended serial passage with pituitary extract. Proc Natl Acad Sci USA 81:5435, 1984

114. Perroteau I, Salomon D, DeBortoli M, et al: Immunological detection and quantitation of alpha transforming growth factors in human breast carcinoma cells. Breast Cancer Res Treat 7:201, 1986

115. King RJB, Wang DY, Daley RJ, et al: Approaches to studying the role of growth factors in the progression of breast tumors from the steroid sensitive to insensitive state. J Steroid Biochem 34:133, 1989

115a. Normanno N, Gullick WJ, et al: Expression of amphiregulin, cripto-1, and herregulin in human breast cancer cells. Int J Oncol 2:903, 1993

116. Knabbe C, Wakefield L, Flanders K, et al: Evidence that TGF beta is a hormonally regulated negative growth factor in human breast cancer. Cell 48:417, 1987

117. Knabbe C, Zugmaier G, Schmal M, et al: Induction of transforming growth factor beta by the antiestrogens droloxifen, tamoxifen, and toremifen in MCF-7 cells. Am J Clin Oncol 14(suppl 2):515, 1991

118. Butta A, MacLennan K, Flanders KC, et al: Induction of transforming growth factor β₁ in human breast cancer in vivo following tamoxifen treatment. Cancer Res 52:4261, 1992

118a. Noguchi S, Motomurak, Inaji H, et al: Down-regulation of transforming growth factor alpha by tamoxifen in breast cancer. Cancer 72:131, 1993

119. Murphy LJ, Sutherland RL, Steed B, et al: Progestin regulation of epidermal growth factor receptor in human mammary carcinoma cells. Mol Endocrinol 1:728, 1986

120. Murphy LC, Murphy LJ, Dubik D, et al: Epidermal growth factor gene expression in human breast cancer cells: Regulation of expression by progestins. Cancer Res 48:4555, 1988

121. Murphy LC, Dotzlau H: Regulation of transforming factor β messenger ribonucleic acid abundance in T47D, human breast cancer cells. Mol Endocrinol 3:611, 1989

122. Musgrove EA, Lee CSL, Sutherland RL: Progestins both stimulate and inhibit breast cancer cell cycle progression while increasing expression of transforming growth factor α, epidermal growth factor receptor, c-fos, and c-myc genes. Mol Cell Biol 11:5032, 1991

123. Krusekopf S, Chauchereau A, Milgrom E, et al: Co-operation of progestational steroids with epidermal growth factor in activation of gene expression in mammary tumor cells. J Steroid Biochem Mol Biol 40:239, 1991

124. Bates SE, McManaway ME, Lippman ME, et al: Characterization of estrogen responsive transforming activity in human breast cancer cell lines. Cancer Res 46:1707, 1986

125. Artega CL, Tandon AK, Von Hoff DD, et al: Transforming growth factor β: Potential autocrine growth inhibitor of estrogen receptor-negative human breast cancer cells. Cancer Res 48:3898, 1988

126. Dickson RB, Lippman ME: Control of human breast cancer by estrogen, growth factors, and oncogenes. In Lippman ME, Dickson RB (eds): Breast Cancer: Cellular and Molecular Biology. Boston, Kluwer, 1988, pp 119–166

127. Saeki T, Cristiano A, Lynch MJ, et al: Regulation by estrogen through the 5'-flanking region of the transforming growth factor α gene. Mol Endocrinol 5:1955, 1991

128. El-Ashry D, Lippman ME, Kern FG: Human TGF-α contains an estrogen responsive element composed of two imperfect palindromes [abstract]. In Proceedings of the Endocrine Society Meeting, 1991

129. Manni A, Wright C, Buck H: Growth factor involvement in the multihormonal regulation of MCF-7 breast cancer cell growth in soft agar. Breast Cancer Res Treat 20:43, 1991

130. Ahmed SR, Badger B, Wright C, et al: Role of transforming growth factor-α (TGF-α) in basal and hormone-stimulated growth by estradiol, prolactin and progesterone in human and rat mammary tumor cells: Studies using TGF-α and EGF receptor antibodies. J Steroid Biochem Mol Biol 38:687, 1991

130a. Kenney N, Sacki T, Gottordis M, et al: Expression of transforming factorα antisense mRNA inhibits estrogen induced production of TGFα and estrogen induced proliferation of estrogen responsive human breast cancer cell. J Cell Physiol 156:497, 1993

131. Colleta AA, Wakefield LM, Howell FV, et al: The growth inhibition of human breast cancer cells by a novel synthetic progestin involves the induction of transforming growth factor beta. J Clin Invest 87:277, 1991

132. Daly RJ, Harris WH, Wang DY, et al: Autocrine production of insulin-like growth factor II using an inducible expression system results in reduced estrogen sensitivity of MCF-7 human breast cancer cells. Cell Growth Differ 2:457, 1991

133. Cullen KJ, Lippman ME, Chow D, et al: Insulin-like growth factor-II overexpression in MCF-7 cells induces phenotypic changes associated with malignant progression. Mol Endocrinol 6:91, 1992

134. Slamon DJ: Role of the Her-2/neu gene in human breast and ovarian cancer [abstract]. In Proceedings of the Cold Spring Harbor Meeting on Genetics and Molecular Biology of Breast Cancer. Cold Spring Harbor, NY, Cold Spring Harbor Laboratory Press, 1992

135. McLeskey SW, Kurebayashi J, Honig SF, et al: Development of an estrogen-independent, antiestrogen resistant, metastatic breast carcinoma line by transfection of MCF-7 cells with fibroblast growth factor-4. Cancer Res 53:2168, 1993

136. Kurebayashi J, McLeskey SW, Johnson MD, et al: Spontaneous metastases of MCF-7 human breast cancer cell line cotransfected with fibroblast growth factor-4 and bacterial lacZ genes. Cancer Res 53:2178, 1993

137. Dickson RB, McManaway M, Lippman ME: Estrogen induced factors of breast cancer cells partially replace estrogen to promote tumor growth. Science 232:1540, 1986

138. Zugmaier G, Paik S, Wilding G, et al: Transforming growth factor beta 1 induces cachexia and systemic fibrosis without an antitumor effect in nude mice. Cancer Res 51:3590, 1991

139. Hurd SD, Johnson MD, Forbes JT, et al: Neutralizing TGFβ antibodies increase natural killer (NK) cell activity and inhibit human breast cancer cell tumorigenicity in athymic mice [abstract]. Proc Annu Meeting Am Assoc Cancer Res, San Diego, 1992

140. Salomon DS, Kidwell WR: Tumor associated growth factors in malignant rodent and human mammary epithelial cells. In Lippman ME, Dickson RB (eds): Breast Cancer: Cellular and Molecular Biology. Boston, Kluwer, 1988, pp 363–390

141. Vonderhaar BK: Regulation of development of the normal mammary gland by hormones and growth factors. In Lippman ME, Dickson RB (eds): Breast Cancer: Cellular and Molecular Biology. Boston, Kluwer, 1988, pp 251–266

142. Oka T, Tsutsumi O, Kurachi H, et al: The role of epidermal growth factor in normal and neoplastic growth of mouse mammary epithelial cells. In Lippman ME, Dickson RB (eds): Breast Cancer: Cellular and Molecular Biology. Boston, Kluwer, 1988, pp 343–362

143. Stampfer MR: Isolation and growth of human mammary epithelial cells. J Tiss Cult Methods 9:107, 1985

144. Osborne CK, Hamilton B, Titus G, et al: Epidermal growth factor stimulation of human breast cancer cells in culture. Cancer Res 40:2361, 1980

145. Davidson NE, Gelmann EP, Lippman ME, et al: Epidermal growth factor receptor gene expression in estrogen receptor-positive and negative human breast cancer cell lines. Mol Endocrinol 1:216, 1987

146. Kurachi H, Okamoto S, Oka T: Evidence for the involvement of the submandibular gland epidermal growth factor in mouse mammary tumorigenesis. Proc Natl Acad Sci USA 81:5940, 1985

147. Salomon DS, Perroteau I, Kidwell WR, et al: Loss of growth responsiveness to epidermal growth factor and enhanced production of alpha-transforming growth factors in ras-transformed mouse mammary epithelial cells. J Cell Physiol 130:397, 1987

148. Liscia DS, Merlo G, Ciardiello F, et al: Transforming growth factor-α messenger RNA localization in the developing adult rat and human mammary gland by an in situ hybridization. Dev Biol 140:123, 1990

149. Snedeker SM, Brown CF, DiAugustine RP: Expression and functional properties of TGFα and EGF during mouse mammary gland ductal morphogenesis. Proc Natl Acad Sci USA 88:276, 1991

149a. Li S, Plowman GD, Buckley SD, et al: Heparin inhibition of autonomous growth implicates amphiregulin as an autocrine growth factor for normal human mammary epithelial cells. J Cell Physiol 153:103–111, 1992

150. Valverius EM, Bates SE, Stampfer MR, et al: Transforming growth factor alpha production and EGF receptor expression in normal and oncogene transformed human mammary epithelial cells. Mol Endocrinol 3:203, 1989

151. Bates SE, Valverius EM, Ennis BW, et al: Expression of the transforming growth factor α/epidermal growth factor receptor pathway in normal human breast epithelial cells. Endocrinology 126:596, 1990

152. Shoyab M, Plowman GD, McDonald VL, et al: Structure and function of human amphiregulin: A member of the epidermal growth factor family. Science 243:1074, 1989

153. Higashigama S, Abraham JA, Miller J, et al: A heparin-binding growth factor secreted by macrophage-like cells that is related to EGF. Science 251:936, 1991

154. Plowman GD, Green JM, McDonald VC, et al: The amphiregulin gene encodes a novel epidermal growth factor-related protein with tumor inhibitory activity. Mol Cell Biol 10:1969, 1990

155. Shankar V, Ciardiello F, Kim N, et al: Transformation of normal mouse mammary epithelial cells following transfection with a human transforming growth factor alpha cDNA. Mol Carcinog 2:1, 1989

156. Ciardiello F, McGready M, Kim N, et al: TGFα expression is enhanced in human mammary epithelial cells transformed by an activated c-Ha-ras but not by the c-neu protooncogene and overexpression of the TGFα cDNA leads to transformation. Cell Growth Differ 1:407, 1990

157. Clarke R, Brunner N, Katz D, et al: The effects of a constitutive production of TGFα on the growth of MCF-7 human breast cancer cells in vitro and in vivo. Mol Endocrinol 3:372, 1989

158. Rosenthal A, Lindquist PB, Bringman TS, et al: Expression in rat fibroblasts of a human transforming growth factor-α cDNA results in transformation. Cell 46:301, 1986

159. Finzi E, Fleming T, Segatto O, et al: The human transforming growth factor type α coding sequence is not a direct-acting oncogene when overexpressed in NIH 3T3 cells. Proc Natl Acad Sci USA 84:3733, 1987

160. Stern DF, Hare DL, Cecchini MA, et al: Construction of a novel oncogene based on synthetic sequences encoding epidermal growth factor. Science 235:321, 1987

161. Gregory H, Thomas CE, Willshire IR, et al: Epidermal and transforming growth factor α in patients with breast tumors. Br J Cancer 59:605, 1989

162. Travers MR, Barrett-Lee PJ, Berger U, et al: Growth factor expression in normal, benign, and malignant breast tissue. BMJ 296:1621, 1988

163. Macias A, Perez R, Hägerström T, et al: Identification of transforming growth factor alpha in human primary breast carcinomas. Anticancer Res 7:1271, 1987

164. Eckert K, Granetzny A, Fischer J, et al: An Mr 43,000 epidermal growth-factor related protein purified from the urine of breast cancer patients. Cancer Res 50:642, 1990

165. Jhappan C, Stahle C, Harkins RN, et al: TGFα overexpression in transgenic mice induces liver neoplasia and abnormal development of the mammary gland and pancreas. Cell 61:1137, 1990

166. Coleman S, Daniel CW: Inhibition of mouse mammary ductal morphogenesis and down regulation of the EGF receptor by epidermal growth factor. Dev Biol 137:425, 1990

167. Sandgren EP, Luetteke NC, Palmiter RD, et al: Overexpression of TGFα in transgenic mice: Induction of epithelial hyperplasia, pancreatic metaplasia and carcinoma of the breast. Cell 61:1121, 1990

168. Matsui Y, Halter SA, Holt JT, et al: Development of mammary hyperplasia and neoplasia in MMTV-TGFα transgenic mice. Cell 61:1147, 1990

169. Ennis BW, Valverius EM, Lippman ME, et al: Anti EGF receptor antibodies inhibit the autocrine stimulated growth of MDA-MB-468 breast cancer cells. Mol Endocrinol 3:1830, 1989

170. Fitzpatrick SL, Brightwell J, Wittliff J, et al: Epidermal growth factor binding by breast tumor biopsies and relationship to estrogen and progestin receptor levels. Cancer Res 44:3448, 1984

171. Sainsbury JRC, Farndon JR, Sherbert GV, et al: Epidermal growth factor receptors and oestrogen receptors in human breast cancers. Lancet 1:364, 1985

172. Klijn JGM, Berns PMJJ, Schmitz PIM, et al: The clinical sig-

nificance of epidermal growth factor receptor (EGF-R) in human breast cancer: A review of 5232 patients. Endocr Rev 13:3, 1992

173. Cohen S, Ushiro H, Stoscheck C, et al: A native 170,000 epidermal growth factor receptor-kinase complex from shed plasma membrane vesicles. J Biol Chem 257:1523, 1982
174. Carpenter G, Cohen S: ^{125}I-labelled human epidermal growth factor (hEGF): Binding, internalization, and degradation in human fibroblasts. J Cell Biol 71:159, 1976
175. Ushiro H, Cohen S: Identification of phosphotyrosine as a product of epidermal growth factor-associated protein kinase in A-431 cell membranes. J Biol Chem 255:8363, 1980
176. Hunter T, Cooper JA: Epidermal growth factor induces rapid tyrosine phosphorylation of proteins in A431 human tumor cells. Cell 24:741, 1981
177. Velu TJ, Beguinot L, Vass WC, et al: Epidermal growth factor dependent transformation by a human EGF receptor proto-oncogene. Science 238:1408, 1987
178. DiFiore PP, Pierce JH, Fleming TP, et al: Overexpression of the human EGF receptor confers an EGF-dependent transformed phenotype to NIH3T3 cells. Cell 51:1063, 1987
179. Downward J, Yarden Y, Mayes E, et al: Close similarity of epidermal growth factor receptor and v-erbB oncogene protein sequence. Nature 307:521, 1984
180. Xu Y-H, Ishii S, Clark AJL, et al: Human epidermal growth factor receptor cDNA is homologous to a variety of RNAs overproduced in A431 carcinoma cells. Nature 309:806, 1984
181. Ullrich A, Coussens L, Hayflick JS, et al: Human epidermal growth factor receptor cDNA sequence and aberrant expression of the amplified gene in A431 epidermoid carcinoma cells. Nature 309:418, 1984
182. Lin CR, Chen WS, Verma IM, et al: Expression cloning of human EGF receptor complementary DNA: Gene amplification and three related messenger RNA products in A431 cells. Science 224:843, 1984
183. Makku VR, Stancel GM: Regulation of epidermal growth factor receptor by estrogen. J Biol Chem 260:9820, 1985
184. Lingham RB, Stancel GM, Loose-Mitchell DS: Estrogen regulation of epidermal growth factor receptor messenger ribonucleic acid. Mol Endocrinol 2:230, 1988
185. Hudson LG, Santon JB, Gill GN: Regulation of epidermal growth factor receptor gene expression. Mol Endocrinol 3:400, 1989
186. Saceda M, Dickson RB, Lippman ME, et al: Regulation of estrogen receptor gene expression in MCF-7 cells by tumor promoting agents [abstract]. In UCLA Symposium on Molecular, Biochemical and Cellular Biology of Breast Cancer, 1990
187. Xu YH, Richert N, Ito S, et al: Characterization of epidermal growth factor receptor gene expression in malignant and normal human cell lines. Proc Natl Acad Sci USA 81:7308, 1984
188. King CR, Kraus MH, Williams LT, et al: Human tumor cell lines with EGF receptor gene amplification in the absence of aberrant sized mRNAs. Nucleic Acids Res 13:8477, 1985
189. Kudlow JE, Cheung C-YM, Bjorge JD: Epidermal growth factor stimulates the synthesis of its own receptor in a human breast cancer cell line. J Biol Chem 261:4134, 1986
190. Bjorge JD, Kudlow JE: Epidermal growth factor receptor synthesis is stimulated by phorbol ester and epidermal growth factor. J Biol Chem 262:6615, 1987
191. Earp HS, Austin KS, Blaisdell J, et al: Epidermal growth factor (EGF) stimulates EGF receptor synthesis. J Biol Chem 261:4777, 1986
192. Kageyama R, Merlino GT, Pastan I: A transcription factor active on the epidermal growth factor receptor gene. Proc Natl Acad Sci USA 85:5016, 1988
193. Clark AJL, Ishii S, Richert N, et al: Epidermal growth factor regulates the expression of its own receptor. Proc Natl Acad Sci USA 82:8374, 1985
194. Johnson AC, Ishii S, Jinno Y, et al: Epidermal growth factor receptor gene promoter: Deletion analysis and identification of nuclear protein binding sites. J Biol Chem 263:5693, 1988
195. Kageyama R, Merlino GT, Pastan I: Epidermal growth factor (EGF) receptor gene transcription: Requirement for Sp1 and an EGF receptor-specific factor. J Biol Chem 263:6329, 1988
196. Merlino GT, Johnson AC, Kageyama R, et al: Isolation and characterization of DNA-binding factors regulating transcription of the EGF receptor proto-oncogene. In Lippman ME, Dickson RB (eds): Growth Regulation of Cancer II: UCLA Symposia on Molecular and Cellular Biology, New Series, Vol 115. New York, Alan R. Liss, 1990, pp 83–98
197. Ishii S, Xu Y-H, Stratton RH, et al: Characterization and sequence of the promoter region of the human epidermal growth factor receptor gene. Proc Natl Acad Sci USA 82:4920, 1985
198. Maekawa T, Imamoto F, Merlino GT, et al: Cooperative function of two separate enhancers of the human epidermal growth factor receptor proto-oncogene. J Biol Chem 264:5488, 1989
199. Coulouscow JM, Plowman GD, Carlton GW, et al: Characterization of a breast cancer cell differentiation factor that specifically activates the HER4/p180^{erbB_4} receptor. J Biol Chem 268:18407, 1993
200. Marchionni MA, Goodearl ADJ, Chen MS, et al: Glial growth factors are alternatively spliced erbB_2 ligands expressed in the nervous system. Nature 362:312, 1993
201. Peles E, Ban-Lerg R, Tzahan E, et al: Cell-type specific interaction of new differentiation factor (NDF/HER) with Neu/HER-2 suggests ligand-receptor interactions. EMBO J 12:961, 1993
202. Dobaski K, Davis JG, Mikami Y, et al: Characterization of a neu/erbB_2 protein-specific activating factor. Proc Natl Acad Sci USA 88:8582, 1991
203. Kern JA, Schwartz DA, Nordberg JE, et al: p185neu expression in human lung adenocarcinomas predicts shortened survival. Cancer Res 50:5184, 1990
204. Hall PA, Hughes CM, Staddon SL, et al: The c-erb B-2 proto-oncogene in human pancreatic cancer. J Pathol 161:195, 1990
205. Berchuck A, Rodriguez G, Kinney RB, et al: Overexpression of HER-2/neu in endometrial cancer is associated with advanced stage disease. Am J Obstet Gynecol 164:15, 1991
206. Semba K, Kamata N, Toyoshima K, et al: A v-erbB-related protooncogene, c-erbB-2, is distinct from the c-erbB-1/epidermal growth factor-receptor gene and is amplified in a human salivary gland adenocarcinoma. Proc Natl Acad Sci USA 82:6497, 1985
207. Coussens L, Yang-Feng TL, Liao YC, et al: Tyrosine kinase receptor with extensive homology to EGF receptor shares chromosomal location with neu oncogene. Science 230:1132, 1985
208. Bargmann CI, Hung MC, Weinberg RA: The neu oncogene encodes an epidermal growth factor receptor-related protein. Nature 319:226, 1986
209. Goldman R, Levy RB, Peles E, et al: Heterodimerization of the erbB-1 and erbB-2 receptors in human breast carcinoma cells: A mechanism for receptor transregulation. Biochemistry 29:11024, 1990
210. Quian XL, Decker SJ, Greene MI: p185-c-neu and epidermal growth factor receptor associate into a structure composed of activated kinases. Proc Natl Acad Sci USA 89:1330, 1992
211. Molina R, Tandon AK, Allred DC, et al: HER-2/neu oncoprotein in breast cancer: A comparison of immunohistochemical and western blot techniques [abstract]. Proc Annu Meeting Am Assoc Cancer Res 31:1012, 1990
212. Slamon DJ, Godolphin W, Jones LA, et al: Studies of the HER-2/neu proto-oncogene in human breast and ovarian cancer. Science 244:707, 1989
213. Paik S, Simpson S, King CR, et al: Quantification of erbB-2/neu levels in tissues. Methods Enzymol 198:290, 1991
214. Paik S, Hazan R, Fisher ER, et al: Pathologic findings from the National Surgical Adjuvant Breast and Bowel Project: Prognostic significance of erbB-2 protein overexpression in primary breast cancer. J Clin Oncol 8:103, 1990
215. Anbazhagen R, Gelber RD, Bettelheim R, et al: Association of c-erbB-2 expression and s-phase fraction in the prognosis of node positive breast cancer. Ann Oncol 2:47, 1991
216. Berchuck A, Kamel A, Whitaker R, et al: Overexpression of HER-2/neu is associated with poor survival in advanced epithelial ovarian cancer. Cancer Res 50:4087, 1990

217. Yonemura Y, Ninomiya I, Yamaguchi A, et al: Evaluation of immunoreactivity for erbB-2 protein as a marker of poor short term prognosis in gastric cancer. Cancer Res 51:1034, 1991

218. Yusa K, Sugimoto Y, Yamori T, et al: Low metastatic potential of clone from murine colon adenocarcinoma 26 increased by transfection of activated c-erbB-2 gene. J Natl Cancer Inst 82:1633, 1990

219. Bouchard L, Lamarre L, Tremblay PJ, et al: Stochastic appearance of mammary tumors in transgenic mice carrying the MMTV/c-neu oncogene. Cell 57:931, 1989

220. Guy C, Schaller M, Parsons T, et al: Induction of mammary tumors in transgenic mice expressing the unactivated c-*neu* oncogene [abstract]. *In* Proceedings of the Keystone Symposia on Breast and Prostate Cancers, Lake Tahoe, 1992

221. van de Vijver MJ, Peterse JL, Mooi WJ, et al: Neu-protein over-expression in breast cancer: Association with comedo-type ductal carcinoma in situ and limited prognostic value in stage II breast cancer. N Engl J Med 319:1239, 1988

222. Harris AC, Nicholson S, Sainsburg JR, et al: Epidermal growth factor receptors in breast cancer: Association with early relapse and death, poor response to hormones and interaction with *neu*. J Steroid Biochem 34:123, 1989

223. Langton BC, Crenshaw MC, Chao LA, et al: An antigen immunologically related to the external domain of gp185 is shed from mouse tumors overexpressing the c-erbB2 (HER-2/neu) oncogene. Cancer Res 51:2593, 1991

224. Drebin JA, Link VC, Greene MI: Monoclonal antibodies specific for the neu oncogene product directly mediate anti-tumor effects in vivo. Oncogene 2:387, 1988

225. King OR, Kraus M, DiFiore PP, et al: Implications of *erbB₂* overexpression for basic science and clinical medicine. Semin Cancer Biol 1:329, 1990

226. Mendelsohn J: The epidermal growth factor receptor as a target for therapy with antireceptor monoclonal antibodies. Semin Cancer Biol 1:339, 1990

227. Siegall CB, Fitzgerald DJ, Pastar I: Selective killing of tumor cells using EGF or TGFα-pseudomonas exotoxin chimeric molecules. Semin Cancer Biol 1:345, 1990

228. Hancock MC, Langton BC, Chan T, et al: A monoclonal antibody against the c-*erbB*-2 protein enhances the cytotoxicity of *cis*-diamminedichloroplatinum against human breast and ovarian tumor cell lines. Cancer Res 51:4575, 1991

229. Van Der Burg B, De Groot RP, Isbruecker L, et al: Oestrogen directly stimulates growth factor signal transduction pathways in human breast cancer cells. J Steroid Biochem Mol Biol 40:215, 1991

230. LeRoy X, Escot C, Browillet JP, et al: Decrease of c-*erbB₂* and c-*myc* mRNA levels in tamoxifen-treated breast cancer. Oncogene 6:431, 1991

231. Chiappetta C, Kirkland JL, Loose-Mitchell DS, et al: Estrogen regulates expression of the *jun* family of protooncogenes in the uterus. J Steroid Biochem Mol Biol 41:113, 1992

232. Murphy LJ: Estrogen induction of insulin-like growth factors and *myc* protooncogene expression in the uterus. J Steroid Biochem Mol Biol 40:223, 1991

233. Rusty AK, Dyson N, Bernards R: Amino terminal domains of c-myc and N-myc proteins mediate binding to the retinoblastoma gene product. Nature 352:541, 1991

234. Watson PH, Pon RT, Shiu RPC: Inhibition of c-*myc* expression by phosphorothioate antisense oligonucleotide identifies a critical role for c-*myc* in the growth of human breast cancer. Cancer Res 51:3996, 1991

235. Berns EMJJ, Klijn JGM, Van Putten WLJ, et al: c-*myc* amplification is a better prognostic factor than *HER2/neu* amplification in primary breast cancer. Cancer Res 52:1107, 1992

236. Escot C, Theillet C, Lideream R, et al: Genetic alterations of the c-myc protooncogene in human breast carcinomas. Proc Natl Acad Sci USA 83:4834, 1986

237. Lee LW, Raymond VW, Tsao MS, et al: Clonal cosegregation of tumorigenicity with overexpression of c-*myc* and transforming growth factor α genes in chemically transformed rat liver epithelial cells. Cancer Res 51:5238, 1991

238. Hall JM, Lee MK, Newman B: Linkage of early onset familial breast cancer to chromosome 17q21. Science 250:1684, 1990

238a. Kamb A, Gruis NA, Weaver-Feldhaus J, et al: A cell cycle regulator potentially involved in genesis of many tumor types. Science 264:436, 1994

238b. Keyomarsi K, Pordee AB: Redundant cyclin overexpression and gene amplification in breast cancer cells. Proc Natl Acad Sci USA 90:1112, 1993

239. Thorlacins S, Jonasdottir O, Eyfjord JE: Loss of heterozygosity at selective sites on chromosome 13 and 17 in human breast carcinoma. Anticancer Res 11:1501, 1991

240. Malkin D, Li FP, Strong LC, et al: Germ line p53 mutations in a familial syndrome of breast cancer, sarcomas, and other neoplasms. Science 250:1233, 1990

241. Marx J: Genetic defect identified in rare cancer syndrome: A mutation in the p53 tumor suppressor gene underlies the high cancer rate in members of Li-Fraumeni families. Science 250:1209, 1990

242. Swift M, Morrell D, Massey RB, et al: Incidence of cancer in 161 families afflicted by ataxia-telangiectasia. N Engl J Med 325:1831, 1991

243. Sato T, Akiyama F, Sakamoto G, et al: Accumulation of genetic alterations and progression of primary breast cancer. Cancer Res 51:5794, 1991

244. Thompson AM, Steel CM, Chetty U, et al: p53 gene mRNA expression and chromosome 17p allele loss in breast cancer. Br J Cancer 61:74, 1990

245. Davidoff AM, Kerns BJM, Pence JC, et al: p53 alterations in all stages of breast cancer. J Surg Oncol 48:260, 1991

246. Osborne RJ, Merlo GR, Mitsudomi T, et al: Mutations in the *p53* gene in primary human breast cancers. Cancer Res 51:6194, 1991

247. Branda RF, O'Neill JP, Sullivan LM, et al: Factors influencing mutation at the *hprt* locus in t-lymphocytes: Women treated for breast cancer. Cancer Res 51:6603, 1991

248. Callahan R, Cropp C, Merlo G, et al: Molecular lesions in sporadic human breast carcinomas [abstract]. *In* Proceedings of the Cold Spring Harbor Symposium on Genetics and Molecular Biology of Breast Cancer. Cold Spring Harbor, NY, Cold Spring Harbor Laboratory Press, 1992

249. Muncaster MM, Cohen BL, Phillips RA, et al: Failure of *RB1* to reverse the malignant phenotype of human tumor cell lines. Cancer Res 52:654, 1992

250. Bevilacqua G, Sobel ME, Liotta LA, et al: Association of low nm23 RNA levels in human primary infiltrating ductal carcinomas with lymph node involvement and other histopathologic indicators of high metastatic potential. Cancer Res 49:5185, 1989

251. Steeg P, Benedict MA, MacDonald NJ, et al: Transfection and biochemical analysis of nm23 function [abstract]. *In* Proceedings of the Cold Spring Harbor Meeting on Genetics and Molecular Biology of Breast Cancer. Cold Spring Harbor, NY, Cold Spring Harbor Laboratory Press, 1992

252. Saito H, Streuli M: Molecular characterization of protein tyrosine phosphatases. Cell Growth Differ 2:59, 1991

253. Fischer EH, Charbonneau H, Tonks NK: Protein tyrosine phosphatases: A diverse family of intracellular and transmembrane enzymes. Science 253:401, 1991

254. Drake JW: Mutation rates. Bioessays 2:137, 1992

255. Cohen SM, Ellwein LB: Genetic errors, cell proliferation, and carcinogenesis. Cancer Res 51:6493, 1991

256. Tlsty TD, White A, Sanchez J: Suppression of gene amplification in human cell hybrids. Science 256:1425, 1992

257. Moffett BF, Baban D, Bao L, et al: Fate of clonal lineages during neoplasia and metastasis studied with an incorporated genetic marker. Cancer Res 52:1737, 1992

258. Ciardiello F, Gottardis M, Basolo F, et al: Additive effects of c-*erbB*-2, c-Ha-*ras*, and transforming growth factor α genes on the *in vitro* transformation of human mammary epithelial cells. Carcinogenesis 6:43, 1992

259. Valverius EM, Ciardiello F, Heldin NE, et al: Stromal influences on transformation of human mammary epithelial cells overexpressing c-myc and SV40T. J Cell Physiol 145:207, 1990

260. Sinn E, Muller W, Pattengale P, et al: Coexpression of MMTV/v-Ha-ras and MMTV/c-myc genes in transgenic mice: Synergistic actions of oncogenes *in vivo*. Cell 49:465, 1987

260a. Amundadottir LT, Johnson MD, Smith GH, et al: The interaction of TGFα and c-myc in mouse mammary gland tumorigenesis. Proceedings of the Keystone Symposium on Breast and Prostate Cancer II. Lake Tahoe, 1994

261. Valles AM, Tucker GC, Thiery JP, et al: Alternative patterns of mitogenesis and cell scattering induced by acidic FGF and a function of cell density in a rat bladder carcinoma cell line. Cell Regul 1:975, 1990

262. Rusciano D, Burger MM: Why do cancer cells metastasize into particular organs? Bioessays 14:185, 1992

263. Strange R, Li F, Friis RR, et al: Mammary epithelial differentiation in vitro: Minimum requirements for a functional response to hormonal stimulation. Cell Growth Differ 2:549, 1991

264. Sommers CL, Thompson EW, Torri JA, et al: Cell adhesion molecule uvomorulin expression in human breast cancer cell lines: Relationship to morphology and invasive capacities. Cell Growth Differ 2:365, 1991

265. Thompson EW, Paik S, Brunner N, et al: Association of increased basement membrane-invasiveness with absence of estrogen receptor and expression of vimentin in human breast cancer cell lines. J Cell Physiol 150:534, 1992

266. Boyer B, Tucker GC, Valles AM, et al: Rearrangements of desmosomal and cytoskeletal proteins during the transition from epithelial to fibroblastoid organization in cultured rat bladder carcinoma cells. J Cell Biol 109:1495, 1989

267. Hendrix MJC, Seftor EA, Chu YW, et al: Coexpression of vimentin and keratins by human melanoma tumor cells: Correlation with invasive and metastatic potential. J Natl Cancer Inst 84:165, 1992

268. Navarro P, Gomez M, Pizarro A, et al: A role for the E-cadherin cell-cell adhesion molecule during tumor progression of mouse epidermal carcinogenesis. J Cell Biol 115:517, 1991

269. Stetler-Stevenson WG, Liotta LA, Brown PD: Role of type IV collagenases in human breast cancer. In Dickson RB, Lippman ME (eds): Genes, Oncogenes and Hormones. Boston, Kluwer, 1992, pp 21–42

269a. Groendahl-Hansen J, Christensen IJ, Rosenquist C, et al: High levels of urokinase-type plasminogen activator and its inhibitor PAI-1 in cytosolic extracts of breast carcinomas are associated with poor prognosis. Cancer Res 53:2513, 1993

270. Rochefort H, Augereau P, Capony F, et al: The 52k cathepsin D of breast cancer: Structure, regulation, function, and clinical value. In Lippman ME, Dickson RB (eds): Breast Cancer: Cellular and Molecular Biology. Boston, Kluwer, 1988, pp 207–222

271. Shi YE, Towi J, Yieh L, et al: Identification and characteristics of a novel matrix-degrading protease from hormone-dependent breast cancer cells. Cancer Res 53:1409, 1993

272. O'Brian CA, Vogel VG, Singletary SE, Ward NE: Elevated protein kinase C expression in human breast tumor biopsies relative to normal breast tissue. Cancer Res 49:3215, 1989

273. Hartwig JH, Thelen M, Rosen A, et al: MARCKS is an actin filament crosslinking protein regulated by protein kinase C and calcium-calmodulin. Nature 356:618, 1992

274. Isakov N, Gopas J, Priel E, et al: Effect of protein kinase C activating tumor promoters on metastases formation by fibrosarcoma cells. Invasion Metastasis 11:14, 1991

275. Liotta LA, Steeg PS, Stetler-Stevenson WA: Cancer metastases and angiogenesis: An imbalance of positive and negative regulation. Cell 64:327, 1991

276. Castronova V, Taraboletti G, Liotta LA, et al: Modulation of laminin receptor expression by estrogen and progestins in human breast cancer. J Natl Cancer Inst 81:781, 1989

277. Hynes RO: Integrins: A family of cell surface receptors. Cell 48:549, 1987

278. Thompson EW, Torri J, Arand G, et al: Basement membrane invasion/migration stimulated by the erbB-2 receptor ligand (gp30) in human breast cancer cell lines [abstract]. In Proceedings of the Keystone Symposium on Breast and Prostate Cancer. Lake Tahoe, 1992

279. Jouanneau J, Gavrilovic J, Caruelle D, et al: Secreted or nonsecreted forms of acidic fibroblast growth factor produced by transfected epithelial cells influence cell morphology, motil-

ity, and invasive potential. Proc Natl Acad Sci USA 88:2893, 1991

280. Rosen EM, Knesel J, Goldberg ID: Scatter factor and its relationship to hepatocyte growth factor and met. Cell Growth Differ 2:603, 1991

281. Thompson EW, Katz D, Shima TB, et al: ICI 164,384: A pure antiestrogen for basement membrane invasiveness and proliferation of MCF-7 cells. Cancer Res 49:6929, 1990

282. Greg AM, Schor AM, Rushton G, et al: Purification of the migration stimulating factor produced by fetal and breast cancer patient fibroblasts. Proc Natl Acad Sci USA 86:2438, 1989

283. Singer C, Smith HS, Lippman ME, Cullen KJ: IGF-1 and IGF-II expression in fibroblasts derived from tumor, normal breast and skin of breast cancer patients [abstract]. In Proceedings of the Keystone Symposium on Breast and Prostate Cancer. Lake Tahoe, 1992

284. Lamacher JM, Podhajcer OL, Chenard MP, et al: A novel metalloproteinase gene specifically expressed in stromal cells of breast carcinomas. Nature 348:699, 1990

285. Sakakura T, Ishihara A, Yatani R: Tenascin in mammary gland development: From embryogenesis to carcinogenesis. In Lippman ME, Dickson RB (eds): Regulatory Mechanisms in Breast Cancer. Boston, Kluwer, 1991, pp 365–382

286. Blood CH, Zetter BR: Tumor interactions with the vasculature: Angiogenesis and tumor metastases. Biochim Biophys Acta 1032:89, 1990

287. Widner N, Semple JP, Welsch WR, et al: Tumor angiogenesis and metastases—correlation in invasive breast carcinoma. N Engl J Med 324:1, 1991

288. Price JE, Polyzos A, Zhang RD, et al: Tumorigenicity and metastases of human breast carcinoma cell lines in nude mice. Cancer Res 50:717, 1990

289. Meschter CL, Connolly JM, Rose DP: Influence of regional location of the inoculation site and dietary fat on the pathology of MDA-MB-435 human breast cancer cell-derived tumors given in nude mice. Clin Exp Metastasis 10:167, 1992

290. Naguchi M, Ohta N, Kifugawa H, et al: Effects of switching from a high fat diet to a low fat diet on tumor proliferation and cell kinetics of DMBA-induced mammary carcinoma in rats. Oncology 49:246, 1992

291. Kandel J, Bossy-Wetzel E, Radvanyi F, et al: Neovascularization is associated with a switch to the export of bFGF in the multistep development of fibrosarcoma. Cell 66:1095, 1991

292. Murakami A, Tanaka H, Matsuzawa A: Association of hst gene expression with metastatic phenotype in mouse mammary tumor cells. Cell Growth Differ 1:225, 1990

293. Dickson C, Fantl A, Lammie S, et al: Growth factor and cell cycle genes implicated in mammary tumorigenesis [abstract]. In Proceedings of the Cold Spring Harbor Meeting on Genetics and Molecular Biology of Breast Cancer, 1992

294. Wellstein A, Fang W, Khatri A, et al: A heparin-binding growth factor secreted from breast cancer cells is homologous to a developmentally regulated cytokine. J Biol Chem 267:2582, 1992

295. Hamm JT, Ross WE: Patterns of recurrence in breast cancer. In Bland KI, Copeland EW (eds): The Breast. Philadelphia, WB Saunders Company, 1991, pp 309–312

296. Powles T, Smith IE (eds): Medical Management of Breast Cancer. London, Martin Dunitz, 1991

297. Horowitz KB: The molecular biology of RU486: Is there a role for antiprogestins in the treatment of breast cancer? Endocr Rev 13:146, 1992

298. Sledge GW, Antman KH: Progression chemotherapy for metastatic breast cancer. Semin Oncol 19:317, 1992

299. Paterson AHG: The natural history of breast cancer and the impact of systemic therapy. In Powles T, Smith IE (eds): Medical Management of Breast Cancer. London, Martin Dunitz, 1992, pp 37–48

300. Clarke R, Brunner N, Thompson EW, et al: The interrelationships between ovarian independent growth, tumorigenicity, invasiveness, and antiestrogen resistance in the malignant progression of human breast cancer. J Endocrinol 122:331, 1989

301. Bronzert DA, Greene GL, Lippman ME: Selection and characterization of a breast cancer cell line resistant to the antiestrogen LY 117018. Endocrinology 117:1409, 1985

302. Osborne CK, Coronado EB, Wiebe VJ, et al: Antiestrogen sensitivity and resistance [abstract]. In Proceedings of the 74th Annual Meeting of the Endocrine Society. San Antonio, 1992

303. Gottardis MM, Jordan VC: Development of tamoxifen-stimulated growth of MCF-7 tumors in athymic mice after long-term antiestrogen administration. Cancer Res 48:5183, 1988

304. Graham ML II, Smith JA, Jewett PB, et al: Heterogeneity of progesterone receptor content and remodeling by tamoxifen characterize subpopulations of cultured human breast cancer cells: Analysis by quantitative dual parameter flow cytometry. Cancer Res 52:593, 1992

305. Jackson IM, Litherland S, Wakeling AE: Tamoxifen and other antiestrogens. In Powles TJ, Smith IE (eds): Medical Management of Breast Cancer. London, Martin Dunitz, 1991, pp 51–59

306. Pastan I, Gottesman MM: Multiple drug resistance in human cancer. N Engl J Med 316:1388, 1987

307. Schneider J, Bak M, Efferth T, et al: P-glycoprotein expression in treated and untreated human breast cancer. Br J Cancer 60:815, 1989

308. DeGregorio MW, Ford JM, Benz CL, et al: Toremifene: Pharmacological and pharmacokinetic basis of reversing multidrug resistance. J Clin Oncol 7:1359, 1989

309. Yang CPH, Depinho SG, Greenberger LM, et al: Progesterone interacts with P-glycoprotein in multidrug resistant cells and in the endometrium of gravid uterus. J Biol Chem 264:782, 1989

310. Vickers PJ, Dickson RB, Shoemaker R, et al: Multidrug resistant MCF-7 human breast cancer cell line which exhibits cross resistance to antiestrogens and hormone independent tumor growth in vivo. Mol Endocrinol 2:886, 1988

311. Clarke R, Currier S, Kaplan O, et al: Effect of expression of the multidrug resistance mdr-1 glycoprotein cDNA on hormone responsivity in human breast cancer cells. J Natl Cancer Inst 84:1506, 1992

312. Page DL, Dupont WD: Management of the patient at high risk. In Bland KI, Copeland EM (eds): The Breast. Philadelphia, WB Saunders Company, 1991, pp 1046–1052

313. Miller AB: Screening and detection. In Bland KI, Copeland EM (eds): The Breast. Philadelphia, WB Saunders Company, 1991, pp 419–425

314. Osborne MP, Telang NT: Primary prevention of breast cancer. In Bland KI, Copeland EM (eds): The Breast. Philadelphia, WB Saunders Company, 1991, pp 246–261

315. Martinez E, Wahli W: Characterization of hormone responsive elements. In Parker MG (ed): Nuclear Hormone Receptors. New York, Academic Press, 1991, pp 125–153

316. White MRA, Hung ME: Cloning and characterization of the mouse new promoter. Oncogene 7:677, 1992

317. Tal M, King CR, Kraus M, et al: Human HER2 (neu) promoter: Evidence for multiple mechanisms for transcriptional initiation. Mol Cell Biol 7:2597, 1987

SECTION IV

MOLECULAR BASIS OF CANCER THERAPY

18

CHEMOTHERAPY SUSCEPTIBILITY AND RESISTANCE

KATHLEEN W. SCOTTO
JOSEPH R. BERTINO

Despite the fact that chemotherapy remains the most successful option for the treatment of many tumor types, drug therapy often fails for several reasons. Perhaps the most serious impediment to the cure of neoplastic disease is drug resistance, either intrinsic or acquired. In *intrinsic* drug resistance, the tumor is not susceptible or barely susceptible to treatment from the outset; this type of resistance may be caused by pharmacologic obstacles or it may be due to *inherent properties* of the tumor cell (Table 18–1). *Acquired* resistance, in contrast, is observed in patients who have relapsed following successful chemotherapy (i.e., there initially had been substantial tumor regression or even complete remission, with no clinical evidence of residual disease). In this case, the new tumor has arisen from a small number of resistant tumor cells that had escaped initial therapy, and is refractory to the same drug regimen originally employed as a result of newly *acquired properties* of the tumor cell.

During the past decade, a large body of information has accumulated as a result of laboratory investigations into cellular drug resistance. Most of these studies have been directed at an understanding of acquired drug resistance, because highly resistant tumor cell lines can be produced easily, allowing mechanisms of resistance to be determined readily. Moreover, the rapid advances in molecular biology, particularly the development of polymerase chain reaction (PCR) and DNA sequencing technologies, has made it possible to identify dominant-acting genes whose altered expression is associated with the drug resistance phenotype. Furthermore, a recent genetic approach described by Roninson and colleagues promises to enable the identification of recessive gene products whose modulation plays a role in the resistance phenotype.[1] Although

less is known about intrinsic drug resistance, in most instances where it has been studied, the mechanisms responsible are similar to those found for acquired resistance. Nevertheless, it is premature at this point to predict the extent of this similarity.

In this chapter, the mechanisms underlying intrinsic and acquired resistance are reviewed in both experimental systems and patient tumors, although information on the latter is limited.[2] In addition, strategies to reverse drug resistance as well as predictive tests for resistance and sensitivity are discussed. Because it is not possible within the scope of this review to describe all known mechanisms of resistance to every drug, examples are used to illustrate principles, and extension to clinical circumstances is mentioned whenever appropriate. During recent years, specialized volumes on cancer drug resistance as well as informative reviews have been published.[3–8]

INTRINSIC RESISTANCE

Apparent Drug Resistance

Often, intrinsic drug resistance is not due to an inherent property of the tumor, but rather is caused by problems with drug administration, such as poor absorption, inadequate dosage, or inadequate clinical trial in terms of duration.[9] For example, following oral drug delivery, a certain level of drug is expected to be achieved in the blood. However, many factors may influence the absorption of a drug, including interaction with food and other drugs, and transit time. Studies in children treated with orally admin-

TABLE 18–1. CAUSES OF APPARENT AND INTRINSIC DRUG RESISTANCE

APPARENT OR SPECIOUS DRUG RESISTANCE
Poor absorption
Inadequate dosage
Wrong treatment schedule
Inadequate clinical trial
Drug interactions
Pharmacologic sanctuaries (brain, testes)
Kinetic resistance
   Large tumor (decreased growth fraction, larger
     number of "G_0" in cells)
   Hypoxic areas of tumor (poor perfusion of drug, cell in G_0)

INTRINSIC CELLULAR RESISTANCE
Poor uptake into tumor cell
Poor drug "activation"
Increased drug catabolism

istered 6-mercaptopurine have shown that there is a wide variation in the blood levels achieved after a standard dose.[10] In addition, a significant number of patients do not absorb orally administered melphalan well enough to achieve therapeutic drug levels.[11] Solid tumors may be inherently sensitive to a drug, but poor localization of a drug may result from factors such as heterogeneous blood supply or elevated interstitial pressure in the tumor.[12]

Pharmacologic Reasons for Inherent Drug Resistance

SANCTUARY SITES

Sanctuary sites that may be protected from exposure to drugs are the brain and the testes. The central nervous system (CNS) is protected by the blood-brain barrier, and cytotoxic concentrations of most antineoplastic drugs are not achieved in the cerebrospinal fluid (CSF) following parenteral administration. There are probably several components involved in creating the barrier, some of which may be specific for a subset of drugs. For example, it has been proposed that the inability of drugs of the multidrug resistance (MDR) phenotype (see later in this chapter) to penetrate the CNS and testes may be due to the presence, in the capillary endothelial cells, of a membrane protein involved in drug efflux (P-glycoprotein).[13]

In an effort to breach sanctuary sites, parenteral administration of some drugs (e.g., methotrexate [MTX]) has been replaced by intrathecal administration or irradiation to treat or prevent disease in the brain, meninges, or testes. It also has been shown that, when tumors arise in the brain, either as primary or metastatic tumors, there may be a partial deterioration of the blood-brain barrier; drugs that do not normally cross the barrier may be effective in these circumstances. In addition, the systemic administration of very high doses of drugs may provide sufficient spillage into the CNS to achieve cytotoxic concentrations in the CSF. For example, intravenous use of MTX in very high doses (>1 gm/sq m) has proven effective for the treatment and prophylaxis of meningeal leukemia and CNS lymphoma.[14]

DRUG SCHEDULING

The importance of the treatment *schedule*, particularly for antimetabolite drugs, has been demonstrated clearly in experimental studies and in some clinical trials. For example, when administered to children with acute lymphocytic leukemia (ALL) in relapse, MTX is much more effective in an intermittent pulse schedule than in a daily schedule.[15] There are also many examples in which the *sequence* of drug administration is critical in terms of therapeutic effect. Perhaps the most striking example of this is in the use of MTX and 1-asparaginase in the treatment of pre-B– or T-cell ALL. When administered together, 1-asparaginase will protect not only the host but the tumor from MTX toxicity. However, if MTX is given 24 hours prior to asparaginase, there is a striking cytotoxic effect on ALL cells, with virtually no normal tissue toxicity, because these tumors are auxotrophic for 1-asparaginase, whereas the bone marrow and gastrointestinal tract stem cells are not.[16,17]

TUMOR CELL KINETICS

Cell kill by many drugs, including antimetabolites, the vinca alkaloids, and topoisomerase inhibitors, is cell cycle dependent (i.e., is maximal when the tumor is growing rapidly and is in cycle). It follows that large tumors with a decreased growth fraction (containing a large number of stationary or "G_0" cells and/or hypoxic or necrotic areas) will be less affected by these drugs; in addition, there may be poor perfusion of the drug into the tumor. Therefore, in an advanced tumor in which growth has plateaued, treatment with antimetabolites may be less effective than would be expected if the same tumor had been treated earlier. For example, MTX has a poor efficacy in the *induction* of remission of ALL. However, when MTX is used as an adjunct treatment *during* remission (when tumors are presumably in log phase growth) there is a high cure rate of this disease.[15]

Cellular Resistance

One of the more recently studied aspects of intrinsic drug resistance is resistance that occurs at the level of the tumor cell. This predicts that a characteristic of the tumor cell, presumably one that is a property of the normal cell from which the malignant cell was derived, renders it resistant to certain chemotherapeutic agents. For example, colon tumors are inherently resistant to chemotherapy, but this resistance cannot be explained by any of the heretofore described mechanisms. It has been proposed, although not yet proven, that resistance may be mediated at least in part by the expression of the MDR-associated protein P-glycoprotein (Pgp).[18] It has been shown that, in normal tissues, Pgp is highly expressed in the differentiated epithelium of the colon; many tumors derived from these cells also have been shown to produce high levels of this protein, which may mediate their resistance to MDR drugs. As is discussed later in this chapter, Pgp also plays a major role in acquired drug resistance, when it is anomalously expressed in tumor cells following drug exposure.

ACQUIRED DRUG RESISTANCE

An increased understanding of the mechanisms of drug action and the availability of cell lines from human as well as animal tumors had led to the elucidation of mechanisms of drug resistance. As might be expected, more than one mechanism of resistance may follow drug selection, especially when the drug challenge and the ensuing degree of drug resistance is high.

In most instances, acquired drug resistance results from the outgrowth of a small group of mutant cells, preexisting in the population, that are resistant to the drug used in treatment and therefore have a growth advantage over the rest of the tumor. The frequency with which such drug-resistant cells can arise in a tumor may depend on the degree of tumor aneuploidy, the relative instability of the genome, and other factors. It follows from theoretical considerations, as described by Goldie and Coldman,[19] that the higher the mutation rate within the cell population the earlier a drug-resistant tumor cell is likely to emerge. The appearance of drug-resistant cells ranges from 1 in 10^4 to 1 in 10^6 doublings in a tumor cell population. Therefore, because human tumors are difficult to detect unless they contain at least 10^9 cells and have undergone a large number of doublings, it is easy to understand why single-agent chemotherapy is not curative (except for some patients with choriocarcinoma or Burkitt's lymphoma). This provides a strong argument for the use of a *combination* of drugs and for the use of drugs in the adjuvant setting (i.e., after surgery or irradiation) in order to eliminate the few remaining cells. However, one caveat of the latter approach is that x-rays and alkylating agents may increase the frequency of mutations and thus the frequency with which drug-resistant populations emerge.[20]

The type of mutation responsible for the acquisition of drug resistance often depends on the cell type, the drug used, and the schedule employed. For example, acquired resistance to the pyrimidine synthesis inhibitor N-phosphonoacetyl-L-aspartate (PALA) has been found to be almost invariably due to gene amplification,[21] whereas resistance to 5-fluorouracil (5FUra) may develop by one of several mechanisms.[22] Different resistance mechanisms also can occur depending on the dose schedule employed. For example, resistance of CEM lymphoblast cells to MTX following pulse (24-hour) exposures at high concentrations was found to be a consequence of decreased retention resulting from a decrease in MTX polyglutamylation, whereas continuous exposure to low doses of MTX selected for a population of drug-resistant cells that were defective in uptake or had high levels of the target enzyme, dihydrofolate reductase (DHFR).[23] Similarly, short-term high-dose exposures of colon carcinoma cells (HCT-8) to 5FUra in high doses resulted in cells resistant to MTX by a mechanism different than what was noted in cells selected by low-dose continuous exposure.[24] These observations may have clinical relevance in that tumors resistant to a certain dosage schedule of a drug still may be sensitive to the same drug administered in a different schedule.

The various mechanisms of acquired drug resistance are listed in Table 18–2 and discussed in the following pages.

Decreased Drug Influx

Some drugs, such as MTX and nitrogen mustards, enter cells via a carrier-mediated transport system. Alterations in the carrier (increase in K_t, decrease in V_{max}), presumably resulting from mutations or decreased synthesis, may limit the entry of the drug, thus resulting in drug resistance.[25,26]

Increased Drug Efflux

Perhaps the most widely studied resistance mediated by an increase in drug efflux is multidrug resistance. Cells resistant to drugs of this class (vinca alkaloids, most anthracyclines, etoposide, actinomycin D) are believed to be effluxed rapidly as a result of the presence of the plasma membrane protein Pgp, which apparently functions as an energy-dependent drug "transporter."[27,28]

A related mechanism also can underlie resistance to drugs such as MTX. In this case, there is not a change in a drug transport mechanism per se, but rather a decrease in the ability of the cell to convert the drug into a more efficiently retained form (by polyglutamulation).[29]

Increased Drug Inactivation

Increased drug inactivation may occur at several levels. In the case of cytosine arabinoside, for example, inactivation can occur at the level of the nucleoside or at the level of the nucleotide.[30] Drug inactivation also may occur via glutathione (GSH) adduct formation. For example, glutathione transferase (GST), which catalyzes the con-

TABLE 18–2. MECHANISMS OF ACQUIRED DRUG RESISTANCE

MECHANISM	EXAMPLES*
Decreased influx	MTX, nitrogen mustard
Increase in efflux	MDR drugs (doxorubicin, vinca alkaloids, etoposide, taxol)
Increase in inactivation of drug, or of activated drug	Ara-C, FUDR, alkylating agents
Decreased activation	5FUra, 6MP, ara-C
Increase in target enzyme	MTX, PALA
Altered target	MTX, etoposide, doxorubicin
Decrease in binding to target, not due to altered target	5FUra
Increased DNA repair	Cisplatin
Adaptation or "induction"	MTX, fluoropyrimidines

*MTX, methotrexate; ara-C, cytosine arabinoside; FUDR, 5-fluoro-deoxyuridine; 5FUra, 5-fluorouracil; 6MP, 6-mercaptopurine; PALA, N-phosphonoacetyl-L-aspartate.

jugation of GSH with free radicals, can inactivate several anticancer drugs, primarily alkylating agents such as chlorambucil, melphalan, and cyclophosphamide, and resistance to these agents has been shown in some cases to be due to increased production of GSTs.[31] Increase in the levels of GST and other GSH-metabolizing enzymes also has been implicated in the development of the MDR phenotype, although this remains to be proven.[32]

Decreased Drug Activation

Many drugs, particularly purine and pyrimidine analogues, are more efficiently taken up by cells when they are administered as the free base or nucleoside. Antitumor activity then depends on the capacity of these cells to convert the bases or nucleosides to the nucleotide forms, which then function as enzyme inhibitors or are incorporated into RNA or DNA, leading to cell death. Thus, drugs like 5FUra, which require activation, may be ineffective against cells that lack activating enzymes.[22]

Quantitative Changes in the Target Enzyme or Receptor

When the mechanism of drug action involves the inhibition of an enzyme or receptor molecule, resistance can be mediated by an *increase* in the level of this target protein, such that sufficient protein will escape drug action and remain available for normal cellular processes. The relative increase needed to confer resistance is dependent on the particular target or enzyme involved. For example, in cases in which the drug uptake is limited by a carrier-mediated process (e.g., MTX), a fairly small increase in the intracellular target protein may result in drug resistance. It is important to keep in mind that, because most therapeutics are administered at the maximum tolerated dose, even a two-fold increase in drug resistance can be clinically significant and render the current drug regimen ineffective.

If the mechanism of drug action involves the formation of a drug-target complex that is toxic to the cell, resistance can be mediated by a *decrease* in the target protein. Such a mechanism has been proposed for cells resistant to inhibitors of DNA topoisomerase II (Topo II)[33] (Table 18–3). Topo II mediates topologic changes in DNA that are essential for a variety of activities, including DNA replication, RNA transcription and chromatin condensation during mitosis. Some Topo II inhibitors, such as teniposide and etoposide (Table 18–3), bind Topo II and stabilize a "cleavable complex," presumably preventing chromosome segregation and DNA synthesis. Although a decrease in Topo II levels as a mechanism of drug resistance has not yet been established firmly, it has been shown that Chinese hamster ovary (CHO) cells that exhibit unusual *sensitivity* to Topo II inhibitors show an increase in enzyme levels. Moreover, it has been suggested that the intrinsic drug resistance of slow-growing tumors may be mediated in part by their inherently low levels of Topo II. However, it must be noted that some cells se-

TABLE 18–3. TOPOISOMERASE INHIBITORS IN CLINICAL USE

Topoisomerase I inhibitors	Camptothecin*
	CPT-11*
	Topotecan*
Topoisomerase II inhibitors	Etoposide
	Doxorubicin
	Daunorubicin
	m-AMSA (Amsacrine)*
	Mitoxantrone
	Actinomycin D
	9-Hydroxyellipticine*

*Investigational drugs.

lected for resistance to alkylating agents have an up-regulation of topoisomerase I, suggesting that multiple mechanisms may come into play.[34]

GENE AMPLIFICATION

When drug resistance in tissue culture cells is due to an overproduction of a target protein, the mechanism most often responsible for this overproduction, and the one most intensely studied to date, is gene amplification. The amplification of genes encoding DHFR first was found in cells highly resistant to MTX as a result of an increase in DHFR. Biedler and Spengler[35] noted that such cells contained chromosomal regions that appeared abnormal following Giemsa staining. They called these regions "abnormal banding regions" (ABRs) or "homogeneously staining regions" (HSRs) and postulated that they were the site of amplified genes. Shortly thereafter, Alt et al.,[36] using molecular hybridization techniques, demonstrated that the increase in DHFR enzyme activity found in these highly MTX-resistant cells was due to amplification of the *DHFR* gene. Subsequent studies have shown that, when gene amplification is "unstable" or reversible in the absence of drug, the amplified genes often are found on extra chromosomal elements called "double minute" chromosomes (DMs).[37] Because these DM chromosomes do not contain a centromere and are not distributed equally after cell division, cells containing these structures can decrease or increase their gene dosage rapidly depending on the selection pressure of the drug. In contrast, when the amplified *DHFR* genes are integrated into the chromosome, these cells are usually stably resistant; that is, even in the absence of the drug, resistance is maintained for long periods of time.

Other resistant cell systems in which amplification has been identified as the genetic mechanism underlying the overproduction of a target protein are listed in Table 18–4. It should be noted that for most drugs, with the possible exception of PALA, amplification is only one of several mechanisms that may be responsible for development of a drug resistance phenotype.

Mechanisms of Gene Amplification[38–43]

The chromosomal manifestations of gene amplification (HSRs and ABRs) usually are detected only when ampli-

TABLE 18–4. GENE AMPLIFICATION AS A MECHANISM OF DRUG RESISTANCE*

SELECTIVE DRUG	AMPLIFIED GENE
Methotrexate	Dihydrofolate reductase
5-fluorodeoxyuridine	Thymidylate synthase
PALA	CAD
Hydroxyurea	Ribonucleotide reductase
Deoxycoformycin	Adenosine deminase
Coformycin and adenine	AMP deaminase
Difluoromethyl ornithine	Ornithine decarboxylase
Doxorubicin, colchicine, vinca alkaloids	p170 glycoprotein
Albizzin	Asparagine synthetase
Hypoxanthine-aminopterin-thymidine	HGPRTase (mutant)
Compactin	Hydroxymethylglutaryl co-enzyme A reductase
6-Azauridine, pyrazofurin	UMP synthetase
Methionine sulfoximine	Glutamine synthetase
Ouabain	Na⁺/K⁺-transporting ATPase
Histidinol	Histidyl-tRNA synthetase
Tunicamycin	n-Acetylglucosaminyltransferase
Berrelidin	Threonyl-tRNA synthetase
Cadium	Metallothionein

*Data from refs. 39–41.

Abbreviations: PALA, N-phosphoacetyl-L-aspartate; CAD, carbamoylphosphate synthetase–aspartate carbamoyltransferase–dihydroorotase; HGPRTase, hypoxanthine-guanine phosphoribosyltransferase.

fication levels are high. Studies of the mechanism of gene amplification have shown that the initial event is a replication of a large segment of the genome (several thousand kilobases).[41] With additional selection, the size of the amplicon usually decreases to several hundred kilobases in length[38,41] and, in highly resistant cell lines, may be present in several hundred copies. Moreover, in addition to an amplification of the gene mediating drug resistance, other genes may be co-amplified. For example, we have reported that the hydroxymethylglutaryl co-enzyme A (HMG CoA) reductase gene is co-amplified in two MTX-resistant human cell lines with high gene copy number for DHFR.[42] Also, the amplification of the Pgp gene in MDR cells often is accompanied by the amplification of other genes, such as that for the calcium-binding protein sorcein.[44] In both instances there is no evidence that these inadvertently co-amplified genes are involved in mediating resistance to the selective agent.

The mechanism by which gene amplification occurs is not yet clear, although several models have been proposed.[38–41] It has been assumed generally that amplification is a random event associated with an error in DNA replication, and drug-resistant tumors arise as a result of the selection of a preexisting population that happens to have amplified a gene that confers a growth advantage in the presence of drug. However, one important observation has been that drugs or treatments that damage DNA can increase the frequency of gene amplification, suggesting that the frequency of amplification may be enhanced by external factors.[41] Furthermore, recent studies suggest that the tendency to amplify may be a characteristic peculiar to, or at least more prevalent in, tumor cells relative to normal cells as a result of a greater plasticity or instability

of their genome. For example, normal cells exposed to MTX do not develop resistance by DHFR gene amplification.[45,46] In our own studies of lethally irradiated mice treated with MTX after receiving marrow transfected with mutated DHFR drug-resistant genes, we have not seen amplification of either the endogenous or a transfected mutant DHFR gene. Recent evidence has linked the increased instability of tumor cell genomes, and hence their tendency to amplify, to mutations of the tumor suppressor gene p53. Cells that lack a wild-type p53 protein are unable to arrest at the G_1/S boundary to repair DNA damage, which could result in either cell death or gene amplification.[47,48]

Gene Amplification in Clinical Tumor Specimens

Surprisingly little information exists as to the frequency of gene amplification as a mechanism of resistance in the clinic. We have examined 38 samples of blast cells from patients with acute lymphocytic leukemia resistant to MTX and have found only a few instances of DHFR gene amplification associated with this resistance.[49] To date, there is no evidence for amplification of the Pgp gene in patients whose tumors exhibit an MDR phenotype.

TRANSCRIPTIONAL/POSTTRANSCRIPTIONAL REGULATION

Although gene amplification is the major genetic mechanism underlying the overexpression of drug targets in resistant tissue culture cells, it is not a major mechanism in clinical drug resistance. For example, increases in the level of Pgp and Pgp RNA have been associated with the development of MDR in several clinical cancers,[27,50,51] yet Pgp gene amplification has not been detected. Although the mechanism underlying the overexpression of Pgp genes in the absence of amplification is unknown, analysis of MDR cell lines suggests that regulation may be imposed at both the transcriptional and posttranscriptional levels, and may be influenced by tissue-specific as well as environmental factors.[52–55] The quantitative changes in Topo II levels observed in many drug-resistant cells (see earlier in this chapter) most likely also are regulated transcriptionally and/or posttranscriptionally. Recently, it has been shown that a reduction in the steady-state level of Topo II in resistant cells can be mediated by an allelic mutation in a Topo II gene[56] or an allelic hypermethylation of the gene,[57] presumably decreasing the amount of gene transcription. Whether these mechanisms play a role in clinical drug resistance is yet to be determined.

TRANSLATIONAL/POSTTRANSLATIONAL REGULATION

Increased activity of a target enzyme can occur in the absence of an increase in the encoding RNA, and most often is due to a posttranslational modification. For example, the function of many proteins is regulated by phosphorylation. Both Pgp and Topo II are examples of resistance-related proteins whose activity appears to be modulated by phosphorylation, although the precise nature of this regulation, and whether it plays a role in the resistance phenotype, has not yet been defined. Recent studies in laboratory models suggest that control at the level of translation also can lead to drug resistance. For example, preliminary evidence indicates that both thymidylate synthase (TS) and DHFR translation are subject to autoregulation—excess protein binds to the mNRA and prevents translation.[58-60]

Qualitative Changes in the Target Enzyme or Receptor

Mutations in target genes that cause drug resistance have been observed now for a large number of clinically useful compounds (Table 18–5). These mutations can result in loss of function (e.g., loss of an activating enzyme for a drug) or can make the target enzyme resistant to drug. The mutations are usually dominant because, although the product of the wild-type allele remains drug sensitive, there is usually a sufficient amount of mutant enzyme to confer resistance. Most mutations identified to date have occurred in the drug-binding site of the target protein.[61,62] Recently, a mutation that lies outside the drug-binding site of DHFR has been described; this mutation most likely interferes indirectly with MTX binding by altering enzyme conformation.[63] In some cases of resistance to Topo II inhibitors, changes have been identified in amino acid composition and phosphorylation pattern of the enzyme that are believed to be associated with the resistance phenotype.[64,65] Recently, resistance to camptothecin, a drug that inhibits topoisomerase I, has been shown to be associated with alterations in this enzyme.[66,67]

Decreased Drug-Target Binding

A relatively uncommon mechanism of drug resistance involves an increase in the amount or availability of the natural substrate for the drug target, which competes for inhibitor binding. Another rare mechanism involves a decrease in a co-enzyme required for the binding of inhibitor to its target. It has been reported recently that a cell line resistant to 5FUra exhibits a decrease in the level of the polyglutamate forms of the co-enzyme 5,10-methylene-tetrahydrofolate, required for the tight binding of the 5FUra metabolite FdUMP to TS.[23]

TABLE 18–5. EXAMPLES OF MUTATIONS IN TARGET ENZYMES GIVING RISE TO DRUG RESISTANCE

SELECTIVE DRUG	ALTERED TARGET
Methotrexate, trimetrexate	Dihydrofolate reductase
5-Fluorodeoxyuridine	Thymidylate synthase
Colchicine	P-glycoprotein
6-Mercaptopurine	HGPRTase
Etoposide, amsacrine	Topoisomerase II
Camptothecin	Topoisomerase I

Increased Repair of Drug Damage

Several anticancer drugs, such as alkylating and intercalating agents, target DNA and cause sublethal as well as lethal damage. Resistance to this class of drugs has been attributed in some circumstances to an increase in the ability to repair this type of damage, presumably as a consequence of increased activities of DNA repair enzymes. Indirect support of the notion that resistance to these agents involves alteration in DNA repair is found in the observation that DNA repair–deficient cells have been shown to be hypersensitive to *cis*-platinum.[68]

MECHANISMS OF RESISTANCE TO SPECIFIC ANTICANCER DRUGS

Mechanisms of resistance to chemotherapeutics have been identified in laboratory models (Table 18–6). In the limited number of cases in which clinical mechanisms have been investigated, they agree in context, but not necessarily in relative importance, with those identified in experimental systems.

Folate Antagonists

Four mechanisms of resistance to folate antagonists have been demonstrated in experimental systems (Fig. 18–1). In tumor cell lines, the most commonly observed mechanisms of resistance to MTX are increased synthesis of DHFR due to gene amplification and/or decreased influx of drug. A decrease in MTX polyglutamate formation or an altered DHFR with decreased affinity for MTX are less common resistance phenotypes.[69] Resistance to trimetrexate, a folate antagonist that most likely enters the cell through passive or facilitated diffusion and does not undergo polyglutamylation, is mediated by increased DHFR activity or mutations in *DHFR* that decrease drug binding. Resistance to trimetrexate also has been reported to be associated, in rare instances, with increased expression of Pgp.[70]

To date, three of the mechanisms of MTX resistance identified in laboratory models have been observed in clinical samples. Both gene amplification and, more commonly, decreased uptake have been found in blasts from patients with ALL who are clinically resistant to MTX.[49,71] Inherent resistance to MTX in patients with soft tissue sarcoma and acute myelocytic leukemia likely is due to lack of polyglutamate formation, resulting in poor drug retention.[72] Mutations in DHFR have not yet been observed in tumor cases resistant to MTX, but the number of patient samples tested for this resistance mechanism has been limited.

Fluorouracil

Both the mechanism of action and, consequently, the mechanism of resistance to 5FUra are complex and may

TABLE 18–6. MECHANISMS OF DRUG RESISTANCE TO THE COMMONLY USED ANTICANCER AGENTS

DRUG	MECHANISM OF RESISTANCE
Methotrexate	Decreased influx Decreased polyglutamylation Increase in polyglutamate hydrolase Increase in DHFR activity Altered DHFR
Fluorouracil	Decreased activation Decreased incorporation in RNA Increase in thymidylate synthase Altered thymidylate synthase Increased breakdown of nucleotide Decreased nucleotide formation
6-Mercaptopurine	Increased breakdown of nucleotide
Cytosine arabinoside	Decreased uptake Increased breakdown Poor nucleotide formation
Alkyating agents	Poor uptake (nitrogen mustard) Increase in catabolism or inactivation Increased repair of DNA damage
Cisplatin	Poor uptake Increase in catabolism or inactivation Increased repair of DNA damage
Doxorubicin	Increased efflux (MDR) Altered toposimerase II binding
Vinblastine, vincristine	Increased efflux (MDR) Decreased binding to tubulin Increased breakdown
Taxol	Increased efflux (MDR) Decreased binding to tubulin
Etoposide	Increased efflux (MDR) Altered topoisomerase II binding
Nitrosoureas	Repair of alkylated DNA (O-methyltransferase)
L-asparaginase	Increase in asparagine synthetase

depend on the dose and schedule employed.[21] Two different dose schedules generally are used to treat neoplastic disease in humans: pulse treatments administered intravenously weekly or daily × 5, or intravenous infusions extending from 24 hours to 3 weeks or greater. Unlike what has been observed with fluorodeoxyuridine, toxicity to 5FUra decreases as the duration of the infusion is lengthened. In laboratory models, several mechanisms of 5FUra resistance have been identified, including decreased anabolism of 5FUra to the nucleotide, decreased incorporation of 5FUra into RNA, altered expression of the target protein TS, and increased breakdown of the 5FUra nucleotide (Fig. 18–2). However, mechanisms of resistance to this drug have not yet been elucidated in the clinic, in part because of the difficulty in obtaining pure populations of tumor cells from patients following treatment. A promising recent study showed that gastric tumors with low levels of TS mRNA responded to treatment with 5FUra, whereas tumors with higher levels of expression did not,[73] supporting the laboratory studies indicating that an increase in TS expression confers 5FUra resistance.

Cytosine Arabinoside

The pyrimidine antagonist cytosine arabinoside (ara-C) is used to treat acute leukemia and intermediate and high-grade lymphoma, usually in combination with daunomycin or MTX, respectively. Drug efficacy has been correlated with efficient intracellular conversion of ara-C to ara-CTP and subsequent incorporation into DNA. Decreased activity of the enzyme responsible for this conversion (deoxycytidine kinase) and increased breakdown of ara-C (via cytosine deaminase) or ara-CMP (via deoxycytidylate deaminase) (Fig. 18–3) are resistance mechanisms commonly observed in experimental tumor models. However, none of these mechanisms appears to play a major role in clinical resistance. One mechanism that does appear to be clinically significant is decreased transport of ara-C,[74] although the transport molecules have not yet been identified.

Alkylating Agents

Table 18–6 lists the various mechanisms of resistance to alkylating agents that have been described in experimental tumors. One mechanism involves the inactivation of these agents through an interaction with thiols, particularly GSH. It is not surprising, then, that an increase in the levels of both GSH and GST has been associated with resistance to alkylating agents.[31] Buthionine sulfoximine (BSO), a compound that lowers GSH levels, presently is being evaluated as a modulating agent in combination with alkylating agents.[75] Another example of increased drug catabolism as a mechanism of resistance has been reported in a cyclophosphamide-resistant cell line. In this case, resistance is mediated by an increased level of aldehyde dehydrogenase, a drug-metabolizing enzyme that converts aldophosphamide, a metabolite of cyclophosphamide, to an inactive compound. Inherent resistance to nitrosoureas is associated with the presence of the enzyme O-methyltransferase,[76] which removes from DNA the alkyl groups found as a consequence of nitrosourea alkylation. Inhibitors of this enzyme are now under investigation in the clinic. The importance of these mechanisms in clinical resistance is not yet known.

Cisplatin

Cisplatin cytotoxicity apparently occurs via the formation of intrastrand DNA cross links, and resistance is multifactorial (Table 18–6). A major mechanism of resistance involves an increased repair of these lesions, probably mediated by an increase in the expression of enzymes involved in DNA synthesis. Reduced intracellular accumulation of cisplatin also has been reported as a component of drug resistance in vitro. Additional mechanisms of resistance include decreased uptake or changes in DNA-binding proteins and metallothioneins.[68]

Vinca Alkaloids and Taxol

Tubulin is the major component of microtubules, which are the primary structural element of mitotic spindles. During mitosis, the segregation of chromosomes is mediated by the synthesis and breakdown of mitotic spindles. The vinca alkaloids exert their cytotoxic effect by binding to tubulin and inhibiting microtubule formation. The binding of taxol, in contrast, increases and stabilizes tubulin polymerization, thereby preventing breakdown.[77] These agents all are excluded rapidly from cells containing Pgp, and overexpression of this protein results in resistance to these compounds (Table 18–6). Alterations in tubulin that decrease binding of these drugs also have been reported to result in cellular resistance to these agents.[78]

MULTIDRUG RESISTANCE

In certain instances of resistance to complex, usually hydrophobic drugs, cell lines selected for resistance to one drug have been found to be resistant to other drugs not sharing the same mechanism of action.[79] For example, cells selected for resistance to colchicine, an inhibitor of

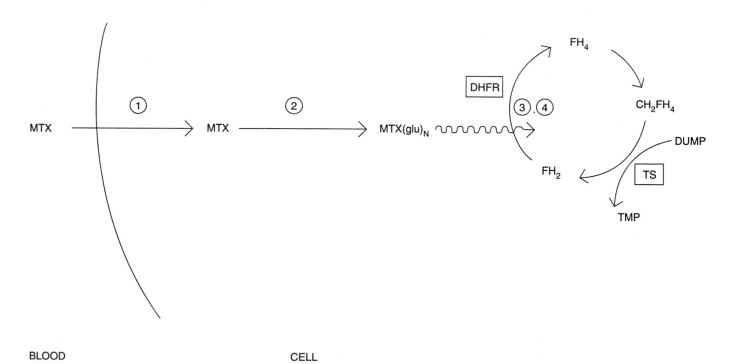

Figure 18–1. Mechanisms of action of MTX and resistance mechanisms. Resistance mechanisms are: (1) transport, (2) polyglutamylation, (3) increase in DHFR, and (4) altered DHFR. FH$_2$, dihydrofolate; FH$_4$, tetrahydrofolate; CH$_2$FH$_4$, 5,10-methylenetetrahydrofolate; TS, thymidylate synthase.

tubulin, have been found to be resistant to doxorubicin, actinomycin D, and the vinca alkaloids (Table 18–7). The biochemical basis of this multidrug resistance was shown by Ling and his coworkers to be due to the overproduction of the cell membrane protein Pgp.[80] The exact mechanism by which this protein acts to exclude drugs from the interior of the cells is not clear and its determination has been complicated by the finding that this protein also may act as a chloride channel.[81] In humans the gene that codes for Pgp is called *mdr-1*. Another homologous gene, *mdr-2*, also has been identified, but the function of this gene has not been elucidated as yet and it is not likely to contribute to the resistance phenotype. In some cell lines, gene amplification has been found to be responsible for the overproduction of this protein; however, Pgp overproduction can occur without a proportional increase in *mdr-1* gene copy number. Indeed, in human cell lines and in the clinic, overexpression of Pgp has not been found to

be associated with gene amplification, and an increase in transcriptional activation has been proposed.[82]

Of interest has been the finding that many normal tissues also express Pgp. The *mdr-1*–encoded Pgp has been found in the gastrointestinal tract, in particular in the canalicular surface of hepatocytes, in the apical surface of the intestinal epithelium, and in the proximal tubules of the kidney[83,84] (Table 18–8). As mentioned previously, Pgp also has been found in the endothelium of the blood-brain barrier and in the testes. This distribution has prompted the suggestion that Pgp is important for protecting organisms from toxic compounds in the environment. The importance of this gene product is underscored by its finding in even simple organisms such as yeast and *C. elegans*. Other tissues (e.g., the adrenal cortex and the pregnant uterus) have high levels of Pgp and may use this efflux pump for specific functions, perhaps to excrete steroids.[85]

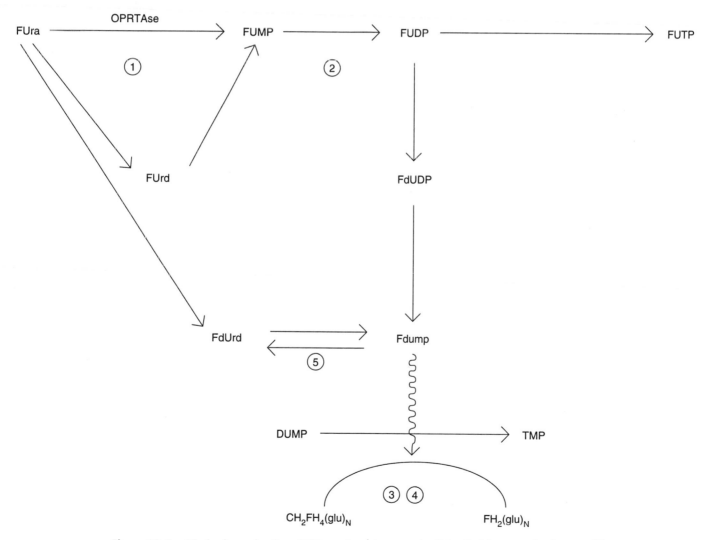

Figure 18–2. Mechanisms of action of FUra and resistance mechanisms. Resistance mechanism are: (1) decreased FUMP formation orotate phospho-tribosyl transferase (OPRTase), (2) decreased triphosphate formation (UMP kinase), (3) increase in TS, (4) altered TS, and (5) increased breakdown of FdUMP. FUra, 5-fluorouracil; FUrd, fluorouridine; FdUrd, deoxyfluorouridine; FUMP, FUDP, FUTP, fluorouridine mono-, di-, and triphosphate; FdUMP, FdUDP, deoxyfluorouridine mono- and diphosphate.

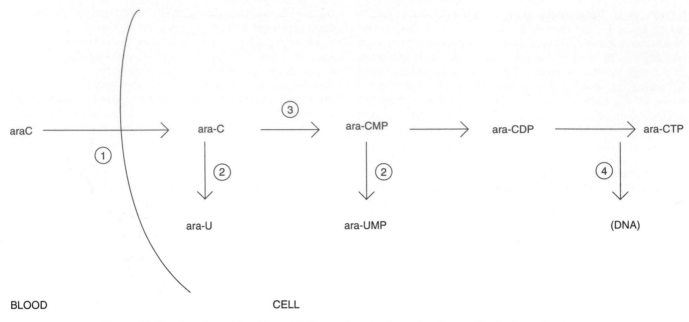

Figure 18–3. Cytosine arabinoside metabolism and mechanisms of resistance. Mechanisms of resistance: (1) transport, (2) deamination to ara-U or ara-UMP, (3) decreased formation of Ara-CMP, and (4) decreased inhibition of DNA polymerase. U, uracil.

The presence of Pgp in normal tissues may explain some cases of intrinsic drug resistance (see later in this chapter).

Multidrug Resistance in the Clinic

The demonstration that many human tumors express Pgp and the identification of several classes of reversal agents has prompted clinical trials of MDR drugs together with a reversal agent in an attempt to restore sensitivity of the tumor to chemotherapy. Neoplasms have been shown to fall into two classes with respect to expression of Pgp. The first group of tumors express this protein at diagnosis (Table 18–9); the second group of tumors infrequently express this protein but, after treatment with MDR drugs and development of resistance, are found to contain Pgp.[83,84]

It is of interest that the former class of tumors are derived from normal tissues that endogenously express the

TABLE 18–7. DRUGS INVOLVED IN THE MDR PHENOTYPE

CLASS	DRUG
Anthracyclines	Doxorubicin
	Daunorubicin
	Mitoxantrone
Tubulin inhibitors	Vincristine
	Vinblastine
	Colchicine
	Taxol
Epipodophyllotoxins	Etoposide
	Teniposide
Antibiotics	Actinomycin D

TABLE 18–8. EXPRESSION OF P-GLYCOPROTEIN IN NORMAL TISSUES*

HIGH EXPRESSION
Bronchial cells
Sweat glands
Kidney proximal tubules
Adrenal cortex
Placenta—trophoblasts
Endothelium of brain, testes, papillary dermis

LOW TO MODERATE EXPRESSION
Stomach
Large intestine
Pancreas ducts, acini
Biliary canaliculi
Prostate
Thyroid
Breast epithelia
Endometrium
Bone marrow stem cells

NO EXPRESSION
Neurons, glial cells, peripheral nerves
Pneumocytes
Esophageal mucosa
Liver hepatocytes
Heart
Keratinocytes, melanocytes
Kidney, glomeruli
Adrenal gland, chromaffin cells
Pancreatic islet cells
Cervical mucosa
Ovary, testis—germ cells
Connective tissues

*From Cardon-Cardo C, O'Brien JP, Boccia J, et al: Expression of the multidrug resistance gene product (p-glycoprotein) in human normal and tumor tissues. J Histochem Cytochem *38*:1277, 1990, with permission.

TABLE 18–9. EXPRESSION OF P-GLYCOPROTEIN IN TUMOR TISSUES*

HIGH LEVELS OF EXPRESSION
Carcinoma of colon
Carcinoma of kidney
Carcinoma of adrenal gland
Carcinoma of pancreas

INTERMEDIATE LEVELS OF EXPRESSION
Carcinoma of esophagus
Carcinoma of stomach
Head and neck cancer
Carcinoma of prostate

LOW LEVELS OF EXPRESSION
Acute leukemia
Lymphoma
Myeloma
Breast cancer
Small-cell lung cancer
Non–small-cell lung cancer
Melanoma

*Data from refs. 83, 84.

mdr gene product. Furthermore, these malignancies are, as expected, intrinsically resistant to MDR drugs. However, clinical trials with various reversal agents in combination with MDR drugs have been unsuccessful against this class of tumors, raising the possibility that other causes for resistance to these drugs exist. It may be argued that these trials have not been optimal with regard to the type and dose of the reversal agent employed. However, even in the case in which high concentrations of the reversal agent verapamil, in combination with doxorubicin, were achieved via hepatic artery delivery, there were no responses noted in patients with colon cancer.[86]

In contrast, somewhat more encouraging results using MDR-modulating agents have been obtained in tumors with acquired resistance to MDR drugs via overexpression of Pgp, particularly hematologic malignancies (acute leukemia, non-Hodgkin's lymphoma, multiple myeloma). However, definitive randomized trials of MDR modulation with appropriate controls are required, as are trials of MDR modulation in other tumors that usually do not express Pgp at diagnosis but frequently express this protein at relapse (i.e., breast cancer, small-cell lung cancer, sarcomas, and ovarian cancer).

The success of MDR modulation in the clinic has been hampered by the toxicity of the reversal agents employed, mainly verapamil and cyclosporin. New, less toxic analogues of these drugs, as well as other new modulating drugs, are now in clinical trial and should be of great value in determining if MDR reversal is clinically achievable.

Multidrug Resistance Not Involving P-Glycoprotein

A number of cell lines also have been described that exhibit a MDR phenotype without a concomitant increase in Pgp. Some of these cells mediate resistance via changes in topoisomerase activity (see earlier in this chapter).

Other cells have been described in which resistance is associated with a change in membrane proteins other than Pgp.[87,88] The significance of these membrane proteins in MDR, both in laboratory models and in the clinic, is under investigation.

Collateral Sensitivity

A potentially attractive but as yet unexplored strategy for the treatment of certain cancers would take advantage of the phenomenon of collateral drug sensitivity. Several examples exist of drug-resistant experimental tumors that are more sensitive than the parent cell line to a second drug. For example, several MDR cell lines are collaterally sensitive to MDR reversal agents administered in the absence of MDR drugs. Unfortunately, the doses of these agents necessary to achieve selective kill are often higher than those needed for reversal, and are clinically unfeasible. A recent report suggests that β-napthoflavone (βNF) and other flavones selectively kill MDR cells, as compared to wild-type cells.[89] Initial studies in animals suggest that these compounds are relatively nontoxic and noncarcinogenic, and in vivo studies evaluating the efficacy of the flavones in treating drug-resistant tumors are now in progress. In another example, MTX-resistant human CEM cells that are defective in the uptake of MTX are collaterally sensitive to 6-thioguanine.[72]

A somewhat related concept exploits natural or acquired resistance to drugs in order to develop selective cytotoxic regimens. For example, we are studying the use of leucovorin (folinic acid) together with trimetrexate to selectively eradicate sarcoma or leukemia cells unable to take up MTX and leucovorin efficiently.[90] The selectivity of this approach is based on the fact that normal renewal tissues (marrow, gastrointestinal tract) are protected from trimetrexate toxicity by leucovorin. In leukemia cells, trimetrexate, a potent antifolate that does not use the reduced folate transporter, is accumulated to toxic levels, whereas the intracellular concentrations of leucovorin achieved are not sufficient to reverse cytotoxicity.

PREDICTIVE TESTS FOR DRUG RESISTANCE/ SENSITIVITY

An important advance in the treatment of patients with chemotherapy would be the ability to predict a priori the drug sensitivity of a given tumor by a rapid in vitro analysis of a tumor biopsy. Thus far, efforts to develop a predictive assay have been hampered by an inability to reliably grow human tumors in vitro under conditions that are comparable to growth in the patient. Nevertheless, various in vitro assays have been described that show some promise. In these assays, cell viability following drug exposure is indirectly measured by quantitating ^{3}H-labeled thymidine incorporation into DNA, ATP levels, or dyes. In general, these assays have the advantage of being simple and rapid, and they measure cell death irrespective of the mechanism of cell killing. They are limited, however, in that they do not measure killing of the tumor stem cell and are not useful in detecting sensitivity to certain antimetabolites (e.g., antifolates, inhibitors of TS) because of the high thymidine levels in the fetal calf serum usually employed in these assays. Nevertheless, there are some reports that indicate that this type of assay may have some value, particularly in detecting high-level intrinsic resistance to a drug.[91]

In contrast, the clonogenic assay assesses cell kill in the important clonogenic population of the tumor. However, it has had limited value in predicting patient outcome, probably because of the low efficiency of tumor cell cloning and the difficulty of obtaining clonogenic cell growth from all tumors.[92–95] Perhaps more valuable has been its use in the screening of new compounds prior to clinical use, thus providing some evidence for sensitivity and blood levels that may be needed in the clinic.[95]

In Vitro Assays for Specific Classes of Drugs

In certain circumstances, when the drug target is known (e.g., DHFR, TS), it is possible to assay the effects of an inhibitor on a tumor cell population by evaluating the effect on the target protein. For example, we have determined resistance or sensitivity to folate antagonists in leukemia blasts,[96] and more recently in fresh human sarcoma cells,[97] by directly measuring the inhibition of TS activity. This type of assay not only allows a determination of cellular resistance but also gives clues to the mechanism of resistance as well.[96] It also is useful in determining the relative efficacy of new analogs that have the same target for inhibition.

In Vivo Studies of Drug Resistance

In vitro studies have the limitations discussed; moreover, the effect of the drug(s) on the host are not assessed. The ability to grow human tumors in relatively privileged sites of the mouse (renal capsule, anterior chamber of the eye) or in "nude" mice with defects in their immune system that allow tumor growth, has provided a model in which to analyze drug effects on both the tumor and host cells.[98] Although these results appear to be useful, there are limitations. The host is the mouse, not humans, and thus drug metabolism, as well as host toxicity, may not be comparable. In addition, the tumors are inoculated subcutaneously and thus differ in natural origin and behavior from the corresponding tumors in humans. Furthermore, the use of nude mice is limited by the cost of the animals and the slow growth of tumors relative to in vitro models, thus making this an unlikely model for drug selection for individual patients. However, as an advanced screen for new compounds, it is probably the most useful of all of the preclinical assays.

A further advance in the use of immunocompromised mice for growth of human tumors for drug sensitivity has been the severe combined immunodeficiency (SCID) mouse. Recent studies have shown that human leukemia blast cells in low numbers (10^6) may be introduced sub-cutaneously into these animals and tumor spread will occur via the blood to the marrow, similar to the clinical situation. This system, although expensive, may be the closest to the clinical situation for evaluating drug therapy. A recent use of SCID mice to test reversal of MDR in human myeloma cells produced very encouraging results that may be clinically applicable.[99]

FUTURE CONSIDERATIONS

As outlined in this chapter, there is already a fair understanding of the mechanism of *acquired* resistance to most of the drugs used to treat cancer, at least in experimental tumor systems. Although less is understood about inherent drug resistance, some progress also is being made in this important area. What emerges is that cancer cells, although not growth regulated, often retain the phenotype of their origin. Perhaps the best example of this is that tumors that derive from organs that express Pgp also express Pgp, and are resistant to MDR drugs. It is clear then, that in addition to determining the tumor phenotype in an effort to understand and ultimately overcome drug resistance, it is critical to consider the impact of tumor origin on the predisposition to drug resistance.

The identification of genes that control cell growth (i.e., oncogenes and tumor suppressor genes) has led to the hypothesis that, in addition to their role in the malignant phenotype, they also may play a role in the development of drug resistance. For example, it has been postulated that the presence of certain oncogenes such as *p53* (see earlier in this chapter) may contribute to the genomic instability characteristic of tumor cells, which in turn could lead to a higher frequency of gene amplification and mutation.[47,48] Moreover, *p53* also has been implicated in the apoptotic pathway that leads to cell death following exposure to cytotoxic drugs.[100] Furthermore, other oncogenes, such as *ras*,[101] also have been implicated recently in the resistance phenotype. Although more studies are needed to define the role of oncogenes in drug resistance, it is intriguing to speculate that drugs directed at oncogenes may someday play a dual role by both halting tumor progression and preventing the emergence of resistant cells.

REFERENCES

1. Cudkov AV, Zelnick CR, Kazarov AR, et al: Isolation of genetic suppressor elements, inducing resistance to topoisomerase II-interactive cytotoxic drugs from human topoisomerase II cDNA. Proc Natl Acad Sci USA 90:3231, 1993
2. Sobrero AF, Bertino JR: Clinical aspects of drug resistance. Cancer Surv 5:93, 1986
3. Fox BW, Fox M (eds): Antitumor Drug Resistance. Berlin, Springer-Verlag, 1984
4. Woolley PV, Tew KD (eds): Mechanisms of Drug Resistance in Neoplastic Cells. San Diego, Academic Press, 1988
5. Twentyman PR, Blechen NM: Cytotoxic drug resistance. Br J Radiol 66(suppl 24):84, 1993
6. Borst P: Genetic mechanisms of drug resistance. Rev Oncol 4:87, 1991

7. Hochauser D, Harris AL: Drug resistance. Br Med Bull 47:178, 1991

8. Hayes JD, Wolf CR: Molecular mechanisms of drug resistance. Biochem J 272:281, 1990

9. McVie JG: Drug disposition and pharmacology. In Fox BW, Fox M (eds): Antitumor Drug Resistance. Springer-Verlag, New York, 1984, pp 39–66

10. Zimm S, Collins JM, Riccardi R: Variable bioavailability of oral 6-mercaptopurine: Is maintenance chemotherapy in acute lymphoblastic leukemia being optimally delivered? N Engl J Med 308:1005, 1983

11. Tattersall MNH, Jarman M, Newlands ES, et al: Pharmacokinetics of melphalan for following oral or intravenous administration in patients with malignant disease. Eur J Cancer 14:507, 1978

12. Jain RK: Determinants of tumor blood flow: A review. Cancer Res 48:2641, 1988

13. Cordon-Cardo C, O'Brien JP, Casals D, et al: Multidrug-resistance gene (P-glycoprotein) is expressed by endothelial cells at blood-brain barrier sites. Proc Natl Acad Sci USA 86:695, 1989

14. De Angelis LM, Yahalom J, Thaler HT, Kher U: Combined modality therapy for primary CNS lymphoma. J Clin Oncol 10:635, 1992

15. Henderson ES, Hoelzer D, Freeman AI: Treatment of Childhood ALL. In Henderson ES, Lister TA (eds): Leukemia. Philadelphia, WB Saunders Company, 1990, pp 452–458

16. Lobel JS, O'Brien RT, McIntosh S, et al: Methotrexate and asparaginase combination chemotherapy in refractory acute lymphoblastic leukemia of childhood. Cancer 43:1089, 1979

17. Yap BS, McCredie KB, Benjamin RS, et al: Refractory acute leukemia in adults treated with sequential colaspase and high-dose methotrexate. BMJ 2:791, 1978

18. Cordon-Cardo C, O'Brien JP: The multidrug resistance phenotype in cancer. Important Adv Oncol 199:19, 1993

19. Goldie JH, Coldman AJ: A mathematical model for relating the drug sensitivity of tumors to their spontaneous mutation rate. Cancer Treat Rep 63:1727, 1979

20. Fanin R, Banerjee D, Volkenandt M, et al: Mutations leading to antifolate resistance in Chinese hamster ovary cells following exposure to the alkylating agent, ethylmethane sulfonate. Mol Pharmacol 44:13, 1993

21. Wahl GM, Padgett RA, Stark GR: Gene amplification causes overproduction of the first three enzymes of UMP synthesis in N(phosphonacetyl)-L-aspartate-resistant hamster cells. J Biol Chem 254:8679, 1979

22. Grem JL: Fluorinated pyrimidines. In Chabner BA, Collins JM (eds): Cancer Chemotherapy: Principles and Practice. Philadelphia, JB Lippincott Company, 1990, pp 180–224

23. Pizzorno G, Mini E, Coronello M, et al: Impaired polyglutamylation of methotrexate as a cause of resistance in CCRF-CEM cells after short-term, high-dose treatment with this drug. Cancer Res 48:2149, 1988

24. Aschele C, Sobrero A, Faderan MA, Bertino JR: Novel mechanism(s) of resistance to 5-fluorouracil in human colon cancer (HCT-8) sublines following exposure to two different clinically relevant dose schedules. Cancer Res 52:1855, 1992

25. Goldenberg GJ, Lee M, Lam HYP, Begleiter A: Evidence for carrier mediated transport of melphalan by 5178Y lymphoblasts in vitro. Cancer Res 37:755, 1977

26. Sirotnak FM: Obligate genetic expression of a fetal membrane property mediating "folate" transport: Biological significance and implications for improved therapy. Cancer Res 45:3992, 1985

27. Rischin D, Ling V: Multidrug resistance in leukemia. In Freireich EJ, Kantarjian HM (eds): Advances in Research and Treament. Boston, Kluwer, 1993, pp 269–293

28. Chin JE, Soffier R, Noonan KE, et al: Structure and expression of the human MDR (P-glycoprotein) gene family. Mol Cell Biol 9:3808, 1989

29. Chabner BA, Allegra CA, Curt GA: Polyglutamylation of methotrexate: Is methotrexate a prodrug? J Clin Invest 76:907, 1985

30. Handschumacher RE, Cheng YC: Purine and pyrimidine antimetabolites. In Holland JF, Frei E III, Bast RC Jr, et al (eds): Cancer Medicine. Philadelphia, Lea & Febiger, 1993, pp 712–732

31. Morrow CS, Cowna KH: Glutathione S-transferase and drug resistance. Cancer Cells 2:15, 1990

32. Clapper ML, Buller AL, Smith TM, Tew KD: Glutathione S-transferase in alkylating agent resistant cells. In Mantle TJ, Pickett CB, Hayes JD (eds): Glutathione S-transferase and Carcinogenesis. London, Taylor and Francis, 1987, pp 213–221

33. Webb CD, Latham MD, Lock RB, Sullivan DM: Attenuated topoisomerase II content directly correlates with a low level of drug resistance in a Chinese hamster ovary cell line. Cancer Res 51:6543, 1991

34. Ferguson PJ, Fischer MH, Stephenson J, et al: Combined modalities of resistance in etoposide-resistant human KB cell lines. Cancer Res 48:5956, 1988

35. Beidler JL, Spangler BD: Metaphase chromosome anomaly association with drug resistance and cell specific products. Science 191:185, 1976

36. Alt FW, Kellems RE, Bertino JR, Schimke RT: Selective multiplication of dihydrofolate reductase genes in methotrexate resistant variants of cultured murine cells. J Biol Chem 253:1357, 1978

37. Kaufman RJ, Brown PC, Schimke RT: Amplified dihydrofolate reductase genes in unstably methotrexate-resistant cells are associated with double-minute chromosomes. Proc Natl Acad Sci USA 76:5669, 1979

38. Hamlin JL, Milbrandt JD, Heintz NH, Azizkhan JC: DNA sequence amplification in mammalian cells. Int Rev Cytol 90:31, 1984

39. Stark GR: DNA amplification in drug resistant cells and in tumors. Cancer Surv 5:1, 1984

40. Stark GR, Debatisse M, Guilotto E, Wahl GM: Recent progress in understanding mechanisms of mammalian DNA amplification. Cell 57:901, 1989

41. Schimke RT: Gene amplification in cultured cells. J Biol Chem 263:5989, 1988

42. Srimatkandada S, Dube SK, Mehlman L, et al: Co-amplification of 3-hydroxy-3-methylglutaryl co-enzyme A reductase and dihydrofolate reductase genes in methotrexate-resistant human leukemia cell lines. (submitted for publication)

43. Wahl GM: The importance of circular DNA in mammalian gene amplification. Cancer Res 49:1333, 1989

44. Van der Bliek AM, Meyers MB, Biedler JL, et al: A 22-kd protein (sorcein/V19) encoded by an amplified gene in multi-drug resistant cells is homologous to the calcium-binding light chain of calpain. EMBO J 5:3201, 1986

45. Tlsty TD, Margolin BH, Lum K: Differences in the rates of gene amplification in non-tumorigenic and tumorigenic cell lines as measured by Luria-Delbruck fluctuation analysis. Proc Natl Acad Sci USA 86:9441, 1989

46. Wright JA, Smith HS, Watt FM, et al: DNA amplification is rare in normal human cells. Proc Natl Acad Sci USA 87:1791, 1990

47. Livingstone LR, White A, Sprouse J, et al: Altered cell cycle arrest and gene amplification potential accompany loss of wild-type p53. Cell 70:923, 1992

48. Yin Y, Tainsky MA, Bischoff FZ, et al: Wild-type p53 restores cell cycle control and inhibits gene amplification in cells with mutant p53 alleles. Cell 70:937, 1992

49. Goker E, Trippett T, Kheradapour A, et al: Gene amplification in resistant ALL blast is associated with p53 mutations. Blood 82:38a, 1993

50. Arceci P: Clinical significance of P-glycoprotein in multidrug resistance malignancies. Blood 81:2125, 1993

51. Sikic BI: Modulation of multidrug resistance: At the threshold. J Clin Oncol 11:1629, 1993

52. Thorgeirsson SS, Huber BE, Sorrell S, et al: Expression of the multidrug-resistant gene in hepato-carcinogenesis and regenerating rat liver. Science 236:1120, 1987

53. Burt RK, Thorgeirsson SS: Coinduction of MDR-1 multi-drug resistance and cytochrome P-450 genes in rat and liver by xenobiotics. J Natl Cancer Inst 80:1383, 1988

54. Fairchild CR, Ivy SP, Rushmore T, et al: Carcinogen-induced MDR overexpression is associated with xenobiotic resistance in rat preneoplastic liver nodules and hepatocellular carcinomas. Proc Natl Acad Sci USA 84:7701, 1987

55. Mariano PA, Gottesman MM, Pastan I: Regulation of the multidrug resistance gene in regenerating rat liver. Cell Growth Differ 1:57, 1990

56. Hochhauser D, Harris AL: The role of topoisomerase II α and β in drug resistance. Cancer Treat Rev 19:181, 1993

57. Tan KB, Mattern MR, Eng W-K, et al: Nonproductive rearrangement of DNA topoisomerase I and II genes: Correlation with resistance to topoisomerase inhibitors. J Natl Cancer Inst 81:1732, 1989

58. Chu E, Voeller D, Koeller DM, et al: Identification of an RNA binding site for human thymidylate synthase. Proc Natl Acad Sci USA 90:517, 1993

59. Keyomarsi K, Samet J, Molnar G, Pardee AB: The thymidylate synthase inhibitor, ICI D1694, overcomes translational detainment of the enzyme. J Biol Chem 268:15142, 1993

60. Ercikan E, Banerjee D, Waltham M, et al: Translational regulation of the synthesis of dihydrofolate reductase. Adv Exp Biol 338:537, 1993

61. Simonsen CC: Drug-resistant dihydrofolate reductases. In Malacmski G, Simonsen CC, Shepard M (eds): The Molecular Genetics of Mammalian Cells. New York, Macmillan, 1986, pp 99–129

62. Melera PN: Acquired vs. intrinsic resistance to methotrexate: Diversity of the drug-resistant phenotype in mammalian cells. Semin Cancer Biol 2:245, 1991

63. Dicker AP, Waltham MN, Volkenandt M, et al: Methotrexate resistance in an in vivo mouse tumor due to an non-active site dihydrofolate reductase mutation. Proc Natl Acad Sci USA 90:11797, 1993

64. Sullivan DM, Latham MD, Rowe TC, Ross WE: Purification and characterization of an altered topoisomerase II from a drug resistant Chinese hamster ovary cell line. Biochemistry 28:5680, 1989

65. Zwelling LA, Hinds M, Chan D, et al: Characterization of an amsacrine-resistant line of human leukemia cells: Evidence for a drug resistant form of topoisomerase II. Biochemistry 28:8154, 1989

66. Andoh T, Tshi K, Susuki Y, et al: Characterization of a mammalian mutant with a campothecin-resistant DNA topoisomerase I. Proc Natl Acad Sci USA 84:5585, 1987

67. Benedetti P, Fiorami P, Capuani L, Wang JC: Campothecin resistance from a single mutation changing glycine 363 of human DNA topoisomerase I to cysteine. Cancer Res 53:4343, 1993

68. Muggia F, Los G: Platinum resistance: Laboratory findings and clinical implications. Stem Cells 11:182, 1993

69. Schweitzer B, Dicker AP, Bertino JR: Dihydrofolate reductase as a therapeutic agent. FASEB J 4:2441, 1990

70. Klohs WD, Steinkampf RW, Besserer JR, et al: Cross-resistance of pleiotropically drug resistant p388 leukemia cells to the lipophilic antifolates trimetrexate and BW 301U. Cancer Lett 31:233, 1986

71. Trippett T, Schlemmer S, Elisseyeff Y, et al: Defective transport as a mechanism of acquired resistance to methotrexate in patients with acute lymphocytic leukemia. Blood 80:1158, 1992

72. Bertino JR: Karnofsky Memorial Lecture: Ode to methotrexate. J Clin Oncol 11:5, 1993

73. Lenz HJ, Leichman C, Danenberg P, et al: Thymidylate synthase gene expression predicts response of primary gastric cancer to 5 fluorouracil leucovorin cisplatin. Proc Am Soc Clin Oncol 12:199, 1993

74. While JC, Rak JP, Capizzi R: Membrane transport influences the rate of accumulation of cytosine arabinoside in human leukemia cells. J Clin Invest 79:380, 1987

75. Meister A: Glutathione deficiency produced by inhibition of its synthesis, and its reversal: Applications in research and therapy. Pharmacol Ther 51:155, 1991

76. Bodie WJ, Tokuda K, Ludlum D: Differences in DNA alkylation products formed in sensitive and resistant glioma cells treated with N-(2-chloroethyl nitrosourea). Cancer Res 48:4489, 1986

77. Horwitz DB, Liao LL, Greenberger L, Lothstein L: Mode of action of taxol and characterization of a multidrug-resistant cell line selected with taxol. In Kessel D (ed): Resistance to Neoplastic Drugs. Boca Raton, FL, CRC Press, 1989, p 109

78. Gupta RS: Taxol resistant mutants of Chinese hamster ovary cells: Genetic, biochemical and cross-resistance studies. J Cell Physiol 114:137, 1983

79. Chin KV, Pastan J, Gottesman MM: Function and regulation of the human multidrug resistance gene. Adv Cancer Res 60:157, 1993

80. Juliano RL, Ling V: A surface glycoprotein modulating drug permeability in Chinese hamster ovary mutants. Biochim Biophys Acta 455:152, 1976

81. Gill DR, Hyde SC, Higgins CF, et al: Separation of drug transport and chloride channel functions of the human multidrug resistance p-glycoprotein. Cell 71:23, 1992

82. Hsu SI, Cohen D, Kirschner LS, et al: Structural analysis of the mouse mdr1a (P-glycoprotein) promoter reveals the basis for differential transcript heterogeneity in multidrug resistant J774.2 cells. Mol Cell Biol 10:3596, 1990

83. Thiebaut F, Tsuro T, Hamada H, et al: Immunohistochemical localization in normal tissues of different epitopes in the multidrug transport protein p170: Evidence for localization in brain capillaries and cross reactivity of one antibody with a muscle protein. J Histochem Cytochem 37:159, 1989

84. Cardon-Cardo C, O'Brien JP, Boccia J, et al: Expression of the multidrug resistance gene product (p-glycoprotein) in human normal and tumor tissues. J Histochem Cytochem 38:1277, 1990

85. Ueda K, Okamura N, Hirai M, et al: Human p-glycoprotein transports cortisone, aldosterone, and dexamethasone, but not progesterone. J Biol Chem 267:24248, 1992

86. Saltz L, O'Brien J, Kemeny N, et al: Phase I study of intrahepatic verapamil and doxorubicin: Regional therapy to overcome multidrug resistance. Proc Am Acad Clin Oncol 11:118, 1992

87. Eijdems EWHM, de Haas M, Versantvoort CHM, et al: Non-p-glycoprotein mediated drug resistance is the major mechanism for low-level resistance to doxorubicin in resistant variants of a human non-small cell lung cancer cell line. Proc Natl Acad Sci USA 89:3498, 1992

88. Cole SPC, Bhardwaj G, Gerlach JH, et al: Overexpression of a transporter gene in a multidrug-resistant human lung cancer cell line. Science 258:1650, 1992

89. Scotto KW, Prochaska HP: Collateral sensitivity of multidrug-resistant cells to a new family of compounds. Proc Am Assoc Cancer Res 34:314, 1993

90. Li WW, Bertino JR: Inability of leucovorin to rescue naturally methotrexate-resistant human soft tissue sarcoma cell line from trimetrexate cytotoxicity. Cancer Res 52:6866, 1992

91. Kern DH, Weisenthal LM: Highly specific prediction of antineoplastic drug resistance with an in vitro assay using suprapharmacologic drug exposures. J Natl Cancer Inst 82:582, 1990

92. Hamburger AW: In vitro evaluation of chemotherapeutic agents. Cancer Invest 9:683, 1991

93. Phillips RM, Bibby MC, Double JA: A critical appraisal of the predictive value of in vitro chemosensitivity assays. J Natl Cancer Inst 82:1457, 1990

94. Hamburger AW, Salmon SE, Soehnlen B: Quantitation of differential sensitivity of human tumor stem cells to anticancer drugs. N Engl J Med 298:1321, 1978

95. Von Hoff DD: In vitro predictive testing—the sulfonamide era. Int J Cell Cloning 5:179, 1987

96. Rodenhuis S, McGuire JJ, Narayanan R, Bertino JR: Development of an assay system for the detection and classification of methotrexate resistance in fresh human leukemic cells. Cancer Res 46:6513, 1986

97. Li WW, Lin JT, Tong WP, et al: Mechanisms of natural resistance to antifolates in human soft tissue sarcomas. Cancer Res 52:1434, 1992

98. Boyd MR: Status of the NCI preclinical antitumor drug discovery screen. Prin Pract Oncol 3(10):1, 1989

99. Bellamy W, Odeleye A, Finley P, et al: An in vivo model of human multidrug-resistant multiple myeloma in SCID mice. Am J Pathol 142:1, 1993

100. Lowe SW, Ruley HE, Jacks T, Housman DE: p53-dependent apoptosis modulates the cytotoxicity of anticancer agents. Cell 74:657, 1993

101. Sklar MD: Increased resistance to cis-diamminedichloro-platinum(II) in NIH 3T3 cells transformed by ras oncogenes. Cancer Res 48:793, 1988

19

RADIATION THERAPY

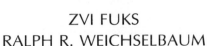

ZVI FUKS
RALPH R. WEICHSELBAUM

The interaction of ionizing radiation with biologic matter generates a variety of molecular lesions that occur in essentially every organelle or subcompartment of the cell. Although every cellular molecule is a potential candidate for damage by ionizing radiation, the lesions most detrimental to cell survival are those involving the structure and function of the DNA. The outcome of damage to the DNA is either cell death or, in the case of surviving cells, repair of the lesions and recovery to a normal state. If misrepair of DNA occurs, the final outcome may be associated with permanent mutations and the induction of carcinogenesis. Therefore, a review of the effects of radiation on tumor and normal cells should include not only a description of the lesions and the metabolic pathways leading to cell death, but also an understanding of the cellular mechanisms involved in repair. At the present time, the molecular basis of radiation damage repair in mammalian cells is only partially known, and there is little information on its control mechanisms at the genetic and epigenetic levels. Several repair genes have been identified in eukaryotic cells that, on transfection into hypersensitive mutant cell lines, restore radiation resistance to the levels observed in the corresponding parental wild-type cells. However, overexpression of such genes has not been found as yet to correlate with clinical radiation resistance. Other studies have reported that the response of mammalian cells to radiation is affected significantly by microenvironmental and tissue factors, but the mechanisms and biologic significance of these effects are only partially known. This chapter discusses some of these issues in the context of their relevance to the clinical effects of radiation on tumor and normal cells. A detailed understanding of the mechanisms and pathways of radiation injury and repair may lead to the design of new biologic response modifiers to improve the therapeutic ratio of radiation treatments in human cancer.

NATURE OF RADIATION LESIONS IN MAMMALIAN CELLS

Interactions of Ionizing Radiation with Biologic Matter

The production of radiation lesions in the molecular infrastructure of the cell involves a sequential multistep process that eventually generates several types of chemically stable lesions.[1-4] The events involved in this process occur within 10^{-18} to 10^{-3} seconds and are initiated by transfer of energy from the incident photon to cellular molecules.[3] The absorption of the photon energy destabilizes the target molecule, leading to permanent molecular breaks or to the release of energetic electrons and secondary energy-attenuated photons. The ejected electrons and the secondary photons interact with other cellular molecules, leading to a chain of reactions that dissipates the original photon energy within the cell and produces a variety of short-lived ions and chemically unstable free radicals.[3,4] There are a variety of biologically relevant free radicals, but the most common radicals are produced from the radiolysis of cellular water[3-6] and include hydroxyl radicals($^{\cdot}$OH), hydrated electrons (e_{aq}), hydrogen atoms (H$^{\cdot}$), and hydrogen peroxide (H_2O_2). Free radicals are extremely unstable and interact nearly instantaneously with neighboring molecules to produce chemically stable lesions.[4] This process can be modified by free radical scavengers or by oxygen, which have opposing effects on the number of stable lesions and on the level of cellular radiosensitivity.[4] However, if all factors remain constant, the permanent damage is linear with dose. At clinically relevant dose levels, the yield of any of the known species of lesions is very low. For instance, the incidence of single-strand breaks (ssb) in DNA is approximately 1000 lesions per gray per cell,[7] which translates to about one ssb per 10^7 bp. Damage to other molecules is approximately the same in terms of the percentage of monomer molecular changes. Thus, the physical process by itself creates only minimal changes in the chemical composition of the cellular matrix irradiated.

Although essentially every cellular molecule is a potential candidate for permanent damage by ionizing radiation, there is evidence that the lesions responsible for cell death involve the structure and function of the DNA.[3] Experiments in which the cell nucleus and the cytoplasm were irradiated selectively[8–10] demonstrated that the doses required in the cytoplasm to kill a cell were larger by orders of magnitude compared to the doses required in the nucleus. Further support for the importance of DNA damage in radiation killing is the observation that incorporation of halogenated pyrimidines into DNA in the place of thymidine sensitizes the cell to radiation.[11] It is thus generally accepted that the target molecules for radiation-induced cell killing are located in the nucleus and involve damage to the DNA.[12]

Types of Radiation Lesions to the DNA

Permanent radiation lesions in the DNA are produced either by a direct deposition of the photon energy in the DNA chain, or indirectly via interaction with radiation-induced free radicals. Studies that used scavengers of free radicals showed that the contribution of the indirect effects to the production of the lethal damage was approximately 70 per cent in oxic cells.[13,14] Both the direct and indirect effects at biologically relevant doses produce in mammalian cell DNA a variety of sugar and base lesions, and also lead to covalent cross links within the DNA strands or with nuclear proteins.[15–19] Damage to the deoxyribose backbone of the DNA frequently disrupts phosphodiester bonds and produces ssb[20–23] (Fig. 19–1). Breaks to single strands are very common and increase in proportion to the radiation dose, but ssb by themselves are not considered as lethal to mammalian cells.[18,20] In general, the efficiency of cell killing by ionizing radiation increases as a direct function of the linear energy transfer (LET) characteristics of the radiation beam,[24] yet the concomitant efficiency of ssb induction decreases.[25] Furthermore, when ssb are induced by H_2O_2 at a level corresponding to 10 Gy, it does not result in killing of Chinese hamster cells.[20] In fact, ssb are considered highly reparable and, under normal growth conditions, their rejoining proceeds exponentially during the early postirradiation period in a first-order kinetics.[26] Most ssb represent simple discontinuities in phosphodiester bonds with 5'-phosphate and 3'-hydroxyl ends[27] that are directly re-ligated (Fig. 19–1). This type of lesion comprises 70 to 90 per cent of ssb and normally is rejoined with a $t_{1/2}$ of 2 to 10 minutes. Some ssb contain a 3'-phosphate or other abnormal structures (Fig. 19–1), or represent virtual gaps created from base loss (apurinic or apyrimidinic lesions).[28] Such lesions are repaired more slowly because the damaged ends require endonuclease-mediated removal before polymerases and ligases can patch the damaged area.

DNA base damage also is frequent in mammalian cells after ionizing radiation exposure.[2,29,30] However, although base damage generally is not considered as lethal to normal mammalian cells, it is regarded as an important process in the genesis of mutations. X-ray base damage is repaired in mammalian cells by excision through enzymatic pathways that are not fully known. In *Escherichia coli*, excision repair following ultraviolet (UV) light exposure is carried out by the UVR-ABC enzyme complex.[31] It is likely, although not yet proven, that a similar (although not an identical) enzymatic complex may operate in eukaryotic cells. Base damage–specific endonucleases and glycosylases apparently are involved in the excision phase,[28] while β-polymerase and type II ligases are believed to participate in the subsequent phase of repair synthesis.[32] The base repair function in mammalian cells is apparently highly efficient, because about 80 per cent of the base damage is removed from the DNA within 15 minutes of irradiation.[33] Damaged base excision repair after x-irradiation in mammalian cells appears to be different from the nucleotide excision repair after UV exposure, because xeroderma pigmentosum fibroblasts that are deficient in the capacity to repair UV base damage repair x-ray–induced base damage at a normal rate.[34,35] The removal of x-ray base damage is impaired in radiation-sensitive cells from ataxia-telangiectasia (AT) patients,[36] although the defect in the excision of damaged bases does not correlate with cellular lethality.

The most important lesions in cell killing by ionizing radiation are heterologous DNA double-strand breaks (dsb).[3,4,10] These lesions can arise either from a single severing event involving both DNA strands simultaneously, or as result of two independent ssb closely apposed on the deoxyribose backbones of the DNA[28] (Fig. 19–1). The structure of the two loose ends of the broken strands may vary within a spectrum of chemical changes, but every dsb is potentially lethal if unrepaired. Freifelder[37] showed that a single DNA dsb can inactivate the bacteriophage T7, and Frankenberg-Schwager and colleagues[38,39] reported that the *rad-54-3* mutant of the budding yeast *Saccharomyces cerevisiae*, which is completely deficient in dsb repair at 36° C, is killed at the restrictive temperature by about one dsb per cell (Fig. 19–2). Similarly, mammalian cell lines partially defective in their ability to repair dsb (e.g., the xrs and XR-1 cells derived from the Chinese hamster ovary [CHO] cell line, or the L517Y/S cells derived from a murine lymphoblastoid cell line) show a significant increase in sensitivity to x-rays as compared to the corresponding parental cell lines,[40–43] although their response to UV light irradiation remains similar to that of the parental cells.[43] These data suggest a specificity to dsb as lethal lesions and indicate that repair can abrogate cell death from dsb. Indeed, Radford,[44] who used the neutral elution technique to study DNA dsb frequency, showed that cell survival in several repair-proficient murine tumor cell lines correlated with the initial number of dsb, and Schwartz et al.[45] reported that the radiosensitivity of human squamous cell carcinoma cell lines correlated with their ability to rejoin dsb (Fig. 19–3). Similarly, studies performed by McMillan et al.[46] on nine human tumor lines showed that the variations in radiosensitivity corre-

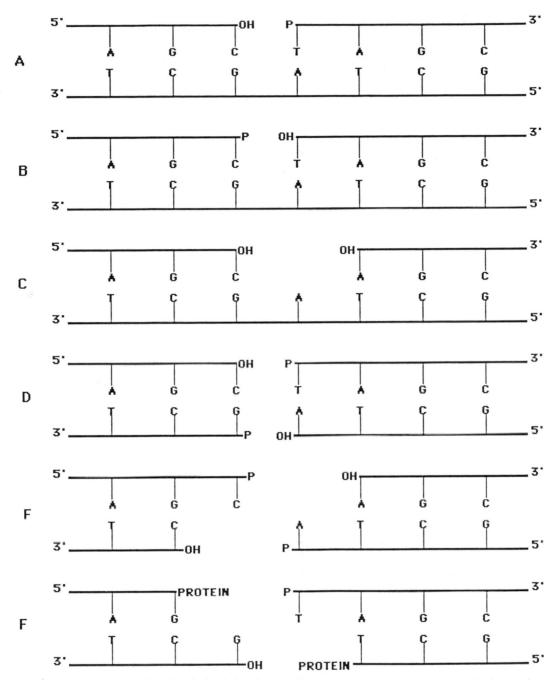

Figure 19-1. Examples of radiation-induced DNA single- and double-strand breaks. *A*, Single-strand breaks containing a 3'-phosphate. *B*, Single-strand breaks containing a 5'-phosphate. *C*, A gap in the damaged deoxyribose with a thymine base loss and a modified 3'-terminus leading to 3'- and 5'-hydroxyl ends. *D*, DNA double-strand breaks created by two adjacent single-strand breaks. *E*, DNA double-strand breaks created by two adjacent gaps. *F*, DNA double-strand breaks created by two adjacent gaps with termini modified by cross linking to protein.

lated with the number of residual DNA dsb remaining after repair is completed. These data indicate that both the initial damage induced and the extent of repair play a role in survival.

Other studies have indicated that, in addition to the ultimate net number of dsb, the structural nature of the dsb also may impact on mammalian cell survival. Several studies showed that, although the initial number of dsb in mammalian cells changes very little relative to LET,[47] there are qualitative differences in the nature of the lesions and in their reparability. High-energy photons or high-LET-particle irradiation were shown to produce complex types of dsb, which involve multiple locally damaged sites consisting of combinations of different types of DNA lesions.[3,4,48] The pattern of energy deposition that produces such lesions, calculated by computer modeling of the pas-

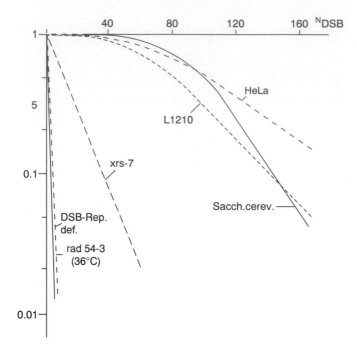

Figure 19–2. Comparison of dose-survival curves of mammalian and yeast cells. The surviving fraction is plotted versus the number of radiation-induced dsb per cell (N_{DSB}). Similar radiation resistance is observed for HeLa, mouse leukemia L1210, and yeast (*Saccharomyces cerevisiae*) cells. The CHO mutant xrs-7, which is partially deficient in dsb rejoining, shows reduced radioresistance. Extreme radiosensitivity (about one dsb per cell leading to a lethal event) is observed for the yeast mutant rad54-3, which is completely deficient in dsb rejoining at 36° C. The hypothetical dose-survival curve of a completely dsb rejoining–deficient mammalian cell mutant (DSB-Rep.def), which may be killed by one dsb per cell, also is shown. (Modified from Frankenberg-Schwager M, Frankenberg D: DNA double-strand breaks: Their repair and relationship to cell killing in yeast. Int J Radiat Biol *58*:569, 1990, with permission.)

ular configurations, may exceed the capacity of conventional DNA repair mechanisms, thus yielding irreparable damage. The dependence of dsb reparability on the chemical nature of the break termini has been demonstrated by experiments in which restriction endonucleases introduced into permeabilized cells produced different biologic effects depending on the nature of the dsb created by each of these enzymes.[49] Thus, the current hypothesis on the lethal effects of ionizing radiation postulates that both the initial number and chemical nature of the DNA dsb and the rate and overall efficiency of the DNA dsb repair determine the ultimate survival after radiation exposure. The final number of lethal lesions consists of lesions that are primarily irreparable and of potentially reparable lesions that for some reason do not undergo repair.[50–53]

REPAIR OF RADIATION DAMAGE IN MAMMALIAN CELLS: RELATION TO CELLULAR RADIOSENSITIVITY

Mechanisms of Cell Death after Irradiation

The reason why mammalian cells that sustain DNA dsb after radiation exposure proceed to die is unknown, nor is there information on the genetic and molecular mechanisms of this process. Cytogenetic studies have revealed a variety of chromosomal aberrations following irradiation, and several studies have reported correlations between the frequency of chromosomal aberrations and cell killing.[54,55] However, it generally is believed that aberrations that lead to cell death are mostly those associated with the loss of essential gene function.[56] In mammalian cells, it is difficult to correlate loss of gene function with metabolic disruptions that might lead to cell death because of the overall size of mammalian genomic DNA and methodologic difficulties in studying mammalian gene function. Even when an apparent structural reconstitution of the DNA is achieved by repair of strand breaks, the fidelity of the functional recovery of the genome may be impaired, as has been demonstrated in AT.[57,58] Further-

sage of photons through water,[48] was described as occurring in spurs that consist of several ionizing events. These spurs have a larger diameter than the width of the DNA strand, thus creating a number of lesions within a short stretch of the DNA.[3,48] The local load of chemical damage in such lesions, or the presence of distorted DNA molec-

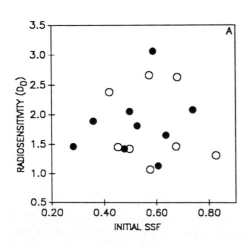

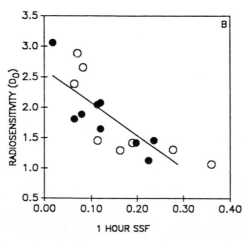

Figure 19–3. Relationship between DNA dsb frequency (SSF) after 100 cGY x-irradiation exposure and radiation sensitivity (expressed as the D_0 of the dose-survival curve) in nine early-passage (●) and eight late-passage (○) human squamous cell carcinoma cell lines. The dsb frequency–D_0 relationship was evaluated immediately after irradiation (A) and after 1 hour incubation at 37° C to permit repair of dsb (B). (Modified from Schwartz JL, Mustafi R, Beckett MA, Weichselbaum RR: Prediction of the radiation sensitivity of human squamous cell carcinoma cells using DNA filter elution. Radiat Res *123*:1, 1990, with permission.)

more, radiation-induced lethality in many types of mammalian cells is not instantaneous, because cells continue to function after x-ray exposure and even undergo one to several cell divisions before viability is lost.[59] Cinephotography studies of irradiated cells showed that a single cell and its pedigrees may undergo up to nine divisions before undergoing cell lysis.[59] These observations suggest that, as the cell progresses through repeated cycles of DNA replication and mitosis, it increasingly produces chromosomal aberrations and genomic dysfunction, leading eventually to metabolic failure and cell death. Not all cells, however, exhibit this pattern of death after irradiation. Noncycling lymphocytes, thymocytes, and hematopoietic cells were shown to undergo an interphase mode of cell death, without progressing through the mitotic phase of the cell cycle.[60–62]

There are two patterns of morphologic changes associated with cell death in mammalian cells. The more commonly recognized pattern is *cell necrosis,* which is degenerative in nature and is the usual outcome of the more severe types of cell damage. Necrotic cell death results from the collapse of cellular metabolism and the depletion of its ATP stores,[63–65] leading to failure of the ionic homeostasis mechanisms of the cell membrane.[66,67] As ATP is depleted, the transmembrane ion pump disintegrates, the cell swells and its internal organelles become distended. Initially, reversible plasma membrane blebbing may be observed, but ultimately the membrane ruptures, spilling out lysosomal enzymes.[67] The final events of necrosis involve degradation of nuclear chromatin and karyolysis. If there is a genetic control mechanism to this process, it is totally unknown. Necrosis occurring in vivo is accompanied by exudative inflammation, and, if large numbers of cells are involved, it often is followed by the development of scar tissue.

The other morphologically defined process of radiation-induced cell death is *apoptosis* (also known as programmed cell death). The typical morphologic features of this process include chromatin condensation and segmentation, fragmentation of the nucleus into apoptotic bodies, cell shrinkage, and loss of cellular contact with neighboring cells.[65,67] An as yet unidentified calcium-magnesium–dependent endonuclease cleaves the chromatin at selective internucleosomal linker sites, yielding the discrete nuclear fragments.[67,68] Concomitant elevation of cell surface transglutaminase activity results in cross linkage of apoptotic cell membrane proteins,[69] generating surface signal molecules. These signals are recognized by infiltrating phagocytes that engulf the apoptotic cells and phagocytize its components.[70] The end result of this process is that the cell dies without inflicting damage to viable neighboring cells. Apoptosis occurs spontaneously in solid tumors of various types[64,66,71,72] and contributes to the balance between tumor cell gain and cell loss. Cancer chemotherapeutic agents enhance apoptosis in tumor cell populations as well as in normal tissues,[73] and certain chemical carcinogens induce apoptosis in their target tissues.[74] Ionizing radiation induces programmed cell death in thymic, lymphoid, and hematopoietic cells[60,61,75,76] and in stem and undifferentiated progenitors of testicular, intestinal, renal, neuronal, and oligodendrocytic cell lineages.[61] Mature and differentiated progenies of nonlymphoid mammalian cells are believed to undergo radiation-induced apoptosis only rarely,[61] although it has been reported in the epithelium of intestinal crypts,[77] the ascini of the protid and lacrimal glands,[78] bovine aortic endothelial cells (BAECs),[79] and several experimental murine mammary, ovarian, and hepatocellular carcinomas.[80,81]

Apoptosis is conceptualized as a preprogrammed pathway of sequential biochemical events that are only partially known, eventually leading to activation of a calcium-magnesium–dependent endonuclease that cleaves the nuclear chromatin at selective internucleosomal linker sites.[68,82] The typical 180-bp oligonucleosomal fragments thus produced can be visualized by electron microscopy[67] or demonstrated as a "DNA ladder" on agarose gel electrophoresis.[68] Radiation-induced apoptosis requires active mRNA and protein synthesis and an obligatory presence of intracellular calcium ions.[61] Presently, there is little information on the genetic mechanisms that control the apoptotic response. In the nematode *Caenorhabditis elegans* the ced-3 and ced-4 genes have been found to regulate apoptosis,[83] but their mammalian homologues are unknown. In mammalian cells, the testosterone-repressed prostatic message 2 (*TRPM*-2) gene is expressed coordinately with the onset of apoptosis of prostatic[84] and several other murine and human tumor[85] cells, but it is not clear whether *TRPM*-2 serves as an effector gene for apoptosis in these or in other cell types. In *C. elegans,* the ced-9 gene inhibits apoptosis,[86] and several investigators have suggested that the mammalian *bcl*-2 gene represents its homologue.[87,88]

There is also little information on signaling mechanisms that initiate apoptosis. Tumor necrosis factor α (TNF-α)[89–91] and transforming growth factor β (TGF-β)[92–94] were found to induce apoptosis via interactions with their specific cell surface receptors. Furthermore, for TNF-α the sphingomyelin pathway was reported to constitute the early events in the apoptotic cascade. TNF-receptor interaction initiated sphingomyelin hydrolysis to ceramide by the sphingomyelinase enzyme, and ceramide was found to act as a second messenger to induce apoptosis.[91] Activation of the sphingomyelin pathway by TNF-α is tightly coupled to its 55-kDa low-affinity receptor,[95] because activation of the sphingomyelin cascade could be produced in isolated membranes of EL4 thymoma cells.[96] As for apoptosis induced by irradiation, most investigators have suggested that the apoptotic signals are triggered by damaged DNA.[62,97,98] However, recent studies have demonstrated that membrane signaling also may induce the apoptotic pathway in some cell types. Haimovitz-Friedman et al.[79] reported that radiation exposure of plateau phase (>90 per cent G_0-G_1) BAECs resulted in a rapid hydrolysis of sphingomyelin to ceramide and apoptosis. Elevation of ceramide with exogenous ceramide analogues was sufficient for induction of apoptosis. Protein kinase C (PKC) activation blocked both radiation-induced sphingomyelin hydrolysis and apoptosis, and apoptosis was restored by ceramide analogues added exogenously. Ionizing radiation acted directly on membrane preparations devoid of nuclei, stimulating sphingomyelin hydrolysis enzymatically through a neutral sphingomyelinase.

Hence, the data indicate that apoptotic signaling can be generated by direct interaction of ionizing radiation with cellular membranes and suggest an alternative to the hypothesis that DNA damage mediates radiation-induced cell kill.

At least two pathways seem to mediate apoptosis in hematopoietic cell lineages.[99–101] One pathway is triggered by exposure of mouse thymocytes to dexamethasone and is independent of *p53*. The second pathway is dependent on the induction of *p53* and follows exposure to ionizing radiation and other agents associated with DNA damage.[99–104] In cells that express *p53,* the level of its protein increases in response to radiation.[98,105] The enhanced p53 protein is associated with G_1/S arrest that permits the repair of damaged DNA by holding the cell in G_1,[98,106] or with cell kill via induction of the apoptotic pathway.[101,107] p53-mediated radiation-induced apoptosis is associated with suppression of the cyclin-cdk2 kinase complex by the suppressor gene product p21[WAF1/CIP1].[107,108] Several other transcriptional factors and proto-oncogenes were shown to be associated with the progression of the apoptotic pathway in different cell systems, including c-*fos*,[109,110] c-*jun*,[109–111] c-*myc*,[112–115] NF-κB,[116,117] and *hsp*-70,[109] but their exact biochemical functions in this cascade are still unknown.

Several cytokines and growth factors, such as interleukin (IL)-2,[118,119] IL-3,[120,121] IL-4,[118,119] and IL-6,[120] insulin growth factor type 1 (IGF-1),[121] and basic fibroblast growth factor (bFGF),[122] were found to inhibit apoptosis via activation of membrane PKC. Both PKC[123–128] and the Bcl-2 protein[87,103,115,129–132] were found to down-regulate the apoptotic cascade. Haimovitz-Friedman et al.[128] reported that the α isoform of PKC mediated the effect of bFGF to inhibit the programmed cell death induced in BAECs by radiation exposure. The mechanism of this effect involves the inhibition of radiation-induced hydrolysis of sphingomyelin to ceramide, which acts as a second messenger in the apoptotic pathway.[79] Hockenbery et al. demonstrated that Bcl-2 functions to protect against programmed cell death by suppression of lipid peroxidation that is produced in the cell by apoptotic signals.[131] Bcl-2 was found to be localized to intracellular sites of oxygen free radical generation, including mitochondria, endoplasmic reticula, and nuclear membranes. Like antioxidants that scavenge peroxides, Bcl-2 protected cells from H_2O_2-induced apoptosis, and overexpression of Bcl-2 functioned to suppress lipid peroxidation completely. Hence, it was suggested that Bcl-2 regulates an antioxidant pathway at sites of free radical generation and thus prevents the triggering of the apoptotic pathway.[132]

In summary, these data suggest that both the interphase apoptotic mechanism and the postmitotic mechanism of cell death contribute to cell killing after exposure of mammalian cells to ionizing irradiation. The relative contribution from each mode of cell death may differ with dose and from one cell type to another, relative to their inherent and inducible capacities to overcome each of these types of lethal radiation damage, thus determining the characteristic level of radiation sensitivity or resistance of each cell type.

Monitoring the Surviving Cell: Radiation Dose-Survival Curves

Whereas a certain proportion of an irradiated cell population will succumb to the lethal effects of radiation, other cells repair the damage and maintain both their morphologic and their functional integrity. One survival function that classically has been studied, which is particularly relevant to cancer therapy, is the clonogenic reproductive capacity. It is measured as the ratio of the ability of the irradiated/control cells to form colonies when seeded in culture dishes at low cellular densities. The survival of progenitor hematopoietic cells, or of epithelial cells of the gastrointestinal mucosa and the skin, also can be evaluated by in vivo clonogenic assays. The net effect of increasing doses of radiation on the clonogenic capacity is described by dose-survival curves.[133] Such curves typically consist of two components, an initial curved component at the low dose range (the threshold shoulder) and a subsequent exponential component that translates into a straight line when plotted on a semilogarithmic scale. Several biophysical models have been suggested to simulate the actual cell survival data and to provide hypotheses on the cellular mechanisms that produce the dose-survival patterns. A commonly used model is the single-hit multitarget model,[134,135] expressed mathematically as

$$Sf = 1 - (1 - e^{-qD})^n$$

where Sf represents the surviving fraction, D is the dose, and $-q$ is the final slope of the survival curve. When plotted on a semilogarithmic scale (Fig. 19–4A), the curve is biphasic and its parameters define the radiosensitivity of the given population of cells and their capacity to repair radiation damage. The D_0 value, which is derived from the slope (slope = $1/D_0$), describes the inherent radiosensitivity, while the exponent n (which also can be derived from extrapolation of the terminal exponential region to its intercepts with the radiation dose axis) and the D_q (the quasi-threshold dose, defined as the point at which the shoulder region transforms into an exponential function) correlate with level of cellular recovery from sublethal radiation injury. Although n and D_q define the width of the shoulder on the dose-survival curve, they do not necessarily indicate its shape, which may be of prime importance in radiotherapy.

Another commonly used model is the linear quadratic model[136] (Fig. 19–4B), expressed mathematically as

$$Sf = e^{-(\alpha D + \beta D^2)}$$

where α describes the initial linear slope dominated by single-hit killing kinetics at the low dose range, and the quadratic component β describes the bending part of the curve at higher doses. The α component represents nonrecoverable damage, while the β component corresponds to reparable lesions and is affected by the repair capacity of the tested cells.[52,53] When cells are exposed to continuous low-dose irradiation (<1 Gy/hr), they have an opportunity to recover from radiation damage during the course of exposure, thus eliminating the β component and creating a dose-survival curve that is linear, with a slope identical to the α coefficient.[52,53] The ratio α/β is the dose

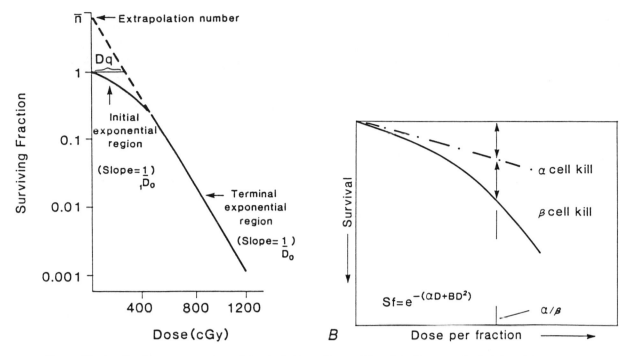

Figure 19–4. Graphic representations of the single-hit multitarget (*A*) and the linear quadratic (*B*) models of radiation dose-survival analysis.

at which the linear and quadratic components of the cell killing are equal. For a given β value, the increasing value of α represent higher sensitivities to ionizing irradiation (Fig. 19–4*B*).

To emphasize the effects of radiation at the dose levels used in human tumor radiotherapy, Fertil and Malaise[137] introduced the mean inactivation dose $\overline{D}$ as a measure of the intrinsic radiation sensitivity of human cells. The calculation of $\overline{D}$ involves a linear quadratic analysis of survival data plotted on linear coordinates. $\overline{D}$ is equal to the area under the curve and is affected significantly by the surviving fractions obtained at the 100 to 300 cGy dose range. Other authors have suggested the surviving fraction at 200 cGy (SF-2) as the most important parameter for describing the clinical radiosensitivity characteristics of human tumor cells, because 200 cGy is a common daily dose used in radiotherapy.[138] Neither the linear quadratic model nor the single-hit multitarget model and other parameters used to describe the radiation sensitivity characteristics of mammalian cells have a firmly established biologic basis. Therefore, they should be viewed only as convenient models for describing survival parameters mathematically. Critical appraisals of dose-survival curve analysis as applied to radiotherapy have been published recently by Elkind and Sutton[135] and by Steel et al.[52,53]

Use of Radiation Survival Parameters In Vitro as Predictors of Response to Radiotherapy

A potential limitation to the use of human tumor cells in culture is the uncertainty as to whether they represent the functional clonogenic cell compartment of the tumor in vivo. Nonetheless, the characterization of human tumor cells that are phenotypically resistant to chemotherapeutic agents in vitro has led to advances in the understanding of the cellular and molecular aspects of chemoresistance. Therefore, investigation of cell lines of differing radiosensitivity may be useful in understanding the mechanistic basis of the radiation response.

The in vitro sensitivity of human tumor cell lines to radiation originally was reported to lie within a fairly narrow range.[139–143] However, many early studies reported no more than four or five cell lines in any individual study.[144–146] Deacon et al.[140] reported a direct relationship between the SF-2 of 51 human tumor cell lines and the known clinical radiosensitivity of the corresponding tumors, although there were significant variations in the individual sensitivities within each category. Weichselbaum et al.[141,147] reported that the D_0 values of 20 tumor cell lines were within the range of those observed in normal fibroblasts, while, in another 9 cell lines established from tumors considered to be clinically radioresistant, the D_0 values exceeded the highest value observed in normal fibroblasts[147] (Fig. 19–5). A more direct correlation between the clinical response to treatment and the in vitro sensitivity was attempted by the same investigators[142,147,148] in 20 early-passage head and neck tumor cells and 13 early-passage soft tissue sarcomas. Both patient groups from whom the cell lines were derived were treated with curative radiotherapy and were followed clinically for extended periods of time. Tumor cells cultured from the head and neck cancer patients exhibited a wide range of radiosensitivity (D_0 of 107 to 333 cGy). Within this group, tumor cells from nine patients had a D_0 of 186 cGy or greater, considered to be within the radioresistant range.

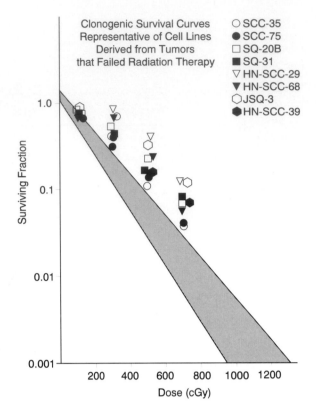

Figure 19–5. Dose-survival curves of head and neck tumor cell lines derived from tumors generally considered to be resistant to cure by radiation therapy. The shaded area represents the distribution of dose-survival curves of normal human diploid cell lines. (Adapted from Weichselbaum RR: Cellular and molecular aspects of human radioresistance. Important Adv Oncol 1991, p 75, with permission.)

Radiotherapy failed to achieve local control in five of these nine patients. The soft tissue sarcoma cell lines were in general more radiosensitive and exhibited less radiobiologic heterogeneity than the head and neck cells. A recent update of the outcome in these patients showed that the D_0 values did not predict local failures as an independent variable (R. R. Weichselbaum, unpublished data).

Brock et al.[149] reported another approach to the use of radiobiologic parameters as predictors of the clinical outcome after radiotherapy. Tumor cells from pretreatment biopsies of 72 patients with head and neck squamous cell carcinomas were cultured in an adhesive tumor cell assay system, and their SF-2 was evaluated. The average SF-2 of cultures derived from the 12 patients who had local recurrences was slightly higher (0.40) than that from those who remained at local tumor control (0.30), but the differences were not statistically significant. The same method was used by West et al.[150] in 51 patients with carcinoma of the uterine cervix. Patients with radioresistant tumors (SF-2 > 0.55) had a significantly lower probability of local control ($p < .001$). When local control was evaluated by stage, the differences remained significant.

Taken together, these data indicate that, although the in vitro parameters of radiosensitivity correlate with the clinical course in some patients, their value as routine predictors of treatment outcome is still unproven. The data do,

however, suggest that tumor cells with inherent radioresistance can be detected by in vitro assays, and that such clones may contribute to the radiotherapeutic failure in some patients. It is not clear whether, in other patients, tumor residual clones that survive the radiation treatments and subsequently lead to local failures are a priori radioresistant, or whether mutations occur during therapy that lead to the conversion of radiosensitive into radioresistant clonogens (Fig. 19–6).

Repair of Sublethal and Potentially Lethal Radiation Damage in Mammalian Cells

Although mammalian cells are proficient in their capacity to repair radiation damage to DNA,[18,51,151,152] not all radiation lesions are repaired.[153–155] Whereas irreparable lesions are lethal,[45,50,153] the fate of sublethal and potentially lethal lesions depends on competing processes of repair versus lethal fixation.[51,153] Thus, the total sum of lethal lesions at a given radiation dose consists of primary nonrepairable lesions and of potentially repairable lesions that undergo a lethal fixation. Because the repair of radiation lesions progresses as a time-dependent function, accumulation of potentially reparable lesions that have not had an opportunity to complete the time-dependent repair may occur in the early postradiation period. If a second radiation fraction is given before repair is completed, residual lesions from the previous exposure may transform into unrepairable lesions, or may combine with new lesions to produce compounded lethal lesions. Sublethal damage repair is observed experimentally as an increase in survival when a dose of radiation is divided into two fractions separated by time intervals sufficient for completion of the repair process. The classic work of Elkind and Sutton[155] has introduced the concept that the shoulder of the dose-survival curve reflects the ability of the cell to accumulate sublethal radiation damage. This work also showed that sublethal recovery usually is completed by 6 hours, and the enhancement in survival is equal to the extrapolation number ($\bar{n}$) of the radiation dose-survival curve.[155] Sublethal damage repair is regarded as important in radiotherapy because the shoulder region is recapitulated in a multifractionated regimen[156] and the small enhancement in survival following a single treatment thus is magnified greatly (Fig. 19–7). Most human fibroblasts and tumor cell lines studied in vitro have relatively small $\bar{n}$ values of less than 2.[154,157,158] However, unusual high values have been reported in some human tumor cell lines. Barranco et al.[159] reported melanoma cell lines with extrapolation numbers as large as 40. Similarly, Carney et al.[160] reported large-cell lung carcinoma cell lines with extrapolation numbers of 5.6 to 11, and Leith et al.[161] reported values of 5.8 to 20.3 in several subclones of human colon and lung carcinoma. It is important to note, however, that a low surviving fraction in the high-dose region of the dose-survival curve may give the appearance of a large $\bar{n}$.[162]

Another important type of repair that affects the survival of irradiated mammalian cells is potentially lethal damage repair (PLDR). Whereas potentially lethal damage (PLD) is reparable, its fate depends on interactions of

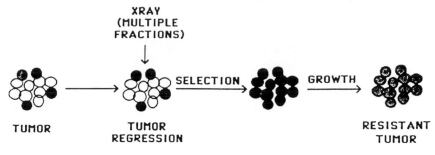

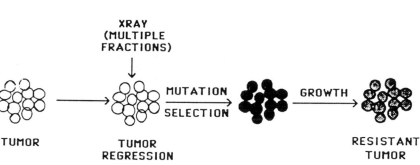

Figure 19–6. Radiation-induced selection of radioresistant cells in a tumor with inherently radiosensitive and radioresistant cell populations, leading to a residual radioresistant tumor (top). An alternative pathway leading to radioresistant tumors is by mutational induction of radioresistance in primarily radiosensitive cells, followed by therapeutic selection of the radioresistant clones (bottom). ○ radiosensitive or wild type cells, ● radioresistant cells, ● killed cells.

○ RADIOSENSITIVE OR WILD TYPE CELLS

● RADIORESISTANT CELLS

● KILLED CELLS

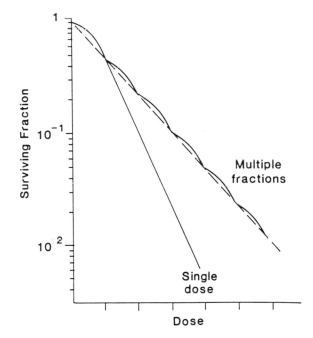

Figure 19–7. Recapitulation of the shoulder region of the dose-survival curve following multiple radiation doses greatly magnifies the surviving fraction of a given total dose over that observed after a similar single dose level.

the irradiated cells with factors present in the culture medium or in the tissue microenvironment. It is the susceptibility to specific environmental stimuli that distinguishes PLD from other types of radiation damage. These definitions of PLDR are operational rather than mechanistic and do not describe the molecular basis of PLD or the metabolic pathways that lead to its repair. There are several postradiation culture conditions that facilitate PLDR, including the postradiation maintenance of irradiated cells in high-density cultures before being subcultured at low densities as required for the colony formation assays, incubation under culture conditions that are suboptimal for progression through the cell cycle, incubation in anisotonic media, or treatment with chemical inhibitors of DNA synthesis.[153,163] These conditions apparently postpone the progression through the mitotic cell cycle, thus permitting the completion of repair of damaged DNA templates before entry into the next S phase.

PLDR occurs mainly in stationary (G_0-G_1) cells, although it has been demonstrated in other phases of the cell cycle.[153] Hahn and Little[164] were the first to study PLDR using stationary-phase cultures, which they considered more analogous to in vivo tumors than exponentially growing cells. PLDR has been demonstrated in human tumor cell lines maintained in vitro (Fig. 19–8) and in experimental tumors irradiated in vivo when explanation of

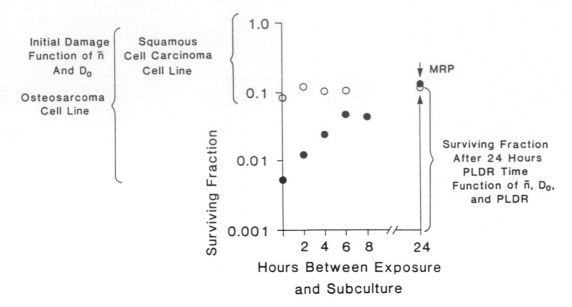

Figure 19–8. PLDR and the maximum recovery potential demonstrated in an osteosarcoma cell line. The survival of osteosarcoma cells in plateau-phase cultures (○) is shown immediately after a single dose of 700 cGy and in cells whose subculture for testing the clonogenic survival was delayed up to 8 hours after irradiation to permit the progress of PLDR. The 24-hour surviving fraction is referred to as the maximum recovery potential (MRP), which is a function of the initial damage (D_0 and n) and the PLDR occurring over time. A similar value of MRP is shown for a head and neck squamous cell carcinoma cell line (●) that does not perform PLDR after radiation exposure. The identical MRP results from a difference in the amounts of the initial lethal damage induced by radiation in each of the cell types, leading to a difference of D^0 and n values of the acute dose-survival curves. (Adapted from Weichselbaum RR: Cellular and molecular aspects of human radioresistance. Important Adv Oncol 1991, p 77, with permission.)

the tumor is delayed.[165–167] The effect in vivo is more pronounced in large tumors, presumably because a large proportion of cells are in G_0 or G_1. Several investigators also have reported proficient repair of potentially lethal damage in a variety of human tumor cell lines in vitro.[168–172]

Sublethal or potentially lethal damage repair is not necessarily expressed under all circumstances in vivo, because cells must be genetically and metabolically competent to repair these types of damage.[173] The tumor paracrine and endocrine microenvironment may affect both the proliferative status of tumor cells and their ability to carry out PLDR.[174] Also, cell kill following radiation therapy induces tumor repopulation, which may involve radiation-damaged cells that have not yet completed PLDR. The induction of mitogenesis in such cells may lead to fixation of PLD, analogous to that observed when cells irradiated in vitro are subcultured immediately after radiation exposure. Therefore, repair of PLD is likely to be significant in tumor cells with prolonged cell cycle times in which such repair is allowed to occur between delivery of dose fractions.

GENES AND ENZYMES INVOLVED IN THE REPAIR OF RADIATION DAMAGE

Biochemical Pathways of DNA Repair in Mammalian Cells

Much of the knowledge of the biochemistry of DNA repair has been obtained from studies with bacteria and

yeast,[31,175] and only more recently has there been progress in studies with mammalian cell systems.[43,176–179] The major DNA repair processes appear to have been conserved through evolution, because both excision and recombinational repair, which are prevalent in bacteria, seem to be operational in mammalian cells. Excision repair, which is responsible in bacteria for removal of UV-induced purine and pyrimidine dimers, bulky chemical adducts, and alkylation lesions, has been reported to exist in mammalian cell systems,[180] but the details of the enzymatic pathways are only partially known. Genetic recombination, which involves the exchange of DNA sequences between DNA strands, has been reported as a mechanism of repair of DNA adducts and DNA strand breaks in yeast, and also has been detected in mammalian cell systems in vitro.[181] As for the recognition and repair of dsb, the predominant lethal radiation lesions in mammalian cells, there are only a few details that are currently available on the actual enzymatic pathways involved in this repair.

One of the factors that affect the initiation of repair of radiation-induced DNA lesions is the accessibility of particular genomic regions to repair enzymes, which depends on the local topology of the nuclear chromatin. In mammalian cells, only a small fraction of the genome is transcribed actively, with active genes packaged in nucleosomal structures.[182] Studies in both rodent and human xeroderma pigmentosum cells have demonstrated the existence of preferential repair of UV damage in transcriptionally active DNA.[178] Extracts from xeroderma pigmentosum cells have demonstrated a capability for removing pyrimidine dimers from purified DNA in vitro, but not from the damaged DNA in the intact cell, suggesting that the enzymes required are expressed but the damaged sites may not be accessible in the intact cell.[183] Although this type of information progressively is becoming available from studies utilizing modern molecular biology techniques, most of the past information has been derived from repair-deficient mutants[43] and from the use of chemical inhibitors of DNA repair.[51,145]

One of the first steps in any putative DNA repair pathway involves a recognition process of the damaged sites. The existence of damage recognition proteins has been demonstrated in UV- and in cisplatin-treated human tumor cells.[184] These recognition systems seem to be defective in certain xeroderma pigmentosum cell lines, while overexpression of such proteins has been described in cisplatin-resistant cells.[185] The involvement of DNA-damage recognition proteins in the initial steps of dsb or base damage repair after ionizing irradiation has not been reported as yet.

Another molecule that binds to damaged sites in the DNA is poly(ADP-ribose), a unique homopolymer produced from NAD by the nuclear enzyme poly(ADP-ribose) transferase (ADPRT).[186] This enzyme is bound naturally to chromatin and is involved in the conversion of NAD to poly(ADP-ribose). It is believed that ADPRT is activated by DNA strand breaks[187] and adds long branched ADPR polymers to a number of proteins, including itself, and to topoisomerase I. The ADP-ribosylation of topoisomerase I inactivates its enzymatic function. The involvement of ADPRT in PLDR has been demonstrated through the inhibition of PLDR by 3-aminobenzamide (3-AB)[163,187,188] a nicotinamide analogue that specifically inhibits ADPRT.[187,189] The mechanism of involvement of ADP-ribosylation of nuclear proteins in PLDR is unknown, although it may be associated with the effects of ADPRT on topoisomerase I. Because neither the incision nor the replication steps involved in DNA repair are inhibited by 3-AB, it has been proposed that 3-AB may inhibit DNA ligase II,[187] thus possibly interfering with the final steps of the enzymatic repair of DNA breaks.

Another target for the inhibitory effect of 3-AB on the repair of DNA damage may be the enzyme topoisomerase I, which was shown to be involved in PLDR. Topoisomerase I modifies the topologic state of the DNA by nicking transient ssb in the deoxyribose backbone, through which the complementary unbroken strand can pass, thus temporarily unwinding the supramolecular coiled structure of the DNA.[190,191] This enzymatic function has an important role in DNA replication,[192] and topoisomerase I is detected at elevated levels in transcriptionally active regions of the DNA.[193] Radiation-induced activation of ADPRT inhibits topoisomerase I by ADP-ribosylation, thus interfering with DNA replication.[194] The metabolic delay in DNA replication may provide the cell with enough time to complete the repair of damaged templates before DNA replication is completed. Accordingly, the metabolic activator of topoisomerase I, β-lapachone, has been shown to abolish PLDR and to enhance the lethality of x-rays in nonproliferating human Hep-2 laryngeal carcinoma cells.[195] In contrast, inhibition of topoisomerase I by its specific inhibitor, the plant alkaloid camptothecin, was found to inhibit PLDR and to sensitize Hep-2 cells.[195] The reason for the latter effect is unclear. Haisang et al.[196] have suggested that camptothecin inhibits topoisomerase I by trapping and fixating the covalent complexes that form between the enzyme and the DNA. This fixation prevents both religation of nicked DNA and the progression of the replication fork, thus in effect producing an unrepaired ssb. If the DNA also is damaged by x-ray exposure, this potentially may lead to the formation of dsb. Furthermore, because of the discontinuous nature of DNA replication, a camptothecin-arrested region may be skipped, thus potentially leaving behind unrepaired dsb in the DNA. The involvement of topoisomerase II in PLDR is less clear, although experiments with radiation-sensitive mutants of mammalian cells suggest such a role.[197]

The exact role of polymerases in the repair of x-ray damage is also unclear, although the use of metabolic inhibitors of polymerases suggest an involvement in this process. The arabinofuranosyl nucleoside analogues β-ara-A and ara-C, known to be competitive inhibitors of DNA α and β polymerases,[198] are inhibitors of PLDR.[152,163] However, the mechanism by which polymerase inhibition leads to lethal fixation of PLD is unknown. Recent experiments showed that there are quantitative differences in the ability of β-ara-A and ara-C to inhibit DNA replication versus PLDR, with DNA replication being an order of magnitude more sensitive to the effects of these agents.[199] Furthermore, inhibition of PLDR in a kinetic pattern similar to that observed with β-ara-A and ara-C was reported with the nucleoside analogue 3′-deoxyadenosine (cordycepin),[200,201] which is an RNA synthesis inhibitor but does not have a direct effect on DNA polymerases. Also, caffeine, when used in high concentrations (>5 nmol/L), produces inhibition of PLDR in a variety of mammalian cells[51,163] The exact mechanism of the caffeine effect is unknown, although it is believed to reverse the radiation-induced inhibition of replicon initiation, enabling replication of damaged DNA templates before repair is completed.[202] Such a mechanism would assume an accelerated polymerase activity rather than its inhibition.

Although the current information on enzymatic pathways of dsb repair is limited, the recent application of modern molecular techniques to quantify repair at functionally relevant levels of genomic organization has provided new opportunities for research in this field. Promising approaches include the isolation of mutants with abnormal sensitivity to ionizing radiation and attempts to restore or complement the defect by transfection of DNA from normal cells,[203] or complementation of repair defects at the biochemical level by microinjection of proteins into an irradiated cell.[180] Other methods include the use of plasmids and DNA vectors to analyze specific repair reactions,[204,205] and the use of cell-free extracts and defined DNA substrates to quantitate the ability of cells to repair defined classes of DNA damage.[58] These and similar assays are beginning to yield new information with a potential for clinical applications.

Genetic Control of Radiation Damage Repair

The introduction of molecular and genetic techniques to the field of DNA repair has revealed that prokaryotic and eukaryotic cells use several genetically defined responses to DNA damage. The most advanced knowledge has been accrued in bacterial systems, in particular with *E. coli,* for which the current state of knowledge on genes and mechanisms that participate in repair and recombination is relatively detailed.[31,34,206-209] In lower eukaryotic systems, such as *S. cerevisiae* and *Drosophila melanogaster,* the genetic analysis of repair systems is less advanced, but several genes that participate in various pathways have been identified and cloned.[175,208-210] Progress has been much slower with mammalian cells because of their larger size of genes, the longer cell doubling times, and other methodologic limitations in performing genetic analysis in such cells. However, the notion that specific genes may be involved in the response to radiation was suggested recently by Cowan et al.,[211] who analyzed the karyotypes of 16 cell lines derived from human squamous cell carcinomas of the head and neck. When the cell lines were grouped according to their in vitro response to radiation, it was observed that recurrent chromosomal changes occurred with differing frequencies between radiation-sensitive and -resistant cells. Radiation resistance was associated with clusters of breakpoints in chromosomes 1p22, 3p21, and 8p11.2 and deletion of distal 14q, whereas radiation sensitivity was associated with a high frequency of breakpoints in chromosome 11q13 and duplication of distal 14q.

More than 40 genes have been associated with cellular responses to DNA damage in yeast, and over 25 of them have been isolated by molecular cloning. Specific biochemical information has been defined for no less than half a dozen of these genes. Some of the genes also are required for meiotic recombination or play other roles related to repair of radiation and UV damage.[175,209] Five of the genes are believed to be involved in the primary biochemical events of damage-specific recognition of UV lesions (*RAD*1, *RAD*2, *RAD*3, *RAD*4, and *RAD*10).[175,209] Of these, only *RAD*3 has been both cloned and functionally characterized as encoding a DNA-dependent ATPase/DNA helicase.[212] The *RAD*7, *RAD*14, *RAD*16, *RAD*23, and *RAD*24 genes apparently are involved in nucleoside excision repair and in checkpoint functions, although the exact roles of their proteins in the process are unknown.[177,212] The *RAD*50 gene series is involved in recombination and repair of x-ray–induced dsb in yeast.[213] The *RAD*6 gene encodes a ubiquitin-conjugating enzyme[177,212] and may be associated with modulation of chromatin conformation by histone ubiquitination. The *REV*3 gene very likely encodes a DNA polymerase,[214] and the *RADH* gene encodes a putative DNA helicase.[215] The *cdc*-9 gene is known to be the structural gene for DNA ligase, an enzyme that is involved in all forms of excision repair.[175,210] Although the number of identified genes involved in the repair of the various classes of radiation lesions in yeast is relatively large, the control mechanisms of damage repair in yeast systems are to a large extent still unknown.

The genetic control of radiation damage repair in mammalian cells is even less clear. Information obtained from yeast systems may be of help, especially if it turns out that a reasonable conservation of the genetic systems has been maintained throughout evolution. Historically, one successful approach to identifying mammalian repair genes has involved complementation techniques, in which mutants deficient in radiation damage repair are fused with normal human cells, usually lymphocytes.[203,216] Examples of radiation-sensitive mutants used for hybridization include human cell lines from xeroderma pigmentosum and AT patients and a variety of rodent cell mutants (i.e., XR-1, xrx5, LY/S, irs1, irs2, irs3, EM9). Extensive segregation of transfected human chromosomes from hybrids then is performed to identify chromosomes with complementing activity by testing for concordance between the yield of repair-proficient transfectants and specific human chromosomes.[203,216] The use of repair-deficient mutants of CHO cells that are defective in the nucleotide excision repair pathway[203,216,217] has led to the identification of five human *ERCC* (excision repair cross-complementing) genes (Table 19–1). These include the *ERCC*1,[218] *ERCC*2,[219,220] *ERCC*3,[221] *ERCC*5,[222] and *ERCC*6[32] genes that are involved in the repair of UV lesions in CHO cells, but whether they also are associated with the defects existing in xeroderma pigmentosum is unknown. The *ERCC*1 and *ERCC*2 genes have been shown to be located on the human chromosome 19q13.2,[223] and the other members of the *ERCC* gene family have been localized to other chromosomes, as shown in Table 19–1. Little information is available on chromosomal loci that carry the xeroderma pigmentosum mutations. Saxon et al.[224] recently have reported that the human chromosome 15 partially corrects the defects in xeroderma pigmentosum cells belonging to the complementation group F. Analysis of the cDNA sequence of the human *ERCC*2 gene showed homology (73 per cent) to the *RAD*3 repair gene in the yeast *S. cerevisiae,*[220] the product of which is known to have ATPase and helicase activities.[212]

Another human DNA repair gene recently cloned is the human apurinic endonuclease (*APE*) gene.[225] The *APE* cDNA encodes the main human nuclear APE, a multifunctional enzyme that removes apurinic lesions from damaged DNA and also removes fragments of deoxyribose from the 3′ termini of DNA strand breaks produced by free radicals.[226,227] The APE protein is a member of a family of DNA repair enzymes that includes two bacterial APEs (the ExoA protein of *Streptococcus pneumoniae* and the exonuclease III of *E. coli*),[228] the yeast Apn1 protein,[227] and the Rrp1 protein of *D. melanogaster.*[229,230] The purified human APE protein lacks the 3′-exonuclease activity against undamaged DNA that is found in the bacterial and *Drosophila* enzymes, and confers significant resistance to killing by methyl methanesulfonate on transfection into *E. coli.*[225] No defects in this gene have been identified in genetic diseases or in tumor tissues, and its role in repair pathways of ionizing radiation damage is unclear.

Several human x-ray cross-complementing (*XRCC*) genes have been identified and localized to different human chromosomes. The *XRCC*1 gene is located on chromosome 19q13.2-q13.3[231] (Table 19–1), and complements a repair defect in the mutagen-sensitive CHO cell line

TABLE 19–1. HUMAN DNA REPAIR GENES MAPPED AND CLONED USING HAMSTER CELL MUTANTS*

GENE NAME	HUMAN CHROMOSOME LOCALIZATION	CLONED	cDNA	HOMOLOGOUS GENE IN *S.cerevisiae*	GENE SIZE (kb)	PROTEIN AMINO ACIDS	ESSENTIAL GENE
ERCC1	19	Yes	Yes	*RAD10*	15	297	Yes
ERCC2	19	Yes	Yes	*RAD3*	19	760	Yes
ERCC3	2	Partly	Yes	Not found	35	782	Yes
ERCC4	16	No	No				Yes
ERCC5	13	Yes	No		32		Yes
ERCC6		Partly	Partly		100		?
XRCC1	19	Yes	Yes	Not found	33	633	
XRCC2	7	No	No				

*Modified from Thompson LH: Properties and applications of human DNA repair genes. Mutat Res *247*:213, 1991, with permission.

EM9.[231] The size of the *XRCC*1 gene is 33 kb, as determined by a restriction endonuclease site mapping of one of its cosmid clones.[231] Its gene product is a 69.5-kDa protein, believed to be involved in the rejoining of DNA ssb following x-irradiation and in regulating sister chromatid exchanges.[231,232] In EM9 cells, the defect slows DNA ssb rejoining,[231,232] increases the rate of sister chromatid exchange,[232] reduces the efficiency of homologous recombination,[233] and increases the radiosensitivity of cells to x-ray exposure by a factor of 2.[231] The cells also exhibits hypersensitivity to the radiomimetic agents ethyl methanesulfonate and methyl methanesulfonate.[231] Inactivation of the *XRCC*1 gene product confers sensitivity to ionizing radiation, monofunctional alkylating agents, and halogenated pyrimidines.[232] Although the gene product encoded by *XRCC*1 is unknown, recent studies have indicated that it may have a regulatory effect on the expression of the DNA ligase III enzyme.[234,235] thus suggesting a major role for this DNA ligase in the repair of radiation-induced damage. However, a recent study designed to investigate whether the levels of the in vitro radiation sensitivity of human squamous cell carcinoma lines correlate with *XRCC*1 gene expression or structure has failed to show any correlation.[236] Using Southern and Northern blotting techniques, 25 human squamous cell carcinoma cell lines with a spectrum of sensitivities to ionizing radiation exhibited *XRCC*1 polymorphism, expressed as six different patterns of the *XRCC*1 Southern blotting with EcoRI-digested genomic DNA. The levels of *XRCC*1 mRNA in the cell lines varied, and the expression levels did not correlate with either the radiobiologic parameters (i.e., n, D_0), the clinical outcome in the patients from whom the tumor cell lines were derived, or the patterns of DNA restriction fragment length polymorphisms as defined by the Southern blots of the EcoRI-digested tumor DNA.[236]

Other human genes that control DNA dsb repair include the *XRCC*4 gene, mapped to chromosome 5,[237] and the *XRCC*5 gene, localized on the human chromosome 2q34-36,[238] but the exact biochemical functions carried out by these gene products remain unknown. A role for homologous recombination in DNA dsb repair has been suggested by recent studies that demonstrated that mutations affecting either site-specific or general recombination are deficient in the repair of DNA dsb.[209] Another promising direction for future research is provided by the newly discovered recombinational defective strains of severe com-

bined immunodeficiency (SCID) mice. These mice carry an autosomal recessive SCID mutation on the mouse chromosome 16. The mutation impairs a common recombinational activity that mediates V(D)J joining for immunoglobulins and for T-cell receptor gene elements.[239,240] Therefore, mice that carry the SCID mutation are severely deficient in both T-cell– and B-cell–mediated immunity.[240] Previous studies showed that mutations that affect either site-specific or general recombination frequently also affect the pathways responsible for the repair of DNA dsb.[209] Recent experiments showed that SCID cells exhibit a profound hypersensitivity to ionizing irradiation.[241–244] Bone marrow stem cells, fibroblasts, intestinal crypt cells, and epithelial skin cells from SCID mice were two- to threefold more sensitive to x-ray exposure than congenic BALB/c cells.[243,244] Measurements of the rejoining of x-ray–induced dsb indicated that SCID mice are defective in dsb repair, but they seem to repair ssb and bulky lesions normally.[242,243] These data suggest that a common factor may participate in both dsb repair after radiation exposure and V(D)J rejoining during lymphocyte differentiation. Therefore, the murine SCID system can provide a useful tool for human gene complementation studies to unravel the radiation-induced DNA dsb repair pathway and its genetic control, as well as to identify human genes that are associated with radiation resistance.

The potential importance of DNA repair genes to radiotherapy is analogous to the discovery of multidrug resistance genes that affect the response to chemotherapeutic agents. For example, modulation of mammalian genes that repair different classes of x-ray–induced DNA damage may be used to improve the therapeutic ratio by increasing tumor cell kill, or possibly by decreasing normal tissue sequelae. When genes that repair x-ray–induced DNA damage are cloned, detection of amplification or overexpression of these genes may lead to a rapid and accurate prediction of tumor radiosensitivity. The ability to define specific alterations that characterize the response in any given individual patient may yield new approaches to the management of human tumors with combined radiation and gene-directed therapies.

Stress Genes Induced by Ionizing Radiation

While details of the genetic basis for radiation resistance in mammalian cells are beginning to emerge, there is also increasing evidence that inductive processes are involved in the regulation of cellular response to radiation damage. Exposure of cells to adverse environmental conditions induces genetically programmed stress responses that involve the activation of specific genes. The types of genes induced depend on the nature of the stress. Heat stress induces a particular set of genes, oxidative stress another, and DNA UV and x-ray damage still another, although there is some overlap between the responses. Gene induction in response to DNA damage has been studied extensively in prokaryotes, but comparatively little is known about this response in mammalian cells.

In E. coli, UV and x-ray damage to DNA induces a well-characterized transcriptional activation of approximately 20 genes and a biochemical pathway known as the SOS response.[206,245,246] Induction of the rec-A gene, which encodes for a protein with a modified proteinase activity, leads to cleavage of the Lex-A repressor protein. The Lex-A protein normally binds to the regulatory regions of SOS genes, and, with its removal, transcription of SOS genes ensues. A cascade of transcriptional activations of downstream genes eventually leads to excision of the DNA lesions and site-specific recombinational repair. In yeast, it has been suggested that more than 80 genes are activated by DNA damage,[247] but a defined SOS-like pathway has not been identified as yet. Induction of the yeast RAD-2 epistasis group of excision repair genes apparently is involved in the recognition and repair of UV DNA lesions,[248] and some of the genes in the epistasis group RAD50 are inducible and play roles in the repair of x-ray–induced damage.[249]

In mammalian cells, DNA damage by genotoxic stress induces a large number of genes, but the search for a specific and well-characterized pathway of response to damage from ionizing radiation has been slowed by the fact that only a few of the DNA repair genes actually are known. Recent studies nonetheless have reported a large number of genes and gene products that are induced, or their expression altered, after exposure to ionizing radiation (Table 19–2). Boothman et al.[250] have demonstrated in human melanoma cell lines the induction of eight polypeptides with molecular weights of 126,000 to 275,000 identified by two-dimensional gel electrophoresis. In addition, a group of peptides with molecular weights of 47,000 to 254,000 were suppressed with increasing x-ray doses. The changes in expression of these proteins were specific for ionizing radiation damage, because heat shock, hypoxia, and alkylating agents failed to alter their synthesis. Singh and Lavin[251] have identified a DNA-binding protein in the nuclei of human cells exposed to ionizing radiation. This protein was present in the cytoplasm of unirradiated cells and was translocated to the nucleus after exposure to ionizing radiation. DNA binding by the protein was dose dependent and did not require de novo protein synthesis. However, no further insight is available regarding the nature of this potential transcription factor, and whether it is associated with an inductive control of radiation damage repair is unknown.

TABLE 19–2.   GENES ACTIVATED BY IONIZING RADIATION IN MAMMALIAN CELLS

GENE	CELL TYPE
Early-Response Genes	
c-fos	Human cell lines[258,260]
c-myc	Human lymphoblastoid cells[257]
c-jun	Human cell lines[258,260]
egr-1	Human cell lines[261]
NF-κB	Human myeloid leukemia cells[116,117]
Cell Cycle–Related Genes	
GADD 45	Human cell lines[106,262]
cyclin B	CHO cells[263]
p34^{cdc2} kinase	CHO cells[315]
p53	Human normal and myeloblastic leukemia cells[99–102,105,106,264]
Growth Factors and Cytokines	
bFGF, PDGF	Endothelial cells[174,252]
TNF-α	Sarcoma[265] and leukemia[256] cells
IL-1	SHE fibroblasts[268]
Cellular Enzymes	
β-PKC	SHE fibroblasts[270]
Heme-oxygenase	Human skin fibroblasts[271]
t-PA, TK	Human melanoma cells[272]
X-ray–Induced Proteins	
''Stress proteins'' (XIP 126-275)	Human melanoma cells[250]
''DNA-binding protein''	Human lymphoblastoid cells[251]

Abbreviations: bFGF, basic fibroblastic growth factor; PDGF, platelet-derived growth factor; TNF-α, tumor necrosis factor α; IL-1, interleukin-1; SHE, syrian hamster embryo; t-PA, tissue-type plasminogen activator; TK, thymidine kinase.

Other evidence for the existence of a programmed stress response to ionizing irradiation was reported by Haimovitz-Friedman et al.[174] The study showed that bFGF serves as a specific inducer of radiation damage repair in BAECs, thus conferring radiation resistance in these cells. When plateau-phase BAECs were irradiated at high culture densities under strict bFGF-free conditions, and incubated after irradiation without medium change and without addition of exogenous bFGF, the cells still exhibited significant PLDR. This repair process was inhibited by a neutralizing monoclonal antibody against bFGF, suggesting that the irradiated cells secreted bFGF into the medium.[174] Nuclear RNA run-on and Northern blot hybridization demonstrated that the bFGF gene was induced and expressed by the radiation exposure, and the newly synthesized bFGF was secreted into the medium[252] and induced the repair of PLD in the radiation-injured cells via an extracellular autocrine loop.[174]

Earlier studies have provided evidence to support the hypothesis that PLDR after x-ray exposure is indeed an inducible process. Conditioned media from irradiated cells were shown to confer PLDR in other irradiated cells.[253–255] One study reported that postradiation conditioned media accumulated an unidentified factor that induced PLDR, and that was temperature labile but both DNAse and RNAse resistant.[255] Hallahan et al.[256] showed that the TNF-α gene is induced by x-irradiation and the secreted cytokine induced PLDR in some tumor cell types, although it enhanced radiation cell killing in most cell types tested. Whereas there may be several classes of radiation-induced ''PLDR stimulating factors,'' it is possible to envision that each cell system would respond to one or to a limited number of such factors, acting via autocrine/paracrine interactions with specific receptors. Signals transduced from a such diverse repair factor/receptor systems may converge to a specific common final pathway that terminates with repair of radiation lesions.

Table 19–2 lists genes known to be induced in mammalian cells after radiation exposure. These include early-response genes (i.e., c-myc,[257] c-fos, c-jun, junB, junD, egr-1,[257–261] and NF-κB[116,117]) cell cycle–related genes (i.e., gadd45,[106,262] cyclin B,[263] and p53[99–102,105,106,264] growth factors and cytokines (i.e., bFGF, platelet-derived growth factor [PDGF][174,252] TNF-α,[256,265–267] and IL-1,[268] and several cellular enzymes (i.e., collagenase,[269] β-PKC,[270] heme-oxygenase,[271] and tissue plasminogen activator [tPA][272]). The exact role of this pleiotropic gene response is not clearly known, but, inasmuch as it represents a programmed stress response to radiation injury to the DNA, the response seem to be specific for ionizing irradiation. The expression of products of the x-ray–induced stress response and the kinetics of their production are essentially distinct from products of the stress responses to heat shock, hypoxia, or alkylation treatment with melphalan,[195,262,269,273,274] although some overlaps do, in fact, exist.

INDUCTION OF EARLY-RESPONSE GENES

Genes that are rapidly induced following serum or growth factor stimulation without involving protein synthesis are referred to as immediate-, early-, or primary-response genes.[275,276] In addition to being induced by growth factors, early-response genes can be activated by phorbol esters, indicating that phosphorylation by PKC may be associated with the induction of some of these genes. The ability of early-response genes to express specific mRNA in the presence of inhibitors of protein synthesis indicates that their transcription is regulated by pre-existing modulators that are activated following growth factor stimulation.[276] The polypeptide products of many early-response genes, such as c-fos, c-jun, egr-1, and NF-κB, are themselves transcription factors[275,276] that bind to specific sites in the DNA and promote or suppress gene activities, leading to specific biologic responses. For example, the c-jun and c-fos genes encode transcription factors that belong to the AP-1 family,[277,278] which are characterized by a leucine zipper motif and a basic amino acid–binding domain.[258,260,279,280] Homodimers or heterodimers of AP-1 proteins bind to the specific DNA consensus sequence 5′-TGAC/GTCA-3′ (AP-1 sequence), which is found in cis promoter–acting elements of several genes.[278,281] Other classes of early-response genes include the egr-1 and the NF-κB/rel gene families, as well as a member of the steroid hormone receptor family.[275,276,282,283]

Sherman, Hallahan, and their colleagues[259,260] have reported that exposure of normal and neoplastic human cells to x-irradiation resulted in transcriptional activation and expression of the c-jun gene. Nuclear run-on analysis in irradiated HL-60 cells showed active c-jun transcription by 30 minutes after radiation exposure, and a peak of c-jun mRNA expression at 3 hours. Induction of c-jun occurred with a dose as low as 2 Gy and varied inversely with dose rate. Radiation exposure also prolonged the half-life of c-jun mRNA in HL-60 cells, suggesting that posttranscriptional effects also occur. Prior treatment with the protein synthesis inhibitor cycloheximide did not inhibit x-ray induction of the c-jun gene, and was associated with superinduction of c-jun transcripts.[259] In normal human diploid fibroblasts, in 293-epithelial kidney cells, and in several sarcoma and epithelial tumor cells, c-jun expression peaked at 0.5 to 3 hours after exposure to x-rays, depending on the cell line studied.[260]

The egr-1 transcription factor also was reported to be associated with activation of early-response genes after x-ray exposure. The egr-1 gene encodes a nuclear transcription phosphoprotein with a zinc finger motif and has partial homology to the Wilms' tumor suppressor gene.[275,276] Hallahan et al.[261] reported that egr-1 mRNA was induced in normal and neoplastic human cell lines after radiation exposure and was superinduced in the presence of both x-rays and cycloheximide. Datta et al.[284] reported that radiation induces egr-1 transcription in HL-525 cells through CArG elements in its promoter. The Egr-1 protein is co-regulated with Fos after serum or tissue plasminogen activator stimulation. Studies with the c-fos promoter showed that CArG sequences serve as binding sites for the serum response factor.[285] The absence of c-fos expression in most irradiated cells[261] suggests that, whereas down-regulation of egr-1 expression by Fos occurs after serum and tissue plasminogen activator stimulation, a different regulatory pathway is involved in control of *egr*-1 expression by x-rays.[277,281]

The third family of early-response transcription factors that are involved in the regulation of stress response to x-rays is the NF-κB/*rel* family. NF-κB protein is a cytoplasmic factor that, in its unstimulated state, is inactivated by a complex formation with the I-κB inhibitory protein.[282,283] On activation of PKC by phorbol ester stimulation, the I-κB moiety is phosphorylated and released from the complex. The free NF-κB then translocates to the nucleus and binds to specific DNA sequences to activate transcription in target genes. Induction of the human immunodeficiency virus type 1 (HIV-1) promoter by UV light is mediated by a nuclear signal that is generated by NF-κB binding to the HIV-1 promoter region.[286] Brach et al.[116] reported that ionizing radiation results in nuclear binding of NF-κB in KG-1 human myeloid leukemia cells. This effect was detectable at doses as low as 2 Gy and reached a maximum at 5 to 20 Gy. At a dose of 20 Gy, the increase in NF-κB binding activity was maximal at 2 to 4 hours and then declined to pretreatment levels. The study also demonstrated that ionizing radiation transiently increased NF-κB mRNA levels. However, the finding that induction of NF-κB binding to DNA occurred in the presence of cycloheximide indicates that ionizing radiation activates preexisting NF-κB protein.

About two dozen genes have been shown to contain NF-κB binding sites and are probable targets for NF-κB or some combinations of its constituent subunits with other cellular proteins.[287,288] The most relevant of these genes for the radiation effects is the TNF-α gene,[283,288] shown to be induced by x-irradiation and to modulate the radiation response in several types of mammalian cells.[256,265–267] Another radiation-inducible activity that may involve NF-κB is programmed cell death. Uckun et al.[117,289] reported that radiation induces in human progenitor B lymphocytes a cascade of protein-tyrosine kinase (PTK) activity that involves downstream the activation of NF-κB and apoptosis.[289] This pathway was effectively abolished by pretreatment with the PTK inhibitors genistein and herbimycin A.[289] Similar to radiation, NF-κB also was found to mediate TNF-induced apoptosis via the sphingomyelin pathway. TNF binding to its cell surface receptors activates a plasma membrane neutral sphingomyelinase that hydrolyzes sphingomyelin to generate ceramide and phosphocholine.[91] Ceramide then serves as a second messenger that activates proline-directed serine-threonine kinases and nuclear translocation of NF-κB, leading eventually to apoptosis.[91] Radiation was reported to induce apoptosis in endothelial cells via activating the sphingomyelin pathway,[79] but the involvement of NF-κB in this response has not been reported as yet.

ROLE OF PKC IN THE ACTIVATION OF EARLY-RESPONSE GENES

The induction of several of the early-response genes by radiation exposure is associated with PKC activity. Data in the literature indicate that growth factor activation of early-response genes can be mimicked by phorbol ester stimulation,[276] suggesting that protein phosphorylation by PKC is associated with the induction of at least some of these genes. Specific interactions between *trans*- and *cis*-acting phorbol ester–response elements, which involve one or more copies of unique sequences in the 5' region of tPA–sensitive genes, were found to be associated with radiation-induced responses. Studies performed with several tPA–sensitive genes have indicated that the various specific *cis* elements are not identical, nor do they interact with the same transcription factors.[274,286,290] The importance of phorbol ester–response elements for the activation of early-response genes has been demonstrated in studies that showed that either deletion of the phorbol ester–response site or site mutations abolished the binding of the respective transcriptional activators and the response to DNA damage.[286,290]

Growth factor–independent stimulation of PKC, occurring within 1 minute after radiation exposure, recently has been reported by Hallahan et al. in HL-60 cells[265] and RIT-3 cells[291] and by Kim et al.[292] who found that radiation activates the ε isoform of PKC in human lung adenocarcinoma A549 cells. The rapid activation of PKC by irradiation in these cell lines is analogous to growth factor–mediated activation of PKC via the PLC-γ–phosphoinositide turnover pathway. In this pathway, activation of the tyrosine kinase domain of receptors for growth factors initiates a cascade of events in which diacylglycerol (DAG) is produced by PLC-γ–mediated hydrolysis of phosphatidylinositol 4,5-biphosphate and activates PKC.[293–295] DAG production via this pathway is normally transient and elicits short-term activation of PKC.[294,295] Although the pathway of PKC induction by radiation exposure was not explored in the studies listed above, Uckun et al.[117,289] reported that radiation induces in human progenitor B lymphocytes a cascade of PTK activity, phosphatidylinositol turnover, and PKC within 30 seconds after exposure. This mode of PKC activation is distinguished from the PLD-mediated hydrolysis of phosphatidylcholine, associated with a more sustained production of DAG and long-term and persistent activation of PKC.[294,295]

Once activated, PKC modifies preexisting Jun protein by phosphorylation of the transcriptional activation domain and dephosphorylation of the DNA-binding domain of Jun.[261] PKC-dependent signaling following x-irradiation also has been demonstrated by the induction of reporter genes, such as the chloramphenicol acetyltransferase (CAT) gene transfected into NIH 3T3 cells and expressed under the influence of Maloney murine sarcoma virus long terminal repeats (LTRs) as a promoter.[296] This induction was blocked by prior depletion of cellular PKC. Radiation-induced activation of PKC also can modulate the level of radiation sensitivity. Hallahan et al.[291] and Kim et al.[292] have reported that inhibition of radiation-induced activation of PKC by staurosporine enhanced the radiation killing of human tumor cells. In both studies, the increase in radiation killing of staurosporine-treated cells was not associated with a measurable difference in the rejoining of DNA dsb as compared to the staurosporine-untreated control cells. Although the investigators did not report the mechanism of this effect, this pattern seemed to be similar to the pattern observed in irradiated endothelial cells treated with the PKC inhibitor H-7.[122,128] In the latter study, the enhanced radiation sensitivity in PKC-inhibited cells was shown to be associated with increased expression of radiation-induced programmed cell death.[128]

INDUCTION OF LATE-RESPONSE GENES

One of the consequences of early-response gene activation is that it apparently leads to activation of several growth factors and cytokines that are induced relatively late in the sequence of responses of mammalian cells to x-irradiation. Recent studies have suggested that these factors play an important role in the overall response of the cell to radiation exposure. Hallahan et al.[256] and Witte et al.[252] were the first to report the release of growth factors and cytokines by irradiated normal and tumor cells and showed that autocrine or paracrine stimulation by these biologically active peptides either induced repair of radiation lesions[174] or enhanced x-ray cell killing.[256] Conditioned media from irradiated human sarcoma cell lines exhibited an acquired cytotoxic activity, which could be inhibited by a neutralizing monoclonal antibody against TNF-α.[256,265,266] The TNF-α peptide mediates a wide range of cellular immune responses, but also has cytotoxic effects in some cell systems, or growth stimulation activity in other cells.[297] In irradiated cells, the cytotoxic effects of TNF synergize with that of radiation damage in some tumor cell lines but have no effect in other cells.[256,265] TNF also was shown to inhibit PLDR in most instances, but was found to enhance PLDR significantly in some cells.[265]

Investigation of TNF-α gene regulation after ionizing radiation showed that signal transduction via a PKC-dependent pathway is required for TNF gene induction[265] (Fig. 19–9). A fivefold increase in TNF-α expression was found 3 hours following a dose of 10 Gy. TNF expression was down-regulated in the presence of the PKC inhibitor H-7 or in PKC-depleted cells by preincubation with TPA for 24 hours. Furthermore, TNF-α induction following x-irradiation was not observed in HL-525 cells, a variant of

HL-60 deficient in both the α and β isoforms of PKC. Nuclear run-on analysis in irradiated HL-60 cells showed that TNF-α was regulated at the level of transcription,[266] leading to an 8.1-fold increase in TNF mRNA by 3 hours following a dose of 20 Gy.[266] The transcription of the TNF gene after irradiation was not affected by the protein synthesis inhibitor cycloheximide,[266] indicating that the transcription factors regulating the expression of the TNF gene already are present within the cell at the time of irradiation. In contrast, measurements of TNF mRNA stability after radiation exposure showed no effect on the transcript levels in the presence of actinomycin D,[266] indicating that the increased expression of the TNF protein results from radiation-related induction of transcription of the TNF gene, rather than from posttranscriptional effects.

Studies performed by Haimovitz-Friedman et al.[174,252] showed that, when BAECs were exposed to x-irradiation, they synthesized and secreted bFGF into the culture media. These investigators also reported that the bFGF secreted into the medium served as a specific inducer of radiation damage repair in BAECs. Nuclear RNA run-on experiments showed a fourfold increase in nuclear bFGF RNA within 20 minutes after the delivery of a single dose of 400 cGy, followed by an increase in bFGF-specific mRNA, with a 6.5-fold increase in the 7.0-kb species, a 3.5-fold increase in the 3.7-kb species, and a 5-fold increase in the 3.0-kb species[298] (Fig. 19–10). These transcripts peaked at 2 to 4 hours after irradiation and returned to normal levels by 8 hours. Dose-response experiments demonstrated a significant increase in bFGF mRNA at doses as low as 125 cGy, peaking at 250 cGy and remaining unchanged at doses up to 5000 cGy. In addition to bFGF, the PDGF-β gene was activated, leading to an increase of its 3.7-kb transcripts, but there was no evidence for radiation induced activation of the TGF-β gene.[298] Radiation activation of the bFGF and PDGF-β genes was accompanied by de novo synthesis of the corresponding peptides and their secretion into the condi-

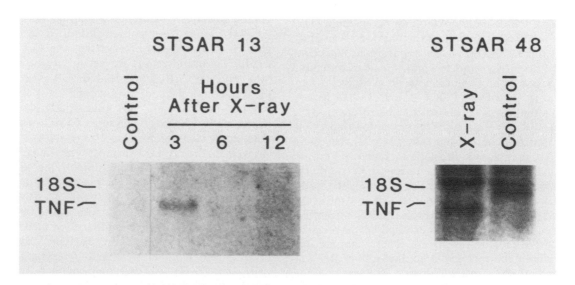

Figure 19–9. Induction of TNF-α mRNA by x-irradiation in two human sarcoma cell lines. (Adapted from Hallahan DE, Virudachalam S, Sherman MA, et al: Tumor necrosis factor gene expression is mediated by protein kinase C following activation by ionizing radiation. Cancer Res *51*:4565, 1991, with permission.)

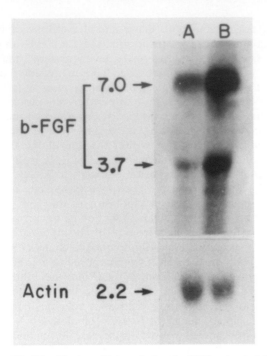

Figure 19–10. Northern blot analysis of mRNA extracted from irradiated bovine aortic endothelial cells (BAECs). The 3.7-kb and 7.0-kb species of bFGF transcriptional mRNA are increased by fourfold in the BAECs irradiated with a single dose of 400 cGy (lane *B*) as compared to control unirradiated cells (lane *A*). (Adapted from Haimovitz-Friedman A, Vlodavsky I, Chaudhuri, A, et al: Autocrine effects of fibroblast growth factor in repair of radiation damage in endothelial cells. Cancer Res *51*:2552, 1991, with permission.)

tioned media of the irradiated cells.[252] The secreted FGF was shown to stimulate PLDR in irradiated BAECs, acting via autocrine/paracrine loops. These effects were inhibited by a monoclonal antibody to bFGF.[174] Based on these data, the investigators suggested that radiation induces in endothelial cells a cycle of an autoregulated damage repair pathway. This cycle involves the induction of the bFGF gene in response to radiation, followed by synthesis and secretion of the cytokine into the medium. The bFGF that thus becomes available to the radiation-damaged cells activates PLDR via an extracellular autocrine loop, and the cycle is completed with repair of radiation lesions and restoration of the clonogenic capacity.[174]

In addition to the bFGF, PDGF-β, and TNF-α genes, ionizing radiation also was shown to induce the IL-1,[268] TGF-β[299] and PKC-β[270] genes. The kinetics of induction and down-regulation of these genes suggests that their transcription is another manifestation of the pleiotropic late-response gene activation that occurs after x-irradiation in mammalian cells. Of particular interest is the study by Woloschak et al.,[270] which demonstrated an expression of the PKC-β gene. Induction of PKC-β mRNA occurred at a time when the total cellular transcription was reduced as a result of the radiation exposure. These data are important in view of the recently described role of PKC in activating several genes after radiation exposure.[261,265,291] We hypothesize that the induction and expression of the PKC gene serves to replenish cytoplasmic stores of PKC, required to promote gene activation.

INVOLVEMENT OF CELL CYCLE REGULATORY GENES

Yamada and Puck reported in 1961 that radiation exposure of HeLa cells delayed the entry of the cells into mitosis.[300] Many studies since have reported that ionizing irradiation temporarily delays the progression of the cell through the G_1/S and G_2/M checkpoints of the mitotic cell cycle.[301–307] These genetically controlled delays are regarded as surveillance mechanisms that detect and facilitate the repair of DNA lesions, thus affecting the ultimate survival of the irradiated cell.[304–308] Progression of eukaryotic cells through the mitotic cell cycle is a genetically controlled process, regulated at two major decision points: the G_1/S boundary, at which cells become committed to DNA replication, and the G_2/M boundary, at which a commitment is made to produce the mitotic spindle and to proceed with the other activities of the M phase.[309–311] Progression through the G_2/M checkpoint is regulated by activation and inactivation of an M-phase inducer, known as the maturation- or mitosis-promoting factor (MPF). Recent studies have shown that MPF consists of a complex between $p34^{cdc2}$ kinase and cyclin B.[309–311] The association with cyclin B was reported to be essential for the expression of the kinase activity of $p34^{cdc2}$.[309–311] Studies in yeast also demonstrated that the *wee*-1 and the *cdc*25 genes control the $p34^{cdc2}$–cyclin B kinase activity by regulating the level of phosphorylation/dephosphorylation of serine, threonine, and tyrosine residues on the $p34^{cdc2}$ subunit.[312,313] Although the kinase function of cdc2–cyclin B appears to be required for cell progression through the G_2/M checkpoint,[309–311] there are reports indicating that transformed cells may bypass this requirement for G_1/S transition, and the involvement of $p34^{cdc2}$ in the regulation of the G_1/S checkpoint remains an open question.[314] The level of $p34^{cdc2}$ protein was shown to be constant throughout the cell cycle, but the cyclin proteins are synthesized and degraded in a cell cycle–dependent manner.[315]

In *S. cerevisiae,* the *RAD*9 gene product is responsible for the G_2/M arrest,[305–307] and mutants at the *RAD*9 locus do not undergo such an arrest and exhibit increased radiation sensitivity. Although a mammalian homologue to the *RAD*9 gene has not been described as yet, treatment with caffeine reduces or abolishes the G_2/M delay after irradiation and increases the sensitivity of cells to radiation exposure.[303] Ionizing irradiation was shown to affect the function of the cdc2-cyclin complex. Lock and Ross[315] reported that the $p34^{cdc2}$ H1 kinase activity was decreased significantly when asynchronous CHO cells were treated with etoposide or exposed to 10-Gy x-rays. Muschel et al. showed that x-ray exposure of synchronized HeLa cells resulted in a delayed expression of the mRNA for the cyclin B gene,[263] although the messenger for cyclin A was not affected.[316] The delay in cyclin B mRNA expression was cell cycle dependent, because it was most significant in S-phase cells but was not affected in the G_2 phase when the messenger levels were already high.[263] Similarly, Datta et al.[317] reported that treatment of asynchronous U-937 cells with 20 Gy was associated with a transient down-regulation of the *cdc*2, cyclin A, cyclin B, and *cdc*25 genes. This effect also was associated with a transient induction of the c-*jun* gene. Messenger RNA stability studies demonstrated that the down-regulation was at least in part due to a decrease in transcript half-life. However, irradiation of elutriation-enriched G_1- or S-phase cells revealed a selective decrease in cyclin B mRNA levels and no detectable changes in the messenger levels of the other associated genes. Taken together, these studies suggest that ionizing irradiation perturbs the normal function of the G_2/M checkpoint. The regulation of this effect at the gene level, and its relation to the repair of radiation-induced DNA lesions and to the activation of x-ray stress response genes, are as yet unknown.

Radiation also affects the function of the G_1/S checkpoint. Recent studies have indicated that cyclin-cdc2 kinase complexes and the suppressor genes Rb, p53, and p21 participate in this function.[107,108,318,319] Kastan et al.[105] recently reported a transient increase in wild-type p53 protein after radiation exposure of leukemic and human normal myeloid progenitor cells, associated with G_1 arrest and with a concomitant temporal inhibition of replicative DNA synthesis. Radiation-induced DNA template alterations have been suggested as the signals for this p53-dependent response pathway.[98] Tumor cells with mutated or absent wild-type p53 genes failed to exhibit a similar G_1 arrest,[105,264] and transfection of these tumor cells with the wild-type p53 genes restored the G_1 arrest after x-ray exposure. Embryonal fibroblasts cultured from p53 knockout mice, in which one or both copies of the endogenous p53 alleles were disrupted by homologous recombination, failed to arrest in G_1 after radiation exposure.[105] El-Deiry et al.[107] recently demonstrated that the p53 effect to arrest irradiated cells at G_1/S is mediated via transcriptional activation of the p21[WAF1/CIP1] gene. Induction of WAF1/CIP1 protein and its transport to the nucleus resulted in association and inhibition of cyclin-dependent kinase complexes. The specific target of the radiation-induced WAF1/CIP1 protein in human foreskin fibroblasts was shown by Dulic et al.[108] to be the cyclin E–cdc2 kinase complex. The latter complex was shown to contribute to the phosphorylation of the retinoblastoma tumor suppressor gene product (pRb) at the G_1/S checkpoint, thus neutralizing the cell cycle–inhibitory effect of pRb and promoting the transition into the S phase.[320] The studies by Dulic et al.[108] showed that radiation-induced inhibition of cyclin E–cdk2 kinase by the p21[WAF1/CIP1] protein dramatically inhibited the phosphorylation of pRb, thus regulating the G_1 arrest after radiation exposure.

Other genes were reported to participate in the regulation of the G_1/S checkpoint after radiation exposure. Several studies have demonstrated that the radiation-induced G_1/S checkpoint function is defective in AT cells.[321,322] Kastan et al.[106] reported that products of the AT gene are, in fact, required for the increased expression of the p53 protein after irradiation. Furthermore, AT cells also were defective in radiation-induced increase of the GADD45 protein.[106] The GADD (growth arrest and DNA damage)–inducible genes were isolated and cloned by Fornace and co-workers, and the GADD-45 gene of this series is induced strongly by x-rays.[308] An interaction between wild-type p53 and the GADD45 gene was described by Kastan et al., who found that p53 binds to a conserved element of the GADD45 gene during the induction of G_1 arrest

after radiation exposure.[106] The complex process of interactions between AT proteins, p53, and the GADD45 gene is not fully understood, but it was suggested[106] that the AT proteins are associated with the recognition of radiation damage. This recognition leads via an unknown signal transduction mechanism to the increased expression of wild-type p53. The induced p53 functions as a transcription factor to up-regulate the expression of GADD45, which subsequently triggers the G_1/S checkpoint.

SUMMARY OF STRESS RESPONSE PATHWAY THAT CONTROLS REPAIR OF RADIATION DAMAGE

The current knowledge of mammalian genes that are induced in response to ionizing radiation indicates a specificity to x-ray damage versus that of other genotoxic responses,[269,273,274,323–327] although some overlap exists. In addition, several x-ray–inducible genes exhibit cell type specificity, because they may be responsive to radiation exposure in one cell type but not in another. The data nonetheless indicate that gene induction after x-irradiation is not a random phenomenon, but rather represents elements of programmed pathways that lead either to cell death or to recovery from potentially lethal radiation damage. A mechanism for recognition of specific DNA-damaged sites seems to be involved in the process, but membrane signaling induced directly by radiation or via reactive oxygen intermediates also plays a role in these pathways and seems to be independent of the DNA damage-recognition process. The activation of PKC by radiation initiates a cascade of successive events that involves transphosphorylation of preexisting cytoplasmic transcription proteins, transcriptional activation of early-response genes, induction of late-response genes, PLDR, and restoration of the structure and function of the DNA (Fig. 19–11). The regulation of the radiation-induced cell cycle–dependent events at the G_1/S and G_2/M checkpoints presumably is associated with a surveillance mechanism that facilitates the identification and repair of radiation-induced DNA lesions, but regulation of programmed cell death also seems to occur at these checkpoints. The fact AT cells do not exhibit normal inhibition at G_1/S suggests that recognition of DNA-damaged sites and genetically regulated effector mechanisms may control this function. With the recent realization that the same factors (i.e., FGF) control both radiation damage repair and cell proliferation, it is possible to conceive the involvement of the cell cycle control genes as a switch-mechanism between proliferative, repair, and programmed cell death pathways, but the signals that control and direct the ultimate expression of one of these pathways over the others are unknown.

GROWTH FACTORS AND CYTOKINES THAT MODULATE THE RESPONSE OF MAMMALIAN CELLS TO IONIZING RADIATION

Hematopoietic Cytokines

The first indirect evidence that cytokines may serve as modulators of the radiation response in mammals was de-

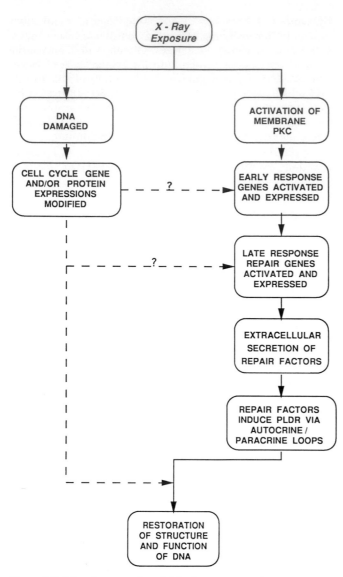

Figure 19–11. A proposed model for the programmed stress response that regulates the recovery of mammalian cells from ionizing radiation damage.

rived from early experiments by Ainsworth and Chase,[328] who showed that mice pretreated with bacterial lipopolysaccharide (LPS) prior to total-body irradiation were protected from the lethal hematopoietic syndrome. LPS induces the production of several cytokines by macrophages, including IL-1, IL-6, granulocyte colony-stimulating factor (G-CSF), granulocyte-macrophage colony-stimulating factor (GM-CSF), TNF-α and TNF-β, interferon (IFN) α and β and TGF-β.[329] Enhanced IL-1 bioactivity was demonstrated following x-irradiation of macrophages by Geiger et al.,[330] and radiation induction of the TNF gene was demonstrated in human monocytes by Sherman et al.[266] Wasserman et al.[331] recently reported increased release of IL-1 from patients receiving breast irradiation. Recent studies also demonstrated that both IL-1 and TNF-α can substitute for LPS and protect bone marrow progenitor cells both in vitro and in vivo.[332] IL-1 gene induction after radiated exposure was described by

Woloschak et al.[268] in Syrian hamster embryo cells. IL-1 mRNA was induced by 3 hours irradiation but decreased to background levels by 7 hours.

Radioprotective effects of IL-1 on colony-forming unit granulocyte-macrophage (CFU-GM) cells were reported as affecting both the D_q and the D_0 of the dose-survival curves.[333] Neta and Oppenheim[332] reported IL-1 radioprotection of hematopoietic progenitor cells in vivo in total-body–irradiated mice. Administration of an antibody to the interleukin 1 receptor (IL-1R) neutralized the in vivo protective effect in mice. Other hematopoietic cytokines also confer radioprotection on progenitor hematopoietic cells in vitro and in vivo. Uckun et al. showed that administration of recombinant G-CSF (rG-CSF) or recombinant GM-CSF (rGM-CSF) protected mice from the lethal effects of total-body irradiation.[334,335] At equivalent doses, rG-CSF was associated with a more potent radioprotective activity than rGM-CSF.

Neta et al.[336] reported that administration of low doses of IL-1α, which by themselves did not have a radioprotective effect in vivo, synergized the protective effects of GM-CSF or G-CSF in total-body–irradiated mice. These findings suggest that interactions between multiple cytokines may be necessary for effective radioprotection of hematopoietic progenitor cells. Similar protection against the lethal effects of total-body irradiation was observed with various other combinations of TNF-α, IL-1, IL-6, GM-CSF, and G-CSF.[332] Administration of an anti–IL-6 antibody to mice greatly enhanced radiation-induced lethality, and a similar effect was observed with anti–IL-6 antibody given to IL-1–treated or TNF-treated mice.[332,337] These data suggest that IL-6 is an important mediator of both IL-1– and TNF-induced hematopoietic radioprotection. Paradoxically, IL-6 given alone before irradiation increased radiation lethality. IL-1 therapy also was shown to protect mice against radiation-induced lung[338] and gastrointestinal[339,340] toxicity. IL-1 protection of jejunal crypt cell depletion in the mouse and the subsequent death of the animals from loss of these cells was dependent on the IL-1 dose and the animal strain.[340] However, the strain dependence of the effect of IL-1 on animal survival at 10 days was attributed to differences in the slopes of the respective crypt cell dose-survival curves and not to different effects of IL-1.[340]

Tumor Necrosis Factor

Similarly to IL-1, TNF-α mediates the radioprotective effects of LPS[332,337] and is secreted from macrophages stimulated by LPS.[329] TNF is a polypeptide mediator of the inflammatory response[297] and has diverse effects on hematopoietic progenitor cells, lymphocytes, fibroblasts, and tumor cells by binding to at least two different cell surface receptors to initiate divergent signaling pathways.[341] As described earlier in this chapter, several sarcoma cell lines synthesize and secrete TNF following exposure to ionizing radiation.[256,265,266] Radiation also induces TNF gene transcription in HL-60 human promyelocytic leukemia cells, U937 human monocytic leukemia cells, and human monocytes, but no TNF protein production was observed in human fibroblasts and epithelial tumor cell lines.[266] Radiation induction of TNF in vivo was demonstrated in monocytes cultured from patients receiving breast irradiation.[331] In addition, an increased serum level of TNF was found in patients receiving total-body irradiation prior to bone marrow transplantation, which was associated with a higher risk of radiation-related complications in these patients.[342,343]

Involvement of TNF in radiation protection of hematopoietic progenitor cells was demonstrated by experiments in which exogenous TNF was injected into mice prior to the delivery of lethal doses of total-body irradiation, while pretreatment of animals with anti-TNF antibody reversed the radioprotective effects of LPS.[337] Conversely, in vitro experiments using human tumor cell lines showed that TNF enhanced tumor cell killing by x-irradiation[256,265] (Fig. 19–12). The enhanced radiation effect in the presence of nontoxic concentrations of TNF was observed in some but not all cell lines tested, provided that the TNF was added 4 to 12 hours prior to irradiation. When added simultaneously with or after irradiation, TNF did not modify the effect of radiation. TNF inhibited PLDR in most instances, but significantly enhanced PLDR occurred in some cells.[265] The mechanism

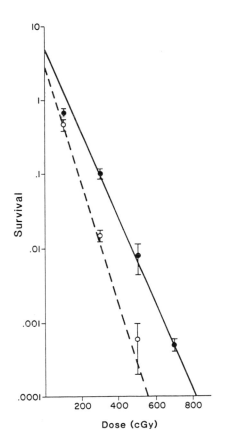

Figure 19–12. Radiation sensitizing effect of TNF-α in the SAS-TAR-33 human Ewing sarcoma cell line. The radiosensitizing effect was obtained with sublethal concentrations of TNF-α. (●) indicate control cells and (○) indicate TNF-treated cells. (Adapted from Hallahan DE, Spriggs DR, Beckett MA, et al: Increased tumor necrosis factor alpha mRNA after cellular exposure to ionizing radiation. Proc Natl Acad Sci USA 86:10104, 1989, with permission.)

by which TNF confers radiation protection is unknown, but its radiosensitizing effect may associated with induction of programmed cell death. Obeid et al.[89] and Jarvis et al.[90] recently have reported that TNF-α induces apoptosis in U937 monoblastic and HL-60 promyelocytic leukemia cell lines, and in L292/LM and WEHI-164/13 human fibrosarcoma cell lines, mediated via activation of sphingomyelin degradation and generation of ceramide. In these studies, TNF stimulated sphingomyelin degradation to ceramide, and elevation of cellular ceramide levels by addition of synthetic ceramide analogues or bacterial sphingomyelinase mimicked TNF action to induce apoptosis. Patterns of signal transduction from TNF–cell surface receptor interactions may underlie the different modes of the effects of the TNF on irradiated cells. Two divergent signaling pathways originating from two immunologically distinct TNF receptors (the 55-kDa TNF R1 and the 75-kDa TNF R2) have been reported.[341,344] The receptors have 20 per cent homology in the extracellular TNF-binding domain and no homology in the intracellular domains. It was suggested that the two receptors are associated with different signal transduction pathways.[341]

Fibroblast Growth Factor

Recent studies carried out by Haimovitz-Friedman et al.[174] demonstrated that bFGF serves as a specific inducer of radiation damage repair in BAECs, thus conferring radiation resistance in these cells. When plateau-phase BAECs were seeded on top of a bFGF-enriched extracellular matrix (the HR9-bFGF/ECM), they exhibited an enhanced repair capacity as compared to cells plated on top of a bFGF-free isotype of this extracellular matrix (the HR9/ECM). Figure 19–13 shows that, although the slopes of the dose-survival curves did not differ significantly, there was a nearly complete elimination of the threshold shoulder in the curves generated on the FGF-free HR9/ECM (D_q of 29 ± 19 cGy, compared to 174 ± 22 cGy in the cells plated on the HR9-bFGF/ECM; $p < .05$). The bFGF effect was observed mainly in G_0-G_1–phase cells, was expressed only if bFGF stimulation was provided during the first several hours after irradiation, and was neutralized by specific monoclonal antibodies against bFGF.[174,345] When BAECs were incubated after irradiation at high cellular densities and under strict bFGF-free conditions (on top of the bFGF-free HR9/ECM in bFGF-free medium), they exhibited significant PLDR, which could be inhibited by a neutralizing monoclonal antibody against bFGF.[174] This experiment indicated the presence of bFGF in the culture media, apparently secreted by the irradiated cells themselves. Taken together, these data suggest that radiation induces in endothelial cells an autoregulated damage repair pathway. This cycle involves the induction of the bFGF gene as a late-response repair gene and the activation of PLDR via an extracellular autocrine loop. The end result is the recovery of damaged DNA and restoration of the cell's clonogenic capacity.

The pattern of the radiation protection conferred by bFGF in endothelial cells could suggest that bFGF, if provided shortly after irradiation, induces or enhances the

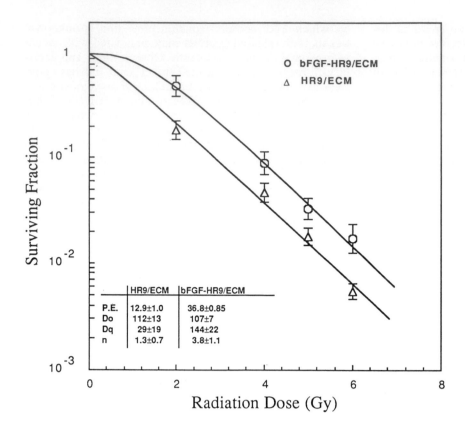

	HR9/ECM	bFGF-HR9/ECM
P.E.	12.9±1.0	36.8±0.85
Do	112±13	107±7
Dq	29±19	144±22
n	1.3±0.7	3.8±1.1

Figure 19–13. Radiation dose-survival curves of plateau-phase BAECs seeded for colony formation assays on top of either the bFGF-enriched bFGF-HR9/ECM (O) or the bFGF-free HR9/ECM (△). The cells seeded on top of the HR9/ECM received a single dose of partially purified bovine brain bFGF (200 ng/ml) 72 hours after irradiation, whereas the cells plated on top of the bFGF-HR9/ECM did not receive exogenous bFGF supplements. (Adapted from Haimovitz-Friedman A, Vlodavsky I, Chaudhuri A, et al: Autocrine effects of fibroblast growth factor in repair of radiation damage in endothelial cells. Cancer Res 51:2552, 1991, with permission.)

repair mechanisms of radiation-induced DNA break. However, studies reported by Fuks et al.[122] demonstrated that the radiation protection conferred by bFGF was not mediated via an effect on the repair of DNA breaks, but rather through inhibition of apoptosis, triggered in endothelial cells by radiation exposure. Radiation exposure produced in endothelial cells heterologous double-stranded DNA breaks, but the cells exhibited a similar competence for repair of this damage in the presence or absence of bFGF. Subsequent to the completion of this repair process, a second process of DNA fragmentation became apparent, which was detected only in the absence of bFGF, and was associated with a DNA ladder of oligonucleosomal fragments characteristic of apoptosis.[122] The radioprotective effect of bFGF to inhibit radiation-induced apoptosis was mediated via activation of membrane PKC.[128] Inhibitors of PKC abrogated the radioprotective effect of bFGF, and nonspecific stimulation of membrane PKC by phorbol esters mimicked the effect of bFGF.[128] Furthermore, the effect of radiation to induce apoptosis in endothelial cells was mediated via the sphingomyelin pathway, and PKC activation blocked both radiation-induced sphingomyelin hydrolysis and apoptosis.[79]

The inhibition of radiation-induced sphingomyelin hydrolysis to ceramide by PKC activation and the associated inhibition of apoptotic DNA degradation in endothelial cells may have important implications for the understanding of mechanisms of radiation resistance in vitro and in vivo. PKC activation may provide an antiapoptotic mechanism in vitro and in vivo and may constitute a generic mechanism of radiation resistance.[122,128] Recent studies have reported that PKC inhibitors sensitized the radiation

killing in several types of cells.[291,292] This sensitization was not associated with direct radiation damage to the DNA or its repair.[291,292] Furthermore, Fuks et al.[122] reported that intravenous bFGF therapy protected mice against radiation-induced tissue damage. C3H/HeJ mice exposed to lethal doses of whole-lung irradiation exhibited apoptotic changes in the endothelial cell lining of the pulmonary microvasculature within 6 to 8 hours after radiation exposure. Intravenous bFGF given immediately before and after irradiation inhibited the development of apoptosis in these cells and protected mice against the development of lethal radiation pneumonitis. Taken together, these observations provide a basis for a hypothesis on the existence of a balance between radiation induction of programmed cell death via the sphingomyelin pathway and its down-regulation by natural suppressor mechanisms through PKC. According to this model, spontaneous radiation activation of membrane PKC or its activation by growth factors, such as bFGF, may play an important role in the homeostatic control of radiation resistance and may have important clinical implications.

Epidermal Growth Factor

Several studies have demonstrated that epidermal growth factor (EGF) sensitizes cells to the effects of radiation. Schmidt-Ulrich et al.[346] reported that the MCF-IR-3 variant of human breast cancer cells was significantly more sensitive to irradiation than the parental MCF-7 cells. The MCF-IR-3 cells exhibited an increase in TGF-α mRNA and decreased estrogen receptor mRNA after radiation exposure. The increased radiosensitivity of the MCF-IR-3 cells may be associated with an autocrine effect of radiation-induced TGF-α, because a similar radiosensitization was observed in TGF-α–treated MCF-7 cells.[346] The role of the down-regulation of the estrogen receptors in mediating this response remains unclear.

Kwok and Sutherland[347,348] described the effect of EGF on the radiation response of several squamous cell carcinoma cell lines, all of which have high-affinity cell surface receptors to EGF and respond to EGF stimulation. The radiation sensitivity of the CsSki, HN5, and A431 cells increased under EGF stimulation, whereas there was no effect on the sensitivity of the SiHa cells and of a mouse 3T3 cell line. In A431 cells, the EGF enhancement of sensitivity was most significant in G_1-phase cells and was associated mainly with a reduction of the shoulder region of the dose-survival curve. Correlations of the number of high-affinity EGF receptors revealed an inverse relationship with the degree of EGF radiosensitization.[347] The investigators concluded that the EGF radiosensitization is EGF receptor density dependent. However, these data do not provide a mechanistic basis for this phenomenon.

An understanding of the various patterns of the modulation of the radiation effect by growth factors may be derived from a recent study by Goldkorn et al.[349] These investigators demonstrated that tyrosine autophosphorylation of the EGF receptor occurs spontaneously after x-ray exposure of A431 cells. Treatment of control cells with 20-nM EGF for 15 minutes resulted in a 4.7-fold increase in tyrosine autophosphorylation, whereas only a 2.7-fold increase was observed after exposure to 500 cGy in the absence of EGF stimulation. Both the binding of EGF to the receptor and receptor stability as measured by quantitative analysis of the receptor immunoprecipitated from metabolically ^{35}S-labeled cells were unaffected by radiation. However, contrary to BAECs stimulated by FGF, there was a decrease in PKC activity after either radiation or EGF stimulation of A431 cells. Treatment with 20-nM EGF reduced membrane PKC activity by twofold within 15 seconds. Similarly, membrane PKC activity of A431 cells dropped within 30 seconds after irradiation with 500 cGy to 0.4 of controls. The fact that the enzymatic activity of PKC decreases after EGF stimulation may underlie the sensitizing effect of EGF on irradiated cells in this system. These results suggest that the level of PKC activation or suppression may determine the ability of growth factors to regulate the level of radiation sensitivity in mammalian cells.

The involvement of EGF-like activity in radiation effects at the tissue level was suggested by recent experiments performed by Rubin et al.[350] The investigators reported that alveolar macrophages obtained by bronchial lavage from irradiated rabbit lungs exhibited enhanced production and release of TGF-α and TGF-β as compared to macrophages obtained from normal lungs. TGF-α is known to stimulate fibroblast proliferation, and TGF-β induces synthesis and secretion of extracellular matrix components. The investigators suggested that the control of fibroblast proliferation and excessive matrix production, which occur in the lung after exposure to damaging levels of radiation, is mediated via these and other growth factors that are released from parenchymal cells as the result of gene activation by the radiation exposure. These observations provide an insight into mechanisms by which messages exchanged between cells via paracrine loops may mediate specific cellular and tissue responses that lead to the eventual manifestations of radiation damage in normal tissues. In the lung, these events occur during a clinically latent but biologically active period, and constitute an early phase in the pathogenesis of radiation injury.

Transforming Growth Factor β

TGF-β is a peptide that has a fundamental role in controlling proliferation of many cell types. Its main biologic effects at the tissue level include the induction of connective tissue hyperplasia inhibition of epithelial cell growth. Radiation induction of the TGF-β gene and its secretion in irradiated tissues have been implicated in the pathogenesis of radiation-induced pneumonitis in the rabbit,[350] radiation hepatitis and hepatic fibrosis in the rat,[351] and radiation-induced damage to porcine skin.[352] Furthermore, a recent study reported that increased serum levels of TGF-β predict the subsequent development of hepatic venous occlusive disease or idiopathic interstitial pneumonitis in patients undergoing autologous marrow transplantation after high-dose chemotherapy (without total-body irradiation) for advanced breast cancer.[353] The correlation between the increased hepatic concentration of TGF-β and radiation injury suggests a role for TGF-β in the pathogenesis of radiation hepatitis. TGF-β also is associated with deleterious effects on irradiated hematopoietic stem cells.[322,337] It sensitizes mice to lethal total-body irradiation, possibly by down-regulating IL-1R expression or reducing IL-1 and TNF production.[337] Thus, attenuation of TGF-β induction during radiotherapy may represent a method for reducing radiation sequelae in normal tissues.

CONCLUDING COMMENTS

Although the basic mechanisms of radiation injury and its repair in normal and tumor tissues remain essentially unknown, significant progress has been made in the field and new discoveries offer increasing opportunities for clinical applications. It is becoming increasingly apparent that molecular events mediated by autocrine, paracrine, and endocrine growth and inhibitory factors play a major role in tissue responses to ionizing radiation. The new information on the role of cytokines, growth factors, and hormones in either regulating the biochemical pathways of radiation damage repair or sensitizing mammalian cells to the effects of radiation may have immediate clinical applications. The release of radiation-induced growth factors into the tissue extracellular space produces multiple opportunities for a variety of secondary genetic and epigenetic events stimulated via autocrine or paracrine loops in cells equipped with specific receptors for the trophic factors that become available. The evolution of radiation injury thus is placed within a cellular and molecular context that provides a biologic background for generating testable experimental hypotheses for the study of tissue damage. This is in contrast to much of the previous descriptive work. As mechanisms of radiation injury syndromes in normal and tumor tissues are unraveled, it may become possible to intervene actively in specific pathways of such processes to alter favorably the therapeutic ratio of tumor versus normal tissue effects in radiation treatments in several types of human cancer.

REFERENCES

1. Chapman JD, Deuvers AP, Borsa J, Greenstock CL: Chemical radioprotection and radiosensitization of mammalian cells growing in vitro. Radiat Res 56:291, 1973
2. Ward JF: Biochemistry of DNA lesions. Radiat Res 104:s103, 1985
3. Ward JF: DNA damage produced by ionizing radiation in mammalian cells: Identities, mechanisms of formation and repairability. Prog Nucleic Acids Mol Biol 35:95, 1988
4. Ward JF: The yield of DNA double-strand breaks produced intracellularly by ionizing radiation: A review. Int J Radiat Biol 57:1141, 1990
5. Painter RB: The role of DNA damage and repair in cell killing induced by ionizing radiation. In Meyn RE, Withers HR (eds): Radiation Biology in Cancer Research. New York, Raven Press, 1980, p 59
6. Von Sonntag C: The Chemical Basis of Radiation Biology. London, Taylor and Francis, 1987
7. Elkind MM, Redpath JL: Molecular and cellular biology of radiation lethality. In Becker FF (ed): Cancer, a Comprehensive Treatise. New York, Plenum, 1977, p 51
8. Warters RL, Hofer KG, Harris CR: Radionuclide toxicity in cultured mammalian cells: Elucidation of the primary site of radiation damage. Curr Top Radiat Res Q 12:389, 1977
9. Munro TR: The relative radiosensitivity of the nucleus and the cytoplasm of the Chinese hamster fibroblast. Radiat Res 42:451, 1990
10. Cole A, Meyn RE, Chen R, et al: Mechanisms of cell injury. In Meyn RE, Withers HR (eds): Radiation Biology in Cancer Research. New York, Raven Press, 1980, p 33
11. Szybalski W: X-ray sensitization by halopyrimidines. Cancer Chemother Rep 58:539, 1974
12. Dizdaroglu M: Measurement of radiation-induced damage to DNA at the molecular level. Int J Radiat Biol 61:175, 1992
13. Roots R, Okada S: Estimation of life times and diffusion distances of radicals involved in X-ray-induced DNA strand breaks or killing of mammalian cells. Radiat Res 64:306, 1975
14. Chapman JD, Gillespie CJ: Chemical radiosensitization studies with mammalian cells growing in vitro. In Nygaard OF, Adler H, Sinclair WK (eds): Radiation Research: Biomedical, Chemical and Physical Perspectives. New York, Academic Press, 1975, p 752
15. Teoule R, Cadet J: Radiation-induced degradation of the base component in DNA and related substances—final products. In Huttermann J, Kohnlein R, Teoule R, Bertinchamps AJ (eds): Effects of Ionizing Radiation on DNA. New York, Springer-Verlag, 1978, p 171
16. Von Sonntag C, Hagen U, Schon-Bopp A, Schulte-Frohlinde D: Radiation-induced strand breaks in DNA: Chemical and enzymatic analysis of end groups and mechanistic aspects. Adv Radiat Biol 9:109, 1981
17. Oleinick NL, Chiu S, Ramakrishnan N, Xue L: The formation, identification, and significance of DNA-protein cross-links in mammalian cells. Br J Cancer 55(suppl VIII):135, 1987
18. Frankenberg-Schwager M: Review of repair kinetics for DNA damage induced in eukaryotic cells in vitro by ionizing radiation. Radiother Oncol 14:307, 1989
19. Dizdaroglu M: Chemical determination of free radical-induced damage to DNA. Free Radical Biol Med 10:225, 1991
20. Ward JF, Blakely WF, Joner EI: Mammalian cells are not killed by DNA single-strand breaks caused by hydroxyl radicals from hydrogen peroxide. Radiat Res 103:383, 1985
21. Ahnstrom G, Edvardsson KA: Radiation induced single-strand breaks in DNA determined by rate of alkaline strand separation and hydroxylapatite chromatography: An alternative to velocity sedimentation. Int J Radiat Biol 26:493, 1974
22. Coquerelle T, Bopp A, Kessler B, Hagen U: Strand breaks and 5'- end groups in DNA of irradiated thymocytes. Int J Radiat Biol 24:397, 1973
23. Kohn KW, Erickson LC, Ewing RAG, Friedman CA: Fractionation of DNA from mammalian cells by alkaline elution. Biochemistry 15:4629, 1976
24. Fowler JF: Nuclear Particles in Cancer Treatment. Bristol, England, Adam Hilger, 1981
25. Sakai K, Suzuki S, Nakamura N, Okada S: Induction and subsequent repair of DNA damage by fast neutrons in cultured mammalian cells. Radiat Res 110:311, 1987
26. Dikomey E, Franzke J: DNA repair kinetics after exposure to X-irradiation and to internal x-rays in CHO cells. Radiat Environ Biophys 25:189, 1986
27. Hansson J, Munn M, Rupp WD, et al: Localization of DNA repair synthesis by human cell extracts to a short region at the site of a lesion. J Biol Chem 264:21788, 1989
28. Wood ML, Dizdaroglu M, Gajewski E, Essigmann JM: Mechanistic studies of ionizing radiation and oxidative mutagenesis: Genetic effects of a single 8-hydroxyguanine (7-hydro-8-oxoguanine) residue inserted at a unique site in a viral genome. Biochemistry 29:7024, 1990
29. Cerutti PA: Base damage induced by ionizing radiation. In Wang SY (ed): Photochemistry and Photobiology of Nucleic Acids, vol II. New York, Academic Press, 1976, p 375
30. Von Sonntag C, Schuchmann HP: The radiolysis of pyrimidines in aqueous solutions: An updating review. Int J Radiat Biol 49:1, 1986
31. Sancar A, Sancar G: DNA repair enzymes. Annu Rev Biochem 57:29, 1988
32. Hoeijmakers JHJ, van Duin M, Weeda G, et al: Analysis of mammalian excision repair: From mutants to genes and gene products. In Friedberg E, Hanawalt PC (eds): Mechanisms and Consequences of DNA Damage Processing. New York, Alan R. Liss, 1988, p 281
33. Mattern MR, Hariharan PV, Cerutti PA: Selective excision of gamma-ray damaged thymine from the DNA of cultured mammalian cells. Biochim Biophys Acta 395:48, 1975
34. Friedberg EC: DNA Repair. New York, WH Freeman, 1985
35. Fornace AJ, Dobson PP, Kinsella TJ: Repair of gamma-ray-induced DNA base damage in Xeroderma pigmentosum cells. Radiat Res 106:73, 1986
36. Paterson MC, Smith PJ: Ataxia telangiectasia: An inherited human disorder involving hypersensitivity to ionizing radiation and related DNA damaging chemicals. Annu Rev Genet 13:291, 1979
37. Freifelder D: Mechanism of in activation of coliphage T7 by x-rays. Proc Natl Acad Sci USA 54:128, 1965
38. Frankenberg D, Frankenberg-Sehwager M, Harbieh R: Interpretation of the shape of survival curves in terms of induction and repair/misrepair of DNA double-strand breaks. Br J Cancer 49(suppl VI):223, 1984
39. Frankenberg-Schwager M, Frankenberg D: DNA double-strand breaks: Their repair and relationship to cell killing in yeast. Int J Radiat Biol 58:569, 1990
40. Kemp LM, Sedgwick SG, Jeggo PA: X-ray sensitive mutants of CHO cells defective in double strand break rejoining. Mutat Res 132:189, 1984
41. Giaccia A, Welnsrein R, Liu J, Stamato TD: Cell cycle dependent repair of double strand DNA breaks in a gamma ray sensitive Chinese hamster cell line. Somatic Cell Mol Genet 11:485, 1985
42. Wlodek D, Hittelman WN: Repair of double-strand DNA breaks correlates with radiosensitivity of L5178Y and L5178Y-R cells. Radiat Res 112:1, 1988

43. Jeggo PA: Studies on mammalian mutants defective in rejoining double-strand breaks in DNA. Mutat Res 239:1, 1990

44. Radford IR: Evidence for a general relationship between the induced level of DNA double-strand breakage and cell-killing after x-irradiation of mammalian cells. Int J Radiat Biol 49:611, 1986

45. Schwartz JL, Mustafi R, Beckett MA, Weichselbaum RR: Prediction of the radiation sensitivity of human squamous cell carcinoma cells using DNA filter elution. Radiat Res 123:1, 1990

46. McMillan TJ, Cassoni AM, Edwards S, et al: The relationship of DNA double-strand break induction to radiosensitivity in human tumour cell lines. Int J Radiat Biol 58:427, 1990

47. Prise KM, Davis S, Michael BD: The relationship between radiation-induced DNA double strand breaks and cell kill in hamster V79 fibroblasts irradiated with 250 kvp x-rays, 2.3 Mev neutrons or ^{238}Pu a-particles. Int J Radiat Biol 52:893, 1987

48. Brenner DJ, Ward JF: Constraints on energy depletion and target size of multiply damaged sites with DNA double-strand breaks. Int J Radiat Biol 61:737, 1992

49. Bryant PE: Use of restriction endonucleases to study relationships between DNA double-strand breaks, chromosomal aberrations and other end points in mammalian cells. Int J Radiat Biol 54:869, 1988

50. Curtis SB: Lethal and potentially lethal lesions induced by radiation—a unified repair model. Radiat Res 106:252, 1986

51. Iliakis G: Radiation-induced potentially lethal damage: DNA lesions susceptible to fixation. Int J Radiat Biol 53:541, 1988

52. Steele GG, McMillan TJ, Peacock JH: The picture has changed in the 1980s. Int J Radiat Biol 56:525, 1989

53. Steele GG, Peacock JH: Why are some human tumors more radiosensitive than others? Radiother Oncol 15:63, 1989

54. Dewey WC, Miller HH, Leeper DB: Chromosomal aberrations and mortality of x-irradiated mammalian cells: Emphasis on repair. Proc Natl Acad Sci USA 68:667, 1971

55. Natarajan AT: Chromosomal aberrations from radiation induced DNA lesions. In Sharma T (ed): Trends in Chromosome Research. Narosa Publishing House, 1990, pp 119–124

56. Cornforth NM, Bedford JS: A quantitative comparison of potentially lethal damage repair and the rejoining of interphase chromosome breaks in low passage normal human fibroblasts. Radiat Res 111:385, 1987

57. Debenham P, Jones N, Webb M: Vector-mediated DNA double strand break repair analysis in normal and radiation sensitive Chinese hamster V79 cells. Mutat Res 199:1, 1988

58. North P, Ganesh A, Thaeker J: The rejoining of double strand breaks in DNA by human cell extracts. Nucleic Acids Res 18:6205, 1990

59. Thompson LH, Suit HD: Proliferation kinetics of x-irradiated mouse L cells studied with time-lapse photography. II. Int J Radiat Biol Relat Stud Phys Chem Med 15:347, 1969

60. Yamada T, Ohyama H: Radiation-induced interphase death of rat thymocytes is internally programmed (apoptosis). Int J Radiat Biol 53:65, 1988

61. Allan DJ: Radiation-induced apoptosis: Its role in a MADCaT (mitosis-apoptosis-differentiation-calcium toxicity) scheme of cytotoxicity mechanisms. Int J Radiat Biol 62:145, 1992

62. Radford IR: Mouse lymphoma cells that undergo interphase death show markedly increased sensitivity to radiation-induced DNA double-strand breakage as compared with cells that undergo mitotic death. Int J Radiat Biol 65:1353, 1991

63. Judah JD, Ahmed K, Mclean AG: Pathogenesis of cell necrosis Fed Proc 24:1217, 1965

64. Wyllie AH: The biology of cell death in tumours. Anticancer Res 5:131, 1985

65. Wyllie AH, Kerr JFR, Currie AR: Cell death: The significance of apoptosis. Int Rev Cytol 68:251, 1980

66. Kerr JFR, Wyllie AH, Currie AR: Apoptosis: A basic biological phenomenon with wide ranging implications in tissue kinetics. Br J Cancer 26:239, 1972

67. Kerr JFR, Harmon BV: Definition and incidence of apoptosis: An historical perspective. In Tomei LD, Cope FO (eds): Apoptosis: The Molecular Basis of Cell Death. Cold Spring Harbor, NY, Cold Spring Harbor Laboratory Press, 1991, p 5

68. Arends MJ, Morris RG, Wyllie AH: Apoptosis: The role of the endonuclease. Am J Pathol 136:593, 1990

69. Fesus L, Thomazy V, Falus A: Induction and activation of tissue transglutaminase during programmed cell death. FEBS Lett 224:104, 1987

70. Duvall E, Wyllie AH, Morris RG: Macrophage recognition of cells undergoing programmed cell death (apoptosis). Immunology 56:351, 1985

71. Kyprianou N, English HF, Isaacs JT: Programmed cell death during regression of PC-82 human prostate cancer following androgen ablation. Cancer Res 50:3748, 1990

72. Szende B, Zalatini A, Schally AV: Programmed cell death (apoptosis) in pancreatic cancers of hamsters after treatment with analogs of both luteinizing hormone-releasing hormone and somatostatin. Proc Natl Acad Sci USA 86:1643, 1989

73. Tritton TR: Cell death in cancer chemotherapy: The case of adriamycin. In Tomei LD, Cope FO (eds): Apoptosis: The Molecular Basis of Cell Death. Cold Spring Harbor, NY, Cold Spring Harbor Laboratory Press, 1991, p 121

74. Ronen A, Heddle JA: Site-specific induction of nuclear anomalies (apoptotic bodies and micronuclei) by carcinogens in mice. Cancer Res 44:1536, 1984

75. Trowell OA: Ultrastructural changes in lymphocytes exposed to noxious agents in vitro. J Exp Physiol 51:207, 1966

76. Urmansky SR: Apoptotic process in radiation-induced death of lymphocytes. In Tomei LD, Cope FO (eds): Apoptosis: The Molecular Basis of Cell Death. Cold Spring Harbor, NY, Cold Spring Harbor Laboratory Press, 1991, pp 193

77. Potten CS: Extreme sensitivity of some intestinal crypt cells to X and γ irradiation. Nature 269:518, 1977

78. Stephens LC, Schultheiss TE, Price RE, et al: Radiation apoptosis of serous ascinar cells of salivary and lacrimal glands. Cancer 67:1539, 1991

79. Haimovitz-Friedman A, Kan C-C, Ehleiter D, et al: Ionizing radiation acts on cellular membranes to generate ceramide and induce apoptosis. J Exp Med, August, 1994

80. Stephens LC, Ang KK, Schultheiss TE, et al: Apoptosis in irradiated murine tumor. Radiat Res 127:308, 1991

81. Meyn RE, Stephens LC, Ang KK, et al: Heterogeneity in the development of apoptosis in irradiated murine tumors of different histologics. Int J Radiat Biol 64:583, 1993

82. Wyllie AH: Glucocorticoid induced thymocyte apoptosis is associated with endogenous endonuclease activation. Nature 284:555, 1980

83. Yuan J, Horvitz HR: The Caenorhabditis elegans genes ced-3 and ced-4 act cell autonomously to cause programmed cell death. Dev Biol 138:33, 1990

84. Buttyan R, Olsson CA, Pintar J, et al: Induction of the TRPM-2 gene in cells undergoing programmed death. Mol Cell Biol 9:3473, 1989

85. Kyprianou N, English HF, Davidson NE, Isaacs JT: Programmed cell death during regression of the MCF-7 human breast cancer following estrogen ablation. Cancer Res 51:162, 1991

86. Hengartner MO, Ellis RE, Horvitz HR: Caenorhabditis elegans gene ced-9 protects cells from programmed cell death. Nature 356:494, 1992

87. Hockenbery DM, Zutter M, Hickey W, et al: Bcl2 protein is topographically restricted in tissues characterized by apoptotic cell death. Proc Natl Acad Sci USA 88:6961, 1991

88. Vaux DL: Toward an understanding of the molecular mechanisms of physiological cell death. Proc Natl Acad Sci USA 90:786, 1993

89. Obeid LM, Linardic CM, Karolak LA, Hannun YA: Programmed cell death induced by ceramide. Science 259:1769, 1993

90. Jarvis DW, Kolesnick RN, Fornari FA, et al: Induction of apoptotic DNA degradation and cell death by activation of the sphingomyelin pathway. Proc Natl Acad Sci USA 91:73, 1994

91. Kolesnick RN, Goldie DW: The sphingomyelin pathway in tumor necrosis factor and interleukin-1 signaling. Cell 77:325, 1994

92. Rotello RJ, Lieberman RC, Purchio AF, Gerschenson LE: Coordinated regulation of apoptosis and cell proliferation by transforming growth factor beta 1 in cultured uterine epithelial cells. Proc Natl Acad Sci USA 88:3412, 1991

93. Oberhammer FA, Pavelka M, Sharma S, et al: Induction of apoptosis in cultured hepatocytes and in regressing liver by transforming growth factor beta 1. Proc Natl Acad Sci USA 89: 5408, 1992

94. Yanagihara K, Tsumuraya M: Transforming growth factor beta 1 induces apoptotic cell cultured human gastric carcinoma cells. Cancer Res 52:4042, 1992

95. Wiegmann K, Schutze S, Kampen E, et al: Human 55-kDa receptor for tumor necrosis factor coupled to signal transduction cascades. J Biol Chem 267:17997, 1992

96. Mathias S, Younes A, Kan C-C, et al: Activation of the sphingomyelin pathway in intact EL4 cells and in a cell-free system by IL-1b. Science 259:519, 1993

97. Warters RL: Radiation-induced apotosis in a murine T-cell hybridoma. Cancer Res 52:883, 1992

98. Nelson WG, Kastan MB: DNA strand breaks: The DNA template alterations that trigger p53-dependent DNA damage response pathways. Mol Cell Biol 14:1815, 1994

99. Clarke AR, Purdie CA, Harrison DJ, et al: Thymocyte apoptosis induced by p53-dependent and independent pathways. Nature 362:849, 1993

100. Lowe SW, Schmitt EM, Smith SW, et al: p53 is required for radiation-induced apoptosis in mouse thymocytes. Nature 62: 847, 1993

101. Lowe SW, Ruley HE, Jacks T, Housman DE: p53-dependent apoptosis modulates the cytotoxicity of anticancer agents. Cell 74:957, 1993

102. Yonish-Rouach E, Resnitzky D, Lotem J, et al: Wild-type p53 induces apoptosis of myeloid leukaemic cells that is inhibited by interleukin-6. Nature 353:345, 1991

103. Lotem J, Sachs L: Regulation by bcl-2, c-myc, and p53 of susceptibility to induction of apoptosis by heat shock and cancer chemotherapy compounds in differentiation-competent and -defective myeloid leukemia cells. Cell Growth Differ 4:41, 1993

104. Yonish-Rouach E, Grunwald D, Wilder S, et al: p53-mediated cell death: Relationship to cell cycle control. Mol Cell Biol 13:1415, 1993

105. Kastan MB, Onyekwere O, Sindarsky D, et al: Participation of p53 in the cellular response to DNA damage. Cancer Res 51: 6304, 1991

106. Kastan MB, Zhan Q, El-Deiry WS, et al: A mammalian cell cycle checkpoint pathway utilizing p53 and GADD45 is defective in ataxia-telangiectasia. Cell 71:587, 1992

107. El-Deiry WS, Harper JW, O'Connor PM, et al: TI WAF1/CIP1 is induced in p53-mediated G1 arrest and apoptosis. Cancer Res 54:1169, 1994

108. Dulic V, Kaufmann WK, Wilson SJ, et al: p53-dependent inhibition of cyclin-dependent kinase activities in human fibroblasts during radiation-induced G1 arrest. Cell 76:1013, 1994

109. Buttyan R, Zakeria Z, Lockshin R, Wolgemut HD: Cascade induction of c-fos, c-myc, and heat shock 70K transcripts during regression of the rat ventral prostate gland. Mol Endocrinol 2: 650, 1988

110. Colotta F, Polentarutti N, Sironi M, Mantovani A: Expression and involvement of c-fos and c-jun protooncogenes in programmed cell death induced by growth factor deprivation in lymphoid cell lines. J Biol Chem 267:18278, 1992

111. Rubin E, Kharbanda S, Gunji H, Kufe D: Activation of the c-jun protooncogene in human myeloid leukemia cells treated with etoposide. Mol Pharmacol 39:697, 1991

112. Shi Y, Glynn JM, Guilbert LJ, et al: Role of c-myc activation-induced apoptotic cell death in T-cell hybrydomas. Science 257:212, 1992

113. Askew DS, Ashmun RA, Simmons BC, Cleveland JL: Constitutive c-myc expression in an IL-3-dependent myeloid line suppresses cell cycle arrest and accelerates apoptosis. Oncogene 6:1915, 1991

114. Evan GI, Wyllie AH, Gilbert CS, et al: Induction of apoptosis in fibroblasts by c-myc protein. Cell 69:119, 1992

115. Bissonnette RP, Echeverri F, Mahboubi A, Green DR: Apoptotic cell death induced by c-myc is inhibited by bcl-2. Nature 359: 552, 1992

116. Brach MA, Hass R, Sherman ML, et al: Ionizing radiation induces expression and binding activity of the nuclear factor kappa B. J Clin Invest 88:691, 1991

117. Uckun FM, Schieven GL, Tuel-Ahlgren LM, et al: Tyrosine phosphorylation is a mandatory proximal step in radiation-induced activation of the protein kinase C signaling pathway in human B-lymphocyte precursors. Proc Natl Acad Sci USA 90:252, 1993

118. Vazquez A, Auffredou MT, Chaouchi N, et al: Differential inhibition of interleukin 2- and interleukin 4-mediated human B cell proliferation by ionomycin: A possible regulatory role for apoptosis. Eur J Immunol 21:2311, 1991

119. Zubiaga AM, Munoz E, Huber BT: IL-4 and IL-2 selectively rescue Th cell subsets from glucocorticoid-induced apoptosis. J Immunol 149:107, 1992

120. Collins MK, Marvel J, Malde P, Lopez-Rivas A: Interleukin 3 protects murine bone marrow cells from apoptosis induced by DNA damaging agents. J Exp Med 176:1043, 1992

121. Rodriguez-Tarduchy G, Collins MK, Garcia I, Lopez-Rivas A: Insulin-like growth factor-I inhibits apoptosis in IL-3-dependent hemopoietic cells. J Immunol 149:535, 1992

122. Fuks Z, Persaud RS, Alfieri A, et al: Basic fibroblast growth factor protects endothelial cells from radiation-induced programmed cell death in vitro and in vivo. Cancer Res 54:2582, 1994

123. Story MD, Stephens LC, Tomasovic SP, Meyn RE: A role for calcium in regulating apoptosis in rat thymocytes irradiated in vitro. Int J Radiat Biol 61:243, 1992

124. Tomey LD, Kanter P, Wenner CE: Inhibition of radiation-induced apopyosis in vitro by tumor promoters. Biochem Biophys Res Commun 155:324, 1990

125. Kizaki H, Tadakuma T, Okada C, et al: Activation of a suicide process of thymocytes through DNA fragmentation by calcium and phorbol esters. J Immunol 143:1790, 1989

126. McConkey DJ, Hartzell P, Jondal M, Orrenius S: Inhibition of DNA fragmentation in thymocytes and isolated thymocyte nuclei by agents that stimulate protein kinase C. J Biol Chem 264:13399, 1989

127. Araki S, Shimada Y, Kaji K, Hayashi H: Role of protein kinase C in the inhibition by fibroblast factor of apoptosis in serum depleted endothelial cells. Biochem Biophys Res Commun 172:1081, 1990

128. Haimovitz-Friedman A, Balaban AN, McLoughlin M, et al: Protein kinase c mediates basic fibroblast growth factor protection of endothelial cells against radiation-induced apoptosis. Cancer Res 54:2591, 1994

129. Sentman CL, Shutter JR, Hockenbery D, et al: bcl-2 inhibits multiple forms of apoptosis but not negative selection in thymocytes. Cell 67:879, 1991

130. Siegel RM, Katsumata M, Miyashita T, et al: Inhibition of thymocyte apoptosis and negative antigenic selection in bcl-2 transgenic mice. Proc Natl Acad Sci USA 89:7003, 1992

131. Hockenbery DM, Oltvai ZN, Yin XM, et al: Bcl-2 functions in an antioxidant pathway to prevent apoptosis. Cell 75:241, 1993

132. Oltvai ZN, Milliman CL, Korsmeyer SJ: Bcl-2 heterodimerizes in vivo with a conserved homolog, Bax, that accelerates programmed cell death. Cell 74:609, 1993

133. Elkind MM: The initial part of the survival curve: Does it predict outcome of fractionated radiotherapy? Radiat Res 114:425, 1988

134. Astwood KC, Norman A: On the interpretation of multihit survival curves. Proc Natl Acad Sci USA 35:697, 1949

135. Elkind MM, Sutton H: Radiation response of mammalian cells grown in culture. Radiat Res 13:556, 1960

136. Kellerer PM, Ross HH: The theory of dual radiation action. Curr Top Radiat Res Q 8:85, 1972

137. Fertil B, Malaise EP: The mean inactivation dose: Experimental versus theoretical. Radiat Res 108:222, 1986

138. Tucker S: Is the mean inactivation dose a good measure of cell radiosensitivity? Radiat Res 105:18, 1986

139. Fertil B, Malaise EP: Inherent cellular radiosensitivity as a basic concept for human tumor radiotherapy. Int J Radiat Oncol Biol Phys 7:621, 1981

140. Deacon JM, Peckham MJ, Steel GG: The radioresponsiveness of

human tumors and the initial slope of the cell survival curves. Radiother Oncol 2:314, 1984

141. Weichselbaum RR, Dahlberg W, Little JB: Inherently radio-resistant cells exist in some human tumors. Proc Natl Acad Sci USA 82:4732, 1985

142. Weichselbaum RR, Dahlberg W, Beckett MA, et al: Radiation resistant and repair proficient human tumor cells may be associated with radiotherapy failure in head and neck cancer patients. Proc Natl Acad Sci USA 83:2683, 1986

143. Weichselbaum RR, Beckett MA: The maximum recovery potential of human tumor cells may predict clinical outcome in radiotherapy. Int J Radiat Oncol Biol Phys 13:709, 1987

144. Gerwick LE, Kornblith P, Burlett P, et al: Radiation sensitivity of cultured glioblastoma cells. Radiology 125:234, 1977

145. Kelland LR, Bingle L, Edwards S, Steele GG: High intrinsic radiosensitivity of a newly established and characterized human embryonal rhabdomyosarcoma cell line. Br J Cancer 59:160, 1989

146. Nilsson S, Carlson J, Larson E, Ponten J: Survival of irradiated glioma cells studied with a new cloning technique. Int J Radiat Biol 37:267, 1980

147. Weichselbaum RR, Beckett MA, Schwartz JL, Dritschilo A: Radioresistant tumor cells are present in head and neck carcinomas that recur after radiotherapy. Int J Radiat Oncol Biol Phys 15:575, 1988

148. Weichselbaum RR, Beckett MA, Vijayakumar S, et al: Radiobiological characterization of head and neck and sarcoma cells derived from patients prior to radiotherapy. Int J Radiat Oncol Biol Phys 19:313, 1990

149. Brock WA, Baker FL, Wike JL, et al: Cellular radiosensitivity of primary head and neck squamous cell carcinomas and local tumor control. Int J Radiat Oncol Biol Phys 18:1283, 1990

150. West CM, Davidson SE, Hendry JH, Hunter RD: Prediction of cervical carcinoma response to radiotherapy (letter). Lancet 338:818, 1991

151. Powell S, McMillan TJ: DNA damage and repair following treatment with ionizing radiation. Radiother Oncol 19:95, 1990

152. Iliakis G: The role of DNA double strand breaks in ionizing radiation-induced killing of eukaryotic cells. Bioessays 13:641, 1992

153. McMillan TJ: Residual DNA damage: What is left over and how does this determine cell fate? Eur J Cancer 28:267, 1992

154. Weichselbaum RR: Cellular and molecular aspects of human radioresistance. Important Adv Oncol 1991, p 73

155. Elkind MM, Sutton HG: X-ray damage and recovery in mammalian cells in culture. Nature 184:1293, 1959

156. Elkind MM: Fractionated dose radiotherapy and its relationship to survival curve shapes. Cancer Treat Rev 3:2, 1976

157. Weichselbaum R, Nove J, Little JB: X-ray sensitivity of 53 human diploid fibroblast cell strains from patients with characterized genetic disorders. Cancer Res 40:920, 1980

158. Weichselbaum RR, Nove J, Little JB: X-ray sensitivity of human tumor cells in vitro. Int J Radiat Oncol Biol Phys 6:437, 1980

159. Barranco SC, Romsdahl NM, Humphrey RM: The radiation response of human malignant melanoma cells grown in vitro. Cancer Res 31:830, 1971

160. Carney DN, Mitchell JB, Kinsella T: In vitro radiation and chemotherapeutic sensitivity of established cell lines in human small cell lung cancer and large cell morphology variants. Cancer Res 43:2806, 1983

161. Leith G, Dexter DL, DeWynagaert J, et al: Differential responses to x-irradiation of subpopulations of two heterogeneous human carcinomas in vitro. Cancer Res 42:2556, 1982

162. Weichselbaum RR, Rotmensch J, Ahmed-Swan S, Beckett MA: Radiobiological characterization of 53 human tumor cell lines. Int J Radiat Biol 56:553, 1989

163. Kelland LR, Steel GG: Inhibition of recovery from damage induced by ionizing radiation in mammalian cells. Radiother Oncol 13:285, 1988

164. Hahn GM, Little JB: Plateau phase cultures of mammalian cells: An in vitro model for human cancer. Curr Top Radiat Res 8:39, 1972

165. Belli JA, Dicus GJ, Nagle W: Repair of radiation damage as a factor in preoperative radiation therapy. Front Radiat Ther Oncol 5:40, 1970

166. Little JB, Hahn GM, Frindel E, Tubian M: Repair of potentially lethal radiation damage in vitro and in vivo. Radiology 106:689, 1973

167. Shipley WV, Stanley JA, Courtenay VD, Field SB: Repair of radiation damage in Lewis lung carcinoma cells following in situ treatment with fast neutrons and gamma rays. Cancer Res 35:932, 1975

168. Weichselbaum RR, Little JB, Nove J: Response of human osteosarcoma in vitro to irradiation: Evidence for unusual cellular repair activity. Int J Radiat Biol 31:295, 1977

169. Weichselbaum RR, Schmit A, Little JB: Cellular repair factors influencing radiocurability of human malignant tumors. Br J Cancer 45:10, 1982

170. Guichard M, Weichselbaum RR, Little JB, Malaise EP: Potential lethal damage as a possible determinant of human tumor radiosensitivity. Radiother Oncol 1:263, 1984

171. Kinsella TJ, Mitchell JB, McPhearson S, et al: In vitro radiation studies on Ewing sarcoma cell lines and human bone marrow: Application to the clinical use of total body irradiation. Int J Radiat Oncol Biol Phys 10:1005, 1984

172. Arundel LM, Leith JT: Effects of nutritional state on expression of radiation injury in two subpopulations obtained from a heterogeneous colon carcinoma. Int J Radiat Oncol Biol Phys 12:559, 1986

173. Weichselbaum RR, Nove J, Little JB: Deficient recovery from potentially lethal radiation damage in ataxia telangiectasia and xeroderma pigmentosum. Nature 27:261, 1978

174. Haimovitz-Friedman A, Vlodavsky I, Chaudhuri A, et al: Autocrine effects of fibroblast growth factor in radiation damage repair in endothelial cells. Cancer Res 51:2552, 1991

175. Friedberg EC: Eukaryotic DNA repair: Glimpses through the yeast Saccharomyces cerevisiae. Bioessays 13:295, 1991

176. Lindahl T: Regulations and deficiencies in DNA repair. Br J Cancer 56:91, 1987

177. Wood RD, Coverly D: DNA excision repair in mammalian cell extracts. Bioessays 13:447, 1991

178. Bohr VA: Gene specific DNA repair. Carcinogenesis 12:1983, 1991

179. Eastman A, Barry MA: The origin of DNA breaks: A consequence of DNA damage, repair, or apoptosis. Cancer Invest 10:229, 1992

180. Hoeijmakers J, Eker APM, Wood RD, Robins P: Use of in vivo and in vitro assays for the characterisation of mammalian excision repair and isolation of repair proteins. Mutat Res 236:223, 1990

181. Lopez B, Rousset S, Coppey J: Homologous recombination intermediates between two duplex DNA catalysed by human cell extracts. Nucleic Acids Res 15:5643, 1987

182. Bohr V, Phillips D, Hanawalt P: Heterogeneous DNA damage and repair in the mammalian genome. Cancer Res 47:6426, 1987

183. Fujiwara Y, Kano Y: Cellular responses to DNA damage. Mol Cell Biol 2:215, 1983

184. Andrews P, Jones J: Characterisation of binding proteins from ovarian carcinoma and kidney tubule cells that are specific for cisplatin-modified DNA. Cancer Commun 3:1, 1991

185. Chu G, Chang E: Xeroderma pigmentosum group E cells lack a number of factors that bind to damaged DNA. Science 242:564, 1989

186. Althaus FR, Richter C: ADP-ribosylation of proteins: Enzymology and biological significance. Mol Biol Biochem Biophys 37:1, 1987

187. Shall S: ADP-ribose in DNA repair: A new component of DNA excision repair. Adv Radiat Biol 11:1, 1984

188. Ben Hur E: Involvement of poly (ADP-ribose) in the radiation response of mammalian cells. Int J Radiat Biol 46:659, 1984

189. Cleaver JE, Morgan WF: 3-Aminobenzamide, an inhibitor of poly(ADP-ribose) polymerase, is a stimulator, not an inhibitor, of DNA repair. Exp Cell Res 172:258, 1987

190. Wang JC: DNA topoisomerases. Annu Rev Biochem 54:665, 1985

191. Liu LF: DNA topoisomerase poisons as antitumor drugs. Annu Rev Biochem 58:351, 1989

192. Trask DK, Muller MT: Stabilization of type I topoisomerase-

DNA covalent complexes by actinomycin D. Proc Natl Acad Sci USA 85:1417, 1988

193. Zhang H, Wang JC, Liu LF: Involvement of DNA topoisomerase I in transcription of human ribosomal RNA genes. Proc Natl Acad Sci USA 85:1060, 1988

194. Krupitza G, Crutti P: ADP-ribosylation of ADPR-transferase and topoisomerase I in intact mouse epidermal cell JB6. Biochemistry 28:2034, 1989

195. Boothman DA, Bouvard I, Hughes EN: Identification and characterization of x-ray-induced proteins in human cells. Cancer Res 49:2871, 1989

196. Haisang YH, Lihou MG, Liu LF: Arrest of replication forks by drug stabilized topoisomerase I-DNA cleavable complexes as a mechanism of cell killing by camptothecin. Cancer Res 49:5077, 1989

197. Hickson ID, Davis SM, Robson CN: DNA repair in radiation sensitive mutants of mammalian cells: Possible involvement of DNA topoisomerases. Int J Radiat Biol 58:561, 1990

198. Muller WEG, Rohde HJ, Beyer R, et al: Mode of action of 9-p-D-arabinofuranosyladenine on the synthesis of DNA, RNA and protein in vivo and in vitro. Cancer Res 35:2160, 1975

199. Iliakis G, Pantelias G, Okayasu R, Seaner R: Comparative studies on repair inhibition by araA, araC and aphidicolin of radiation induced DNA and chromosome damage in rodent cells: Comparison with fixation of PLD. Int J Radiat Biol Oncol Phys 16:1261, 1989

200. Koval TM, Kazmar ER: DNA double-strand break repair in eukaryotic cell lines having radically different radiosensitivities. Radiat Res 113:268, 1988

201. Van Ankeren SC, Murray D, Meyn R: Induction and rejoining of gamma-ray-induced DNA single and double-strand breaks in Chinese hamster AA8 cells and in two radiosensitive clones. Radiat Res 116:511, 1988

202. Painter RB: Effect of caffeine on DNA synthesis in irradiated and unirradiated mammalian cells. J Mol Biol 143:289, 1980

203. Thompson LH: Properties and applications of human DNA repair genes. Mutat Res 247:213, 1991

204. Thaeker J: The use of recombinant DNA techniques to study radiation-induced damage, repair, and genetic exchange in mammalian cells. Int J Radiat Biol 50:1, 1986

205. Thaeker J: The use of integrating DNA vectors to analyse the molecular defects in ionising radiation-sensitive mutants of mammalian cells including ataxia telangectasia. Mutat Res 220:187, 1989

206. Walker GC: Mutagenesis and inducible responses to deoxyribonucleic acid damage in Escherichia coli. Microbiol Rev 48:60, 1984

207. Walker GC, Marsh L, Dobson LA: Genetic analysis of DNA repair: Inference and extrapolation. Annu Rev Genet 19:103, 1985

208. Myles GM, Sancar A: DNA repair. Chem Res Toxicol 2:197, 1989

209. Friedberg EC: Deoxyribonucleic acid repair in the yeast Saccharomyces cerevisiae. Microbiol Rev 52:70, 1988

210. Boyd JB, Mason JM, Yamamoto AH, et al: A genetic and molecular analysis of DNA repair in Drosophila. J Cell Sci Suppl 6:39, 1987

211. Cowan JM, Beckett MA, Weichselbaum RR: Chromosome changes characterizing in vitro response to radiation in human squamous cell carcinoma lines. Cancer Res 53:5542, 1993

212. Harosh I, Naumovski L, Friedberg EC: Purification and characterization of the Rad3 ATPase/DNA helicase from Saccharomyces cerevisiae. J Biol Chem 264:20532, 1989

213. Alani E, Subbiah S, Kleckner N: The yeast RAD50 gene encodes a predicted 153kD protein containing a purine nucleotide-binding domain and two large heptad repeat regions. Genetics 122:47, 1989

214. Morrison A, Christensen RB, Alley J, et al: REV3, a yeast gene whose function is required for induced mutagenesis, is predicted to encode a nonessential DNA polymerase. J Bacteriol 171:5659, 1990

215. Aboussekhra A, Chanet R, Zgaga Z, et al: RADH, a gene of Saccharomyces cerevisiae encoding a putative DNA helicase involved in DNA repair: Characteristics of RadH mutants and sequence of the gene. Nucleic Acids Res 17:7211, 1989

216. Thompson LH: Somatic cell genetics approach to dissecting mammalian DNA repair. Environ Mol Mutagen 14:264, 1989

217. Zdzienicka MZ, Tran Q, van der Shans GP, Simons JWIM: Characterization of an X-ray-hypersensitive mutant of V79 Chinese hamster cells. Mutat Res 194:239, 1988

218. Westerveld AJ, Hoeijmakers JHJ, van Duin M, et al: Molecular cloning of a human DNA repair gene. Nature 310:425, 1984

219. Weber CA, Salazar SA, Stewart SA, Thompson LH: Molecular cloning and biological characterization of a human gene, ERCC2, that corrects the nucleotide excision repair defect in CHO UV5 cells. Mol Cell Biol 8:1137, 1988

220. Weber CA, Salazar EP, Stewart SA, Thompson LH: ERCC2: cDNA cloning and molecular characterization of a human nucleotide excision repair gene with high homology to yeast RAD3. EMBO J 9:1437, 1990

221. Weeda G, van Ham RCA, Masurel R, et al: Molecular cloning and biological characterization of the human excision repair gene ERCC-3. Mol Cell Biol 10:2570, 1990

222. MacInnes MA, Mudgett JS: Cloning of the functional human excision repair gene ERCC-5: Potential gene regulatory features conserved with other human repair genes. Prog Clin Biol Res 340:265, 1990

223. Mohrenweiser HW, Carrano AV, Fertitta A, et al: Refined mapping of the three DNA repair genes, ERCC1, ERCC2, and XRCC1, on human chromosome 19. Cytogenet Cell Genet 52:11, 1989

224. Saxon PJ, Schultz RA, Stanbridge EJ, Friedberg EC: Human chromosome 15 confers partial complementation of phenotypes to xeroderma pigmentosum group F cells. Am J Hum Genet 44:474, 1989

225. Demple B, Herman T, Chen DS: Cloning and expression of APE, the cDNA encoding the major human apurinic endonuclease: Definition of a family of DNA repair enzymes. Proc Natl Acad Sci USA 88:11450, 1991

226. Demple B, Johnson AW, Fung D: Endonuclease III and endonuclese IV remove 3' blocks from DNA synthesis primers in H_2O_2-damaged Eschericia coli. Proc Natl Acad Sci USA 83:7731, 1986

227. Ramotar D, Popoff SC, Gralla EB, Demple B: Cellular role of yeast Apn1 apurinic endonuclease/3'-diesterase: Repair of oxidative and alkylation DNA damage and control of spontaneous mutation. Mol Cell Biol 11:4537, 1991

228. Puyet A, Greenberg B, Lacks S: The exoA gene of Streptococcus pneumoniae and its product, a DNA exonuclease with apurinic endonuclease activity. J Bacteriol 171:2278, 1988

229. Saporito SM, Smith-White BJ, Cunningham RP: Nucleotide sequence of the xth gene of Escherichia coli K-12. J Bacteriol 170:4542, 1988

230. Sander M, Lowenhaupt K, Rich A: Drosophila Rrp1 protein: An apurinic endonuclease with homologous recombination activities. Proc Natl Acad Sci USA 88:6780, 1991

231. Thompson LH, Brookman KW, Jones NJ, et al: Molecular cloning of the human XRCCI gene, which corrects defective DNA strand-break repair and sister chromatid exchange. Mol Cell Biol 10:6160, 1990

232. Thompson LH, Brookman KW, Minkler JL, et al: DNA-mediated transfer of a human DNA repair gene that controls sister chromatid exchange. Mol Cell Biol 5:881, 1985

233. Hoy CA, Fuscoe JC, Thompson LH: Recombination and ligation of transfected DNA in CHO mutant EM9, which has high levels of sister chromatid exchange. Mol Cell Biol 7:2007, 1987

234. Caldecott KW, McKeown CK, Tucker JD, et al: An interaction between the mammalian DNA repair protein XRCC1 and DNA ligase III. Mol Cell Biol 14:68, 1994

235. Ljungquist S, Kenne K, Olsson L, Sandstrom M: Altered DNA ligase III activity in the CHO EM9 mutant. Mutat Res 314:177, 1994

236. Dunphy EJ, Beckett MA, Thompson LH, Weichselbaum RR: Expression of the polymorphic human DNA repair gene XRCC1 does not correlate with radiosensitivity in the cells of human head and neck tumor cell lines. Radiat Res 130:166, 1992

237. Giaccia AJ, Denko N, MacLaren R, et al: Human chromosome 5 complements the DNA double-strand break-repair deficiency

and gamma-ray sensitivity of the XR-1 hamster variant. Am J Hum Genet 47:459, 1990

238. Hafezparast M, Kaur GP, Zdzienicka M, et al: Subchromosomal localization of a gene (XRCC5) involved in double strand break repair to the region 2q34-36. Somat Cell Mol Genet 19:413, 1993

239. Bosma GC, Custer RP, Bosma MJ: Severe combined immunodeficiency in the mouse. Nature 301:527, 1983

240. Schuler W, Bosma MJ: Nature of the scid defect: A defective VDJ recombinase system. Curr Top Microbiol Immunol 152:55, 1989

241. Fulop GM, Phillips RA: The scid mutation in mice causes a general defect in DNA repair. Nature 347:479, 1990

242. Biedermann KA, Sun JR, Giaccia AJ, et al: Scid mutation in mice confers hypersensitivity to ionizing radiation and a deficiency in DNA double-strand break repair. Proc Natl Acad Sci USA 88:1394, 1991

243. Hendrickson EA, Qin XQ, Bump EA, et al: A link between double-strand break-related repair and V(D)J recombination: The scid mutation. Proc Natl Acad Sci USA 88:4061, 1991

244. Disney JE, Barth AL, Shultz LD: Defective repair of radiation-induced chromosomal damage in scid/scid mice. Cytogenet Cell Genet 59:39, 1992

245. Little JW, Mount DW: The SOS regulatory system of escherichia coli. Cell 29:11, 1982

246. Quillaret P, Frelet G, Nguyen UD, Hofnung M: Detectio of ionizing radiations with SOS Chemotest. Mutat Res 216:251, 1989

247. Ruby SW, Szostak JW: Specific Saccharomyces cerevisiae genes are expressed in response to DNA-damaging agents. Mol Cell Biol 5:75, 1985

248. Robinson GW, Nicolet CM, Kalainov D, Friedberg EC: A yeast excision repair gene is inducible by DNA damaging agents. Proc Natl Acad Sci USA 83:1842, 1986

249. Cole G, Schild D, Lovett S, Mortimer RK: Regulation of RAD-54 and RAD-52 Lac-Z gene fusions in Saccharomyces cervisiae in response to DNA damage. Mol Cell Biol 7:1078, 1987

250. Boothman DA, Trask DK, Pardee AB: Inhibition of potentially lethal DNA damage repair in human tumor cells by beta-lapachone, an activator of topoisomerase I. Cancer Res 49:605, 1989

251. Singh SP, Lavin MF: DNA-binding protein activated by gamma radiation in human cells. Mol Cell Biol 10:5279, 1990

252. Witte L, Fuks Z, Haimovitz-Friedman A, et al: Effects of radiation on the release of growth factors from cultured bovine, porcine and human endothelial cells. Cancer Res 49:5066, 1989

253. Hetzel FW, Kruuv J, Frey HE: Repair of potentially lethal damage in irradiated V79 cells. Radiat Res 68:308, 1976

254. Horowitz IA, Norwint H, Hall EJ: Conditioned media from plateau phase cells: Effect on growth of proliferative cells and on repair of potentially lethal radiation damage. Radiology 114:723, 1975

255. Little JB: Factors influencing the repair of potentially lethal radiation damage in growth-inhibited human cells. Radiat Res 56:320, 1973

256. Hallahan DE, Spriggs DR, Beckett MA, et al: Increased tumor necrosis factor alpha mRNA after cellular exposure to ionizing radiation. Proc Natl Acad Sci USA 86:10104, 1989

257. Sullivan NF, Willis AE: Elevation of c-myc protein by DNA strand breakage. Oncogene 4:1497, 1989

258. Sherman ML, Datta R, Hallahan DE, et al: Ionizing radiation regulates expression of the c-jun protooncogene. Proc Natl Acad Sci USA 87:5663, 1990

259. Sherman ML, Stone RM, Datta R, et al: Transcriptional and post-transcriptional regulation of c-jun expression during monocytic differentiation of human myeloid leukemic cells. J Biol Chem 265:3320, 1990

260. Hallahan DE, Virudachalam S, Beckett ML, et al: Mechanism of x-ray mediated protooncogene c-jun expression in radiation-induced human sarcoma cell lines. Int J Radiat Oncol Biol Phys 21:1677, 1991

261. Hallahan DE, Sukatme VP, Sherman ML, et al: Protein kinase C mediates x-ray inducibility of nuclear signal transducers EGR1 and JUN. Proc Natl Acad Sci USA 88:2156, 1991

262. Papathanasiou MA, Ker NCK, Robbins JH, et al: Induction by ionizing radiation of the gadd 45 gene in cultured human cells: Lack of mediation by protein kinase-C. Mol Cell Biol 11:1009, 1991

263. Muschel RJ, Zhang HB, Iliakis G, McKenna G: Cyclin B in HeLa cells during the G_2 block induced by ionizing irradiation. Cancer Res 51:5113, 1991

264. Kuerbitz SJ, Plunkett BS, Walsh WV, Kastan MB: Wild-type p53 is a cell cycle checkpoint determinant following irradiation. Proc Natl Acad Sci USA 89:7491, 1992

265. Hallahan DE, Virudachalam S, Sherman MA, et al: Tumor necrosis factor gene expression is mediated by protein kinase C following activation by ionizing radiation. Cancer Res 51:4565, 1991

266. Sherman ML, Datta R, Hallahan D, et al: Tumor necrosis factor gene expression is transcriptionally and post-transcriptionally regulated by ionizing radiation in human myeloid leukemia cells and peripheral blood monocytes. J Clin Invest 87:1794, 1991

267. Hallahan DE, Beckett ML, Kuff DW, Weichselbaum RR: The interaction between recombinant human tumor necrosis factor and radiation in 13 human tumor cell lines. Int J Radiat Oncol Biol Phys 19:69, 1990

268. Woloschak GE, Chang-Liu CM, Shearin-Jones P, Jones CA: Modulation of gene expression in Syrian hamster embryo cells following ionizing irradiation. Cancer Res 50:339, 1990

269. Kaina B, Stein B, Schonthal A, et al: An update of the mammalian UV response: Gene regulation and induction of a protective function. In Lambert MW, Laval J (eds): DNA Repair Mechanisms and Their Biological Implications in Mammalian Cells. New York, Plenum, 1990, p 149

270. Woloschak GE, Chang-Liu CM, Shearin-Jones P, Jones CA: Regulation of protein kinase C by ionizing irradiation. Cancer Res 50:3963, 1990

271. Applegate LA, Luscher P, Tyrrell RM: Induction of hemeoxygenase: A general response to oxidant stress in cultured mammalian cells. Cancer Res 51:974, 1991

272. Boothman DA, Wang M, Lee SW: Induction of tissue type plasminogen activator by ionizing radiation in human malignant melanoma cells. Cancer Res 51:5587, 1991

273. Herrlich P, Angel P, Rahmsdorf HJ, et al: The mammalian genetic stress response. Adv Enzym Regul 25:458, 1986

274. Holbrook NJ, Fornace AJ: Response to adversity: Molecular control of gene activation following genotoxic stress. New Biol 3:825, 1991

275. Sukhatme VP: Early events in cell growth. J Am Soc Nephrol 1:859, 1990

276. Herschman HR: Primary response genes induced by growth factors and tumor promoters. Annu Rev Biochem 60:281, 1992

277. Angel P, Hattori K, Smeal T, Karin M: The jun proto-oncogene is positively autoregulated by its product. Cell 55:875, 1988

278. Lamph WW, Wamsley P, Sassone-Corsi P, Verma IM: Induction of proto-oncogene JUN/AP-1 by serum and TPA. Nature 334:629, 1988

279. Halazonetis TD, Georgopoulos K, Greenberg ME, Leder P: c-Jun dimerizes with itself and with c-Fos, forming complexes of different DNA binding affinities. Cell 55:917, 1988

280. Turner R, Tjian R: Leucine repeats and an adjacent DNA binding domain mediate the formation of functional cFos-cJun heterodimers. Science 243:1689, 1989

281. Rauscher FJ, Sambucetti LC, Curran T, et al: Common DNA binding site for Fos protein complexes and transcription factor AP-1. Cell 52:471, 1988

282. Ghosh S, Baltimore D: Activation in vitro of of NF-kB by phosphorylation of its inhibitor IkB factor. Nature 344:540, 1990

283. Rushlow C, Warrior R: The rel family of proteins. Bioessays 14:89, 1992

284. Datta R, Hallahan DE, Kharbanda SM, et al: Involvement of reactive oxygen intermediates in the induction of c-jun gene transcription by ionizing radiation. Biochemistry 31:8300, 1992

285. Dalton S, Treisman R: Characterization of SAP-1, a protein recruited by serum response factor to the c-fos serum response element. Cell 68:597, 1992

286. Stein B, Rahmsdorf F, Steffen A, et al: UV induced DNA damage is an intermediate step in UV-induced expression of human immunodeficiency virus, type I collagenase, c-fos, and metallothionein. Mol Cell Biol 9:5169, 1989

287. Sen R, Baltimore D: Multiple nuclear factors interact with the immunoglobulin enhancer sequences. Cell 46:705, 1986

288. Lenardo MJ, Baltimore D: NF-kb: A pleiotropic mediator of inducible and tissue specific gene control. Cell 58:227, 1989

289. Uckun FM, Tuel-Hahlgren L, Song CW, et al: Ionizing irradiation stimulates unidentified tyrosine-specific protein kinases in human B-lymphocyte precursors, triggering apoptosis and clonogenic cell death. Proc Natl Acad Sci USA 89:9005, 1992

290. Devary Y, Gottlieb RA, Lau LF, Karin M: Rapid and preferential activation of the cjun gene during the mammalian UV response. Mol Cell Biol 11:2804, 1991

291. Hallahan DE, Virudachalam S, Schwartz JL, et al: Inhibition of protein kinases sensitizes human tumor cells to ionizing radiation. Radiat Res 129:345, 1992

292. Kim CY, Giaccia AJ, Strulovici B, Brown JM: Differential expression of protein kinase C epsilon protein in lung cancer cell lines by ionising radiation. Br J Cancer 66:844, 1992

293. Ullrich A, Schlessinger J: Signal transduction by receptors with tyrosine kinase activity. Cell 61:203, 1990

294. Nishizuka Y: Studies and perspectives of protein kinase C. Science 233:305, 1986

295. Nishizuka Y: Intracellular signalling by hydrolysis of phospholipids and activation of protein kinase C. Science 258:607, 1992

296. Lin CS, Goldthwait DA, Samols D: Induction of transcription from the long terminal repeat of Moloney murine sarcoma provirus by UV-irradiation, x-irradiation, and phorbol ester. Proc Natl Acad Sci USA 87:36, 1990

297. Fiers W: Tumor necrosis factor. FEBS Lett 285:199, 1991

298. Haimovitz-Friedman A, Witte L, Chaudhuri A, et al: Induction of the bFGF, PDGF and TGFb genes and their transcription by irradiation of endothelial cells. (submitted for publication)

299. Canney P, Dean S: Transforming growth factor beta: A promotor of late connective tissue injury following radiotherapy? Br J Radiol 63:620, 1990

300. Yamada M, Puck TT: Actions of radiation in mammalian cells. IV. Reversible mitotic lag in the S3 HeLa cell produced by low doses of x-rays. Proc Natl Acad Sci USA 47:1181, 1961

301. Whitmore GF, Stanners CP, Till JE, Gulyas S: Nucleic acid synthesis and division cycle in x-irradiated L-strain mouse cells. Biochim Biophys Acta 47:66, 1961

302. Terasima T, Tolmach LJ: Variations in several responses of HeLa cells to x-irradiation during the cell cycle. Biophys J 3:11, 1963

303. Tolmach LJ, Busse PM: The action of caffeine on X-irradiated HeLa cells. IV. Progression delays and enhanced cell killing at high caffeine concentrations. Radiat Res 82:374, 1980

304. Carlson JG: Chinese hamster ovary cell mitosis and its response to ionizing irradiation: A morphological analysis. Radiat Res 118:311, 1989

305. Weinert TA, Hartwell LH: The RAD9 gene controls the cell cycle response to DNA damage in Saccharomyces cerevisiae. Science 241:317, 1988

306. Weinert TA: Dual cell cycle checkpoints sensitive to chromosome replication and DNA damage in the budding yeast Saccharomyces cerevisiae. Radiat Res 132:141, 1992

307. Rowley R: Radiation-induced mitotic delay: A genetic characterization in the fission yeast. Radiat Res 132:144, 1992

308. Fornace AJJ, Nebert DW, Hollander MC, et al: Mammalian genes coordinately regulated by growth arrest signals and DNA-damaging agents. Mol Cell Biol 9:4196, 1989

309. Hartwell LH, Weinert TA: Checkpoints: Controls that ensure the order of the cell cycle events. Science 246:629, 1989

310. Nurse P: Universal control mechanism regulating onset of M-phase. Nature 344:503, 1990

311. Pines J, Hunter T: p34cdc2: The S and M kinase? New Biol 2:389, 1990

312. Clarke PR, Karsenti E: Regulation of p34^{cdc2} protein kinase: New insights into phosphorylation and the cell cycle. J Cell Sci 100:400, 1991

313. Rowley R, Hudson J, Young PG: The Wee-1 protein kinase is required for radiation-induced mitotic delay. Nature 356:353, 1992

314. Crissman HA, Gadbois DM, Tobey RA, Bradbury EM: Transformed mammalian cells are deficient in kinase-mediated control of proggression through the G$_1$ phase of the cell cycle. Proc Natl Acad Sci USA 88:7580, 1991

315. Lock RB, Ross WE: Inhibition of p34cdc2 kinase activity by etoposide or irradiation as a mechanism of G2 arrest in Chinese hamster ovary cells. Cancer Res 50:3761, 1990

316. Muschel RJ, Zhang HB, McKenna G: Differential effect of ionizing radiation on the expression of cyclin A and cyclin B in HeLa cells. Cancer Res 53:1128, 1993

317. Datta R, Hass R, Gunji H, et al: Down-regulation of cell cycle control genes by ionizing radiation. Cell Growth Differ 3:637, 1992

318. Sager G: Tumor suppressor genes in the cell cycle. Curr Opin Cell Biol 4:155, 1992

319. Mercer E: Cell cycle regulation and the p53 tumor suppressor gene. Crit Rev Eukary Gene Express 2:251, 1992

320. DeCaprio JA, Furukawa Y, Ajchenbaum F, et al: The retinoblastoma-susceptibility gene product becomes phosphorylated in multiple stages during cell cycle entry and progression. Proc Natl Acad Sci USA 89:1795, 1992

321. Painter RB, Young BR: Radiosensitivity in ataxia-telangiectasia: A new explanation. Proc Natl Acad Sci USA 77:7315, 1980

322. Rudolph NS, Latt SA: Flow cytometric analysis of x-ray sensitivity in ataxia telangiectasia. Mutat Res 211:31, 1989

323. Fornace AJJ, Alamo I, Hollander MC: DNA damage-inducible transcripts in mammalian cells. Proc Natl Acad Sci USA 85:8800, 1988

324. Fornace AJJ, Smudzka B, Hollander MC, Wilson SH: Induction of b-polymerase by DNA damaging agents in Chinese hamster cells. Mol Cell Biol 9:851, 1989

325. Hollander MC, Fornace AJJ: Induction of fos RNA by DNA-damaging agents. Cancer Res 49:1687, 1989

326. Luethy JD, Holbrook NJ: Activation of the gadd 153 promoter by genotoxic agents: A rapid and specific response to DNA damage. Cancer Res 52:5, 1992

327. Woloschak GE, Shearin-Jones P, Chang-Liu C-M: Effect of ionizing radiation on expression of genes encoding cytoskeletal elements: Kinetics and dose effects. Mol Carcinog 3:374, 1990

328. Ainsworth EJ, Chase HB: Effect of microbial antigens on irradiation mortality in mice. Proc Soc Exp Biol Med 102:483, 1959

329. Vogel SN, Hogan M: Role of cytokines in endotoxin-mediated host responses. *In* Oppenheim JJ, Sugahara T (eds): Immunophysiology: Role of Cells and Cytokines in Immunity and Inflammation. London, Oxford University Press, 1990, p 238

330. Geiger B, Galily R, Gery I: The effect of irradiation on the release of lymphocyte activating factor (LAF). Cell Immunol 7:177, 1973

331. Wasserman J, Petrini B, Wolk G, et al: Cytokine release from mononuclear cells in patients irradiated for breast cancer. Anticancer Res 11:461, 1991

332. Neta R, Oppenheim JJ: Radioprotection with cytokines—learning from nature to cope with radiation damage. Cancer Cells 3:391, 1991

333. Uckun FM, Gillis S, Souza L, Song CW: Effects of recombinant growth factors on radiation survival of human bone marrow progenitor cells. Int J Radiat Oncol Biol Phys 16:415, 1989

334. Uckun FM, Souza L, Waddick KG, et al: In vivo radioprotective effects of recombinant human granulocyte colony-stimulating factor in lethally irradiated mice. Blood 75:638, 1990

335. Waddick KG, Song CW, Souza L, et al: Comparative analysis of the in vivo radioprotective effects of recombinant granulocyte colony-stimulating factor (G-CSF), recombinant granulocyte-macrophage CSF, and their combination. Blood 77:2364, 1991

336. Neta R, Oppenheim JJ, Douches SD: Interdependence of the radioprotective effects of human recombinant interleukin 1 alpha, tumor necrosis factor alpha, granulocyte colony-stimulating factor, and murine recombinant granulocyte-macrophage colony-stimulating factor. J Immunol 140:108, 1988

337. Neta R, Oppenheim JJ, Schreiber RD, et al: Role of cytokines

interleukin 1, tumor necrosis factor, and transforming growth factor beta in natural and lipopolysaccharide-enhanced radioresistance. J Exp Med 173:1177, 1991

338. Dorie MJ, Kallman RF, Cebulska-Wasilewska A: Interleukin-1 modification of the effects of cyclophosphamide and fractionated irradiation. Int J Radiat Oncol Biol Phys 20:311, 1991

339. Hancock SL, Chung RT, Cox RS, Kallman RF: Interleukin 1 beta initially sensitizes and subsequently protects murine intestinal stem cells exposed to photon radiation. Cancer Res 51:2280, 1991

340. Roberts DB, Travis EL, Tucker SL: Interleukin-1 dose, mouse strain, and end point as they affect protection of mouse jejunum. Radiat Res 135:56, 1993

341. Tartaglia LA, Weber RF, Figari IS, et al: The two different receptors for tumor necrosis factor mediate distinct cellular responses. Proc Natl Acad Sci USA 88:9292, 1991

342. Bianco J, Applebaum F, Nemunaitis J: Phase I-II trial of pentoxifylline for the prevention of transplant-related toxicities following bone marrow transplantation. Blood 78:1205, 1991

343. Holler E, Kolb H, Moller A, et al: Increased serum levels of TNF precede major complications of bone marrow transplantation. Blood 75:1011, 1990

344. Naume B, Shalaby R, Lesslauer W, Espevik T: Involvement of the 55- and 75-kDa tumor necrosis factor receptors in the generation of lymphokine-activated killer cell activity and proliferation of natural killer cells. J Immunol 146:3045, 1991

345. Fuks Z, Vlodavsky I, Andreeff M, et al: Effects of extracellular matrix on the response of endothelial cells to radiation in vitro. Eur J Cancer 28/A:725, 1992

346. Schmidt-Ulrich RK, Valerie K, Chan W, et al: Expression of oestrogen receptor and transforming growth factor-alpha in MCF-7 cells after exposure to fractionated irradiation. Int J Radiat Biol 61:405, 1992

347. Kwok TT, Sutherland RM: Differences in EGF related radiosensitisation of human squamous carcinoma cells with high and low numbers of EGF receptors. Br J Cancer 64:251, 1991

348. Kwok TT, Sutherland RM: Cell cycle dependence of epidermal growth factor induced radiosensitization. Int J Radiat Oncol Biol Phys 22:525, 1992

349. Goldkorn T, Haimovitz-Friedman A, Balaban AN, et al: Radiation modulation of epidermal growth factor receptor phosphorylation in A431 cells: Evidence that radiation modulates signal transduction. Proc Am Assoc Cancer Res 33:90, 1992

350. Rubin P, Finkelstein J, Shapiro D: Molecular biology mechanisms in radiation induction of pulmonary injury syndrome: Interrelationship between the alveolar macrophage and septal fibrosis. Int J Radiat Oncol Biol Phys 24:93, 1992

351. Anscher M, Crocker I, Jirtle R: Transforming growth factor-beta 1 expression in irradiated liver. Radiat Res 122:77, 1990

352. Martin M, Lefaix JL, Pinton P, et al: Temporal modulation of TGF-b1 and b-actin gene expression in pig skin and muscular fibrosis after ionizing radiation. Radiat Res 134:63, 1993

353. Anscher MS, Peters WP, Risenbichler H, et al: Transforming growth factor b as a predictor of liver and lung fibrosis after autologous bone marrow transplantation for advanced breast cancer. N Engl J Med 328:1592, 1993

20

GROWTH FACTORS IN MALIGNANCY

JOHN MENDELSOHN
JANICE GABRILOVE

The capacity to coordinate and regulate cellular activities is essential for the life of multicellular organisms. This is because complex processes such as an embryologic development, tissue differentiation and repair, and inflammatory responses to invading organisms require large numbers of cells to perform widely differing activities, with critical timing and with the necessity of ceasing these activities when they have accomplished their mission. Growth factors are polypeptides that play a major role in coordinating these activities. Bioregulatory processes mediated by growth factors are central both to routine activities, such as replenishment of circulating blood cells by their progenitors in the bone marrow, and to unprogrammed challenges, such as restoration of normal tissue architecture following trauma.

Cancer is a disorder characterized by inappropriate division and function of cells that have escaped from the normal orderly coordination of their activities in the body. Elucidation of the mechanisms by which malignant cells bypass regulatory pathways has been one of the most interesting areas of scientific exploration during the past decade. Knowledge of the normal regulatory activities of growth factors and of the abnormalities discovered in malignancy has profoundly altered our understanding of the molecular machinery and communication systems that enable cells to function.

The growth factors that activate receptor tyrosine kinase activity have been described in Chapter 7. In this chapter we discuss the role of growth factors and their receptors in the pathogenesis and treatment of neoplastic disease. This represents a large area of investigation. Considerations related to the historic development of the field, as well as the complex interrelations between these regulatory molecules, suggest that the subject is best approached by considering, separately, two large categories of growth factors: those acting primarily on epithelial, endothelial,

and mesenchymal cells (which form the "solid" tumors), and those acting on hematopoietic cells and lymphocytes (which are the sources of the hematologic malignancies).

GROWTH FACTORS FOR THE SOLID TUMORS

More than three dozen growth factors have been described to date. Research has demonstrated that their presence is remarkably consistent across phyla, suggesting that they control regulatory pathways that are fundamental to the living process. Table 20–1 lists many of the nonhematopoietic growth factors and receptors found in normal and malignant cells. The information in the table is derived from a number of excellent reviews and monographs that are highly recommended for more detailed discussions of this field.[1-6]

Functions of Growth Factors and Receptors

MOLECULAR STRUCTURE OF RECEPTORS FOR GROWTH FACTORS

The great majority of nonhematopoietic growth factors mediate their effects by means of receptors containing an intrinsic tyrosine kinase (reviewed in refs. 7,8). These receptors are transmembrane glycoproteins which have an extracellular ligand-binding domain and an intracellular tyrosine kinase domain that mediates signal transduction into growth regulatory pathways (Fig. 20–1). The binding of growth factor to monomeric receptors activates formation of homodimers, or oligomers[9] (Fig. 20–2). In a manner that remains to be explained, this stimulates the tyrosine kinase domains on receptor molecules to carry

TABLE 20–1. PROPERTIES OF POLYPEPTIDE GROWTH FACTORS*

GROWTH FACTORS†	DESCRIPTION	KNOWN LOCALIZATION/ SOURCES	KNOWN TARGETS	RECEPTORS
PDGF AA, AB, and BB	Dimers of A (17 kDa) and B (16 kDa) chains. B chain is product of c-*sis* proto-oncogene.	Platelets, placenta, preimplantation embryos, endothelial cells.	Mesenchymal cells, glial cells, smooth muscle, placental trophoblasts.	Two species of glycoprotein. Both tyrosine kinases. Type α (170 kDa) binds all PDGF dimers. Type β (180 kDa) binds PDGF BB and AB weakly.
EGF and TGF-α	Major forms 6 kDa. Some larger species detected. EGF and TGF-α proteins are 40% identical. Both released by proteolysis of membrane-bound precursors.	EGF: submaxillary gland, Brunner's gland, mRNA (but not 6-kDa protein) in variety of newborn mouse tissues. TGF-α: Preimplantation mouse embryos, later embryos, placenta. Common in transformed cells.	Epithelial, mesenchymal, and glial cells.	Protein tyrosine kinase (175 kDa). Product of the c-*erbB* proto-oncogene. Receptor for EGF, TGF-α, and vaccinia virus growth factor.
TGF-β1, -β2, and -β3	25-kDa homodimers. Secreted as latent complexes.	Preimplantation mouse embryos, later embryos. Widespread throughout adult tissues and cultured cells.	Wide variety of cell types.	Type 1 50 kDa, type 2 70 kDa, type 3 280–330 kDa. Each type binds TGF-β1, -β2, and -β3. Types 1 and 2 are main mediators of responses.
IGF-1 and -2	7 kDa. Related to each other and to proinsulin.	IGF-1 mainly produced in liver. IGF-2 mRNA in variety of cells, including some tumor cells, but protein sometimes undetectable. Both present in plasma, in association with specific binding proteins.	Wide variety of cell types.	IGF-1 receptor (130 kDa + 90 kDa)₂ protein tyrosine kinase, binds IGF-1 and -2. IGF-2 receptor (250 kDa) binds IGF-2, identical to mannose 6-phosphate receptor.
FGF-1 and -2	"Acidic" and "basic" FGF, respectively. 16–17 kDa. Occasionally larger forms. No consensus signal peptide. 55% identical. Also related to other FGFs and interleukin 1 family.	Low mRNA levels in wide range of normal and transformed cells. Proteins widely distributed, associated with extracellular matrix.	Variety of endothelial, epithelial, mesenchyme, and neuronal cell types.	(150-kDa) FGF-1 and (130-kDa) FGF-2 receptors both protein tyrosine kinases. High cross reactivity of FGF-1 and -2 binding.
FGF-3	27-kDa alternative translation products of *int-2* proto-oncogene.	mRNA in mouse embryonic tissues, brain, testes, mouse mammary tumor, and teratocarcinoma cells.	Unknown.	Unknown.
FGF-4	19-kDa glycoprotein product of *hst* (human) or *ks3* (mouse) proto-oncogenes.	Unknown.	Vascular endothelial cells, fibroblasts.	Unknown.
FGF-5	26-kDa glycoprotein.	Unknown.	Fibroblasts.	Unknown.

*From Cross M, Dexter TM: Growth factors in development, transformation, and tumorigenesis. Cell *64*: 271, 1991, with permission.

†PDGF, platelet-derived growth factor; EGF, epidermal growth factor; TGF, transforming growth factor; IGF, insulin-like growth factor; FGF, fibroblast growth factor.

out transphosphorylation on selected tyrosine residues of their paired partners. The dimeric receptors, with phosphorylated tyrosine residues, are now ready to bind with high affinity to substrates for their activated intrinsic tyrosine protein kinases.

The primary amino acid sequences of the extracellular domains of growth factor receptors are known in most cases. The spacing of cysteine residues in these domains allows predictions of tertiary structure in one of two major categories: immunoglobulin-like domains, in which a series of looped structures is created by formation of disulfide bonds between cysteines; and cysteine-rich domains,

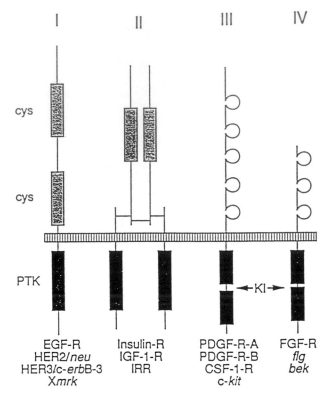

Figure 20–1. Growth factor receptor subclasses. Cys, cysteine-rich region; PTK, protein tyrosine kinase; KI, kinase insert region. (Adapted from Ullrich A, Schlessinger J: Signal transduction by receptors with tyrosine kinase activity. Cell *61*: 203, 1990, with permission.)

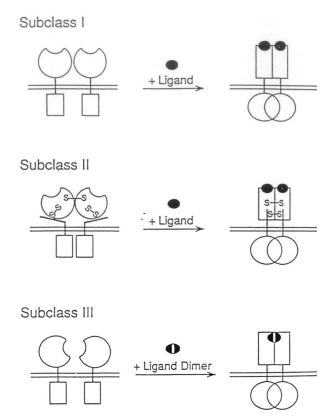

Figure 20–2. Models of receptor subclass-specific variations of the mechanism of activation by dimerization. Receptor activation may occur by binding of monomeric ligands, resulting in a conformational change of the extracellular domain and dimer formation (subclass I); by interaction of the ligand with a disulfide-stabilized receptor dimer and subsequent intracomplex conformational change (subclass II); or by mediation of dimer formation through a dimeric ligand (subclass III). (Adapted from Ullrich A, Schlessinger J: Signal transduction by receptors with tyrosine kinase activity. Cell *61*:203, 1990, with permission.)

in which complex tertiary folding results from the formation of disulfide bonds, creating pockets into which ligands can bind with high affinity (reviewed in ref. 7) (Fig. 20–1). There is intensive effort to resolve the molecular details of growth factor–binding sites, because this would allow the design of specific pharmacologic agonists and antagonists.

SUBSTRATES OF TYROSINE PROTEIN KINASES

The binding of growth factors to their specific receptors and activation of autophosphorylation stimulates a cascade of biochemical reactions collectively referred to as signal transduction pathways (reviewed in refs. 2,7). These pathways can initiate cell cycle traversal and differentiation. The substrates for activated receptors and the molecular pathways for signal transduction are described in Chapters 6 and 7, respectively.

RECEPTOR KINETICS AND MODULATION

The binding of a growth factor to its receptor does not permanently activate a signal transduction pathway. Both the receptor and its bound ligand are efficiently internalized, typically within less than an hour.[10] In the endosomes, the reduced pH may shift the binding equilibrium and release the ligand. Receptors (and ligands) eventually are transported to the lysosomes, where they are catabolized. However, prior to this event, recycling of receptors

to the surface of the cell may occur, permitting further rounds of activation before they are metabolized. It also is possible that receptors may have direct interactions with nuclear components.

Whereas activation of particular substrates occurs within minutes following binding of growth factors to receptors, the stimulation of receptor tyrosine kinase activity must be maintained for 5 to 6 hours in order to activate movement into the active phases of the cell cycle that lead to cell division.[11,12] The half-life of a receptor after exposure to growth factor is typically less than 4 hours. Thus, in order to maintain an active receptor-mediated signal through a period longer than a few hours, new receptors must be synthesized and put into place in the plasma membrane. In parallel, new growth factor molecules must be synthesized, in order to make contact with the new receptors and activate them. In response to a variety of external stimuli, cells have the capacity to alter the quantity of a particular receptor expressed on their surface membranes.

An important mechanism for modulating the activity of growth factor receptors involves tyrosine phosphatases.[13,14] These enzymes can efficiently dephosphorylate tyrosine residues on the cytoplasmic portions of receptors. Phosphatases can be expressed in the surface membranes of cells. In some cases, the extracellular portions of tyrosine phosphatases are structurally similar to cell surface molecules known to mediate interactions between cells in tissues and during embryonic development (integrins; see Chapter 9). It has been postulated that the well-described phenomenon of contact inhibition in cell cultures may be mediated by the interaction between cell surface proteins and the external segments of tyrosine phosphatase molecules, thereby activating intracellular phosphatase activity, which could deactivate proliferation signals that depend on tyrosine kinases.[15] Some phosphatases have extracellular domains reminiscent of growth factor receptors, raising the possibility that they can be activated by polypeptides. Tyrosine phosphatases may be inserted into the cell membrane adjacent to growth factor receptors and regulate their levels of tyrosine phosphorylation. Establishment of the contribution of tyrosine phosphatases to the regulation of receptor function requires further exploration.

OTHER RECEPTOR MECHANISMS

Activation of signal transduction pathways also can be accomplished by binding of growth factors to receptors with biochemical characteristics entirely different from tyrosine kinases. These are presented in Chapter 7.

GROWTH FACTOR SYNTHESIS AND RELEASE

Growth factors are produced by cells in all tissues of the body. Typically, the growth factors that act on particular cells are produced and released by other cells in the microenvironment. This arrangement establishes the pathways whereby one cell can regulate the activity of another cell. Interactions of this type have been demonstrated in angiogenesis, wound repair, and many other physiologic situations.

Many growth factors are synthesized as portions of larger precursor molecules which contain hydrophobic sequences that anchor them in the plasma membrane (reviewed in ref. 16). After synthesis and transport in the endoplasmic reticulum and Golgi apparatus, these molecules are expressed on the cell surface. The soluble growth factor polypeptide is released into the extracellular environment by proteolytic cleavage from the precursor molecule.

It has been discovered that the membrane-bound form of transforming growth factor α (TGF-α) also can activate receptors.[17,18] Using a mutated form of TGF-α, which encodes a noncleavable form of the precursor molecule, pro–TGF-α, variants can be made to accumulate on the cell surface. These can bind to receptors on adjacent cells and activate tyrosine phosphorylation.[19] It is possible that receptor activation might commonly occur through cell-to-cell contact mediated by membrane-bound factor acting on a receptor on an adjacent cell, termed juxtacrine stimulation[19] (Fig. 20–3).

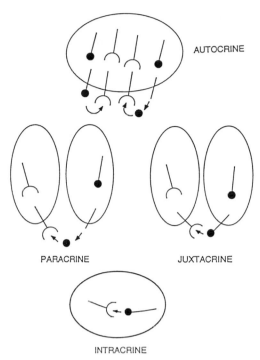

Figure 20–3. Interactions between cells producing growth factors and receptors. ●—, precursor for growth factor; ●, soluble growth factor released into extracellular space; —c, receptor. (From Mendelsohn J, Lippman M: Principles of Molecular Biology of Cancer: Growth Factors. *In* DeVita VT Jr, Hellman S, Rosenberg SA (eds): Cancer: Principles and Practice of Oncology. Philadelphia, JB Lippincott Company, 1993, pp 114–133, with permission.)

AUTOCRINE PRODUCTION OF GROWTH FACTORS

The concept that simultaneous production of a growth factor and expression of its specific receptor by the same cell could result in self-stimulation first was formulated by DeLarco and Todaro, in their landmark description of the autostimulatory pathway of epidermal growth factor (EGF) receptor activation in cultured tumor cells.[20] These and other observations were expanded into a generalized hypothesis of *autocrine* growth regulation by Sporn and Todaro.[21,22] They postulated that autoproduction of growth factors essential for proliferation could provide a mechanism by which a cell could escape from the requirement for those particular growth factors in its environment, resulting in unregulated cell growth (Fig. 20–3). Escape from growth regulation is one of the primary characteristics of malignant cell transformation.

Receptors and their growth factors frequently are co-expressed in both primary tumor tissues and human cancer cell lines, as is detailed in the discussion of individual growth factors later in this chapter. Evidence for the existence of autostimulatory growth factor pathways comes from many studies with tumor cell lines cultured in the absence of an exogenous supply of growth factors, and studies of comparable cultures grown in the presence of monoclonal antibodies that bind to either receptors or growth factors.[23] By blocking the capacity of the growth factor to activate the receptor, these antibodies can prevent receptor activation and thereby inhibit cell proliferation.

Blood levels of most growth factors are low, although platelets are a repository of growth factors such as TGF-α, platelet-derived growth factor (PDGF), and TGF-β that are released subsequent to platelet activation at a wound or inflammatory site (reviewed in ref. 24). In physiologic situations, the growth factors that act on a particular cell are thought to be produced primarily in the immediate vicinity, either in an autocrine fashion by the cell itself, or by adjacent cells.[25] The latter form of stimulation has been called *paracrine* (Fig. 20–3), and it has been shown that this type of interaction can occur between cells of the same or different histologic type.[21] For example, breast cancer cell lines may be stimulated by insulin-like growth factor type II (IGF-II), which has been shown to be produced by fibroblasts in malignant lesions but not by fibroblasts in normal tissues.[26] PDGF produced by breast cancer cells can activate the fibroblasts, which bear PDGF receptors, but not breast cancer cells, because they do not express PDGF receptors.[27]

INTRACELLULAR RECEPTOR ACTIVATION

Because both the receptor and its growth factor may be produced by the same cell, it is possible that the union of growth factor and receptor could occur intracellularly, prior to expression of either of the molecules on the cell surface (*intracrine*; Fig. 20–3). This has been shown to occur in a cell line transformed with the v-*sis* oncogene,[28,29] but whether this is a generalized physiologic mechanism mediating responses to PDGF is not known. Evidence from other studies suggests that the receptor for PDGF must be expressed on the cell surface in order to mediate signal transduction through its activated tyrosine kinase.[30] Exploration of the autocrine pathway for EGF/TGF-α in A431 cells, which express both the EGF receptor and TGF-α, suggests that the major pathway of autocrine activation occurs extracellularly, mediated by binding of growth factor to receptors that are expressed on the cell surface.[31]

GROWTH FACTORS REGULATE PROLIFERATION OF CELLS

When growth factors activate their receptors, cells in the resting or G_0 phase of the cell cycle are stimulated to enter the proliferative phases of the cycle, leading to mitosis. In the case of some intensively studied cell lines, the resting cells are stimulated to enter the G_1 phase by growth factors controlling "competence" for cell cycle traversal, and subsequently are stimulated to become committed to completion of G_1 and the other phases of the cell cycle (S, G_2, M) when stimulated by "progression" factors.[32,33] For example, PDGF might serve as a competence factor to initiate entry into G_1, and subsequent addition of IGF during G_1 might stimulate progression of cells to entry into S phase. The point at which a progression factor acts may coincide with the "restriction point," beyond which cells assemble the DNA polymerase complex in preparation for initiating replication of the genome.[34] It is believed that the majority of growth factors that act by stimulation of an intrinsic tyrosine kinase regulate the cell cycle through mechanisms that act on G_1-phase progression. In some cases, such as stimulation of fibroblasts by EGF, the differentiation of competence and progression is not apparent.

Other mechanisms for growth factor–mediated regulation of cells have been described. One, utilized by TGF-β, may involve pathways that antagonize progression from G_1 into S phase. In the case of hematopoietic cells, withdrawal of a growth factor has been shown to activate the apoptosis pathway, which leads to programmed cell death.

Serum is a source of growth factors, many of which, as noted, are released by platelets during the clotting process. The requirement for serum in synthetic cell culture media is believed to be attributable primarily to its content of growth factors and hormones.[35] Many cells can be cultured in chemically defined medium in the absence of serum if they produce the growth factors required for proliferation, or if these agents are provided in the culture medium. Characteristically, tumor cells in serum-free cultures have reduced requirements for growth factors, indicating that they produce the factors or have bypassed the need for them.[25]

Although the receptor for a particular growth factor is not known to differ from one cell type to another, the group or constellation of receptors expressed does vary between cells from different tissues. Cells from different tissues require individually tailored "cocktails" of growth factor supplements, typically between three and five, in order to grow optimally in serum-free cultures. When deprived of these essential growth-promoting agents, cells proliferate at reduced rates or are prevented from dividing.[36] The differences in growth factor requirements provide some potential for selectivity and specificity in the application of antireceptor agents to cancer therapy.

Role of Growth Factors in Malignancy

Many converging lines of evidence accumulated over the past decade indicate that growth factors play a central role in malignant transformation of human cells.

AUTOCRINE GROWTH FACTOR PATHWAYS

The original observation of autostimulation of proliferation in cells expressing both a growth factor and its receptor has been followed by a large number of studies showing that many primary human tumors and human tumor cell lines express high levels of growth factor receptors and are capable of producing the relevant growth factors, thereby establishing conditions conducive to autocrine or paracrine stimulation. It must be stressed that normal cells also have the capacity to produce growth factors that can activate autostimulatory pathways.

MANY PROTO-ONCOGENES ACT BY GROWTH FACTOR PATHWAYS

In the early 1980s, a number of laboratories were able to establish that protein tyrosine kinase activity was a property of both the EGF receptor and the oncogenic pp60[src] protein, and that the two molecules were antigenically related.[37-39] Then, in 1983 and 1984, the discovery was made that three viral oncogenes shared extensive amino acid sequence homology with growth factors and receptors: v-*sis* with the B chain of PDGF,[40,41] v-*erbB* with the EGF receptor,[42-44] and v-*fms* with the receptor for macrophage colony-stimulating factor.[45] It had been shown previously that viral oncogenes were derived from cellular genes (termed proto-oncogenes), and the new information pinpointed growth factor/receptor pathways as sources in the cellular genome for the virally transmitted oncogenic activity. Because expression of viral oncogenes is, alone, sufficient to induce malignant transformation of some cells, the conclusion was drawn that unregulated growth factor activity could mediate malignant transformation.

Experimental evidence has accumulated indicating that many oncogenes are analogues of cellular proto-oncogenes that code for growth factors, their receptors, soluble protein tyrosine kinases, or biochemical pathways mediated by tyrosine kinase activation (reviewed in refs. 1–5). A partial list of oncogenes that are related to proto-oncogenes for growth factors and receptors is presented in Table 20–2.

The mechanisms by which these oncogenes mediate malignant transformation vary. The v-*sis* oncogene encodes a polypeptide that shares 90 per cent homology with its proto-oncogene (B chain of PDGF).[27,40,41] The product of v-*sis* can form a homodimer that activates PDGF receptors, and the unregulated activation of proliferation mediated by this receptor can result in malignant behavior in certain cells that are susceptible (presumably as a result of biochemical pathways active in these cells or of their particular stage of differentiation). In contrast, the oncogene v-*erbB* is a defective version of its proto-oncogene, the EGF receptor, and two modifications in its structure have been characterized.[42-44] The oncogene encodes a protein that lacks the extracellular domain of the receptor (binding site for EGF), and it also lacks the carboxy-terminal residues that are presumed to have a regulatory function. Another example is provided by the *neu* oncogene, originally isolated from a carcinogen-induced neuroblastoma in rats. In this case, conversion of the proto-oncogene to an oncogene involves a single nucleotide change, resulting in alteration of one amino acid in the transmembrane region.[46] However, the search for mutated receptors and growth factors in primary human tumor specimens has revealed only a modest number of examples.

OVEREXPRESSION OF GROWTH FACTOR PATHWAYS MAY BE ONCOGENIC

Experiments using recombinant molecular technology have demonstrated that constitutive overexpression of cellular oncogenes encoding growth factors and/or their receptors can cause nonmalignant cells to display a malignant phenotype. Typically, this is measured by anchorage-independent growth in soft agar culture, and by the capacity to form successful xenografts in nude mice. For example, experiments have shown that malignant properties can be conferred merely by overexpression of proto-oncogenes HER-2, TGF-α, or PDGF (see later in this chapter). Unregulated expression of TGF-α can result in mammary carcinogenesis in transgenic mice, indicating that this proto-oncogene can be oncogenic without modification, but only in certain tissues.[47-49] In these animals the only other malignant tumor observed was hepatocellular carcinoma.

TABLE 20–2. ONCOGENES RELATED TO PROTO-ONCOGENES WHICH ENCODE GROWTH FACTORS OR RECEPTORS

ONCO-GENE	PROTO-ONCOGENE	ORIGINAL SOURCE
v-*sis*	PDGF (B chain)	Simian retrovirus
v-*erbB*	EGF receptor†	Avian retrovirus
neu/HER-2/ v-*erbB2*	Heregulin receptor†	Rat neuroblastoma
v-*fms*	CSF-1 receptor	Feline retrovirus
v-*ros*	Insulin receptor, β chain	Avian retrovirus
met	Hepatocyte growth factor receptor†	Human osteosarcoma
k-*fgf*/*hst*	FGF-4†	Human stomach cancer, Kaposi's sarcoma
int-2	Related to FGF-3	Murine mammary tumors
trk family	NGF receptor family†	Human colon carcinoma
v-*kit*	Kit ligand receptor	Feline retrovirus
v-*sea*	Related to insulin receptor	Avian erythroblastosis/ sarcoma virus
v-*erbA*	Thyroid hormone receptor	Avian retrovirus

*From Leutz A, Graf T: Relationships between oncogenes and growth control. *In* Sporn MB, Roberts AB (eds): Peptide Growth Factors and Their Receptors, Vol II. Berlin, Springer-Verlag, 1990, pp 655–703, and Mendelsohn J, Lippman M: Principles of Molecular Biology of Cancer: Growth Factors. *In* DeVita VT Jr, Hellman S, Rosenberg SA (eds): Cancer: Principles and Practice of Oncology. Philadelphia, JB Lippincott Company, 1993, pp 114–133, with permission.

†Indicates evidence for involvement in human cancer.

CLINICAL EVIDENCE FOR ONCOGENESIS BY GROWTH FACTOR PATHWAYS

A number of recent reports document high levels of growth factor receptor expression in primary human tumor specimens. In many cases, overexpression of receptors is correlated with a poor clinical prognosis in these patients. Increased expression of *neu/HER-2/c-erbB2* is associated with a worse prognosis in adenocarcinoma of the breast and ovary.[50-54] High EGF receptor levels are prognostically adverse in adenocarcinoma of the breast,[55,56] transitional bladder cancer,[55,57] and squamous cell lung carcinoma.[58,59]

From this accumulation of observations, it is reasonable to postulate that expression of high levels of growth factor receptors or the relevant growth factors causes the formation of autocrine or paracrine activation pathways that give a selective advantage to malignant human cells. This could result in enhancement of tumor cell growth and survival. Such tumor cells might be better able to withstand an environment in which exogenous essential growth factors are in low abundance. The capacity to subvert growth regulation by bypassing the requirement that certain essential growth factors be provided in the extracellular environment may, in itself, be sufficient for oncogenesis. In other situations, enhanced activation of growth factor/receptor pathways can play an important supporting rule in a series of oncogenic events that also may include other regulatory pathways.

Specific Growth Factors and Their Receptors

TGF-α/EGF FAMILY

Epidermal growth factor was described first by Cohen, who purified it using accelerated eyelid opening and tooth eruption in newborn mice as an assay.[60] Subsequently it was demonstrated that EGF stimulates proliferation of cultured cells and that it activates a specific high-affinity membrane receptor with protein tyrosine kinase activity, which mediates its proliferative effects on cells (reviewed in refs. 10, 11, 61). The receptor for EGF is activated by a family of growth factors, which are described in Chapter 7.

Transforming growth factor α is produced by many tumor cell lines and by cells transformed by retroviruses and oncogenes. It was first discovered when conditioned medium from cultures of transformed cells was found to stimulate growth of fibroblasts in soft agar.[7] Later, it was found that this particular stimulatory property required concurrent exposure to a pair of ligands, TGF-α and TGF-β, both of which were present in the conditioned medium.[62] Many normal adult and embryonic tissues have been shown to express the messenger RNA for TGF-α and the growth factor protein.[61]

Although TGF-α and EGF act primarily by stimulating cell proliferation, it should be noted that they also can have inhibitory effects. For example, they can inhibit the growth of hair follicle cells.[63] This property has been used to cause de-epilation of wool from sheep. These two growth factors in high concentrations also inhibit the growth of cultured tumor cell lines that express extraordinarily high levels of EGF receptors. Activation of EGF receptors by amphiregulin can stimulate proliferation in some types of cells and inhibit others.[64] The mechanisms that determine these two opposed pathways are not yet determined.

Introduction of TGF-α cDNA into cells is transforming,[65] but weaker than some other cellular protooncogenes in that these cells have less capacity to form xenografts in athymic mice. Expression of vectors carrying EGF receptors can transform cells, but this usually is dependent on addition of exogenous ligand.[66-68]

Role of EGF Receptor Pathways in the Common Malignancies

Many types of epithelial malignancies display increased EGF receptors on their cell surface membranes. Examples include cancer of the lung,[69-71] glioblastoma,[72] breast cancer,[55,56] head and neck cancer,[73] and cancer of the bladder.[57] Gene amplification is not a commonly reported finding in these tumors, with the exception of the glioblastomas.[71] Only in the case of high-grade glioblastomas have mutant EGF receptors been described.[74] Increased receptor expression often is associated with increased production of TGF-α by the same tumor cells.[75] This establishes conditions conducive to receptor activation by an autocrine stimulatory pathway.

The role of the EGF receptor in breast cancer has been under study for more than a decade. High levels of the receptor are observed in 30 per cent of breast cancer specimens.[55,56] Aside from one cell line, MDA 468, the gene for the EGF receptor is not amplified, and increased transcription is believed to explain the high levels of receptors observed in many mammary cell lines.[76]

Messenger RNA for TGF-α was expressed in more than half of primary breast adenocarcinoma specimens examined,[77,78] and immunoreactive and biologically active TGF-α was significantly higher in malignant effusions from breast cancer patients than in effusions from non–cancer patients.[78] Studies with breast cell lines also have demonstrated TGF-α production.[79] The level of TGF-α may be regulated by estrogen, which can induce increased TGF-α production in a number of breast cancer cell lines.[77,80]

TGF-α and EGF have a role in normal breast growth and development. They have been shown to stimulate the lobular-alveolar development of the mouse mammary gland in explant cultures and in vivo.[81] Normal breast tissues express EGF receptors,[82] and nonmalignant human mammary cell lines express the EGF receptor[83,84] and express and secrete TGF-α.[84] Furthermore, TGF-α is a growth-promoting factor for nontransformed breast cell lines in serum-free culture.[83,84]

Clinical studies of primary breast cancer specimens have revealed important correlations between the levels of EGF receptors and both prognosis and response to therapy. Both relapse-free survival and total survival are significantly shorter for EGF receptor–positive as compared with EGF receptor–negative tumors.[55,56] There also is evidence for lack of response to endocrine therapy in patients with EGF receptor–positive tumors.[85] From these observations, it is clear that EGF receptors play a regulatory role in a significant subpopulation of breast cancer patients.

Further data in support of this conclusion are derived from studies using anti–EGF receptor monoclonal antibodies (MAbs) as reagents to explore for the presence of autocrine-stimulating pathways in cultured human cells. Studies have been performed with nonmalignant and malignant breast cell lines, using anti–EGF receptor MAbs that can block activation of signal transduction mediated by the receptor. The data from these experiments indicate that many breast cell lines produce TGF-α (or EGF), which is required for their optimal growth in culture.[77] Treatment of cultures with MAbs against TGF-α also can inhibit growth of EGF/TGF-α-dependent mammary epithelial cells.[86]

EGF receptors are expressed on normal bowel epithelium, and TGF-α appears to be a growth factor for cultured colon cells.[87] Anti–EGF receptor MAbs can inhibit the proliferation of cultured nonmalignant and malignant colon cell lines.[87,88]

Examination of primary specimens of human lung cancer tissue using immunohistochemical techniques have demonstrated that high levels of EGF receptors are displayed on nearly all squamous cell carcinomas, the majority of adenocarcinomas, and none of the small-cell lung cancers.[69–71] There was a high expression of TGF-α in nearly all squamous cell cancers and adenocarcinomas of the lung (J. Baselga, J. Mendelsohn, and C. Cordon-Cardo, unpublished observations). As with breast cancer, high levels of EGF receptor expression in lung cancer tissue are associated with a poor survival.[58,59] In addition, a correlation was found between high expression of TGF-α and reduced 5-year survival.[59] The proliferation of cultured lung cancer cell lines of both the squamous cell carcinoma and adenocarcinoma types can be inhibited by addition of anti–EGF receptor MAb.[89,90] In parallel, antibody against TGF-α can inhibit proliferation of adenocarcinoma cell lines known to produce TGF-α and express EGF receptors.[91]

Clinical Trials with Anti–EGF Receptor Monoclonal Antibodies

A number of laboratories have produced anti–EGF receptor MAbs that block EGF/TGF-α binding and prevent activation of tyrosine kinase. These include MAbs 225 and 528,[92,93] 425,[94,95] and 108.[96] Studies of nude mouse xenografts of breast,[97] bowel,[98] and lung cancer[90] cell lines expressing high levels of EGF receptors also have demonstrated the antitumor effects of anti–EGF receptor MAbs in vivo, when administered for a 3-week period. The cell lines studied were dependent on TGF-α for optimal growth in culture, and it is likely that they require TGF-α for optimal growth in vivo. The results of these series of studies involving the three most common human malignancies, and others, provide convincing evidence that EGF receptor blockade is worthy of clinical trials.

Pilot clinical trials with anti–EGF receptor MAb therapy have explored targeted radiotherapy, using labeled antibody 425[99] and antibody R1, which does not block EGF binding.[100] A recent phase I dose escalation trial was carried out with a single dose of MAb 225 in patients with advanced squamous cell lung carcinoma, which invariably expresses high levels of EGF receptors. The antibody was labeled with ^{111}In for visualization by nuclear scanning. There were two important conclusions: (1) doses of 120 mg produced concentrations of antibody in the blood that were saturating for EGF receptors, for a period of more than 3 days, without any toxicity; and (2) primary lung tumors and metastases 1 cm or larger in diameter were visualized with doses of 40 mg or more.[101] Studies with repeated injections of MAb 225, in a chimerized or humanized form, are the next step in testing EGF receptor blockade therapy.

HEREGULINS

There is no uniform nomenclature for this group of growth factors and their receptors. The three names given to the receptor reflect the three experimental systems in which it was identified: *neu* as an oncogene in rat neuroblastomas,[102] *HER-2* as a homologue to the human *EGF* receptor,[103] and *erbB2* as a homologue to the *erbB* oncogene.[104]

The *erbB2* receptor is a 185-kDa transmembrane glycoprotein, with close homology to the receptor for EGF. Its capacity to induce transformation can derive from a single point mutation in the transmembrane portion, in the case of *neu*, or from overexpression. The intracellular portion of the receptor contains a tyrosine kinase, which has the capacity to autophosphorylate the molecule.[105,106] Activated EGF receptors also can phosphorylate *erbB2* on tyrosine residues.[107]

Specific ligands called heregulins have been identified, which can activate the *erbB2* receptor tyrosine kinase.[105,108–110] The heregulins have the capacity to stimulate proliferation and differentiation of breast cancer cell lines. Recent reports have identified two additions to the EGF receptor family, designated *erbB3* and *erbB4*, both of which serve as receptors for heregulin.[110a,110b] Furthermore, there is evidence that the targets for heregulin actually are heterodimers of *erbB2* and *erbB3*, or *erbB2* and *erbB4*, since heregulin does not bind directly to *erbB2* even though it activates the *erbB2* tyrosine kinase.[110c]

erbB2 is amplified or overexpressed in a number of adenocarcinomas. The most extensive studies have been with adenocarcinoma of the breast. Nearly 30 per cent of these cancers express elevated levels of *HER-2*, and this is correlated with a poorer prognosis in patients with involved axillary lymph nodes at the time of diagnosis.[50,51,54] High expression of *HER-2* also is associated with a poorer prognosis in ovarian and lung adenocarcinomas.[50]

Monoclonal antibodies have been produced against both the rat *neu* and the human HER-2 receptors. These can inhibit the proliferation of cells expressing the receptor.[111–113] Recent phase I trials with humanized MAb 4D5 against the HER-2 receptor have demonstrated lack of toxicity, and a phase II trial examining the efficacy of repeated doses of this antibody is ongoing.

PLATELET-DERIVED GROWTH FACTOR

Platelet-derived growth factor[4,27,114] first was described as a constituent of α-granules in platelets, with the capacity to stimulate proliferation of smooth muscle cells and fibroblasts. The growth factor and its receptor are described in Chapter 7. Receptors for PDGF are prominent on mesenchymal cells, including fibroblasts and smooth muscle cells.[24] The release of PDGF from platelets during the conversion of plasma to serum suggests a role for this growth factor in the connective tissue proliferation associated with inflammation and tissue repair. PDGF also has been implicated in the proliferation of periendothelial smooth muscle cells, which is a prominent feature of the pathology of atherogenesis.[115]

The observation that the v-sis oncogene product shares close homology with the B chain of PDGF[40,41] stimulated gene transfer experiments, which demonstrated that constitutive expression of the B chain or A chain of PDGF proto-oncogenes can cause cell transformation, although the A chain is less efficient.[116–118] In addition, PDGF is produced by some tumor cell lines that lack receptors for the growth factor—for example, mammary carcinoma cell lines.[119] In the case of breast cancer, it has been suggested that the tumor cells may stimulate adjacent nonmalignant fibroblasts, resulting in the fibrosis that is commonly an accompanying feature of breast malignancy.[26]

INSULIN-LIKE GROWTH FACTORS

Insulin is a hormone that serves as a regulator of glucose metabolism. However, it has long been known that insulin also has the capacity to facilitate the growth and proliferation of a large number of normal and malignant cultured cell lines under serum-free conditions.[35] This activity may be mediated by cross reactivity with the receptor for a related polypeptide growth factor, known as insulin-like growth factor type I (IGF-I). In its mature form, IGF-I is identical to the earlier described molecule somatomedin C, which was shown to occur in the circulation and to mediate the stimulatory effects of pituitary growth hormone on skeletal cartilage and bone growth.[120] The growth factor is a 70–amino acid polypeptide that is produced in the liver and in a wide variety of tissues throughout the body.[121] The IGF-I receptor is a transmembrane heterotetramer that is expressed on a large number of normal and malignant cell types. IGF-II has a primary structure similar to IGF-I.[121] It binds to an unrelated, specific IGF-II receptor, which is a single transmembrane molecule that lacks tyrosine kinase activity and is homologous with the mannose 6-phosphate receptor.[122]

The presence of IGFs in the serum, in some malignant cells, and in the connective tissue of some malignancies suggests that these growth factors may regulate cell function and proliferation by endocrine, paracrine, or autocrine pathways. The assessment of the physiologic role of the IGF family of growth factors in complicated by the presence of multiple IGF-binding proteins in serum, which stabilize and prevent degradation of IGF-I and IGF-II but may inhibit their capacity to activate receptors.[123]

An example of the potential role of IGFs in malignant cell proliferation has been described in studies of breast cancer. IGF-I and IGF-II both are able to stimulate proliferation of breast cancer cells. Fibroblasts from breast tissue have the capacity to produce these growth factors. Interestingly, IGF-I is produced by fibroblasts in benign portions of the breast tissue surrounding the tumor,[124] whereas IGF-II is synthesized by fibroblasts in the malignant breast tissue.[26] Monoclonal antibody αIR3 against the IGF-I receptor has been shown to inhibit the mitogenic effects of IGF-I and IGF-II, suggesting that this receptor mediates the stimulatory activity of both growth factors.[125,126] In view of the frequent expression of IGFs and their receptors in both normal and malignant cells, it is likely that they play a major role in regulating cell proliferation and function in many tissues of the body.

FIBROBLAST GROWTH FACTOR FAMILY

The fibroblast family of growth factors (FGFs) primarily consists of two closely related isoforms, bFGF (basic isoelectric point) and aFGF (acidic).[127] These molecules control cell proliferation and differentiation in a wide variety of tissues. Their activities originally were characterized as embryonic inducers. As such, they would be expected to act over short distances. FGFs do not circulate in the blood, but are integrated with the basement membranes of cells that produce them, where they can function locally.[128] In addition to FGFs, there are a number of other growth factors with the capacity to stimulate fibroblast proliferation, including PDGF, TGF-α, and tumor necrosis factor.

Once it had been shown that FGFs bind tightly to heparins, it was possible to use affinity chromatography with immobilized heparin to isolate FGF-like activity from many tissues.[129] Presently, seven heparin-binding growth factors that have been isolated from tissues and cultured cells are included in the FGF family (see Chapter 7).

There is strong experimental evidence that FGFs play a physiologic role in angiogenesis, wound healing, tissue regeneration, embryonic development and differentiation, and nerve growth.[130] Their activity in the malignant transformation process in human cancers is not well defined. Perhaps a major role in tumor growth is in angiogenesis (see Chapter 10).[131] The fact that overexpression of FGFs can cause cellular transformation, and their identity as proto-oncogenes, both suggest that they could play a primary role in at least some cancers. Recent careful analysis of pathologic specimens has demonstrated that the amount of angiogenesis in breast cancer tissue is highly correlated with a poorer prognosis.[132]

Pharmacologic agents with the capacity to block the activity of FGFs are of major interest. Heparin stabilizes FGF-1, enhancing its effects on angiogenesis, but does not affect FGF-2.[127] The antiparasitic drug suramin can bind to FGFs and block their interactions with receptors.[133] This agent has undergone extensive clinical trials in patients with advanced prostate cancer, with demonstration of activity in a significant minority of the cases.[134] However, suramin has a number of direct effects on cellular metabolism, and also can interfere with the binding of other growth factors, including PDGF, EGF, and TGF-β.

These agents, and others such as fumagillin,[135] may either turn out to be clinically useful, or point the way to the development of more effective blocking agents.

BOMBESIN

Bombesin is a 14–amino acid peptide, originally isolated from frog skin, that is a homologue of the mammalian gastrin-releasing peptide.[136] Administration of either of these peptides intravenously stimulates gastric acid secretion, via the secretion of gastrin. Some small-cell carcinoma cell lines produce bombesin and are stimulated by it.[137,138] Bombesin can enhance the growth of normal human bronchial epithelial cells in serum-free cultures. The peptide is also mitogenic for Swiss 3T3 murine embryonal fibroblasts, and this effect is potentiated by insulin, PDGF, or EGF.[139] A MAb has been produced that binds to bombesin, and this in turn has been shown to inhibit proliferation of non–small-cell carcinoma cells in culture and in nude mouse xenografts.[138] A trial of antibombesin MAb therapy for small-cell carcinoma has been initiated.

TRANSFORMING GROWTH FACTOR β

Transforming growth factor β is the prototypic member of a family of polypeptide regulatory molecules that includes activins, inhibins, bone morphogenic proteins, and the müllerian inhibitory substance in mammals (reviewed in refs. 140–142). It originally was identified as a transforming component (with TGF-α) of the factors present in conditioned medium of certain tumor cell line cultures, which had the capacity to stimulate the growth of fibroblasts in soft agar.[7,62] Although its name is based on the transforming properties that initially were identified, this growth factor has an array of functions that regulate many normal cellular processes involved in morphogenesis, differentiation, and wound healing.

TGF-β-1 is the best characterized molecule of the group of growth factors that act primarily to *inhibit* cell proliferation. It is synthesized as the carboxy-terminal domain of a precursor molecule that is a secretory polypeptide.[143] After secretion, the pro-region remains attached to the TFG-β-1 domain, and two such precursor molecules form a dimer that has only latent biologic activity. This latent complex originally was found in platelets,[144] but it may be released directly into the environment, where it is bound to the extracellular matrix and to specific binding proteins. Cleavage by proteolytic digestion or by alterations in pH can release an active TGF-β dimer from the latent complex.[145] Most cells have been shown to synthesize TGF-β in one of its molecular forms. In the TGF-β family, there are four additional molecular forms that are closely related to TGF-β-1, each of which forms dimers that express biologic activity.

The effects of TGF-β, activins, and probably all members of this family are mediated by a pair of membrane-spanning receptors: type I, with a molecular mass of 53 kDa, and type II, with a molecular mass of 70 kDa.[140] Each can bind ligand with high affinity, and each has a cytoplasmic portion which is a serine-threonine kinase.[146–148] It appears that signal transduction via these kinases is activated when different portions of a single TGF-β molecule bind to both a type I and a type II receptor, creating an active heterodimer.[148a] Another protein with the capacity to bind TGF-β is betaglycan, previously designated as the type III receptor.[140] Betaglycan can exist as a transmembrane protein or can be released into the extracellular space in a soluble form. It is speculated that these abundant molecules could function as a reservoir or a clearance system for bioactive TGF-β.[140]

The capacity of TGF-β to inhibit proliferation of a variety of malignant epithelial tumor cell lines has attracted attention to its possible use as an anticancer agent. However, it also inhibits the proliferation of normal epithelial cells in the breast, liver, bronchus, kidney, skin, and intestine.[141] In fact, it has been postulated that TGF-β may be the major biologic regulator of normal cells that have the capacity to repopulate tissues.[141] In this model, tumorigenesis could involve escape from cellular regulation by TGF-β. For example, whereas retinal cells bear receptors for TGF-β, retinoblastoma cells lack these receptors, and this may permit the cell to escape regulation by TGF-β in the retina.[149] Although loss of receptors is an unusual event, other mechanisms such as alteration in intracellular signal transduction pathways or suppressor genes might deactivate the regulatory capacity of the TGF-β receptor.

The inhibitory effects of TGF-β on cell proliferation extend beyond the epithelium. Remarkable growth-inhibiting activity has been observed in endothelial, fibroblast, neuronal, lymphoid, and hematopoietic cell types. The degree of inhibition varies. The responding cells display delayed progression through, or arrest in, the late G_1 phase of the cell cycle.[150,151] These observations have led to the hypothesis that TFG-β may have utility in inhibiting the immune system, or in temporarily arresting the production of bone marrow stem cells, to protect them from chemotherapy.[142] In the case of T cells, it has been shown that lymphocyte activation can increase the production of TGF-β and that TGF-β can inhibit the IL-2–induced upregulation of IL-2 receptors. These events might physiologically dampen the IL-2–mediated proliferative response of these immune cells.[152]

Analysis of the effects of TGF-β is complicated by its capacity to activate opposite responses (e.g., growth stimulation and suppression), sometimes in the same target cells. This may depend on the particular growth conditions. The mechanism of growth enhancement in some types of fibroblasts is believed to be an indirect one, through induction of expression of PDGF, which in turn can activate the growth of the fibroblasts by autocrine stimulation.[150,153] Osteoblasts also are stimulated to proliferate in culture by TGF-β. Exposure of cells to TGF-β results in changes in the phenotype that may play a major role in differentiation and embryologic morphogenesis (reviewed in ref. 140,141). Sites of intense development and morphogenesis in the connective tissues of the embryo are known to express high levels of TGF-β, suggesting a role in function and remodeling of embryonic structures.

The mechanism of growth inhibition by TGF-β remains to be fully understood. One line of evidence suggests a role for TGF-β in inhibiting the expression of c-*myc*, which could reduce the transcription of genes key to proliferation.[154] An alternative mechanism involves the demonstrated capacity of TGF-β stimulation to result in a reduced capacity to phosphorylate the retinoblastoma (Rb) protein.[152] Because Rb phosphorylation is required to release bound nuclear transcription regulators and allow entry into S phase, this observation could provide an explanation for the arrest of cells in late G_1 phase after exposure to TGF-β.

TGF-β may play a role in inflammation and repair in a number of ways (reviewed in refs. 140,141). It is a potent chemotactic factor and activator of macrophages. It stimulates the production of components of extracellular matrix such as collagen and fibronectin. In addition, it inhibits expression of proteolytic enzyme activity that could destroy newly formed connective tissue, by reducing the production of enzymes such as collagenase and stromalysin, and by up-regulating the production of protease inhibitors. In parallel, TGF-β up-regulates expression of integrin receptors for molecules such as collagen and fibronectin, thereby increasing the adhesion of cells to matrix proteins.[140] The regulation of integrin expression could modulate the capacity of cells into interact with other cells, by altering cell-to-cell adhesion (see Chapter 9).

Activins and inhibins are growth factors consisting of hetero- and homodimeric molecules related to the TGF-β family.[155] These growth factors originally were recognized as gonadal protein hormones that can modulate follicle-stimulating hormone (FSH) production by the anterior pituitary. The activin and inhibin molecules share a common β chain and differ in the second chain, which could be an α chain (inhibins) or another β chain (activins).[155,156] In addition to regulating pituitary function, activins and inhibins regulate hormone production in gonadal tissues and differentiation of erythroid and neural cells.

Müllerian-inhibiting substance (MIS) also has a structure and biochemical function related to TGF-β.[157] It is expressed in the testes, and this causes regression of the müllerian duct during fetal development. It also is expressed transiently and at low levels in the ovary. MIS inhibited the colony growth of a number of primary ovarian and endometrial cancers from patients, as well as cell lines derived from these sources.[158,159]

INTERFERONS

The interferons (IFNs) are a family of secreted proteins that were discovered as biologic agents interfering with virus replication.[160] Subsequently, it has been found that they have numerous functions, including modulation of the immune system and regulation of cell proliferation and differentiation. The reader is referred to recent reviews of the IFNs for more detailed discussions of the complex actions of these cytokines.[161,162]

The superfamily of IFNs consists of at least 18 IFN-α genes and 6 IFN-γ (IFN-α2) genes expressed in leukocytes, plus a single IFN-β gene expressed in fibroblasts.[161,162] These bind to a class of receptors that are not yet well characterized.

Binding of IFN to receptor can activate signal trans-

duction pathways which regulate nuclear events. The first step appears to be activation of *Jak*, a cytoplasmic protein which contains an intrinsic tyrosine kinase. This, in turn, results in activation of latent cytoplasmic proteins known as STATs (signal transducers and activators of transcription). The activated STAT molecules are translocated to the nucleus where, alone or in combination with other proteins, they bind to specific DNA sequences known as ISREs (interferon-stimulated response elements), thereby stimulating transcription of target genes.[162a] Exposure of cells to IFN thereby activates production of more than 30 proteins, which vary widely in their function. Among the most well-characterized is the (2′,5′)-oligo A synthetase family of enzymes, which convert ATP into 2′,5′(A)n, where n ranges from 2 to 15.[163] This enzyme, which is stimulated by double-stranded RNA, activates RNase L, which cleaves single-stranded RNA and may interfere with virus replication. Other IFN-induced proteins include the major histocompatibility complex class I and class II antigens, which are involved in cell recognition and the processing of antigens.

IFNs can inhibit the proliferation of a wide variety of cells. Their action is generally cytostatic rather than cytotoxic, and inhibition of progression through cell cycle phases has been demonstrated. Therapeutic utility of IFN administration has been demonstrated for hairy-cell leukemia and the chronic leukemias, as well as Kaposi's sarcoma.

By activating immune and inflammatory cells, and regulating immunoglobulin secretion, IFNs exert an important influence on the physiologic processes involved in host defense mechanisms. Alternatively, they could play a role in the pathogenesis of chronic inflammatory and autoimmune diseases.

TUMOR NECROSIS FACTOR

Tumor necrosis factor (TNF) is a protein containing 157 amino acids that is produced by activated macrophages and other cells (reviewed in refs. 164–166). It binds to specific receptors with molecular weights of 55 and 75 kDa. Activation of a G protein may be an important pathway of signal transduction. TNF released at the site of inflammation acts on receptors on endothelial cells, T and B lymphocytes, and granulocytes to stimulate immune and inflammatory responses. In these processes, there is overlap with the functions of both interleukin 1 and the INFs. It is believed that many of the physiologic changes associated with endotoxemia are activated by TNF and related cytokines.

TNF and a related molecule, lymphotoxin, now are known as TNF-α and TNF-β. They have been shown to have cytotoxic effects on a variety of tumor cells in experimental systems. In contrast, TNF can stimulate the proliferation of certain fibroblast lines. The mechanisms of these effects remain to be clarified.

Detection of new members of the TNF family and their receptors continues. The *fas* protooncogene is particularly interesting because its activation on the surface of T lymphocytes results in apoptosis (programmed cell death).[166a]

Future Directions

In addition to antibodies and other extracellular receptor-blocking molecules, a number of new pharmacologic agents have been developed with selective potential for blocking signal transduction pathways mediated by activated receptors. These are presented in Chapters 6 and 7.

GROWTH FACTORS FOR HEMATOPOIETIC CELLS

The development and functional activation of mature blood cells and their respective precursors are regulated by hematopoietic growth factors (Fig. 20–4). These cytokines include the classic colony-stimulating factors as well as the interleukins. The number of regulatory proteins that recently have been identified to control the proliferation, differentiation, and functional activation of hematopoietic elements would appear to be ever increasing; however, for the purpose of this review, we discuss those molecules that have been the most extensively studied (Table 20–3).

Biochemistry and Biology of Hematopoietic Growth Factors

GRANULOCYTE COLONY-STIMULATING FACTOR

Human granulocyte colony-stimulating factor (G-CSF) was purified to homogeneity from the human bladder carcinoma cell line 5637,[167] and subsequently the gene was cloned.[168] The amino acid sequence has no significant homology to human or murine granulocyte-macrophage colony-stimulating factor (GM-CSF), interleukin 3 (IL-3), or macrophage colony-stimulating factor (M-CSF). A region of amino acid homology exists between G-CSF and interleukin 6 (IL-6), suggesting that there may be some similarity in the tertiary structure. Analysis of messenger RNA isolated from 5637 cells using a G-CSF–specific probe has revealed a single species of mRNA migrating at 1650 Da.[168,169] Human G-CSF also has been cloned, from a squamous cell carcinoma cell line[170]; however, this clone contains nine additional bases, giving rise to a protein with three additional amino acids. Furthermore, this 177–amino acid species was 100-fold less biologically active in vitro.[169] Analysis of genomic sequence has indicated that formation of this 177–amino acid species occurs as the result of splicing at an alternative splice donor site between exons 2 and 3.[169]

The gene for G-CSF has been expressed successfully in *Escherichia coli*.[168] The recombinant protein has a molecular weight of 18,000, reflecting the lack of O-glycosylation in the bacterially derived product, which is not required for in vitro or in vivo biologic activity.

Human G-CSF is not species specific in its action. It stimulates the growth of neutrophil granulocyte precursors (colony-forming units, granulocyte [CFU-G]),[167,168,171] supports the survival and expansion in vitro of immature precursors of colony-forming cells (pre-CFU), and stimulates

the proliferation of promyelocytes and myelocytes.[171] Originally, human G-CSF was thought to be a pluripoietin, because it appeared to support the growth of human burst-forming unit, erythroid (BFU-E) and uncommitted progenitors; however, with further depletion of accessory cells and enrichment of progenitors, G-CSF was found to no longer support the growth of erythroid or multilineage progenitors from this target cell population.[172] G-CSF has been shown to support the growth of megakaryocyte colonies in conjunction with IL-3.[173] For cells of the mature, postmitotic compartment, G-CSF has been shown to enhance the specific binding of the chemotactic bacterial peptide formylmethionyl-leucyl-phenylalanine (MLP),[174] to promote chemotaxis,[171] and to augment neutrophil-mediated antibody-dependent cellular cytotoxicity (ADCC).[174]

GRANULOCYTE-MACROPHAGE COLONY-STIMULATING FACTORS

Human GM-CSF was first purified[175] and then molecularly cloned and expressed in mammalian cells.[176] The molecule is highly and variably glycosylated, accounting for a wide range in reported molecular weights. The role of variable glycosylation with regard to cell-specific production, biologic activity, or half-life remains to be determined. Although no formal comparison has been performed, both glycosylated and nonglycosylated GM-CSF are biologically active in vitro and in vivo in humans.

Recombinant human GM-CSF (rhGM-CSF) supports the growth of both granulocytic and monocytic colonies in semisolid culture[175]; however, it also is active at much earlier stages of myeloid development, as evidenced by its ability to produce colonies containing myeloid, erythroid, and megakaryocytic cells when combined with erythropoietin, a late-acting promoter of erythroid development.[176,177] In the presence of rhGM-CSF, mature macrophages and neutrophils demonstrate enhanced tumoricidal and phagocytic activity, intracellular killing, ADCC, superoxide production, complement-mediated (opsonized) phagocytosis, and responsiveness to chemotactic factors.[178] Mature eosinophils also respond to rhGM-CSF with increased ADCC activity.[178] GM-CSF is an extremely potent inducer of Mo-1, a molecule involved in granulocyte cell-to-cell adhesion, and induces increased granulocyte aggregation in vitro[179] and in vivo.[180] The clinical significance of this remains to be determined.

MACROPHAGE COLONY-STIMULATING FACTOR

Macrophage colony-stimulating factor, or CSF-1, is a heavily glycosylated dimer. Two forms of the glycoprotein exist, as a result of differential splicing of the gene.[181] The larger form encodes a 70,000-Da glycoprotein that is the major form of M-CSF in human urine.[181] A smaller form was cloned first from a human pancreatic cell line.[181] Both forms of M-CSF are biologically active. Recombinant human M-CSF (rhM-CSF) promotes the growth and maturation of monocyte and macrophage precursors. In addition, M-CSF enhances the phagocytic and tumoricidal activity of human monocytes/macrophages and induces

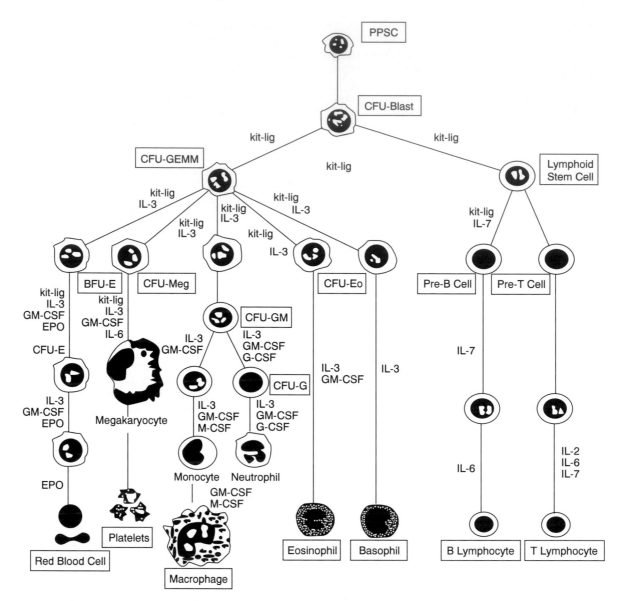

Figure 20–4. The regulation of hematopoiesis. There is a hierarchy of development, with kit ligand and interleukin 3 (IL-3) acting on early multipotential progenitors and erythropoietin (EPO), granulocyte colony-stimulating factor (G-CSF), and macrophage colony-stimulating factor (M-CSF) acting on later progenitors. The effects of kit ligand and IL-3 on lineage-specific progenitors are seen primarily in synergy with late-acting factors such as EPO, G-CSF, and M-CSF. Kit ligand primarily acts on a subset of multipotent stem cells, enhancing their proliferative response to other hematopoietic growth factors. PPSC, pluripotent stem cell; CFU, colony-forming unit; BFU-E, burst-forming unit, erythroid; E, erythroid; Meg, megakaryocytic; Eo, eosinophilic. (Adapted from Investigators Brochure: r-met HuSCF–AMGEN.)

them to secrete a variety of cytokines, including TNF-α, interleukin 1 (IL-1), and CSFs.[182]

ERYTHROPOIETIN

Erythropoietin (EPO) is a primary regulator of erythropoiesis in humans and other mammals. The cloning of the EPO gene[183] has permitted large-scale production of human EPO. EPO appears to act almost exclusively on the committed erythroid progenitor and precursor cells, allowing these cells to proliferate and enter into terminal erythroid maturation, thereby expanding the production of red blood cells.[184] The human EPO gene encodes a mature protein that has a calculated molecular mass of 18,400 Da. Posttranslational glycosylation is required for in vivo function, giving the protein a molecular mass of 30,400 Da, 40 per cent of which is carbohydrate. The EPO receptor has been detected only on erythroid progenitor cells and has sequence homology with receptors for GM-CSF, IL-3, interleukin 4, interleukin 6, interleukin 7, and the β subunit of the interleukin 2 receptor.[184] Little is known regarding the second messenger or molecular events following the binding of EPO to its receptor that lead to the proliferation and differention of erythroid cells.

TABLE 20–3. SUMMARY OF THE BIOCHEMICAL AND MOLECULAR CHARACTERISTICS, CELL SOURCES, AND TARGETS OF THE HEMATOPOIETIC COLONY-STIMULATING FACTORS

FACTOR CELL LINEAGE*	CHROMOSOMAL LOCATION	CELL SOURCE	PROTEIN SIZE (kDa)	RECEPTOR MASS (kDa)
GM-CSF	5q23–q32	Monocyte Fibroblast Endothelial T lymphocyte Epithelial	14–35	50,000 130,000– 180,000
G-CSF (n)	17q11–123	Monocyte Endothelial Epithelial	18	150,000
M-CSF (CSF-1) (m)	5q23–q31	Monocyte Fibroblast Endothelial	35–45 ($\times$2) 18–26 ($\times$2)	160,000
IL-3 (multi-CSF) (n,m,e,b,E,M)	5q23–q31	T lymphocyte Brain: (?)	14–28	140,000
IL-6 (stem cells)	7q15–p21	Monocyte Fibroblasts T cells B cells Endothelial	26	80,000
Erythropoietin	7q11–q22	Kidney: ? Peritubular cells Liver: ? Cell type	30.4	100,000 85,000
Kit ligand	12q14.3–12qter	Endothelial cells Bone marrow stromal cells	31 36	145,000

*GM-CSF, granulocyte-macrophage colony-stimulating factor; G-CSF, granulocyte colony-stimulating factor; M-CSF, macrophage colony-stimulating factor; IL, interleukin; n, neutrophil; m, monocyte; e, eosinophil; b, basophil; E, erythrocyte; M, megakaryocyte.

INTERLEUKINS

Interleukin 1

Interleukin 1 is a mediator involved in numerous inflammatory, immunologic, and hematologic responses.[185] Two forms of IL-1 have been characterized, IL-1α and IL-1β, although few differences in their respective biologic activities have been observed and both species apparently bind to the same receptor. IL-1 is a 17,500-Da protein that is produced by activated monocytes, as well as a variety of other cell types.[185] IL-α and -β have pleiotropic effects, including the induction of fever, production of acute-phase proteins, co-activation of lymphocytes, and proliferation of fibroblasts, endothelial cells, osteoclasts, and hepatocytes. In hematopoiesis, IL-1 also has been shown to stimulate the proliferation of resting stem cells in vitro and induce expression of the M-CSF, G-CSF, and GM-CSF receptors.[185] In addition, IL-1 induces the expression of other CSFs and cytokines from monocytes, fibroblasts, and endothelial cells.[185]

Interleukin 2

Interleukin 2 (IL-2) is a lymphokine produced by activated T lymphocytes in response to antigen or mitogen stimulation. First described as T-cell growth factor, IL-2 is essential for the growth of these cells. Native IL-2 is a 133–amino acid glycoprotein with a molecular mass of 14,000 to 16,000 Da by sodium dodecyl sulfate–polyacrylamide gel electrophoresis and a calculated molecular mass of 15,420 Da. Glycosylation is not required for biologic activity, but an intrachain disulfide bond from residues 58 to 105 is needed. The IL-2 receptor is comprised of two molecules, a 55,000-Da chain known as Tac, or the α chain, and a 75,000-Da β chain. Since its initial discovery, IL-2 has been shown to have pleotrophic effects on immunologic effector cells, including natural killer cells and B lymphocytes. Culture of peripheral blood lymphocytes in the presence of IL-2 results in the outgrowth of lymphocyte-activated killer (LAK) cells, which possess the capability of lysing and destroying fresh noncultured tumor cells.[186]

Interleukin 3 (Multi-CSF)

Murine IL-3 first was purified and characterized by Ihle et al. and subsequently was shown to support the formation of multilineage colonies in vitro.[187] Gibbon and human IL-3 have been cloned recently using expression-cloning techniques.[188] IL-3 is a complex glycoprotein, ranging in size from 14,000 to 28,000 Da. The expected size of the polypeptide is 14,000 to 15,000 Da.[188] The homology between murine IL-3 and human Il-3 at the amino acid level is only 29 per cent, compared with a 93 per cent homology between gibbon and human IL-3.

Recombinant IL-3 supports the growth of single-lineage, as well as multilineage, colonies and blast cell colonies by CD34 (My10)–positive bone marrow cells in the presence of EPO. These data suggest that IL-3 is probably the least restricted of the CSFs with regard to cell lineage. IL-3 also affects the functional activity of mature granulocytes[189] and monocytes.

Interleukin 4

As with most lymphokines, interleukin 4 (IL-4) has been found to be multifunctional in its regulation of the immune response, acting on different cell lineages and at different stages of development and differentiation.[190] More recently, it has been shown to have both direct and indirect effects on the regulation of hematopoiesis. As a hematopoietin, IL-4 affects the proliferation of eosinophil and basophil granulocytes; in addition, it appears to promote degranulation of the mature basophil granulocyte.

Interleukin 5

Interleukin 5 (IL-5) is the product of activated T lymphocytes.[191] It initially was observed that culture supernatants from parasite-specific, antigen-stimulated T lymphocytes induced eosinophil colony formation. This eosinophil differentiation factor was found to be distinct from IL-3, appearing as a single band of 45,000 Da on gel filtration. Independently, others identified a B-cell growth factor (BCGF II) produced by T cells that was distinct from IL-4. These two activities subsequently were demonstrated to be derived from the same protein. IL-5 exists as a dimer and exhibits species cross reactivity. The gene for IL-5 encodes a 134–amino acid polypeptide, which includes a terminal leader sequence. The core protein contains at least two glycosylation sites.

Interleukin 6

Human IL-6 (B-cell–stimulating factor 2 [BSF-2]) originally was identified as a factor in the culture supernatants of mitogen- or antigen-stimulated mononuclear cells, which induced immunoglobulin production in either Epstein-Barr virus (EBV)–transformed B cell lines or *Staphylococcus aureus* Cowan 1 (SAC)–stimulated normal B cells,[192,193] but which now has been shown to exhibit a critical role in hematopoiesis. It is produced by T and B cells, as well as a variety of mesenchymal cells and endothelial cells.[192] The molecular cloning of the cDNA of IL-6 revealed that this factor is identical to a number of other well-described regulatory molecules with a variety of biologic activities.

IL-6 has been shown to stimulate the growth of early hematopoietic progenitor cells and support the formation of multilineage blast colonies in culture. In addition, the synergistic activity of IL-1 with IL-3 in promoting the proliferation of hematopoietic stem cells may be secondary to the induction of IL-6 by IL-1.[194] IL-6 also has been shown to induce differentiation of murine myelomonocytic leukemic cells into macrophages and to enhance phagocytosis and the expression of Fc and C3d receptors on these same targets.

KIT LIGAND (STEM CELL FACTOR, STEELE FACTOR)

Kit ligand is a hematopoietic and tissue growth factor that serves as the ligand for the c-*kit* oncogene. The naturally occurring form of the kit ligand is a 165–amino acid polypeptide, heavily N- and O-glycosylated, that exists as a dimer. The initial gene product is a 248–amino acid precursor that is cleaved during processing to the mature protein. Alternate splicing of the gene also results in a membrane-bound form of kit ligand. Unlike most hematopoietic growth factors, kit ligand circulates at relatively high concentrations in human plasma. Recently, a synthetic gene for human kit ligand has been constructed and transfected into E. coli; this nonglycosylated form of kit ligand exhibits biologic activity similar to the native glycosylated moiety. Kit ligand stimulates little colony growth when used alone, but has been shown to augment the in vitro proliferation of both myeloid and lymphoid hematopoietic progenitor cells[195–202] in the presence of EPO, G-CSF, IL-3, or GM-CSF. It has been proposed that this growth factor, produced locally at high concentrations by marrow stromal cells, acts as an "anchor" factor and permits stem cells to respond to physiologic concentrations of other cytokines. Kit ligand also promotes the activation of purified human skin mast cells and basophils. In addition, in the presence of immunoglobulin E, kit ligand induces the release of histamine and prostaglandin D_2 from mast cells and basophil granulocytes. CD34+ bone marrow cells cultured in the presence of both kit ligand and IL-3 give rise to cultures containing increased numbers of basophil granulocytes as well as mast cells.

Receptors for Hematopoietic Growth Factors

The receptors for hematopoietic growth factors fall into two categories. The receptors for M-CSF and kit ligand belong to the classic tyrosine kinase receptor family described earlier in this chapter. Receptors for the other CSFs and ILs belong to a new family of "cytokine" receptors.[203,204] The extracellular portions of these receptors share, to a greater or lesser extent, a number of structural features: an amino-terminal immunoglobulin-like domain, a region with four conserved cysteine residues, a conserved sequence of tryptophan-serine-X-tryptophan-serine, and a fibronectin type III–like domain (Fig. 20–5). The intracellular portions have varying sizes and no described functional properties.

Several of these receptors bind their ligands with low affinity, unless they are coupled with a second accessory molecule. One such molecule, gp130, appears to couple with IL-6; another molecule, GM-CSF-β (or KH97) can couple with GM-CSF, IL-3, or IL-5.

Some features of interest have emerged with regard to the structure of certain hematopoietic cytokine receptors. A portion of the extracellular domain of the G-CSF receptor exhibits a striking similarity to the prolactin receptor and some similarity to the neural cell adhesion mole-

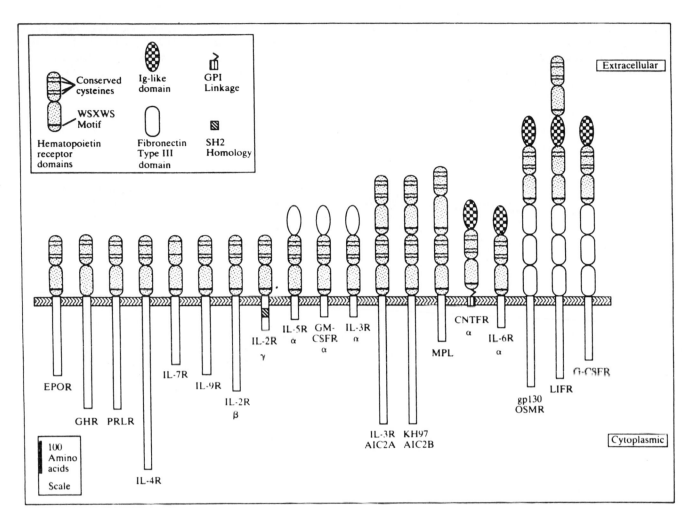

Figure 20-5. Receptors for hematopoietic growth factors. Modular elements are represented as shown in the box. It should be noted that homologies in the cytoplasmic domains are generally very limited and confined to short stretches of amino acid sequence. For those receptors that exist in more than one isoform with different length cytoplasmic domains, the longer is depicted. Abbreviations: R, receptor; EPO, erythropoietin; GH, growth hormone; PRL, prolactin; IL, interleukin; KH-97, beta subunit of GM-CSF and IL-3 receptor; MPL, thrombopoietin; CNTF, ciliary neurotrophic factor; OSM, oncostatin M; LIF, leukemia inhibitory factor. (From Cosman D: The hematopoietic receptor superfamily. Cytokine 5:95, 1993, with permission).

cule family, suggesting that the receptor may play a role in the adhesiveness of early hematopoietic cells to microenvironmental sites.

Binding of hematopoietic growth factors to their receptors leads to activation of many of the signal transduction pathways described earlier in this chapter for the nonhematopoietic growth factors. The cytoplasmic portions of these receptors presumably mediate this process, but the mechanism remains to be determined, since the cytoplasmic domains of the receptors show no tyrosine kinase motifs. Many biochemical changes have been observed following receptor activation, and two general pathways of signal transduction from receptor to nucleus have been defined. In the first, receptor-mediated activation of a tyrosine kinase leads to elevation of *ras* via GRB-2/SOS followed by phosphorylation of *raf* and the MAP kinase cascade.[203a] In the second, activation of one or more Jak-

family tyrosine kinases results in phosphorylation of STAT family proteins and their translocation to the nucleus, where they act as specific transcription factors. There is an intense research effort investigating the mechanisms that activate these signaling pathways.[204]

Evidence for the Role of Hematopoietic Growth Factors in Malignant Transformation

Hematopoietic growth factors not only may be important physiologic regulators in maintaining hematopoiesis and augmenting host defense, but also may play a role in the pathogenesis and/or growth advantage of malignant cells. In this regard, IL-2, IL-7, and IL-6 have been identified as proliferative factors for malignant lymphocytes[205] and plasma cells.[192] In addition, GM-CSF can synergize with IL-6 in supporting the proliferation of human myeloma cells. Hematopoietic growth factors also have been implicated in the pathogenesis of leukemia.[182,206–213] In this regard, the enhanced or unimpaired expression of specific hematopoietic growth factors in vivo, via the introduction of these genes into murine bone marrow cells by means of infection with retroviruses expressing GM-CSF[212] and or IL-3,[213] has been shown to give rise to myeloproliferative disorders. Intriguing data also suggests that, under certain conditions, hematopoietic growth factors contribute to the growth advantage of the leukemic clone, resulting from an inherent hypersensitivity of the leukemic clone to the growth-promoting effects of a particular hematopoietic growth factor.[213] Colony-stimulating factors[206,207] and interleukins[207,209] also have been shown to be constitutively produced by leukemic blasts and have been proposed to play a pathogenic role in hematopoietic malignancies through the activation of an autocrine loop. The autocrine loop hypothesis has been expanded further to include the possibility that abnormal cellular proliferation of blood cell elements may result from the loss of normal inhibitory mechanisms or known suppressor molecules, which counteract the stimulatory effects of the hematopoietic growth factors.[214]

Preclinical and Clinical Studies

Hematopoietic growth factors and interleukins have been shown to have direct clinical use in the management of patients with both malignant and nonmalignant conditions. The clinical applications of these cytokines in the treatment of disease lie in four general areas: (1) the restoration of normal hematopoiesis, (2) augmentation of host defense against infection, (3) stimulation and production of functionally primed effector cells with antitumor capability, and (4) clonal extinction of malignant disease by differentiation induction.

The most extensively studied hematopoietic growth factors in clinical practice include G-CSF, GM-CSF, and EPO. We discuss these cytokines in the greatest detail here. More recently, early-acting hematopoietic growth factors, such as IL-3, IL-1, IL-6, and kit ligand, have been introduced into the clinical arena in hopes of better affecting hematopoietic reconstitution in the setting of disease-related or iatrogenically induced myelosuppression. These studies are highlighted. Studies of IL-2 and M-CSF have been designed to take advantage of the ability of these respective cytokines to enhance effector cell function. Such strategies may be useful in developing novel therapeutic approaches to the treatment of cancer and infectious disease. These results are discussed briefly in this context.

GRANULOCYTE COLONY-STIMULATING FACTOR

Preclinical studies demonstrated early on the ability of G-CSF to augment the number of functionally normal neutrophil granulocytes in normal and tumor-bearing rodents and nonhuman primates. This neutrophil granulocytosis results from an augmentation in the number of divisions in precursor cells and a reduction (from 96 to 24 hours) in the time required for the maturing neutrophil granulocyte precursors to develop into terminally differentiated cells.[215] This particular biologic effect is unique to G-CSF. G-CSF has been shown to reduce the period of neutropenia in cynomolgus primates treated with high-dose cyclophosphamide,[216] busulfan,[217] or total-body irradiation with autologous marrow reinfusion,[218] and in dogs given a DLA-identical littermate transplant.[219] G-CSF also has been shown to be radioprotective and to augment survival in both murine and canine models of supralethal irradiation, in the absence of bone marrow rescue.[219]

Three initial studies in humans revealed that an intravenous bolus, continuous intravenous infusion, subcutaneous injection, or continuous subcutaneous infusion of G-CSF, administered in the absence of myelosuppression, results in a dose-dependent increase in the circulating neutrophil granulocyte count.[220–222] This increase in absolute neutrophil count is due primarily to an increase in mature, functionally normal segmented polymorphonuclear leukocytes and is associated with an expansion of the bone marrow myeloid compartment. On discontinuation of G-CSF, neutrophil counts decreased by one half daily and generally return to baseline within 4 days of discontinuing treatment. The administration of G-CSF also results in a 10- to 100-fold increase in the number of circulating hematopoietic progenitors.[220,223]

Neutropenia in cancer patients is a major cause of morbidity and mortality and results from malignant disease as well as its treatment. Phase I/II clinical studies using a broad spectrum of commonly employed chemotherapeutic regimens initially demonstrated the ability of G-CSF to accelerate recovery from chemotherapy-induced neutropenia.[220–222,224–226] In all of these studies, G-CSF was administered 24 hours following cessation of chemotherapy. Optimization of timing and duration has been investigated in patients receiving high-dose melphalan.[226] This study demonstrated accelerated recovery from neutropenia even when G-CSF treatment was begun 8 days after chemotherapy.

The ability to delay the use of G-CSF but not GM-CSF, and commence treatment close to the time of expected nadir in the neutrophil count, most likely results from the ability of G-CSF to rapidly mobilize neutrophil granulocytes from the bone marrow mitotic compartment. In addition, these data support the hypothesis that the rate-limiting factor in G-CSF–induced recovery from neutropenia is the availability of G-CSF–responsive progenitors.

Based on the results of the phase I and II trials, a randomized, double-blind, placebo-controlled phase III trial of G-CSF was designed to evaluate definitively the incidence of infection as manifested by fever with neutropenia (temperature >38.2° C and absolute neutrophil count <1000 cells/μL), in patients treated with one of the standard aggressive chemotherapeutic regimens for small-cell carcinoma of the lung.[227] In this trial, the placebo group exhibited a 57 per cent incidence of febrile neutropenia, as compared to only a 28 per cent incidence observed in the G-CSF–treated group. The design of the study allowed patients who developed an episode of febrile neutropenia on placebo to cross over to open-label G-CSF, rather than receive a reduced dose of chemotherapy, which normally would be required. Similarly, patients on blinded G-CSF who developed febrile neutropenia crossed over to open-label G-CSF.

The efficacy of G-CSF was demonstrated in many ways in this study. Only 18/110 patients (16 per cent) starting on placebo continued to receive placebo for the six cycles of chemotherapy, as compared to 41/101 patients (41 per cent) who started on blinded G-CSF and remained on blinded G-CSF for six cycles of chemotherapy. The patients receiving G-CSF had a 47 per cent and 45 per cent reduction in the number of days on antibiotics and the time spent in the hospital, respectively. The benefit of G-CSF treatment was sustained throughout the six cycles of therapy. The importance of this study was that it showed that G-CSF–induced neutrophils were clinically functional, and early neutrophil recovery led to easily measurable clinical benefits.

This pivotal phase III trial, as well as earlier studies, led to Food and Drug Administration (FDA) approval of G-CSF to reduce the incidence of infection as manifested by febrile neutropenia, in adult and pediatric patients with nonmyeloid malignancies receiving myelosuppressive chemotherapy. Although only limited data exist regarding the use of G-CSF for myelosuppressive chemotherapy in a pediatric population, considerable data exist to show a comparable safety profile of G-CSF for children and adults. A recent European trial in patients with small-cell lung cancer has confirmed these findings.[228]

Preservation of intended dose intensity also has been demonstrated recently in a randomized trial in non-Hodgkin's lymphoma.[229] Febrile neutropenia occurred in 22 per cent of the G-CSF–treated patients, as compared to 44 per cent of the nontreated group. Doses of chemotherapy were reduced in only 10 per cent of the group treated with G-CSF and in 51 per cent of the group treated without G-CSF. Fifty-nine per cent of the G-CSF–treated group received over 95 per cent of their intended chemotherapy, compared with 25 per cent of the group treated without G-CSF. This trial confirmed the observation that chemotherapy dose intensity can be preserved with G-CSF treatment, as originally suggested in a phase I trial.[224,227] These studies, in turn, have provided the groundwork for pursuing chemotherapy dose escalation trials with G-CSF in a wide variety of cancers.

In this regard, several trials now have been completed supporting the capacity of G-CSF, with and without the addition of G-CSF–primed peripheral blood progenitors, to enable the successful implementation of dose-intensified regimens.[230–234] At the present time, chemotherapy dose escalation trials are ongoing in patients with non–small-cell lung cancer,[235] non-Hodgkin's lymphoma,[236] and advanced breast cancer.[237] These studies will be of considerable import with regard to the ability of a hematopoietic growth factor such as G-CSF to improve responses in patients with cancer, and, it is hoped, to increase survival.

G-CSF has been used to promote hematologic recovery following bone marrow–ablative intensive chemotherapy followed by allogeneic[238] or autologous bone marrow reinfusion in patients with Hodgkin's disease,[239] non-Hodgkin's lymphoma,[240] breast carcinoma, and melanoma.[241]

The use of G-CSF following myeloablative chemotherapy for acute myelogenous leukemia is more controversial. A prospective randomized trial of G-CSF was conducted in patients with either de novo acute myelogenous leukemia, leukemic transformation from myelodysplastic syndrome, acute lymphocytic leukemia, or blastic phase of chronic myelogenous leukemia following chemotherapy.[242] It is important to note that, in this study, G-CSF was started on day 14, 2 days after the completion of induction therapy. In addition, patients were documented to have hypoplastic bone marrow prior to commencing G-CSF treatment. With this schedule employed, the administration of G-CSF significantly accelerated the recovery of neutrophils, reduced the incidence of documented infection, and did not preferentially promote the regrowth of leukemic cells.

Pilot studies of G-CSF in patients with hairy-cell leukemia[243] and myelodysplastic syndrome[244,245] have demonstrated improvements in circulating neutrophil counts, associated in some instances with a decrease in the incidence of or enhanced recovery from active infection. In addition, no evidence of treatment-induced proliferation of the malignant clone has been observed. G-CSF, administered alone or in combination with EPO, has been shown to ameliorate zidovudine-induced myelotoxicity in patients with acquired immunodeficiency syndrome (AIDS), without stimulating p24 antigen expression.[246] Finally, initial pilot studies of G-CSF in patients with primary neutropenic disorders[247–251] (cyclic neutropenia, congenital neutropenia, and idiopathic neutropenia) demonstrated the ability of G-CSF to augment circulating neutrophil counts, reduce the incidence of infection and mucositis, and improve quality-of-life parameters. These preliminary findings have been confirmed by a phase III randomized trial of G-CSF in patients with severe chronic neutropenia, suggesting that this hematopoietic growth factor can play an important role in the management and treatment of these disorders. Recently, G-CSF also has been shown to reduce infection and therefore to be of therapeutic benefit in the treatment of myelokathexis[252] and to correct the neutropenia associated with glycogen storage disease type Ib.[253]

GRANULOCYTE-MACROPHAGE COLONY-STIMULATING FACTOR

In preclinical studies, the administration of human GM-CSF to normal rhesus monkeys resulted in a dramatic leukocytosis consisting initially of only neutrophil granulocytes and monocytes followed by an additional substantial increase in eosinophil granulocytes as well.[254] Treatment also was associated with a significant reticulocytosis; however, no changes in hemoglobin or hematocrit were observed. A model of pancytopenia induced by simian type D retrovirus in rhesus monkeys provided data supporting the clinical application of GM-CSF in patients with AIDS, bone marrow failure states, and infectious disease.[254] Models investigating the utility of GM-CSF following total-body irradiation and autologous bone marrow reinfusion demonstrated the myelorestorative effect of

GM-CSF in the transplant setting and provided the framework for designing clinical trials in humans.[255]

The initial clinical investigation of GM-CSF, which was the first clinical study of a hematopoietic growth factor in humans, was conducted in 16 relatively well patients with AIDS and leukopenia.[256] Continuous intravenous infusion of recombinant GM-CSF derived from hamster cells resulted in a dramatic augmentation in circulating granulocytes found to exhibit improved phagocytosis and antibody-dependent cellular cytotoxicity, and in a lesser increase in monocytes. Additional studies evaluating the safety of bacteria-derived GM-CSF, as well as the chronic subcutaneous administration of hamster cell–derived GM-CSF, showed improved leukocyte counts and enhanced monocyte function in treated patients with AIDS. However, treatment has been associated with an increase in serum human immunodeficiency virus (HIV) p24 antigen in some cases, suggesting stimulation of HIV replication.[257] Furthermore, in patients randomized to receive GM-CSF following chemotherapy for HIV-associated non-Hodgkin's lymphoma, a more than twofold increase in HIV p24 was noted as compared to controls.[258] In contrast, the subcutaneous administration of either nonglycosylated GM-CSF to HIV patients receiving antiviral therapy (gancyclovir), or yeast-derived GM-CSF to patients with AIDS-associated Kaposi's sarcoma receiving antiviral therapy (zidovudine and interferon α), has not been associated with a discernable stimulation of HIV replication, and has resulted in the abrogation of therapy-associated neutropenia.[259] Similarly, the administration of zidovudine alternating with GM-CSF in patients previously treated with GM-CSF alone is associated with a return to baseline of serum HIV p24 values, and has permitted patients to receive zidovudine who otherwise could not tolerate conventional doses of antiviral medication. These data suggest that, although GM-CSF holds promise for use in AIDS in combination with antiviral agents, there are a number of complex interactions that will require investigation. The impressive leukocyte responses observed in these studies also underscore the remarkable sensitivity of leukopenic AIDS patients to low doses of GM-CSF. Although these patients are highly responsive to GM-CSF, they also seem to be more sensitive to toxic effects and often do not tolerate chronic administration well.

In hematologically normal and leukopenic cancer patients, a dose-dependent increase in neutrophils is observed following short or continuous intravenous infusion as well as subcutaneous injection of hamster cell–, yeast-, and bacterially derived GM-CSF[260–264]; an intravenous bolus of nonglycosylated GM-CSF appears to be less efficacious.[260,261] Patients who have received extensive prior chemotherapy or radiotherapy exhibit the smallest elevation in circulating leukocytes in response to GM-CSF treatment. The neutrophils produced in response to GM-CSF appear to function normally as measured by phagocytosis and generation of superoxide. However, impaired migration in vivo has been reported in patients receiving continuous intravenous infusions of hamster cell–derived GM-CSF,[264] but not bacterially derived GM-CSF administered as a 4-hour infusion.[265]

In addition to neutrophilia, treatment with GM-CSF results in an augmentation of circulating monocytes with, in some instances, enhanced tumoricidal activity. Eosinophils also increase after 7 days of treatment with GM-CSF. No consistent effects on hemoglobin, reticulocyte, or platelet counts have been noted following treatment with GM-CSF. However, the occurrence of thrombocytopenia secondary to reactivation of idiopathic thrombocytopenic purpura has been reported. The augmentation in circulating leukocyte counts following glycosylated and nonglycosylated GM-CSF administration also is associated with an 18- and 8-fold increase in circulating myeloid and erythroid hematopoietic precursor cells, respectively.[266] Additional studies in chemotherapy-naive patients have demonstrated impressive mobilization of peripheral blood progenitors (up to 1000-fold) when GM-CSF is administered following myelosuppressive chemotherapy.[267]

Several studies have explored the role of glycosylated and nonglycosylated GM-CSF in ameliorating the myelosuppression associated with autologous bone marrow transplantation for breast carcinoma,[268] melanoma,[268] lymphoid malignancies,[269,270] and non-Hodgkin's lymphoma.[269,270] The first trial in this clinical setting demonstrated that hamster cell–derived GM-CSF, administered as a continuous intravenous infusion beginning 3 hours following autologous marrow infusion, resulted in accelerated recovery of circulating leukocyte counts as well as reduced bacteremia, hepatotoxicity, and nephrotoxicity, when compared to historic controls.[268] Subsequent trials in a variety of bone marrow transplantation settings have confirmed the efficacy of GM-CSF to hasten the recovery of neutrophils in the blood.[269,270] Based on these data, yeast-derived GM-CSF was approved by the FDA to reduce infection in the setting of autologous bone marrow transplantation.

The therapeutic utility of glycosylated and nonglycosylated GM-CSF in ameliorating myelosuppressive toxicity of chemotherapy, in the absence of marrow reinfusion, has been investigated in patients with sarcoma,[271] small-cell carcinoma of the lung,[272] non-Hodgkin's lymphoma,[273] myeloma,[274] ovarian carcinoma,[275] and urithelial tumors[275] and other advanced tumors. The results of these nonrandomized trials suggest that treatment with GM-CSF hastens the recovery of granulocytes, but not platelets or red cells, when administered immediately following the completion of chemotherapy. One study compared granulocyte recovery when hamster cell–derived GM-CSF was administered 1 day or 5 days following high-dose chemotherapy.[267] No accelerated leukocyte recovery was observed when GM-CSF treatment was delayed, suggesting that the immediate administration of GM-CSF following completion of chemotherapy is critical if a therapeutic benefit is to be preserved. Several studies have examined the therapeutic contribution of GM-CSF to the successful implementation of dose-intensified chemotherapeutic regimens, with generally negative results.[276–284]

GM-CSF may be quite useful as a direct anticancer agent by stimulating enhanced effector cell function either alone or in conjunction with MAbs. Combination trials exploring the use of GM-CSF in conjunction with the MAb R24 are being carried out.[285] By enhancing monocyte macrophage killing of tumor cells, GM-CSF may facilitate the presentation of tumor antigens to cytolytic T cells, thereby promoting an immune antitumor response. New approaches will employ the introduction of specific cytokine genes, such as GM-CSF, into vaccines of irradiated tumor cells, thereby allowing for the subsequent local production of cytokines and stimulation of local immune progenitor cells. This approach already has been demonstrated to be efficacious with regard to tumor cell killing in vivo in murine models, employing the transduction of tumor cells with the gene for IL-2.[286] The ability of GM-CSF to enhance the number and functional capacity of effector cells within a localized cavity such as the peritoneum also has implications for future therapeutic approaches to the treatment of malignant disease confined to peritoneal and/or pleural spaces.

Nonrandomized clinical trials investigating the role of yeast- and bacterially derived GM-CSF in patients with myelodysplastic syndrome have reported similar increases in granulocyte counts, without consistent improvements in other hematopoietic lineages.[287–291] In patients with more advanced disease (refractory anemia with excess blasts or refractory anemia with excess blasts in malignant transformation) or chronic myelomonocytic leukemia, treatment is associated with an increase in circulating and bone marrow blasts, although in the majority of cases the blast count returned toward pretreatment values on discontinuation of treatment. A phase III randomized trial in patients with refractory anemia and severe neutropenia receiving 6 months of GM-CSF or no treatment has demonstrated that GM-CSF accelerates transformation to acute leukemia within the time frame studied and augments neutrophil counts. Whether treatment results in a significant reduction in serious infection in this category of patients remains to be determined.

GM-CSF also has been used in patients with acute myeloid leukemia following myelosuppressive chemotherapy,[292] to enhance recovery from granulocytopenia,[292] without evidence of significant predilection to regrowth of the malignant leukemic clone. In addition, GM-CSF has been utilized to recruit cells from G_0 into S, to attempt to render leukemic cells more sensitive to cell cycle–specific killing with chemotherapy.[293] Although in vitro data appeared quite promising for this approach,[294] the clinical data are far from impressive, with very little evidence of significant recruitment from G_0 being accomplished with 3 days of priming prior to introduction of chemotherapy.[293] Additional data will be needed to evaluate this approach further.

UTILITY OF OTHER HEMATOPOIETIC GROWTH FACTORS IN CANCER TREATMENT

Interleukin 3 administration to normal primates results in a modest and delayed leukocytosis with increases in neutrophil, eosinophil, and basophil granulocytes and a dose-dependent increase in intracellular and plasma histamine levels.[295] Increases in corrected reticulocyte counts and variable increases in platelets have been observed. The administration of IL-3 to cynomolgus monkeys after treatment with chemotherapy significantly reduced the du-

ration of severe neutropenia (neutrophil count <500 cells/μL).[296] Platelet recovery appears to occur earlier in animals treated with IL-3.

The ability of glycosylated and nonglycosylated IL-3 to abrogate chemotherapy-induced myelosuppression, alone or in combination with more lineage-specific factors, is under investigation in humans. Several trials explored the therapeutic utility of IL-3 in correcting the pancytopenia associated with aplastic anemia or myelodysplastic syndrome.[297,298] In these studies, IL-3 administration resulted in an increase in neutrophil and eosinophil granulocyte counts, with increases in basophil granulocytes, erythrocytes, and platelets being more variable.

Studies have explored the use of stem cell growth factors, such as IL-1, IL-6, and kit ligand, in an attempt to augment hematopoietic reconstitution further following a myeloablative insult. In patients receiving myelosuppressive doses of chemotherapy, IL-1β administration did not reduce the number of days of neutropenia[299]; however, in another study, 5 days of IL-1α accelerated the recovery from thrombocytopenia following chemotherapy.[300] Recent clinical trials of IL-6 following myelosuppressive chemotherapy and in patients with myelodysplastic syndrome suggest that this hematopoietic growth factor will be quite useful in stimulating the production of platelets. Initial phase I studies of kit ligand have demonstrated that the molecule can be administered safely, with only local erythema and itching observed at the site of subcutaneous administration.[301] Kit ligand by itself following myelosuppressive chemotherapy, does not accelerate the recovery from neutropenia and thrombocytopenia; however, when administered prior to chemotherapy, it appears to be an excellent mobilizing agent for collection of peripheral blood progenitor cells.[301,301a]

ERYTHROPOIETIN

A glycosylated recombinant human EPO has been used successfully to treat the anemia caused by renal disease[302] and has been FDA approved for this indication. In addition, recent studies have demonstrated that erythropoietin administration can correct anemia of chronic disease seen in patients with malignancy[303] and rheumatoid arthritis,[304] as well as that observed in transfusion-dependent patients with AIDS receiving zidovudine.[305] Recent studies suggest that EPO also may be useful in the setting of anemia associated with myelodysplastic syndrome.

ENHANCEMENT OF EFFECTOR CELL FUNCTION WITH GROWTH FACTORS

In vivo, M-CSF increases circulating monocytes that are functionally activated and exhibit enhanced tumoricidal cytotoxicity.[306] There is an associated expansion of bone marrow monocytic elements. M-CSF protects mice from lethal infection after challenge with Candida albicans.[307] The administration of recombinant glycosylated and nonglycosylated M-CSF in cancer patients stimulates a prominent increase in the number of circulating monocytes.[308] Monocytes induced by M-CSF display enhanced antibody-dependent cellular cytotoxicity, respiratory burst activity, migration, and degranulation and ingestion of *Candida*. The ability of M-CSF to augment intracellular killing of fungal organisms prompted a trial designed to evaluate the ability of M-CSF to enhance recovery from invasive fungal infection in marrow transplant recipients receiving conventional antifungal therapy.[309] The results suggest that M-CSF may be useful in this setting, but further investigation is needed to establish its therapeutic benefit. Administration of glycosylated M-CSF also has been associated with marked reduction in serum cholesterol. Additional studies designed to explore this biologic property should prove informative.

IL-2 can produce antitumor activity by two pathways. Elevated levels of circulating natural killer cells, known as LAK cells, are observed after administration of IL-2. In addition, IL-2–activated lymphocytes produce a variety of secondary cytokines, including IL-1, TNF, and IFN, which in turn may act as immune effector molecules.[310] Clinical studies have evaluated the administration of IL-2 alone, or in combination with LAK cells that were obtained by activating and stimulating lymphocytes from the patient and grown in cell cultures. These trials have demonstrated only modest benefits in patients with renal cell carcinoma and malignant melanoma, and the accompanying toxicities were considerable.[310] At the present time, intensive investigation continues to explore methods to ''prime'' autologous lymphocytes by exposing them to growth factors and cytokines in culture.

FUTURE DIRECTIONS

It is becoming increasingly clear that the regulation of hematopoietic cell development is very delicately controlled by an intricate network of positive and negative regulation. In order to take advantage of this complex cascade and to better affect more complete hematopoietic reconstitution, we more than likely will need to employ a combination of regulatory factors that act at different levels along the pathway of blood cell development. Considerable evidence already exists in vitro to suggest that synergism is achieved when hematopoietic growth factors that control the proliferative state of primitive hematopoietic progenitors and augment enhanced effector cell function are used in combination. The use of these growth factors in combination with purified specific stem cell populations may permit expansion of hematopoietic progenitor cell populations in culture, prior to reinfusion into patients. Together, these approaches hold great promise for enabling even more intensive treatment of cancer, without the risk of bone marrow failure.

REFERENCES

1. Cross M, Dexter TM: Growth factors in development, transformation, and tumorigenesis. Cell *64*:271, 1991
2. Aaronson SA: Growth factors and cancer. Science *254*:1146, 1991
3. Leutz A, Graf T: Relationships between oncogenes and growth control. *In* Sporn MB, Roberts AB (eds): Peptide Growth Factors and Their Receptors, Vol II. Berlin, Springer-Verlag, 1990, pp 655–703
4. Heldin C-H, Westermark B: Growth factors as transforming proteins. Eur J Biochem *184*:487, 1989
5. Varmus H: An historical overview of oncogenes. *In* Weinberg RA (ed): Oncogenes and the Molecular Origins of Cancer. Cold Spring Harbor, NY, Cold Spring Harbor Laboratory Press, 1989, pp 3–44
6. Sporn MB, Roberts AB (eds): Peptide Growth Factors and Their Receptors, Vols I & II. Berlin, Springer-Verlag, 1990
7. Ullrich A, Schlessinger J: Signal transduction by receptors with tyrosine kinase activity. Cell *61*:203, 1990
8. Hunter T: A thousand and one protein kinases. Cell *50*:823, 1987
9. Honegger AM, Kris RM, Ullrich A, Schlessinger J: Evidence that autophosphorylation of solubilized EGF-receptors is mediated by intermolecular cross phosphorylation. Proc Natl Acad Sci USA *86*:925, 1989
10. Carpenter G: Receptors for epidermal growth factor and other polypeptide mitogens. Annu Rev Biochem *56*:881, 1987
11. Carpenter G: Epidermal growth factor. Annu Rev Biochem *48*:193, 1979
12. Fox CF, Das M: Internalization and processing of the EGF receptor in the induction of DNA synthesis in cultured fibroblasts: The endocyte activation hypothesis. J Supramol Struct *10*:199, 1979
13. Marx J: Biologists turn on to ''off-enzymes.'' Science *251*:744, 1991
14. Hunter T: Protein-tyrosine phosphatases: The other side of the coin. Cell *58*:1013, 1989
15. Kreuger NX, Streuli M, Saito H: Structural diversity and evolution of human receptor-like tyrosine phosphatases. EMBO J *9*:3241, 1990
16. Massagué J: Transforming growth factor-α. J Biol Chem *265*:21393, 1990
17. Brachmann R, Lindquist PB, Nagashima M, et al: Transmembrane TGF-α precursors activate EGF/TGF-α receptors. Cell *56*:691, 1989
18. Wong ST, Winchell LF, McCune BK, et al: The TGF-α precursor expressed on the cell surface binds to the EGF receptor on adjacent cells, leading to signal transduction. Cell *56*:495, 1989
19. Anklesaria P, Teixido J, Laiho M, et al: Cell-cell adhesion mediated by binding of membrane-anchored transforming growth factor alpha to epidermal growth factor receptors promotes cell proliferation. Proc Natl Acad Sci USA *87*:3289, 1990
20. DeLarco JE, Todaro GJ: Growth factors from murine sarcoma virus-transformed cells. Proc Natl Acad Sci USA *75*:4001, 1978
21. Sporn MB, Todaro GJ: Autocrine secretion and malignant transformation of cells. N Engl J Med *308*:878, 1980
22. Sporn MB, Todaro GJ: Autocrine growth factors and cancer. Nature *313*:747, 1985
23. Mendelsohn J: Antibodies to growth factors and receptors. *In* DeVita VT Jr, Hellman S, Rosenberg SA (eds): Biologic Therapy of Cancer. Philadelphia, JB Lippincott Company, 1991, pp 601–612
24. Deuel TF: Polypeptide growth factors: Roles in normal and abnormal cell growth. Annu Rev Cell Biol *3*:443, 1987
25. Goustin AS, Leof EB, Shipley GD, Moses HL: Growth factors and cancer. Cancer Res *46*:1015, 1986
26. Cullen KJ, Smith HS, Hill S, et al: Growth factor mRNA expression by human breast fibroblasts from benign and malignant lesions. Cancer Res *51*:4978, 1991
27. Heldin C-H, Westermark B: Platelet-derived growth factor: Mechanism of action and possible in vivo function. Cell Regul *1*:555, 1990
28. Huang JS, Huang SS, Deuel TF: Transforming protein of simian sarcoma virus stimulates autocrine cell growth of SSV-transformed cells through platelet-derived growth factor cell surface receptors. Cell *39*:79, 1984
29. Keating MT, Williams LT: Autocrine stimulation of intracellular PDGF receptors in v-*sis*-transformed cells. Science *239*:914, 1988

30. Hannink M, Donoghue DJ: Autocrine stimulation by the v-*sis* gene product requires a ligand-receptor interaction at the cell surface. J Cell Biol *107*:287, 1988

31. Van de Vijver M, Kumar R, Mendelsohn J: Ligand-induced activation of A431 cell EGF receptors occurs primarily by an autocrine pathway that acts upon receptors on the surface rather than intracellularly. J Biol Chem *266*:7503, 1991

32. Pledger WJ, Stiles CD, Antoniades HN, Scher CD: Induction of DNA synthesis in BALB/c 3T3 cells by serum complements: Reevaluation of the commitment process. Proc Natl Acad Sci USA *74*:4481, 1977

33. Pledger WJ, Stiles CD, Antoniades HN, Scher CD: An ordered sequence of events is required before BALB/c 3T3 cells become committed to DNA synthesis. Proc Natl Acad Sci USA *75*:2839, 1978

34. Pardee AB: G1 events and regulation of cell proliferation. Science *246*:603, 1989

35. Barnes D, Sato G: Serum-free cell culture: A unifying approach. Cell *22*:649, 1980

36. Sato G, Pardee AB, Sibasku D: Growth of cells in hormonally defined media. Cold Spring Harbor Conferences on Cell Proliferation, Vol 9. Cold Spring Harbor, NY, Cold Spring Harbor Laboratory Press, 1982

37. Chinkers M, Cohen S: Purified EGF receptor-kinase interacts specifically with antibodies to Rous sarcoma virus transforming protein. Nature *290*:516, 1981

38. Erikson E, Shealy DJ, Erikson RL: Evidence that viral transforming gene products and epidermal growth factor stimulate phosphorylation of the same cellular protein with similar specificity. J Biol Chem *256*:11381, 1981

39. Cooper JA, Hunter T: Similarities and differences between the effect of epidermal growth factor and Rous sarcoma virus. J Cell Biol *91*:878, 1981

40. Doolittle RF, Hunkapiller MW, Hood LE, et al: Simian sarcoma virus oncogene, v-*sis*, is derived from the gene (or genes) encoding a platelet-derived growth factor. Science *221*:275, 1983

41. Waterfield MD, Scrace GT, Whittle N, et al: Platelet-derived growth factor is structurally related to the putative transforming protein p28^sis of simian sarcoma virus. Nature *304*:35, 1983

42. Downward J, Yarden Y, Mayes E, et al: Close similarity of epidermal growth factor receptor and v-*erb*-B oncogene protein sequences. Nature *307*:521, 1984

43. Young-Hua X, Ishii S, Clark AJL, et al: Human epidermal growth factor receptor cDNA is homologous to a variety of RNAs overproduced in A431 carcinoma cells. Nature *309*:806, 1984

44. Lin CR, Chen WS, Kruiger W, et al: Expression cloning of human EGF receptor complementary DNA: Gene amplification and three related messenger RNA products in A431 cells. Science *224*:843, 1984

45. Sherr CJ, Rettenmeier CW, Sacca R, et al: The c-*fms* proto-oncogene product is related to the receptor for the mononuclear phagocyte growth factor, CSF-1. Cell *41*:665, 1985

46. Stern DF, Heffernan PA, Weinberg RA: p185^HER2, a product of the *neu* proto-oncogene, is a receptor-like protein associated with tyrosine kinase activity. Mol Cell Biol *6*:1729, 1986

47. Sandgren EP, Luetteke NC, Palmiter RD, et al: Overexpression of TGF α in transgenic mice: Induction of epithelial hyperplasia, pancreatic metaplasia, and carcinoma of the breast. Cell *61*:1121, 1990

48. Jhappan C, Stahle C, Harkins RN, et al: TGF α overexpression in transgenic mice induces liver neoplasia and abnormal development of the mammary gland and pancreas. Cell *61*:1147, 1990

49. Matsui Y, Halter SA, Holt JT, et al: Development of mammary hyperplasia and neoplasia in MMTV-TGF α transgenic mice. Cell *61*:1147, 1990

50. Slamon DJ, Godolphin W, Jones LA, et al: Studies of the HER-2/*neu* proto-oncogene in human breast and ovarian cancer. Science *244*:707, 1989

51. Wright C, Angus B, Nicholson S, et al: Expression of c-*erb*B-2 oncoprotein: A prognostic indicator in human breast cancer. Cancer Res *49*:2087, 1989

52. King Cr, Swain SM, Porter L, et al: Heterogeneous expression of *erb*B-2 messenger RNA in human breast cancer. Cancer Res *49*:4185, 1989

53. Van de Vijver MJ, Peterse JL, Mooi WJ, et al: *Neu*-protein overexpression in breast cancer: Association with comedo-type ductal carcinoma in situ and limited prognostic value in Stage II breast cancer. N Engl J Med *319*:1239, 1988

54. Gullick WJ: The role of the epidermal growth factor receptor and the c-*erb*B-2 protein in breast cancer. Int J Cancer Suppl *5*:55, 1990

55. Harris AL, Nicholson S, Sainsbury JRC, et al: Epidermal growth factor receptor: A marker of early relapse in breast cancer and tumor stage progression in bladder cancer; interactions with *neu*. In Furth M, Greaves M (eds): The Molecular Diagnostics of Human Cancer, Vol 7. Cold Spring Harbor, NY, Cold Spring Harbor Laboratory Press, 1989, pp 353–357

56. Sainsbury JRC, Malcolm AJ, Appleton DR, et al: Presence of epidermal growth factor receptor as an indicator of poor prognosis in patients with breast cancer. J Clin Pathol *38*:1225, 1985

57. Neal DE, Bennett MK, Hall RR, et al: Epidermal growth factor receptors in human bladder cancer: Comparison of invasive and superficial tumors. Lancet *1*:366, 1985

58. Hendler F, Shum-Siu A, Nanu L, et al: Increased EGF receptors and the absence of an alveolar differentiation marker predict a poor survival in lung cancer. Proc Am Soc Clin Oncol *8*:223 (abstract 869), 1989

59. Veale D, Ashcroft T, Marsh C, et al: Epidermal growth factor receptors in non-small cell lung cancer. Br J Cancer *55*:513, 1987

60. Cohen S: Isolation of a mouse submaxillary gland protein accelerating incisor eruption and eyelid opening in the new born animal. J Biol Chem *237*:1555, 1962

61. Carpenter G, Wahl MI: The epidermal growth factor family. In Sporn MB, Roberts AB (eds): Peptide Growth Factors and Their Receptors, Vol I. Berlin, Springer-Verlag, 1990, pp 69–171

62. Anzano M, Roberts AB, Meyers CA, et al: Sarcoma growth factor from conditioned medium of virally transformed cells is composed of both type alpha and type beta transforming growth factors. Proc Natl Acad Sci USA *80*:6264, 1983

63. Thorburn GD, Waters MJ, Dolling M, Young IR: Fetal maturation and epidermal growth factor. Proc Aust Phys Pharmacol Soc *12*:11, 1981

64. Shoyab M, Plowman GD, McDonald VL, et al: Structure and function of human amphiregulin: A member of the epidermal growth factor family. Science *243*:1074, 1989

65. Rosenthal A, Lindquist PB, Bringman TS, et al: Expression in rat fibroblasts of a human transforming growth factor-alpha cDNA results in transformation. Cell *46*:301, 1986

66. Riedel H, Massoglia S, Schlessinger J, Ullrich A: Ligand activation of overexpressed epidermal growth factor receptors transforms NIH 3T3 mouse fibroblasts. Proc Natl Acad Sci USA *85*:1477, 1988

67. Di Fiore PP, Pierce JH, Fleming TP, et al: Overexpression of the human EGF receptor confers an EGF-dependent transformed phenotype to NIH 3T3 cells. Cell *51*:1063, 1987

68. Velu TJ, Beguinot L, Vass WC, et al: Epidermal growth factor-dependent transformation by a human EGF receptor proto-oncogene. Science *238*:1408, 1987

69. Ozanne B, Richards CS, Hendler F, et al: Over-expression of the EGF receptor is a hallmark of squamous cell carcinomas. J Pathol *149*:9, 1986

70. Sobol RE, Astarita RW, Hofeditz C, et al: EGF receptor expression in human lung carcinomas defined by a monoclonal antibody. J Natl Cancer Inst *79*:403, 1987

71. Veale D, Kerr N, Gibson GH, Harris AL: Characterization of epidermal growth factor receptor in primary human non-small cell lung cancer. Cancer Res *49*:1313, 1989

72. Libermann TA, Razon N, Bartal AD, et al: Expression of epidermal growth factor receptors in human brain tumors. Cancer Res *44*:753, 1984

73. Eisbruch A, Blick M, Lee JS, et al: Analysis of the epidermal

growth factor receptor gene in fresh human head and neck tumors. Cancer Res 47:3603, 1984

74. Humphrey PA, Wong AJ, Vogelstein B, et al: Anti-synthetic peptide antibody reacting at the fusion junction of deletion-mutant epidermal growth factor receptors in human glioblastoma. Proc Natl Acad Sci USA 87:4207, 1990

75. Derynck R, Goeddel DV, Ullrich A, et al: Synthesis of messenger RNAs for transforming growth factors α and β and the epidermal growth factor receptor by human tumors. Cancer Res 47:707, 1987

76. Davidson NE, Gelmann EP, Lippman ME, Dickson RB: Epidermal growth factor receptor gene expression in estrogen receptor-positive and negative human breast cancer cell lines. Mol Endocrinol 1:216, 1987

77. Bates SE, Davidson NE, Valverius EM, et al: Expression of transforming growth factor-α and its messenger ribonucleic acid in human breast cancer: Its regulation by estrogen and its possible functional significance. Mol Endocrinol 2:543, 1988

78. Ciardiello F, Kim N, Liscia DS, et al: mRNA expression of transforming growth factor-α in human breast carcinomas and its activity in effusions of breast cancer patients. J Natl Cancer Inst 81:1165, 1989

79. Dickson RB, Bates SE, McManaway ME, Lippman ME: Characterization of estrogen responsive transforming activity in human breast cancer cell lines. Cancer Res 46:1707, 1986

80. Dickson RB, Huff KK, Spencer EM, Lippman ME: Induction of epidermal growth factor-related polypeptides by 17β-estradiol in MCF-7 human breast cancer cells. Endocrinology 118:138, 1985

81. Vonderhaar BK: Local effects of EGF, α-GF and EGF-like growth factors on lobuloalveolar development of the mouse mammary gland in vivo. J Cell Physiol 132:581, 1987

82. Travers MT, Barrett-Lee PJ, Berger U, et al: Growth factor expression in normal, benign, and malignant breast tissue. BMJ 296:1621, 1988

83. Fitzpatrick SL, LaChance MP, Schultz GS: Characterization of epidermal growth factor receptor and action on human breast cancer cells in culture. Cancer Res 44:3442, 1984

84. Valverius EM, Bates SE, Stampfer ME, et al: Transforming growth factor-α production and epidermal growth factor receptor expression in normal and oncogene transformed human mammary epithelial cells. Mol Endocrinol 3:203, 1989

85. Nicholson S, Halcrow P, Farndon JR, et al: Expression of epidermal growth factor receptors associated with lack of response to endocrine therapy in recurrent breast cancer. Lancet 1:182, 1989

86. Ciardiello F, McGeady ML, Kim N, et al: TGF-α expression is enhanced in human mammary epithelial cells transformed by an activated c-Ha-ras proto-oncogene but not by the c-neu proto-oncogene and overexpression of the TGF-α cDNA leads to transformation. Cell Growth Differ 1:407, 1990

87. Markowitz SD, Molkentin K, Gerbic C, et al: Growth stimulation by coexpression of transforming growth factor α and epidermal growth factor-receptor in normal and adenomatous human colon epithelium. J Clin Invest 86:356, 1990

88. Karnes WE Jr, Walsh JH, Wu SV, et al: Autocrine stimulation of EGF receptors by TGF-α regulates autonomous proliferation of human colon cancer cells. Gastroenterology 102:474, 1992

89. Reiss M, Stash EB, Vellucci VF: Activation of the autocrine transforming growth factor alpha pathway in human squamous carcinoma cells. Cancer Res 51:6254, 1991

90. Lee M, Kris RM, Bellot F, et al: EGF receptor monoclonal antibodies inhibit the growth on non-small cell lung cancer in vitro and in vivo. Proc Am Assoc Cancer Res 31:41 (abstract 243), 1990

91. Imanish K, Yamaguchi K, Kuranami M, et al: Inhibition of growth of human lung adenocarcinoma cell lines by anti-transforming growth factor-α monoclonal antibody. J Natl Cancer Inst 81:220, 1989

92. Kawamoto T, Sato JD, Le A, et al: Growth stimulation of A431 cells by EGF: Identification of high affinity receptors for epidermal growth factor by an anti-receptor monoclonal antibody. Proc Natl Acad Sci USA 80:1337, 1983

93. Sato JD, Kawamoto T, Le AD, et al: Biological effect in vitro of monoclonal antibodies to human EGF receptors. Mol Biol Med 1:511, 1983

94. Rodeck U, Herlyn M, Herlyn D, et al: Tumor growth modulation by a monoclonal antibody to the epidermal growth factor receptor: Immunologically mediated and effector cell-independent effects. Cancer Res 47:3692, 1987

95. Rodeck U, Williams N, Murthy U, Herlyn M: Monoclonal antibody 425 inhibits growth stimulation of carcinoma cells by exogenous EGF and tumor-derived EGF/TGF-α. J Cell Biochem 44:69, 1990

96. Aboud-Pirak E, Hurwitz E, Pirak ME, et al: Efficacy of antibodies to epidermal growth factor receptor against KB carcinoma in vitro and in nude mice. J Natl Cancer Inst 80:1605, 1988

97. Mendelsohn J: Potential clinical applications of anti-EGF receptor monoclonal antibodies. In Furth M, Greaves M (eds): The Molecular Diagnostics of Human Cancer, Vol 7. Cold Spring Harbor, NY, Cold Spring Harbor Laboratory Press, 1989, pp 359–362

98. Masui H, Boman B, Hyman J, et al: Treatment with anti-EGF receptor monoclonal antibody causes regression of DiFi human colorectal carcinoma xenografts. Proc Am Assoc Cancer Res 32:394 (abstract 2340), 1991

99. Brady LW, Woo DV, Marko A, et al: Treatment of malignant gliomas with ^{125}I-labeled monoclonal antibody against epidermal growth factor receptor. Antibody Immunoconjugates and Radiopharmaceuticals 3:169, 1990

100. Kalofonos HP, Pawlikowska TR, Hemingway A, et al: Antibody guided diagnosis and therapy of brain gliomas using radiolabeled monoclonal antibodies against epidermal growth factor receptor and placental alkaline phosphatase. J Nucl Med 30:1636, 1989

101. Divgi CR, Welt C, Kris M, et al: Phase I and imaging trial of indium-111 labeled anti-EGF receptor monoclonal antibody 225 in patients with squamous cell lung carcinoma. J Natl Cancer Inst 83:97, 1991

102. Schecter AL, Stern DF, Vaidyanathan L, Decker SJ: The neu oncogene: An erbB-related gene encoding a 185,000 Mr tumour antigen. Nature 312:513, 1984

103. Huziak RM, Schlessinger J, Ullrich A: Increased expression of the putative growth factor receptor p 185 (HER2) causes transformation and tumorigenesis of NIH3T3 cells. Proc Natl Acad Sci USA 84:7159, 1987

104. Fukushige SI, Matsubaru K, Yoshida M: Localization of a novel v-erbB-related gene, c-erbB-2, on chromosome-17 and its amplification in a gastric cell line. Mol Cell Biol 6:955, 1986

105. Lupu R, Colomer R, Zugmaier G, et al: Direct interaction of a ligand for the erbB2 oncogene product with the EGF receptor and p185erbB2. Science 249:1552, 1990

106. Kumar R, Shephard HM, Mendelsohn J: Regulation of phosphorylation of the c-erbB-2/HER2 gene product by a monoclonal antibody and serum growth factor(s) in human mammary carcinoma cells. Mol Cell Biol 11:979, 1991

107. Stern DF, Kamps MP: EGF-stimulated tyrosine phosphorylation of p185neu: A potential model for receptor interactions. EMBO J 7:995, 1988

108. Peles E, Bacus SS, Koski RA, et al: Isolation of the neu/HER-2 stimulatory ligand: A 44 kd glycoprotein that induces differentiation of mammary tumor cells. Cell 69:205, 1992

109. Holmes WE, Sliwkowski MX, Akita RW, et al: Identification of heregulin, a specific activator of p185erbB2. Science 256:1205, 1992

110. Lupu R, Colomer R, Kannan B, Lippman ME: Characterization of a growth factor that binds exclusively to the erbB2 receptor and induces cellular responses. Proc Natl Acad Sci USA 89:2287, 1992

110a. Carraway KL, Sliwkowski MX, Akita R, et al: The erbB3 gene product is a receptor for heregulin. J Biol Chem 269:14303, 1994

110b. Plowman GD, Green JM, Culouscou J-M, et al: Heregulin induces tyrosine phosphorylation of HER4/p180^{erbB4}. Nature 366:473, 1993

110c. Sliwkowski MX, Schaefer G, Akita R, et al: Coexpression of *erbB2* and *erbB3* proteins reconstitutes a high affinity receptor for heregulin. J Biol Chem *269*:14661, 1994

111. Hancock MC, Langton BC, Chan T, et al: A monoclonal antibody against c-*erb*B2 protein enhances the cytotoxicity of cis-diaminine dichoroplatinum against human breast and ovarian tumor cell lines. Cancer Res *51*:4575, 1991

112. Hudziak R, Lewis G, Winget M, et al: pl85HER2 monoclonal antibody has antiproliferative effects in vitro and sensitizes human breast tumor cells to tumor necrosis factor. Mol Cell Biol *9*:1165, 1989

113. Drebin J, Link V, Stern D, et al: Down-modulation of an oncogene protein product and reversion of the transformed phenotype by monoclonal antibodies. Cell *41*:695, 1985

114. Raines EW, Bowen-Pope DF, Ross R: Platelet-derived growth factor. *In* Sporn MB, Roberts AB (eds): Peptide Growth Factors and Their Receptors, Vol I. Berlin, Springer-Verlag, 1990, pp 174–262

115. Ross R: The pathogenesis of atherosclerosis: An update. N Engl J Med *314*:488, 1986

116. Clarke MF, Westin E, Schmidt D, et al: Transformation of NIH 3T3 cells by a human c-*sis* cDNA clone. Nature *308*:464, 1984

117. Gazit A, Igarashi H, Chiu I-M, et al: Expression of the normal human *sis*/PDGF-2 coding sequence induces cellular transformation. Cell *39*:80, 1984

118. Beckmann MP, Betsholtz C, Heldin C-H, et al: Human PDGF-A and -B chains differ in their biological properties and transforming potential. Science *241*:1346, 1988

119. Rozengurt E, Sinnett-Smith J, Taylor-Papadimitriou J: Production of PDGF-like growth factor by breast cancer cell lines. Int J Cancer *36*:247, 1985

120. Salmon WD, Daughaday WH: A hormonally controlled serum factor which stimulates sulfate incorporation by cartilage in vitro. J Lab Clin Med *49*:825, 1957

121. Humbel RE: Insulin-like growth factors, somatomedins, and multiplication-stimulating activity: Chemistry. *In* Li CH (ed): Hormonal Proteins and Peptides, Vol 12. New York, Academic Press, 1984, p 57

122. Morgan DO, Roth RA: Acute insulin action requires insulin receptor kinase activity: Introduction of an inhibitory monoclonal antibody into mammalian cells blocks the rapid effects of insulin. Proc Natl Acad Sci USA *84*:41, 1987

123. Baxter RC, Martin JL: Binding proteins for the insulin-like growth factors: Structure, regulation and function. Prog Growth Factor Res *1*:49, 1989

124. Yee D, Paik S, Lebovic G, et al: Analysis of IGF-I gene expression in malignancy—evidence for a paracrine role in human breast cancer. Mol Endocrinol *3*:509, 1989

125. Cullen KJ, Yee D, Sly WS, et al: Insulin-like growth factor receptor expression and function in human breast cancer. Cancer Res *50*:48, 1990

126. Osborne CK, Coronado EB, Kitten LJ, et al: Insulin-like growth factor-II (IGF-II): A potential autocrine/paracrine growth factor for human breast cancer acting via the IGF-I receptor. Mol Endocrinol *3*:1701, 1989

127. Burgess W, Maciag T: The heparin-binding (fibroblast) growth factor family of proteins. Annu Rev Biochem *58*:575, 1989

128. Baird A, Walicke PA: Fibroblast growth factors. Br Med Bull *45*:438, 1989

129. Gospodarowicz D, Cheng J, Lui GM, et al: Isolation of brain fibroblast growth factor by heparin-Sepharose affinity chromatography: Identity with pituitary fibroblast growth factor. Proc Natl Acad Sci USA *81*:6963, 1984

130. Baird A, Klagsbrun M: The fibroblast growth factor family: An overview. Ann NY Acad Sci *638*:xi, 1991

131. Folkman J, Klagsbrun M: Angiogenic factors. Science *235*:442, 1987

132. Weidner N, Semple J, Welch W, Folkman J: Tumor angiogenesis correlates with metastasis in invasive breast carcinoma. N Engl J Med *324*:108, 1991

133. Coffey R, Leci E, Shipley G, Moses H: Suramin inhibition of growth factor receptor binding and mitogenicity in AKR-2B cells. J Cell Physiol *132*:143, 1987

134. Myers C, Cooper M, Stein CA, et al: Suramin: A novel growth factor antagonist with activity in hormone-refractory metastatic prostate cancer. J Clin Oncol *10*:881, 1992

135. Ingber D, Fujita T, Kishimoto S, et al: Synthetic analogs of fumagillin that inhibit angiogenesis and suppress tumor growth. Nature *348*:555, 1990

136. Lebacq-Verheyden A-M, Trepel J, Sausville EA, Battey JF: Bombesin and gastrin-releasing peptide: Neuropeptides, secretogogues, and growth factors. *In* Sporn MB, Roberts AB (eds): Peptide Growth Factors and Their Receptors, Vol II. Berlin, Springer-Verlag, 1990, pp 71–124

137. Carney DN, Bunn PA, Gazdar AF, et al: Selective growth in serum-free hormone-supplemented medium of tumor cells obtained by biopsy from patients with small cell carcinoma of the lung. Proc Natl Acad Sci USA *78*:3186, 1981

138. Cuttitta F, Carney DN, Mulshine J, et al: Bombesin-like peptides can function as autocrine growth factors in human small-cell lung cancer. Nature *316*:823, 1985

139. Rozengurt E, Sinnett-Smith J: Bombesin stimulation of DNA synthesis and cell division in cultures of Swiss 3T3 cells. Proc Natl Acad Sci USA *80*:2936, 1983

140. Massagué J: The transforming growth factor-β family. Annu Rev Cell Biol *6*:597, 1990

141. Sporn MB, Roberts AB: Transforming growth factor-β: Multiple actions and potential clinical applications. JAMA *262*: 938, 1989

142. Lyons RM, Moses HL: Transforming growth factors and the regulation of cell proliferation. Eur J Biochem *187*:467, 1990

143. Derynck R, Jarrett JA, Chen EY, et al: Human transforming growth factor-β complementary DNA sequence and expression in normal and transformed cells. Nature *316*:701, 1985

144. Assoian RK, Komoriya A, Meyers CA, et al: Transforming growth factor-β in human platelets. J Biol Chem *258*:7155, 1983

145. Gentry LE, Lioubin MN, Purchio AP, Marquardt H: Molecular events in the processing of recombinant type 1 pre-pro-transforming growth factor beta to the mature polypeptide. Mol Cell Biol *8*:4162, 1988

146. Mathews LS, Vale WW: Expression cloning of an activin receptor, a predicted transmembrane serine kinase. Cell *65*.: 973, 1991

147. Attisano L, Wrana JL, Cheifetz S, Massagué J: Novel activin receptors: Distinct genes and alternative mRNA splicing generate a repertoire of serine/threonine kinase receptors. Cell *68*:97, 1992

148. Lin HY, Wang X-F, Ng-Eaton E, et al: Expression cloning of the TGF-β type II receptor, a functional transmembrane serine/threonine kinase. Cell *68*:775, 1992

148a. Massagué J, Attisano L, Wrana JL: The TGF-β family and its composite receptors. Trends in Cell Biology *4*:172, 1994

149. Kimchi A, Wang X-F, Weinberg RA, et al: Absence of TGF-β receptors and growth inhibitory responses in retinoblastoma cells. Science *240*:196, 1988

150. Shipley GD, Tucker RF, Moses HL: Type β-transforming growth factor/growth inhibitor stimulates entry of monolayer cultures of AKR-2B cells into S-phase after prolonged prereplicative interval. Proc Natl Acad Sci USA *82*:4147, 1985

151. Laiho M, DeCaprio JA, Ludlow JW, et al: Growth inhibition by TGF-β linked to suppression of retinoblastoma protein phosphorylation. Cell *62*:175, 1990

152. Kehrl JH, Wakefield LM, Roberts AB, et al: Production of transforming growth factor beta by human T lymphocytes and its potential role in the regulation of T cell growth. J Exp Med *163*:1037, 1986

153. Leof EB, Proper JA, Goustin AS, et al: Induction of c-*sis* mRNA and activity similar to platelet-derived growth factor β: A proposed model for indirect mitogenesis involving autocrine activity. Proc Natl Acad Sci USA *83*:2453, 1986

154. Pietenpol JA, Stein RW, Moran E, et al: TGF-β1 inhibition of c-myc transcription and growth in keratinocytes is abrogated by viral transforming proteins with pRB binding domains. Cell *61*:777, 1990

155. Vale W, Hsueh A, Rivier C, Yu J: The inhibin/activin family of hormones and growth factors. *In* Sporn MB, Roberts AB (eds): Peptide Growth Factors and Their Receptors, Vol II. Berlin, Springer-Verlag, 1990, pp 211–248

156. Burger HG, Igarashi M: Inhibin: Definition and nomenclature, including related substances [letter to the editor]. J Clin Endocrinol Metab 66:885, 1988

157. Cate RL, Donahoe PK, MacLaughlin DT: Müllerian-inhibiting substance. In Sporn MB, Roberts AB (eds): Peptide Growth Factors and Their Receptors, Vol II. Berlin, Springer-Verlag, 1990, pp 179–210

158. Donohoe PK, Fuller AF Jr, Scully RE, et al: Müllerian inhibiting substance inhibits growth of a human ovarian cancer in nude mice. Ann Surg 194:472, 1981

159. Fuller AF Jr, Guy SR, Budzik GP, Donohoe PK: Müllerian-inhibiting substance inhibits colony growth of a human ovarian carcinoma cell line. J Clin Endocrinol Metab 54:1051, 1982

160. Isaacs A, Lindenmann J: Virus interference. I. The interferon. Proc R Soc Lond [Biol] 147:258, 1957

161. Vilček J: Interferons. In Sporn MB, Roberts AB (eds): Peptide Growth Factors and Their Receptors, Vol II. Berlin, Springer-Verlag, 1990, pp 3–38

162. Sen GC, Lengyel P: The interferon system. J Biol Chem 267:5017, 1992

162a. Darnell Jr JE, Kerr IM, Stark GR: Jak-STAT pathways and transcriptional activation in response to IFNs and other extracellular signalling proteins. Science 264:1415, 1994

163. Chebath J, Benech P, Hovanessian A, et al: Four different forms of interferon-induced 2′,5′-oligo(a) synthetase identified by immunoblotting in human cells. J Biol Chem 262:3852, 1987

164. Old LJ: Tumor necrosis factor. Sci Am 258:59, 1988

165. Beutler B: Cachetin/tumor necrosis factor and lymphotoxin. In Sporn MB, Roberts AB (eds): Peptide Growth Factors and Their Receptors, Vol II. Berlin, Springer-Verlag, 1990, pp 39–70

166. Spriggs DR: Tumor necrosis factor: Basic principles and preclinical studies. In DeVita VT Jr, Hellman S, Rosenberg SA (eds): Biologic Therapy of Cancer. Philadelphia, JB Lippincott Company, 1991, pp 354–377

166a. Smith CA, Farrah T, Goodwin RG: The TNF receptor superfamily of cellular and viral proteins: Activation, costimulation, and death. Cell 76:959, 1994

167. Welte K, Platzer E, Lu L, et al: Purification and biochemical characterization of human pluripotent hematopoietic colony stimulating factor. Proc Natl Acad Sci USA 82:1526, 1985

168. Souza LM, Boone TC, Gabrilove J, et al: Recombinant pluripotent human granulocyte colony stimulating factor: Effects on normal and leukemic myeloid cells. Science 232:61, 1986

169. Zsebo KM, Cohen AM, Murdock DC, et al: Recombinant human granulocyte colony stimulating factor: Molecular and biological characterization. Immunobiology 172:175, 1986

170. Nagata S, Tsuchinya M, Asano S, et al: Molecular cloning and expression of cDNA for human granulocyte colony stimulating factor. Nature 319:415, 1986

171. Platzer E, Welte K, Gabrilove J, et al: Biological activities of a human pluripotent hematopoietic colony stimulating factor on normal and leukemic cells. J Exp Med 162:1788, 1985

172. Strife A, Lambeck C, Wisniewski D, et al: Activities of four purified growth factors on highly enriched human hematopoietic progenitor cells. Blood 69:1508, 1987

173. McNiece IK, McGrath HE, Quesenberry PJ: Granulocyte colony stimulating factor augments in vitro megakaryocyte colony stimulating formation by interleukin-3. Exp Hematol 16:807, 1988

174. Platzer E, Oez S, Welte K, et al: Human pluripotent hematopoietic colony stimulating factor: Activities on human and murine cells. Immunobiology 172:185, 1986

175. Gasson JC, Weisbart RH, Kaufman S, et al: Purified human granulocyte macrophage colony stimulating factor: Direct action on neutrophils. Science 226:1339, 1984

176. Wong GG, Witek JS, Temple PA, et al: Human GM-CSF: Molecular cloning of complementary DNA and purification of the natural and recombinant proteins. Science 228:810, 1985

177. Metcalf D, Begley CG, Johnson GR: Biologic properties in vitro of a recombinant human granulocyte-macrophage colony stimulating factor. Blood 67:37, 1986

178. Lopez AF, Williamson J, Gamble JR, et al: Recombinant human granulocyte-macrophage colony-stimulating factor stimulates in vitro mature human neutrophil and eosinophil function, m-surface receptor expression and survival. J Clin Invest 78:1220, 1986

179. Arnaout MA, Wang EA, Clark SC, Sieff CA: Human recombinant granulocyte-macrophage colony-stimulating factor increases cell-to-cell adhesion and surface expression of adhesion-promoting surface glycoproteins on mature granulocytes. J Clin Invest 78:597, 1986

180. Peters WP, Stuart A, Affronti ML, et al: Neutrophil migration is defective during recombinant human granulocyte-macrophage colony stimulating factor infusion after autologous bone marrow transplantation in humans. Blood 72:1310, 1988

181. Rettenmier CW, Sherr CJ: Hematol Oncol Clin North Am 3:479, 1988

182. Griffin JD: Clinical applications of colony stimulating factors. Oncology 2:15, 1988

183. Lun FK, Sygs S, Lun CH, et al: Cloning and expression of the human EPO gene. Proc Natl Acad Sci USA 82:7580, 1985

184. Graber SE, Krantz SB: Erythropoietin: Biology and clinical use. Hematol/Oncol Clin North Am 3:369, 1989

185. Dinarello CA: Biology of interleukin-1. FASEB J 2:108, 1988

186. Bradley EC, Grimm E: Interleukins. In Hollan JF, Frei E, Bast RC, et al (eds): Cancer Medicine. Philadelphia, Lea & Febinger, 1993, pp 941–948

187. Ihle JN, Keller J, Henderson L, et al: Procedures for the purification of interleukin-3 to homogeneity. J Immunol 129:2431, 1982

188. Yang C, Claretta AB, Temple PA, et al: Human IL-3: Identification by expression cloning of a novel hematopoietic growth factor related to murine IL-3. Cell 47:3, 1986

189. Leary AG, Yang YC, Clark SC, et al: Recombinant gibbon IL-3 supports function of human multilineage colonies and blast cell colonies in culture: Comparison with human granulocyte macrophage colony stimulating factors. Blood 70:1343, 1987

190. Peschel C, Paul WE, O'Hara J, Green J: Effects of B-cell stimulatory factor-1 + interleukin-4 on hematopoietic progenitor cells. Blood 70:254, 1987

191. Sanderson CJ, Warren DJ, Stich M: Identification of a lymphokine that stimulates eosinophil differentiation in vitro. J Exp Med 16:60, 1985

192. Kishimoto T: The biology of interleukin-6. Blood 74:1, 1989

193. Muraguchi A, Kishimoto T, Miki Y, et al: T cell replacing factor (TRF). J Immunol 127:412, 1987

194. Leary AG, Ikebuchi K, Herai Y, et al: Synergism between IL-6 and IL-3 in supporting proliferation of human hematopoietic stem cells: Comparison with IL-1. Blood 71:1759, 1988

195. Anderson DM, Lyman S, Baird A, et al: Molecular cloning of mast cell growth factor, a hemopoietin that is active in both membrane bound and soluble forms. Cell 63:235, 1990

196. Williams DE, Eisenman J, Baird A, et al: Identification of a ligand for the c-kit proto-oncogene. Cell 63:167, 1990

197. Zsebo K, Wypych J, McNiece I, et al: Identification, purification and biological characterization of hematopoietic stem cell factor from buffalo rat liver-conditioned medium. Cell 63:195, 1990

198. Nocka H, Huang E, Beier DR, et al: The hematopoietic growth factor KL is encoded by the S1 locus and is the ligand of the c-kit receptor, the gene product of the W locus. Cell 63:225, 1990

199. Martin FH, Suggs S, Langley K, et al: Primary structure and functional expression of rat and human stem cell factor DNAs. Cell 63:203, 1990

200. Flanagan JG, Leder P: The kit ligand: A cell surface molecule altered in steel mutant fibroblasts. Cell 63:185, 1990

201. Bernstein ID, Andrews RG, Zsebo KM: Recombinant human stem cell factor enhances the formation of colonies by CD34+ and CD34+lin− cells, and the generation of colony forming cell progeny from CD34+lin− cells cultured with interleukin-3, granulocyte colony stimulating factor or granulocyte-macrophage colony-stimulating factor. Blood 77:2316, 1991

202. McNiece I, Langley K, Zsebo K: Recombinant human stem cell

facotr (rhSCF) synergizes with GM-CSF, G-CSF, IL-3 and Epo to stimulate human progenitor cells of the myeloid and erythroid lineages. Exp Hematol 19:226, 1991

203. Kacmauski RS, Mufti GJ: The cytokine receptor superfamily. Blood Rev 5:193, 1991

203a. Cosman D: The hematopoietic receptor superfamily. Cytokine 5:95, 1993

204. Taga T, Kishimoto T: Cytokine receptors and signal transduction. FASEB J 6:3387, 1992

205. Touw I, Pouwels K, Agtoven TY, et al: Interleukin-7 is a growth factor of precursor B and T acute lymphoblastic leukemia. Blood 75:2097, 1990

206. Lange B, Valtieri M, Santoli D, et al: Growth factor requirements of childhood acute leukemia: Establishment of GM-CSF dependent cell lines. Blood 70:192, 1987

207. Miyauchi J, Kelleher CA, Yang Y-C, et al: The effects of three recombinant growth factors, IL-3, GM-CSF and G-CSF, on blast cells of acute myeloblastic leukemia maintained in short term suspension culture. Blood 70:657, 1987

208. Kelleher C, Miyauchi J, Wong G, et al: Synergism between recombinant growth factors, GM-CSF and G-CSF, acting on the blast cells of acute myeloblastic leukemia. Blood 69:1498, 1987

209. Griffin JD, Rambaldi A, Vallenga E, et al: Secretion of interleukin-1 by acute myeloblastic leukemia cells in vitro induces endothelial cells to secrete colony stimulating factors. Blood 70:1218, 1987

210. Griffin JD, Young DC, Herrmann D, et al: Effects of recombinant human GM-CSF on proliferation of clonogenic cells in acute myeloblastic leukemia. Blood 67:1448, 1986

211. Le Bousse-Kerdiles M-C, Souyri M, Smadja-Joffe F, et al: Enhanced hematopoietic growth factor production in an experimental myeloproliferative syndrome. Blood 79:3179, 1992

212. Johnson GR, Gonda TJ, Metcalf D, et al: A lethal myeloproliferative syndrome in mice transplanted with bone marrow cells infected with a retrovirus expressing granulocyte-macrophage colony-stimulating factor. EMBO J 8:441, 1989

213. Wong PMC, Chung S-W, Dunbar CE, et al: Retrovirus-mediated transfer and expression of the interleukin-3 gene in mouse hematopoietic cells result in a myeloproliferative disorder. Mol Cell Biol 9:798, 1989

214. Dai CH, Krantz SB, Dessypris EN, et al: Polycythemia vera. II. Hypersensitivity of bone marrow erythroid, granulocyte-macrophage and megakaryocyte progenitor cells to interleukin-3 and granulocyte-macrophage colony-stimulating factor. Blood 80:891, 1992

215. Lord BI, Molineux G, Pojda Z, et al: Myeloid cell kinetics in mice treated with recombinant interleukin-3, granulocyte-macrophage CSF in vivo. Blood 77:2154, 1991

216. Welte K, Bonilla MA, Gillio AP, et al: Recombinant G-CSF: Effects on hematopoiesis in normal and cyclophosphamide treated primates. J Exp Med 165:941, 1987

217. Welte K, Bonilla MA, Gillio AP, et al: In vivo effects of recombinant human G-CSF in therapy induced neutropenias in primates. Exp Hematol 15:72, 1987

218. Gillio AP, Bonilla MA, Potter GK, et al: Effects of recombinant human granulocyte colony stimulating factor on hematopoietic reconstitution following autologous transplantation in primates. Transplant Proc XIX(suppl 7):153, 1988

219. Schuening FG, Storb R, Goehle A, et al: Recombinant human granulocyte colony-stimulating factor accelerates hematopoietic recovery after DLA-identical littermate marrow transplants in dogs. Blood 76:636, 1990

220. Gabrilove JL, Jakubowski A, Fain K, et al: Phase I study of granulocyte colony-stimulating factor in patients with transitional cell carcinoma of the urothelium. J Clin Invest 82:1454, 1988

221. Morstyn G, Souza LM, Keech J, et al: Effects of granulocyte colony-stimulating factor on neutropenia induced by cytotoxic chemotherapy. Lancet 1:667, 1988

222. Bronchud MH, Potter MR, Morgenstern G, et al: In vitro and in vivo analysis of the effects of recombinant human granulocyte colony-stimulating factor in patients receiving intensive chemotherapy for small cell lung cancer. Br J Cancer 58:64, 1988

223. Duhren U, Villeval JL, Boyd J, et al: Effects of recombinant human granulocyte colony-stimulating factor on hematopoietic progenitor cells in cancer patients. Blood 72:2074, 1988

224. Gabrilove JL, Jakubowski A, Scher H, et al: Granulocyte colony stimulating factor reduces neutropenia and associated morbidity of chemotherapy for transitional cell carcinoma of the urothelium. N Engl J Med 318:1414, 1988

225. Bronchud MH, Scarffe JH, Thatcher N, et al: Phase I/II study of recombinant human granulocyte colony-stimulating factor in patients receiving intensive chemotherapy for small cell lung cancer. Br J Cancer 56:809, 1987

226. Morstyn G, Campbell I, Lieschke G, et al: Treatment of chemotherapy-induced neutropemia by subcutaneously administered granulocyte colony-stimulating factor with optimization of dose and duration of therapy. J Clin Oncol 7:1554, 1989

227. Crawford J, Ozer H, Stoller R, et al: Reduction by granulocyte colony-stimulating factor of fever and neutropenia induced by chemotherapy in patients with small cell lung cancer. N Engl J Med 325:164, 1991

228. Trillet Lenoir V, Green J, Manegold C, et al: Recombinant granulocyte colony-stimulating factor reduces the infectious complications of cytotoxic chemotherapy. (in press)

229. Pettengell R, Gurney H, Radford J, et al: A randomized trial of recombinant human granulocyte colony-stimulating factor to preserve dose intensity in non-Hodgkins lymphoma (NHL). Proc Am Soc Clin Oncol 11:1083, 1992

230. Bronchud MH, Howell A, Crowther D, et al: The use of granulocyte colony-stimulating factor to increase the intensity of treatment with doxorubicin in patients with advanced breast and ovarian cancer. Br J Cancer 60:121, 1989

231. Neidhart J, Mangalik A, Kohler W, et al: Granulocyte colony-stimulating factor stimulates recovery of granulocytes in patients receiving dose-intensive chemotherapy without bone marrow transplantation. J Clin Oncol 7:1685, 1989

232. Demetri GD, Horowitz J, McGuire GW, et al: Dose intensification of mitoxantrone with adjunctive G-CSF in patients with advanced breast carcinoma. Proc Am Soc Clin Oncol 11:370, 1992

233. Sarosy G, Kohn E, Link C, et al: Taxol dose intensification in patients with recurrent ovarian cancer. Proc Am Soc Clin Oncol 11:716, 1992

234. Seidman A, Reichman B, Crown J, et al: Activity of taxol with recombinant granulocyte colony stimulating factor (G-CSF) as first chemotherapy (c) of patients (pts) with metastatic breast carcinoma. Proc Am Soc Clin Oncol 11:64, 1992

235. Johnson D, Belani C, Mason B, et al: A phase II trial of recombinant granulocyte colony stimulating factor as an adjunct to cisplatin and etoposide chemotherapy for locally advanced or metastatic non-small cell lung carcinoma. Proc Am Soc Clin Oncol 11:1000, 1992

236. Parker BA, Anderson JR, Canellos GP, et al: Dose escalation study of CHOP plus etoposide (CHOPE) without and with G-CSF in untreated non-Hodgkin's lymphoma. Blood (in press)

237. Budd GT, Silver RT, Wile AC, et al: Neupogen as an adjunct to CNF chemotherapy in advanced breast carcinoma. Proc Am Soc Clin Oncol 11:1346, 1992

238. Masoka T, Takaku F, Kato S, et al: Recombinant human granulocyte colony-stimulating factor for allogeneic bone marrow transplantation. Proc Am Assoc Cancer Res 31:1028, 1990

239. Taylor KM, Jagannath S, Spitzer G, et al: Recombinant human granulocyte colony-stimulating factor hastens granulocyte recovery after high-dose chemotherapy and autologous bone marrow transplantation in Hodgkin's disease. J Clin Oncol 7:1791, 1989

240. Sheridan WP, Wolf M, Lusk J, et al: Granulocyte colony-stimulating factor and neutrophil recovery after high-dose chemotherapy and autologous bone marrow transplantation. Lancet 1:891, 1989

241. Peters WP, Risner G, Ross M, et al: Comparative effects of granulocyte-macrophage colony-stimulating factor (GM-CSF) and granulocyte colony-stimulating factor (G-CSF) on primary peripheral blood progenitor cells for use with auto-

logous bone marrow after high-dose chemotherapy. Blood *81*:1709, 1993

242. Ohno R, Tomonaga M, Kobayaski T, et al: Effect of granulocyte colony-stimulating factor after intensive induction therapy in relapsed or refractory acute leukemia. N Engl J Med *323*: 871, 1990

243. Chao NJ, Schriber JR, Grimes K, et al: Granulocyte colony stimulating factor "mobilized" peripheral blood progenitors accelerate granulocyte and platelet recovery after high-dose chemotherapy. Blood *81*:2031, 1993

244. Greenberg P, Negrin R, Nagler A, et al: Effects of prolonged treatment of myelodysplastic syndromes with recombinant human granulocyte colony-stimulating factor. Int J Cell Cloning *8*:293, 1990

245. Kojima S, Fukuda M, Miyajima Y, et al: Cyclosporine and recombinant granulocyte colony-stimulating factor in severe aplastic anemia. N Engl J Med *323*:920, 1990

246. Miles SA, Mitsuyasu RT, Lee K, et al: Recombinant human granulocyte colony-stimulating factor increases circulating burst forming unit-erythron and red blood cell production in patients with severe human immunodeficiency virus infection. Blood *75*:2137, 1990

247. Hammond WP, Price TH, Souza LM, et al: Treatment of cyclic neutropenia with granulocyte colony-stimulating factor. N Engl J Med *320*:1306, 1989

248. Bonilla MA, Gillio AP, Ruggeiro M, et al: Effects of recombinant human granulocyte colony-stimulating factor on neutropenia in patients with congenital agranulocytosis. N Engl J Med *320*:1574, 1989

249. Jakubowski AA, Souza L, Kelly F, et al: Effects of human granulocyte colony-stimulating factor in a patient with idiopathic neutropenia. N Engl J Med *320*:38, 1989

250. Welte K, Zeidler C, Reuther A, et al: Correction of neutropenia and associated clinical symptoms with G-CSF in children with severe congenital neutropenia. Blood *72*:465, 1988

251. Dale DC, Bonilla MA, Davis MW, et al: A randomized controlled phase III trial of recombinant human granulocyte colony-stimulating factor (Filgrastim) for treatment of severe chronic neutropenia. Blood *81*:2469, 1993

252. Weston B, Axtell RA, Todd RF, et al: Clinical and biological effects of granulocyte colony stimulating factor in the treatment of myelokathexis. J Pediatr *118*:229, 1992

253. Wang WC, Crist WM, Ihle JN, et al: Granulocyte colony stimulating factor corrects the neutropenia associated with glycogen storage disease type 1b. Leukemia *5*:347, 1991

254. Donahue RE, Wang EA, Stone DK, et al: Stimulation of haematopoiesis in primates by continuous infusion of recombinant human GM-CSF. Nature *321*:872, 1986

255. Monroy RL, Skelly RR, MacVittie TA, et al: The effect of recombinant GM-CSF on the recovery of monkeys transplanted with autologous bone marrow. Blood *70*:1696, 1987

256. Groopman JE, Mitsuyasu RT, DeLeo MJ, et al: Effects of recombinant human granulocyte colony-stimulating factor on myelopoiesis in the acquired immunodeficiency syndrome. N Engl J Med *317*:593, 1987

257. Pluda JM, Yarchoan R, Smith PD, et al: Subcutaneous recombinant granulocyte colony-stimulating factor used as a single agent and in an alternating regimen with azidothymidine in leukopenic patients with severe immunodeficiency virus infection. Blood *76*:463, 1990

258. Kaplan LD, Kahn JO, Crowe S, et al: Clinical and virologic effects of recombinant human granulocyte-macrophage colony-stimulating factor in patients receiving chemotherapy for human immunodeficiency virus-associated non-Hodgkins lymphoma: Results of a randomized trial. J Clin Oncol *9*: 929, 1991

259. Scadden DT, Bering HA, Levine JD, et al: Granulocyte-macrophage colony-stimulating factor mitigates the neutropenia of combined interferon alpha and zidovudine treatment of acquired immune deficiency syndrome-associated Kaposi's sarcoma. J Clin Oncol *9*:802, 1991

260. Herrman F, Schultz G, Lindemann A, et al: Hematopoietic responses in patients with advanced malignancies treated with recombinant granulocyte colony-stimulating factor. J Clin Oncol *7*:159, 1989

261. Leischke GJ, Maher D, Cebon J, et al: Bacterially synthesized recombinant human granulocyte-macrophage colony stimulating factor in patients with advanced malignancy. Ann Intern Med *110*:357, 1989

262. Phillips N, Jacob S, Stoller R, et al: Effect of recombinant human granulocyte-macrophage colony-stimulating factor on myelopoiesis in patients with refractory cancer. Blood *74*:26, 1989

263. Steward WP, Scarffe JH, Austen R, et al: Phase I study of recombinant DNA granulocyte colony-stimulating factor. Proc Am Soc Clin Oncol *7*:614, 1988

264. Peters WP, Stuart A, Affronti ML, et al: Neutrophil migration is defective during recombinant human granulocyte-macrophage colony-stimulating factor infusion after autologous bone marrow transplantation in humans. Blood *72*:1310, 1988

265. Toner GC, Gabrilove JL, Gordon M, et al: Phase I/II study of intraperitoneal and intravenous granulocyte-macrophage colony-stimulating factor. Proc Am Assoc Cancer Res *31*:1042, 1990

266. Socinski MA, Elias A, Schnipper L, et al: Granulocyte-macrophage colony-stimulating factor expands the circulating haematopoietic progenitor cell compartment in man. Lancet *1*:1194, 1988

267. Gianni AM, Bregni M, Stern AC, et al: Granulocyte-macrophage colony-stimulating factor to harvest circulating hematopoietic stem cells for autotransplantation. Lancet *1*:580, 1989

268. Brandt SJ, Peters WP, Atwater SK, et al: Effect of recombinant human granulocyte-macrophage colony-stimulating factor on hematopoietic reconstitution after high-dose chemotherapy and autologous bone marrow transplantation. N Engl J Med *319*:869, 1988

269. Nemunaitis J, Singer JW, Buckner CD, et al: Use of recombinant human granulocyte-macrophage colony-stimulating factor in autologous marrow transplantation for lymphoid malignancies. Blood *72*:834, 1988

270. Nemunaitis J, Rabinowe SN, Singer JW, et al: Recombinant granulocyte-macrophage colony-stimulating factor after autologous marrow transplantation for lymphoid cancer. N Engl J Med *324*:1773, 1991

271. Antman KS, Griffin JD, Elias A, et al: Effect of recombinant human granulocyte-macrophage colony-stimulating factor on chemotherapy-induced myelosuppression. N Engl J Med *319*: 593, 1988

272. Morstyn G, Stuart-Harris R, Bishop J, et al: Optimal scheduling of granulocyte-macrophage colony-stimulating factor (GM-CSF) for the abrogation of chemotherapy-induced neutropenia in small cell lung cancer (SCLC). Proc Am Soc Clin Oncol *8*:850, 1989

273. Gianni AM, Bregni M, Siena S, et al: Recombinant human granulocyte-macrophage colony-stimulating factor reduces hematologic toxicity and widens clinical applicability of high-dose cyclophosphamide treatment in breast cancer and non-Hodgkin's lymphoma. J Clin Oncol *8*:768, 1990

274. Barlogie B, Jagamath S, Dixon DO, et al: High-dose melphalan and granulocyte-macrophage colony-stimulating factor for refractory multiple myeloma. Blood *76*:677, 1990

275. de Vries EGE, Biesma B, Willemse PHB, et al: A double-blind placebo controlled study with granulocyte-macrophage colony-stimulating factor during chemotherapy for ovarian carcinoma. Cancer Res *51*:116, 1991

276. Logothelis L, Dexeus F, Sella A, et al: Escalated (ESC) M-VAC (MTX 30 −g/m²) with recombinant human granulocyte-macrophage colony-stimulating factor (rhGM-CSF) for patients with advanced and chemotherapy refractory urothelium tumors: A phase I study. Proc Am Soc Clin Oncol *8*:514, 1989

277. Herrmann F, Schultz G, Weiser M, et al: Effect of granulocyte-macrophage colony-stimulating factor on neutropenia and related morbidity induced by myelotoxic chemotherapy. Am J Med *88*:619, 1990

278. Hoekman K, Wagstaff J, van Groeningen CJ, et al: Effects of recombinant human granulocyte-macrophage colony-stimulating factor on myelosuppression induced by multiple cycles

of high-dose chemotherapy in patients with advanced breast cancer. J Natl Cancer Inst 83:1546, 1991

279. Rodriguez MA, Swan F, Hagemeister F, et al: High-dose ES-HAP with GM-CSF vs. prophylactic antibiotics. Blood 76(suppl 1):10, 1990

280. Bunn PA, Crowley J, Hazuka M, et al: The role of GM-CSF in limited stage SCLC: A randomized phase III study of the Southwest Oncology Group. Proc Am Soc Clin Oncol 11:974, 1992

281. Favoretto A, Paccagnella A, Chiarion Sileni V, et al: Correlation between GM-CSF administration and dose intensity of chemotherapy in SCLC. Proc Am Soc Clin Oncol 11:1022, 1992

282. Gill I, Parker R, Reed E, et al: GM-CSF in combination with weekly etoposide and cisplatin. Proc Am Soc Clin Oncol 11:350, 1992

283. Minniti C, O'Dwyer PJ, Padavic-Shaller K, et al: Phase I trial of etoposide, doxorubicin and cisplatin (EAP) in combination with GM-CSF. Proc Am Soc Clin Oncol 11:364, 1992

284. Krigel R, Haas N, Padavic K, et al: ICE + GM-CSF: A phase I study with apparent activity in non-small cell lung cancer (NSCLC) demonstrating the limitations of hematopoietic growth factor (HGF). Proc Am Soc Clin Oncol 11:1048, 1992

285. Chachoua A, Oratz R, Caron D, et al: A phase IB trial of GM-CSF with murine monoclonal antibody R24 in patients with metastatic melanoma. Proc Am Soc Clin Oncol 11:1188, 1992

286. Gansbacher B, Zier K, Daniels B, et al: Interleukin 2 gene transfer into tumor cells abrogates tumorigenicity and induces protective immunity. J Exp Med 172:1217, 1990

287. Vadhan-Raj S, Keating M, LeMaistre A, et al: Effects of recombinant human granulocyte-macrophage colony-stimulating factor in patients with myelodysplastic syndromes. N Engl J Med 317:1545, 1987

288. Ganser A, Volkers B, Greher J, et al: Recombinant human granulocyte-macrophage colony-stimulating factor in patients with myelodysplastic syndromes: A phase I/II trial. Blood 73:31, 1989

289. Rifkin RM, Hersh EM, Hultquist KN, et al: Therapy of the myelodysplastic syndrome (MDS) with subcutaneously (SC) administered recombinant human granulocyte-macrophage colony-stimulating factor. Proc Am Soc Clin Oncol 8:178, 1989

290. Thompson JA, Lee DJ, Kidd P, et al: Subcutaneous granulocyte-macrophage colony-stimulating factor in patients with myelodysplastic syndrome: Toxicity, pharmacokinetics, and hematological effects. J Clin Oncol 7:629, 1989

291. Herrmann F, Lindemann A, Klein H, et al: Effect of recombinant human granulocyte-macrophage colony-stimulating factor in patients with myelodysplastic syndrome with excess blasts. Leukemia 3:335, 1989

292. Buchner T, Hiddemann W, Koenigsmann M, et al: Chemotherapy followed by recombinant human granulocyte-macrophage colony-stimulating factor (GM-CSF) for acute leukemias at higher age or after relapse. Proc Am Soc Clin Oncol 8:770, 1989

293. Bettelheim P, Valent P, Andreef M: Recombinant human granulocyte-macrophage colony-stimulating factor in combination with standard induction chemotherapy in de novo acute myeloid leukemia. Blood 77:700, 1991

294. Taffuri A, Hegewisch S, Souza LM: Stimulation of leukemic blast cells in vitro by colony-stimulating: Evidence of recombinant and increased cell killing with cytosine arabinoside. Blood 72:329, 1988

295. Mayer P, Valent P, Schmidt G, et al: The in vivo effects of recombinant human interleukin-3: Demonstration of basophil differentiation factor, histamine producing activity, and priming of GM-CSF–responsive human granulocyte-macrophage colony-stimulating factor. Blood 75:2305, 1990

296. Gillio AP, Laver J, Abboud M, et al: IL-3 prevents neutropenia following 5-fluorouracil and cyclophosphamide induced myelosuppression in cynomolgus primates. Blood 72(suppl 1):117 (abstract 380), 1988

297. Ganser A, Seipelt G, Lindemann A, et al: Effects of recombinant human interleukin-3 in patients with myelodysplastic syndromes. Blood 76:455, 1990

298. Ganser A, Lindemann A, Seipelt G, et al: Effects of recombinant human interleukin-3 in aplastic anemia. Blood 76:1287, 1990

299. Crown J, Jakubowski A, Kemeny N, et al: A phase I trial of recombinant human interleukin-1β alone and in combination with myelosuppressive doses of 5-fluorouracil in patients with gastrointestinal cancer. Blood 78:1420, 1991

300. Smith JW, Long DL, Alvord WG, et al: The effects of treatment with interleukin-1α on platelet recovery after high-dose carboplatin. N Engl J Med 328:756, 1993

301. Crawford J, Lau D, Erwin R, et al: A phase I trial of recombinant methionyl human stem cell factor (SCF) in patients (PTS) with advanced non-small cell lung carcinoma (NSCLC). J Clin Oncol 12:338, 1993

301a. Briddell R, Glaspy J, Shpell EJ: Mobilization of myeloid, erythroid and megakaryocyte progenitors by recombinant human stem cell factor plus Filgrastim in patients with breast cancer. Proc ASCO 13:109, 1994

302. Winearls CG, Pippard MJ, Downing MR, et al: Effect of human erythropoietin derived from recombinant DNA on the anaemia of patients maintained by chronic haemodialysis. Lancet 2:1311, 1986

303. Oster W, Hermmann F, Gamm H, et al: Erythropoietin for the treatment of anemia of malignancy associated with neoplastic bone marrow infiltration. J Clin Oncol 8:956, 1990

304. Means RT Jr, Olsen NJ, Krantz SB, et al: Treatment of the anemia of rheumatoid arthritis with recombinant erthryopoietin: Clinical and in vitro studies. Arthritis Rheum 32:638, 1989

305. Fischl M, Galpin JE, Levine JD, et al: Recombinant human erthryopoietin for patients with AIDS treated with zidovudine. N Engl J Med 322:1488, 1990

306. Munn DH, Garnick MB, Cheung N-KV: Effects of parenteral recombinant human macrophage colony-stimulating factor on monocyte number, phenotype, and antitumor cytotoxicity in nonhuman primates. Blood 75:2042, 1990

307. Cenci E, Bartocci A, Puccetti P, et al: Macrophage colony stimulating factor in murine candidiasis: Serum and tissue levels during infection and protective effect of exogenous administration. Infect Immunol 59:868, 1991

308. Bajorin DF, Jakubowski A, Cody B, et al: Phase I trial of recombinant macrophage colony stimulating factor (rhM-CSF) in patients (PTS) with metastatic melanoma. Proc Am Soc Clin Oncol 9:707, 1990

309. Nemunaitis J, Meyers JD, Buckner CD, et al: Phase I trial of recombinant human macrophage colony stimulating factor in patients with invasive fungal infections. Blood 78:907, 1991

310. Rosenberg S: Principles and applications of biologic therapy. In DeVita VT Jr, Hellman S, Rosenberg SA (eds): Cancer: Principles and Practice of Oncology. Philadelphia, JB Lippincott Company, 1993, pp 293–324

21

MONOCLONAL ANTIBODY THERAPY

DAVID G. MALONEY

RONALD LEVY

MICHAEL J. CAMPBELL

The use of antibodies in cancer therapy dates back to the early 20th century. Antisera derived from animals that were immunized with human cancer tissues or cancer extracts or putative cancer-causing microorganisms were administered to patients having various types of cancers. Although some regressions were observed, most of these studies lacked adequate documentation or follow-up.[1,2] Throughout the early and mid-1900s the search for heteroantisera that reacted specifically with cancer cells continued. Time and time again, however, the long-sought-after cancer antigen turned out to be a normal differentiation antigen, generally with aberrant expression in cancer cells. Because it was difficult to distinguish these normal differentiation antigens from tumor-specific antigens using heteroantisera, the search for tumor-specific antigens shifted in the 1960s to examination of the sera of cancer patients.

The search for cancer-specific immunity in patient sera was inspired by the increased incidence of cancer in immunosuppressed individuals, the observation of spontaneous regressions, and the presence of lymphoid infiltrates in solid tumors. One of the first examples of an antibody response against a human tumor was in a patient with gastric cancer who was given an incompatible blood transfusion. The transfusion elicited an antibody response against the P1 blood group antigen. Although the patient was homozygous for the p antigen, the patient's tumor was found to express a P1-related determinant.[3] The patient remained tumor free for 25 years, possibly as a result of the cytotoxic effects of the anti-P1 antibody on the tumor cells. Antibodies reactive with aberrantly expressed Forssman antigen in gastric and colon cancers[4] and ABH in lung cancer[5] also have been found and implicated in tumor regressions. Serologic analyses of patients with Burkitt's lymphoma have revealed the presence of antibodies directed against antigens produced by Epstein-Barr virus (EBV), the causitive agent of Burkitt's lymphoma.[6,7] Subsequently, numerous studies have examined cancer patients' sera for reactivity with established cancer cell lines.[8-14] Because reactive antibodies were found more often in cancer patients' sera than in normal control sera, it was thought that the sera of patients who had a spontaneous regression or a treatment-related regression contained anticancer antibodies. Thus, a number of attempts were made to treat other cancer patients with blood, serum, or plasma thought to contain these anticancer antibodies.[15-20] Disappointingly, there were no clear therapeutic effects observed in these studies.

In 1975, Kohler and Milstein described the production of a monoclonal antibody from a B cell hybridoma,[21] a technique for which they received the Nobel Prize in Medicine in 1984, inspiring once again the search for human tumor-specific antigens. Rather than discovering the much-sought-after tumor-specific antigens, however, an abundance of new differentiation antigens have been found. Although not tumor specific, these antigens tend to have a restricted expression on normal cells. Monoclonal antibodies against these tumor-associated markers, used alone or as carriers of drugs, toxins, radionuclides, and the like, along with recent advances in genetic engineering of antibody molecules, are providing promising new approaches to the classification, diagnosis, localization, and treatment of human cancers.

MONOCLONAL ANTIBODY STRUCTURE AND PRODUCTION

Antibody molecules are multichain proteins composed of two identical heavy (H) and two identical light (L) chains forming a Y-shaped structure, stabilized and cross-linked by intrachain and interchain disulfide bonds (Fig. 21–1). The tips of the arms contain the variable regions that bind antigen and hence differ markedly from one antibody molecule to the next. The stem of the Y contains the constant region, or Fc, which is involved in binding to cell-surface receptors and fixing complement. Each chain of an immunoglobulin (Ig) molecule is divided into structural domains. The light chain folds into two domains, a variable (VL) and a constant (CL) domain. The heavy chain folds to form VH, CH1, hinge, CH2, and CH3 domains (in an IgG molecule). The hinge region is the flexible portion of the molecule. The antigen-binding site of an antibody is formed from six hypervariable loops, three from the VL domain and three from the VH domain. Within each variable-region domain, the loops are connected to relatively conserved β-sheet framework regions that provide supportive scaffolding. The specificity and

affinity of the antigen-binding site are determined primarily by these six hypervariable loops, which are termed the complementarity-determining regions (CDRs).

The domain structure of the antibody molecule is mirrored at the genetic level. Each constant- and variable-region domain is coded for by a separate exon. The variable-region domains are themselves derived from separate exons that recombine during lymphocyte differentiation. The first and second CDRs in both the heavy chain and the light chain are encoded within the germline variable-region genes. In contrast, CDR3 is produced by the combination of V and J elements for the light chain and V, D, and J elements for the heavy chain. This combination of multiple elements yields a hypervariable loop that is generally longer and more diverse than the other loops.

Most antitumor monoclonal antibodies (MAbs) are of murine origin, produced by fusing an immortal myeloma

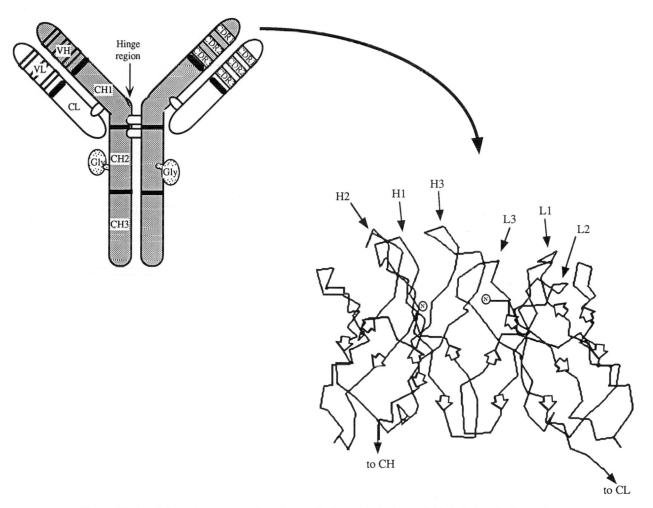

Figure 21–1. Schematic representation of an antibody molecule (upper left) depicting the four-polypeptide-chain structure (two identical heavy and two identical light chains). The heavy chains are glycosylated. The hinge region is a part of the heavy chain, which contains the inter–heavy chain disulfide bonds and confers flexibility on the arms of the antibody molecule. Each chain is divided into domains as illustrated (VL and CL for the light chain; VH, CH1, CH2, and CH3 for the heavy chain). These domains are globular regions of the protein that consist of three to four loops stabilized by β-pleated sheet secondary structure. The structure of the VH and VL domains are depicted at the bottom right. Three variable loops in the light chain (L1 through L3) and three in the heavy chain (H1 through H3) comprise the complementarity-determining regions (CDRs), which together form the antigen binding site.

cell line with antibody-producing B cells from mice that were immunized with whole tumor cells, cell extracts, or purified antigen. A variety of agents have been utilized to fuse the two cell populations, including Sendai virus, as originally used by Kohler and Milstein[21]; polyethylene glycol (PEG), the most commonly used agent for cell fusions[22,23]; and electric current.[24–26] Fusion results in the formation of heterokaryons that possess two or more nuclei. The nuclei fuse at the next cell division, resulting in a "hybridoma." Because fusion is a relatively rare event when using virus or PEG, a selection strategy is used to ensure the growth of the hybridomas and inhibit the growth of the myeloma cells. Generally, this involves the use of a myeloma cell line that lacks hypoxanthine-guanine phosphoribosyltransferase (HGPRT) or thymidine kinase (TK), two enzymes that are important in the salvage pathway of purine and pyrimidine biosynthesis. In the presence of aminopterin, which blocks the main biosynthetic pathways for purines and pyrimidines, these mutants are unable to synthesize DNA. However, fusion to spleen cells (which possess TK and HGPRT but will die in culture) supplies the missing enzyme, allowing growth of the resulting hybridomas. Hybridoma cell lines are capable of producing from 1 to 50 µg of MAb per milliliter of culture medium. Production can be scaled up to obtain gram quantities of monoclonal antibody by growing the hybridoma cells in vivo as ascites in mice or by large-scale in vitro production using hollow fiber cartridges, microencapsulation, or large fermenters.

Production of human MAbs has been more difficult, in part as a result of the lack of a human myeloma cell line that routinely yields stable, producing hybridomas when fused with human B cells. Nonetheless, several groups have generated human MAbs reactive with human tumors by fusing lymph nodes from cancer patients with murine or human myeloma cells or by immortalizing these lymph node cells by infection with EBV, sometimes followed by fusion with myeloma cells.[27–33] Theoretically, human MAbs may identify tumor antigens or epitopes that are not recognized by immunized mice. In addition, human MAbs will not elicit the anti–mouse immunoglobulin response observed in most patients receiving repeated administration of murine antibodies, although some immune response directed against the unique (idiotypic) regions of the MAb still can be seen.

Genetically Engineered Antibodies

The domain structure of an antibody molecule allows for the engineering of a variety of novel fragments by swapping, replacing, and/or deleting various domains (Fig. 21–2). Genetic engineering provides several ways to improve various properties of MAbs, including: (1) reducing human antimouse response by generating chimeric or humanized MAb, (2) enhancing effector functions, (3) altering the pharmacokinetics of plasma and whole-body clearance, (4) increasing penetration into tumor masses, (5) increasing affinity, and (6) developing more efficient delivery of drugs, toxins, or biologic response modifiers.

Mouse/human chimeric antibodies have been produced by swapping the constant region domains of a murine MAb with those from a human antibody.[34–43] These chimeras should demonstrate less immunogenicity when used in humans, and the human Fc portion should interact more effectively with human Fc receptor–bearing effector cells and/or human complement. Taking chimeric MAbs one step further, "humanized" MAbs have been produced in which only the CDRs from the parent rodent MAb were retained.[44–49] However, some humanized antibodies produced by simply grafting murine CDRs into human framework regions demonstrated reduced affinity compared to the parent MAb. This problem is being addressed by choosing a human framework that is as homologous as possible to the original murine MAb in an effort to reduce conformational changes in the grafted CDRs. In addition, computer modeling of the murine MAb is being used to identify framework residues that, although not part of the CDRs, might interact with CDR residues or with antigen. These specific murine framework residues then are grafted along with the murine CDRs to generate the humanized antibody.[50,51]

Antibodies may be genetically engineered to act as efficient vehicles for the delivery of antitumor drugs, toxins, radionuclides, enzymes, or biologic response modifiers. Genetically engineered antibody carriers have the potential of overcoming some of the difficulties associated with chemical conjugation techniques, such as the production of heterogeneous products or the inadvertent chemical alteration of antigen-binding affinity or cytotoxic activity. Recombinant immunotoxins have been produced in which a single genetic construct encodes an antibody fragment joined to a toxin by a peptide linker. This strategy employs the observation that the heavy and light chain variable-region genes of an antibody molecule can be cloned in tandem with a linker sequence in between. This results in the expression of a single polypeptide chain containing both variable regions connected by a flexible linker peptide. These single-chain Fv (scFv) fragments are able to fold into a structure that retains antigen-binding activity.[52–55] By cloning a toxin gene in tandem with a scFv genetic construct, one can produce a single-chain immunotoxin. Both *Pseudomonas* endotoxin 40 (PE40) and diphtheria toxin (DT) have been used in such constructs.[56,57] Several antibodies have been used to construct single-chain immunotoxins with PE40 or DT, including anti-Tac,[58,59] anti–transferrin receptor,[60] OVB3,[61] and B3.[62] The scFv anti-Tac–PE40 has been shown to have potent cytotoxic activity against cells from adult T-cell leukemia patients.[63] In vivo administration of the anti-B3 single-chain toxin, which recognizes a pancarcinoma carbohydrate antigen, to animals bearing human tumor xenografts has resulted in complete tumor regressions.[62] In addition to toxins, genetically engineered antibodies have been constructed as carriers of cytokines such as interleukin 2[64] and tumor necrosis factor.[65,66]

The pharmacokinetics of an antibody also may be altered genetically to prolong its half-life or to increase its clearance. Pharmacokinetic properties can be altered by chimerization or humanization, by size alterations, or by altering glycosylation. Humanized MAbs have been shown to have prolonged survival, compared to their mu-

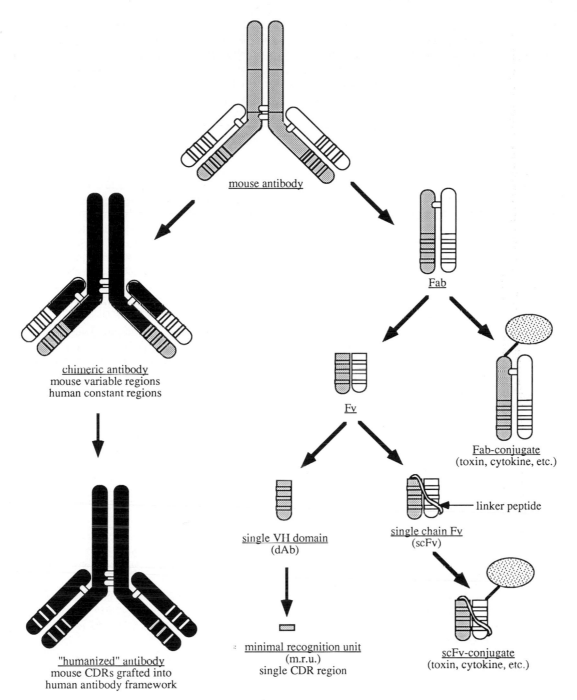

Figure 21–2. Genetically engineered monoclonal antibodies and fragments. A murine MAb can be altered to yield a variety of novel antigen-binding molecules. Chimeric MAbs are produced by swapping the Fc region of the murine MAb with that of a human antibody. Humanized MAbs can be made by grafting the CDRs (along with some framework residues) from the murine MAb into a human antibody framework. The murine MAb also can be fragmented into smaller and smaller units (either chemically or through molecular biology techniques). Fab fragments, containing a light chain disulfide-linked to a truncated heavy chain (C_H1 and V_H regions), and Fv fragments, consisting of a V_H segment associated with a V_L segment (created as two separate chains or as a single-chain Fv), contain the MAb's original antigen-binding site. In contrast, individual V_H domains (dAb) and single CDR segments contain only a portion of the original MAb's binding site, yet some of these fragments have been shown to retain antigen-binding capabilities.

rine counterparts, in monkeys and in humans.[37,67] Because the catabolic rate of an antibody molecule is determined by the CH2 domain, the increased half-life of humanized antibodies is probably due to the presence of the human IgG CH2 replacing the murine IgG CH2.[68,69] In contrast, increased clearance might be desirable when a radiolabeled MAb is used for immunoscanning. Small antigen-binding fragments such as Fab, F(ab')2, Fv, or scFv have half-lives of less than 5 hours. In addition, small fragments probably will penetrate tumor tissue more readily than intact antibody molecules. Rapid clearance of a MAb also has been achieved by deletion of the CH2 domain.[70] Finally, the serum pharmacokinetic patterns of immunoglobulins can be altered by minor changes in glycosylation.[71]

Some antitumor MAbs lack sufficient affinity or avidity to be clinically useful. Increasing the affinity of such a MAb would have the advantage of more efficient tumor binding and possibly prolonged binding time at the tumor site. The affinity of a MAb can be increased through site-directed mutagenesis of the hypervariable regions[72] or by altering variable-region glycosylation.[73]

Finally, a major advantage of utilizing genetic engineering in developing diagnostic or therapeutic MAbs is that, once a modification has been made for one MAb, the same construct can be used with virtually any other antibody. Thus, enzymatic digestion to yield antibody fragments or immunochemistry to link drugs or toxins to MAbs does not have to be repeated for each MAb of interest.

Repertoire Cloning

Recently, an alternative approach to the production of MAbs has been developed. By using molecular genetic techniques to clone and express antibody genes directly, this new method, "repertoire cloning," eliminates the need for cell fusion. Immunoglobulin variable-region genes are amplified using the polymerase chain reaction (PCR) and then cloned into an appropriate expression vector. The resulting antibody fragments can be produced as secreted products from bacteria or expressed on the surface of a bacterium or phage.[74–76] Using repertoire cloning, several murine as well as human antibodies have been produced from immune donor cells.[77–81] Whereas hybridoma technology immortalizes the antibody-producing cell of interest, repertoire cloning immortalizes the antibody genes of interest. Both techniques, however, rely on an immunized animal to invent the specific antibody molecule.

Taking repertoire cloning one step further, investigators are examining the possibility of making new antibodies totally in vivo, thus bypassing animals altogether. This strategy would attempt to mimic and even improve on the way the immune system develops and selects high-affinity antibodies from an initial pool of low-affinity molecules.[82] An initial primary library of variable-region genes would be produced, either from naive lymphocytes or by in vitro synthesis and recombination of new V, D, and J gene segments. This latter approach has the potential advantage of being totally random, whereas a "natural" repertoire, which is probably biased toward the recognition of pathogens and against self-reactivity, is likely to be highly redundant. This primary library ideally would contain low-binding-affinity antibodies capable of recognizing all possible epitopes. Theoretically, a primary repertoire of 10^7 different antibodies would react with more than 99 per cent of all conceivable epitopes with low-affinity binding (at least 10^5 M^{-1}).[83] Thus, once cloned and expressed, millions of clones would need to be screened for antigen binding. An alternative to screening large numbers of clones would be to express the library of antibody fragments on the surface of phage and then to bind the phage to antigen in order to select for the desired V gene segment combinations. Once variable regions that bind antigen have been obtained from the primary library, a secondary library is produced by mutating these genes. Mutations can be introduced during PCR amplification of the variable-region genes by using error-prone polymerases, by amplifying for a large number of cycles, by varying the ratios of nucleotide triphosphates, or by utilizing mutated oligonucleotide primers. These mutated genes are reexpressed, with subsequent selection for antibody fragments with increased affinity. The whole process is repeated several times until high-affinity antibodies are obtained. The feasibility of this approach has been demonstrated recently.[84] Using a phage expression system, specific MAbs to progesterone were isolated from a naive combinatorial antibody library. These isolates then were subjected to random mutagenesis and specific antibodies with increased affinities were obtained.

TUMOR ANTIGENS

A large number of MAbs have been generated against a wide variety of tumor-associated antigens (TAAs). In general, these TAAs fall into one of several classes. The oncofetal antigens include carcinoembryonic antigen (CEA),[85–89] α-fetoprotein (AFP),[90] and tumor-associated glycoprotein 72 (TAG-72).[91,92] MAbs that react with oncofetal antigens can demonstrate either pancarcinoma reactivity, binding a range of carcinomas (e.g., anti–TAG-72) or more specific reactivity (e.g., anti-CEA, which reacts predominantly with gastrointestinal tumors). Another class of TAAs includes antigens that are expressed on cells at a given state of differentiation, such as the human milk fat globule antigen,[93] common acute lymphoblastic leukemia antigen (CALLA),[94] and anti–colon-associated antigen (CAA).[95] An interesting group of TAAs that is emerging as our understanding of the molecular basis of tumorigenesis improves is that of growth factor receptors[96] and oncogene products. MAbs directed against the receptors for transferrin,[97–101] epidermal growth factor,[102–104] platelet-derived growth factor,[105,106] several B- and T-cell growth factors such as interleukin 2 (anti-Tac),[107,108] and cell surface oncogene products such as HER-2/Neu/c-ErbB-2[109–116] have been shown to inhibit tumor cell proliferation in vitro and in vivo. A few MAbs have been produced that react with a specific tissue type. For example, the antibody D612 reacts with malignant and normal gastrointestinal tissues but not with other normal or cancer tissues.[117] Finally, like their normal counterparts, the surface immunoglobulin expressed on malignant B cells and the T-cell receptor (TCR) molecule expressed on the surface of malignant T cells contain unique antigenic determinants known as idiotopes (collectively, the idiotype). Because the idiotype of a given malignant clone of cells is unique, it provides a very tumor-specific marker. Anti-idiotypic antibodies directed against the idiotype on tumor cells have been shown to inhibit tumor growth in animal models.[118–122] One major problem with anti-idiotypic treatment of B-cell tumors is that rearrangement or mutation of immunoglobulin genes within the tumor cells can lead to altered receptors that may no longer be recognized by the antibody.[123–128]

STRATEGIES FOR USING MONOCLONAL ANTIBODIES AGAINST CANCER

Monoclonal antibodies have been applied to the treatment of cancer in a variety of ways. They have been used alone, in conjunction with other agents such as cytokines or chemotherapeutic drugs, and as carriers of numerous cytotoxic agents. In addition, recent advances in molecular biology are yielding novel recombinant antibody constructs. Each of these strategies has a different mode of action along with a different set of strengths and weaknesses, as is discussed in the following pages.

Immunotherapy with Monoclonal Antibodies Alone

Many studies have used MAbs alone to treat cancer. These approaches have relied on indirect antitumor effects involving immune effector functions, direct antiproliferative effects of the MAb itself, or the induction of immunity against the tumor cells via an idiotype/anti-idiotype network. The main advantage of using MAbs alone is their minimal toxicity and their relative ease of production. However, not all MAbs are effective alone and, furthermore, because of antigenic heterogeneity within the population of tumor cells, not all cells will be recognized by a given MAb, thus rendering these approaches less effective.

Antibodies can kill tumor cells indirectly by two main processes, both of which involve the Fc portion of the molecule. These are complement-dependent cytotoxicity (CDC) and antibody-dependent cellular cytotoxicity (ADCC). The complement cascade is activated on fixation of complement to the immunoglobulin Fc region, resulting in the enzymatic piercing of the tumor cell membrane and, ultimately, cell death. ADCC involves effector cells such as monocytes, macrophages, granulocytes, and some lymphocytes that express receptors that bind to the Fc portion of an immunoglobulin molecule. These effector cells bind to antibodies adhering to tumor cells and subsequently lyse the tumor cells.

Because the Fc region must be present for CDC or ADCC, only intact antibody molecules will be effective in this strategy. In addition, differences in the Fc regions of different antibodies will affect their ability to mediate CDC or ADCC. The majority of MAbs used in human clinical trials have been of murine origin. The different classes of murine heavy chains have different affinities for human complement and Fc receptors. Although murine IgM antibodies are the most effective at complement fixation, their large size restricts their ability to penetrate tissues effectively. IgG3 antibodies are good at mediating CDC with human complement, whereas IgG2a, IgG2b, and IgG1 are ineffective. For ADCC with human effector cells, murine IgG2a and IgG3 have demonstrated the best results. Studies with human antibodies or mouse/human chimeric antibodies have ranked IgM > IgG1 > IgG3 > IgG2 > IgG4 for CDC and IgG1 and IgG3 as the best classes for ADCC.

Direct antiproliferative effects of MAbs on tumor cells can occur via inhibition of growth factor and growth factor receptor interaction, via transduction of an inhibitory signal into the cell, or via catalytic action of the MAb. Tumor cells often express various growth factor receptors, many of which are oncogene products. Expression of these receptors often leads to autocrine- or paracrine-stimulated growth. As previously mentioned, MAbs against cell surface receptors have demonstrated the ability of this strategy to inhibit tumor growth.

Signal transduction pathways in cells are only just beginning to be unraveled. A variety of molecules, including kinases, phosphatases, G proteins, and others, play a role in transducing stimulatory as well as inhibitory signals from the cell surface to the nucleus. Some of these molecules are integral membrane proteins and others are cytoplasmic or nuclear proteins. Theoretically, a MAb raised against a cell surface molecule that induces an inhibitory signal to the cell could be used against tumor cells to inhibit their proliferation.

The third and still theoretical approach for direct antitumor cytotoxicity with MAbs utilizes catalytic antibodies. MAbs have been produced that catalyze a variety of enzymatic reactions.[129–131] Catalytic antibodies could be designed to induce hydrolysis of the cell membrane, cellular proteins, or nucleic acids. Such MAbs, if specific for tumor cell membranes or proteins, could have direct cytotoxicity against the tumor cells and prove useful for cancer treatment.

In addition to these strategies for using MAbs alone against cancer, several investigators have examined the use of MAbs to induce antitumor immunity. These studies have their basis in the immune network theory proposed by Jerne.[132] As an example (see Fig. 21–3), when murine MAb (Ab1) is injected into humans, a human antimouse antibody response often is generated. Some of this antibody is directed toward the idiotype of the mouse MAb. This human anti-idiotype (Ab2) could in turn induce an anti–anti-idiotype (Ab3) response. If the Ab2 mimics the original antigen, the resulting Ab3 could mimic the Ab1; that is, a human antibody has been induced that binds the same antigen as the original mouse antibody. Such anti-idiotype antibody responses have been observed in pa-

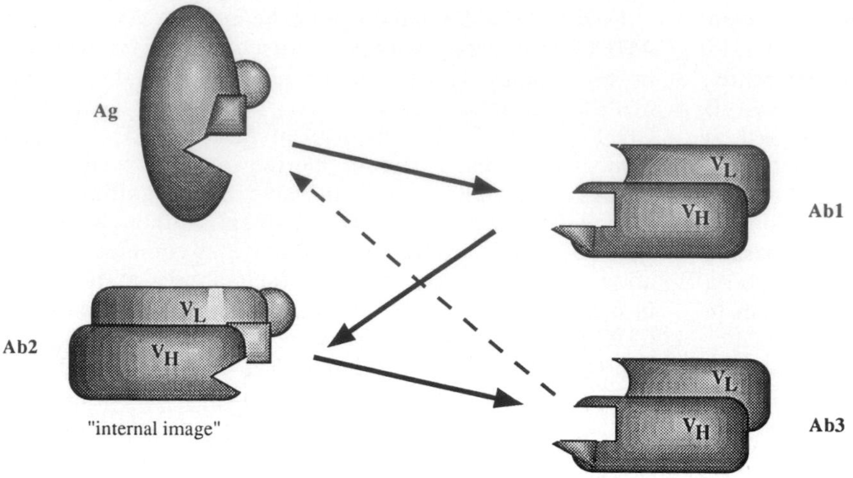

Figure 21–3. Idiotype network concept. Jerne's concept of an "internal image" is one of a three-dimensional shape mimicry in which the interactions between antigen and Ab1 and between Ab1 and Ab2 are dependent on specific shape complementarities. This yields an Ab2 anti-idiotype antibody whose structure resembles the shape of the antigen and that can induce Ab3 that binds antigen.

tients receiving murine MAbs and have been implicated in their antitumor responses.[133,134] In an analogous approach, the Ab1 is bypassed and an anti-idiotype against Ab1 (Ab2) is used for immunization, resulting in an endogenously produced anti–anti-idiotype (Ab3) that binds the tumor antigen.[135–140]

According to Jerne's network hypothesis, the internal image Ab2 is presumed to have a three-dimensional structure that resembles the shape of the antigen[132] (as depicted in Fig. 21–3). However, recent experimental data suggest that this may not be the case. The crystal structures of an antibody complexed with its antigen or with an anti-idiotype antibody display relatively flat contacting surfaces.[141,142] These antibody interactions apparently are governed more by the affinities and types of interactions of their surface-accessible side chains than by the three-dimensional relationship of their contacting surfaces. In addition, some "noninternal image" Ab2 anti-idiotype antibodies can induce specific immune responses against the original antigen, whereas some "internal image" Ab2s are ineffective.[136,143,144] Therefore, the concept of antigen mimicry by Ab2 antibodies may operate functionally, but may not be easy to explain on a structural level.

CLINICAL TRIALS OF ANTIBODIES ALONE

Leukemia and Lymphoma

Of all the clinical trials of MAbs, those performed in patients with lymphoma have shown the most promising results. Unconjugated MAbs directed against a wide variety of antigens have been used in the therapy of patients with lymphoma and leukemia. Representative studies are detailed in Table 21–1. Early studies in the 1980s focused on the use of antigens such as CD5 and CALLA. The CD5 antigen is expressed on the surface of cutaneous T-cell lymphomas (CTCLs) such as mycosis fungoides and on the surface of B-cell chronic lymphocytic leukemia (B-CLL). Therapeutic trials with several MAbs against CD5 demonstrated that murine MAbs could be given safely to humans and that the antibodies localized to the tumor cells in vivo.[145–152] In patients with CTCL, impressive but brief

antitumor effects were seen. These early trials identified several factors that limit the effectiveness of MAb therapy. These include antigenic modulation, free antigen, and the development of human antimouse antibody (HAMA). In B-CLL, responses consisted of transient reductions in the number of circulating tumor cells,[149–152] which rapidly returned following discontinuation of the antibody infusion. Antigenic modulation was demonstrated in these trials of B-CLL, but HAMA was infrequent.[153] In general, HAMA responses have been seen more often in patients with T-cell malignancies than in those with B-cell malignancies. In a similar fashion, antibody therapy of ALL directed against the CALLA antigen produced transient decreases in tumor cells without long-term benefit.[154] Again, antigenic modulation was considered to contribute to the failure of the antibody therapy.[155] Toxicities of antibody infusions included fever, chills, rigors, urticaria, dyspnea, and occasional hypotension, which often were related to the first infusions and could be managed by medication and slowing or temporarily stopping the antibody infusion.

Additional studies using murine antibodies directed against B-cell antigens such as CD19 and CD20 in the treatment of patients with B-cell non-Hodgkin's lymphoma also demonstrated some significant clinical responses.[156,157] In both of these studies, murine antibodies of the IgG2a isotype were used. Once again, HAMA was rarely seen. Biopsies demonstrated localization of antibody into tumor-bearing lymph nodes, especially at cumulative doses of greater than 1000 mg given over 4 to 10 days.[157] In several instances, nonmodulated cells coated with the treatment antibody were observed to persist in the peripheral blood. Trials targeting a human lymphocyte antigen (HLA) class II antigen (LYM-1) also demonstrated minor antitumor responses, but biopsies of tumors failed to demonstrate saturating binding even at doses of more than 450 mg/week for 4 weeks.[158]

Antibodies against the T-cell subset antigen CD4 also have been used to treat patients with CTCL. In an early study, transient depletions of circulating tumor cells were noted, and more significant antitumor effects, including the clearing of generalized erythroderma and decreases in tumor plaques, were observed in a trial of a mouse/human chimerized antibody.[159] The substitution of the human antibody constant region in this trial was associated with a very low incidence of immune response even in these T-cell lymphoma patients.

The effect of antibody isotype on the therapeutic effect of MAbs was addressed in a series of studies using rat antibodies directed against the CAMPATH-1 antigen (CDw52).[160] This nonmodulating antigen is present on lymphoid cells and monocytes and on a wide variety of lymphoid malignancies.[161] In early-phase clinical trials, the IgM and IgG2a rat MAbs caused only transient decreases in circulating tumor cells that were attributed to sequestration, whereas the class switch variant IgG2b (CAMPATH-1G) had a more lasting effect by clearing tumor in the blood, spleen, and bone marrow in the majority of cases.[160] Complete remissions occurred in nine patients who had tumor limited to blood or bone marrow. Interestingly, in contrast to the trials using anti-idiotype antibodies (see later in this chapter), only rarely were effects seen on areas of bulk tumor, such as lymphnodes or tumor masses. This difference may be due to the lower doses of antibody employed. The antibody was ineffective when given intrathecally.[160] All of the rat IgM, IgG2a, and IgG2b antibodies effectively killed cells in vitro utilizing human complement. The unique effectiveness of the rat IgG2b at killing tumor cells in vivo was attributed to its ability to bind to human Fc receptors and to activate ADCC.[162] Toxicity was greater than that reported in trials of more specific antibodies, but manageable, with fever, rigors, bronchospasm, hypotension, and mild elevations of liver enzymes noted in many patients. Antirat immune responses were seen in a minority of patients.[160] Antitumor efficacy in patients with non-Hodgkin's lymphoma (NHL) appeared to be increased using the humanized CAMPATH-1H antibody (human IgG1 [k] construct with rat hypervariable regions).[163] Human antibodies of the IgG1 isotype have demonstrated significant ability to kill cells through complement-mediated lysis as well as ADCC.[164] Antibody responses to the humanized antibody were not observed, and further clinical trials using this antibody are ongoing.

In the above trials, the antitumor effect is thought to be delivered via host effector systems through ADCC or CDC. A different approach has been taken in the therapy of human T-cell leukemia virus type I (HTLV-1)–induced adult T-cell leukemia (ATL). This disease is characterized by the proliferation of malignant T cells that express high levels of the interleukin 2 (IL-2) receptor Tac. Tac also is present on activated normal T cells, and anti-Tac antibodies block the binding of IL-2 to the high-affinity IL-2 receptor and can block various T-cell functions.[108] Thus therapy with anti-Tac antibodies may kill cells using mechanisms of ADCC or CDC but also may interfere with cellular function by inhibition of the IL-2 receptor. In a clinical trial of anti-Tac antibodies in patients with ATL, three of nine patients had clinical benefit, including one complete response of more than 8 months' duration.[165] In a follow-up to this trial, three complete, three partial, and one mixed response occurred following therapy with anti-Tac antibody in the treatment of 20 patients with ATL.[166]

Special Case of Antibodies against Immunoglobulin Idiotype

Stevenson first proposed that the idiotype of the clonal immunoglobulin present on the surface of B-cell tumors could be exploited as a target for antibody-directed therapy.[167,168] Several groups have since made anti-idiotype antibodies that reacted uniquely with a given patient's tumor and have used them as sensitive probes for the detection of the malignant clone or its immunoglobulin product. The detection of rare tumor cells or the idiotype bearing immunoglobulin in the patient's blood often heralded the eventual clinical relapse following conventional therapy.[169] Treatment of patients with these murine monoclonal anti-idiotype antibodies demonstrated limited toxicity and significant antitumor activity, including prolonged complete remissions. Shown in Table 21–2 are the results from a single institution with three clinical trials of anti-idiotype antibodies used alone or in combination with α-interferon or a pulse of chlorambucil.[170–174] In these three trials, 45 patients have been treated with custom-made monoclonal anti-idiotype antibodies. The majority of patients had relapsed disease with extensive prior chemotherapy. The overall tumor rate was 68 per cent. Most importantly, 18 per cent of patients had complete remissions of their disease, with five of six of these patients free of tumors for more than 5 years. These responses occurred in patients with low-grade and intermediate-grade lymphomas, including those that had transformed from low to intermediate grade.

A number of problems associated with anti-idiotype antibody therapy were identified in these trials. High levels of idiotype protein in the serum proved to be a barrier to antibody therapy in some patients. Attempts to decrease the serum idiotype level by plasmapheresis prior to antibody therapy were only transiently effective.[170,171] In some patients with significant tumor regressions, regrowth of the tumor with cells no longer reactive with the anti-idiotype antibody, but with continued expression of surface immunoglobulin, occurred. Analysis of these idiotype-negative cells revealed somatic mutations in the immunoglobulin variable-region genes leading to the expression of an altered idiotype.[175] Re-treatment with the original anti-idiotype antibody was not effective, although, in some cases, treatment with a second antibody reactive with the altered idiotype induced further tumor regression.[173] The addition of a short pulse of chemotherapy combined with the monoclonal anti-idiotype antibody therapy at a time when idiotype-negative cells may have been proliferating failed to decrease the emergence of idiotype-negative variant tumors.[174]

The mechanisms of tumor regression seen in these trials are not known. There was no correlation with the isotype of the anti-idiotype antibody. Tumor regressions occurred with murine IgG1, IgG2a, and IgG2b isotypes.[176] The presence of large numbers of host T cells in the pretreatment tumor biopsy of patients with low-grade lymphomas was correlated with a positive antitumor effect of the antibody therapy.[177] Infrequently, a direct antiproliferative activity of the anti-idiotype antibody on tumor cells in vitro could be demonstrated.[176] A trial combining anti-

TABLE 21–1. CLINICAL TRIALS OF UNCONJUGATED MONOCLONAL ANTIBODIES IN LYMPHOID MALIGANCIES

ANTIBODY	ANTIGEN	DISTRIBUTION	DISEASE	# PATIENTS	DOSE/SCHED
L17F12 (lgG2a)	CD5 67kDa glycoprotein	T cells, B-CLL	ATL	1	1-, 5-mg dose
L17F12	CD5	T cells, B-CLL	CTCL	1	10–20 mg q 3–4 d (164 mg) over 10 wk
L17F12	CD5	T cells, B-CLL	CTCL	7	0.25–100 mg × 4–17 over 14–75 d
T101 (lgG1)	CD5	T cells, B-CLL	CTCL and B-CLL	13	1–500 mg weekly × 4
T101	CD5	T cells, B-CLL	B-CLL	2	10–15 mg
T101	CD5	T cells, B-CLL	B-CLL (6) CTCL (10)	16	10–500 mg 24–hr infusion
T101	CD5	T cells, B-CLL	B-CLL (4) CTCL (4)	8	1–100 mg multiple schedules, 1–16 infusions
T101	CD5	T cells, B-CLL	B-CLL	13	1–140 mg over 1 wk
UCHT1	CD4	T cells	T-CLL	1	3 mg 3× each wk
J-5	CD10 CALLA 100 kDa glycoprotein	ALL, some CML in blast crisis	ALL	4	0.1–10 mg/kg for 3–4 d
Ab 89	?	B-cell NHL	B-cell NHL	1	25 mg–1.5 gm
LYM-1 (lgG2a)	HLA-DR polymorphic variant	B cells	B-cell NHL	10	58–465 mg q wk ×4
CAMPATH-1M (rat lgM) CAMPATH-1G (rat lgG2b class switch variant of YTH34.5 rat lgG2a)	CDw52	Lymphoid cells, monocytes	NHL, B-CLL, PLL, HCL, cALL	18	to 300 mg/10-d course
CAMPATH-1H (rat hypervariable regions onto human lgG1)	CDw52	Lymphoid cells, monocytes	NHL, low grade	2	1–20 mg/d × 43 d— 2 courses give to 1 pt
1F5 (lgG2a)	CD20 35-kDa antigen	B cells	B-cell NHL	4	52–2380 mg over 5–10 d
CLB-CD19 (lgG2a)	CD19 90-kDa glycoprotein	B cclls	B-cell NHL	6	15–250 mg on 4 d of therapy
ALB9 (lgG1) BL13 (lgG1)	CD24 CD21 EBV receptor on B cells	B cells and granulocytes B cells	B-cell lymphoproliferative syndrome following organ transplantation	26	0.2 mg/kg/d ×10
BL13 (lgG1)	CD21	B cells	B-cell lymphoproliferation following heart transplant	1 (peripheral and CNS lesions)	1.4–2.8 mg/d for 35 d, 0.15–1.5 mg intrathecally for 1 mo

Table continued on following page

EFFECT	HAMA	TOXICITY	MAb IN TUMOR	REF.
Transient decrease in WBC; modulation, free antigen noted	1/1 lgM HAMA	Transient decrease in renal function	Modulation of PBL tumor	145
PR blood, skin, lymph nodes for 7 wk; modulation of CD5	None	None	Yes on PBL tumor	146
5 pts with improvement 1.5–4 mo	4 HAMA, some pts with anti-ld	Dyspnea 1 pt	Yes	147
1 CR (MF) for 6 wk; 1 PR (MF) for 3 mo	3/13 HAMA	Pruritus, hives, flushing, dyspnea, cardiac arrhythmias with initial doses of 100 mg or more	Yes	148
Transient decrease in WBC	None	Rigors, fever, hypotension	Yes on PBL tumor	151
Transient responses in 6 pts (greater in CTCL than CLL)	0/6 CLL 5/10 CTCL	Fever, chills, allergic symptoms	Yes	149
Transient responses in decreased WBC (tumor)	2/4 CTCL 0/4 CLL	Fever, chills, allergic symptoms	Yes, on PBL tumor and on CTCL skin Bx; modulation of antigen noted	150
Transient decrease in WBC, no effect in nodes, spleen, or liver	0/13	Fever, urticaria, dyspnea, chest tightness, hypotension	PBL and BM tumor positive, lymph node negative, modulation	152
Transient decrease in WBC	1/1 HAMA	Fever	Low levels on PBL tumor	461
Transient decrease in WBC, but cells returned completely modulated for antigen	None	Fever	Transiently on blood and BM tumor	154
Transient decrease in WBC	None	Decreased creatinine clearance	Low density on blood WBC, antibody excess not obtained due to free antigen	462
3 minor responses	0/10	Fever, rash	3/3 tumor Box positive, although not saturated at highest dose	158
lgM and lgG2a transient decreases in blood tumor; lgG2b caused longer lasting clearing of blood, BM, and splenomegaly; tumor masses and CNS disease not affected	At least 3 anti-rat responses	Fever, rigors, bronchospasm, mild increase in LFTs	Yes, not saturating in BM	160
1 ?CR and 1 PR	None	Fever, hypotension, rash, malaise	Not done	163
1 PR 6 wk	None	Fever, transient thrombocytopenia	PBL coated, but BM and nodes only positive at highest dose	156
1 pt with PR × 2 (3 mo and 9 mo); coated cells in blood not quickly cleared	0 HAMA	Mild	Blood and BM tumor positive, lymph node saturated at doses of >1000 mg over 4 d	157
CR 16/26 (only in oligaclonal disease; N=18); no effect in CNS disease (pts also allowed to have acyclovir, ganciclovir and steroids)	1/26 HAMA	Transient neutropenia	Not done	463, 464
CR, peripheral infusion not effective in CNS, intrathecal injection caused rapid remission of disease	Not done	None	Not done	465

Table continued on following page

TABLE 21–1. *Continued*

ANTIBODY	ANTIGEN	DISTRIBUTION	DISEASE	# PATIENTS	DOSE/SCHED
Anti-Tac (lgG2a)	IL-2 binding site of p55 receptor complex	ATL and activated T cells, various other	ATL caused by HTLV-I	9	100–220 mg over 5–16 d	1 CR (5 mo), PR (6 wk) on retreatment; 1 PR for 8 mo
PMN 6, PMN 29, PM-81 (lgM) AML-2-23 (lgG2b)	?	Granulocytes and monocytes	AML	3	Multiple doses of 20–600 mg
Anti-CD4 chimeric Ab (human lgG1K with murine Leu 3a variable regions)	CD4	T cell, helper subset	CTCL	7	10–80 mg 2 × each week ×3
OKB7 (lgG2b)	CR2 EBV receptor	B cells	NHL	18	0.1–40 mg trace labeled with $_{131}$I
M195	CD33	Myeloid blasts (not on stem cell)	AML	10	1–76 mg trace labeled with $_{131}$I

Abbreviations: HAMA, human antimouse antibody; B-CLL, B-cell chronic lymphocytic leukemia; ATL, adult T-cell leukemia; WBC, white blood cell; PBL, peripheral blood lymphocytes; CTCL, cutaneous T-cell lymphoma; PR, partial response; pt, patient; anti-Id, anti-idiotype; CR, complete response; CLL, chronic lymphocytic leukemia; Bx, biopsy; BM, bone marrow; T-CLL, T-cell chronic lymphocytic leukemia; CALLA, common acute lymphoblastic leukemia antigen; ALL, acute lymphoblastic leukemia; CML, chronic myelogenous leukemia; HLA-DR, human histocompatibility leukocyte antigen; NHL, non-Hodgkin's lymphoma; HLA, human lymphocyte antigen; PLL, prolymphocytic leukemia; HCL, hairy-cell leukemia; cALL, childhood acute lymphoblastic leukemia; CNS, central nervous system; LFT, liver function test; EBV, Epstein-Barr virus; IL-2, interleukin 2; HTLV-I, human T-cell leukemia virus type I; AML, acute myelogenous leukemia.

idiotype antibody therapy with α-interferon was based on the synergistic effect of these two agents in a mouse B-cell tumor model. In this clinical trial, significant tumor remissions occurred in a high fraction of patients.[173] In the murine model, the synergistic activity of antibody and interferon was associated with increased ADCC activity.[178,179]

Recently, a panel of anti-idiotype antibodies reactive with shared idiotypic determinants has been developed.[180] Using this panel, lymphoma tissues have been screened for antibody binding, and antibodies have been selected for immediate therapeutic use. Early-phase clinical trials are underway and clinical activity has been reported.[181]

Published trials using anti-idiotype antibodies are detailed in Table 21–3. With the exception of the series of trials described above, the majority of other trials with anti-idiotype antibodies have been done in patients with CLL or NHL with large numbers of circulating lymphoma cells present in the peripheral blood. Monoclonal[182–188] and polyclonal[189,190] antibodies have been used. In general, responses have been minimal and have consisted of transient decreases in the number of tumor cells present in the peripheral blood. High levels of circulating idiotype and modulation of the surface idiotype have been reported to interfere with the therapeutic effect of the anti-idiotype antibodies. Murine Fab′ fragments of anti-idiotype antibodies have been chemically coupled to normal human IgG1 to create a univalent chimeric antibody and used as therapy in one patient with NHL.[191] A tumor flare with tenderness and swelling was observed 4 days after therapy followed by a partial response of disease at 6 weeks after therapy.

Solid Tumors

Whereas the earliest clinical trials utilizing MAbs for the therapy of human malignancies focused on the treatment of lymphomas and leukemias, a large body of information now has been generated in the therapy of solid tumors such as gastrointestinal carcinomas and malignant melanoma. Representative trials are outlined in Table 21–4. In a variety of clinical trials that have been reviewed recently,[192–196] more than 600 patients were treated with the murine IgG2a antibody MAb 17-1A. This MAb reacts with a 37,000-Da glycoprotein of unknown function with wide distribution throughout the gastrointestinal tract that is expressed on the cell surface of most carcinomas arising from the stomach, pancreas, and colorectal tissues. Rare tumor responses have been documented; however, the majority of patients with advanced cancer have not had significant tumor responses. Moreover, other concurrent or subsequent therapies often have clouded the interpretation of clinical responses. Numerous doses and schedules of antibody delivery have been explored, with no single method clearly superior. In general, large quantities of the antibody (doses greater than 400 mg) have been necessary to achieve significant antibody binding to tumor.[196] Cumulative doses as high as 12 gm have been administered. Infusion-related symptoms have been mild and include diarrhea, nausea, vomiting, abdominal pain, and fever. On repeat infusions of the antibody, anaphylactic reactions were noted in some patients.

The majority of these trials have been performed in patients with bulky disease, and survival has not been compared directly with a randomized control group. A trial has been performed in patients with Dukes B2 and

EFFECT	HAMA	TOXICITY	MAb IN TUMOR	REF.
1 CR (5 mo), PR (6 1 wk) on retreatment; 1 PR for 8 mo	1	Minimal	PBL tumor positive, but not lymph node	165, 108
Transient decrease in WBC	1/3	Fever, back pain, arthralgias and myalgias	Minimal	466
Transient responses all pts; 2 PR, 1 minor response, and 3 mixed responses; antibody-coated cells in blood not cleared.	Low-level anti–variable region antibodies, without clinical significance	Minimal toxicity; 2 pts with infections	Antibody found in tumor biopsies at higher doses	159
None	5/18 HAMA	None	Tumors imaged, especially in pts with minimal disease	292
None	Not done	None	Saturation with > 5mg/m^2	467

C resected colorectal carcinoma, with approximately 180 patients randomized to treatment with MAb 17-1A versus no treatment. Although not yet published, preliminary results of this trial with a median follow-up of nearly 5 years demonstrate a decrease in the occurrence of metastatic disease and a significant prolongation of survival in patients receiving the antibody (G. Riethmuller, personal communication, August 1992).

Universal to these antibody trials, and in contrast to the experience in the treatment of patients with B-cell lymphoma, has been the rapid generation of a HAMA response. An IgM-based immune response can be seen in patients as early as 5 to 7 days, and an IgG response by day 10.[192] In some trials, repeated antibody infusions given in rapid succession or at high doses delayed the onset of the immune response.[197]

It has been proposed that the lack of clinical effect seen in many patients may be due to the limited availability of mononuclear cells at the tumor site, which are needed for ADCC. To explore this possibility, isolated autologous mononuclear cells were precoated ex vivo with MAb 17-1A and then infused.[197–203] However, this "arming" maneuver has resulted in only sporadic and unconfirmed clinical activity.

In an attempt to increase the cytotoxicity of the antibody therapy, agents that increase ADCC activity have

been tested in clinical trials. Antibody therapy combined with a course of interferon-γ demonstrated minor antitumor responses in one trial that were not confirmed in others.[204–206] Antibody combined with a course of granulocyte-macrophage colony-stimulating factor (GM-CSF) also has demonstrated preliminary evidence of increased antitumor activity.[192] In this trial, increased ADCC activity has been demonstrated in the blood, and tumor biopsies taken from patients following therapy demonstrated an increase in the number of mononuclear cells. Of 15 patients treated, one complete and one partial response have been reported. An increased incidence of allergic reactions also was reported, prompting revision of the treatment schedule for subsequent doses.[192]

A phase I trial of chimeric mouse/human MAb 17-1A demonstrated prolonged α and β half-lives of 18 and 126 hours, respectively, in the serum of patients treated with 10 to 40 mg of the antibody every 2 weeks for one to three doses. However, in this trial, no objective clinical responses were seen in any of ten patients with metastatic colorectal cancer.[37] No significant toxicity was seen and decreased immunogenicity was noted, with only a single patient making an antibody response against the murine variable region. It remains to be seen if higher doses or combination with additional agents will result in clinical activity.

TABLE 21–2. CLINICAL TRIALS AT STANFORD UNIVERSITY USING CUSTOM, PRIVATE MONOCLONAL ANTI-IDIOTYPE ANTIBODIES IN PATIENTS WITH B-CELL LYMPHOMA

TRIAL/REF	NO. PATIENTS	CLINICAL RESPONSE		MEDIAN TIME TO TUMOR PROGRESSION (mo)
		PARTIAL	COMPLETE*	
MAb alone[171]	14	8	2	6
MAb/IFN[173]	11	5	3	7
MAb/CHL[174]	13	8	1	7
TOTAL	34	17 (50%)	6 (18%)	

*Five of six complete responses lasted more than 5 years, with three of six ongoing at 66, 69, and 72 months.

TABLE 21–3. CLINICAL TRIALS OF UNCONJUGATED MONOCLONAL ANTIBODIES DIRECTED AGAINST B-CELL TUMOR IMMUNOGLOBULIN IDIOTYPE

ANTIBODY	DISEASE	# PATIENTS	DOSE/ SCHEDULE	EFFECT	HAMA	TOXICITY	MAb IN TUMOR?	COMMENTS	REF.
Monoclonal anti-Id	B-cell NHL	11	400–3183 mg over 2–3 wk	5/11 (1 CR, 4 PR)	5/11	Fever, rigor, rash	Yes (6/8 tumor Bx, 3/3 on tumor in blood)	Toxicity in patients with HAMA or circulating idiotype; plasmapheresis to decrease idiotype prior to Rx minimally effective	170, 171
Monoclonal anti-Id combined with course of α-IFN	B-cell NHL	11	1680–8400 mg over 2–3 wk in 6–12 doses	8/11 (3 CR, 5 PR)	2/11	Fever, rigor, rash	Not done	4/8 Bx with evidence of idiotype-negative variant cells posttherapy	173
Monoclonal anti-Id combined with pulse of chlorambucil	B-cell NHL	13	2 courses of 1920–5757 mg over 2–3 wk in 6–12 doses	9/13 (1 CR, 8 PR)	0/13	Fever, rigor, rash	Not done	Chlorambucil did not affect outcome or prevent emergence of idiotype-negative variants	174
Anti-Id (IgG2a)	B-cell NHL	2	3.8 and 5.8 gm over 65 and 16 d, various schedules	Transient decreases in PBL tumor	0/2	Minimal	Yes in blood, BM, ascites and lymph node	Indium-labeled tumor cells went to liver following MAb therapy	182, 183
Polyclonal sheep anti-Id (IgG1 fraction)	PLL	1	480 mg × 1, 750 and 420 mg × 1	Transient decrease in PBL tumor	None noted	Fever, rigor, bronchospasm	Not at 16 hr post-Rx	Plasmapheresis to decrease idiotype prior to Rx; complement consumption	189
Polyclonal sheep anti-Id (IgG1 fraction)	CLL	4	1.5–2.5 gm over 1–2 d	Transient decrease in WBC (tumor)	None noted	Minimal	Partial saturation and modulation of the surface Ig noted post-Rx	Plasmapheresis to decrease idiotype prior to Rx; FFP given to replace complement	190
Monoclonal anti-Id (IgM)	CLL	1	1–500 mg/d for 10 d	No effect	None noted	Minimal	Minimal	Unable to clear idiotype level of 400 μg/ml	185
Monoclonal anti-Id (IgG1)	CLL	1	5 gm over 18 d, 10 gm over 17 d, 5.5 gm over 14 d	Transient response in nodes, spleen, PBL tumor	None noted	Mucosal edema	Modulation	Decreased clearance of antibody-coated erythrocytes in pt vs control	184
Monoclonal anti-Id (IgG1)	CLL	1	773 mg over 44 d	PR (90% reduction at 2 wk lasting 3 mo)	None noted	Fever, chills, nausea, vomiting diarrhea	Minimal	Increased serum TNF post therapy; tumor cells stimulated in vitro by the anti-Id; not seen in vivo	186, 187

Table continued on following page

TABLE 21–3. *Continued*

ANTIBODY	DISEASE	# PATIENTS	DOSE/ SCHED- ULE	EFFECT	HAMA	TOXICITY	MAb IN TUMOR?	COMMENTS	REF.
Monoclonal anti-Id (IgG1)	CLL	1	24.5 gm over 1 y (four 3-wk courses)	Transient response in PBL tumor and spleen	None noted	None noted	Increasing modulation	BCGF stimulation of tumor cells in vitro blocked by the anti-Id	186, 187
Chimeric univalent murine fab′γ linked to normal human IgG	B-cell NHL	1	380–580 mg in 4 infusions over 11 wk	PR at 6 wk	None	None noted	Not in lymph nodes	Tumor flare with tenderness, swelling 4 d post-Rx	191

Abbreviations: IFN, interferon; FFP, fresh frozen plasma; TNF, tumor necrosis factor; BCGF, B cell growth factor; other abbreviations as in Table 21–1.

Early-phase clinical trials with other antibodies directed against tumor-associated antigens, such as 19-9, a murine IgG2a directed against a monosialoganglioside antigen present in the serum and on gastrointestinal carcinomas, failed to demonstrate tumor binding following injection.[207] A similar study with GA733, a murine IgG2a directed against another epitope of the CO 17-1A antigen, demonstrated tumor penetration and in vivo binding, but with the increased toxicities of abdominal cramps, diarrhea, and nausea at the highest doses used.[207] No clinical effect was seen with either antibody.

Therapeutic trials with L6, a murine IgG2a directed against an antigen expressed on breast, colon, ovary, and non–small-cell lung cancers, demonstrated detection of antibody in saturating amount in tumor biopsies following doses of more than 100 mg.[208] One complete response occurred late after the antibody treatment in a patient with metastatic breast cancer. Biopsies of regressing tumor documented an intense mononuclear infiltrate. The majority of patients in this trial mounted a HAMA response. On the theory that tumor regression in this patient was caused by the induction of an antitumor immune response, a subsequent trial was performed with the addition of IL-2.[209] Increased toxicity attributed to the IL-2 was noted, and, although increased ADCC activity was documented, minimal clinical activity was observed, with one partial and one mixed response in 15 patients. The IL-2 did not augment or suppress the HAMA response. The antibody BW494 (murine IgG1) has been used to treat patients with pancreatic cancer, with minimal effects noted in patients with gross disease.[210,211] An adjuvant trial of this antibody in patients with resected pancreatic carcinoma also failed to demonstrate any beneficial effect on relapse or survival when compared to the randomized control group.[212]

Hybridomas secreting human antibodies against antigens on colorectal tumor cells have been obtained from peripheral blood lymphocytes of patients immunized with autologous tumor.[213] The antibody 16.88 is a human IgM directed against an altered cytokeratin antigen expressed on colorectal cells. Metastatic tumors have been detected by immunoscintigraphy, and a longer half-life observed, though no antitumor activity has been seen.[214–217]

Clinical activity using unconjugated MAbs also has been reported in the treatment of patients with malignant melanoma and neuroblastoma. These trials are detailed in Table 21–5. Target antigens include the gangliosides GD2 and GD3 present on cells of neuroectodermal origin. Antibody R24 is a murine IgG3 reactive with GD3. Several trials of this antibody have been reported in melanoma patients and a number of partial responses have been observed.[218–220] Antibody, together with an inflammatory cellular infiltrate, has been noted in posttreatment tumor biopsies. Toxicities have included urticaria, nausea, vomiting, and diarrhea. HAMA responses have been universal. Antibody combined with a course of interferon (rHu-IFNa2a) demonstrated no clinical responses in 15 patients,[221] whereas antibody combined with a course of IL-2 showed one partial and two minor responses in 20 patients.[222] In both trials, enhanced toxicity attributed to the cytokines was seen, and, in the IL-2 trial, enhanced HAMA formation as early as day 5 was observed.

Two antibodies against GD2 have entered clinical trials. Clinical activity has been demonstrated in patients with neuroblastoma and melanoma with antibody 3F8, although significant toxicity, including severe abdominal pelvic pain, hypertension and urticaria, was observed.[223–225] Melanoma patients treated with 14G2a (a murine IgG2a class switch variant of the IgG3 antibody 14.18) experienced neurotoxicity and severe pain at the higher doses, with one partial and one mixed response in 12 patients.[226] Significant effects in patients with neuroblastoma also have been reported, with similar toxicity.[227] Early trials with 5- to 100-mg doses of a chimeric 14.18 antibody also demonstrated in vivo tumor binding at doses greater than 45 mg; however, significant abdominal/pelvic pain again was seen and no clinical antitumor responses were noted.[228] Interestingly, 8 of 13 patients mounted a weak immune response against the variable region of the chimeric antibody. Intralesional injection of a human IgM anti-GD2 antibody (L72)[229] and a murine IgM antimonosialoganglioside antibody[230] induced regressions of injected lesions.

TABLE 21–4. CLINICAL TRIALS OF UNCONJUGATED MONOCLONAL ANTIBODIES IN CARCINOMAS (Ca)

MAb	ANTIGEN	DISTRIBUTION	DISEASE	# PATIENTS	DOSE/SCHED
17-1A	37-kDa glycoprotein	GI tissues	Colorectal Ca	4	15–200 mg
17-1A	37-kDa glycoprotein	GI tissues	GI Ca	20	15–1000 mg × 1
17-1A	37-kDa glycoprotein	GI tissues GI Ca	GI Ca	20 (phase I) 20 (phase II) 20	15–1000 mg 100 or 700 mg followed by 100 mg 2×/mo × 4 mo
17-1A	37-kDa glycoprotein	GI tissues	GI Ca: gastric (2), pancreas (2), colorectal (21)	25	400 mg IV 1–4 times over 1–2 wk
17-1A	37-kDa glycoprotein	GI tissues	Colorectal Ca	20	200–850 mg single dose
17-1A with Monos	37-kDa glycoprotein	GI tissues	Colorectal and various	22	200 mg with monos
CO17-1A with or without monos	37-kDa glycoprotein	GI tissues	Pancreatic Ca	25	400 mg × 1 (10 pts) or 400 mg × 1 with monos (15 pts)
17-1A alone or with FAM chemotherapy	37-kDa glycoprotein	GI tissues	Pancreatic Ca	8 MAb alone 8 MAb/FAM	400 mg × 1
17-1A with monos	37-kDa glycoprotein	GI tissues	Colorectal Ca	24	200–500 mg by various schemes to 12 gm over 8–18 wk
17-1A with monos	37-kDa glycoprotein	GI tissues	Colorectal Ca	8	400 mg with monos then 200 mg with monos q 6 wk × 3
17-1A with monos (following hepatic XRT)	37-kDa glycoprotein	GI tissues	Colorectal, pancreas, lung Ca met to liver	13	540–2160 mg over 3–10 cycles q 2 wk (following XRT)
17-1A with or without autologous monos; (6 trials); E-17-1A 73-3, 19-9, 55-2 (all IgG2a)	37-kDa glycoprotein	GI tissues	Colorectal Ca	A—25 met disease B—8 met disease C—30 pts (various) D—11 pts E—21 pts F—B2/C pts post resection, 89 pts rand to Rx/control/Rx & 5FU	500 mg with monos × 1 500 mg day 1 and 100 mg day 7 500 mg with monos day 1, 100 mg day 7 150 mg day 1, 50/d × 4 d 150–200 mg each Ab + monos 500 mg + monos or no Rx or Rx + weekly 5FU × 6 mo
17-1A with monos	37-kDa glycoprotein	GI tissues	Pancreatic Ca	18	400 mg with monos × 1

Table continued on following page

EFFECT	HAMA	TOXICITY	MAb IN TUMOR	COMMENTS	REF.
None	3/4	Allergic symptoms with multiple doses	Inflammatory infiltrate in one Bx		194
2 responses ?	11/20	Minimal, except with multiple doses	Not done		195
? 2 responses	10/20 17/20	Minimal in single dose Minor, except anaphylaxis following HAMA response	Yes at large dose		468
1 CR in patient with liver mets (56 mo)	21/25	Diarrhea, nausea, vomiting; anaphylaxis in 2 pts Rx at day 15	Not done	Median survival of 57 wk; HAMA and toxicity if Rx > day 15	196, 469, 470
1 CR, 1 decrease in liver lesions but increase in abd wall tumor	10/20	Urticaria, nausea, diarrhea all mild	Fab scan positive in liver mets, but not in abd wall mass	Prior studies had included some pts also receiving other Rx	193
None	5/8 (anti-Id)	None	Not done		198
4 PR/19 evaluated pts	23/25 11/25 (anti-Id)	None	Not done	Median survival all pts 12 wk; no difference between pts making HAMA vs anti-Id response	199
None MAb alone, 2 PR in MAb/FAM group	Not done	None	Not done		471
Not reported	24/24	Mild GI symptoms; allergic reactions with later doses	Not done	HAMA did not affect pharmacokinetics at this dose level	197
1CR, 1PR	8/8 HAMA	Anaphylaxis with later doses	Yes by Bx		472
1 CR in pt with minimal liver disease; one other minor response	Not done	Mild anaphylaxis in 2 pts on retreatment	Not done	5 other PR responses not seen in CT evaluations	200
1/20 CR, 3/20 MR No response	11/19 6/7 HAMA	Mild toxicity None	Not done Not done	Trial F is a randomized trial of 17-1A with monos (500 mg) vs nothing vs Rx with weekly 5FU for 6 mo (the 5FU arm was closed early) in pts with Dukes B2/C colorectal CA	201
1 MR/26	24/26 HAMA				
No response	5/8 HAMA	None	Not done		
2 CR/16	9/11 HAMA	Increased GI toxicity with 73-3	Not done		
No data	No data	No data	No data		
0/18 responses	13/16 HAMA	No significant toxicity seen	Not done		202

Table continued on following page

TABLE 21–4. *Continued*

MAb	ANTIGEN	DISTRIBUTION	DISEASE	# PATIENTS	DOSE/SCHED
17-1A with monos	37-kDa glycoprotein	GI tissue	Met colorectal Ca	10	200–400 mg with monos q 6 wk $\times$ 1–5
17-1A with γ-IFN	37-kDa glycoprotein	GI tissues	Colorectal and pancreas Ca	27	400 mg MAb following 4 d of γ-IFN
17-1A with γ-IFN	37-kDa glycoprotein	GI tissues	Colorectal Ca	15	MAb 400 mg on days 5, 7, 9, 12; IFN γ 0.1 mg/m^2, days 1–15
17-1A with γ-IFN and monos; phase II trial	37-kDa glycoprotein	GI tissues	Pancreatic Ca with measurable disease	30	MAb 150 mg with monos on days 2, 3, 4 following IFN; IFN-γ 1 $\times$ 10^6 − 6/m^2 IV days 1–4
17-1A with γ-IFN and monos; phase II trial	37-kDa glycoprotein	GI tissues	Met colorectal CA met	19	MAb 150 mg following IFN; IFN-γ 1 $\times$ 10 − 6/m^2 IV days 1–4
BW 494 (IgG1)	?	?	Pancreatic Ca	3	90, 30, 30 mg over 3 d
494/32 (IgG1) adjuvant randomized trial in resectable pancreatic Ca	Carbohydrate structure	Pancreas	Pancreatic Ca	61 (29 Rx, 32 control)	370 mg total over 10 d within 1 mo of complete resection
16.88 and 28A32 human IgM	? altered cytokeratin	Expressed on colon cancer more than normal colorectal tissues	Colorectal Ca	26	8–200 mg weekly (1–5 wk)
16.88	? altered cytokeratin	Expressed on colon Ca more than normal colorectal tissues	Colorectal Ca	10	8 mg with 5 mCi^{131} I
16.88	? altered cytokeratin	Expressed on colon Ca more than normal colorectal tissues	Colorectal Ca	20	8 mg labeled with 5 mCi^{131} I followed by 200–1000 mg
L6 (IgG2a)	? (Tapa family)	Breast, colorectal, lung, ovarian Ca	Colon (2), breast (5), ovary (9), lung (3)	19	5–400 mg/m^2/d $\times$ 7 IV bolus over 4 hr
L6 with IL-2	? (Tapa family)	Breast, colorectal, lung, ovarian Ca	Breast (5), colon (5), lung (5)	15	200 mg/m^2/d$\times$7 Il-2 at 2–4.5 $\times$ 10^6/M^{2}SC for 4 d/wk $\times$ 3, starting at day 15

Table continued on following page

EFFECT	HAMA	TOXICITY	MAb IN TUMOR	COMMENTS	REF.
1 CR in pt with abd lymph nodes (positive node at 2nd look, removed—continues in CR at 33 mo)	10/10 HAMA	Mild except anaphylactoid in pts retreated with a positive skin test	Not done	Responders' (4) median survival 19 mo; non-responders' (6) median survival 7 mo	203
None	8/11 HAMA 7/8 (anti-Id)	Fever, rigors, malaise mostly related to IFN	Not done	Monocytes not activated by high-dose in vivo γ-IFN, ? activated by a lower dose	206
No CR/PR	13/14 HAMA, 11/13 anti-Id	Fever, mild constitutional symptoms; mild nausea/vomiting	Not done	Median survival 56 wk, no correlation between response/survival and development of anti-Id; no difference from trial with MAb alone	473
25 evaluated; 1 CR for 4 mo/25 pts	Not done	CHF to IFN in 1 pt, other mild toxicities	Not done	Improved natural cytotoxicity and mono ADCC noted; not able to demonstrate increase in HLA-DR on monos; median survival 5 mo for entire group	204
All progressed within 2 mo	Not done	Fever, mild constitutional symptoms, increased liver transaminases in 6 pts	8/16 pts imaged; 3/9 Bx + for MAb	Antibody delivery to several antigen-positive tumor masses not seen; too low a dose vs the low O^2 tension in the tumor?	205
Not noted	Not done	Not noted	3 pts Bx by laproscopy; minimal MAb in some of the tumor, not saturated but abundant antigen present		210
No effect on survival or relapse compared with randomized control group	Not done	Mild nausea/vomiting in few pts	Not done (adjuvant therapy)	Randomized adjuvant trial in pancreatic Ca, with no effect seen	212
None	None to 16.88, weak to 28A32	None	9/12 with 16.88, 12/16 with 28A32 7–23 d post-injection	$t^{1/2}$ whole body clearance of MAb 16.88 of 51 hr	217
Not noted	? one case	None	6/10 imaged (tumor >4 cm)		214, 216
Not noted	None	None	16/20 imaged some tumor at 5–7 d	No change in pharmacokinetics with larger doses	215
1 CR in met breast cancer (highest dose level), took 14 wk to achieve; serial Bx revealed an intense mononuclear infiltrate	13/18 HAMA, 8/13 (anti-Id)	Mild fever, chills; fall in serum C3 and C4	Yes by Bx; some in 20–100 mg/m² dose; saturated in vivo by > 100 mg/m²		208
1 PR (colon), 1 mixed transient response (breast)	9/14 HAMA	Fever, chills with MAb; fatigue, malaise, pulmonary capillary leak syndrome with IL-2; decreased C3 and C4	Not done	Demonstrated enhanced ADCC, no change in NK activity; IL-2 did not augment or suppress HAMA formation	209

Table continued on following page

TABLE 21–4. *Continued*

MAb	ANTIGEN	DISTRIBUTION	DISEASE	# PATIENTS	DOSE/SCHED
CO-19-9 (IgG2a class switch variant)	Monosialo-ganglioside	Colorectal, pancreas, and gastric tissues	Advanced GI Ca	11	10–600 mg
GA 733	Different epitope of 17-1A antigen, not shed	Same			10–300 mg
Chimeric 17-1A; human IgG1K	41-kDa glycoprotein	GI cells	Met colon Ca	10	10–40 mg q 2 wk × 1–3
MAb 225 (IgG1)	EGF receptor	Variety	Non–small-cell lung Ca	19	1–300 mg trace-labeled with ^{111}In

Abbreviations: GI, gastrointestinal; abd, abdominal; mets, metastases; monos, mononuclear cells; FAM, 5-fluorouracil; Adriamycin, and mitomycin; XRT, radiation therapy; CT, computerized tomography; 5FU, 5-fluorouracil; CHF, congestive heart failure; ADCC, antibody-dependent cell-mediated cytotoxicity; NK, natural killer cell; EGF, epidermal growth factor; HACA, human anti-chimeric antibody; other abbreviations as in Tables 21–1 and 21–3.

Antibodies targeted to growth factors or their receptors also are entering clinical trials. An antibody to the epidermal growth factor (EGF) receptor that blocks EGF binding and inhibits EGF activation of tyrosine kinase activity and cell proliferation in vitro has been administered to patients with squamous cell carcinoma of the lung.[231] Using trace-labeled antibodies, tumors were imaged successfully; however, no clinical responses were observed using 1 to 300 mg of antibody. Similar trials using antibodies against the *her-2* proto-oncogene[232] and against gastrin-releasing peptide (GRP) are underway.[233] Anti–IL-6 antibodies have been used in a single patient with plasma cell leukemia in an effort to deprive/block the growth stimulatory effect of the factor. A transient decrease in bone marrow myeloma cell proliferation and a decrease in IL-6–related side effects without significant toxicity were demonstrated.[234]

In the evaluation of clinical responses in these trials of antibody therapy of solid tumors, late clinical responses have been observed, prompting investigators to propose that immune mechanisms have been induced by the antibody therapy. Most of the proposed mechanisms involve the induction of a host anti-idiotype antibody (Ab2, carrying the internal image of antigen) response to the murine antibody and the subsequent induction of an anti–anti-idiotype antibody response (Ab3), which would be capable of binding to and destroying the tumor cells. This idiotype cascade originally was proposed by Jerne as a natural mechanism of regulating the immune response.[132] In several studies, the induction of an (Ab2) humoral immune response to the murine immunoglobulin was correlated with improved survival,[133,235] but the nearly universal induction of an Ab2 response in other studies and the overall lack of clinical efficacy make such gross correlations doubtful.[134,236,237] More refined studies looking for the generation of Ab3 (capable of binding to the original tumor antigen) have shown that a higher proportion of patients with Ab3 have demonstrated clinical antitumor responses than those who failed to make an Ab3 response.[236,238] Grouping patients into Ab3-positive and Ab3-negative groups demonstrated a survival advantage for those patients in the Ab3-positive cohort.[236] These results await confirmation by additional studies.

Immunization with anti-idiotype antibodies (Ab2) in attempts to induce an antitumor effect also has been pursued actively. Polyclonal goat anti-idiotype (Ab2) against the 17-1A antigen has been used to immunize patients with colorectal carcinoma.[135,239,240] Production of Ab3 capable of binding antigen-positive colorectal tumor cells has been demonstrated.[240] Human Ab2 has been isolated from immortalized cells obtained from the blood of patients treated with MAb 17-1A. In one study of patients treated with MAb 17-1A and GM-CSF, delayed-type hypersensitivity responses to skin tests with pooled human Ab2 have been demonstrated.[241] Active immunization of patients with these anti-idiotype antibodies to test for immunogenicity and for therapeutic effect is underway. In a similar fashion, patients have been immunized with a human IgG1 monoclonal anti-idiotype antibody (105AD7) raised from lymphocytes from a patient given the anti-gp72 murine antibody (79IT/36) for immunoscintigraphy.[242] The antibody was administered in an aluminum hydroxide gel precipitate as a single intramuscular dose. Although no antitumor or anti–anti-idiotype antibodies were seen, proliferative responses to gp72-positive tumor cells and to the 105AD7 anti-idiotype antibody were seen using isolated mononuclear cells in vitro.

Murine anti-idiotype antibodies also have been used in attempts to induce active immunity in patients with melanoma. In two clinical trials, patients were immunized with anti-idiotype antibody MF11-30 to induce an immune response to the high-molecular-weight melanoma-associated antigen (HMW-MAA).[243] Nearly all patients produced a HAMA response, and most produced a component directed against the binding site of the immunizing antibody. A complete response was seen in one patient and minor responses were seen in six patients. In a subsequent trial, patients were immunized with antibody MK2-23 conjugated to keyhole limpet hemocyanin and mixed with Calmette-Guerin bacillus.[244] Antibodies reac-

EFFECT	HAMA	TOXICITY	MAb IN TUMOR	COMMENTS	REF.
No objective responses	8/11 HAMA (most anti-Id)	Elevation LFTs, elevated lipase, proteinuria	No detection of 19-9 in tumor tissue		207
No objective response		Abd cramps, pain, diarrhea, nausea, vomiting at highest doses (500 mg)	All cases had GA 733 in tumors, most at saturating doses with the highest dose) (normal colon also saturated)		207
No objective responses	1 HACA to murine variant region	None	Not done	$\alpha\ t^{1/2}$ of 18 hr; $\beta\ t^{1/2}$ of 126 hr	37
No objective responses	19/19 HAMA by day 8	None	Imagining at greater than 20 mg dose		231

tive with HMW-MAA were seen in 14/25 patients, and three partial responses were observed in these 14 patients. These patients also had prolonged survival compared with the patients not making an immune response to HMW-MAA.

Targeting Cytotoxic Agents

In the early 1900s, Paul Ehrlich postulated the use of antibodies as "magic bullets" for the treatment of cancer, and this has been the dream of immunotherapists ever since.[245] The design and production of MAbs armed with radionuclides, toxins, and chemotherapeutic drugs has helped keep this dream alive. The rationale behind the use of immunoconjugates is to carry a toxic agent to the tumor site, where it can effect its toxicity on the tumor cells while minimizing toxic effects to nontarget tissue. In contrast, antibody therapy that relies on immunologic mechanisms for tumor destruction may be limited by its inability to recruit sufficient numbers of effector cells, especially in solid tumors. In addition, effector cells may be absent or ineffective as a result of prior therapy, tumor-induced immunosuppression, or the tumor being in an immunoprivileged site. The use of MAbs conjugated to cytotoxic agents bypasses this need for host effector functions.

There are several strategies for targeting cytotoxic agents to tumor cells. These include:

1. Targeting agents that have cytotoxic properties on their own but lack selectivity for tumor cell unless coupled to an antibody. Radiolabeled MAbs, immunotoxins, and MAb-drug conjugates fall under this strategy.

2. Targeting agents that are not cytotoxic on their own but can be activated by external irradiation. Photodynamic therapy with MAbs coupled to photosensitizers that are photoactivated to generate toxic oxygen radicals is one such approach. Utilizing MAbs coupled to the nonradioactive isotope ^{10}B, which releases cytotoxic α particles on irradiation with thermal neutrons, is another.[246-249]

3. Utilizing two-stage systems such as a bispecific MAb that recognizes both tumor antigen and a cytotoxic agent or, alternatively, a MAb-enzyme conjugate to target to the tumor an enzyme that catalyzes the conversion of a nontoxic prodrug to a cytotoxic agent in situ.

RADIOLABELED ANTIBODIES

The first demonstrations of tumor targeting with a radiolabeled antibody were reported in the early 1950s.[250,251] A radiolabeled antiserum against a rat sarcoma was shown to enhance the specific uptake of radioactivity in the tumors of sarcoma-bearing rats. Unfortunately, the difficulties in producing good radiolabeled antisera against human tumors made early clinical trials ineffective.[252] With the advent of hybridoma technology and the continued advancements in conjugation chemistry, however, the use of radiolabeled MAbs in the diagnosis and therapy of cancer is becoming a reality.

There are a number of radioisotopes to choose from for the production of a radiolabeled antibody. Although the killing effect of these different radionuclides on tumor cells is generally by damage to the DNA, each has a characteristic type and rate of decay that must be considered for its applicability to radioimmunotherapy. The most commonly used radionuclide, ^{131}I, has a half-life of 8 days and undergoes β-minus decay with associated γ emissions. γ-Rays are highly energetic and are able to penetrate tens of centimeters of tissue; thus γ-rays produced from localized ^{131}I-MAb will not have much of an effect on the local tumor tissue but will affect more distant tissues. In contrast, β-minus particles, which are basically electrons, only travel up to a few centimeters and affect a more local region of tissue. Other radionuclides with β-minus decay modes include ^{212}Bi, ^{67}Ga, ^{186}Re, and ^{90}Y. Some of these, such as ^{90}Y, lack the associated γ emissions of ^{131}I and hence radiation effects at distant sites are minimized with these isotopes. Positron emitters, such as ^{124}I, decay with the release of a positively charged particle with the same mass as an electron. When a positron come to rest in tissue, it combines with an electron, resulting in the emission of two γ photons at 180 degrees from each other. Another mode of decay is by α-particle emission. α Particles are composed of four protons and release large amounts of energy over a very short distance (~50 mm). These α particles are probably the most efficient at local tumor killing without damage to distant tissues.[253,254]

^{211}At and ^{212}Bi are two α emitters being considered for radioimmunotherapy. Finally, there are some radionuclides that decay by electron capture (e.g., ^{124}I and ^{125}I). In this decay process, several low-energy electrons are emitted over a very short range, around 20 nm, resulting in very intense local radiation effects.

The chemistry involved in conjugating radioisotopes to MAbs is as varied as the radioisotopes themselves. Several, in particular the radioiodine isotopes ^{131}I and ^{125}I, can be directly conjugated to the MAb. Others involve attaching chelating groups to the MAb and then binding the radioisotope to these groups. Radiometals such as ^{90}Y and ^{111}In frequently are coupled to MAbs by this technique.

As with all conjugation techniques, be they for radioisotopes, toxins, or drugs, chemical alteration of the antibody's binding region must be avoided to ensure optimal tumor targeting.

One of the main therapeutic advantages of radiolabeled MAbs lies in their potential to overcome the problem of antigenic heterogeneity. Because several radionuclides, namely the β emitters, can penetrate up to several centimeters of tissue, emissions from a radiolabeled MAb bound to an antigen-positive tumor cell theoretically could kill surrounding antigen-negative tumor cells. In addition, unlike most toxin or drug conjugates, radiolabeled MAbs do not need to be internalized to kill cells. However,

TABLE 21–5. CLINICAL TRIALS OF UNCONJUGATED MONOCLONAL ANTIBODIES IN MELANOMA AND NEUROBLASTOMA (NB)

MAb	ANTIGEN	DISTRIBUTION	DISEASE	# PATIENTS	DOSE
9.2.27 (IgG2a)	250-kDa glyco-protein	Various epidermal cells, melanoma	Melanoma	8	1–200 mg 2×/wk
14G2a (IgG2a class switch of 14.18 IgG3)	GD2 disialogan-glioside	Neuroectodermal origin	Melanoma	12	10–120 mg in 4 doses over 8 d
14G2a	GD2	Neuroectodermal origin	NB	9	20–60 mg/m^2 qd × 5–10 (total 100–400 mg/m^2)
Chimeric 14.18 (Human IgG1 with murine variable regions)	GD2	Neuroectodermal origin	Melanoma	13	5–100 mg
3F8 (IgG3)	GD2	Neuroectodermal origin	Melanoma (9) NB (8)	17	5–100 mg/m^2
3F8	GD2	Neuroectodermal origin	NB	15	10 mg/m^2 each day × 5 for 1–4 cycles
L72 human IgM, intra-lesional injection	GD2	Neuroectodermal region	Melanoma	8	100 μg/1 mm of tumor diameter, multiple injections
MAb 96.5 (IgG2a)	p97	Melanoma	Melanoma	5	1–50 mg q d, 7–10 d (212–424 mg total)
MAb 48.7 (IgG1)	Proteoglycan antigen				
R24 (IgG3)	GD3	Neuroectodermal origin	Melanoma	21	1–50 mg/m^2 days 1–5, 8–12
R24	GD3	Neuroectodermal origin	Melanoma	12	8, 80, 240 mg/m^2/over 2 wk
R24 with IL-2	GD3	Neuroectodermal origin	Melanoma	20	1–12 mg/m^2 days 8–12 IL-2 at 1 × 10^6/m^2/ days 1–5 and days 8–12 over 6 hr
R24 with rHu llFNa2a	GD3	Neuroectodermal origin	Melanoma	15	8 mg/m^2 days 1–5, 8–12; IFN IM to 50,000 on day of Rx

Abbreviations: SIADH, syndrome of inappropriate secretion of antidiuretic hormone; other abbreviations as in Tables 21–1 and 21–3.

radiolabeled MAbs are not without their disadvantages. These include difficulties in production, storage, and handling, and a variety of safety considerations. In addition, circulating labeled MAb or free radiolabel that has been released from the MAb conjugate can lead to bone marrow toxicity.

Clinical Trials of Radiolabeled MAbs

Recent studies demonstrating the diagnostic power of radiolabeled MAbs directed against a variety of tumor-specific and oncofetal tumor antigens to detect metastatic or recurrent tumors have been the subject of multiple symposia, conferences, and reviews. Selected published therapeutic clinical trials using radiolabeled antibodies are detailed in Table 21–6. The majority of clinical trials of radioisotope-labeled antibodies have utilized directly conjugated radioiodine isotopes such as ^{131}I or the indirectly chelated isotopes ^{111}In or [90]Y.

Polyclonal antibodies against ferritin and CEA have shown activity in the treatment of patients with hepatoma, intrahepatic cholangiocarcinoma, and Hodgkin's lymphoma.[255–259] Order and colleagues have combined ^{131}I-labeled antiferritin antibodies with external beam radiotherapy and chemotherapy to treat patients with unresectable hepatoma.[255,256] Additional delivered radia-

EFFECT	HAMA	TOXICITY	IMAGING ? MAb IN TUMOR ?	REF.
None	3/8	Fever, mild nausea	Bx positive at doses of 50 mg or greater (not saturating)	474
1 PR, 1 mixed response	12/12	Abdominal pelvic pain, SIADH, neurotoxicity, delayed extremity pain	8/11 MAb localized to tumor by imaging	226
2/6 CR, 2/6 PR	9/9	Abdominal and joint pain, allergic reactions, urticaria, hypertension	Yes in selected cases	227
None	8/13 weak	Abdominal, pelvic pain syndrome	Bx positive for MAb at doses > 45 mg	228
2 CR (NB) 7–14 mo 2 PR (melanoma) 5–12 mo	17/17	Pain, hypertension, urticaria	Majority imagined, 4 Bx—all positive	223, 225
3 CR, 1 PR 6/10 (best responses in marrow disease only with small volume disease)	6/10	Pain, hypertension, urticaria	11/15 imaged	224
Regression of many lesions, no effect in control injections	5/8 pts made an immune response, 2/5 anti-Id	None	Not done	229
No response	4/4	Minimal symptoms	Bx positive and saturated posttherapy, minimal at day 10 posttherapy	475, 476
4 PR lasting 1–11 mo	20/21	Urticaria, pruritus, nausea, vomiting, diarrhea	MAb with inflammatory response noted at Bx sites	219
5/12 PR	12/12	Urticaria, pruritus, nausea, vomiting	Yes at 80 mg/m²/or greater dose, inflammatory infiltrate with complement also noted	218 220
1 PR 6 mo	20/20 earlier HAMA, some by day 5	Urticaria, rashes, and IL-2 effects	Not known	222
No response	15/15	Urticaria rashes, hematologic fever, & flu-like symptoms	5/12 Bx positive	221

TABLE 21–6. CLINICAL TRIALS USING RADIOLABELED MONOCLONAL ANTIBODIES

ANTIBODY/ISOTOPE	ANTIGEN	DISTRIBUTION	DISEASE	# PATIENTS	DOSE MAb	DOSE RADIATION
LL2 (^{131}I) (IgG2a)	?	B cells (similar to CD20)	B-cell NHL	16 (7 Rx)	0.2–3.9 mg, 2–3 courses given	6.2–58.2 mCi
T101 (^{131}I) (IgG2a)	CD5	T cells, B-CLL	CTCL	3 reRx	10 mg	100 mCi
T101 ^{131}I)	CD5	T cells, B-CLL	CTCL	6	Dx 10 mg, Rx 10–17 mg	Dx 5–13 mCi, Rx 100–150 mCi
MB-1 (^{131}I) (IgG1) with autologous BM support	CD37	B cells	B-cell NHL	10 Dx, 5 high-dose Rx	2.5–10 mg/kg	232–608 mCi
MB-1 (^{131}I); nonmarrow ablative doses	CD37	B cells	B-cell NHL	12 Dx, 10 Rx	40 mg trace labeled, 40 mg for Rx dose	3–7 mCi for Dx, 25–161 mCi for Rx
Lym-1 (^{131}I) (IgG2a)	HLA-DR polymorphic variant	B cells	B-cell NHL	18	4–49 mg cold with 1 mg labeled	30–60 mCi q 2–6 wk to toxicity or 300 mCi total
Anti-Id (^{90}Y)	Private Ig idiotype	B cell tumor	B-cell NHL	1	2.3 gm	10 mCi
OKB7 (^{131}I) (IgG2b)	CR2 EBV receptor	B cells	B-cell NHL	18	0.1–40 mg	2 mCi
3F8 (^{131}I) (IgG3) with ABMT	GD2	Neuroepithelial origin	Neuroblastoma	12	2–10 μCi/μg	6–12 mCi/kg
Multiple (^{131}I) (IgG1, IgG2b and IgG2a)	?	Leptomenangeal tumor	Leptomeningeal tumor	6	2.5–10 mg IT	11–45 mCi
UJ181.4 (^{131}I)	?	Medullo-, neuro-, and retino-blastomas, pineal tumors, fetal brain	Pineo-blastoma	1	3 mg IT	870 MBq
Various (^{131}I)	?	Various	Malignant meningitis	15	? IT	11–60 mCi
HD37 (IgG1) WCMH 15.14 (IgG1) (^{131}I)	CD19, CD10	ALL, B cells	ALL	6		629–1480 MBq
B72.3 (^{131}I) (IgG1)	TAG-72 glycoprotein	Epithelial-derived tumors, colon, breast, lung, ovary, pancreas, stomach	Colorectal Ca	10	6–11 mCi/mg	10 mCi IP prior to surgery
B72.3 (^{131}I) (chimeric human IgG4)	TAG-72 glycoprotein	Epithelial-derived tumors, colon, breast, lung, ovary, pancreas, stomach	Colorectal Ca	12	3.4–6.7 mg	18–36 mCi/m^2
Fab of 8.2 (IgG1) and 96.5 (IgG2a) (^{131}I)	p97 and high-molecular-weight protein	Melanoma	Melanoma	50 Dx, 10 Rx	Rx 4–20 mg, Fab repeated 1–3 times	30–342 mCi (132–861 mCi total)

Table continued on following page

EFFECT	TOXICITY	HAMA	IMAGING ?	$t_{1/2}$	REF.
1 CR, 2PR, 1 mixed	Myelotoxicity at greater than 50 mCi	3/8	82% of known sites	α 2 hr, β 32 hr; IgG and f(ab')2	288
1 PR in patient with low HAMA	Fever, pruritis	All pre	2/3 pts	Decreased	280
2 PR 3 mixed	Fever, tachycardia, myelosuppression	6/6	Yes	α 1 hr, β 15–20 hr	291
4CR, 1PR	Minor, except planned marrow ablation at higher doses	0/10	5/10	Whole-body $t_{1/2}$ 43–59 hr	477, 123, 286
1 CR, 1 PR	Myelosuppression	2/12	11/12		287
2 Cr, 8 PR	Mild myelosuppression	3/18	Yes	ND	289, 290
1 PR	Mild decrease in platelets	0/1	Yes with ^{111}In, Bx nonsaturating	ND	293
None	None	5/18	Yes, 7/13 evaluated	α 2 hr, β 22 hr	292
2 PR	Pain syndrome, diarrhea, pancytopenia	ND	ND	ND	478
4/5 improved	Fever	ND	Yes	ND	265, 266
CR (22 mo)	Mild	ND	Paired label concentrated 20:1 at 2 d postinjection	ND	264
5/9 improved clinically	Headache, nausea, vomiting, fever, myelosuppression, seizures	ND	Yes	ND	267
4/6 CR (1–2 mo)	Headache, nausea, vomiting, fever	ND	ND	ND	263
None	None	ND	Yes	Whole-body $t_{1/2}$ 72 hr	479
None	MTD 36 mCi/m^2 because of myelotoxicity	7/12 HACA	50% tumors > 2 cm, most >4 cm; late imaging 8–23 d postinjection	242-hr plasma $t_{1/2}$	283, 284
1/3 evaluated pts with PR	Mild except thrombocytopenia and neutropenia	7/9 Rx with IgG, 8/17 Rx with Fab	88% of lesions > 1.5 cm imaged	ND	261

Table continued on following page

TABLE 21–6. *Continued*

ANTIBODY/ISOTOPE	ANTIGEN	DISTRIBUTION	DISEASE	# PATIENTS	DOSE MAb	DOSE RADIATION
Fab of 8.2 (IgG1) and 96.5 (IgG2a) (^{131}I)	p97 and high-molecular weight protein	Melanoma	Melanoma	26 Dx, 7 Rx	Dx 1 mg, Fab Rx 5–10 mg, Fab repeated up to 4 times	Dx 5 mCi, Rx 34–197 mCi
HMFG1 (^{90}Y) (IgG1)	300-kDa glycoprotein	Lactating breast, some epithelial tissues (weak), 90% ovarian Ca	Ovarian Ca	30	?	5–30 mCi IP
HMFG1 (^{90}Y) (IgG1)	300-kDa glycoprotein	Lactating breast, some epithelial tissues (weak), 90% ovarian Ca	Ovarian Ca	25	14.6–34.6 mg given IP	5–25 mCi
HMFG1 (^{131}I) given IP with IV HAMA	300-kDa glycoprotein	Lactating breast, some epithelial tissues, (weak), 90% ovarian Ca	Ovarian Ca	5	10–15 mg	112–130 mCi
HMFG1, HMFG2 AUA1; Hi17E2 (all IgG1) (^{131}I)	300-kDa glycoprotein; 40-kDa glycoprotein on adeno-carcinomas, placental-like alkaline phosphatase	Wide-range ovarian Ca	Ovarian Ca	24	? 4–8 mCi/mg Rx 1–4 times IP	20–205 mCi
HMFG1, HMFG2, AUA1, H17E2 (IgG1) (^{131}I)	40-kDa glycoprotein on adeno-carcinomas, placental-like alkaline phosphatase	Wide-range ovarian Ca	Ovarian Ca	36	4–8 mCi/mg given IP	20–158 mCi
HMFG2, AUA1 (IgG1) (^{131}I)	40-kDa glycoprotein on adeno-carcinomas, placental-like alkaline phosphatase	Wide-range ovarian Ca	Ovarian Ca	12	10 mg	75–170 mCi
HMFG1, HMFG2, AUA1, (IgG1) (^{131}I)	40-kDa glycoprotein on adeno-carcinomas, placental-like alkaline phosphatase	Wide-range ovarian Ca	Carcinomas causing malignant pleural or pericardial effusions	11	4–8 mCi/mg	20–86 m/Ci into pleural or pericardial space following removal of effusion
Polyclonal antiferritin (^{131}I) (rabbit, pig, monkey)	Ferritin	Hepatoma, Hodgkin's, neuroblastoma, lung, breast, pancreas Ca, AML	Hodgkin's disease	37	? 8–10 mCi/mg	30 mCi day 0, 20 mCi day 5; responders got repeated cycles with different species Ab Q 2 mo

Table continued on following page

EFFECT	TOXICITY	HAMA	IMAGING ?	$t_{1/2}$	REF.
None	Mild, fever, tachycardia, skin rash, myelotoxicity	3/7	20/33 pts imaged	Whole-body $t_{1/2}$ 28 hr	262
? most Rx adjuvant	Myelotoxicity at greater than 15 mCi decreased when EDTA given systemically	ND	ND	ND	268
1 PR/10 pts < 2 cm disease; no response in tumor > 2 cm	Myelosuppression, (thrombocytopenia), less following Rx with EDTA post-RIT (at 15–20 mCi); also abdominal pain, fever	25/25	ND	$t_{1/2}$ ^{90}Y in blood of 50 hr	271, 269
None	Rigor, flushing with HAMA, else minimal, except myelosuppression	5/5	ND	Decreased following HAMA	272
9/16 with disease < 2 cm; 0/8 with > 2 cm	Abdominal pain, fever, nausea, vomiting, diarrhea, mild myelotoxicity	Most with multiple doses	ND	Whole-body $t_{1/2}$ 38–60 hr	274
0/8 disease > 2 cm; 2/15 PR with < 2 cm; 3/6 CR in microscopic disease	Severe myelosuppression at doses > 120 mCi	36/36	ND	Effective $t_{1/2}$ of 50 hr	270
Minimal control of ascites	Nausea, dysphagia thrombocytopenia	ND	ND	Longer in pts with ascites	273
3/3 pericardial and 7/10 pleural effusions did not recurr during follow-up	Mild	ND	ND	ND	480
1 CR, 14 PR (PR 40%, symptomatic response 77%)	Myelotoxicity, platelets > leukeopenia	ND	Yes	ND	259

Table continued on following page

TABLE 21-6. *Continued*

ANTIBODY/ISOTOPE	ANTIGEN	DISTRIBUTION	DISEASE	# PATIENTS	DOSE MAb	DOSE RADIATION
Polyclonal antiferritin (^{90}Y) (rabbit, pig, baboon) with autologous marrow support	Ferritin	Hepatoma, Hodgkin's neuroblastoma, lung, breast, pancreas Ca, AML	Hodgkin's disease	6	5–40 mCi/mg	10–30 mCi, 1–3 courses
Polyclonal antiferritin (^{90}Y) (rabbit, pig, baboon) with autologous marrow support	Ferritin	Hepatoma, Hodgkin's, neuroblastoma, lung, breast, pancreas Ca, AML	Hodgkin's disease	45	5–40 mCi/mg	20–50 mCi
Polyclonal antiferritin (^{131}I) (rabbit, pig, monkey, horse) with low-dose chemotherapy	Ferritin	Hepatoma, Hodgkin's, neuroblastoma, lung, breast, pancreas Ca, AML	Hepatoma	180 induced (50 in each randomized ram)	8–10 mCi/mg	30 mCi day 0, 20 mCi day 5; responders got repeated cycles with different species Ab q 2 mo
Polyclonal antiferritin (^{131}I) with XRT and chemotherapy; review of 3 protocols	Ferritin	Hepatoma, Hodgkin's, neuroblastoma, lung, breast, pancreas Ca, AML	Hepatoma	105	8–10 mCi/mg	30 mCi day 0, 20 mCi day 5; Rx q 2 mo if possible
Multiple (IgG1) (^{131}I)	CEA and others	Various tissues	Gastrointestinal, lung, breast, and others	500 Dx, 12 Rx	?	100 mCi via IV, IP, or intrapleural
Anti-CEA (^{131}I) with XRT and chemotherapy (rabbit, pig, monkey, bovine antibodies)	CEA	Various	Intrahepatic cholangio-carcinoma	37	8–10 mCi/mg	20 mCi day 0 and 10 mCi day 5 with repeat q 2 mo with different species of Ab (1–4 times)
BC-2 (^{131}I) (IgG1) intralesional injection	Tenascin	Various tissues	Glioblastoma	10	0.8–5.8 mg intralesional injection, 1–3 cycles	111–1147 MBq per cycle (average=551 Mbq)
EGFR1 (IgG1) (^{131}I), H17E2 (IgG1)	Epidermal growth factor receptor Placental alkaline Phosphatase	Vulvar, colorectal cervical Ca, melanoma, astrocytomas	Gliomas	27 Dx, 10 Rx	?	40–140 mCi IV or IC
Anti-EGFR-425 (^{125}I) (IgG2) (adjuvant to surgery, XRT)	Epidermal growth factor receptor, placental alkaline phosphatase	Vulvar, colorectal, cervical Ca, melanoma, astrocytomas	Malignant astrocytomas	25	10–15 mCi/mg IV or IC	35–90 mCi, multiple injections (151 mCi average total)
Anti-EGFR-425 (^{125}I) (IgG2)	Epidermal growth factor receptor, placental alkaline phosphatase	Vulvar, colorectal, cervical Ca, melanoma, astrocytomas	Gliomas	15	10 mCi/mg IV or IC	8–75 mCi, multiple injections, total dose of 25–130 mCi

Table continued on following page

EFFECT	TOXICITY	HAMA	IMAGING ?	$t_{1/2}$	REF.
3 CR, 1 PR	Myelotoxicity	None	6/7	3.3 d whole body in CR	257
9/29 PR, 9/29 CR	Severe myelo-toxicity, 3 pts with persistant aplasia despite ABMT	None	89%	Blood $t_{1/2}$ of 1–2 d, tumor $t_{1/2}$ of 3 d	258
Equal response (PR of 25%) and survival; AFP− patients better than AFP+	Myelosuppression	ND	ND	ND	256
7% CR, 41% PR	Myelotoxicity, platelets > leukopenia esophagitis	ND	Yes	Tumor $t_{1/2}$ of 3–5 d	255
2 PR, 1 CR	Mild	12/12	Yes	2 d for IV, 3–5 d for local-regional Rx	481
27% PR rate	Myelotoxicity, platelets > leukopenia esophagitis	ND	ND	ND	260
2 PR, 1 CR	No systemic, headache, seizure	2/10	Yes	49 hr for specific MAb, 23 hr for irrelevant	278
6/10 improved, 2/6 with decreased tumor on CT	No acute toxicity, mild myelotoxicity	1/10	18/27, 5/11 with nonspecific MAb	ND	275
Median survival 15.6 mo	None noted	0/25	ND	ND	277
1 CR (83 mCi/3 doses), 2 PR	Minor toxicity	ND	Majority	ND	276

Table continued on following page

TABLE 21–6. *Continued*

ANTIBODY/ISOTOPE	ANTIGEN	DISTRIBUTION	DISEASE	# PATIENTS	DOSE MAb	DOSE RADIATION
A5B7 (^{131}I) (IgG1), +/− cyclosporin	CEA	Various	Lung, colorectal, gastric Ca	6	5–7.5 mg, 2–4 doses/pt	40–80 mCi
NR-LU-10 (IgG2b)	40-kDa molecule	Epithelial tissue	Lung, colorectal, breast, ovarian, renal Ca	15	40 mg	25–120 mCi/m^2
NR-CO-02 (IgG1 Fab′2) (^{189}Re)	CEA	Various		31	46 mg	25–200 mCi/m^2

Abbreviations: ND, not done; ABMT, autologous bone marrow transplant; IT, intra-thecal; Ca, carcinoma; MTD, maximum tolerated dose, HACA, human anti-chimeric antigen; EDTA, ethylenediaminetetra-acetic acid; RIT, radioimmunotherapy; AFP, α-fetoprotein; CEA, carcinoembryonic antigen; XRT, radiation therapy; CT, computerized tomography; CSA, cyclosporin A; other abbreviations as in Tables 21–1 and 21–2.

tion doses to the tumor of up to 1200 rad have been achieved by saturating quantities of antiferritin antibodies (30 mCi administered, with activity of 8 to 10 mCi/mg protein). Higher doses of isotope or antibody lead to increased bone marrow toxicity without an increase in the delivered radiation dose to the tumor. Repeated courses of treatment have been given in the face of immune responses by alternating the source of polyclonal antisera from rabbit, pig, monkey, or bovine species. Overall, a 48 per cent response rate to the combined-modality therapy has been seen. In these and other similar trials, radiolabeled antibody alone or in combination with additional agents has converted non resectable tumors to resectable tumors by the antitumor effect of the therapy.[256] Toxicity has been primarily hematopoietic, with decreases in platelets and neutrophils. These antibodies also have been used in the treatment of patients with Hodgkin's lymphoma, with a 40 per cent response rate.[259] The majority of responding patients in this trial did not respond further to subsequent radiolabeled antibody infusions. The use of ^{90}Y-labeled polyclonal antibodies in patients with end-stage Hodgkin's lymphoma resulted in increased antitumor activity (18/29 partial plus complete response rate) but with marked myelosuppression, requiring autologous marrow support above 20 mCi, with persistent marrow aplasia seen in some patients following 50 mCi.[257,258] Similar clinical antitumor activity also has been seen with polyclonal antibodies directed against CEA in the treatment of patients with intrahepatic cholangiocarcinoma.[260] The majority of other trials have used murine MAbs.

Other solid tumors that have responded to radioimmunotherapy include melanoma, neuroblastoma, and ovarian cancer. A trial of Fab fragments of anti-p97 antibodies in the treatment of patients with melanoma demonstrated that 88 per cent of lesions greater than 1.5 cm imaged.[261] Ten patients with the most intense imaging were selected and treated with 4 to 20 mg of Fab conjugated with 30 to 342 mCi of ^{131}I given in repeated courses. One partial response was seen. In a similar trial, tumor doses of 1040 rad with liver doses of 325 rad/100 mCi were achieved, although there were no responses in any of the seven treated patients.[262]

Treatment of localized disease has been attempted by infusing radiolabeled antibodies directly into the peritoneal, thecal, and pleural spaces. Malignant meningitis has responded to a variety of radiolabeled antibodies given intrathecally. Reduction in cerebrospinal fluid cell count and abnormal protein concentration with clinical improvement have been achieved with limited toxicity in patients with ALL,[263] pineoblastoma,[264] and other carcinomatous meningitides.[265–267] Antitumor responses were seen in ovarian cancer patients with limited (<2 cm bulk) or microscopic residual disease treated intraperitoneally with a variety of antibodies conjugated with ^{131}I or ^{90}Y.[268–274] No responses were seen in patients with bulky disease. The initial attempts to use ^{90}Y-conjugated antibodies resulted in severe myelosuppression at doses of only 15 mCi that was found to be due to the release of free ^{90}Y from the DTPA chelating group.[268] Subsequent dose escalation to 25 to 30 mCi was possible following intravenous treatment with EDTA to clear the released ^{90}Y.[268,269,271] In a similar fashion, human antimouse antibodies have been used to clear the blood pool more rapidly following labeled antibody infusions.[272]

Antibodies to EGF receptor that bind to the receptor and are internalized, but do not stimulate tyrosine kinase activity, have been radiolabeled and used to target intracranial tumors such as glioblastoma and astrocytoma.[275–277] Intravenous administration appears safer and as effective as intra-arterial infusion.[276,277] In one study, tumors of 18/27 patients imaged with the radiolabeled specific antibody, and those of 5/11 patients studied with an inactive antibody also imaged, illustrating the difficulties in determining the effect of the binding properties of the antibody.[275] Hematologic toxicity has not been reported. Direct intralesional injection of radiolabeled antitenascin antibodies in patients with glioblastoma resulted in a particularly high percentage of injected dose per gram of tumor tissue, with better distribution throughout the tumor.[278] Prolonged intratumor half-life of the specific antibody versus a nonspecific control antibody also was demonstrated.

As seen previously with unlabeled antibodies, the treatment of patients with solid tumors results in the nearly universal appearance of a HAMA immune response. Decreased tumor binding, decreased serum half-life, and increased dehalogination with decreased tumor imaging following the appearance of a HAMA have been reported.[270] Attempts to decrease HAMA formation by cyclophosphamide[279] or reduce existing HAMA titers to allow multiple courses of therapy by plasmapheresis[280] have been

EFFECT	TOXICITY	HAMA	IMAGING ?	$t_{1/2}$	REF.
None	Allergic reaction with multiple doses, myelosuppression	All, but decreased with CSA	Yes when HAMA < 6 μg/ml	Shorter with increasing HAMA	281, 282
None 1 PR (7 mo)	Myelosuppression at highest doses	All 80%	Yes Yes	$t_{1/2}$ 25 hr	482

generally ineffective. Co-administration of high doses of cyclosporin A delayed and decreased the emergence of HAMA, allowing multiple courses of therapy in patients treated with a murine anti-CEA antibody; however, all patients eventually became HAMA positive.[281,282] The immune response to ^{131}I-labeled chimeric B72.3 in patients with metastatic colon cancer was decreased compared to the intact murine antibody; however, 7/12 patients eventually mounted a weak immune response to the murine variable region.[283,284] The use of the chimeric antibody also was associated with a longer half-life (240 hr), delayed tumor imaging (8 to 23 days postinjection), and increased marrow toxicity with doses of 36 mCi/m[2]. Increased whole-body radiation as a result of the prolonged half-life was demonstrated.

Not surprisingly, the most promising antitumor activity with radiolabeled antibodies has been in the treatment of the relatively radiation-sensitive NHL. A variety of tumor antigens have been targeted. One of the most illustrative trials has been performed by Press and colleagues with the antibody MB-1 directed against the B-cell antigen CD37.[156,285,286] Patients first were given labeled antibody combined with various amounts of unlabeled antibody. The dose of radiation that would be delivered from a therapeutic dose of ^{131}I-labeled antibodies to each organ and to all of the tumor sites was estimated. Patients were selected for treatment only if the tumor was imaged and if the dose delivered to the tumor in all sites was greater than that to normal organs. A progressive dose escalation trial then was undertaken, searching for the maximum tolerated dose. Bone marrow suppression was overcome by infusing autologous marrow following antibody therapy. Of the first five patients treated with up to 608 mCi, there were four complete and one partial response. Durable remissions have been seen in some patients. As expected, the major toxicity was myelosuppression. The presence of splenomegaly and of significant tumor bulk were correlated with unsuccessful imaging. In a similar trial with non–marrow ablative doses of ^{131}I-labeled anti-CD37 antibody, grade III myelosuppression consisting primarily of thrombocytopenia was encountered at doses estimated to give a whole-body radiation dose of 50 cGy.[287] Antitumor responses were seen in two of ten patients. Trials with lower doses of ^{131}I conjugated to the antibodies LL2,[288] LYM-1,[289,290] T101,[280,291] and OKB7[292] also have demonstrated antitumor effects. ^{90}Y-conjugated anti-idiotype antibodies induced a partial response in one patient

following the administration of more than 2 gm of unlabeled antibody in an effort to clear blocking circulating idiotype.[293] Minimal toxicity was reported; however, the impact of the ^{90}Y is difficult to sort out because anti-idiotype antibodies alone in other trials have demonstrated significant antitumor effects.[173,174] In most of these trials, successful targeting of the labeled antibody has been demonstrated by imaging or by biopsy. However, even in the best circumstances with systemic injection, only 0.05 per cent of the injected radioactivity per gram of tumor tissue has been achieved. In the previously mentioned trial of OKB7, which targeted B cells, significant B-cell but not T-cell depletion was noted in the peripheral blood of treated patients; however, the identical effect was seen in patients receiving a labeled irrelevant (anti-CEA) antibody. In this case, selective B-cell depletion represented increased radiation sensitivity of the B versus T cells and could not be attributed to the selective binding of the antibody.[292] In radiation-sensitive tumors, the contribution of antitumor activity from the whole-body radiotherapy obtained from the slow decay of the labeled antibody is not clear.[294]

IMMUNOTOXINS

Another immunoconjugate strategy involves the use of immunotoxins. An immunotoxin consists of a monoclonal antibody and a toxin linked via a chemical cross linker, natural peptide, or disulfide bond. The antibody targets the immunotoxin to the tumor cell and the toxin then enters the cell and irreversibly blocks an essential metabolic process. A variety of toxins derived from plants or bacteria have been used to produce immunotoxins. These include ricin, abrin, gelonin, saporin, DT, and *Pseudomonas* exotoxin A (PE). These toxins are among the most potent cell poisons known; no more than ten molecules in the cytosol are needed to kill a cell.

Most toxins, as depicted in Figure 21–4, contain a binding domain, a catalytic domain, and a translocation domain or region. Native toxins act by attaching to a cell surface receptor via their binding domain and then are endocytosed into endosomes. The toxin then is processed to release the catalytic domain, which is translocated to the cytosol, where it acts to inhibit protein synthesis. By removing or modifying the cell-binding domain and replacing it with the binding specificity of an antitumor

MAb, the cytotoxic action of these toxins can be redirected specifically toward tumor cells.

Ricin and abrin are the most frequently used plant toxins for the production of immunotoxins. These toxins consist of two disulfide-bonded polypeptide chains. The A chain contains the catalytically active domain. This polypeptide chain is essentially a ribosome-inactivating protein (RIP) that catalyzes a specific *N*-glycosidic cleavage of the 28S rRNA, resulting in the irreversible inactivation of the eukaryotic 60S ribosomal subunit. The B chain is a galactose-specific lectin that binds various galactose-containing glycolipids and glycoproteins. In addition, the B chain contains a region that is involved in promoting A chain translocation from an intracellular vesicle into the cytosol.

Another group of plant toxins, the single-chain RIPs, also have been used to construct immunotoxins. Single-chain RIPs, such as gelonin and saporin, are analogous to the A chain of ricin or abrin and inactivate ribosomes in a similar manner.[295] Because they lack a B chain, they have no intrinsic cell-binding properties and hence demonstrate very low toxicity to cells on their own. However,

when coupled to a cell-binding moiety such as an antibody, they can demonstrate powerful cytotoxicity. Another group of single-chain RIPs that includes α-sarcin and restrictocin has been identified in the *Aspergillus* mold. Like their plant counterparts, these also may prove useful in the production of immunotoxins.[296]

Pseudomonas exotoxin A and DT have been the most frequently used bacterial toxins for the construction of immunotoxins. Both toxins arrest protein synthesis by catalyzing ADP ribosylation and inactivation of elongation factor 2. DT is synthesized as a single polypeptide that subsequently is cleaved to form an A chain and a B chain, held together by a disulfide linkage. Like the plant toxins ricin and abrin, the A chain of DT contains the catalytic domain and the B chain contains both the binding domain and a region that facilitates translocation of the A chain into the cytosol. In contrast, PE is a single polypeptide chain that is arranged into three structural domains. Each domain has been shown to contain a different function.[297] Domain I contains the cell-binding region, domain II contains the translocation region, and domain III is the catalytic domain.

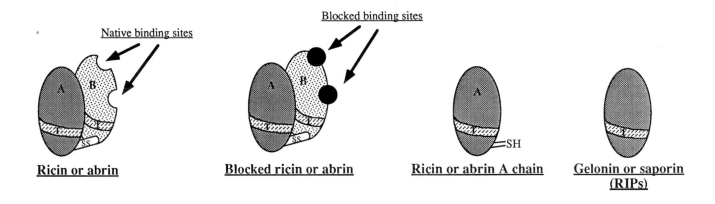

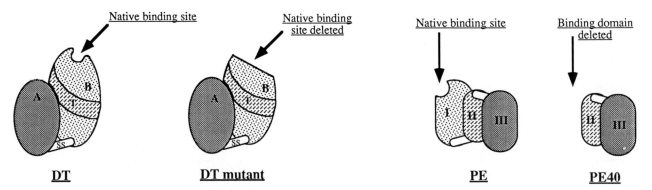

Figure 21–4. Schematic representations of toxins used in the construction of immunotoxins. DT, diphtheria toxin; DT mutant, DT from which the native binding site has been genetically deleted; PE, *Pseudomonas* exotoxin; PE40, PE with binding domain deleted; A, catalytic domain; B, binding domain; T, translocation domain; I, PE-binding domain; II, PE translocation domain; III, PE catalytic domain; SS, disulfide bond; SH, free sulfhydryl.

A number of other toxins have been examined for use in immunotoxin studies. These include pokeweed antiviral protein,[298-301] mistletoe lectin,[302-305] trichokirin,[306] momordin,[307-309] and a sea anemone hemolytic toxin.[310,311] The latter has phospholipase activity and is of interest in that it acts at the cell surface. Such surface-acting immunotoxins may prove useful for directing cytotoxicity toward tumor antigens that are not readily internalized.

The linkage of a toxin molecule to an antibody must provide a stable interaction while the immunotoxin is traveling through the body, but also must allow the release of the toxin into the cytosol after being internalized into a tumor cell. A variety of linkers have been used to prepare immunotoxins.[312] Intact toxins can be linked to an antibody molecule via a thioether linkage.[313,314] This linkage is stable to reduction, limiting the toxicity resulting from dissociation of the toxin from the antibody. The toxin retains the natural linkage between the A and B chain, which can be cleaved for release of the A chain inside the cell. The main drawback to using intact toxins is that not only can they bind to cells that express the antigen against which the antibody portion of the immunotoxin is directed, but they also can bind to nontarget cells via the natural cell-binding site of the toxin.[315,316]

One strategy to circumvent the problem of nontarget cell binding is to attach a toxin's A chain, separated from the B chain, to the antibody molecule. Linkers that have been used to couple A chains to MAbs introduce a disulfide bond between the two molecules; they include *N*-succinimidyl-3-(2-pyridyldithio)propionate (SPDP), *N*-succinimidyl-*S*-thioacetate (SATA), 2-iminothiolane (2-IT), and *N*-succinimidyloxycarbonyl-*α*-methyl-*α*(2-pyridyldithio)toluene (SMPT). These heterobifunctional reagents introduce one or two activated thiol groups into the antibody. The toxin molecule is reduced to separate the A and B chains and the free thiol group on the A chain is reacted with the derivatized antibody to form the disulfide linkage. One problem with these heterobifunctional reagents is that they potentially link the A chain anywhere on the antibody molecule, including the antigen-binding site, which would render the immunotoxin ineffective. As an alternative, Fab' fragments have a free cysteine residue near the hinge region that can be disulfide linked to the free thiol group on an A chain.[317] Because the free cysteine residue on the Fab' is near the hinge region, which is distant from the antigen-binding site, these constructs in general retain full antigen-binding activity. Initial studies using immunotoxins produced with 2-IT or SPDP as cross linkers demonstrated a marked degree of instability in vivo. The antibody and A chain were being broken down, probably by thiol-containing molecules in the body, with a half-life of 6 to 8 hours.[318] Subsequently, immunotoxins have been prepared with cross linkers such as SMPT that contain bulky phenyl or methyl groups adjacent to the disulfide bond. These immunotoxins are more stable in vivo and demonstrate improved antitumor activity.[319,320] The A chain–like RIPs, such as gelonin and saporin, are linked to antibody molecules in much the same way as free A chains. A free thiol group first must be introduced into the RIP because, unlike A chains, these proteins lack a natural thiol group. The thiolating reagent, however, potentially can create the disulfide linkage at or near the catalytic site of the RIP, reducing or abolishing its activity.[312,321]

Immunotoxins produced with isolated A chains or RIPs are generally very specific because their only binding is via the antibody molecule. However, these immunoconjugates display variable cytotoxic activity. Some of this variability is due to differences in antibody affinity.[322-324] High-affinity MAbs make more effective immunotoxins than do low-affinity MAbs, and Fab' immunotoxins tend to be less effective than intact molecules. In addition, antibodies raised against tumor antigens that are poorly internalized or that are internalized into lysosomes make poor immunotoxins. The specific A chain or RIP also determines, in part, the efficacy of the particular immunotoxin. For example, DT A chain immunoconjugates are generally less effective than ricin or abrin A chain or RIP immunotoxins. Presumably the latter A chains or RIPs all contain a translocation region that facilitates entry into the cytosol, whereas the DT A chain lacks such a region.[315]

The cytotoxicity of A chain– or RIP-containing immunotoxins often can be improved dramatically by the addition of ionophores such as monensin,[325,326] lysosomotropic amines,[325,327] free B chains,[328] or antibody-conjugated B chains.[329,330] The ionophores and lysosomotropic amines probably act by decreasing the fusion of endosomes with lysosomes, thus reducing the degradation of the A chain. The B chains probably also protect the A chains from degradation and in addition facilitate their translocation into the cytosol.

Another technique for attenuating binding of immunotoxins to nontarget cells relies on blocking or modifying the binding domain of the toxin either chemically or genetically. An initial approach was to prepare immunotoxins with intact native ricin or abrin and then to select for those molecules that do not bind galactose. This approach was based on the principal that, during the conjugation procedure, some toxin molecules will be bound to the antibody in such a way that the antibody sterically blocks the toxins' binding site. Such sterically blocked immunotoxins have demonstrated specific cytotoxicity in vitro.[331] The nonspecific binding of ricin or abrin immunotoxins also can be blocked in vitro by adding large amounts of galactose.[313,332,333] However, the inability to administer large enough doses of the competing sugar in vivo limits this approach. The binding sites on ricin also have been specifically blocked using a chemically reactive galactose-containing oligosaccharide that binds to the ricin B chain and becomes covalently attached.[334,335] This approach is limited to ricin and abrin immunotoxins, because the binding ligands for PE and DT have not been identified. Finally, genetically engineered recombinant immunotoxins have been produced in which the toxin's cell-binding domain is mutated or deleted. For PE this involved deleting domain I (amino acids 1 through 252) and coupling the antibody to domain II.[336] The resulting toxin, denoted PE40, has been used to construct immunotoxins that demonstrate marked antitumor activity in vitro and in vivo.[337-339] DT binding also has been genetically altered by mutating a key residue in the binding domain or by deleting this binding region.[340,341]

Nonspecific cell binding can occur by mechanisms other than binding via the toxin's binding domain. Both ricin A and B chains are glycosylated proteins.[342] Cells in the liver and the reticuloendothelial system express receptors for the sugars on these chains,[343,344] resulting in rapid clearance and liver toxicity. Deglycosylation of ricin A chain reduces its nonspecific binding without adversely affecting its cytotoxic activity.[320,345] Deglycosylation of ricin B chain, however, reduces the ability of the B chain to facilitate A chain translocation.[346] Immunotoxins constructed with the RIP saporin also demonstrate liver toxicity even though saporin is not glycosylated.[295,347,348] Liver cells apparently bind saporin via a specific cell surface receptor. Immunotoxins containing PE, another nonglycosylated toxin, also are recognized by liver cells.[349]

There are a number of studies using antitumor immunotoxins in animal tumor models. In several of these, animals are injected with tumor cells and the immunotoxin is administered shortly thereafter.[350,351] In a more clinically relevant model, animals bearing advanced tumors have been treated with immunotoxins alone or in combination with cytoreductive therapy.[352-354] Marked antitumor effects, including some cures, have been obtained with limited toxicity. Regressions of hematopoietic tumors as well as solid tumors have been observed. These antitumor effects can be potentiated by the co-administration of the ionophore monensin[355] and by the co-administration of β-adrenergic blockers, which increases access of the immunotoxin to solid tumors.[356]

Because immunotoxins must bind to the tumor cell and be internalized to effect their cytotoxicity, antigen-negative tumor cells will be unaffected. For this reason, cocktails of immunotoxins with different antigen specificities probably will be more effective. In addition to antigen-negative mutants, tumor cells that have lost the ability to transport the toxic moiety into the cytosol have been observed.[357] One strategy to address this problem is to administer immunotoxins in conjunction with other cytotoxic agents that have different modes of action, such as conventional chemotherapy or radiotherapy.

Clinical Trials of Immunotoxins

Shown in Table 21–7 are details from published clinical trials using antibody-based immunotoxins in patients with a variety of malignancies. In general, the amount of antitumor activity has been low and the toxicity moderately high. Clinical responses in a variety of malignancies have been reported. These have been most frequently in the therapy of patients with B- or T-cell lymphomas[358-360] or Hodgkin's disease.[361] Most of these responses have been minor or partial in nature and transient. Antitumor effects in patients with solid malignancies have been the exception rather than the rule, although occasional partial or mixed responses have been seen in patients with melanoma, neuroblastoma, and a variety of gastrointestinal malignancies.[362-365] Further complicating the interpretation of these trials is the fact that occasional responses have been seen in similar trials using unconjugated antibodies, although often at a higher dose.

Significant toxicity has been seen in a number of these trials. Most prominently, a vascular or capillary leak syndrome consisting of weight gain, edema, hypoalbuminia, dyspnea, and in some cases pulmonary edema has been encountered.[358] The etiology of this toxicity is unknown, but the symptoms are similar to the syndrome seen with high-dose IL-2 or γ-interferon therapy and may reflect the release of cytokines.[366] In other trials, hepatic damage has been the most significant toxicity.[360]

In several cases, unknown cross reactions between the treatment antibody and normal host tissues have led to significant toxicity and morbidity. In a trial of antibody 260F9 conjugated to recombinant ricin A chain, significant neurotoxicity was encountered that was not predicted by preclinical tests.[367] Subsequent testing revealed antibody reactivity with monkey Schwann cells.[367] Likewise, unexpected central nervous system toxicity was seen in a trial of OVB3-PE given intraperitoneally to patients with ovarian cancer.[368]

A universal finding in the use of murine immunotoxins in a wide variety of human malignancies, including B-cell lymphomas, has been the rapid development of a human antitoxin antibody response as well as a HAMA response. In most cases a significant amount of the HAMA is directed at the murine antigen binding site, resulting in blocked binding of the immunotoxin to the tumor target.[359] Studies have demonstrated a more rapid half-life and lower serum levels of the immunotoxins in patients developing an immune response. In some cases, retreatment in the face of a nonblocking immune response has yielded continued antitumor responses.[359] The development of a HAMA occurs in nearly all patients with nonlymphoid malignancies. The inclusion of a high dose of cyclophosphamide immediately following the administration of the immunotoxin failed to decrease the induction of a strong HAMA and human antirat antibody (HARA) response in patients with colorectal malignancies.[364] Attempts are being made to induce specific immunosuppression following the administration of the immunotoxin.

It should be noted that the majority of these early trials were performed with first-generation immunotoxins in patients with a wide variety of advanced malignancies often refractory to other therapies. However, the use of these agents in minimal disease as an adjuvant to other therapies to maintain or improve significant disease-free remissions remains to be tested. Adjuvant trials of a number of these agents are underway. It is hoped that the use of the newer methods of toxin preparation and conjugation will further decrease the host toxicity and improve tumor killing.

ANTIBODY-DRUG CONJUGATES

Chemotherapeutic agents have a limited therapeutic index because of their nonspecific cytotoxicity against normal cells. The use of MAbs to deliver drug molecules specifically to the tumor could decrease their toxicity and increase their efficacy. In addition, the use of an antibody-drug conjugate may alter subsequent resistance to the drug by decreasing efflux of free drug.[369] A variety of chemotherapeutic agents have been conjugated to MAbs, including methotrexate,[370-373] vinblastine,[374-377] daunomycin,[378] daunorubicin,[379,380] doxorubicin,[381,382] and mitomycin C.[383-385]

Initial MAb-drug conjugates were prepared by simple covalent coupling procedures that generally resulted in low yields, cross-linking of drug molecules, reduced immunoreactivity of the MAb, and limited specific cytotoxicity. Subsequently, a variety of linkers such as glutaraldehyde, albumin, and short peptides have been tried. Linkage to carbohydrate groups in the Fc portion of the antibody molecule also has been examined.[386] Some linker strategies are based on the knowledge that cytotoxicity is achieved after an antibody-drug conjugate binds to the target cell and is internalized, and the free active drug is released within the cell by lysosomal digestion. These MAb-drug conjugates contain a neutralized drug that becomes activated on acid hydrolysis within the cell or in the acidic environment around hypoxic tumor cells.[378,387,388]

One of the major advantages of antibody-drug conjugates for cancer treatment is the ability to take a wide range of agents with known antitumor activity and pharmacology and enhance their relative tumor uptake. However, there are a number of drawbacks to the use of MAb-drug conjugates. Many MAb-drug conjugates are of low potency, partly as a result of alterations in both the MAb and the drug during the conjugation process, and partly because of physiologic barriers preventing uniform distribution of the MAb-drug within the tumor mass. In addition, like immunotoxins, most MAb-drug reagents must be internalized to effect their cytotoxicity. However, many tumor antigens are stable, cell surface molecules, not readily internalized. Finally, because these agents must be internalized, antigen-negative tumor cells will not be affected by such therapy. One potential solution to the problems of internalization and of antigenic heterogeneity lies in the use of a labile chemical bond to attach the drug to the MAb. This bond would permit dissociation at the tumor cell periphery, allowing transport into the antigen-positive tumor cell, or into a nearby antigen-negative cell.[377,389]

Several drug-conjugated antibody trials have been published. Oldham reported on the use of a cocktail of up to six antibodies conjugated with Adriamycin or mitomycin C in patients with a variety of malignancies.[390] Antitumor effects were seen in patients given the Adriamycin-conjugated, but not the mitomycin C—conjugated, antibodies. Dissociation of active Adriamycin from the antibody was seen in some patients and caused hematologic toxicity. A high incidence of HAMA was observed.[391] The mitomycin C conjugates also caused dose-limiting thrombocytopenia.[392] Drug-induced colitis was observed and believed to be caused by radioactivity with normal colonic epithelium. Large doses of antibody (up to 4200 mg) were administered in these trials. Although minor responses were seen in some Adriamycin-treated patients, the relative contribution to this effect of antibody alone, free drug, and antibody specificity remains to be determined. Methotrexate-conjugated antibodies have been shown to localize to tumor tissues in ratios similar to those of unconjugated antibodies.[393] The antibody KS1/4 conjugated to desacetylvinblastine (four to six molecules per antibody)

has been given to patients with adenocarcinoma.[394] The majority of patients mounted HAMA immune responses as well as anti—vinca alkaloid antibody responses.[395] The same antibody (KS1/4), alone or conjugated to methotrexate, was given to patients with non—small-cell lung cancer.[396] A total dose of 28 mg of methotrexate and 1661 mg of antibody were administered. Antibody was detected on postinfusion tumor biopsies and on biopsies of normal colon. Toxicities were similar between the antibody alone and the antibody-methotrexate conjugate groups.

PHOTODYNAMIC THERAPY

Other cytotoxic agents that have been conjugated to monoclonal antibodies in attempts to develop a "magic bullet" against cancer are the photosensitizers. These molecules, most of which are porphyrin- or phthalocyanine-related compounds, are accumulated somewhat selectively in malignant cells as compared to normal cells.[397,398] They are activated by exposure to light of specific wavelengths and their cytotoxicity is mediated primarily by the generation of free-radical singlet oxygen. Thus, unlike chemotherapeutic agents, which are mainly cell cycle specific, the cytotoxic activity of photosensitizers is independent of cell proliferation.

Numerous investigators have conjugated photosensitizers to MAbs to increase their selectivity. Selective in vitro destruction of tumor cells has been demonstrated with hematoporphyrin conjugates,[399,400] chlorin-e6 conjugates,[401,402] benzoporphyrin derivative monoacid ring A (BPD) conjugates,[403] and MAb-coupled liposomes containing phthalocyanine.[404] In vivo administration of a hematoporphyrin-MAb conjugate directed against a murine myosarcoma was shown to inhibit tumor growth in mice following exposure to incandescent light.[405] Treatment with control conjugates, hematoporphyrin, or antibody alone demonstrated no significant suppression of tumor growth.

As previously mentioned, MAbs that are not readily internalized are ineffective as carriers of toxins and chemotherapeutic agents, which act intracellularly. Such antibodies may be good candidates for conjugation with photosensitizers, which are effective at the cell surface. As yet, there have been no clinical trials of antibody-directed photodynamic therapy.

BISPECIFIC ANTIBODIES

As described earlier in this chapter, numerous immunoconjugates have been produced by covalently attaching toxins, radionuclides, or cytotoxic drugs to MAbs. However, there are several disadvantages to the direct coupling of cytotoxic agents to antibodies. Chemical conjugation can alter both the antibody-binding site and the cytotoxic compound, resulting in an ineffective immunoconjugate. Additionally, for its full biologic action, the cytotoxic agent may need to be free from the antibody and the covalent bonds formed between the antibody and the cytotoxic compound may not be easily split. Bispecific antibodies, which have two different antigen-specific binding sites, have been developed as an alternative to direct cou-

TABLE 21–7. CLINICAL TRIALS USING IMMUNOTOXIN (IT) CONJUGATED MONOCLONAL ANTIBODIES

MAb	ANTIGEN	LINKER	TOXIN	DISEASE	# PATIENTS Rx
260F9 (IgG1)	55-kDa on 50% of breast Ca cells	Disulfide bond	Recombinant ricin A chain (no carbohydrate)	Breast Ca	4
260F9 (IgG1)	55-kDa on 50% of breast Ca cells	Disulfide bond	Recombinant ricin A chain (no carbohydrate)	Breast Ca	5
OVB3 (IgG2b)	? mice were immunized with OVCAR-3 human ovarian Ca cell line	Thioether bond	PE	Ovarian Ca	23
RFB4 Fab' (IgG1) M_r=80,000	CD22	Disulfide bond (cystine)	Chemically deglycosylated ricin A chain	B-cell NHL	15
T101-RTA (lgG2a)	CD5	Disulfide linked	Ricin A chain	B-CLL	5
T101-RTA (lgG2a)	CD5	Disulfide linked	Ricin A chain	B-CLL	4
T101-RTA (IgG2a)	CD5	Disulfide linked	Ricin A chain	B-CLL/T-ALL	2
XOMAZYME-MEL (IgG2a)	220-kDa and >500-kDa melanoma-associated antigens	SPDP	Ricin A chain	Melanoma	20
XOMAZYMEMEL (IgG2a)	220- and > 500-kDa melanoma-associated antigens	SPDP	Ricin A chain	Melanoma	22
H65-RTA (lgG1)	CD5	?	Ricin A chain	CTCL (phase I)	14
XMMME-001-RTA (IgG2a)	220 and >500-kDa	SPDP	Ricin A chain	Melanoma (phase II with cytoxan given in single dose of 1000 mg/m² following the IT)	20

Table continued on following page

DOSE GIVEN	RESPONSE TO Rx	TOXICITY	HAMA/ HARA	TUMOR BINDING?	REF.
2 at 10 µg/kg/d × 8, 2 at 50 µg/kg/d × 6, IV bolus	1 PR in pulmonary nodule (3.5 mo)	VLS with increased weight, edema, dyspnea, decreased albumin; ? FC γ on monocytes as cause	4/4 anticonjugate; some anti-Id at 8–14 days into Rx	IT not found in tumor Bx (though tumors were antigen positive)	367
50 µg/kg d×8, 100 µg/kgd × 8 continuous IV infusion	None	VLS, neurotoxic in 3/5 pts; plexopathy and neuropathies severe with drop in KPS 80–40%; motor recovered but persistent sensory deficit; later found that Ab reacts with Schwann cells on monkey nerve Bx	4/5 HARA, 3/5 HAMA	No IT found in tumor biopsies despite higher levels in blood	483
1–10 µg/kg× 2–3 days IP	None	Dose-limiting CNS toxicity at 5–10 µ/kg	23/23 anti-PE at < 14 d, 12/23 with HAMA at 14–28 d	Not done	368
12.5–75 mg/m² q 48 hr × 2–6 doses I V bolus	40% PR of 1–4 mo duration	VLS, expressive aphasia, rhabdomyolysis	4/14 (29%) with immune response	Not done	358
7, 14 mg/m² 2 × per wk × 8, IV bolus	None < 24 hr response	Mild toxicity (no VLS)	No HARA, no HAMA	Tumor cells saturated in vivo, but not killed in vitro even at 10^{-8} molar concentration; in vitro killing improved by HSA-monensin	484
3 mg/m² 2× per wk × 8, IV bolus	None < 24 hr response	Mild toxicity (no VLS)	1/4 HARA- no HAMA	Tumor cells saturated in vivo but not killed	485
13.5 mg × 2, 25 mg × 3, IV bolus	None (< 24 hr)	None	None in 1 pt	Saturated in 1 pt	486, 487
0.6–1.6 mg/kg × 1 dose IV bolus	1 CR	Fatigue, arthralgias, fever, VLS	ND	ND	362
0.01 mg/kg/d × 5 to 1.0 mg/kg/d × 4 IV bolus	1 CR (pulmonary mets lasting 13+ mo), 4 mixed responses	VLS, mild liver toxicity	22/22 HAMA, 22/22 HARA	Tumor Bx positive for ricin A chain in vivo	363
0.2–0.5 mg/kg/d × 10 q mo 0–3 cycles given IV bolus; 6/14 pts more than one cycle; MTD 0.33 mg/kg	4 PR lasting 3–8 mo; mostly skin, but 1 pt with decrease retroperitoneal nodes; many other minor responses	VLS at higher doses	10/12 HARA, 7/11 blocking HAMA	?	359
0.4 mg/kg × 1, IV bolus; with cytoxan, 1000 mg/m² IV × 1	4 PR lasting 1.5–4 mo, 2 mixed responses	Mild VLS, nausea and vomiting from Cytoxan	13/13 HARA, 12/13 HAMA	?	364

Table continued on following page

TABLE 21–7. *Continued*

MAb	ANTIGEN	LINKER	TOXIN	DISEASE	# PATIENTS Rx
XomaZyme-791, 791T/36 (IgG2b)	72-kDa	SPDP	Ricin A chain	Colon Ca	17
Anti-B4-bR (IgG1)	CD19	SMCC	Blocked ricin	B-cell NHL	25
Anti-B4-bR (IgG1)	CD19	SMCC	Blocked ricin	B-cell NHL	43
Ber-H2	CD30	?	Saporin	Hodgkin's lymphoma	4

Abbreviations: Ca; carcinoma; VLS, vascular leak syndrome; IT, immunotoxin; KPS, Karnofsky's performance status; PE, *Pseudomonas* endotoxin; CNS, central nervous sytem; HARA, Human anti-ricin antibody; HSA, human serum albumin; T-ALL, T-cell acute lymphocytic leukemia; SPDP, *N*-succinimidyl-3-(2-pyridyldithio) propionate; MTD, maximum tolerated dose; SMCC, succinimidyl 4-(N-maleimidomethyl) cyclohexane carboxylate; other abbreviations as in Tables 21–1 and 21–2.

pling of antibodies and effector compounds. Bispecific antibodies consist of a target binding arm, specific for the tumor cell, and an effector binding arm, specific for the cytotoxic agent. Unlike direct conjugates, bispecific MAbs avoid the potential chemical damage of the coupling process and the cytotoxic agent can be released without having to break covalent bonds. Although specific MAbs (at least those produced by hybrid hybridomas, as described later in this chapter) are structurally bivalent, they are functionally monovalent. Thus they may be less likely to induce antigenic modulation.[406,407]

Bispecific antibodies have been produced by fusing two different hybridoma cell lines, by chemically linking two antibody molecules, or by gene transfection.[408] The fusion of two different hybridoma cell lines, one producing an antitumor antibody and the other an anti–cytotoxic agent antibody, results in a hybrid hybridoma secreting a variety of antibody molecules. If total random association of heavy and light chains occurs, the hybrid hybridoma will produce ten different combinations of immunoglobulin molecules, only one of which has the desired bispecific activity (Fig. 21–5). Several bispecific antibodies have been produced using this technique. One advantage to this fusion technique is that the bispecific antibodies are produced by the same process as normal antibodies and therefore should have similar stability and pharmacokinetics. In addition, a hybrid hybridoma cell line theoretically provides an unending supply of bispecific antibody. There are disadvantages, however, including the difficulty of fusing hybridoma cells, instability of the resulting hybrid hybridoma cell lines, low yields, and difficulty in purification of the bispecific antibodies.

The advantages of chemically coupling two different antibodies to produce bispecific antibodies includes not requiring cell fusion, efficient production, and relatively easy purification. Several conjugation techniques have been employed.[409–413] A disadvantage to this approach is that chemically coupled antibodies have different physical and biologic properties compared to native antibody molecules and, as with direct chemical conjugation of cytotoxic agents to monoclonal antibodies, chemically produced bispecific antibodies frequently are altered with respect to their antigen-binding sites.[414]

One strategy for the use of bispecific MAbs is to administer the antibody first, allowing enough time for it to target specifically to the tumor site and for any nonspecifically bound antibody to be cleared. Then the toxin, drug, or radionuclide is administered, is recognized by the second half of the bispecific antibody, and becomes localized at the tumor site. Using an anti-CEA-anti–vinca alkaloid bispecific antibody, Corvalan and co-workers[415–417] demonstrated tumor localization of radiolabeled vinblastine sulfate. Compared to radiolabeled drug alone, background levels in liver and spleen with the bispecific antibody were much lower. They also found that, in a human colorectal tumor xenograft system in nude mice, the combination of bispecific antibody and vinblastine had a greater antitumor effect than did the free drug alone. Tsukada et al.[418] prepared a bispecific antibody to anthracyclines and a hepatoma-associated membrane glycoprotein. This bispecific antibody was shown to be more effective than a direct antibody-drug conjugate in a rat tumor model.

Bispecific antibodies also have been used to direct toxin molecules to tumor cells. Anti–ricin A chain antibodies have been incorporated effectively into bispecific antibodies.[414,419] A bispecific anti-idiotype/antisaporin has been used to deliver saporin toxin to lymphoma cells with encouraging results.[420,421]

A second therapeutic strategy using bispecifics involves linking a tumor-specific antibody to an anti–T-cell antibody, producing a bispecific antibody that can bypass the normal specificity of the TCR and redirect cytotoxic T lymphocytes to lyse tumor cells.[422,423] A number of investigators have reported the production of bispecific antibodies with effector binding specificity for the TCR/CD3

DOSE GIVEN	RESPONSE TO Rx	TOXICITY	HAMA/ HARA	TUMOR BINDING?	REF.
0.02–0.2 mg/kg/d × 5 d IV bolus	5 mixed responses (short)	VLS, proteinuria	15/17 HARA, 16/ 17 HAMA (blocking)	Not known	365
1–60 μg/kg/d × 5 d IV bolus	1 CR (21 mo), 2 PR (BM only)	Hepatotoxicity, hypoalbumin without VLS	9/25 HAMA, 9/25 HARA	Not known	360
10–70 μg/kg/d × 7 d via continuous IV infusion	Not reported	Toxicity varied from lot to lot of the drug; hepatoxicity was dose limiting	Not reported	Not reported	488
0.8 mg/kg × 1–2 doses	3 PR	Fever, malaise, anorexia, fatigue, increased LFTs	4/4 HAMA, 4/4 antisaporin	2/4 in vivo binding demonstrated	361

complex (reviewed in refs. 423–426). These bispecific antibodies can bind to target cells, cross link the target cell to the T cell, and activate the T cell to kill the target cell. Most in vivo studies with antitumor/anti–T-cell bispecifics have been neutralization studies in tumor xenograft models involving immunoincompetent animals. In these studies, the bispecific antibody as well as exogenous effector cells are administered to animals inoculated with tumor cells. Although inhibition of tumor growth was observed in several of these studies, the clinical relevance of such models remains speculative.

There are, however, three recently described murine tumor models that provide potentially valuable systems for studying the efficacy of redirecting T cells with bispecific antibodies in immunocompetent animals. One model is that of a murine melanoma transfected with a human melanoma antigen, p97. When injected intravenously, these cells grow as pulmonary metastases. Treatment with a bispecific reagent consisting of an anti-CD3 antibody cross linked to an anti-p97 antibody resulted in a significant decrease in the number of pulmonary metastases.[427] The other models are two murine B cell lymphomas treated with anti-CD3/anti-idiotype bispecific antibody.[428–430] In vitro binding of these bispecific antibodies to tumor cells and T cells was shown to induce T-cell proliferation and lymphokine production and to redirect lysis by the T cells toward the tumor cells. In addition, in vivo studies demonstrated the ability of bispecific antibodies to target T cells toward the lymphoma cells, resulting in the long-term survival and cure of tumor-bearing mice.

Finally, bispecific antibodies have been produced in which one arm is directed against Fc receptors (e.g., FcgRI [CD64], FcgRII [CD32], or FcgRIII [CD16]) to target Fc receptor–positive effector cells against tumor

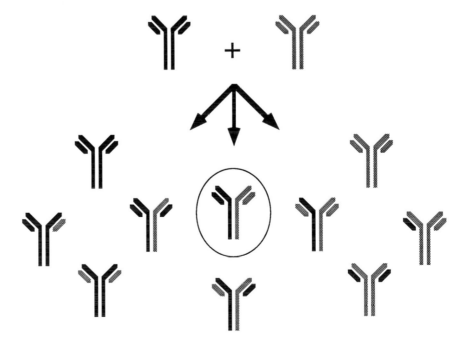

Figure 21–5. Schematic representation of the random association of heavy and light chains from a hybrid hybridoma. Theoretically, ten different antibody molecules will be produced, only one of which (circled) will display bispecific binding activity.

cells.[410,431–433] In one such study, an anti-CD16/antitumor bispecific antibody effectively targeted resting natural killer (NK) cells to lyse an NK-resistant ovarian carcinoma cell line.[434]

Clinical trials utilizing bispecific antibodies are underway. Lymphocyte-activated killer (LAK) cells have been targeted to malignant gliomas by a bispecific antibody composed of anti-CD3 and antiglioma antibody (NE150) activity.[435] The armed versus untreated LAK cells were infused intrathecally into 20 patients. There were no clinical responses in the ten LAK-treated patients, and mean recurrence time following initial diagnosis was less than 1 year. In contrast, partial regression was seen in four targeted LAK-treated patients, and tissue necrosis on biopsy and CT scans was noted in four additional patients. There was minimal toxicity, and, of the eight responding patients, no recurrence was detected in 10 to 18 months of follow-up. In a similar fashion, T cells have been targeted to intraperitoneal ovarian carcinoma using anti-CD3/MOv18 bispecific antibodies.[436] Toxicity was minimal; however, four of four patients developed HAMA to the idiotype of MOv18. Bispecific antibodies also have been used to image colorectal malignancies.[437]

ANTIBODY-DIRECTED ENZYME-MEDIATED CYTOTOXICITY

One of the drawbacks to directly attaching cytotoxic agents such as toxins or chemotherapeutic drugs to MAbs is that the effective dose that can be delivered to the tumor is directly proportional to the amount of antibody that can localize there. An alternative approach might utilize MAbs to deliver enzymes that have no direct cytotoxicity against the tumor cells but can catalyze reactions at the tumor cell surface that lead to cell killing.

The role of enzymes in tumor cell cytotoxicity has been demonstrated in some animal models of chemotherapy. There are very few animal models in which administration of chemotherapeutic agents results in complete regression of advanced transplantable tumors. Examples include the regression of advanced lymphosarcoma in mice by asparaginase,[438] dinitrobenzene treatment of Walker tumors,[439] and the regression of established plasma cell tumors in mice by aniline mustard.[440] Interestingly, in each of these tumor model systems, the cytotoxic effect of the chemotherapeutic agent is dependent on either the increased expression of or the lack of a particular enzyme in the tumor cells. The murine lymphosarcoma lacks the enzyme asparagine synthase, resulting in increased sensitivity to the effects of asparaginase. The Walker tumor expresses high levels of DT diaphorase, which converts the relatively weak dinitrobenzene into a potent alkylating agent. Finally, the plasma cell tumor expresses high levels of β-glucuronidase, which creates a toxic agent from aniline mustard.

Although most tumors do not express such drug-activating enzymes, strategies using MAbs have been developed by which enzymes can be localized at the tumor site. One class of enzymes that have been investigated for this strategy are oxidases, which generate toxic metabolites. MAb-oxidase conjugates have been shown to be cytotoxic

to tumor cells in vitro.[441–443] Another class includes enzymes that deprive the tumor cells of essential nutrients. Carboxypeptidase, which hydrolyzes folate, has been conjugated to an anti–chorionic gonadotropin MAb and was shown to be cytotoxic to a choriocarcinoma cell line in vitro.[444]

An alternative strategy, termed antibody-directed enzyme prodrug therapy (ADEPT) involves coupling an antitumor antibody to an enzyme that can convert a relatively nontoxic drug precursor (prodrug) into an active, cytotoxic agent.[445–447] The antibody-enzyme conjugate is injected and allowed to localize to the tumor. The prodrug then is administered and an active, cytotoxic drug is produced at the tumor site. The active drug is able to penetrate and kill surrounding tumor cells, even those inaccessible to the antibody-enzyme conjugate. Thus this strategy potentially can overcome several of the limitations associated with antibody-drug or antibody-toxin conjugates, namely, low drug potency, nonuniform distribution within the tumor mass, the requirement for internalization, and antigenic heterogeneity.

Several enzyme-prodrug combinations have been prepared and tested in vitro and in vivo. Alkaline phosphatase–MAb conjugates have been used to convert phosphorylated drug derivatives, including etoposide phosphate, doxorubicin phosphate, and mitomycin phosphate, into active chemotherapeutic agents.[448–450] In vitro, these phosphorylated drugs are less toxic to tumor cells than their activated counterparts, probably because of their inability to penetrate cell membranes. In vitro treatment of tumor cells with a specific MAb–alkaline phosphatase conjugate enhanced the cytotoxicity of these prodrugs up to 100-fold. In addition, regression of established tumor xenografts was observed when the prodrug was administered 18 to 24 hours after injection of the MAb–alkaline phosphatase conjugate. The antibody-enzyme conjugate alone or the prodrug alone had little effect on the tumors.

Carboxypeptidase-MAb conjugates have been used for the activation of a nitrogen mustard prodrug to an active benzoic acid mustard.[451] This conjugate, given before the prodrug, demonstrated pronounced antitumor effects in a nude mouse tumor xenograft model. Carboxypeptidase enzyme conjugates also have been used to convert relatively inactive α-peptidyl methotrexate prodrugs into active methotrexate.[452–454] These conjugates, along with various prodrugs, also have proven effective in a nude mouse tumor xenograft model system.[455] Two other enzymes that may prove useful in ADEPT therapy are penicillin-V amidase and cytosine deaminase. Penicillin-V amidase cleaves phenoxyacetamide-containing molecules.[456] Phenoxyacetamide derivatives of doxorubicin and melphalan have been examined as potential prodrugs for penicillin-V amidase–MAb conjugates.[457] Cytosine deaminase hydrolyzes cytosine to uracil and has been shown to convert the antifungal agent 5-fluorocytosine (5-FC) into the anticancer drug 5-fluorouracil (5-FU). Implantation of cytosine deaminase capsules near subcutaneous tumors in rats resulted in local conversion of 5-FC to 5-FU and significant antitumor effects.[458] A MAb–cytosine deaminase conjugate has been shown to be specifically cytotoxic to a human lung cancer cell line in the presence of 5-FC.[459]

5-FC was not cytotoxic on its own, and the cytotoxicity generated by the MAb-enzyme-prodrug combination was equivalent to that of 5-FU.

A pilot trial of ADEPT therapy was reported recently in six patients with advanced colorectal cancer using the prodrug *para-N*-(mono-2-chloroethylmonomesyl)aminobenzoyl glutamic acid. The prodrug caused minimal symptoms, except at high doses. Following administration of an antibody-enzyme conjugate, and clearing of circulating antibody with an antienzyme antibody, increasing doses of the prodrug were given. Myelosuppression at higher doses was noted.[460] Further clinical trials are in progress.

CONCLUSIONS

It is clear at the end of a decade and a half of work on MAbs as therapeutic agents for cancer that the goal has not been reached. Despite use and progress in detection and imaging of malignant disease, there is still no approved therapy for cancer based on MAbs. The appeal of antibodies remains their potential for specific recognition and the possibility of targeting the therapeutic attack against the cancer cell, avoiding the toxicity to normal cells that is the hallmark of our current therapeutic modalities. Problems associated with the use of the antibodies include: (1) picking a suitable target, (2) their immunogenicity, and (3) their low efficacy in killing tumor cells.

The most successful clinical outcome to date is the use of antibodies directed at the idiotypic structures on the surface of B-cell lymphomas.[170,171,173,174] A cohort of patients failing conventional therapy now has been rendered free of lymphoma for greater than 5 years after therapy with custom-made monoclonal anti-idiotype antibodies. The creation of a new monoclonal antibody for each patient is not practical by current technology, however, and probably will not be made available despite its salutary effect. It is possible, however, with the development of rapid screening techniques applied to phage libraries of antibodies, that the production of custom antibodies will be made more practical and that this approach will re-emerge.[74–76]

The importance of this positive result for the field is that it establishes the principal that, if the antibody is specific for the tumor cell and if it is directed against a functional receptor that regulates the growth of the cell, then therapeutic benefit can be obtained. Analogous approaches using noncustomized antibodies against known growth factor receptors on other tumors are being tried. If receptors can be found in solid tumors that are critical regulators of growth, then targeting these receptors by antibodies should lead to similar therapeutic benefit.

Attempts to improve the cytotoxicity of antibodies by using them as delivery agents for drugs, toxins, enzymes, or radionuclides raises a whole set of new problems. Aside from the chemistry of attachment of these cytotoxic substances, which has not yet been optimized in any case, the issues of specificity, toxicity, and immunogenicity loom larger. In each case, the balance of these problems is slightly different. For instance, with immunotoxins, the overriding issues have been hepatotoxicity and vascular leak syndrome resulting from the toxin, as well as enhanced immunogenicity also resulting from the toxin. With radiolabeled antibodies, the best results have been obtained in lymphoma patients who were treated with doses of radiation that ablated the normal bone marrow and, therefore, required rescue of the patient with bone marrow stem cells. In both of these examples, interpretation of the clinical effects ultimately will require sorting out the independent contributions of the antibodies themselves from that of the toxin or radiation delivered either specifically or nonspecifically. These problems are not insurmountable, however, and we can predict rapid progress as these clinical trials proceed.

With rare exceptions, MAbs have had limited antitumor effect when given to patients with bulky disease. The extension of these early studies to the adjuvant setting, using antibodies alone or conjugated to other effector molecules such as toxins or radionuclides, is rapidly underway with promising results.

The most rapid progress in the field has been in the engineering of antibody genes and their derived molecules. The problem of immunogenicity of naked antibodies, although not solved completely, has been ameliorated greatly by chimerization or humanization of antibodies. The great contributions of the new technology, however, will come from the orders of magnitude of power in screening for antibodies with desired binding properties, and in the construction of new molecules containing the recognition units of antibodies and effector functions that are yet to be discovered.

REFERENCES

1. Berkeley WN: Results of three years' observation on a new form of cancer treatment. Am J Obstet 69:1060, 1914
2. Vaughan JW: Cancer vaccine and anticancer globulin as an aid in the surgical treatment of malignancy. JAMA 63:1258, 1914
3. Levine P, Bobbit OB, Waller RK, et al: Isoimmunization by a new blood factor in tumor cells. Proc Soc Exp Biol Med 77:403, 1951
4. Hakomori S, Wang SM, Young WW: Isoantigenic expression of Forssman glycolipid in human gastric and colonic mucosa: Its possible identity with "A-like antigen" in human cancer. Proc Natl Acad Sci USA 74:3023, 1977
5. Kabat EA, Liao J, Shyong J, et al: A monoclonal IgMλ macroglobulin with specificity for lacto-N-tetraose in a patient with bronchogenic carcinoma. J Immunol 128:540, 1982
6. Henle G, Henle W: Immunofluorescence in cells derived from Burkitt's lymphoma. J Bacteriol 91:1248, 1966
7. Klein G, Clifford P, Klein E, et al: Search for tumor specific immune reactions in Burkitt lymphoma patients by the membrane immunofluorescence reaction. Proc Natl Acad Sci USA 55:1628, 1966
8. Giraldo G, Beth E, Hirshaut Y, et al: Human sarcomas in culture: Foci of altered cells and a common antigen: induction of foci and an antigen in human fibroblasts by filtrates. J Exp Med 133:454, 1971
9. Lewis MG, Ikonopisov RL, Nairn RC, et al: Tumor-specific antibodies in human malignant melanoma and their relationship to the extent of disease. BMJ 3:547, 1969
10. Morton DL, Malmgren RA, Holmes EC, et al: Demonstration of antibodies against human malignant melanoma by immunofluorescence. Surgery 64:233, 1968
11. Morton DL, Malmgren RA: Human osteosarcomas: Immunolog-

ical evidence suggesting an associated infectious agent. Science *162*:1279, 1969

12. Morton DL, Malmgren RA, Hall WT, et al: Immunologic and virus studies with human sarcomas. Surgery *66*:152, 1969

13. Muna N, Marcus S, Smart C: Detection of immunofluorescence of antibodies specific for human malignant melanoma cells. Cancer *23*:88, 1969

14. Rosenberg SA: Lysis of human normal and sarcoma cells in tissue culture by normal human serum: Implications for experiments in human tumor immunology. J Natl Cancer Inst *58*:1233, 1977

15. Sumner WC, Foraker AG: Spontaneous regression of human melanoma; clinical and experimental studies. Cancer *13*:79, 1960

16. Teimouraian B, McCune WS: Surgical management of malignant melanoma. Am Surg *29*:515, 1963

17. Ngu VA: Clinical evidence of host defences in Burkitt tumor. *In* JH Burchenal, Burkitt D (eds): Treatment of Burkitt's Tumor. New York, Springer, 1967, p 204

18. Horn L, Horn HL: An immunological approach to the therapy of cancer. Lancet *2*:466, 1971

19. Skurkovich SV, Makhonova LA, Reznichenko FM, et al: Treatment of children with acute leukemia by passive cyclic immunization with autologous and autoleukocytes operated during the remission period. Blood *33*:186, 1969

20. Fass L, Herberman RB, Ziegler J, et al: Evaluation of the effect of remission plasma on untreated patients with Burkitt's lymphoma. J Natl Cancer Inst *44*:145, 1970

21. Kohler G, Milstein C: Continuous culture of fused cells secreting antibody of predefined specificity. Nature *236*:495, 1975

22. Pontecorvo G: Production of indefinitely multiplying mammalian somatic cell hybrids by polyethylene glycol (PEG) treatment. Somatic Cell Genet *1*:397, 1976

23. Galfre G, Milstein C: Preparation of monoclonal antibodies: Strategies and procedures. Meth Enzymol *73*:3, 1981

24. Vienken J, Zimmermann U: Electric field-induced fusion: Electro-hydraulic procedure for production of heterokaryon cells in high yield. FEBS Lett *137*:11, 1982

25. Karsten U, Stolley P, Walther I, et al: Direct comparison of electric field-mediated and PEG-mediated cell fusion for the generation of antibody producing hybridomas. Hybridoma *7*:627, 1988

26. Zimmermann U, Klock G, Gessner P, et al: Microscale production of hybridomas by hypo-osmolar electrofusion. Hum Antibodies Hybridomas *3*:14, 1992

27. Gallagher G, al-Azzawi F, Walsh LP, et al: 14C1, an antigen associated with human ovarian cancer, defined using a human IgG monoclonal antibody. Clin Exp Immunol *83*:92, 1991

28. Gallagher G, al-Azzawi, F, Walsh LP, et al: Multiple epitopes of the human ovarian cancer antigen 14C1 recognised by human IgG antibodies: Their potential in immunotherapy. Br J Cancer *64*:35, 1991

29. Posner MR, Elboim HS, Tumber MB, et al: An IgG human monoclonal antibody reactive with a surface membrane antigen expressed on malignant breast cancer cells. Hum Antibodies Hybridomas *2*:74, 1991

30. Posner MR, Elboim HS, Tumber MB, et al: Human monoclonal antibodies reactive with cell surface antigens on human leukemia cell lines: Many antibodies are (auto)antibodies. Hybridoma *9*:97, 1990

31. Inoue H, Hirohashi S, Shimosato Y, et al: Establishment of an anti-A human monoclonal antibody from a blood group A lung cancer patient: Evidence for the occurrence of autoimmune response to difucosylated type-2 chain A. Eur J Immunol *19*:2197, 1989

32. Jansson B, Borrebaeck CA: The human repertoire of antibody specificities against Thomsen-Friedenreich and Tn-carcinoma-associated antigens as defined by human monoclonal antibodies. Cancer Immunol Immunother *34*:294, 1992

33. Kudo T, Asao A, Tachibana T: Highly efficient procedure for production of human monoclonal antibodies: Establishment of hybrids between Epstein-Barr virus-transformed B lymphocytes and heteromyeloma cells by use of GIT culture medium. Tohoku J Exp Med *154*:345, 1988

34. Hosono M, Endo K, Sakahara H, et al: Human/mouse chimeric antibodies show low reactivity with human anti-murine antibodies (HAMA). Br J Cancer *65*:197, 1992

35. Shin SU: Chimeric antibody: Potential applications for drug delivery and immunotherapy. Biotherapy *3*:43, 1991

36. Liao SK, Horton L, Flahart RE, et al: Binding and functional properties of a mouse-human chimeric monoclonal antibody of the human IgG1 subclass with specificity for human carcinomas. Hum Antibodies Hybridomas *1*:66, 1990

37. LoBuglio AF, Wheeler RH, Trang J, et al: Mouse/human chimeric monoclonal antibody in man: Kinetics and immune response. Proc Natl Acad Sci USA *86*:4220, 1989

38. Colcher D, Milenic D, Roselli M, et al: Characterization and biodistribution of recombinant and recombinant/chimeric constructs of monoclonal antibody B72.3. Cancer Res *49*:1738, 1989

39. Stevenson GT, Pindar A, Slade CJ: A chimeric antibody with dual Fc regions (bisFabFc) prepared by manipulations at the IgG hinge. Anticancer Drug Des *3*:219, 1989

40. Shaw DR, Harrison G, Sun LK, et al: Human lymphocyte and monocyte lysis of tumor cells mediated by a mouse/human IgG1 chimeric monoclonal antibody. J Biol Response Mod *7*:204, 1988

41. Shaw DR, Khazaeli MB, LoBuglio AF: Mouse/human chimeric antibodies to a tumor-associated antigen: Biologic activity of the four human IgG subclasses. J Natl Cancer Inst *80*:1553, 1988

42. Steplewski Z, Sun LK, Shearman CW, et al: Biological activity of human-mouse IgG1, IgG2, IgG3, and IgG4 chimeric monoclonal antibodies with antitumor specificity. Proc Natl Acad Sci USA *85*:4852, 1988

43. Fogler WE, Sun LK, Klinger MR, et al: Biological characterization of a chimeric mouse-human IgM antibody directed against the 17-1A antigen. Cancer Immunol Immunother *30*:43, 1989

44. Carter P, Presta L, Gorman CM, et al: Humanization of an anti-p185HER2 antibody for human cancer therapy. Proc Natl Acad Sci USA *89*:4285, 1992

45. Kelley RF, O'Connell MP, Carter P, et al: Antigen binding thermodynamics and antiproliferative effects of chimeric and humanized anti-p185HER2 antibody Fab fragments. Biochemistry *31*:5434, 1992

46. Woodle ES, Thistlethwaite JR, Jolliffe LK, et al: Humanized OKT3 antibodies: Successful transfer of immune modulating properties and idiotype expression. J Immunol *148*:2756, 1992

47. Shalaby MR, Shepard HM, Presta L, et al: Development of humanized bispecific antibodies reactive with cytotoxic lymphocytes and tumor cells overexpressing the HER2 protooncogene. J Exp Med *175*:217, 1992

48. Junghans RP, Waldmann TA, Landolfi NF, et al: Anti-Tac-H, a humanized antibody to the interleukin 2 receptor with new features for immunotherapy in malignant and immune disorders. Cancer Res *50*:1495, 1990

49. Co MS, Queen C: Humanized antibodies for therapy. Nature *351*:501, 1991

50. Foote J, Winter G: Antibody framework residues affecting the conformation of the hypervariable loops. J Mol Biol *224*:487, 1992

51. Queen C, Schneider WP, Selick HE, et al: A humanized antibody that binds to the interleukin 2 receptor. Proc Natl Acad Sci USA *86*:10029, 1989

52. Bird RE, Hardman KD, Jacobson JW, et al: Single-chain antigen-binding proteins. Science *242*:423, 1988

53. Johnson S, Bird RE: Construction of single-chain Fv derivatives of monoclonal antibodies and their production in *Escherichia coli*. Meth Enzymol *203*:88, 1991

54. Huston JS, Mudgett-Hunter M, Tai M-S, et al: Protein engineering of single-chain Fv analogs and fusion proteins. Meth Enzymol *203*:46, 1991

55. Davis GT, Bedzyk WD, Voss EW, et al: Single chain antibody (SCA) encoding genes: One-step construction and expression in eukaryotic cells. Biotechnology *9*:165, 1991

56. Murphy JR: Diphtheria-related peptide hormone gene fusions: A molecular genetic approach to chimeric toxin development. Cancer Treat Res *37*:123, 1988

57. Pastan I, FitzGerald D: Pseudomonas exotoxin: Chimeric toxins. J Biol Chem 264:15157, 1989

58. Chaudhary VK, Queen C, Junghans RP, et al: A recombinant immunotoxin consisting of two antibody variable domains fused to Pseudomonas exotoxin. Nature 339:394, 1989

59. Chaudhary VK, Gallo MG, FitzGerald DJ, et al: A recombinant single-chain immunotoxin composed of anti-Tac variable regions and a truncated diphtheria toxin. Proc Natl Acad Sci USA 87:9491, 1990

60. Batra JK, Fitzgerald DJ, Chaudhary VK, et al: Single-chain immunotoxins directed at the human transferrin receptor containing Pseudomonas exotoxin A or diphtheria toxin: Anti-TFR(Fv)-PE40 and DT388-anti-TFR(Fv). Mol Cell Biol 11: 2200, 1991

61. Chaudhary VK, Batra JK, Gallo MG, et al: A rapid method of cloning functional variable-region antibody genes in Escherichia coli as single-chain immunotoxins. Proc Natl Acad Sci USA 87:1066, 1990

62. Brinkmann U, Pai LH, FitzGerald DJ, et al: B3(Fv)-PE38KDEL, a single-chain immunotoxin that causes complete regression of a human carcinoma in mice. Proc Natl Acad Sci USA 88: 8616, 1991

63. Kreitman RJ, Chaudhary VK, Waldmann T, et al: The recombinant immunotoxin anti-Tac(Fv)-Pseudomonas exotoxin 40 is cytotoxic toward peripheral blood malignant cells from patients with adult T-cell leukemia. Proc Natl Acad Sci USA 87: 8291, 1990

64. Fell HP, Gayle MA, Grosmaire L, et al: Genetic construction and characterization of a fusion protein consisting of a chimeric F(ab') with specificity for carcinomas and human IL-2. J Immunol 146:2446, 1991

65. Hoogenboom HR, Volckaert G, Raus JC: Construction and expression of antibody-tumor necrosis factor fusion proteins. Mol Immunol 28:1027, 1991

66. Hoogenboom HR, Raus JC, Volckaert G: Targeting of tumor necrosis factor to tumor cells: Secretion by myeloma cells of a genetically engineered antibody-tumor necrosis factor hybrid molecule. Biochim Biophys Acta 1096:345, 1991

67. Brown PJ, Parenteau GL, Dirbas FM, et al: Anti-Tac H, a humanized antibody to the interleukin 2 receptor, prolongs primate cardiac allograft survival. Proc Natl Acad Sci USA 88: 2663, 1991

68. Waldmann TA, Strober W: Metabolism of immunoglobulins. Prog Allergy 13:1, 1969

69. Yasmeen D, Ellerson JR, Dorrington KJ, et al: The structure and function of immunoglobulin domains. IV. The distribution of some effector functions among the Cγ2 and Cγ3 homology regions of human immunoglobulin G. J Immunol 116:518, 1976

70. Mueller BM, Reisfeld RA, Gillies SD: Serum half-life and tumor localization of a chimeric antibody deleted of the CH2 domain and directed against the disialoganglioside GD2. Proc Natl Acad Sci USA 87:5702, 1990

71. Mattes MJ: Biodistribution of antibodies after intraperitoneal or intravenous injection and effect of carbohydrate modifications. J Natl Cancer Inst 79:855, 1987

72. Roberts JC, Cheetham JC, Rees AR: Generation of an antibody with enhanced affinity and specificity for its antigen by protein engineering. Nature 328:731, 1987

73. Wallick SC, Kabat EA, Morrison SL: Glycosylation of a VH residue of a monoclonal antibody against α(1 → 6) dextran increased its affinity for antigen. J Exp Med 168:1099, 1988

74. McCafferty J, Griffiths AD, Winter G, et al: Phage antibodies: Filamentous phage displaying antibody variable domains. Nature 348:552, 1990

75. Kang AS, Barbas CF, Fanda KD, et al: Linkage of recognition and replication functions by assembling combinatorial antibody Fab libraries along phage surfaces. Proc Natl Acad Sci USA 88:4363, 1991

76. Huse WD, Sastry L, Iverson SA, et al: Generation of a large combinatorial library of the immunoglobulin repertoire in phage lambda. Science 246:1275, 1989

77. Persson MAA, Caothien RH, Burton DR: Generation of diverse high-affinity human monoclonal antibodies by repertoire cloning. Proc Natl Acad Sci USA 88:2432, 1991

78. Mullinax RL, Gross EA, Amberg JR, et al: Identification of human antibody fragment clones specific for tetanus toxoid in a bacteriophage λ immunoexpression library. Proc Natl Acad Sci USA 87:8095, 1990

79. Hawkins RE, Winter G: Cell selection strategies for making antibodies from variable gene libraries: Trapping the memory pool. Eur J Immunol 22:867, 1992

80. Caton AJ, Koprowski H: Influenza virus hemagglutinin-specific antibodies isolated from a combinatorial expression library are closely related to the immune response of the donor. Proc Natl Acad Sci USA 87:6450, 1990

81. Clackson T, Hoogenboom HR, Griffiths AD, et al: Making antibody fragments using phage display libraries. Nature 352: 624, 1991

82. Winter G, Milstein C: Man-made antibodies. Nature 349:293, 1991

83. Perelson AS: Immune network theory. Immunol Rev 110:5, 1989

84. Gram H, Marconi L-A, Barbas CF, et al: In vitro selection and affinity maturation of antibodies from a naive combinatorial immunoglobulin library. Proc Natl Acad Sci USA 89:3576, 1992

85. Hammarstrom S, Shively JE, Paxton RJ, et al: Antigenic sites in carcinoembryonic antigen. Cancer Res 49:4852, 1989

86. Kuroki M, Kuroki M, Koga Y, et al: Monoclonal antibodies to carcinoembryonic antigen: A systematic analysis of antibody specificities by using related normal antigens and evidence for allotypic determinants on carcinoembryonic antigen. J Immunol 133:2090, 1984

87. Kuroki M, Greiner JW, Simpson JF, et al: Serologic mapping and biochemical characterization of the carcinoembryonic antigen epitopes using fourteen distinct monoclonal antibodies. Int J Cancer 44:208, 1989

88. Muraro R, Wunderlich D, Thor A, et al: Definition by monoclonal antibodies of a repertoire of epitopes on carcinoembryonic antigen differentially expressed in human colon carcinomas versus normal adult tissues. Cancer Res 45:5769, 1985

89. Primus FJ, Newel KD, Blue A, et al: Immunological heterogeneity of carcinoembryonic antigen: Antigenic determinants on carcinoembryonic antigen distinguished by monoclonal antibodies. Cancer Res 43:686, 1983

90. Abelev GI, Perova SD, Khramkova NI, et al: Production of embryonal beta-globulin by transplantable mouse hepatomas. Transplantation 1:174, 1963

91. Muraro R, Kuroki M, Wunderlich D, et al: Generation and characterization of B72.3 second generation monoclonal antibodies reactive with the tumor-associated glycoprotein 72 antigen. Cancer Res 48:4588, 1988

92. Thor A, Ohuchi N, Szpak CA, et al: Distribution of oncofetal antigen tumor-associated glycoprotein-72 defined by monoclonal antibody B72.3. Cancer Res 46:3118, 1986

93. Hilkens J, Buijs F, Hilgers J, et al: Monoclonal antibodies against human milk-fat globule membranes detecting differentiation antigens of the mammary gland and its tumors. Int J Cancer 34:197, 1984

94. Griffin JD, Linch D, Sabbath K, et al: A monoclonal antibody reactive with normal and leukemic human myeloid progenitor cells. Leuk Res 8:521, 1984

95. Muraro R, Wunderlich D, Thor A, et al: Immunological characterization of a novel human colon associated antigen (CAA) by a monoclonal antibody. Int J Cancer 39:34, 1987

96. Mendelsohn J: Growth factor receptors as targets for antitumor therapy with monoclonal antibodies. Prog Allergy 45:147, 1988

97. Hopkins CR, Trowbridge IS: Internalization and processing of transferrin and the transferrin receptor in human carcinoma A431 cells. J Cell Biol 97:508, 1983

98. Sauvage CA, Mendelsohn JC, Lesley JF, et al: Effects of monoclonal antibodies that block transferrin receptor function on the in vivo growth of a syngeneic murine leukemia. Cancer Res 47:747, 1987

99. Taetle R, Honeysett JM: Effects of monoclonal anti-transferrin antibodies on in vitro growth of human solid tumors. Cancer Res 47:2040, 1987

100. Thompson CH, Jones SL, Whitehead RH, et al: A human breast tissue-associated antigen detected by a monoclonal antibody. J Natl Cancer Inst 70:409, 1983

101. Trowbridge IS: Transferrin receptor as a potential therapeutic target. Prog Allergy 45:121, 1988

102. Masui H, Kawamoto T, Sato JD, et al: Growth inhibition of human tumor cells in athymic mice by anti-epidermal growth factor receptor monoclonal antibodies. Cancer Res 44:1002, 1984

103. Rodeck U, Herlyn M, Herlyn D, et al: Tumor growth modulation by a monoclonal antibody to the epidermal growth factor receptor: Immunologically mediated and effector cell-independent effects. Cancer Res 47:3692, 1987

104. Sato JD, Kawamoto T, Le AD, et al: Biological effects in vitro of monoclonal antibodies to human epidermal growth factor receptors. Mol Biol Med 1:511, 1983

105. Ronnstrand L, Terracio L, Claesson WL, et al: Characterization of two monoclonal antibodies reactive with the external domain of the platelet-derived growth factor receptor. J Biol Chem 263:10429, 1988

106. Vassbotn FS, Langeland N, Hagen I, et al: A monoclonal antibody against PDGF B-chain inhibits PDGF-induced DNA synthesis in C3H fibroblasts and prevents binding of PDGF to its receptor. Biochim Biophys Acta 1054:246, 1990

107. Waldmann TA: The structure, function, and expression of interleukin-2 receptors on normal and malignant lymphocytes. Science 232:727, 1986

108. Waldmann TA: Multichain interleukin-2 receptor: A target for immunotherapy in lymphoma. J Natl Cancer Inst 81:914, 1989

109. Bacus SS, Stancovski I, Huberman E, et al: Tumor-inhibitory monoclonal antibodies to the HER-2/Neu receptor induce differentiation of human breast cancer cells. Cancer Res 52:2580, 1992

110. Drebin JA, Link VC, Weinberg RA, et al: Inhibition of tumor growth by a monoclonal antibody reactive with an oncogene-encoded tumor antigen. Proc Natl Acad Sci USA 83:9129, 1986

111. Drebin JA, Link VC, Greene MI: Monoclonal antibodies specific for the neu oncogene product directly mediate anti-tumor effects in vivo. Oncogene 2:387, 1988

112. Drebin JA, Link VC, Greene MI: Monoclonal antibodies reactive with distinct domains of the neu oncogene-encoded p185 molecule exert synergistic anti-tumor effects in vivo. Oncogene 2:273, 1988

113. Hudziak RM, Lewis GD, Winget M, et al: p185HER2 monoclonal antibody has antiproliferative effects in vitro and sensitizes human breast tumor cells to tumor necrosis factor. Mol Cell Biol 9:1165, 1989

114. Stancovski I, Hurwitz E, Leitner O, et al: Mechanistic aspects of the opposing effects of monoclonal antibodies to the ERBB2 receptor on tumor growth. Proc Natl Acad Sci USA 88:8691, 1991

115. Tagliabue E, Centis F, Campiglio M, et al: Selection of monoclonal antibodies which induce internalization and phosphorylation of pl85HER2 and growth inhibition of cells with HER2/NEU gene amplification. Int J Cancer 47:933, 1991

116. Wada T, Myers JN, Kokai Y, et al: Anti-receptor antibodies reverse the phenotype of cells transformed by two interacting proto-oncogene encoded receptor proteins. Oncogene 5:489, 1990

117. Muraro R, Nuti M, Natali PG, et al: A monoclonal antibody (D612) with selective reactivity for malignant and normal gastro-intestinal epithelium. Int J Cancer 43:598, 1989

118. Kaminski MS, Kitamura K, Maloney DG, et al: Importance of antibody isotype in monoclonal anti-idiotype therapy of a murine B cell lymphoma: A study of hybridoma class switch variants. J Immunol 136:1123, 1986

119. Perek Y, Hurwitz E, Burowski D, et al: Immunotherapy of a murine B cell tumor with antibodies and F(ab')2 fragments against idiotypic determinants of its cell surface IgM. J Immunol 131:1600, 1983

120. Maloney DG, Kaminski MS, Burowski D, et al: Monoclonal anti-idiotype antibodies against the murine B cell lymphoma 38C13: Characterization and use as probes for the biology of the tumor in vivo and in vitro. Hybridoma 4:191, 1985

121. Krolick KA, Isakson PC, Uhr JW, et al: BCL1, murine model for chronic lymphocytic leukemia: Use of the surface immunoglobulin idiotype for the detection and treatment of tumor. Immunol Rev 48:81, 1979

122. George AJT, McBride HM, Glennie MJ, et al: Monoclonal antibodies raised against the idiotype of the murine B cell lymphoma BCL1, act primarily with heavy chain determinants. Hybridoma 10:219, 1991

123. Berinstein N, Campbell MJ, Lam K, et al: Idiotypic variation in a human B lymphoma cell line. J Immunol 144:752, 1990

124. Carroll WL, Starnes CO, Levy R, et al: Alternative V kappa gene rearrangements in a murine B cell lymphoma: An explanation for idiotypic heterogeneity. J Exp Med 168:1607, 1988

125. Levy S, Mendel E, Kon S, et al: Mutational hot spots in Ig V region genes of human follicular lymphomas. J Exp Med 168:475, 1988

126. Roth MS, Weiner GJ, Allen EA, et al: Molecular characterization of anti-idiotype antibody-resistant variants of a murine B cell lymphoma. J Immunol 145:768, 1990

127. Starnes CO, Carroll WL, Campbell MJ, et al: Heterogeneity of a murine B cell lymphoma: Isolation and characterization of idiotypic variants. J Immunol 141:333, 1988

128. Weiner GJ, Kaminski MS: Idiotype variants emerging after anti-idiotype monoclonal antibody therapy of a murine B cell lymphoma. J Immunol 142:343, 1989

129. Jacobs JW: New perspectives on catalytic antibodies. Biotechnology 9:258, 1991

130. Lerner RA, Benkovic SJ, Schultz PG: At the crossroads of chemistry and immunology: Catalytic antibodies. Science 252:659, 1991

131. Shokat KM, Schultz PG: Catalytic antibodies. Annu Rev Immunol 8:335, 1990

132. Jerne NK: Towards a network theory of the immune system. Ann Immunol Inst Pasteur 125:373, 1974

133. Koprowski H, Herlyn D, Lubeck M, et al: Human anti-idiotype antibodies in cancer patients: Is the modulation of the immune response beneficial for the patient? Proc Natl Acad Sci USA 81:216, 1984

134. Traub UC, DeJager RL, Primus FJ, et al: Antiidiotypic antibodies in cancer patients receiving monoclonal antibody to carcinoembryonic antigen. Cancer Res 48:4002, 1988

135. Herlyn D, Ross AH, Iliopoulos D, et al: Induction of specific immunity to human colon carcinoma by anti-idiotypic antibodies to monoclonal antibody C017-1A. Eur J Immunol 17:1649, 1987

136. Raychaudhuri S, Saeki Y, Fuji H, et al: Tumor-specific idiotype vaccines. I. Generation and characterization of internal image tumor antigens. J Immunol 137:1743, 1986

137. Raychaudhuri S, Kohler H, Saeki Y, et al: Potential role of anti-idiotype antibodies in active tumor immunotherapy. Crit Rev Oncol Hematol 9:109, 1989

138. Raychaudhuri S, Kang CY, Kaveri SV, et al: Tumor idiotype vaccines. VII. Analysis and correlation of structural, idiotypic, and biologic properties of protective and nonprotective Ab2. J Immunol 145:760, 1990

139. Chattopadhyay P, Starkey J, Raychaudhuri S: Analysis of anti-tumor antibodies in mice and rabbits induced by monoclonal anti-idiotope antibodies. J Immunol 147:2055, 1991

140. Chattopadhyay P, Starkey J, Morrow WJ, et al: Murine monoclonal anti-idiotope antibody breaks unresponsiveness and induces a specific antibody response to human melanoma-associated proteoglycan antigen in cynomolgus monkeys. Proc Natl Acad Sci USA 89:2684, 1992

141. Amit AG, Mariuzza RA, Phillips SEV, et al: Three-dimensional structure of an antigen-antibody complex at 2.8 A resolution. Science 233:747, 1986

142. Bentley GA, Boulot G, Riottot MM, et al: Three-dimensional structure of an idiotope-anti-idiotope complex. Nature 348:254, 1990

143. Huang J-H, Ward RE, Kohler H: Idiotope antigens (Ab2α and Ab2β) can induce in vitro B cell proliferation and antibody production. J Immunol 137:770, 1986

144. Schick MR, Dreesmann GR, Kennedy RC: Induction of an anti-hepatitis B surface antigen response in mice by noninternal

image (Ab2α) anti-idiotypic antibodies. J Immunol *138*:3419, 1982

145. Miller RA, Maloney DG, McKillop J, et al: In vivo effects of murine hybridoma monoclonal antibody in a patient with T-cell leukemia. Blood *58*:78, 1981

146. Miller RA, Levy R: Response of cutaneous T cell lymphoma to therapy with hybridoma monoclonal antibody. Lancet *2*:226, 1981

147. Miller RA, Oseroff AR, Stratte PT, et al: Monoclonal antibody therapeutic trials in seven patients with T-cell lymphoma. Blood *62*:988, 1983

148. Bertram JH, Gill PS, Levine AM, et al: Monoclonal antibody T101 in T cell malignancies: A clinical, pharmacokinetic, and immunologic correlation. Blood *68*:752, 1986

149. Dillman RO, Beauregard J, Shawler DL, et al: Continuous infusion of T101 monoclonal antibody in chronic lymphocytic leukemia and cutaneous T-cell lymphoma. J Biol Resp Mod *5*:394, 1986

150. Dillman RO, Shawler DL, Dillman JB, et al: Therapy of chronic lymphocytic leukemia and cutaneous T-cell lymphoma with T101 monoclonal antibody. J Clin Oncol *2*:881, 1984

151. Dillman RO, Shawler DL, Sobol RE, et al: Murine monoclonal antibody therapy in two patients with chronic lymphocytic leukemia. Blood *59*:1026, 1982

152. Foon KA, Schroff RW, Bunn PA, et al: Effects of monoclonal antibody therapy in patients with chronic lymphocytic leukemia. Blood *64*:1085, 1984

153. Shawler DL, Miceli MC, Wormsley SB, et al: Induction of in vitro and in vivo antigenic modulation by the anti-human T-cell monoclonal antibody T101. Cancer Res *44*:5921, 1984

154. Ritz J, Pesando JL, Sallan SE, et al: Serotherapy of acute lymphoblastic leukemia with monoclonal antibody. Blood *58*:141, 1981

155. Ritz J, Schlossman SF: Utilization of monoclonal antibodies in the treatment of leukemia and lymphoma. Blood *59*:1, 1982

156. Press OW, Appelbaum F, Ledbetter JA, et al: Monoclonal antibody 1F5 (anti-CD20) serotherapy of human B cell lymphomas. Blood *69*:584, 1987

157. Hekman A, Honselaar A, Vuist WM, et al: Initial experience with treatment of human B cell lymphoma with anti-CD 19 monoclonal antibody. Cancer Immunol Immunother *32*:364, 1991

158. Hu E, Epstein AL, Naeve GS, et al: A phase 1a clinical trial of LYM-1 monoclonal antibody serotherapy in patients with refractory B cell malignancies. Hematol Oncol *7*:155, 1989

159. Knox SJ, Levy R, Hodgkinson S, et al: Observations on the effect of chimeric anti-CD4 monoclonal antibody in patients with mycosis fungoides. Blood *77*:20, 1991

160. Dyer MJ, Hale G, Hayhoe FG, et al: Effects of CAMPATH-1 antibodies in vivo in patients with lymphoid malignancies: Influence of antibody isotype. Blood *73*:1431, 1989

161. Hale G, Xia MQ, Tighe HP, et al: The CAMPATH-1 antigen (CDw52). Tissue Antigens *35*:118, 1990

162. Hale G, Clark M, Waldmann H: Therapeutic potential of rat monoclonal antibodies: Isotype specificity of antibody-dependent cell-mediated cytotoxicity with human lymphocytes. J Immunol *134*:3056, 1985

163. Hale G, Dyer MJ, Clark MR, et al: Remission induction in non-Hodgkin lymphoma with reshaped human monoclonal antibody CAMPATH-1H. Lancet *2*:1394, 1988

164. Bruggemann M, Williams GT, Bindon CI, et al: Comparison of the effector functions of human immunoglobulins using a matched set of chimeric antibodies. J Exp Med *166*:1351, 1987

165. Waldmann TA, Goldman CK, Bongiovanni KF, et al: Therapy of patients with human T-cell lymphotrophic virus I-induced adult T-cell leukemia with anti-Tac, a monoclonal antibody to the receptor for interleukin-2. Blood *72*:1805, 1988

166. Waldmann TA: Monoclonal antibodies in diagnosis and therapy. Science *252*:1657, 1991

167. Stevenson GT, Stevenson FK: Antibody to molecularly defined antigen confined to a tumor cell surface. Nature *254*:714, 1975

168. Stevenson GT, Elliot EV, Stevenson FK: Idiotypic determinants on the surface immunoglobulin of neoplastic lymphocytes: A therapeutic target. Fed Proc *36*:2268, 1977

169. Hatzubai A, Maloney DG, Levy R: The use of a monoclonal anti-idiotype antibody to study the biology of a human B cell lymphoma. J Immunol *126*:2397, 1981

170. Miller RA, Maloney DG, Warnke R, et al: Treatment of B cell lymphoma with monoclonal anti-idiotype antibody. N Engl J Med *306*:517, 1982

171. Meeker TC, Lowder J, Maloney DG, et al: A clinical trial of anti-idiotype therapy for B cell malignancy. Blood *65*:1349, 1985

172. Lowder JN, Meeker TC, Levy R: Monoclonal antibody therapy of lymphoid malignancy. Cancer Surv *4*:359, 1985

173. Brown SL, Miller RA, Horning SJ, et al: Treatment of B-cell lymphomas with anti-idiotype antibodies alone and in combination with alpha interferon. Blood *73*:651, 1989

174. Maloney DG, Brown S, Czerwinski DK, et al: Monoclonal anti-idiotype antibody therapy of B cell lymphoma: The addition of a short course of chemotherapy does not prevent the emergence of idiotype negative variant cells. Blood *80*:1502, 1992

175. Meeker T, Lowder J, Cleary ML, et al: Emergence of idiotype variants during treatment of B-cell lymphoma with anti-idiotype antibodies. N Engl J Med *312*:1658, 1985

176. Lowder JN, Meeker TC, Campbell M, et al: Studies on B lymphoid tumors treated with monoclonal anti-idiotype antibodies: Correlation with clinical responses. Blood *69*:199, 1987

177. Garcia CF, Lowder J, Meeker TC, et al: Differences in "host infiltrates" among lymphoma patients treated with anti-idiotype antibodies: Correlation with treatment response. J Immunol *135*:4252, 1985

178. Basham TY, Kaminsky M, Kitamura K, et al: Synergistic antitumor effect of interferon and anti-idiotype monoclonal antibody in murine lymphoma. J Immunol *137*:3019, 1986

179. Basham YT, Race ER, et al: Synergistic antitumor activity with IFN and monoclonal anti-idiotype for murine B cell lymphoma: Mechanism of action. J Immunol *141*:2855, 1988

180. Miller RA, Hart S, Samouszuk M, et al: Shared idiotypes expressed by human B cell lymphomas. N Engl J Med *321*:851, 1989

181. Maloney DG, Levy R, Miller RA: Monoclonal anti-idiotype antibody therapy of B-cell lymphoma. *In* DeVita VT, Hellman S, Rosenberg SA (eds): Biologic Therapy of Cancer Update. Philadelphia, Lippincott Healthcare Publications, 1992, pp 1–10

182. Rankin EM, Hekman A, Somers R, et al: Treatment of two patients with B cell lymphoma with monoclonal anti-idiotypic antibodies. Blood *65*:1373, 1985

183. Rankin EM, Hekman A, Hardeman MR, et al: Dynamic studies of lymphocytes labelled with indium-111 during and after treatment with monoclonal anti-idiotype antibody in advanced B cell lymphoma. BMJ *289*:1097, 1984

184. Capel PJA, Preijers WMB, Allebes WA, et al: Treatment of chronic lymphocytic leukemia with monoclonal anti-idiotypic antibody. Neth J Med *28*:112, 1985

185. Caulfield MJ, Murthy S, Tubbs RR, et al: Treatment of chronic lymphocytic leukemia with an anti-idiotypic monoclonal antibody. Cleve Clin J Med *56*:182, 1989

186. Allebes WA, Preijers FW, Haanen C, et al: The development of non-responsiveness to immunotherapy with monoclonal anti-idiotypic antibodies in a patient with B-CLL. Br J Haematol *70*:295, 1988

187. Allebes WA, Knops R, Bontrop RE, et al: Phenotypic and functional changes of tumour cells from patients treated with monoclonal anti-idiotypic antibodies. Scand J Immunol *32*:441, 1990

188. Allebes W, Knops R, Herold M, et al: Immunotherapy with monoclonal anti-idiotypic antibodies: Tumour reduction and lymphokine production. Leuk Res *15*:215, 1991

189. Hamblin TJ, Stevenson FK, Abdul-Ahad AK, et al: Preliminary experience in treating lymphocytic leukaemia with antibody to immunoglobulin idiotypes on the cell surface. Br J Cancer *42*:495, 1980

190. Gordon J, Abdul-Ahad AK, Hamblin TJ, et al: Mechanisms of tumor cell escape encountered in treating lymphocytic leukaemia with anti-idiotype antibody. Br J Cancer *49*:547, 1984

191. Hamblin TJ, Cattan AR, Glennie MJ: Initial experience in treat-

ing human lymphoma with a chimeric univalent derivative of monoclonal anti-idiotype antibody. Blood 69:790, 1987

192. Mellstedt H, Frodin JE, Masucci G, et al: The therapeutic use of monoclonal antibodies in colorectal carcinoma. Semin Oncol 18:462, 1991

193. Sears HF, Herlyn D, Steplewski Z: Phase II clinical trial of a murine monoclonal antibody cytotoxic for gastrointestinal adenocarcinoma. Cancer Res 45:5910, 1985

194. Sears HF, Atkinson B, Mattis J, et al: Phase I clinical trial with monoclonal antibody in the treatment of gastrointestinal tumors. Lancet 1:762, 1982

195. Sears HF, Herlyn D, Steplewski Z, et al: Effects of monoclonal antibody immunotherapy on patients with gastrointestinal adenocarcinoma. J Biol Resp Mod 3:138, 1984

196. LoBuglio AF, Saleh MN, Lee J, et al: Phase I trial of multiple large doses of murine monoclonal antibody CO17-1A. I. Clinical aspects. J Natl Cancer Inst 80:932, 1988

197. Frodin JE, Lefvert AK, Mellstedt H: Pharmacokinetics of the mouse monoclonal antibody 17-1A in cancer patients receiving various treatment schedules. Cancer Res 50:4866, 1990

198. Verrill H, Goldberg M, Rosenbaum R, et al: Clinical trial of Wistar Institute 17-1A monoclonal antibody in patients with advanced gastrointestinal adenocarcinoma: A preliminary report. Hybridoma 5:S175, 1986

199. Sindelar WF, Maher MM, Herlyn D, et al: Trial of therapy with monoclonal antibody 17-1A in pancreatic carcinoma: Preliminary results. Hybridoma 5:S125, 1986

200. Amendola BE, Brady LW, Woo D, et al: Monoclonal antibodies in the treatment of metastatic carcinoma to the liver: Report of a pilot study including leukopheresis. Am J Clin Oncol 13:144, 1990

201. Douillard JY, Lehur PA, Vignoud J, et al: Monoclonal antibodies specific immunotherapy of gastrointestinal tumors. Hybridoma 5:S139, 1986

202. Tempero MA, Pour PM, Uchida E, et al: Monoclonal antibody CO17-1A and leukapheresis in immunotherapy of pancreatic cancer. Hybridoma 5:S133, 1986

203. Frodin JE, Harmenberg U, Biberfeld P, et al: Clinical effects of monoclonal antibodies (MAb 17-1A) in patients with metastatic colorectal carcinomas. Hybridoma 7:309, 1988

204. Tempero MA, Sivinski C, Steplewski Z, et al: Phase II trial of interferon gamma and monoclonal antibody 17-1A in pancreatic cancer: Biologic and clinical effects. J Clin Oncol 8:2019, 1990

205. Weiner LM, Moldofsky PJ, Gatenby RA, et al: Antibody delivery and effector cell activation in a phase II trial of recombinant gamma-interferon and the murine monoclonal antibody CO17-1A in advanced colorectal carcinoma. Cancer Res 48:2568, 1988

206. Weiner LM, Steplewski Z, Koprowski H, et al: Biologic effects of gamma interferon pre-treatment followed by monoclonal antibody 17-1A administration in patients with gastrointestinal carcinoma. Hybridoma 5:S65, 1986

207. Herlyn D, Sears HF, Ernst CS, et al: Initial clinical evaluation of two murine IgG2a monoclonal antibodies for immunotherapy of gastrointestinal carcinoma. Am J Clin Oncol 14:371, 1991

208. Goodman GE, Hellstrom I, Brodzinsky L, et al: Phase I trial of murine monoclonal antibody L6 in breast, colon, ovarian, and lung cancer. J Clin Oncol 8:1083, 1990

209. Ziegler LD, Palazzolo P, Cunningham J, et al: Phase I trial of murine monoclonal antibody L6 in combination with subcutaneous interleukin-2 in patients with advanced carcinoma of the breast, colorectum, and lung. J Clin Oncol 10:1470, 1992

210. Bosslet K, Keweloh HC, Hermentin P, et al: Percolation and binding of monoclonal antibody BW494 to pancreatic carcinoma tissues during high dose immunotherapy and consequences for future therapy modalities. Br J Cancer Suppl 10:37, 1990

211. Schulz G, Buchler M, Muhrer KH, et al: Immunotherapy of pancreatic cancer with monoclonal antibody BW 494. Int J Cancer Suppl 2:89, 1988

212. Buchler M, Friess H, Schultheiss KH, et al: A randomized controlled trial of adjuvant immunotherapy (murine monoclonal antibody 494/32) in resectable pancreatic cancer. Cancer 68:1507, 1991

213. Haspel MV, McCabe RP, Pomato N, et al: Generation of tumor cell-reactive human monoclonal antibodies using peripheral blood lymphocytes from actively immunized colorectal carcinoma patients. Cancer Res 45:3951, 1985

214. Haisma HJ, Kessel MA, Silva C, et al: Human IgM monoclonal antibody 16.88: Pharmacokinetics and distribution in mouse and man. Br J Cancer Suppl 10:40, 1990

215. Haisma HJ, Pinedo HM, Kessel MA, et al: Human IgM monoclonal antibody 16.88: Pharmacokinetics and immunogenicity in colorectal cancer patients. J Natl Cancer Inst 83:1813, 1991

216. Steis RG: An evaluation of the toxicity, immunogenicity, and tumor radioimmunodetecting ability of two human monoclonal antibodies in patients with metastatic colorectal carcinoma. Cancer Invest 8:291, 1990

217. Steis RG, Carrasquillo JA, McCabe R, et al: Toxicity, immunogenicity, and tumor radioimmunodetecting ability of two human monoclonal antibodies in patients with metastatic colorectal carcinoma. J Clin Oncol 8:476, 1990

218. Houghton AN, Mintzer D, Cordon CC, et al: Mouse monoclonal IgG3 antibody detecting GD3 ganglioside: A phase I trial in patients with malignant melanoma. Proc Natl Acad Sci USA 82:1242, 1985

219. Vadhan RS, Cordon CC, Carswell E, et al: Phase I trial of a mouse monoclonal antibody against GD3 ganglioside in patients with melanoma: Induction of inflammatory responses at tumor sites. J Clin Oncol 6:1636, 1988

220. Houghton AN, Bajorin DF, Lonberg M, et al: Treatment of human metastatic melanoma with mouse monoclonal antibodies against GD3 ganglioside. Prog Clin Biol Res 288:383, 1989

221. Caulfield MJ, Barna B, Murthy S, et al: Phase Ia-Ib trial of an anti-GD3 monoclonal antibody in combination with interferon-alpha in patients with malignant melanoma. J Biol Response Mod 9:319, 1990

222. Bajorin DF, Chapman PB, Wong G, et al: Phase I evaluation of a combination of monoclonal antibody R24 and interleukin 2 in patients with metastatic melanoma. Cancer Res 50:7490, 1990

223. Cheung NK, Lazarus H, Miraldi FD, et al: Ganglioside GD2 specific monoclonal antibody 3F8: A phase I study in patients with neuroblastoma and malignant melanoma. J Clin Oncol 5:1430, 1987

224. Cheung NK, Burch L, Kushner BH, et al: Monoclonal antibody 3F8 can effect durable remissions in neuroblastoma patients refractory to chemotherapy: A phase II trial. Prog Clin Biol Res 366:395, 1991

225. Cheung NV, Lazarus H, Miraldi FD, et al: Reassessment of patient response to monoclonal antibody 3F8. J Clin Oncol 10:671, 1992

226. Saleh MN, Khazaeli MB, Wheeler RH, et al: Phase I trial of the murine monoclonal anti-GD2 antibody 14G2a in metastatic melanoma. Cancer Res 52:4342, 1992

227. Handgretinger R, Baader P, Dopfer R, et al: A phase I study of neuroblastoma with the anti-ganglioside GD2 antibody 14.G2a. Cancer Immunol Immunother 35:199, 1992

228. Saleh MN, Khazaeli MB, Wheeler RH, et al: Phase I trial of the chimeric anti-GD2 monoclonal antibody ch14.18 in patients with malignant melanoma. Hum Antibodies Hybridomas 3:19, 1992

229. Irie RF, Morton DL: Regression of cutaneous metastatic melanoma by intralesional injection with human monoclonal antibody to ganglioside GD2. Proc Natl Acad Sci USA 83:8694, 1986

230. Hamanaka S, Ota T, Nakayasu K, et al: Strong anti-tumor effect of monosialoganglioside specific monoclonal antibody 202: A clinical trial in a cancer patient with melanoma. J Dermatol 16:480, 1989

231. Divgi CR, Welt S, Kris M, et al: Phase I and imaging trial of indium 111-labeled anti-epidermal growth factor receptor monoclonal antibody 225 in patients with squamous cell lung carcinoma. J Natl Cancer Inst 83:97, 1991

232. Shepard HM, Lewis GD, Sarup JC, et al: Monoclonal antibody therapy of human cancer: Taking the HER2 protooncogene to the clinic. J Clin Immunol 11:117, 1991

233. Mulshine JL, Avis I, Treston AM, et al: Clinical use of a monoclonal antibody to bombesin-like peptide in patients with lung cancer. Ann NY Acad Sci 547:360, 1988

234. Klein B, Wijdenes J, Zhang XG, et al: Murine anti-interleukin-6 monoclonal antibody therapy for a patient with plasma cell leukemia. Blood 78:1198, 1991

235. Herlyn D, Sears H, Iliopoulos D, et al: Anti-idiotypic antibodies to monoclonal antibody CO17-1A. Hybridoma 5(suppl 1):S51, 1986

236. Frodin JE, Faxas ME, Hagstrom B, et al: Induction of anti-idiotypic (ab2) and anti-anti-idiotypic (ab3) antibodies in patients treated with the mouse monoclonal antibody 17-1A (ab1): Relation to the clinical outcome—an important antitumoral effector function? Hybridoma 10:421, 1991

237. Wettendorff M, Iliopoulos D, Tempero M, et al: Idiotypic cascades in cancer patients treated with monoclonal antibody CO17-1A. Proc Natl Acad Sci USA 86:3787, 1989

238. Courtenay LN, Epenetos AA, Sivolapenko GB, et al: Development of anti-idiotypic antibodies against tumour antigens and autoantigens in ovarian cancer patients treated intraperitoneally with mouse monoclonal antibodies. Lancet 2:894, 1988

239. Herlyn D, Wettendorff M, Schmoll E, et al: Anti-idiotype immunization of cancer patients: Modulation of the immune response. Proc Natl Acad Sci USA 84:8055, 1987

240. Herlyn D, Benden A, Kane M, et al: Anti-idiotypic cancer vaccines: Pre-clinical and clinical studies. In Vivo 5:615, 1991

241. Mellstedt H, Frodin JE, Biberfeld P, et al: Patients treated with a monoclonal antibody (ab1) to the colorectal carcinoma antigen 17-1A develop a cellular response (DTH) to the "internal image of the antigen" (ab2). Int J Cancer 48:344, 1991

242. Robins RA, Denton GW, Hardcastle JD, et al: Antitumor immune response and interleukin 2 production induced in colorectal cancer patients by immunization with human monoclonal anti-idiotypic antibody. Cancer Res 51:5425, 1991

243. Mittelman A, Chen ZJ, Kageshita T, et al: Active specific immunotherapy in patients with melanoma: A clinical trial with mouse antiidiotypic monoclonal antibodies elicited with syngeneic anti-high-molecular-weight-melanoma-associated antigen monoclonal antibodies. J Clin Invest 86:2136, 1990

244. Mittelman A, Chen ZJ, Yang H, et al: Human high molecular weight melanoma-associated antigen (HMW-MAA) mimicry by mouse anti-idiotypic monoclonal antibody MK2-23: Induction of humoral anti-HMW-MAA immunity and prolongation of survival in patients with stage IV melanoma. Proc Natl Acad Sci USA 89:466, 1992

245. Ehrlich P: On immunity with specific reference to cell life. Proc R Soc Lond 66:424, 1900

246. Varadarajan A, Sharkey RM, Goldenberg DM, et al: Conjugation of phenyl isothiocyanate derivatives of carborane to antitumor antibody and in vivo localization of conjugates in nude mice. Bioconjug Chem 2:102, 1991

247. Tamat SR, Moore DE, Patwardhan A, et al: Boronated monoclonal antibody 225.28S for potential use in neutron capture therapy of malignant melanoma. Pigment Cell Res 2:278, 1989

248. Hersey P: Preclinical and phase I studies of monoclonal antibodies in melanoma: Application to boron neutron capture therapy of melanoma. Pigment Cell Res 2:264, 1989

249. Alam F, Soloway AH, Barth RF, et al: Boron neutron capture therapy: Linkage of a boronated macromolecule to monoclonal antibodies directed against tumor-associated antigens. J Med Chem 32:2326, 1989

250. Pressman D, Korngold L: The in-vivo localization of anti-Wagner-osteogenic-sarcoma antibodies. Cancer 6:619, 1953

251. Pressman D, Day ED, Blau M: The use of paired labeling in the determination of tumor-localizing antibodies. Cancer Res 17:845, 1957

252. Bale WF, Spar IL: Studies directed toward the use of antibodies as carriers of radioactivity for therapy. Adv Biol Med Phys 5:285, 1957

253. Goldenberg DM: Future role of radiolabeled monoclonal antibodies in oncological diagnosis and therapy. Semin Nucl Med 19:332, 1989

254. Goldenberg DM: Challenges to the therapy of cancer with monoclonal antibodies. J Natl Cancer Inst 83:78, 1991

255. Order SE, Stilwagon GB, Klein JL, et al: Iodine-131 antiferritin: A new treatment modality in hepatoma. A Radiation Therapy Oncology Group study. J Clin Oncol 3:1573, 1985

256. Order S, Pajak T, Leibel S, et al: A randomized prospective trial comparing full dose chemotherapy to 131I antiferritin: An RTOG study. Int J Radiat Oncol Biol Phys 20:953, 1991

257. Vriesendorp HM, Herpst JM, Leichner PK, et al: Polyclonal 90Yttrium labeled antiferritin for refractory Hodgkin's disease. Int J Radiat Oncol Biol Phys 17:815, 1989

258. Vriesendorp HM, Herpst JM, Germack MA, et al: Phase I-II studies of yttrium-labeled antiferritin treatment for end-stage Hodgkin's disease, including Radiation Therapy Oncology Group 87-01. J Clin Oncol 9:918, 1991

259. Lenhard RJ, Order SE, Spunberg JJ, et al: Isotopic immunoglobulin: A new systemic therapy for advanced Hodgkin's disease. J Clin Oncol 3:1296, 1985

260. Stillwagon GB, Order SE, Klein JL, et al: Multi-modality treatment of primary nonresectable intrahepatic cholangiocarcinoma with 131I anti-CEA—a Radiation Therapy Oncology Group Study. Int J Rad Oncol Biol Phys 13:687, 1987

261. Carrasquillo JA, Krohn KA, Beaumier P, et al: Diagnosis of and therapy for solid tumors with radiolabeled antibodies and immune fragments. Cancer Treat Rep 68:317, 1984

262. Larson SM, Carrasquillo JA, Krohn KA, et al: Localization of 131I-labeled p97-specific Fab fragments in human melanoma as a basis for radiotherapy. J Clin Invest 72:2101, 1983

263. Pizer B, Papanastassiou V, Hancock J, et al: A pilot study of monoclonal antibody targeted radiotherapy in the treatment of central nervous system leukaemia in children. Br J Haematol 77:466, 1991

264. Coakham HB, Richardson RB, Davies AG, et al: Neoplastic meningitis from a pineal tumour treated by antibody-guided irradiation via the intrathecal route. Br J Neurosurg 2:199, 1988

265. Richardson RB, Kemshead JT, Davies AG, et al: Dosimetry of intrathecal iodine 131 monoclonal antibody in cases of neoplastic meningitis. Eur J Nucl Med 17:42, 1990

266. Lashford LS, Davies AG, Richardson RB, et al: A pilot study of 131I monoclonal antibodies in the therapy of leptomeningeal tumors. Cancer 61:857, 1988

267. Moseley RP, Davies AG, Richardson RB, et al: Intrathecal administration of 131I radiolabelled monoclonal antibody as a treatment for neoplastic meningitis. Br J Cancer 62:637, 1990

268. Hird V, Stewart JS, Snook D, et al: Intraperitoneally administered 90Y-labelled monoclonal antibodies as a third line of treatment in ovarian cancer. A phase 1-2 trial: Problems encountered and possible solutions. Br J Cancer Suppl 10:48, 1990

269. Stewart JS, Hird V, Snook D, et al: Intraperitoneal 131I- and 90Y-labelled monoclonal antibodies for ovarian cancer: Pharmacokinetics and normal tissue dosimetry. Int J Cancer Suppl 3:71, 1988

270. Stewart JS, Hird V, Snook D, et al: Intraperitoneal radioimmunotherapy for ovarian cancer: Pharmacokinetics, toxicity, and efficacy of I-131 labeled monoclonal antibodies. Int J Radiat Oncol Biol Phys 16:405, 1989

271. Stewart JS, Hird V, Snook D, et al: Intraperitoneal yttrium-90-labeled monoclonal antibody in ovarian cancer. J Clin Oncol 8:1941, 1990

272. Stewart JS, Sivolapenko GB, Hird V, et al: Clearance of 131I-labeled murine monoclonal antibody from patients' blood by intravenous human anti-murine immunoglobulin antibody. Cancer Res 50:563, 1990

273. Ward B, Mather S, Shepherd J, et al: The treatment of intraperitoneal malignant disease with monoclonal antibody guided 131I radiotherapy. Br J Cancer 58:658, 1988

274. Epenetos AA, Munro AJ, Stewart S, et al: Antibody-guided irradiation of advanced ovarian cancer with intraperitoneally administered radiolabeled monoclonal antibodies. J Clin Oncol 5:1890, 1987

275. Kalofonos HP, Pawlikowska TR, Hemingway A, et al: Antibody guided diagnosis and therapy of brain gliomas using radiolabeled monoclonal antibodies against epidermal growth factor receptor and placental alkaline phosphatase. J Nucl Med 30:1636, 1989

276. Brady LW, Markoe AM, Woo DV, et al: Iodine 125 labeled anti-

epidermal growth factor receptor-425 in the treatment of malignant astrocytomas: A pilot study. J Neurosurg Sci *34*:243, 1990

277. Brady LW, Miyamoto C, Woo DV, et al: Malignant astrocytomas treated with iodine-125 labeled monoclonal antibody 425 against epidermal growth factor receptor: A phase II trial. Int J Radiat Oncol Biol Phys *22*:225, 1992

278. Riva P, Arista A, Sturiale C, et al: Treatment of intracranial human glioblastoma by direct intratumoral administration of 131I-labelled anti-tenascin monoclonal antibody BC-2. Int J Cancer *51*:7, 1992

279. Thistlethwaite JRJ, Cosimi AB, Delmonico FL, et al: Evolving use of OKT3 monoclonal antibody for treatment of renal allograft rejection. Transplantation *38*:695, 1984

280. Zimmer AM, Rosen ST, Spies SM, et al: Radioimmunotherapy of patients with cutaneous T-cell lymphoma using an iodine-131-labeled monoclonal antibody: Analysis of retreatment following plasmapheresis. J Nucl Med *29*:174, 1988

281. Ledermann JA, Begent RH, Bagshawe KD, et al: Repeated antitumour antibody therapy in man with suppression of the host response by cyclosporin A. Br J Cancer *58*:654, 1988

282. Ledermann JA, Begent RH, Massof C, et al: A phase-I study of repeated therapy with radiolabelled antibody to carcinoembryonic antigen using intermittent or continuous administration of cyclosporin A to suppress the immune response. Int J Cancer *47*:659, 1991

283. Meredith RF, Khazaeli MB, Plott WE, et al: Phase I trial of iodine-131-chimeric B72.3 (human IgG4) in metastatic colorectal cancer. J Nucl Med *33*:23, 1992

284. Khazaeli MB, Saleh MN, Liu TP, et al: Pharmacokinetics and immune response of 131I-chimeric mouse/human B72.3 (human gamma 4) monoclonal antibody in humans. Cancer Res *51*:5461, 1991

285. Bernstein ID, Eary JF, Badger CC, et al: High dose radiolabeled antibody therapy of lymphoma. Cancer Res *50*:1017s, 1990

286. Eary JF, Press OW, Badger CC, et al: Imaging and treatment of B-cell lymphoma. J Nucl Med *31*:1257, 1990

287. Kaminski MS, Fig LM, R. Zasadny KR, et al: Imaging, dosimetry, and radioimmunotherapy with iodine 131-labeled anti-CD37 antibody in B-cell lymphoma. J Clin Oncol *10*:1696, 1992

288. Goldenberg DM, Horowitz JA, Sharkey RM, et al: Targeting, dosimetry, and radioimmunotherapy of B-cell lymphomas with iodine-131-labeled LL2 monoclonal antibody. J Clin Oncol *9*:548, 1991

289. DeNardo SJ, DeNardo GL, O'Grady LF, et al: Treatment of B cell malignancies with 131I Lym-1 monoclonal antibodies. Int J Cancer Suppl *3*:96, 1988

290. DeNardo GL, DeNardo SJ, O'Grady LF, et al: Fractionated radioimmunotherapy of B-cell malignancies with 131I-Lym-1. Cancer Res *50*:1014s, 1990

291. Rosen ST, Zimmer AM, Goldman LR, et al: Radioimmunodetection and radioimmunotherapy of cutaneous T cell lymphomas using an 131I-labeled monoclonal antibody: An Illinois Cancer Council Study. J Clin Oncol *5*:562, 1987

292. Scheinberg DA, Straus DJ, Yeh SD, et al: A phase I toxicity, pharmacology, and dosimetry trial of monoclonal antibody OKB7 in patients with non-Hodgkin's lymphoma: Effects of tumor burden and antigen expression. J Clin Oncol *8*:792, 1990

293. Parker BA, Vassos AB, Halpern SE, et al: Radioimmunotherapy of human B-cell lymphoma with 90Y-conjugated antiidiotype monoclonal antibody. Cancer Res *50*:1022s, 1990

294. Knox SJ, Levy R, Miller RA, et al: Determinants of the antitumor effect of radiolabeled monoclonal antibodies. Cancer Res *50*:4935, 1990

295. Stirpe F, Gasperi-Campani A, Barbieri L, et al: Ribosome-inactivating proteins from the seeds of Saponaria officinalis L. (soapwort), of Agrostemma githago L. (corn cockle) and of Asparagus officinalis L. (asparagus), and from the latex of Hura crepitans L. (sandbox tree). Biochem J *216*:617, 1983

296. Wawrzynczak EJ, Henry RV, Cumber AJ, et al: Biochemical, cytotoxic and pharmacokinetic properties of an immunotoxin composed of a mouse monoclonal antibody Fib75 and the ribosome-inactivating protein alpha-sarcin from Aspergillus giganteus. Eur J Biochem *196*:203, 1991

297. Hwang J, FitzGerald DJ, Adhya S, et al: Functional domains of Pseudomonas exotoxin identified by deletion analysis of the gene expressed in E. coli. Cell *48*:129, 1987

298. Myers DE, Irvin JD, Smith RS, et al: Production of a pokeweed antiviral protein (PAP)-containing immunotoxin, B43-PAP, directed against the CD19 human B lineage lymphoid differentiation antigen in highly purified form for human clinical trials. J Immunol Meth *136*:221, 1991

299. Uckun FM, Chelstrom LM, Finnegan D, et al: Effective immunochemotherapy of CALLA+C mu+ human pre-B acute lymphoblastic leukemia in mice with severe combined immunodeficiency using B43 (anti-CD19) pokeweed antiviral protein immunotoxin plus cyclophosphamide. Blood *79*:3116, 1992

300. Uckun FM, Chelstrom LM, Irvin JD, et al: In vivo efficacy of B43 (anti-CD19)-pokeweed antiviral protein immunotoxin against BCL-1 murine B-cell leukemia. Blood *79*:2649, 1992

301. Uckun FM, Manivel C, Arthur D, et al: In vivo efficacy of B43 (anti-CD19)-pokeweed antiviral protein immunotoxin against human pre-B cell acute lymphoblastic leukemia in mice with severe combined immunodeficiency. Blood *79*:2201, 1992

302. Tonevitsky AG, Toptygin AY, Pfuller U, et al: Immunotoxin with mistletoe lectin I A-chain and ricin A-chain directed against CD5 antigen of human T-lymphocytes; comparison of efficiency and specificity. Int J Immunopharmacol *13*:1037, 1991

303. Schutt C, Pfuller U, Siegl E, et al: Selective killing of human monocytes by an immunotoxin containing partially denatured mistletoe lectin I. Int J Immunopharmacol *11*:977, 1989

304. Wiedlocha A, Sandvig K, Walzel H, et al: Internalization and action of an immunotoxin containing mistletoe lectin A-chain. Cancer Res *51*:916, 1991

305. Jonas L, Walzel H, Bremer H, et al: Comparative studies on internalization of gold labelled mistletoe lectin I (MLI), its subunits, and of an immunotoxin into mouse L 1210V leukemia cells. Acta Histochem *92*:46, 1992

306. Casellas P, Dussossoy D, Falasca AI, et al: Trichokirin, a ribosome-inactivating protein from the seeds of Trichosanthes kirilowii Maximowicz: Purification, partial characterization and use for preparation of immunotoxins. Eur J Biochem *176*:581, 1988

307. Bolognesi A, Barbieri L, Carnicelli D, et al: Purification and properties of a new ribosome-inactivating protein with RNA N-glycosidase activity suitable for immunotoxin preparation from the seeds of Momordica cochinchinensis. Biochim Biophys Acta *993*:287, 1989

308. Dinota A, Barbieri L, Gobbi M, et al: An immunotoxin containing momordin suitable for bone marrow purging in multiple myeloma patients. Br J Cancer *60*:315, 1989

309. Wawrzynczak EJ, Cumber AJ, Henry RV, et al: Pharmacokinetics in the rat of a panel of immunotoxins made with abrin A chain, ricin A chain, gelonin, and momordin. Cancer Res *50*:7519, 1990

310. Avila AD, Mateo de Acosta C, Lage A: A new immunotoxin built by linking a hemolytic toxin to a monoclonal antibody specific for immature T lymphocytes. Int J Cancer *42*:568, 1988

311. Avila AD, Mateo de Acosta C, Lage A: A carcinoembryonic antigen-directed immunotoxin built by linking a monoclonal antibody to a hemolytic toxin. Int J Cancer *43*:926, 1989

312. Wawrzynczak EJ, Thorpe PE: Methods for preparing immunotoxins: Effects of the linkage on activity and stability. *In* Vogel CW (ed): Immunoconjugates: Antibody conjugates in radioimaging and therapy of cancer. New York, Oxford University Press, 1987, p 28

313. Youle RJ, Neville JDM: Anti-Thy 1.2 monoclonal antibody linked to ricin is a potent cell-type-specific toxin. Proc Natl Acad Sci USA *77*:5483, 1980

314. Houston LL, Nowinski RC: Cell-specific cytotoxicity expressed by a conjugate of ricin and murine monoclonal antibody directed against thy 1.1 antigen. Cancer Res *41*:3913, 1981

315. Thorpe PE, Ross WC: The preparation and cytotoxic properties of antibody-toxin conjugates. Immunol Rev *62*:119, 1982

316. Blakey DC, Thorpe PE: An overview of therapy with immunotoxins containing ricin or its A chain. Antibody Immunoconj Radiopharm *1*:1, 1988

317. Raso V, Griffin T: Specific cytotoxicity of a human immunoglobulin directed Fab'-ricin A conjugate. J Immunol 125:2610, 1980

318. Fulton RJ, Tucker TF, Vitetta ES, et al: Pharmacokinetics of tumor-reactive immunotoxins in tumor-bearing mice: Effect of antibody valency and deglycosylation of the ricin A chain on clearance and tumor localization. Cancer Res 48:2618, 1988

319. Thorpe PE, Wallace PM, Knowles PP, et al: New coupling agents for the synthesis of immunotoxins containing a hindered disulfide bond with improved stability in vivo. Cancer Res 47:5924, 1987

320. Thorpe PE, Wallace PM, Knowles PP, et al: Improved antitumor effects of immunotoxins prepared with deglycosylated ricin A-chain and hindered disulfide linkages. Cancer Res 48:6396, 1988

321. Blakey DC, Wawrzynczak EJ, Wallace PM, et al: Antibody toxin conjugates: A perspective. Prog Allergy 45:50, 1988

322. Bjorn MJ, Ring D, Frankel A: Evaluation of monoclonal antibodies for the development of breast cancer immunotoxins. Cancer Res 45:1214, 1985

323. Engert A, Burrows F, Jung W, et al: Evaluation of ricin A chain-containing immunotoxins directed against the CD30 antigen as potential reagents for the treatment of Hodgkin's disease. Cancer Res 50:84, 1990

324. Shen GL, Li JL, Ghetie MA, et al: Evaluation of four CD22 antibodies as ricin A chain-containing immunotoxins for the in vivo therapy of human B-cell leukemias and lymphomas. Int J Cancer 42:792, 1988

325. Casellas P, Bourrie BJP, Gros P, et al: Kinetics of cytotoxicity induced by immunotoxins: Enhancement by lysosomotropic amines and carboxylic ionophores. J Biol Chem 259:9359, 1984

326. Raso V, Lawrence J: Carboxylic ionophores enhance the cytotoxic potency of ligand- and antibody-delivered ricin A chain. J Exp Med 160:1234, 1984

327. Ramakrishnan S, Houston LL: Inhibition of human acute lymphoblastic leukemia cells by immunotoxins: Potentiation by chloroquine. Science 223:58, 1984

328. McIntosh DP, Edwards DC, Cumber AJ, et al: Ricin B chain converts a noncytotoxic antibody-ricin A chain conjugate into a potent and specific cytotoxic agent. FEBS Lett 164:17, 1983

329. Vitetta ES, Cushley W, Uhr JW: Synergy of ricin A chain-containing immunotoxins and ricin B chain-containing immunotoxins in in vitro killing of neoplastic human B cells. Proc Natl Acad Sci USA 80:6332, 1983

330. Vitetta ES, Fulton RJ, Uhr JW: Cytotoxicity of a cell-reactive immunotoxin containing ricin A chain is potentiated by an anti-immunotoxin containing ricin B chain. J Exp Med 160:341, 1984

331. Thorpe PE, Ross WC, Brown ANF, et al: Blockade of the galactose-binding sites of ricin by its linkage to antibody: Specific cytotoxic effects of the conjugates. Eur J Biochem 140:63, 1984

332. Thorpe PE, Mason DW, Brown ANF, et al: Selective killing of malignant cells in a leukaemic rat bone marrow using an antibody-ricin conjugate. Nature 297:594, 1982

333. Thorpe PE, Cumber AJ, Williams N, et al: Abrogation of the non-specific toxicity of abrin conjugated to anti-lymphocyte globulin. Clin Exp Immunol 43:195, 1981

334. Houston LL: Inactivation of ricin using 4-azidophenyl-beta-D-galactopyranoside and 4-diazophenyl-beta-D-galactopyranoside. J Biol Chem 258:7208, 1983

335. Moroney SE, D'Alarcao LJ, Goldmacher VS, et al: Modification of the binding site(s) of lectins by an affinity column carrying an activated galactose-terminated ligand. Biochemistry 26:8390, 1987

336. Kondo T, FitzGerald D, Chaudhary VK, et al: Activity of immunotoxins constructed with modified Pseudomonas exotoxin A lacking the cell recognition domain. J Biol Chem 263:9470, 1988

337. Batra JK, Jinno Y, Chaudhary VK, et al: Antitumor activity in mice of an immunotoxin made with anti-transferrin receptor and a recombinant form of Pseudomonas exotoxin. Proc Natl Acad Sci USA 86:8545, 1989

338. Pai LH, Batra JK, FitzGerald DJ, et al: Anti-tumor activities of immunotoxins made of monoclonal antibody B3 and various forms of Pseudomonas exotoxin. Proc Natl Acad Sci USA 88:3358, 1991

339. Pai LH, Gallo MG, FitzGerald DJ, et al: Antitumor activity of a transforming growth factor alpha-Pseudomonas exotoxin fusion protein (TGF-alpha-PE40). Cancer Res 51:2808, 1991

340. Colombatti M, Greenfield L, Youle RJ: Cloned fragment of Diphtheria toxin linked to T cell-specific antibody identified regions of B chain active in cell entry. J Biol Chem 261:3030, 1986

341. Greenfield L, Johnson VG, Youle RJ: Mutations in Diphtheria toxin separate binding from entry and amplify immunotoxin selectivity. Science 238:536, 1987

342. Kimura Y, Hase S, Kobayashi Y, et al: Structures of sugar chains of ricin D. J Biochem (Tokyo) 103:944, 1988

343. Blakey DC, Skilleter DN, Price RJ, et al: Uptake of native and deglycosylated ricin A-chain immunotoxins by mouse liver parenchymal and non-parenchymal cells in vitro and in vivo. Biochim Biophys Acta 968:172, 1988

344. Skilleter DN, Paine AJ, Stirpe F: A comparison of the accumulation of ricin by hepatic parenchymal and non-parenchymal cells and its inhibition of protein synthesis. Biochim Biophys Acta 677:495, 1981

345. Blakey DC, Watson GJ, Knowles PP, et al: Effect of chemical deglycosylation of ricin A chain on the in vivo fate and cytotoxic activity of an immunotoxin composed of ricin A chain and anti-Thy 1.1 antibody. Cancer Res 47:947, 1987

346. Vitetta ES, Thorpe PE: Immunotoxins containing ricin A or B chains with modified carbohydrate residues act synergistically in killing neoplastic B cells in vitro. Cancer Drug Deliv 2:191, 1985

347. Blakey DC, Skilleter DN, Price RJ, et al: Comparison of the pharmacokinetics and hepatotoxic effects of saporin and ricin A-chain immunotoxins on murine liver parenchymal cells. Cancer Res 48:7072, 1988

348. Stirpe F, Derenzini M, Barbieri L, et al: Hepatotoxicity of immunotoxins made with saporin, a ribosome-inactivating protein from Saponaria officinalis. Virchows Arch B Cell Pathol 53:259, 1987

349. Jinno Y, Chaudhary VK, Kondo T, et al: Mutational analysis of domain I of Pseudomonas exotoxin: Mutations in domain I of Pseudomonas exotoxin which reduce cell binding and animal toxicity. J Biol Chem 263:13203, 1988

350. FitzGerald DJ, Willingham MC, Pastan I: Antitumor effects of an immunotoxin made with Pseudomonas exotoxin in a nude mouse model of human ovarian cancer. Proc Natl Acad Sci USA 83:6627, 1986

351. Thorpe PE, Brown ANF, Bremner JAG, et al: An immunotoxin composed of monoclonal anti-Thy 1.1 antibody and a ribosome-inactivating protein from Saponaria officinalis: Potent antitumor effects in vitro and in vivo. J Natl Cancer Inst 75:151, 1985

352. Bernhard MI, Foon KA, Oeltmann TN, et al: Guinea pig line 10 hepatocarcinoma model: Characterization of monoclonal antibody and in vivo effect of unconjugated antibody and antibody conjugated to diphtheria toxin A chain. Cancer Res 43:4420, 1983

353. Hwang KM, Foon KA, Cheung PH, et al: Selective antitumor effect on L10 hepatocarcinoma cells of a potent immunoconjugate composed of the A chain of abrin and a monoclonal antibody to a hepatoma-associated antigen. Cancer Res 44:4578, 1984

354. Krolick KA, Uhr JW, Slavin S, et al: In vivo therapy of a murine B cell tumor (BCL1) using antibody-ricin A chain immunotoxins. J Exp Med 155:1797, 1982

355. Ramakrishnan S, Bjorn MJ, Houston LL: Recombinant ricin A chain conjugated to monoclonal antibodies: Improved tumor cell inhibition in the presence of lysosomotropic compounds. Cancer Res 49:613, 1989

356. Smyth MJ, Pietersz GA, McKenzie IF: Use of vasoactive agents to increase tumor perfusion and the antitumor efficacy of drug-monoclonal antibody conjugates. J Natl Cancer Inst 79:1367, 1987

357. Thorpe PE, Blakey DC, Brown ANF, et al: Comparison of two

anti-Thy 1.1-abrin A-chain immunotoxins prepared with different cross-linking agents: Antitumor effects, in vivo fate, and tumor cell mutants. J Natl Cancer Inst 79:1101, 1987

358. Vitetta ES, Stone M, Amlot P, et al: Phase I immunotoxin trial in patients with B-cell lymphoma. Cancer Res 51:4052, 1991

359. LeMaistre CF, Rosen S, Frankel A, et al: Phase I trial of H65-RTA immunoconjugate in patients with cutaneous T-cell lymphoma. Blood 78:1173, 1991

360. Grossbard ML, Freedman AS, Ritz J, et al: Serotherapy of B-cell neoplasms with anti-B4-blocked ricin: A phase I trial of daily bolus infusion. Blood 79:576, 1992

361. Falini B, Bolognesi A, Flenghi L, et al: Response of refractory Hodgkin's disease to monoclonal anti-CD30 immunotoxin. Lancet 339:1195, 1992

362. Gonzalez R, Salem P, Bunn PJ, et al: Single-dose murine monoclonal antibody ricin A chain immunotoxin in the treatment of metastatic melanoma: A phase I trial. Mol Biother 3:192, 1991

363. Spitler LE, Del RM, Khentigan A, et al: Therapy of patients with malignant melanoma using a monoclonal antimelanoma antibody-ricin A chain immunotoxin. Cancer Res 47:1717, 1987

364. Oratz R, Speyer JL, Wernz JC, et al: Antimelanoma monoclonal antibody-ricin A chain immunoconjugate (XMMME-001-RTA) plus cyclophosphamide in the treatment of metastatic malignant melanoma: Results of a phase II trial. J Biol Response Mod 9:345, 1990

365. Byers VS, Rodvien R, Grant K, et al: Phase I study of monoclonal antibody-ricin A chain immunotoxin XomaZyme-791 in patients with metastatic colon cancer. Cancer Res 49:6153, 1989

366. Rosenberg SA, Lotze MT: Cancer immunotherapy using interleukin-2 and interleukin-2-activated lymphocytes. Annu Rev Immunol 4:681, 1986

367. Weiner LM, O'Dwyer J, Kitson J, et al: Phase I evaluation of an anti-breast carcinoma monoclonal antibody 260F9-recombinant ricin A chain immunoconjugate. Cancer Res 49:4062, 1989

368. Pai LH, Bookman MA, Ozols RF, et al: Clinical evaluation of intraperitoneal Pseudomonas exotoxin immunoconjugate OVB3-PE in patients with ovarian cancer. J Clin Oncol 9:2095, 1991

369. Uadia P, Blair AH, Ghose T, et al: Uptake of methotrexate linked to polyclonal and monoclonal antimelanoma antibodies by a human melanoma cell line. J Natl Cancer Inst 74:29, 1985

370. Singh M, Ghose T, Kralovec J, et al: Inhibition of human renal cancer by monoclonal-anti-body-linked methotrexate in an ascites tumor model. Cancer Immunol Immunother 32:331, 1991

371. Shih LB, Goldenberg DM: Effects of methotrexate-carcinoembryonic-antigen-antibody immunoconjugates on GW-39 human tumors in nude mice. Cancer Immunol Immunother 31:197, 1990

372. Rowland AJ, Harper ME, Wilson DW, et al: The effect of an anti-membrane antibody-methotrexate conjugate on the human prostatic tumour line PC3. Br J Cancer 61:702, 1990

373. Affleck K, Embleton MJ: Monoclonal antibody targeting of methotrexate (MTX) against MTX-resistant tumour cell lines. Br J Cancer 65:838, 1992

374. Apelgren LD, Zimmerman DL, Briggs SL, et al: Antitumor activity of the monoclonal antibody-vinca alkaloid immunoconjugate LY203725 (KS1/4-4-desacetylvinblastine-3-carboxhydrazide) in a nude mouse model of human ovarian cancer. Cancer Res 50:3540, 1990

375. Johnson DA, Baker AL, Laguzza BC, et al: Antitumor activity of L/1C2-4-desacetylvinblastine-3-carboxhydrazide immunoconjugate in xenografts. Cancer Res 50:1790, 1990

376. Schrappe M, Bumol TF, Apelgren LD, et al: Long-term growth suppression of human glioma xenografts by chemoimmunoconjugates of 4-desacetylvinblastine-3-carboxyhydrazide and monoclonal antibody 9.2.27. Cancer Res 52:3838, 1992

377. Starling JJ, Maciak RS, Law KL, et al: In vivo antitumor activity of a monoclonal antibody-vinca alkaloid immunoconjugate directed against a solid tumor membrane antigen characterized by heterogeneous expression and noninternalization of antibody-antigen complexes. Cancer Res 51:2965, 1991

378. Lavie E, Hirschberg DL, Schreiber G, et al: Monoclonal antibody L6-daunomycin conjugates constructed to release free drug at the lower pH of tumor tissue. Cancer Immunol Immunother 33:223, 1991

379. Liu J, Zhu Z, Liu J, et al: Specific binding and internalization of monoclonal antibody HI98-daunorubicin conjugate by human leukemic cells (HL60). Chinese Med Sci J 6:157, 1991

380. Page M, Thibeault D, Noel C, et al: Coupling a preactivated daunorubicin derivative to antibody: A new approach. Anticancer Res 10:353, 1990

381. Sinkule JA, Rosen ST, Radosevich JA: Monoclonal antibody 44-3A6 doxorubicin immunoconjugates: Comparative in vitro anti-tumor efficacy of different conjugation methods. Tumour Biol 12:198, 1991

382. Yeh MY, Roffler SR, Yu MH: Doxorubicin: Monoclonal antibody conjugate for therapy of human cervical carcinoma. Int J Cancer 51:274, 1992

383. Noguchi A, Takahashi T, Yamaguchi T, et al: Tumor localization and in vivo antitumor activity of the immunoconjugate composed of anti-human colon cancer monoclonal antibody and mitomycin C-dextran conjugate. Jpn J Cancer Res 82:219, 1991

384. Li S, Zhang XY, Zhang SY, et al: Preparation of antigastric cancer monoclonal antibody MGb2-mitomycin C conjugate with improved antitumor activity. Bioconjugate Chem 1:245, 1990

385. Li S, Zhang XY, Chen XT, et al: Specific targeting of mitomycin C to tumors by anti-gastric cancer monoclonal antibody. Chinese Med J 104:358, 1991

386. Rodwell JD, Alvarez VL, Lee C, et al: Site-specific covalent modification of monoclonal antibodies: In vitro and in vivo evaluations. Proc Natl Acad Sci USA 83:2632, 1986

387. Diener E, Diner UE, Sinha A, et al: Specific immunosuppression by immunotoxins containing daunomycin. Science 231:148, 1985

388. Dillman RO, Johnson DE, Shawler DL, et al: Superiority of an acid-labile daunorubicin-monoclonal antibody immunoconjugate compared to free drug. Cancer Res 48:6097, 1988

389. Laguzza BC, Nichols CL, Briggs SL, et al: New antitumor monoclonal antibody-vinca conjugates LY203725 and related compounds: Design, preparation, and representative in vivo activity. J Med Chem 32:548, 1989

390. Oldham RK: Custom-tailored drug immunoconjugates in cancer therapy. Mol Biother 3:148, 1991

391. Avner B, Swindell L, Sharp E, et al: Evaluation and clinical relevance of patient immune responses to intravenous therapy with murine monoclonal antibodies conjugated to Adriamycin. Mol Biother 3:14, 1991

392. Orr D, Oldham R, Lewis M, et al: Phase I trial of mitomycin C immunoconjugates cocktails in human malignancies. Mol Biother 1:229, 1989

393. Ballantyne KC, Perkins AC, Pimm MV, et al: Biodistribution of a monoclonal antibody-methotrexate conjugate (791T/36-MTX) in patients with colorectal cancer. Int J Cancer Suppl 2:103, 1988

394. Schneck D, Butler F, Dugan W, et al: Disposition of a murine monoclonal antibody vinca conjugate (KS1/4-DAVLB) in patients with adenocarcinomas. Clin Pharmacol Ther 47:36, 1990

395. Petersen BH, DeHerdt SV, Schneck DW, et al: The human immune response to KS1/4-desacetylvinblastine (LY256787) and KS1/4-desacetylvinblastine hydrazide (LY203728) in single and multiple dose clinical studies. Cancer Res 51:2286, 1991

396. Elias DJ, Hirschowitz L, Kline LE, et al: Phase I clinical comparative study of monoclonal antibody KS1/4 and KS1/4-methotrexate immunoconjugate in patients with non-small cell lung carcinoma. Cancer Res 50:4154, 1990

397. Manyak MJ, Russo A, Smith PD, et al: Photodynamic therapy. J Clin Oncol 6:380, 1988

398. Dougherty TJ: Therapy and detection of malignant tumors. Photochem Photobiol 45:879, 1987

399. Donald PJ, Cardiff RD, He DE, et al: Monoclonal antibody-porphyrin conjugate for head and neck cancer: The possible magic bullet. Otolaryngol Head Neck Surg 105:781, 1991

400. Mew D, Lum V, Wat C-K, et al: Ability of specific monoclonal antibodies and conventional antisera conjugated to hematoporphyrin to label and kill selected cell lines subsequent to light activation. Cancer Res 45:4380, 1985

401. Goff BA, Bamberg M, Hasan T: Photoimmunotherapy of human ovarian carcinoma cells ex vivo. Cancer Res 51:4762, 1991

402. Oseroff AR, Ohuoha D, Hasan T, et al: Antibody-targeted photolysis: Selective photodestruction of human T-cell leukemia

cells using monoclonal antibody-chlorin e6 conjugates. Proc Natl Acad Sci USA 83:8744, 1986

403. Jiang FN, Liu DJ, Neyndorff H, et al: Photodynamic killing of human squamous cell carcinoma cells using a monoclonal antibody-photosensitizer conjugate. J Natl Cancer Inst 83:1218, 1991

404. Morgan J, Gray AG, Huehns ER: Specific targeting and toxicity of sulphonated aluminium phthalocyanine photosensitised liposomes directed to cells by monoclonal antibody in vitro. Br J Cancer 59:366, 1989

405. Mew D, Wat C-K, Towers GHN, et al: Photoimmunotherapy: Treatment of animal tumors with tumor-specific monoclonal antibody-hematoporphyrin conjugates. J Immunol 130:1473, 1983

406. Gordon J, Stevenson GT: Antigenic modulation of lymphocytic surface immunoglobulin yielding resistance to complement-mediated lysis. II. Relationship to redistribution of the antigen. Immunology 42:13, 1981

407. Gordon J, Robinson DSF, Stevenson GT: Antigenic modulation of lymphocytic surface immunoglobulin yielding resistance to complement-mediated lysis. I. Characterization with syngeneic and xenogeneic complements. Immunology 42:7, 1981

408. Songsivilai S, Clissold PM, Lachmann PJ: A novel strategy for producing chimeric bispecific antibodies by gene transfection. Biochem Biophys Res Commun 164:271, 1989

409. Glennie MJ, McBride HM, Worth AT, et al: Preparation and performance of bispecific F(ab'γ)2 antibody containing thioether-linked Fab'γ fragments. J Immunol 139:2367, 1987

410. Karpovsky B, Titus JA, Stephany DA, et al: Production of target-specific effector cells using hetero-cross-linked aggregates containing anti-target cell and anti-Fcγ receptor antibodies. J Exp Med 160:1686, 1984

411. Liu MA, Kranz DM, Jurnick JT, et al: Heteroantibody duplexes target cells for lysis by cytotoxic T lymphocytes. Proc Natl Acad Sci USA 82:8648, 1985

412. Lansdorp PM, Aalberse RC, Bos R, et al: Cyclic tetramolecular complexes of monoclonal antibodies: A new type of cross-linking reagent. Eur J Immunol 16:679, 1986

413. Brennan M, Davison PF, Paulus H: Preparation of bispecific antibodies by chemical recombination of monoclonal immunoglobulin G1 fragments. Science 229:81, 1985

414. Webb KS, Ware JL, Parks SF, et al: Evidence for a novel hybrid immunotoxin recognizing ricin A-chain by one antigen-combining site and a prostate-restricted antigen by the remaining antigen-combining site: Potential for immunotherapy. Cancer Treat Rep 69:663, 1985

415. Corvalan JRF, Smith W, Gore VA, et al: Specific in vitro and in vivo drug localisation to tumour cells using a hybrid-hybrid monoclonal antibody recognising both carcinoembryonic antigen (CEA) and vinca alkaloids. Cancer Immunol Immunother 24:133, 1987

416. Corvalan JRF, Smith W: Construction and characterisation of a hybrid-hybrid monoclonal antibody recognising both carcinoembryonic antigen (CEA) and vinca alkaloids. Cancer Immunol Immunother 24:127, 1987

417. Corvalan JRF, Smith W, Gore VA: Tumor therapy with vinca alkaloids targeted by a hybrid-hybrid monoclonal antibody recognising both CEA and vinca alkaloids. Int J Cancer 2:22, 1988

418. Tsukada Y, Ohkawa K, Hibi N, et al: The effect of bispecific monoclonal antibody recognizing both hepatoma-specific membrane glycoprotein and anthracycline drugs on the metastatic growth of hepatoma AH66. Cancer Biochem Biophys 10:247, 1989

419. Raso V, Griffin T: Hybrid antibodies with dual specificity for the delivery of ricin to immunoglobulin-bearing targets. Cancer Res 41:2073, 1981

420. Glennie MJ, Brennand DM, Bryden F, et al: Bispecific F(ab'γ)2 antibody for the delivery of saporin in the treatment of lymphoma. J Immunol 141:3662, 1988

421. French RR, Courtenay AE, Ingamells S, et al: Cooperative mixtures of bispecific F(ab')2 antibodies for delivering saporin to lymphoma in vitro and in vivo. Cancer Res 51:2353, 1991

422. Perez P, Hoffman RW, Titus JA, et al: Specific targeting of human peripheral blood T cells by heteroaggregates containing anti-T3 cross linked to anti-target cell antibodies. J Exp Med 163:166, 1986

423. Lanzavecchia A, Scheidegger D: The use of hybrid hybridomas to target human cytotoxic T lymphocytes. Eur J Immunol 17:105, 1987

424. Nelson H: Targeted cellular immunotherapy with bifunctional antibodies. Cancer Cells 3:163, 1991

425. Bolhuis RLH, Sturm E, Braakman E: T cell targeting in cancer therapy. Cancer Immunol Immunother 34:1, 1991

426. Nolan O, O'Kennedy R: Bifunctional antibodies: Concept, production, and applications. Biochim Biophys Acta 1040:1, 1990

427. Reid I, Lundy J, Monson J, et al: Heteroconjugated antibodies enhance lymphocyte-mediated tumour cell lysis in vitro and in vivo. Br J Surg 79:628, 1992

428. Weiner GJ, Hillstrom JR: Bispecific anti-idiotype/anti-CD3 antibody therapy of murine B cell lymphoma. J Immunol 147:4035, 1991

429. Brissinck J, Demanet C, Moser M, et al: Treatment of mice bearing BCL1 lymphoma with bispecific antibodies. J Immunol 147:4019, 1991

430. Demanet C, Brissinck J, Van Mechelen M, et al: Treatment of murine B cell lymphoma with bispecific monoclonal antibodies (anti-idiotype x anti-CD3). J Immunol 147:1091, 1991

431. de Palazzo IG, Gercel-Taylor C, Kitson J, et al: Potentiation of tumor lysis by a bispecific antibody that binds to CA19-9 antigen and the Fcγ receptor expressed by human large granular lymphocytes. Cancer Res 50:7123, 1990

432. Shen L, Guyre PM, Anderson CL, et al: Heteroantibody-mediated cytotoxicity: Antibody to the high affinity Fc receptor for IgG mediates cytotoxicity by human monocytes that is enhanced by interferon-γ and is not blocked by human IgG. J Immunol 137:3378, 1991

433. Greenman J, Hogg N, Nikoletti S, et al: Comparative efficiencies of bispecific F(ab'γ)2 and chimeric mouse/human IgG antibodies in recruiting cellular effectors for cytotoxicity via Fcγ receptors. Cancer Immunol Immunother 34:361, 1992

434. Ferrini S, Prigione I, Miotti S, et al: Bispecific monoclonal antibodies directed to CD16 and to a tumor-associated antigen induce target-cell lysis by resting NK cells and by a subset of NK clones. Int J Cancer 48:227, 1991

435. Nitta T, Sato K, Yagita H, et al: Preliminary trial of specific targeting therapy against malignant glioma. Lancet 335:368, 1990

436. Mezzanzanica D, Canevari S, Colnaghi MI: Retargeting of human lymphocytes against human ovarian carcinoma cells by bispecific antibodies: From laboratory to clinic. Int J Clin Lab Res 21:159, 1991

437. Gridley DS, Stickney DR: Changes in leucocyte populations following murine bifunctional antibody infusion in colon cancer patients. Clin Exp Immunol 84:289, 1991

438. Connors TA: The effect of asparaginase on some animal tumors. Rec Results Cancer Res 33:181, 1970

439. Connors TA: The need for additional alkylating agents. Cancer Res 29:2443, 1969

440. Connors TA, Whisson ME: Cure of mice bearing advanced plasma cell tumours with aniline mustard: The relationship between glucuronidase activity and tumour sensitivity. Nature 210:866, 1966

441. Battelli MG, Abbandonza A, Tazzari PL, et al: Selective cytotoxicity of an oxygen-radical-generating enzyme conjugated to a monoclonal antibody. Clin Exp Immunol 73:128, 1988

442. Philpott GW, Shearer WT, Bower RW, et al: Selective cytotoxicity of hapten-substituted cells with an antibody-enzyme conjugate. J Immunol 111:921, 1973

443. Stanislawski M, Rousseau V, Goavec M, et al: Immunotoxins containing glucose oxidase and lactoperoxidase with tumoricidal properties: In vitro killing effectiveness in a mouse plasmacytoma cell model. Cancer Res 47:5497, 1989

444. Searle F, Bier C, Buckley RG, et al: The potential of carboxypeptidase G2-antibody conjugates as anti-tumor agents: Preparation of antihuman chorionic gonadotropin-carboxypeptidase G2 and cytotoxicity of the conjugate against JAR choriocarcinoma cells in vitro. Br J Cancer 53:377, 1986

445. Bagshawe KD: Antibody directed enzymes revive anti-cancer prodrugs concept. Br J Cancer 56:531, 1987

446. Bagshawe KD: Towards generating cytotoxic agents at cancer sites. Br J Cancer 60:275, 1989

447. Bagshawe KD: Antibody-directed enzyme/prodrug therapy (ADEPT). Biochem Soc Trans 18:750, 1990

448. Haisma HJ, Boven E, van Muijen M, et al: Analysis of a conjugate between anticarcinoembryonic antigen monoclonal antibody and alkaline phosphatase for specific activation of the prodrug etoposide phosphate. Cancer Immunol Immunother 34:343, 1992

449. Senter PD, Saulnier MG, Schreiber GJ, et al: Anti-tumor effects of antibody-alkaline phosphatase conjugates in combination with etoposide phosphate. Proc Natl Acad Sci USA 85:4842, 1988

450. Senter PD, Schreiber GJ, Hirschberg DL, et al: Enhancement of the in vitro and in vivo antitumor activities of phosphorylated mitomycin c and etoposide derivatives by monoclonal antibody-alkaline phosphatase conjugates. Cancer Res 49:5789, 1989

451. Bagshawe KD, Springer CJ, Searle F, et al: A cytotoxic agent can be generated selectively at cancer sites. Br J Cancer 58:700, 1988

452. Haenseler E, Esswein A, Vitols KS, et al: Activation of methotrexate-alpha-alanine by carboxypeptidase A-monoclonal antibody conjugate. Biochemistry 31:891, 1992

453. Kuefner U, Lohrmann U, Montejano YD, et al: Carboxypeptidase-mediated release of methotrexate from methotrexate α-peptides. Biochemistry 28:2288, 1989

454. Springer CJ, Antoniw P, Bagshawe KD, et al: Novel prodrugs which are activated to cytotoxic alkylating agents by carboxypeptidase G2. J Med Chem 33:677, 1990

455. Springer CJ, Bagshawe KD, Sharma SK, et al: Ablation of human choriocarcinoma xenografts in nude mice by antibody-directed enzyme prodrug therapy (ADEPT) with three novel compounds. Eur J Cancer 27:1361, 1991

456. Lowe DA, Romancik G, Elander RP: Enzymatic hydrolysis of penicillin-V to 6-aminopenicillanic acid by Fusarium oxysporum. Biotech Lett 8:151, 1986

457. Kerr DE, Senter PD, Burnett WV, et al: Antibody-penicillin-V-amidase conjugates kill antigen-positive tumor cells when combined with doxorubicin phenoxyacetamide. Cancer Immunol Immunother 31:202, 1990

458. Nishiyama T, Kawamura Y, Kawamoto K, et al: Antineoplastic effects in rats of 5-fluorocytosine in combination with cytosine deaminase capsules. Cancer Res 45:1753, 1985

459. Senter PD, Su PC, Katsuragi T, et al: Generation of 5-fluorouracil from 5-fluorocytosine by monoclonal antibody-cytosine deaminase conjugates. Bioconjug Chem 2:447, 1991

460. Bagshawe KD, Sharma SK, Springer CJ, et al: Antibody directed enzyme prodrug therapy (ADEPT): Clinical report. Dis Markers 9:233, 1991

461. Linch DC, Beverey PCL, Newland A, et al: Treatment of low grade T cell proliferation with monoclonal antibody. Clin Exp Immunol 51:244, 1983

462. Nadler LM, Stashenko P, Hardy R, et al: Serotherapy of a patient with a monoclonal antibody directed against a human lymphoma associated antigen. Cancer Res 40:3147, 1980

463. Fischer A, Blanche S, Le BJ, et al: Anti-B-cell monoclonal antibodies in the treatment of severe B-cell lymphoproliferative syndrome following bone marrow and organ transplantation. N Engl J Med 324:1451, 1991

464. Blanche S, Le DF, Veber F, et al: Treatment of severe Epstein-Barr virus-induced polyclonal B-lymphocyte proliferation by anti-B-cell monoclonal antibodies: Two cases after HLA-mismatched bone marrow transplantation. Ann Intern Med 108:199, 1988

465. Stephan JL, Le DF, Blanche S, et al: Treatment of central nervous system B lymphoproliferative syndrome by local infusion of a B cell-specific monoclonal antibody. Transplantation 54:246, 1992

466. Ball ED, Bernier GM, Cornwell GG III, et al: Monoclonal antibodies to myeloid differentiation antigens: In vivo studies of three patients with acute myelogenous leukemia. Blood 62:1203, 1983

467. Scheinberg DA, Lovett D, Divgi CR, et al: A phase I trial of monoclonal antibody M195 in acute myelogenous leukemia: Specific bone marrow targeting and internalization of radionuclide. J Clin Oncol 9:478, 1991

468. Sears HF, Herlyn D, Steplewski Z, et al: Initial trial use of murine monoclonal antibodies as immunotherapeutic agents for gastrointestinal adenocarcinoma. Hybridoma 5(suppl 1):S109, 1986

469. Khazaeli MB, Saleh MN, Wheeler RH, et al: Phase I trial of multiple large doses of murine monoclonal antibody CO17-1A. II. Pharmacokinetics and immune response. J Natl Cancer Inst 80:937, 1988

470. Lobuglio AF, Saleh M, Peterson L, et al: Phase I clinical trial of CO17-1A monoclonal antibody. Hybridoma 5(suppl 1):S117, 1986

471. Paul AR, Engstrom PF, Weiner LM, et al: Treatment of advanced measurable or evaluable pancreatic carcinoma with 17-1A murine monoclonal antibody alone or in combination with 5-fluorouracil, Adriamycin and mitomycin (FAM). Hybridoma 5:S171, 1986

472. Frodin JE, Biberfeld P, Christensson B, et al: Treatment of patients with metastasizing colo-rectal carcinoma with mouse monoclonal antibodies (Moab 17-1A): A progress report. Hybridoma 5(suppl 1):S151, 1986

473. Saleh MN, LoBuglio AF, Wheeler RH, et al: A phase II trial of murine monoclonal antibody 17-1A and inteferon-gamma: Clinical and immunological data. Cancer Immunol Immunother 32:185, 1990

474. Oldham RK, Foon KA, Morgan AC: Monoclonal antibody therapy of malignant melanoma: In vivo localization in cutaneous metastasis after intravenous administration. J Clin Oncol 2:1235, 1984

475. Goodman GE, Beaumier P, Hellstrom I, et al: Pilot trial of murine monoclonal antibodies in patients with advanced melanoma. J Clin Oncol 3:340, 1985

476. Murray JL, Lamki LM, Shanken LJ, et al: Immunospecific saturable clearance mechanisms for indium-111-labeled anti-melanoma monoclonal antibody 96.5 in humans. Cancer Res 48:4417, 1988

477. Press OW, Eary JF, Badger CC, et al: Treatment of refractory non-Hodgkin's lymphoma with radiolabeled MB-1 (anti-CD37) antibody. J Clin Oncol 7:1027, 1989

478. Larson SM, Cheung NV, Liebel SA: Radioisotope conjugates. In DeVita VT, Hellman S, Rosenberg SA: Biologic Therapy of Cancer. Philadelphia, JB Lippincott Company, 1991, p 496

479. Larson SM, Carrasquillo JA, Colcher DC, et al: Estimates of radiation absorbed dose for intraperitoneally administered iodine-131 radiolabeled B72.3 monoclonal antibody in patients with peritoneal carcinomatoses. J Nucl Med 32:1661, 1991

480. Pectasides D, Stewart S, Courtenay LN, et al: Antibody-guided irradiation of malignant pleural and pericardial effusions. Br J Cancer 53:727, 1986

481. Riva P, Moscatelli G, Paganelli G, et al: Antibody-guided diagnosis: An Italian experience on CEA-expressing tumours. Int J Cancer Suppl 2:114, 1988

482. Breitz HB, Weiden PL, Vanderheyden JL, et al: Clinical experience with rhenium-186-labeled monoclonal antibodies for radioimmunotherapy: Results of phase I trials. J Nucl Med 33:1099, 1992

483. Gould BJ, Borowitz MJ, Groves ES, et al: Phase I study of an anti-breast cancer immunotoxin by continuous infusion: Report of a targeted toxic effect not predicted by animal studies. J Natl Cancer Inst 81:775, 1989

484. Hertler AA, Schlossman DM, Borowitz MJ, et al: An anti-CD5 immunotoxin for chronic lymphocytic leukemia: Enhancement of cytotoxicity with human serum albumin-monensin. Int J Cancer 43:215, 1989

485. Hertler AA, Schlossman DM, Borowitz MJ, et al: A phase I study of T101-ricin A chain immunotoxin in refractory chronic lymphocytic leukemia. J Biol Response Mod 7:97, 1988

486. Laurent G, Pris J, Farcet JP, et al: Effects of therapy with T101 ricin A-chain immunotoxin in two leukemia patients. Blood 67:1680, 1986

487. Laurent G, Frankel AE, Hertler AA, et al: Treatment of leukemia patients with T101 ricin A chain immunotoxins. Cancer Treat Res 37:483, 1988

488. Grossbard ML, Lambert JM, Goldmacher VS, et al: Correlation between in vivo toxicity and preclinical in vitro parameters for the immunotoxin anti-B4-blocked ricin. Cancer Res 52:4200, 1992

22

CELLULAR IMMUNITY

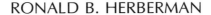

RONALD B. HERBERMAN

Cellular immunity or cell-mediated immunity in tumor-bearing individuals has been a topic of intense interest and extensive investigations. It has been considered from two main standpoints. The first of these is the overall function of the cellular immune system in tumor-bearing individuals. Cancer, particularly in advanced stages, frequently has been shown to be associated with substantial deficiencies in the function of various aspects of the cellular immune system. Various aspects of T-cell–mediated immunity have been shown to be deficient in tumor-bearing individuals. A recent study has suggested that this may be due to a deficit in the ability of T cells to transduce signals on stimulation.[1] Natural killer (NK) cell activity also has been found to be depressed in some patients with cancer, and there have been some indications that this may have prognostic significance, with low NK activity associated with poor prognosis. For example, pretreatment NK activity in the blood of patients with head and neck tumors was inversely related to the development of distant and regional metastases and to death from progressive disease.[2] Also, decreased NK activity appears to be an important predisposing factor in recurrent melanoma.[3] Similarly, a marked and sudden decrease in NK activity has been reported to signal rather accurately relapse of leukemia.[4]

Cellular immunity also is of interest in the defense against development or progression of cancer. The potential of the cellular immune system to recognize and resist tumor growth is clearly of primary interest in the context of this section on cancer therapy, and these aspects are the predominant focus of this chapter.

IMMUNE SURVEILLANCE HYPOTHESIS

Many investigators have proposed that the immune system has a general role in preventing or limiting tumor growth. The central concept, known as the *immune surveillance* hypothesis, postulates that the immune system is a key factor in resistance against the development of detectable tumors. The first known suggestion along these lines came from Paul Ehrlich in 1909; the modern formulation of the hypothesis originated from MacFarlane Burnet and Lewis Thomas. When information about thymus-dependent immunity became known, and particularly when T cells were found to play a central role in homograft rejection, Burnet modified the immune surveillance hypothesis to stress the key role of this effector mechanism in antitumor resistance.

The immune surveillance hypothesis has since generated many experimental studies and much discussion and controversy. One of the reasons for the controversy is that the concept leads to a series of predictions; most available evidence relates to tests of one or more of these predictions:

1. Tumor cells have transplantation-type antigens.
2. Resistance against tumors is T-cell dependent and analogous to the homograft reaction.
3. There is a close evolutionary link between malignancy and the development of an immune system with capability for rejection of tumors.
4. Immune depression is associated with, and must precede, development of detectable tumors.
5. A requisite action of carcinogens and/or tumor promoters might be immunosuppression.

The main support for the immune surveillance hypothesis has come from evidence related to prediction 4, because naturally occurring or induced immunodepression has been associated with a higher incidence of some types of tumors. In experimental animal systems, this has been demonstrated most clearly with tumors induced by oncogenic viruses. Neonatal thymectomy and other forms of immune suppression have been shown to lead to increased susceptibility to polyoma virus–induced tumors in mice and Marek's disease in chickens.

Considerable clinical evidence shows that immune deficiency diseases are associated with a much higher incidence of lymphomas and leukemia. Allograft recipients receiving immunosuppressive agents, either prednisone and azathioprine or, more recently, cyclosporine A and/or other immunosuppressive drugs, also have been found to have an increased incidence (approximately 100-fold) of lymphoproliferative disease or other tumors.[5] Patients with cancer, arthritis, or other diseases who received chemotherapeutic (mainly alkylating) agents have been found to develop a relatively high frequency of subsequent primary malignancies, mainly leukemias and lymphomas. The recent observations of a remarkably high incidence of Kaposi's sarcoma or B-cell lymphoma in young adults with acquired immunodeficiency syndrome (AIDS) are yet another indication of the association of malignancy with immunodepression.

Although such data support the concept of immune surveillance, the original hypothesis had several major problems or limitations:

1. The majority of human tumors associated with immunodepression have been leukemias and lymphoproliferative diseases, rather than a complete array of the common types of malignancy. The lymphoproliferative disease occurring in immunosuppressed patients after organ transplantation has been shown to be associated closely with infection by Epstein-Barr virus,[6] derived in at least some cases from the donor organs.
2. There has not been a consistent association between immunodepression and tumors.
3. Neonatally thymectomized mice have been found to have a decreased incidence of mammary tumors, and nude and euthymic mice have similar incidences of spontaneous and carcinogen-induced tumors.
4. Most spontaneous tumors of experimental animals lack detectable tumor-associated transplantation antigens.[7]
5. There appears to be an evolutionary dissociation between the development of tumors and the appearance of a sophisticated immune system and T cells.

These hypotheses have led to the suggestion[8] that immune surveillance may be operative only against tumors induced by oncogenic viruses, which have strong transplantation antigens and for which immune T cells have been shown to be important in resistance. The major exceptions to the central role of immune T cells in resistance to tumor growth have even led Richmond Prehn to formulate a countertheory of immunostimulation, suggesting that the immune system may have mainly enhancing effects on tumor induction and growth.

A more likely explanation for many of the discordant results is that a variety of effector mechanisms may be involved in host resistance. In the past several years, it has become apparent that natural immunity, as well as specifically induced immune responses, may contribute to host defenses (see later in this chapter). When T-cell–mediated immunity is viewed as only one of a series of possible host defense mechanisms, the evidence summarized above need not be viewed in such a negative light. Target cell structures other than tumor-associated transplantation antigens might be involved in recognition by other types of effector cells; and in T-cell–deficient individuals, natural immunity still might be functional and capable of resisting tumor growth. This is the basis for an updated immune surveillance hypothesis: Transformed cells express surface antigens or other structures that one or more

components of the immune system can recognize; one or more components of the natural and/or induced immunologic effector mechanisms can eliminate the transformed cells or impede the progression and spread of tumors.

This broader hypothesis leads to a somewhat different set of predictions:

1. Tumor cells have surface structures recognized by one or more effectors.
2. Tumor cells will be susceptible to lysis or growth inhibition by one or more effector mechanisms.
3. One or more of the relevant effector cells should be able to enter the site of tumor growth.
4. Augmentation of relevant effector mechanism(s) will decrease the incidence of tumors or metastases.
5. Depression of relevant effector mechanism(s), either by carcinogens or by immunosuppressive treatment, will increase the incidence of tumors or metastases.
6. Restoration of depressed effector activity will decrease the incidence of tumors or metastases.

In addition to the immune system's postulated role in surveillance against the development of tumors, there is considerable evidence for involvement of both the classic and natural immune responses in host resistance against the progression and metastatic spread of tumors once they arise. In fact, the evidence for an important role of some components of the immune system (e.g., NK cells) is much more compelling in regard to antimetastatic effects than for immune surveillance.

T-CELL–MEDIATED IMMUNITY

There is substantial evidence that thymus-dependent immune responses are important in resistance to tumors induced by oncogenic viruses. However, the absence of the thymus has not been associated with increased susceptibility to other types of tumors, suggesting a limited role for T-cell immunity in immune surveillance. Furthermore, the inability to detect tumor-associated transplantation antigens on most spontaneous rodent tumors argues against a major involvement of specific immune responses. Recent evidence indicates, however, the importance of distinguishing between *immunogenicity* and *antigenicity*. Immunogenicity refers to the ability of a tumor-associated antigen (TAA) to induce an immune response and appears to depend on the degree of expression of the antigen on the tumor cells as well as the expression of major histocompatibility complex (MHC) antigens and the immunologic responsiveness. Ultraviolet (UV) light–induced tumors in mice have been found to express strong TATAs but are usually nonimmunogenic in UV-irradiated animals because of a specific form of immune suppression.[9] Some other tumors in mice appear to be nonimmunogenic because they lack expression of MHC antigens. Immunogenicity and MHC antigen expression can be induced by treatment of the tumor cells with a chemical mutagen or UV irradiation.[10]

The reactivity of specifically immune cytotoxic T lymphocytes (CTLs) against TAAs or other cell surface antigens usually is restricted by the MHC, with cytotoxicity only detectable against target cells that share class I MHC determinants with the CTLs. There has been considerable recent progress in elucidating the basis for the close association between immunogenicity and MHC expression. Some TAAs or other exogenous antigens must be presented to T cells by macrophages or other antigen-presenting cells in physical association with class II MHC molecules. Before presentation, the antigenic molecules are endocytosed and degraded into short peptides, and a physical complex between such peptides and class II molecules is transported to the cell surface. The T-cell receptors on helper (CD4$^+$) T cells can specifically bind to and recognize these MHC-peptide complexes. TAAs also may be degraded into short peptides, eight to ten amino acids in length, by proteosomes within the tumor cells themselves, which then complex with class I MHC molecules.[11] Such peptide–class I complexes can specifically bind to T-cell receptors on CD8$^+$ CTLs.

Although most TAAs can be recognized by T cells only when physically associated with MHC molecules, a notable exception recently has been characterized in detail.[12] In the regional lymph nodes of some patients with pancreatic cancer, CTLs have been detected that can specifically recognize and lyse not only autologous tumor cells, but also MHC-unrelated pancreatic and breast tumor cells. This lack of MHC restriction has been shown to be due to recognition of repeating peptide subunits on mucin molecules that are preferentially expressed on the tumor cells.

During the past few years, there has been increasing evidence that many tumors, despite their progressive growth and metastasis, contain specifically immune T cells, which are termed tumor infiltrating lymphocytes (TILs). In studies of human tumors, cultures of TILs from some malignant melanomas or, less frequently, other tumor types have been shown to contain CTLs with specific antitumor reactivity. These findings not only provide indications for the immunogenicity of some human tumors but, as discussed later in this chapter, also provide a basis for specific adoptive therapy with such immune cells.

Antitumor CTLs derived from a melanoma patient also have been utilized to identify and characterize the gene (MAGE-1) encoding the recognized TAA.[13] This gene was shown to be expressed selectively on some tumor cells and not in normal cells, and CTLs appeared to recognize the encoded antigen in the context of a particular class I human lymphocyte antigen molecule, HLA-A1.

NATURAL KILLER CELLS AND EVIDENCE FOR THEIR ROLE IN ANTITUMOR DEFENSES

Natural killer cells were discovered about 20 years ago,[14,15] during studies of cell-mediated cytotoxicity. Although investigators expected to find specific cytotoxic activity of tumor-bearing individuals against autologous tumor cells or against allogeneic tumors of similar or the same histologic type, appreciable cytotoxic activity was observed with lymphocytes from normal individuals. With the wide array of recent studies related to natural cell-mediated cytotoxicity, there has been considerable diversity in the terminology related to the effector cells; this has led to confusion in the literature. However, at a recent workshop devoted to the study of NK cells, a consensus definition for these effector cells was developed.[16] NK cells were defined as effector cells with spontaneous cytotoxicity against various target cells; these effector cells lack the properties of classic macrophages, granulocytes, or CTLs, and the observed cytotoxicity does not show restriction related to the MHC. This definition is sufficiently broad to include not only "classic" NK cells but also the natural effector cells such as natural cytotoxic (NC) cells. The workshop participants agreed that the observations relating to the development of cytotoxic cells in culture (e.g., lymphokine-activated killer [LAK] cells, anomalous killer [AK] cells) were difficult to interpret. However, more recently it has become rather clear that most LAK activity of blood or splenic lymphocytes can be attributed to interleukin 2 (IL-2)–stimulated NK cells.

Cells Responsible for NK Activity

Until recently, the cells responsible for NK activity could be defined in a negative way—that is, by distinguishing them from typical T cells, B cell, or macrophages. However, it is now possible to isolate highly enriched populations and show that the NK activity is closely associated with a subpopulation of lymphocytes, morphologically identified as large granular lymphocytes (LGLs),[17] that comprise about 5 per cent of peripheral blood lymphocytes and 1 to 3 per cent of total mononuclear cells. LGLs have been found in all vertebrates tested (e.g., human, mouse, hamster, rat, chicken, guinea pig, and miniature swine). Cells with similar morphology and with spontaneous cytotoxic reactivity also have been identified in several invertebrate species, suggesting that NK cells represent a phylogenetically ancient effector mechanism.[18] LGLs, which contain azurophilic cytoplasmic granules, can be isolated by discontinuous density-gradient centrifugation on Percoll. LGLs are nonphagocytic, nonadherent cells that lack surface immunoglobulin or receptors for the third component of complement but contain cell surface receptors for the Fc portion of immunoglobulin G (IgG).[17] This latter quality allows them to bind antibody-coated target cells and mediate the phenomenon termed "antibody-dependent cellular cytotoxicity" (ADCC),[19] a function previously attributed to the killer (K) cell. Hence, the same cells (i.e., NK/K cells) seem able to mediate both forms of cytotoxicity, with NK activity due to NK receptors discrete from the Fc receptors that interact with target cell–bound antibody.[19,20]

The levels of NK activity have a characteristic organ distribution. Studies first performed with mouse and rat cells,[14,21] and more recently with human cells,[17,21,22] have demonstrated (1) high levels of NK activity in the peripheral blood and spleen; (2) intermediate to low levels of activity present in the lymph nodes, peritoneal cavity, and bone marrow; and (3) undetectable levels present in the tonsils or thymus. Recently, studies in the rat[21,22] have demonstrated a high degree of association of LGLs with mucosal epithelial tissues, especially with the bronchial-associated lymphoid tissue and epithelium of the gut. Mucosal LGLs have been isolated from the small intestine of mice and shown to possess intermediate to high levels of NK activity. In addition, precursors of NK cells have been shown by transplantation experiments to be derived from the bone marrow.

NK cells have been found to be mainly nonadherent, nonphagocytic, surface immunoglobulin–negative cells that are positive for β-glucuronidase and acid phosphatase and negative for nonspecific esterases.[21,22] No diversity in the cytochemical features of these cells has been reported, with virtually all cells in the population showing the same pattern of cytoplasmic enzymes.

Although LGLs appear to account for most NK activity in humans, other primates, and rodents, not all LGLs possess measurable NK activity.[17,21,22] One possible explanation for the lack of detectable cytotoxic activity in some LGLs is that the array of target cells tested has not been sufficient to reflect the entire repertoire, and that some LGLs may recognize and lyse only a limited variety of target cells. Despite this potential limitation, tests of human LGLs against several NK-susceptible target cell lines in a single-cell cytotoxicty assay enable us to estimate that, in most normal individuals, after activation of the cells with interferon, 75 to 85 per cent[23] of the LGLs are capable of killing at least one NK-susceptible target cell line. The nature of the other 15 to 25 per cent of the LGLs, with no detectable cytolytic activity, is unclear. In addition, at least some of these LGLs are CD3[+] T cells, also with the potential for mediating cytotoxic activity.[24]

Most LGLs have surface receptors for the Fc portion of IgG (mainly Fc receptor III, or CD16), and both NK activity and K-cell–mediated ADCC have been closely associated with LGLs.[17,21,22] Approximately 50 per cent of human NK cells and LGLs express detectable receptors for sheep erythrocyte, as measured by rosette formation at 4° C. However, some monoclonal antibodies to the sheep erythrocyte receptor react with a considerably higher proportion of LGLs.[25] Analogously, a proportion of mouse NK cells express Thy 1 antigens,[26] and most rat NK cells express CD8 and some other T-cell–associated markers.[27]

Thus, although NK cells clearly are not thymus dependent (because high levels of activity have been detected in thymic nude mice or in neonatally thymectomized mice),[14,21,22] they share many characteristics associated with CTLs and other T cells.

In both rat and human spleens, and to a lesser extent in other organs, large agranular lymphocytes (LALs) have been detected that possess morphologic characteristics similar to those of LGLs but that lack detectable azurophilic granules.[21,22] Aside from their lack of cytoplasmic granules, LALs have been indistinguishable from LGLs. They co-purify in the lower density fractions of Percoll density gradients. They have the same morphology, and their cytoplasm has the same appearance with Wright-Giemsa stain. Also, no cell surface markers have been found to distinguish between LGLs and LALs. In studies with purified populations of human LGLs plus LALs, a high proportion of both LALs and LGLs binds to NK-susceptible target cells. It appears that LGLs and LALs are directly related and differ only in their stages of granule maturation.[28] A range of granule development has been reported in LGLs that is detectable by electron microscopy.[21,22] It has been suggested that the earliest forms of LGL are in bone marrow, with immature granules, and that differentiation of this cell population is reflected by increasing development of mature, typical granules. According to this hypothesis, LGLs in the peripheral blood, with high NK activity and usually few cells without readily detectable granules, would represent the most differentiated cells in this lineage. Cells in the spleen and lymph nodes with lower NK activity and less prominent granules might be at an intermediate stage of differentiation. It is possible that the cytoplasmic granules are more closely related to cytolytic capability, and it appears that LALs are pre-NK cells, with the ability to bind but not lyse NK-susceptible targets.[28] This hypothesis is consistent with a body of evidence for the existence of pre-NK cells,[22] which can be induced to develop NK activity after treatment with interferon or other activating stimuli.

Overall, the results to date indicate that a discrete, small subpopulation of lymphoid cells, LGLs, is responsible for most NK activity (at least 90 per cent). These findings seem to rule out the possibility that diverse cell types share the NK function. Rather, the observed heterogeneity remains mainly within the LGL and related populations.

NK Cell Phenotype

Some cell surface antigens, particularly those detected by monoclonal antibodies (MAbs), have been found on virtually all NK cells. They therefore help to characterize the phenotype of these effector cells. For example, most human NK cells react with the following antibodies: (1) several monoclonal antibodies (B73,1, 3G8, Leu11)[29] reactive with the CD16 FcIII receptors for IgG on LGLs (these antigens also are strongly expressed on granulocytes [polymorphonuclear leukocytes]); (2) rabbit antisera to the glycolipid asialo-GM$_1$, which also reacts with monocytes and granulocytes[25]; (3) OKT10, which also reacts with most thymocytes and activated lymphocytes[25]; (4) OKM1, which also reacts with monocytes/macrophages, polymorphonuclear leukocytes, and platelets[25]; and (5) CD56, which is quite selective for NK cells but also is expressed on a small percentage of T cells.[30] Removal of cells bearing any of these markers, either by treatment with antibody plus complement or by negative selection immunoaffinity procedures, results in a depletion of most or all detectable NK activity.

In the rat, a monoclonal antibody, OX8, which also reacts with the subpopulation of T cells with suppressor activity (the antigen detected is homologous with human CD8),[27] reacts with most NK cells and LGLs. Recently, monoclonal antibody 3.2.3 has been shown to react quite selectively with virtually all rat NK cells[31] and detects NKR-PI, a molecule involved in signal transduction for which the gene has been cloned.[32] Antisera to asialo-GM$_1$ also react with virtually all rat and mouse NK cells.[27] NK cells also can be characterized by a lack of expression of certain cell surface markers. For example, human NK cells have no detectable surface reactivity with monoclonal antibodies to pan–T-cell antigens (such as CD5 and CD3) or to the CD4 T-helper antigen.[22,25] Human NK cells also do not express surface antigens detected by a number of monocyte-specific reagents such as M02 and Leu-M1.[22,25]

In contrast to a pattern of features common to most or all CTLs, NK cells and also LGLs in general are rather heterogeneous with respect to other MAb-defined markers. Human NK cells react to a variable extent with MAbs directed against the sheep erythrocyte receptor CD2 (Lyt 3, OKT11, Leu 5),[25] with only about half of the NK cells in some experiments giving positive results. Only a portion of human NK cells has been shown to react with a variety of other MAbs, including 3A1 (on most CTLs and other T cells and 50 to 60 per cent of LGLs), CD57 (or Leu 7, on 40 to 60 per cent of NK cells), and CD8 (on the suppressor/cytotoxic T lymphocytes and 10 to 30 per cent of LGLs); about 25 per cent of the LGLs react with MAbs against Ia framework (human histocompatibility leukocyte antigen [HLA-DR]) determinants.[25]

Similarly, in the mouse, only about half of the NK cells[26] express Thy 1, and only 20 per cent express readily detectable Lyt 1.[21,22] In addition, the allelic markers NK1.1 and NK2.1[21,22] are expressed on at least 50 to 60 per cent of mouse NK cells.

In contrast to classic mouse NK cells, NC cells appear to be devoid of most lymphoid surface markers, being Lyt 1$^-$, Thy1$^-$, asialo-GM$_1^-$, and H$_2$K$^-$D$^-$.[21,22] All attempts to phenotype NC cells have failed to define a characteristic marker on these cells. However, despite such indications that NC cells might be completely distinct from typical NK cells, NC cells and typical mouse NK cells co-purify in Percoll density gradients.[33] Thus NC cells also may be LGLs—either a subset of NK cells or at a stage of differentiation associated with poor expression of cell surface markers and altered receptors for target cells.

Although most NK cells and LGLs are nonadherent to plastic or nylon wool, a subset of these cells shows some adherence. For instance, when isolating human myelomonocytic cells by means of their adherence to plastic, the small percentage of contaminating cells is disproportionately comprised of LGLs.[34] In addition, after in vivo stimulation of NK cells with microbial agents such as *Corynebacterium parvum* or after in vitro stimulation of allogeneic cells with lectins or interferon, a substantial proportion of NK cells adheres either to plastic or nylon wool columns.[21,22] Although this subpopulation of cells shares the adherence property with myelomonocytic cells, it retains the morphology and cell surface characteristics of LGLs. The phenotype of human adherent NK cells has been shown to be OKT3$^-$, OKT10$^+$, OKT11$^+$, OKM1$^+$, Leu-M1$^-$, and B73.1$^-$.[34] Such cells thus contrast with typical adherent monocytes, which only react with OKM1 and Leu M1.

In summary, NK cells have a characteristic phenotype. For example, most human NK cells and LGLs can be described as CD3$^-$, CD4$^-$, OKT10$^+$, CD16$^+$, CD56$^+$, CD11b$^+$, and Leu-M1$^-$. Thus, these cells have a readily definable and general phenotype, which sets them apart from all other lymphoid cell types. The heterogeneity in cell surface phenotypes extends to only a few markers, for example, with human NK cells: OKT8, CD57, Ia, and CD2.

The observed heterogeneity in surface marker expression on NK cells has not been explained. However, recent studies using a new method to examine intracellular expression of MAb-defined markers in NK and T cells have indicated the need for caution in conclusions about the ability of lymphoid cell subpopulations to express particular antigens.[35] By means of this new procedure, all human T cells have been shown to express CD4 (only on the surface of the helper T-cell subset), B$_2$ (considered to be B-cell associated), and M02 (expressed on the surface of only myelomonocytic cells). Most LGLs also were found to have internal M02 and B$_2$ and to contain CD5 (pan-T) antigen. Although the mechanisms responsible for expression of markers intracellularly and/or on the cell surface remain to be determined, expression of a variety of markers may depend on many factors. One must be cautious in using marker data to draw conclusions about the degree of divergence among subsets of NK cells or other lymphoid cells.

Taken together, the above data may indicate discrete subsets of NK cells that vary in their cell surface markers and adherence properties. However, an alternative explanation for such data is that cell surface markers and adherence properties of NK cells vary with the stage of activation or maturation of the cells. In regard to this possibility, one notes that most of these markers do not change after stimulation with interferon[23] or other NK simulators such as IL-2 or *C. parvum*. In contrast, such treatments induce substantial changes in the levels of expression of Fc receptors and β$_2$-microglobulin on a variety of lymphoid cells.

Effect of Interferon on NK Cells

In addition to the spontaneous levels of cytotoxicity expressed by NK cells, these cells have been found to be very sensitive to rapid up-regulation by several cytokines, including interferon (IFN). All three types of IFN (α, β, γ) have been shown to augment the activity of NK cells potently.[23,36,37] In vivo administration to mice or rats of a variety of IFN inducers,[38] or of IFN itself, led to rapid boosting of NK activity. Similarly, in vitro incubation of lymphoid cells or of purified LGLs with IFN induced considerable augmentation of NK activity.[23,36,37]

To determine the role of IFN more definitively, experiments were performed with a variety of IFN species, most of which were purified to homogeneity. Almost all of the proteins with antiviral activity that have been studied, including various species of IFN-α, IFN-β, and IFNγ, have had the ability to increase NK activity significantly.[39] The one exception found to date has been IFN-αJ: Although it was apparently able to bind to LGLs, it induced no boosting of NK activity after treatment of human NK cells for several hours and induced low levels of boosting after overnight incubation.[40] In addition, there have been considerable quantitative differences in the efficacy of boosting by the various species.[39] Some IFN species have been shown to be high-level boosters, with greater than 50 per cent increase in NK activity by less than 50 units, whereas other species have been found to have low-level boosting activity, with an increase in NK activity by 50 per cent only seen with 500 units or more.

Several groups of investigators have been interested in determining the mechanisms by which IFN augments NK activity. Such studies have been facilitated considerably by the ability to identify morphologically and purify human and rat NK cells. One question was whether purified LGLs after pretreatment with IFN acquire an increased ability to recognize and bind to NK-susceptible targets.[23] When such studies were done with K562 or other suspension target cells, pretreatment with IFN was not found to result in an increased percentage of LGLs forming conjugates. In contrast, when various monolayer target cells were studied, IFN pretreatment of LGLs resulted in an increased proportion of binding cells. Thus, with some target cells but not with others, one action of IFN is to convert pre-NK cells into cells able to recognize and bind to the targets. To determine the possible effects of IFN on postbinding interactions with target cells, a single-cell agarose cytotoxicity assay was utilized.[23] With K562 targets, pretreatment of LGLs with IFN was shown to result primarily in an accelerated rate of lysis of bound target cells. In contrast, with G-11 monolayer target cells, IFN pretreatment of LGLs resulted in a substantial increase in the proportion of bound targets that were lysed. In addition, IFN pretreatment caused an acceleration in the kinetics of lysis. IFN also has been shown to increase interactions with target cells by increasing the degree of recycling (i.e., facilitating the interaction with, and lysis of, multiple target cells during the cytotoxicity assay). IFN-induced augmentation of recycling was demonstrated directly by observation of the dissociation of LGLs from bound targets and their subsequent rebinding.[23] When LGLs were pretreated with IFN, the dissociation was decreased and rebinding occurred considerably more rapidly. Yet another aspect of the effect of IFN on the interactions between NK cells and targets has been the demonstration of the ability of IFN to protect certain target cells from lysis by NK cells.[41] Thus IFN can have opposite effects on effector cell–target interactions, depending on the cell exposed to the IFN.

Effect of Interleukin 2 on NK Cells

Interleukin 2 has been shown to have two types of effects on NK cells: the stimulation of both proliferation and augmentation of cytotoxicity. In parallel with the potent ability of IL-2 to act as a growth factor for T cells, it also has been shown to promote the growth of NK cells.[42] As with T cells, this proliferative effect of IL-2 is detected by anti-Tac (IL-2 receptor α chain) MAbs.[43] Proliferating LGLs have been shown to express Tac, and anti-Tac completely interfered with the growth of the cells and

their maintenance of cytotoxic activity. However, as a major divergence from the data obtained with cells in which IL-2 receptors had to be induced by mitogens or antigens in order for the cells to become responsive to IL-2,[44] IL-2 alone has been shown to promote the growth of human or murine NK cells.[43,45] Quite unexpectedly, fresh IL-2–responsive human LGLs have been found to have no detectable high-affinity IL-2 receptors, as measured either by flow cytometry with anti-Tac or by binding studies with radiolabeled anti-Tac.[43] In addition, messenger RNA for IL-2 receptor α chain was not detectable in fresh human LGLs.[43] However, most NK cells express the intermediate-affinity β chain of the IL-2 receptor. On exposure to IL-2 alone, message for the α chain became detectable within 2 days of culture, and this was accompanied by detectable high-affinity IL-2 receptors on the cells and the onset of proliferation. Thus, it appears that IL-2 alone can induce the up-regulation of the α chain of the IL-2 receptor at the transcriptional level,[43] and this appears to account for the ability of this lymphokine by itself to promote the growth of NK cells.

In contrast to the dependence of NK cell proliferation on the expression of detectable levels of high-affinity IL-2 receptors, the ability of IL-2 to induce augmented levels of cytolytic activity rapidly has been found to be independent of entry into the cell cycle or the detectable expression of Tac.[46] Overnight incubation of LGLs with IL-2 could stimulate NK activity strongly, despite the presence in the culture medium of high concentrations of antibodies to Tac. These observations are now attributed to expression of the β chain of the IL-2 receptor on most NK cells, which allows this cytotoxic reactivity to be stimulated. In addition, such interaction of IL-2 with Tac-independent p75 receptors for IL-2 may provide the signal for induction of expression of Tac and the consequent proliferative response to IL-2.

NK-Like Cells

In addition to clear-cut situations in which cell cultures are initiated with highly purified LGLs that retain their morphologic and cytotoxic characteristics,[47] cultures usually have been initiated with unseparated lymphoid populations and cytolytic activity has been observed against NK-susceptible target cells.[48] Because the relationship of the generated cytotoxic effector cells to NK cells has been difficult to determine, such activities have been referred to as ''NK-like'' or as ''activated killer cells.'' Under some conditions, cells with broad, NK-like reactivity can be generated in cultures from precursors lacking NK activity and having a somewhat different phenotype than NK cells.[49] Furthermore, NK-like cytotoxic activity has developed in cultures of thymocytes or highly purified T cells or T-cell clones in the presence of IL-2, especially when the concentrations of IL-2 have been high.[50–54]

Lymphokine-activated killer cells have been described[55] that share many of the characteristics of the above-discussed culture-activated NK-like cells. LAK cells have been activated after a short period of culture in vivo with highly purified or recombinant IL-2 and display cytotoxic activity against a variety of autologous, allogenic, and xenogeneic tumors. These cells initially were thought to lack markers typical of fresh NK cells, to be devoid of cytolytic activity prior to culture, and to develop T cell marker activation.[56] However, more recent studies in several laboratories have indicated that most LAK activity developing from blood or splenic lymphocytes is attributable to NK cells, and their progenitors have a phenotype characteristic of NK cells but not T cells.[57]

Role of NK Cells in Inhibition of Metastasis

In the initial descriptions of LAK cells, much emphasis was placed on the observations that fresh solid tumor target cells appeared to be insusceptible to lysis by NK cells.[55] However, susceptibility or resistance of target cells to lysis by NK cells appears to be a relative rather than an absolute distinction. Under some circumstances, "NK-resistant" targets can be lysed to a significant extent by unstimulated NK cells. Regarding the possibility of NK activity against fresh noncultured tumor cells, low but significant levels of cytotoxic activity against fresh human leukemia cells were observed in the earliest studies of human NK cells.[15] Similarly, some of the "NK-resistant" culture cell lines that are being used as good targets for assessing LAK activity, particularly the Raji cell line, were used in early studies of NK activity,[58,59] prior to the discovery of more sensitive targets such as K562. Clearly, the increase of NK activity by various agents, including IFN as well as IL-2, not only can increase the levels of reactivity against NK-sensitive target cells, but also can induce detectable levels of lysis of targets that seemed refractory to unstimulated NK cells. The artificiality of the distinction between NK-sensitive and NK-resistant target cells has been emphasized by a series of in vivo studies of the role of NK cells in resistance to metastatic spread of tumors. Much of the strong evidence for the potent ability of NK cells in vivo to eliminate tumor cells from the circulation rapidly and to prevent the subsequent development of metastases in the lungs and other organs has come from studies with tumor cell lines that appear to be highly resistant to NK activity in vitro.[60–62]

Even when it has not been possible to detect lysis of fresh leukemia or solid tumor target cells by unseparated blood or splenic lymphocytes, significant levels of NK activity could be detected simply after purification of the effector cells. Human LGLs, purified by Percoll density-gradient centrifugation, have been shown to have significant cytotoxic activity against the majority of fresh solid tumor cells or fresh leukemia cells tested. The effector cells for solid tumor targets appeared to be a subset of LGLs,[63] but in conjugate assays with two target cells it was shown that the effector cells lysing autologous tumor cells also could lyse the NK-sensitive K562 cell line.[64] The effector cells reactive against human leukemia targets were further shown to be CD16[+] and NKH1[+] (CD56[+]).[65,66] In contrast to such lytic activity of LGLs against human "NK-resistant" targets, LGL-depleted populations of small T cells were without detectable activity.

During the last 15 years, there has been an increasing body of evidence to indicate that NK cells play a major role in the resistance of the host to metastatic spread of tumors and that they may contribute to immune surveillance. As the initial indication for the involvement of NK cells in metastasis, it was found that NK cells play an important role in the intravascular elimination of tumor cells.[67–71] Numerous experimental data demonstrated that 90 to 99 per cent of intravenously (IV) inoculated tumor cells were eliminated during the first 24 hours. The small fraction of surviving tumor cells (often <0.1 per cent) then were able to form tumor metastases.[72–74] Recent investigations have provided some insight into the mechanisms of intravascular death of tumor cells. The ability to eliminate the tumor cells in vivo was found to correlate directly with the level of NK activity in the recipients, with selective inhibition of NK activity resulting in survival of a large proportion of the tumor cells.

More direct evidence for the involvement of NK cells in intravascular tumor cell destruction and inhibition of metastasis formation has come from experiments with adoptively transferred NK-enriched or -depleted lymphoid cell populations. NK reactivity of mice depressed by cyclophosphamide (Cy) treatment could be reconstituted by adoptive transfer of lymphoid cells.[71] In parallel, adoptively transferred lymphoid cells were able to abrogate the metastasis-augmenting effects of Cy treatment.[75] The cells responsible for reconstitution of antimetastatic activity of Cy-treated mice were shown to be distinct from T or B lymphocytes or macrophages, and exerted NK activity in vitro. The NK activity of transfused spleen cells was depleted by pretreatment of donors with Cy or by direct incubation of spleen cells with anti-NK 1 serum and complement. Spleen cells with depleted NK cell activity failed to restore antimetastatic defense in Cy-treated recipients.[75]

Treatment of rats with anti–asialo-GM$_1$ has been associated with elimination of LGLs as well as NK activity.[61] The NK activity of peripheral blood lymphocytes (PBLs) and spleen cells of rats treated with anti–asialo-GM$_1$ could be reconstituted by IV transfusion of purified populations of LGLs. Furthermore, rats reconstituted with LGLs recovered their ability to eliminate IV-inoculated radiolabeled tumor cells and inhibited the formation of experimental metastases.[60,61]

These experimental data strongly support the concept that NK cells can be extremely efficient in the intravascular elimination of tumor cells and in prevention of metastasis formation, although it is impossible to exclude the involvement of other cells, such as neutrophils and monocytes, or of humoral factors, such as natural antibodies or complement, in these processes.[76–78] In order to evaluate adequately the role of NK cells in antimetastatic defenses, it is necessary also to assess their involvement in the formation of spontaneous metastases in tumor-bearing hosts: Metastatic spread can be assessed by comparing metastatic growth in animals with high or low NK cell activity. Treatment with C. parvum of mice bearing 3LL tumors protected against the development of postoperative pulmonary metastases. However, the antimetastatic effect of C. parvum was observed when treatment was performed at least 3 to 4 days before, but not after, local tumor excision.[79] Inoculation of polyI:C into mice bearing B16 melanoma, at 4 to 5 days before tumor removal, also inhibited the formation of postoperative pulmonary metastases. In contrast, no effect was found when polyI:C treatment was started 1 day after surgery (E. Gorelik, unpublished observation.)

These data suggest that the antimetastatic effect of *C. parvum* or polyI:C was mediated by the increase in tumor cell elimination rather than by inhibition of the proliferation of tumor cells and delay in the appearance of the visible metastatic foci. Indeed, the differences in numbers of postoperative metastases in the control and *C. parvum*–treated mice did not diminish when metastases were observed at various periods after surgery.[79]

When the formation of spontaneous metastases was investigated in mice with low or depressed NK reactivity, an increase in the number of visible metastases was found.[67,79,80] In beige mice bearing B16 melanoma cells, the number of pulmonary metastases was significantly higher than in the control mice.[81] Low levels of NK cell activity could be maintained by multiple (every 4 to 5 days) injections of anti–asialo-GM_1 serum into C57BL/6 mice with transplanted B16 melanoma or 3LL carcinoma cells. After surgical removal of the established local B16 melanoma or 3LL carcinoma, there was a substantial increase in the number of postoperative pulmonary metastases in these mice.[67] Similar effects on the formation of spontaneous pulmonary metastases in mice were observed when NK reactivity of tumor-bearing mice was depressed by implantation of pellets containing 17-β-estradiol.[82] Thus, these data demonstrate that NK cells can play an important role in the prevention of the metastatic spread and formation of tumor metastases.

MACROPHAGES AND EVIDENCE FOR THEIR ROLE IN ANTITUMOR DEFENSES

Macrophages have been suggested as important factors in antitumor defenses and might be primarily responsible for immune surveillance against tumors.[83–85] This possibility is supported by several lines of evidence:

1. Macrophages can accumulate in considerable numbers in a variety of transplantable tumors[86] and in many primary tumors.[87]
2. Macrophages have natural[88] as well as rapidly activatable ability to lyse or inhibit the growth in vitro of a wide variety of transformed cells.
3. Several treatments that can depress the function of macrophages (e.g., silica or carrageenan) have been associated with an increased incidence of tumors and metastases.[89]
4. Adoptive transfer of in vitro– or in vivo–activated macrophages was shown to inhibit the metastatic spread of some tumor cell lines.[90,91]
5. Some carcinogens (e.g., methylcholanthrene, acetylaminofluorene) have been shown to depress reticuloendothelial function.[92]
6. Stimulation of macrophage function by various im-

munomodulators has been associated with decreased tumor growth or a decreased incidence of tumors.[89]

However, there are some major limitations to such evidence:

1. There is remarkably little evidence that macrophages have cytotoxic activity against primary, freshly harvested tumor cells, as opposed to established tumor cell lines.
2. Silica and carrageenan, and virtually all of the other depressive treatments that have been used, may not be entirely selective in their effects. In fact, they may increase some functions, particularly suppressor activity, by macrophages or other cells. The treatment effects on tumor growth are not always in the same direction, even with the same tumor. For example, Mantovani et al.[93] found that treatment of mice with silica or carrageenan increased the incidence of pulmonary metastases but inhibited the growth of the primary tumors.
3. The carcinogens shown to depress reticuloendothelial function also may have affected a variety of effector mechanisms, and other carcinogens have had no detectable effects on macrophage or reticuloendothelial function.[94]
4. In experiments with some transplantable tumors in mice, adoptive transfer of macrophages facilitated the development of metastases rather than conferring resistance to metastasis.[95,96]

As with specific T-cell–mediated immunity, some recent evidence suggesting an important antitumor defense role for macrophages has come from therapeutic studies. An immunostimulatory agent, based on the minimal immunomodulatory unit in mycobacteria and shown to be a quite selective activator of macrophages, has had substantial therapeutic efficacy against metastatic tumors in mice and dogs and also has appeared to have activity against lung metastases of patients with osteosarcoma.[97]

TUMOR-INFILTRATING LYMPHOCYTES AND EFFECTOR CELL–TUMOR CELL INTERACTIONS

Human solid tumors often contain numerous mononuclear cells (MNCs) situated either around the tumor or in the tumor stroma. From an immunologic point of view, large infiltrations with MNCs into a solid tumor might indicate a vigorous local inflammatory response, an immune response, or both. Histology has been useful in providing clues regarding cellular identity, localization, and intensity of these infiltrates. Indeed, it was on the basis of histologic observations that, in the mid-1970s, Underwood[98] and then Ioachim[99] first proposed that MNC infiltrations into human tumors may bear a direct relationship to improved prognosis and may represent an expression of immune surveillance. Over the years, this notion has gained ground and support from studies by Svennevig et al.,[100] Watt and House,[101] and many others.[102–105] But even today, the role of lymphocytic infiltrations in and around solid tumors remains controversial. In human tumors for which correlations between the intensity of lymphoid infiltrates and prognosis or survival exist (e.g., melanoma,[106] carcinomas of colon,[100,101] breast,[107] and head and neck[105]), the infiltrating cells could be viewed as effectors of local antitumor immunity. In contrast, in many cases, it has not been possible to establish such correlations (see, e.g., ref. 108), and infiltrating lymphocytes are viewed as inflammatory cells mediating nonspecific rather than tumor-specific interactions.

Histology and Immunohistology of TILs

Until recently, in situ studies of TILs have been limited to histology and immunohistology. As indicated previously, much of what is known about TIL localization, distribution, and density in human tumors has been derived from examination of biopsy sections stained with conventional histologic reagents or with labeled MAbs to surface antigens on MNCs. A great deal of variability exists among different solid tumors, even with the same histopathologic type, in the distribution of MNC infiltrates.[109–111] In general, MNCs are located around the tumor, surrounding it like a wreath, and in the tumor stroma.[112,113] In some tumors MNCs also may be found in between or in touch with tumor cells. The intensity of MNC infiltrates is equally variable from one tumor to another regardless of the tumor histology. There are, however, certain notable exceptions. For example, human primary melanomas are almost always well infiltrated, and a greater degree of infiltrations has been reported to indicate good prognosis.[106] Human squamous cell carcinomas of the head and neck often contain large MNC infiltrates in the tumor stroma, and the presence as well as intensity of the infiltrates have been linked to improved survival in this group of patients.[114,115] In ovarian carcinoma, tumors of low malignant potential contain few MNCs, whereas malignant ovarian carcinomas, whether serous or mucinous, are often very well infiltrated.[116] Among breast carcinomas, those that produce and secrete mucins appear to be better infiltrated than those that do not.[117]

An argument could be made that, if TILs represent antitumor effector cells, then local accumulations of such cells in the tumor stroma or parenchyma should be beneficial to the host, and more intensely infiltrated tumors should have a better prognosis than poorly infiltrated ones. With few exceptions,[100,101,105–107] however, it has not been possible to make this type of correlation between TILs in the tumor and prognosis. There may be several reasons for this lack of correlation. Most human tumors are in advanced stages by the time they come to surgery, and it is possible that TIL infiltrations observed may be different from those present during early disease not only in density but also in composition. Also, TILs that have remained in the tumor for a period of time are likely to be influenced by the tumor and various immunoinhibitory factors known to be produced by human tumors.[110,118,119] But most important is the fact that careful prospective studies with long follow-up are necessary to seek the correlation be-

tween the degree of infiltration and prognosis or survival, and few such studies have been done.

Immunohistology also has contributed to phenotypic characterization of TIL subpopulations in situ.[107,115,120–122] The proportions of lymphocytes to monocytes and of various lymphoid subpopulations of TILs in the stroma and parenchyma were determined in many tumors.[113,123] In spite of a large degree of individual variability, it has been possible to conclude that T (CD3+) lymphocytes are the main component of infiltrates,[109,124] although in many tumors monocytes also are prominent.[123] B lymphocytes rarely are found, with the exception of melanoma,[125] and NK cells are present but in relatively small numbers.[113] In the tumor stroma, the CD4/CD8 ratios tend to be higher than in the parenchyma, which means that CD8+ T cells are more likely to be found in close contact with tumor cells than CD4+ T cells.[113,126] The latter are seen mainly in the stroma.[114] In addition, variable but often substantial numbers of T cells in the tumor appear to be activated, because they express HLA-DR antigens.[14,34,127,128] In contrast, CD25+ (i.e., expressing Tac, the α chain of the IL-2 receptor) T cells are found less frequently among TILs than are HLA-DR antigens,[111] although proportions of CD25+ T cells are generally higher in TILs than in autologous PBLs.[129] It is important to realize that the above conclusions do not apply to every solid tumor but represent a consensus derived from many different immunohistologic studies.

In situ immunohistology of solid tumors also has contributed insights into interactions between TILs and tumor cells, especially in regard to the expression of the MHC antigens and adhesion molecules on tumor cells.[130] Attempts have been made to relate the expression of these antigens on tumor cells with the intensity of MNC infiltrates into the tumor. However, although some evidence supporting the presence of large MNC infiltrates enriched in CD8+ T cells in tumors expressing the class I MHC antigens has been provided,[131–133] associations between these parameters remain largely unconfirmed.

Immunohistology has a number of limitations that must be recognized. It is performed on fragments of tumor tissues especially sampled for this purpose, and its results cannot be generalized to the rest of tumor tissue, because local differences in composition (e.g., between the parenchyma and stroma; tumor periphery versus interior) and intensity of infiltrates are known to exist. Certain lymphocyte surface antigens (e.g., the CD56 antigen) appear to be sensitive to the air drying and fixation necessary for immunostaining in situ, and no accurate information about the phenotype of cells expressing these antigens can be obtained.[134] Immunohistology is also subjective, and a bias introduced by examination of serial sections, each stained with different MAbs, must be considered in interpreting results. Finally, although immunohistology characterizes TILs and tumor cells phenotypically and topographically, it offers no clues about their functional status.

Functional Characterization of TILs

Recently, in situ hybridization technology with labeled cDNA probes has been applied to analysis of TILs. Of special interest is the ability to determine the expression of cytokine genes in TILs using ^{35}S-labeled cDNA probes for cytokine mRNA. This approach offers a unique opportunity to assess the functional potential of TILs in situ. Studies have been performed to determine the proportions of TIL-expressing genes for cytokines in frozen tissue sections of various types of human solid tumors.[135] TILs in the stroma of ovarian carcinomas or most invasive ductal breast tumors only rarely expressed mRNA for tumor necrosis factor α (TNF-α), IL-2, or IFN-γ. The intensity of MNC infiltrates in these tumors correlated with the percentage of cells that expressed mRNA for IL-2, TNF-α, or IL-2 receptor α (p55) or β (p75) chains. In those invasive ductal breast carcinomas that contained intracellular or intraductal mucins, up to 30 per cent of lymphoid cells in the tumor stroma were positive for IL-2, TNF-α, IFN-γ, and IL-2 receptor. TILs in other invasive ductal breast carcinomas or in mucinous ovarian tumors did not express genes for cytokines as measured by in situ hybridization. These observations led to the conclusion that human solid tumors differ in the ability to modulate gene expression for cytokines in TILs and that both the immunogenicity of a tumor and its immunoinhibitory potential may determine the state of TIL activation in situ.

One other new approach to in situ characterization of TILs involves determination of the T-cell receptor (TCR) Vβ chain repertoire using the polymerase chain reaction (PCR). The rationale is to seek restriction in the utilization of the TCR Vβ genes in fresh TILs in order to confirm their clonal nature. This approach has been utilized previously with IL-2–expanded TILs.[136] However, based on a likely possibility that IL-2–expanded TILs represent a selected, IL-2–responsive population, it seemed preferable to look for the TCR Vβ restriction in freshly isolated TILs. Recent improvements in methods for RNA extraction from very small (e.g., 1×10^6) numbers of cells[137] made it possible to probe for the TCR Vβ chain restriction in fresh tumor tissues. Although MAbs to Vβ-chain antigens on human lymphocytes could be used for assessing TIL clonality by, for example, immunohistology, only five such specificities are currently available, not enough to probe for the over 50 specificities detectable with labeled oligonucleotide probes by PCR.[138,139] This approach has been used recently in our laboratory to probe TILs freshly isolated from human primary liver tumors. In several hepatocellular carcinomas studied, restriction in the expression of Vβ genes in TILs was observed.[140] These preliminary results indicated that TILs obtained from different hepatocellular carcinomas might use preferentially only a limited number of the TCR Vβ genes and, thus, probably recognize the same or a related antigen expressed on the tumor in different patients. These observations are of more than just basic significance; they give support to the idea that human TILs might be restricted in their specificity and that this restriction extends to tumors other than melanoma. Because future therapy with TILs may depend on the use of autotumor-specific effector cells, the demonstration that such effectors exists in a variety of human tumors is essential from the therapeutic point of view.

Functional characterization of human TILs has been limited by their small numbers. Using microassays, it has been ascertained several years ago that both proliferative and cytotoxic responses of freshly isolated TILs are impaired (reviewed in refs. 113,141). Not only antitumor cytotoxicity against NK-sensitive or NK-resistant tumor cell targets,[142,143] but also profoundly reduced proliferative responses to mitogens, alloantigens, and low doses of IL-2, of TILs, and, especially, of CD8$^+$ TILs have been well documented in the literature.[144,145] Functional characteristics of freshly isolated TILs at a clonal level have been examined using a limited dilution assay in several types of human solid tumors.[109,146,147] Clonal analysis of TILs is thought to be important for the demonstration of CTLs, because tumor-specific responses mediated by CTLs may be difficult to differentiate from LAK activity in IL-2–driven bulk cultures of TILs.[148,149] The clonogenic potential of T-lymphocyte TILs (TIL-Ts) was significantly reduced in limiting dilution assays (LDAs), which permit calculations of the frequency of proliferating and cytolytic T-lymphocyte precursors among TILs. In LDAs performed with TILs from different types of solid tumors, only about 1 in 20 T cells was able to proliferate under culture conditions allowing every normal T-lymphocyte PBL to grow.[150] Another function of lymphocytes, that of locomotion, has been described recently to be deficient in TILs obtained from human melanomas and renal cell carcinomas and tested for ability to migrate through collagen gel.[151] The functional deficiencies of TILs were not an all-or-none phenomenon. On the contrary, some preparations of fresh TILs retained considerable functional activities and, especially, those isolated from primary tumors often were more active than those from metastatic tumors.[112,152]

These observations regarding functional deficiencies of TILs did not appear to be in agreement with the presence of activated or ''committed'' memory T cells in TILs, as described earlier in this chapter. In order to find a reasonable explanation for this behavior of TILs, several alternative hypotheses have been advanced; (1) TIL-Ts are intrinsically incapable of normal responses; (2) activated suppressor T lymphocytes are present among TILs, and (3) the microenvironment in human tumors does not foster TIL functions but rather contributes to functional paralysis of TILs.

Currently available evidence supports the hypothesis that human TILs, and especially CD8$^+$ TILs, have an intrinsic and selective defect in the antigen-dependent activation pathway that leads to proliferation.[144,150] Other functional activities of TILs (e.g., cytokine production or cytotoxicity) may be normal or only partially affected. It appears quite likely that tumor-derived immunoinhibitory factors, which may be different in various human tumors, are responsible for this intrinsic defect of CD8$^+$ TILs.[110,119,153–155] The phenotypic expression of activation and memory markers (CD25, HLA-DR, or CD29/CD45RO) on TILs indicates that functional, or more specifically proliferative, paralysis of TILs, might take place after they reach the activated state at the tumor site.

TILs cultured in the presence of IL-2 acquire the ability to proliferate and to kill tumor cell targets.[156,157] Thus, IL-2 at high concentrations (>100 Cetus U/mL) appears to be the best and fairly ''universal'' agent for activating TILs and overcoming tumor-induced inhibition of proliferation as extensive as that described for TILs from human melanomas.[111,157] For example, TILs obtained from metastatic disease were significantly less responsive to IL-2 in bulk cultures than were those from primary cancers.[111]

The major issue has been the nature of cytotoxic antitumor effector cells generated in these cultures. Two-color cytometry analyses showed that TILs cultured in IL-2 were as heterogeneous as LAK cell cultures established from PBLs, comprising CD3+CD56−, CD3+CD56+, and CD3−CD56+ cell subsets in various proportions.[148,149,158] The ratios of CD4+/CD8+ T cells were equally variable in these cultures, with the only exception of TILs from melanomas, which often, but certainly not always, outgrew more homogeneous populations of CD3+/CD8+ effectors with autotumor cytotoxicity.[156,159,160] In a great majority of TIL preparations grown in the presence of IL-2 by our group and others, effector cells generated in bulk cultures were identical to autologous LAK cells in the peripheral blood.[121,158,161,162] The anticipated enrichment in autotumor-specific CD3+CD8+ effector cells was difficult to achieve in TIL cultures, even after an initial enrichment in CD8+ T cells by, for example, negative selection on MAb-coated flasks and expansion in IL-2.[163]

To improve the feasibility of outgrowing CD3+CD8+ class 1 MHC-restricted effector cells rather than CD3−CD56+ NK cells or CD3+CD56+ non–MHC-restricted T cells from TIL preparations, mixtures of IL-2 with other cytokines have been employed.[164–166] The rationale for this approach came from studies with murine TILs, which showed that additions at optimal concentrations of IFN-γ, TNF-α or IL-4[167–169] to culture media containing IL-2 enhanced the development of cytotoxic T cells. Synergistic antitumor interactions of IL-2, IFN-α, and TILs have been described in mice and led to a concept of combination immunotherapy for cancer.[170] Based on these studies in animal models, combinations of various cytokines (e.g., IL-2 and TNF-α[166] or IL-2 and IL-4[171]) have been used recently to obtain TIL cultures enriched in autotumor-reactive T lymphocytes in patients with solid tumors. For example, in our laboratory, the combination of IL-2 (100 U/mL) and TNF-α (1000 U/mL) was quite effective in promoting enrichment of autotumor-reactive CD3+/CD8+ T lymphocytes in long-term cultures of TILs obtained from human ovarian carcinomas[166,172] or primary liver tumors.[152] IL-2 alone induced growth of effectors with non–MHC-restricted cytotoxicity.[152] Additions of IFN-γ or IL-4 to these TIL cultures did not result in improved selected growth of autotumor-reactive CD3+CD8+ T cells. In agreement with the generally poorer growth of TILs from metastatic than primary tumors referred to earlier, TILs from colon adenocarcinomas metastatic to liver showed both limited expansion and less cytotoxicity against autologous tumor cells regardless of which cytokine or cytokine combinations were used in culture.[152] The precise mechanism involved in preferential outgrowth of CD3+CD8+ T lymphocytes from TILs in the presence of IL-2 and TNF-α or other cytokines is not understood. It has been proposed that TNF-α might reverse inhibition of CTLs induced in vivo by tumor-derived transforming growth factor β.[173] An alternative explanation might be that TNF-α increases immunogenicity of a tumor by, for

example, up-regulating the expression of class 1 MHC antigens on its surface.[174] Not all combinations of cytokines are equally effective for TILs from different tumors; for example, in melanoma, IL-2 and IL-4 were reported to augment the growth and cytotoxicity of TILs specific for autologous tumor[171] but the same combinations of cytokines did not have augmenting effects in cultures of TILs from primary liver tumors.[152] Nevertheless, certain cytokine combinations promote outgrowth of populations of T lymphocytes with restricted specificity from TILs obtained from a variety of human solid tumors, and this seems to indicate that autotumor-specific CD8+ T lymphocytes are a component of these TILs in situ.

Perhaps the most critical single parameter that determines the presence of CTLs in the tumor is its immunogenicity, or ability to evoke and sustain the host immune response specifically directed at the tumor. That is, human tumors that express immunogenic TAAs in the context of class I MHC antigens and present these antigens effectively to the immune system are expected to be well infiltrated with CTLs. Such appears to be the case in human melanomas, where both the existence of CTLs in the circulation[175,176] and in cultured TILs[159,160] and the existence of melanoma antigens capable of evoking development of CTLs in vitro[177] have been documented clearly. In melanoma, class 1 MHC molecules are well expressed in most of the primary and metastatic lesions.[178,179] Guerry and his collaborators showed that melanoma cells effectively process antigen, present it to T cells, and secrete IL-1,[180] leaving little doubt that melanomas, especially in early disease stages, are immunogenic. Recently, Weber and Rosenberg reported that, in a murine system, TILs obtained from the class I MHC–deficient B16-BL6 melanoma had no autotumor cytotoxicity in vitro after growth in the presence of IL-2, whereas those from B16-BL6 tumors transfected with the class 1 gene specifically lysed the autologous tumor and caused its regression in vitro.[181]

These studies convincingly show that immunogenicity, association with class 1 MHC antigens on the tumor surface, and processing of TAAs are prerequisite for development of CTLs in patients with solid tumors. However, even in patients with melanoma, antimelanoma-specific reactions develop in vitro in only 30 to 50 per cent of cases when using lymph node lymphocytes, PBLs, or TILs, as sources of effector cells.[182] In other solid tumors, generation of autotumor-specific responses seems to occur even less frequently,[183] and it has been confirmed that human TILs are a better source of CTLs than are circulating T lymphocytes.

THERAPEUTIC STRATEGIES RELATED TO CELLULAR IMMUNITY

The building evidence for the immune system's participation in resistance against the progression and spread of cancer has raised expectations that manipulation of the immune system also might serve as a valuable approach to therapy. A variety of strategies have been explored, with the common objective of augmenting the activity of the host's T cells, NK cells, and/or macrophages. The use of tumor vaccines to actively and specifically induce endogenous T-cell–mediated immunity against tumors recently has been attracting much attention. Much of the experience with active specific immunotherapy has been reviewed recently.[184] The most recent and innovative studies with tumor vaccines have utilized tumor cells transfected with genes for various cytokines, and the experience to date is summarized in chapter 23. A wide variety of cytokines also have been utilized for therapy of tumor-bearing individuals, with the objective at least in part being to stimulate the cellular immunity of the host. This approach is reviewed in detail in Chapter 20. Yet another strategy for immunotherapy is based on the adoptive transfer of antitumor effector cells into the tumor-bearing host.

During the past several years, several preclinical[101,185–195] and clinical[20,196–198] studies have indicated that adoptive cellular immunotherapy, particularly in combination with IL-2, can have substantial therapeutic efficacy. In the clinical studies, complete or partial regressions of large, advanced metastatic lesions in some patients with malignant melanoma or renal cell carcinoma have been particularly encouraging. However, the results to date have been less than optimal. In many of the preclinical studies, significant decreases in the number of experimental metastases often have not been accompanied by cures or substantial prolongation of survival. Similarly, in the clinical studies, at least 70 to 80 per cent of the treated patients have not shown objective responses from such therapy. There clearly appears to be a pressing need to improve on the promising first-generation results and to devise approaches to increase the rate and duration of therapeutic responses. In addition, the use of very high numbers of adoptively transferred cells together with high doses of IL-2 has resulted in appreciable toxicity, and it would be very desirable to develop effective strategies that would be accompanied by decreased or no toxicity.

Recent studies at our center have been based on the hypothesis that such objectives of improved efficacy and decreased toxicity might be achieved by the use of purified effector cells. Almost all of the previous preclinical and clinical studies have utilized unfractionated populations of IL-2–cultured lymphocytes, among which the effector cells would be expected to represent only a minor subpopulation. Highly purified effector cells might be expected to have a substantially greater therapeutic potency, with fewer cells needed to confer therapeutic effects. In parallel, one might anticipate the requirement for lower amounts of IL-2 to support the viability and activity of the adoptively transferred cells.

Rationale for Therapy of Cancer with Activated NK Cells

The above-cited study of Barlozzari et al.[60] indicated that transfer of purified LGLs could restore NK activity in rats that had had their effector activity selectively depleted by anti–asialo-GM$_1$. As an extrapolation from such results, coupled with the above evidence for the important role of NK cells in resistance to tumor growth, one would predict that adoptive transfer of large numbers of highly activated NK cells would be useful for the therapy of tumors.

THERAPY IN EXPERIMENTAL TUMORS WITH IL-2–ACTIVATED EFFECTOR CELLS

The initial studies with normal lymphocytes cultured in the presence of IL-2 indicated that such cells could have significant antitumor effects.[199] Normal murine lymphocytes cultured for 3 days in the presence of a high concentration of human recombinant IL-2 were shown to have significant therapeutic activity against metastases from various syngeneic sarcomas when injected intravenously at 3 and 6 days after tumor challenge, along with repeated high doses of human recombinant IL-2 (25,000 units intraperitoneally three times a day from days 3 through 8). This treatment with high doses (10^8 cells) of LAK cells significantly reduced the number of metastases detectable in the lungs and liver but did not result in complete elimination of metastases or cures of the mice. Mule et al.[189,190] then began a series of focused efforts to optimize the parameters for effective therapy of syngeneic murine sarcomas by this approach. They examined several of the parameters of the treatment protocol to gain some insight into the requirements for effective therapy.

Two injections of LAK cells, 3×10^7 or 10^8, were found to be more effective than one dose of cells. The cells cultured for 3 days in the presence of IL-2 were shown to have optimal therapeutic effects, and it is of interest that this length of culture also resulted in peak levels of cytotoxic reactivity. Therapeutic effects were seen in recipients pretreated with 400 rad of radiation, suggesting that the therapeutic effects were not due to a major host component. In contrast, irradiation of the LAK cells with 3000 rad resulted in a loss of efficacy, suggesting that the transferred cells had to not only remain viable but also be able to proliferate. However, because the transfer of allogeneic LAK cells appeared to be as effective as that of syngeneic cells, long-term survival and proliferation in the recipients probably was not required. The administration of recombinant IL-2 along with LAK cells appeared to be required, with the presumption that the lymphokine treatment was needed for in vivo stimulation of proliferation of the donor cells. The use of 6000 units of recombinant IL-2 per dose, without administration of LAK cells, had no detectable effect on tumor metastases when the treatment was initiated on day 3 after tumor challenge. However, 20,000 units of IL-2 per dose was effective by itself in significantly reducing established pulmonary metastases when treatment was initiated on day 10 after tumor challenge. On both days 3 and 10, a total of 1 million units per dose of IL-2 was appreciably more effective.

To understand the possible basis for the therapeutic effects of high doses of IL-2 by itself and also to assess the hypothesis regarding the need for administration of IL-2 to support in vivo proliferation of transferred LAK cells, studies have been performed on the ability of various doses of recombinant IL-2 to sustain the proliferation of lymphocytes in vivo. As a parallel to the dose of IL-2 shown to be required for significant therapeutic effects of LAK cells, 6000 units of IL-2 administered intraperitoneally three times per day was found to increase significantly the uptake of radiolabeled iododeoxyuridine as a measure of proliferating lymphocytes in a variety of organs, including the lungs, liver, kidneys, and mesenteric lymph nodes.[200] Substantially higher levels of proliferation in these organs were observed after administration of 1 million units of IL-2 per dose. Although the cellular composition of the proliferating lymphocytes was not studied in detail, it is of note that augmented levels of cytotoxic reactivity against NK-resistant target cells were observed after the in vivo treatment with IL-2. As a further study along these lines, uptake of radiolabeled iododeoxyuridine was examined in mice treated with 6000 units of IL-2 per dose, alone or in combination with transferred LAK cells.[201] The combination of both treatments gave higher levels of proliferation in the lungs and liver, but, in other organs such as spleen, kidneys, and lymph nodes, the maximal uptake of radiolabeled material was observed with IL-2 alone. As another correlation with the therapy studies, expansion of lymphocytes also was seen in recipients pretreated with 500 rad of radiation.

In the above series of studies, although adoptive immunotherapy could induce an impressive reduction in established metastases of murine sarcomas, the therapeutic effects were usually transient, and few, if any, complete cures were achieved. To explore further this approach to therapy and to explore the treatment conditions that might be required for curative results, a model of transplantable murine adenocarcinoma of the kidney (Renca) was developed.[192] By inoculation of Renca cells under the kidney capsule, a course of tumor progression was initiated that closely mimicked the progression of human renal cell carcinoma, with spontaneous metastases to regional lymph nodes in the peritoneal cavity, liver, and lungs. This model has become of particular interest because of the recent clinical studies[202] indicating that adoptive immunotherapy with LAK cells plus recombinant IL-2 may be particularly effective for metastatic renal cell carcinoma. In the initial therapy experiments, treatment was initiated at 7 days after tumor challenge, when only occult metastases were present. Administration of cytotoxic lymphocytes, after 24 hours of incubation with human recombinant IL-2 (rIL-2), plus IL-2, resulted in a significant increase in survival but only a low percentage of cures. Similarly, treatment at this time with chemotherapy, either doxorubicin or Cy, gave a low percentage of cures. In contrast, combination chemoimmunotherapy with doxorubicin and IL-2–stimulated cytotoxic lymphocytes plus IL-2 resulted in a cure of two thirds of the tumor-bearing mice. These results are quite interesting from several standpoints. First, they demonstrate that treatment with a combination of modalities may be considerably more effective than immunotherapy alone, with cytoreduction or other effects of chemotherapy leading to synergistic interactions with adoptive immunotherapy. Second, the protocol for immunotherapy that was required for these impressive results was considerably less intensive than those utilized by Mule and his colleagues.[192] The lymphocytes utilized for transfer were cultured with only 200 units of IL-2 for a shorter period (only 24 hours), because these conditions were sufficient to induce strong cytotoxicity in vitro against Renca cells. The immunotherapy itself consisted of three daily IV inoculations of 3.5×10^7 cultured lymphocytes plus three daily IV inoculations of 10,000 units of IL-2. These doses were lower than those utilized in the above-described experiments, indicating that, under some circumstances, effective therapy can be achieved with relatively modest doses of IL-2 and cytotoxic lymphocytes.

Similar results were achieved when a combination of doxorubicin and IL-2–stimulated lymphocytes plus IL-2 was used for treatment of intraperitoneal Renca cell tumor.[193] Administration of chemotherapy into the peritoneal cavity resulted in cures of 90 per cent of the tumor-bearing mice. Based on such encouraging results, attempts were made to treat this transplantable tumor at a more advanced stage of disease, beginning at 3 weeks after tumor inoculation under the kidney capsule, when visible peritoneal and systemic metastases already were present. It was possible to achieve cures in up to 80 per cent of tumor-bearing mice by chemoimmunotherapy, but only when the treatment was administered by both the intraperitoneal and intravenous routes.[191] In addition, removal of the tumor-bearing kidney was required for effective therapy. Such impressive results with advanced disease are quite encouraging and suggest that maximal reduction of tumor burden by surgery and chemotherapy, as well as administration of immunotherapy into the regions of metastases, may be required for complete elimination of advanced metastatic tumors.

CLINICAL ADOPTIVE IMMUNOTHERAPY BY IL-2–STIMULATED LYMPHOCYTES

Based on the results of these adoptive immunotherapy studies in mice with LAK cells plus IL-2, Rosenberg[202] performed an analogous clinical trial on patients with advanced, metastatic solid tumors. Large numbers of peripheral blood mononuclear cells were isolated from the patients by leukapheresis and cultured for 3 to 4 days in the presence of 1000 U/mL of IL-2. The resultant LAK cells then were infused into the autologous patient, with greater than 10^{10} cells being administered. In addition, each patient received high doses of IV IL-2, between 10,000 and 100,000 U/kg of body weight every 8 hours, before and continuing for about 1 week beyond the course of LAK cell infusions. With the first 25 treated patients, 10 had partial progressions of detectable tumor and 1 had a prolonged complete regression.[202] Most of the responses occurred in patients with renal cell carcinoma, melanoma, and colon carcinoma.

Extensions of this trial have been performed at the National Cancer Institute and several other institutions.[20,198] Although some clinical results have been very encouraging, with marked or even complete regression of metastatic lesions in some patients with advanced solid tumors that are refractory to conventional chemotherapy, there have been several major limitations. First, the tumor responses occurred in only a minority of the patients, and those have in most cases been rather transient, with subsequent progression of disease. In addition, the currently utilized protocol has been associated with severe toxic side effects in most patients. These toxic reactions appear to be attributable to the very high doses of IL-2 that have been utilized. The most striking side effect has been a capillary leak syndrome, with hypotension and accumulation of large volumes of fluid, that results in greater than 10 per cent increases in weight in the majority of patients. In addition, severe respiratory distress and cardiac problems have been observed in a few patients, and such life-threatening toxic side effects have required very close monitoring of the patients in intensive care units.

Therapy with Purified IL-2–Activated NK Cells

The extensive preclinical data and also clinical observations indicate that adoptive immunotherapy with IL-2–stimulated lymphocytes plus IL-2 can induce substantial antitumor effects, even when treatment is initiated after metastases are established. However, there are several major problems with the current generation of therapeutic protocols. Most of the therapeutic effects have been partial and transient, the processing of the cells for therapy is very expensive and labor intensive, and the high doses utilized for treatment have been associated with serious toxic side effects. Thus, many parameters involved in this therapeutic approach should be investigated to develop more effective and simpler therapeutic strategies.

It seems important to consider seriously whether the rather cumbersome process of harvesting large numbers of lymphocytes, culturing them in the presence of IL-2, and then reinfusing them is indeed necessary or whether it might be possible to reproduce the same effects in vivo by administration of IL-2 alone. Administration of high doses of IL-2 has been shown to induce substantial proliferation of lymphocytes in vivo.[200,203,204] As discussed previously, high doses of IL-2 alone have been therapeutically effective in some situations in the mouse therapy experiments, and some clinical responses have been observed in trials with IL-2 alone.[20,198] It is of interest that the clinical responses to IL-2 alone tended to occur in the same tumor types as those found to be responsive to therapy with LAK cells plus IL-2. It would seem that, if the optimal dose, schedule, and route of administration of IL-2 could be found for expansion of the relevant lymphocytes in vivo, it might be possible to obviate the need for the more cumbersome in vitro stimulation and expansion of effector cells, and adoptive transfer, to achieve therapeutic results. However, the optimal dose and schedule for IL-2 is not as yet known, especially for clinical studies. Until the full potential of IL-2 alone is known or realized, it seems very desirable to continue the major efforts with adoptive therapy, in which the effector cells can be more directly manipulated. A fundamental limitation to therapy by IL-2 administration in vivo may be the inability to achieve sufficiently selective expansion of the desired effector cells. In contrast, in vitro, one has the ability to separate and highly purify the desired effector cells and to remove undesired suppressive or inhibitory factors that may strongly interfere with the generation of high levels of effector cell activity. It is also unclear whether it will be possible to achieve the desired optimal in vivo expansion of effector cells by the administration of IL-2 alone, without incurring serious toxic side effects. In some circumstances, it appears that this should be possible. For example, Riccardi et al.[205] observed that rather low doses of IL-2 were able to stimulate substantially the generation of NK cells from bone marrow precursors in chimeric mice. Also, Talmadge et al.[206] observed that quite low doses of IL-2 as well as much higher doses of IL-2 could have therapeutic effects in T-cell–competent mice. Administration into the region of tumor growth may be a useful strategy to expand effector cells more selectively in the region of the tumor without inducing severe systemic toxic reactions.

The number of effector cells actually required for therapeutic effects is not clear. The adoptive therapy studies performed to date have utilized unfractionated mononuclear cells. It may be possible to achieve a substantially more favorable situation if effector cells are first isolated and purified. This should decrease substantially the requirement for the total number of cells and also may help to eliminate suppressor cells as well as irrelevant T cells. This also might alter substantially the requirement for IL-2, because the dose needed to stimulate and expand a relatively small number of cells may be considerably less than that required for effects on a much larger number of total responding lymphocytes.

Recently, a new and simple procedure for the purification and rapid expansion of IL-2–activated NK cells from peripheral blood and splenic LGLs has been developed.[207] This procedure exploits the observation made in our laboratory that rat LGL/NK cells initially respond to IL-2 by adhering to plastic surfaces. As soon as 2 hours after the addition of IL-2, a small portion of LGLs adhere to plastic. These adherent cells are 94.97 per cent LGLs and express surface markers characteristic of rat NK cells, including OX8, asialo-GM$_1$, and laminin. The cells did not express pan–T-cell (CD5), helper T-cell (CD4), or B-cell (immunoglobulin) markers, nor did they express the rat T-cell–associated IL-2 receptor OX39. Whereas 2-hr adherent cells show high levels of cytotoxic activity against YAC-1 targets only (NK activity), 48-hr adherent cells already demonstrate the development of high levels of LAK activity. The adherent LGL cells exhibiting LAK activity have been designated adherent NK (A-NK) cells.

When 48-hr A-NK cells were separated from the non-adherent cells, washed, and refed with conditioned medium, they rapidly expanded over the next 3 to 4 days, with expansion indices often reaching 90-fold in this time period. These expanding cells generated very high levels of cytotoxic LAK activity. When compared to the levels of cytotoxic LAK activity generated in standard bulk cultures, the adherent cultures generated between 20 and 50 times more total lytic units per culture.

Studies of the phenotype of the rat A-NK cells after expansion for 5 days or more in culture indicated that these cells are LGLs and do not express surface markers (CD5) or helper T-cell (CD4) markers or significant levels of rat IL-2 receptor (Tac type), as detected by the OX39 MAb. These activated lymphocytes display cytolytic activity against neoplastic cells from a wide variety of tumors. Cytolytic activity could be demonstrated against tumor lines from different tissues and cell preparations, including ascites tumors, solid tumors, and neoplastic cell lines grown in vitro or in vivo.

In a series of studies, A-NK cells have been utilized for therapy of experimental animal tumors, in both rats[208] and mice (E. Gorelik and H. Gunji, unpublished observations). The initial results of these studies have been highly encouraging, indicating that the purified A-NK cells have substantially stronger antimetastatic effects than unpurified LAK cells obtained by culturing mononuclear cells in the presence of IL-2. Utilizing the MCA-105 sarcoma in BALB/c mice, the same metastatic tumor model used by Rosenberg and his colleagues for most of their experimental therapy studies, A-NK cells gave strong antimetastatic effect at cell numbers considerably less than those needed to produce significant effects with standard LAK cells. With the B16-BL6 melanoma, a mouse tumor that is quite resistant to therapeutic effects of standard LAK cells, relatively low numbers of purified A-NK cells produced considerable reduction in lung metastases when administered with a modest dose of IL-2. Strong therapeutic effects with A-NK cells also have been seen with a rat experimental breast cancer, MADB106.[208] Even when the same total amount of in vivo measured cytotoxic activity (i.e., same total lytic units) was transferred to the recipient tumor-bearing rats, purified effector cells were considerably more active therapeutically, against both pulmonary and hepatic metastases, than standard unpurified LAK cells.

Conditions similar to those that have been effective for isolating rat and mouse A-NK cells have been successful for obtaining purified human A-NK cells with the characteristics of NK cells.[209] Based on the promising preclinical therapy and the ability to isolate A-NK cells from cancer patients as well as normal human donors, a phase I clinical trial with A-NK cells, for patients with malignant melanoma and renal cell carcinoma, has been initiated in my institute (M. Ernstoff and J.M. Kirkwood, principal investigators). The results to date have been encouraging and consistent with those obtained in the experimental animal tumors. Patients on this phase I trial received a single intravenous infusion of A-NK cells along with continuous infusion of a moderate dose of human rIL-2 (10^6 U/m²/day × 5). An additional 5-day course of IL-2 was given on day 28. In patients who showed clinical response, a cycle of A-NK cells and rIL-2 was repeated one to three times. Escalating doses of A-NK cells (the dosage was based on the cytolytic potential of A-NK cells equivalent to that of 10^{10} autologous LAK cells determined in vitro) were administered to three groups of ten patients per group. Before and during therapy, patients were monitored for immunologic parameters, including antitumor cytotoxicity and cytokine levels. Of the first ten patients treated, five received one cycle of therapy, two received two cycles, and three received three cycles. There were three clinical responses, two patients remained in a stable condition, and five progressed. One of the three patients who responded achieved complete remission after excision of a residual subcutaneous mass. This complete remission lasted for 6 to 7 months; the

patient subsequently relapsed with brain metastases. It should be noted that A-NK cells in cultures established from the leukapheresed blood of these patients were variably enriched in CD3⁻CD56⁺ effector cells and that the highest number of A-NK cells given per cycle was 40 × 10^6. Thus, the number of infused effector cells was considerably lower that the total of 10 × 10^{10} LAK cells used by Rosenberg et al.[20] All ten patients treated with A-NK cells and IL-2 were monitored for selected immunologic functions before and serially during therapy. Possible immunologic correlates of clinical response included pretreatment NK activity and ability to generate LAK cells in vitro as well as the increased percentage of CD56⁺ and CD56⁺HLA-DR⁺ cells in the circulation of responders versus patients who did not respond to immunotherapy. This phase I clinical trial is one of the first in which effector cells enriched in NK cells rather than heterogeneous LAK cells were administered to patients with metastatic disease. It is encouraging that clinical responses have been seen with the relatively low doses of cells transferred in comparison with conventional LAK cell trials[198,202] (about 10^9 versus about 10^{11}, respectively).

Adoptive Therapy with TILs

A rationale for cancer immunotherapy with human TILs has been derived largely from experiments performed in animals, in which eradication of established metastases of strongly or weakly immunogenic tumors was obtained by transfer of activated T lymphocytes.[210,211] Studies of Rosenberg and his collaborators showed that TILs derived from murine tumors and grown in rIL-2 were 50 to 100 times more effective than LAK cells in eradicating established lung metastases of sarcoma after pretreatment with Cy.[212] From these and other animal studies,[213] a notion has developed that immunotherapy with T cells specifically primed against autotumor may be more effective than that with non–MHC-restricted effectors such as LAK[20] or A-NK[214] cells. In vitro studies with TILs isolated from melanoma and other human solid tumors, as described earlier in this chapter, have confirmed that T lymphocytes at the tumor site might be a better source of tumor-specific T lymphocytes than PBLs. The excellent results with TILs and IL-2 for treatment of metastatic deposits of immunogenic murine tumors[212] provided the basis for the first clinical trials with human TILs in patients with metastatic melanoma and renal cell carcinoma.[197,215] Several protocols, with human TILs obtained from melanoma or renal cell carcinoma have been completed to date,[214,216–220] mainly at the Surgery Branch of the National Cancer Institute (NCI). The results have indicated clear regression of measurable metastases in some patients, but the frequency of such responses has not been unequivocally higher than that obtained with cytokines alone, LAK cells, or more conventional therapies. Although the response rate, in an initial report from the NCI,[197] was 55 per cent in 20 patients with metastatic melanoma, including several who failed previous LAK therapy, it has been noted that the response rate calculated on the basis of intent to treat (20 additional patients were biopsied for TIL cultures but were not treated because of a rapid disease progression [or inadequate TIL growth]) was only 28 per cent.[216] This figure was not statistically different from results obtained in LAK/IL-2 studies, in which all patients entered could be treated.

There are several concerns that confound objective evaluation of the TIL trials conducted to date:

1. The bulk of patients treated with TILs were at the Surgery Branch, NCI, and received cells prepared by the intramural laboratory. It remains uncertain how well TIL preparation and administration to patients can be duplicated at extramural sites.

2. Nearly all of the patients with TILs had either metastatic melanoma or renal cell carcinoma, and the effectiveness of TIL therapy in a broader array of tumors has not been determined.

3. Criteria for evaluating responses may not have been applied uniformly in different clinical trials.

4. Duration of responses has not been specified clearly, and it may be too early to evaluate survival in these relatively recent trials.

5. It remains unclear whether patients who responded to TIL therapy were treated with TIL populations enriched in autotumor-reactive CD8$^+$ T cells or effectors with broad non–MHC-restricted cytotoxicity.

6. Responses to therapy have not been correlated to changes in the immune function of patients treated with TIL infusions.

These concerns arise because there is a paucity of information about adoptive immunotherapy with TILs for patients with cancer. Only a handful of NCI intramural or extramural clinical trials have been completed to date. Other groups (e.g., Parmiani and colleagues in Italy and Murthy et al. in the United States) reportedly have treated considerable numbers of patients with melanoma or renal cell carcinoma, respectively, but the results of these trials have not yet been published. There is therefore a great need for information about the therapeutic efficacy of human TILs and about mechanisms that might mediate or influence clinical responses. The most recent report from the NCI[220] describes 67 melanoma patients (55 were treated and evaluable) enrolled into TIL/IL-2 immunotherapy trials. The response rate was 40 per cent of the evaluated or 33 per cent of the initially enrolled patients. Based on the limited clinical experience to date, it appears that immunotherapy with TILs and IL-2 can lead to regression of tumor in patients with cancers that are resistant to conventional therapies, and it may be considered a promising novel approach to therapy of human solid tumors.

The issue of TIL preparation and cost associated with it has been one aspect of this form of therapy that deserves further attention and where improvements are needed. As used by Rosenberg et al., this therapy calls for administration of 10^{10} to 10^{11} TILs and, therefore, requires in vitro expansion of TILs for 4 to 8 weeks.[221,222] Several independent groups now have acquired experience in culturing TILs on a large scale for therapy.[217,220,223–225] Although the feasibility of a large-scale TIL culture for therapy has been sufficiently established, at least for TILs from melanoma and renal cell carcinoma, optimal conditions for expansion of autotumor-specific T cells remain to be determined. Also, it remains unconfirmed that TILs from other solid tumors can be expanded similarly, and, of course, not all TILs, especially those obtained from metastatic tumors, are able to grow in vitro.[152] The expense, largely related to long-term in vitro culture, currently is estimated to be about \$10,000 to \$15,000 per patient. Attempts are being made to improve and optimize TIL culture by, for example, application of hollow-fiber technology,[223] panning,[163] or additions of growth factors, which might selectively facilitate outgrowth of therapeutically active TIL cell populations. Against these expenditures in cost and effort for the culturing of TILs, it is necessary to balance significant gains already achieved in: (1) the clinical arena (e.g., evaluation of side effects, which seem to be mostly attributable to concurrently administered cytokines, or confirmation of feasibility, safety, and efficacy of TIL immunotherapy, which did result in complete responses in a small number of patients with metastatic disease who did not respond to conventional therapy); (2) basic scientific investigations of biologic properties of human TILs, their antitumor properties, their movement through vasculature into tumors, or the mechanisms involved in elimination by TILs of tumor metastases; and (3) increased awareness of clinicians and the scientific community of a possible new approach to cancer therapy with the potential for developing into a major modality in the future.

Two other major issues concerning therapy with TILs must be considered. The first relates to the criteria that must be developed and applied for the optimal use of TIL therapy. Although it might be premature to set firm guidelines, recent developments suggest that clinical response might correlate ($p<.005$) with the ability of cultured TILs to lyse autologous tumor in vitro.[220] If this observation could be extended to TILs from tumors other than melanoma and confirmed, it would provide a strong argument for therapy with TIL-Ts cultured under conditions selecting for growth of autotumor-specific effectors. In respect to potential positive correlation between autotumor cell–killing activity of effectors and prognosis in patients with cancer in general, a recent report by Uchida et al.[226] deserves attention. Fifty patients with primary localized lung cancer were tested at the time of surgery for ability of their PBLs to kill autotumor cells.[226] Most patients (85 per cent) whose PBLs were effective in vitro against autotumor remained alive and were tumor free 5 years after curative surgery, whereas all patients whose PBLs showed no autotumor-killing activity relapsed within 18 months of surgery and died within 42 months. These data indicated that autotumor-killing ability of PBLs was an important predictive factor for survival. This type of analysis has not been applied to TILs, but should autotumor killing by fresh or cultured TILs prove to be an equally significant prognostic parameter for survival, then both a rationale for therapy with TIL-Ts and a choice of cancer patients most likely to benefit from such therapy might be strengthened.

Studies to Explore Mechanisms and Optimize Antitumor Therapeutic Effects of Adoptively Transferred Effector Cells

In addition to the expected value of purified cells for use in therapy, the availability of more defined cell populations permits more detailed examination of the mechanism by which such cells might mediate their therapeutic effects. The first issue to be considered is the in vivo distribution of the adoptively transferred cells. One would predict that therapeutic effects would be dependent on these cells reaching the tumor site or at least accumulating in the vicinity of the tumor. Although in vivo distribution of LAK cells, prepared in the usual manner, has been examined previously, interpretation of the results with such unpurified, heterogeneous cell populations is fraught with difficulty. The concern is that the in vivo distribution information would reflect mainly the distribution of the predominant cell type in the population rather than that of the effector cells. Furthermore, if uptake of some transferred cells were demonstrated in the tumor lesions, it would be unclear which cells were represented and whether they included cells with antitumor effector function. Based on such considerations, my laboratory has been utilizing A-NK cells to study the in vivo distribution of these defined cells with therapeutic potential.

Our initial studies were performed with a radiolabel as a marker for the distribution of the cells in vivo. Studies performed with ^{51}Cr-labeled rat A-NK cells revealed initial uptake of most of the label in the lungs after intravenous inoculation, followed by redistribution mainly to the liver and the spleen by 24 hours.[227] In contrast to T cells, A-NK cells showed no ability to accumulate in lymph nodes.[228] More recent studies have indicated that ^{51}Cr as a cellular label may provide an overestimate of uptake of cells in the liver, presumably by accumulation of released free metal, and that ^{125}I-labeled deoxyuridine is a more reliable indicator of in vivo distribution.[229] However, with either label, there has been little indication of a significant uptake of labeled cells in primary or metastatic tumors, above that measured in normal tissues or in the same organ uninvolved by tumor. We considered the possibility that failure to detect significant accumulation of effector cells in tumors, especially in tumor models showing therapeutic effects by the transferred cells, might be due to insufficient sensitivity of the radioisotopic technique. If there were accumulation of only small numbers of effector cells at the tumor site, the levels of associated radioactivity might not be detectable above background levels.

To explore this issue, we have utilized fluorescent dyes to label mouse A-NK cells and have studied their distribution in mice with experimental metastases induced by the B16-F1 melanoma. Intravenous inoculation of tumor cells induces experimental pulmonary metastases, and liver metastases can be induced by left ventricular inoculation of a liver-homing variant of B16-F1 cells. After intravenous inoculation of fluorescent A-NK cells, at 1 hour the uptake of cells in normal lungs was similar to that detectable in tumor-bearing mice.[230] At this time point, there was no indication of selective uptake by tumor metastases; however, by 16 to 18 hours, there appeared to be a redistribution of cells within the lungs of tumor-bearing mice, with an average 20-fold greater localization in pulmonary metastases relative to normal lung tissue. However, very few cells per metastases were observed, with some metastases showing no detectable uptake of fluorescent cells in other major organs, including the liver. After intraportal inoculation, there was much higher uptake in the liver, and a substantial proportion of metastases contained fluorescent A-NK cells.[231]

The failure of transferred cells to accumulate appreciably in the metastases may account for the only partial therapeutic efficacy that has been observed for adoptive immunotherapy with A-NK cells in this B16 tumor model. However, a further major question raised by these results is how might the small number of effector cells that accumulate in at least some of the tumor lesions result in complete regression of some metastases. Although one might have expected that in vivo therapeutic results might be due to direct cytotoxicity, as measured with the effector cells in vitro, this seems quite unlikely because the apparent effector cell–target cell ratios in the experimental metastases were very low, usually less than 1:1. An alternative explanation for therapeutic efficacy might be local cytokine production by the A-NK cells. A-NK cells have been shown to produce substantial levels of TNF-α and IFN-γ. Perhaps small numbers of cells at the tumor site could secrete sufficient amounts of these and possibly other factors to amplify their effects and to enlist the involvement of other effector cells. Consistent with this possibility has been the observation that A-NK cells (mouse and rat) produce a variety of proteolytic enzymes, similar to those associated with the invasive properties of basement membranes.[232]

One major unanswered question, which is quite relevant to the above considerations, is whether the adoptively transferred cells are able to emigrate out of the microvasculature into tumor tissues and then directly interact with tumor cells. To examine this issue, we recently have utilized a novel animal model that permits visualization of the microvasculature of normal and tumor-bearing tissues.[233] These studies have involved vital videomicroscopy of the microvasculature of chambers in the ears of rabbits, containing granulation tissue or the VX2 carcinoma, a transplantable rabbit tumor that induces extensive neovascularization. Human A-NK cells have been inoculated into the artery of the ears of normal or tumor-bearing rabbits. As in the studies of A-NK cell distribution in mice, only a very small proportion of the inoculated cells were retained in the microvasculature of either normal or tumor-bearing ears. However, it was possible to observe selective and longer retention of transferred A-NK cells in the tumor microvasculature, and this retention appeared to be confined to adherence in the postcapillary venules. Over a period of observation of up to 25 hours, there was no indication that these cells retained in the microvasculature emigrated into the tumor tissues. Despite this apparent failure of the transferred cells to interact directly with tumor cells, focal necrosis of tumors has been observed to occur in this model system. Histologic sections of treated tumors taken at about 1 week after inoculation showed not only evidence of necrosis, but also substantial accumulation of a variety of inflammatory cells, including macrophages and eosinophils in addition to lymphocytes.

These recent results indicate involvement of a novel mechanism for the therapeutic effects, which had not been previously considered. From this study as well as from the studies with mouse tumor cells, direct cytotoxic effects seem unlikely to account for the therapeutic efficacy that has been observed. Production of cytokines by a small number of effector cells seems to be a real possibility, but this would appear to occur at some distance from the tumor cells. In addition to the possibility of cytokines directly inhibiting the growth of tumor cells, the hemostasis and focal necrosis seen in the rabbit ear model strongly suggest that the antitumor effects may be indirect, via changes in the microvasculature. It is intriguing to consider the possibility that one or a few A-NK cells might have major effects after attaching to the tumor microvasculature, perhaps by secreting cytokines such as TNF that might induce attachment of granulocytes to endothelial cells and also induce coagulation; or the attached effector cells might damage or activate the endothelial cells, with this in turn leading to the observed changes. Further studies are needed to distinguish among these possibilities and also to determine the basis for the selective retention of A-NK cells in the postcapillary venules of the tumor microvasculature. Also, detailed studies with TILs and CTLs that are analogous to the studies with A-NK cells are needed. Insights into these and related issues may help to explain the basis for therapeutic efficacy and allow the rational development of improved strategies for adoptive cellular therapy.

REFERENCES

1. Ochoa AC: Alterations in signal transduction molecules in T lymphocytes from tumor-bearing mice. Science 258:1795, 1992
2. Schantz SV, Goepfert HG: Multimodality therapy in distant metastasis: The impact of natural killer cell activity. Arch Otolaryngol Head Neck Surg 112:545, 1987
3. Hersey P, Hobbs A, Edwards A, et al: Tumor related changes and prognostic significance of natural killer cell activity in melanoma patients. In Herberman RB (ed): NK Cells and Other Natural Effector Cells. New York, Academic Press, 1982, pp 1167–1174
4. Lotzova E, Savary CA, Herberman RB: Induction of NK cell activity against fresh human leukemia in culture with interleukin-2. J Immunol 138:2718, 1987
5. Penn I, Starzl TR: A summary of the status of de novo cancer in transplant recipients. Transplant Proc 4:719, 1993
6. Ho M, Jaffe R, Miller G, et al: The frequency of Epstein-Barr virus infection and associated lymphoproliferative syndrome after transplantation and its manifestations in children. Transplantation 45:719, 1993
7. Hewitt HB: Animal tumor models and their relevance to human tumor immunology. J Lab Clin Med 1:107, 1982
8. Klein G, Klein E: Rejectability of virus induced tumors and non-rejectability of spontaneous tumors—a lesson in contrasts. Transplant Proc 9:1095, 1988
9. Kripke ML: Immunologic mechanisms in UV radiation carcinogenesis. Adv Cancer Res 34:69, 1981
10. Peppoloni S, Herberman RB, Gorelik E: Lewis lung carcinoma (3LL) cells treated in vitro with ultraviolet radiation show reduced metastatic ability due to an augmented immunogenicity. Clin Exp Metastasis 5:43, 1987
11. Ljunggren H-G, Stam NJ, Öhlen C, et al: Empty MHC class I molecules come out in the cold. Nature 346:476, 1990
12. Jerome KR, Varnd DL, Boyer CM, et al: Cytotoxic T-lymphocytes derived from patients with breast adenocarcinoma recognize an epitope present on the protein core of a mucin molecule preferentially expressed by malignant cells. Cancer Res 51:2908, 1991
13. van der Bruggen P, Traversari C, Chomez P, et al: A gene encoding an antigen recognized by cytolytic T lymphocytes on a human melanoma. Science 254:1643, 1991
14. Herberman RB, Nunn ME, Lavrin DH: Natural cytotoxic reactivity of mouse lyphoid cells against syngeneic and allogeneic tumors. I. Distribution of reactivity and specificity. Int J Cancer 16:216, 1975
15. Rosenberg EB, Herberman RB, Levine PH, et al: Lymphocyte cytotoxicity reactions to leukemia-associated antigens in identical twins. Int J Cancer 9:648, 1972
16. Koren HS, Herberman RB: Natural killing—present and future (summary of workshop on natural killer cells). J Natl Cancer Inst 70:785, 1983
17. Timonen T, Ortaldo JR, Herberman RB: Characteristics of human large granular lymphocytes and relationship to natural killer and K cells. J Exp Med 153:569, 1981
18. Savary CA, Lotzova E: Phylogeny and ontogeny of NK cells. In Herberman RB, Lotzova E (eds): Immunobiology of Natural Killer Cells. Boca Raton, FL, CRC Press, 1986, pp 45–61
19. Kay HD, Bonnard GD, Herberman RB: Evaluation of the role of IgG antibodies in human natural cell-mediated cytotoxicity against the myeloid cell line K562. J Immunol 122:675, 1979
20. Rosenberg SA, Lotze MT, Muul LM, et al: Progress report on the treatment of 157 patients with advanced cancer using lymphokine-activated killer cells and interleukin-2 or high-dose interleukin-2 alone. N Engl J Med 316:889, 1987
21. Herberman RB: Natural Cell-Mediated Immunity against Tumors. New York, Academic Press, 1980
22. Herberman RB (ed): NK Cells and Other Natural Effector Cells. New York, Academic Press, 1982
23. Timonen T, Ortaldo JR, Herberman RB: Analysis by a single cell cytotoxicity assay of NK cell frequencies among human large granular lymphocytes and of the effects of interferon on their activity. J Immunol 128:2514, 1982
24. Phillips JH, Lanier LL: Dissection of the lymphokine-activated killer phenomenon: Relative contribution of peripheral blood natural killer cells and T lymphocytes to cytolysis. J Exp Med 164:814, 1986
25. Ortaldo JR, Sharrow SO, Timonen T, et al: Determination of surface antigens on highly purified human NK cells by flow cytometry with monoclonal antibodies. J Immunol 127:2401, 1981
26. Mattes MJ, Sharrow SO, Herberman RB, et al: Identification and separation of thy-1 positive mouse spleen cells active in natural cytotoxicity and antibody-dependent cell mediated cytotoxicity. J Immunol 123:2851, 1979
27. Reynolds CW, Sharrow SO, Ortaldo JR, et al: Natural killer (NK) activity in the rat. II. Analysis of surface antigens on LGL by flow cytometry. J Immunol 127:2204, 1981
28. Maghazachi AA, Vujanovic NL, Herberman RB, et al: Lymphokine-activated killer cells in rats. IV. Developmental relationships among large agranular lymphocytes and lymphokine-activated killer cell. J Immunol 140:2846, 1988
29. Perussia B, Acuto O, Terhorst C, et al: Human natural killer cells analyzed by B73l.1.1, a monoclonal antibody blocking Fc receptor functions. J Immunol 130:2142, 1983
30. Hercend T, Griffin JD, Bensussan A, et al: Generation of monoclonal antibodies to a human natural killer clone characterization of 2 natural killer-associated antigens NKH1A and NKH2 expressed on subsets of large granular lymphocytes. J Clin Invest 75:932, 1985
31. Chambers WH, Vujanovic NL, DeLeo AB, et al: Monoclonal antibody to a triggering structure expressed on rat natural killer cells in adherent-lymphokine activated killer cells. J Exp Med 169:1373, 1989

32. Giorda R, Rudert WA, Vavassori C, et al: NKR-P1, a novel signal transduction molecule on natural killer cells. Science 249:1298, 1990

33. Herberman RB, Mason L, Ortaldo JR: Studies on the possible relationship of NC cells to mouse NK cells. In Hoshino T, Koren HS, Uchida A (eds): Natural Killer Activity and Its Regulation. Tokyo, Excerpta Medica, 1984, pp 16–21

34. Chang ZL, Hoffman T, Bonvini E, et al: Spontaneous cytotoxicity by monocyte-enriched subpopulations of human peripheral blood mononuclear cells against human or mouse anchorage-dependent tumor cells lines: Contribution of NK-like cells. Scand J Immunol 18:439, 1983

35. Morgan AC, Schroff RW, Klein RA, et al: Occult (non-surface expression) of T, B and monocyte markers in human large granular lymphocytes. Mol Immunol 24:117, 1987

36. Herberman RB, Ortaldo JR, Djeu JY, et al: Role of interferon in regulation of cytotoxicity by natural killer cells and macrophages. Ann N Y Acad Sci 350:63, 1980

37. Reynolds CW, Timonen TT, Holden HT, et al: Natural killer (NK) cell activity in the rat: Analysis of effector cell morphology and effects of interferon on NK cell function in the athymic (nude) rat. Eur J Immunol 12:577, 1982

38. Oehler JR, Lindsay LR, Nunn ME, et al: Natural cell-mediated cytotoxicity in rats. II. In vivo augmentation of NK-cell activity. Int J Cancer 21:210, 1978

39. Herberman RB, Ortaldo JR, Riccardi C, et al: Interferon and NK cells. In Merigan TC, Friedman RM (eds): Interferons. UCLA Symposium on Molecular and Cellular Biology, 25th ed. New York, Academic Press, 1982, pp 287–293

40. Ortaldo JR, Herberman RB, Harvey C, et al: A species of human-interferon which lacks the ability to boost human natural killer (NK) activity. Proc Natl Acad Sci USA 81:4926, 1984

41. Karre K, Ljunggren H, Piontek G, et al: Activation of cell mediated immunity by absence or deleted expression of normal cellular gene products, i.e., by "no-self" rather than "non-self." Immunobiology 167:43, 1984

42. Timonen T, Ortaldo JR, Stadler BM, et al: Cultures of purified human natural killer cells: Growth in the presence of interleukin 2. Cell Immunol 72:178, 1982

43. Yamada S, Ruscetti FW, Overton WR, et al: Regulation of human large granular lymphocytes and T cell growth and function by recombinant interleukin 2. I. Induction of interleukin 2 receptor and promotion of growth of cells with enhanced cytotoxicity. J Leukocyte Biol 41:505, 1987

44. Bonnard GD, Yasaka K, Jacobson D: Ligand-activated T cell growth factor-induced T-cell proliferation: Absorption of T cell growth factor by activated T cells. J Immunol 123:2704, 1979

45. Talmadge JE, Wiltrout RH, Counts DF, et al: Proliferation of human peripheral blood lymphocytes induced by recombinant human interleukin 2: Contribution of large granular lymphocytes and T lymphocytes. Cell Immunol 102:262, 1986

46. Ortaldo JR, Mason AT, Gerard JP, et al: Effects of natural and recombinant IL-2 on regulation of IFN production and natural killer activity: Lack of involvement of the Tac antigen for these immunoregulatory effects. J Immunol 133:779, 1984

47. Allavena P, Ortaldo JR: Specificity and phentotype of IL2 expanded clones and human large granular lymphocytes. Diagn Immunol 1:162, 1983

48. Kedar BL, Ikerjiri B, Sredni B, et al: Propagation of mouse cytoxic clones with characteristics of natural killer (NK) cells. Cell Immunol 69:305, 1982

49. Ortaldo JR, Bonnard GD, Kind PD, et al: Cytotoxicity by cultured human lymphocytes: Characteristics of effector cells and specificity of cytotoxicity. J Immunol 122:1489, 1979

50. Brooks CG: Reversible induction of natural killer cell activity in clonal murine cytotoxic T lymphocytes. Nature 305:155, 1983

51. Gray JD, Torten M, Golub SH: Generation of natural killer-like cytotoxicity from human thymocytes with interleukin-2. Nat Immun Cell Growth Regul 3:124, 1983

52. Hiserodt JC, Vujanovic NL, Reynolds CW, et al: Studies on lymphokine activated killer cells in rats: Analysis of precursor and effector cell phenotype and relationship to natural killer cells. In Truitt RL, Gale RP, Bortin MM (eds): Cellular Immuno-therapy of Cancer. New York, Alan R. Liss, 1987, pp 137–146

53. Shortman K, Wilson A, Scollay R: Loss of specificity in cytolytic T lymphocyte clones obtained by limited dilution culture of Lyt2⁺ T cells. J Immunol 132:584, 1984

54. Torten M, Sidell N, Golub SH: Interleukin-1 and stimulator lymphoblastoid thymocytes to bind and kill K562 targets. J Exp Med 156:1545, 1982

55. Grimm EA, Mazumder A, Zhang HZ, et al: Lymphokine activated killer cell phenomenon. I. Lysis of natural killer resistant fresh solid tumor cells by interleukin-2-activated autologous human peripheral blood lymphocytes. J Exp Med 155:823, 1982

56. Grimm EA, Ramsey KM, Mazumder A, et al: Lymphokine activated killer cell phenomenon. II. Precursor phenotype is serologically distinct from peripheral T lymphocytes and natural killer cells. J Exp Med 157:884, 1983

57. Herberman RB: Adoptive therapy of cancer with interleukin 2 (IL2) activated killer cells. Cancer Bull 39:6, 1987

58. McCoy JL, Herberman RB, Rosenberg EB, et al: 51-Chromium release assay for cell-mediated cytotoxicity of human leukemia and lymphoid tissue culture cells. Natl Cancer Inst Monogr 37:59, 1973

59. Rosenberg EB, McCoy JL, Green SS, et al: Destruction of human lymphoid tissue culture cell lines by human peripheral lymphocytes in 51-Cr-release cellular cytotoxicity assay. J Natl Cancer Inst 52:345, 1974

60. Barlozzari T, Leonhardt J, Wiltrout R, et al: Direct evidence for the role of LGL in the inhibition of experimental tumor metastases. J Immunol 134:2783, 1985

61. Barlozzari T, Reynolds CW, Herberman RB: In vivo role of natural killer cells: Involvement of large granular lymphocytes in the clearance of tumor cells in anti-asialo GM₁-treated rats. J Immunol 131:1024, 1983

62. Gorelik E, Wiltrout RH, Okomura K, et al: Role of NK cells in the control of metastatic spread and growth of tumor cells in mice. Int J Cancer 30:107, 1982

63. Uchida A, Micksche M: Lysis of fresh human tumor cells by autologous peripheral blood lymphocytes and pleural effusion lymphocytes activated by OK-432. J Natl Cancer Inst 71:673, 1983

64. Uchida A, Yangawa E: Natural killer cell activity and autologous tumor killing activity in cancer patients: Overlapping involvement of effector cells as determined in two target conjugate cytotoxicity assay. J Natl Cancer Inst 73:1093, 1984

65. Lotzova E, Savary CA, Herberman RB, et al: Induction of NK cell activity against fresh human leukemia in culture with interleukin-2. Nat Immun Cell Growth Regul 5:61, 1986

66. Lotzova E, Savary CA, Herberman RB, et al: Induction of NK cell activity against fresh human leukemia in culture with interleukin-2. J Immunol 138:2718, 1987

67. Gorelik E: Role of NK cells in the control of metastatic spread and growth of tumor cells in mice. Int J Cancer 30:107, 1982

68. Hanna N, Fidler IJ: The role of natural killer cells in the destruction of circular tumor emboli. J Natl Cancer Inst 65:801, 1980

69. Hanna N, Fidler IJ: Expression of metastatic potential of allogeneic and xenogenic neoplasms in young nude mice. Cancer Res 1:438, 1981

70. Riccardi C, Puccetti P, Santoni A, et al: Rapid in vivo assay of mouse NK cell activity. J Natl Cancer Inst 3:1041, 1979

71. Riccardi C, Barlozzari T, Santoni A, et al: Transfer to cyclophosphamide treated mice of natural killer (NK) cells and in vivo natural reactivity against tumors. J Immunol 126:1284, 1981

72. Brown J, Parker E: Host treatments affecting artificial pulmonary metastases: Interpretation of loss of radioactivity labelled cells from lungs. Br J Cancer 40:677, 1979

73. Fidler IJ: Metastasis: Quantitative analysis of distribution and fate of tumor emboli labeled with ¹²⁵1–5-iodo-s deoxyuridine. J Natl Cancer Inst 45:773, 1970

74. Hofer K, Prensky W, Hughes WL: Death and metastatic distribution of tumor cells in mice monitored with 125-iododeoxyuridine. J Natl Cancer Inst 43:763, 1969

75. Hanna N, Burton R: Definitive evidence that natural killer (NK)

cells inhabit experimental tumor metastasis in vivo. Br J Gen Pract 127:1754, 1981

76. Chow D: NK cell and NAB antitumor activity in vivo. In Herberman RB (ed): NK Cells and Other Natural Effector Cells. New York, Academic Press, 1982, pp 114–1047

77. Gale RP, Zighelboim J: Polymorphonuclear leukocytes in antibody-dependent cellular cytotoxicity. J Immunol 114:1047, 1975

78. Korec S: The role of granulocytes in host defense against tumors. In Herberman RB (ed): Natural Cell-Mediated Immunity against Tumors. New York, Academic Press, 1980, pp 1301–1307

79. Sadler T, Cestro J: The effects of Corynebacterium parvum and surgery on the Lewis lung carcinoma and it metastases. Br J Surg 63:292, 1976

80. Hanna N: Role of natural killer cells in control of cancer metastasis. Cancer Metastasis Rev 1:45, 1982

81. Talmadge JE, Meyers KM, Prieur DJ, et al: Role of NK cells in tumour growth and metastasis in beige mice. Nature 284:622, 1980

82. Hanna N, Schneider M: Enhancement of tumor metastasis and suppression of natural killer cell activity by β-estradiol treatment. J Immunol 130:974, 1983

83. Hibbs JB, Chapman HA, Weinberg JB: The macrophage as an antineoplastic surveillance cell: Biological perspectives. Pharm Times 24:549, 1978

84. Adams DO, Snyderman R: Do macrophages destroy nascent tumors? J Natl Cancer Inst 62:1341, 1979

85. Whitworth PW, Pak CC, Esgro J, et al: Macrophages and cancer. Cancer Metastasis Rev 8:319, 1989

86. Evans CH: Macrophages in syngeneic animal tumors. Transplantation 14:468, 1972

87. Gauci CL, Alexander P: The macrophage content of some human tumors. Cancer Lett 1:20, 1975

88. Keller R: Macrophage-mediated natural cytotoxicity against various target cells in vitro. I. comparison of tissue macrophages from diverse anatomic sites and from different strains of rats and mice. Br J Cancer 37:732, 1978

89. Norbury KC, Kripke ML: Ultraviolet-induced carcinogenesis in mice treated with silica, trypan blue or pyran copolymer. Pharm Times 26:827, 1979

90. Herberman RB, Balch C, Bolhius R, et al: Lymphokine activated killer cell activity: Characteristics of effector cells and their progenitors in blood and spleen. Immunol Today 8:178, 1987

91. Sones PDE, Castro JE: Immunological mechanisms in metastatic spread and the antimetastatic effect of C. parvum. Br J Cancer 35:519, 1977

92. Stern K: Control of tumors by the RES. In Herberman RB, Friedman H (eds): The Reticuloepithelial System: A Comprehensive Treastise. New York, Plenum Press, 1983, pp 59–153

93. Mantovani A, Giavazzi R, Polentarutti N, et al: Divergent effects of macrophage toxins on growth of primary tumors and lung metastasis. Int J Cancer 25:617, 1980

94. Zwilling BS, Filippi JA, Chorpenning FW: Chemical carcinogenesis and immunity: Immunologic studies of rats treated with methylnitrosourea. J Natl Cancer Inst 61:731, 1978

95. Gorelik E, Wiltrout RH, Brunda MJ, et al: Augmentation of metastasis formation by thioglycollate-elicited macrophages. Int J Cancer 29:575, 1982

96. Gorelik E, Wiltrout RH, Copeland D, et al: Modulation of formation of tumor metastases by peritoneal macrophages elicited by various agents. Cancer Immunol Immunother 19:35, 1985

97. Kleinerman ES, Raymond AK, Bucana CD, et al: Unique histological changes in lung metastases of osteocarcoma patients following therapy with liposomal muramy tripeptide (CGP 19835A lipid). Cancer Immunol Immunother 34:211, 1992

98. Underwood JC: Lymphoreticular-cell infiltration in human tumors: Prognostic and histological immplications. A review. Br J Cancer 30:538, 1974

99. Ioachim HL: The stroma reaction of tumors: An expression of immune surveillance. J Natl Cancer Inst 57:465, 1976

100. Svennevig JL, Lunde OC, Holter J, et al: Lymphoid infiltration and prognosis in colorectal carcinoma. Br J Cancer 49:375, 1984

101. Watt AG, House AK: Colonic carcinoma: A quantitated assessment of lymphocyte infiltration at the periphery of colonic tumors related to prognosis. Cancer 41:279, 1978

102. Lauder I, Ahern EW: The significance of lymphocytic infiltration in neuroblastoma. Br J Cancer 26:321, 1972

103. Kreider JW, Bartlett GL, Butkiewicz BL: Relationship of tumor leukocyte infiltration to host defense mechanisms and prognosis. Cancer Metastasis Rev 3:53, 1984

104. Haskill S: Some historical perspectives on the relationship between survival and mononuclear cell infiltration. In Haskill S (ed): The Role of Mononuclear Cell Infiltration. New York, Marcel Dekker, 1982, pp 1–10

105. Wolf GT, Hudson JL, Peterson KA, et al: Lymphocyte subpopulations infiltrating squamous carcinomas of the head and neck: Correlations with extent of tumor and prognosis. Otolaryngol Head Neck Surg 95:142, 1986

106. Poppema S, Brocker EB, Deleij L, et al: In situ analysis of the mononuclear cell infiltrate in primary malignant melanoma of the skin. Clin Exp Immunol 51:77, 1983

107. Bhan AK, Des Marais CL: Immunohistology characterization of major histocompatibility antigens and inflammatory cellular infiltrate in human breast cancer. J Natl Cancer Inst 71:507, 1983

108. Brocker EB, Kolde G, Steinhausen D, et al: The pattern of the mononuclear infiltrate as a prognostic parameter in flat superficial spreading melanomas. J Cancer Res Clin Oncol 107:48, 1984

109. Whiteside TL, Miescher S, Hurlimann J, et al: Clonal analysis and in situ characterization of lymphocytes infiltrating human breast carcinomas. Cancer Immunol Immunother 23:169, 1986

110. Wrann M, Bodmer S, deMartin R, et al: T-cell suppressor factor from human glioblastoma cells is a 12.5 Kd protein closely related to transforming growth factor β. EMBO J 6:1633, 1987

111. Takagi S, Chen K, Schwarz R, et al: Functional and phenotypic analysis of tumor infiltrating lymphocytes isolated from human primary and metastatic liver tumors and cultured in recombinant IL2. Cancer 63:102, 1989

112. Whiteside TL: Human tumor-infiltrating lymphocytes and their characterization. In Lotzova E, Herberman RB (eds): Interleukin-2 and Killer Cells in Cancer. Boca Raton, FL, CRC Press, 1990, pp 130–151

113. Vose BM, Moore M: Human tumor-infiltrating lymphocytes: A marker of host response. Semin Hematol 22:27, 1985

114. Whiteside TL, Heo DS, Chen K, et al: Expansion of tumor-infiltrating lymphocytes from human solid tumors in interleukin 2. In Truitt RL, Gale RP, Bortin MM (eds): Cellular Immunotherapy of Cancer. New York, Alan R. Liss, 1987, pp 213–222

115. Snyderman CH, Heo DS, Chen K, et al: T cell tumor-infiltrating lymphoctyes of head and neck cancer. Head Neck 11:331, 1989

116. Vaccarello L, Kanbour A, Kanbour-Shakir A, et al: Tumor-infiltrating lymphocytes from ovarian tumors of low malignant potential. Int J Gynecol Pathol 12:41, 1993

117. Vitolo D, Zerbe T, Kanbour A, et al: Expression of mRNA for cytokines in tumor-infiltrating mononuclear cells in ovarian adenocarcinoma and invasive breast cancer. Proc Am Assoc Cancer Res 32:237, 1991

118. Snyderman R, Cianciolo GJ: Immunosuppressive activity of retroviral envelope protein p15E and its possible relationship to neoplasia. Immunol Today 5:240, 1984

119. Botha JH, Robinson KM, Ramchurren N, et al: Human esophageal carcinoma cell lines: Prostaglandin production, biologic properties, and behavior in nude mice. J Natl Cancer Inst 76:1053, 1986

120. Kornstein MJ, Brooks JS, Elder DE: Immunoperoxidase localization of lymphocyte subsets in the host response to melanoma and nevi. Cancer Res 43:2749, 1983

121. Finke JH, Tubbs R, Connely B, et al: Tumor infiltrating lymphocytes in patients with renal cell carcinoma. Ann N Y Acad Sci 532:387, 1988

122. Bilik R, Mor C, Hazaz B, et al: Characterization of T lymphocyte subpopulations infiltrating primary breast cancer. Cancer Immunol Immunother 28:143, 1989

123. Svenneig J-L, Svaar H: Content and distribution of macrophages and lymphocytes in solid malignant human tumors. Int J Cancer 24:754, 1979

124. Rowe DJ, Beverly PCL: Characterization of breast cancer infiltrates using monoclonal antibodies to human leukocyte antigens. Br J Cancer 49:149, 1984

125. Ruiter DJ, Bhan AK, Harrist TJ, et al: Major histocompatibility antigens and mononuclear inflammatory infiltrate in benign neuromelanocytic proliferations and malignant melanoma. J Immunol 129:2808, 1982

126. Cardi G, Mastrangelo MJ, Berd D: Depletion of T-cells with the CD4+CD45+ phenotype in lymphocytes that infiltrate subcutaneous metastases of human melanoma. Cancer Res 49:6562, 1989

127. Binz H, Fenner M, Frei D, et al: Two independent receptors allow selective target lysis by T cell clones. J Exp Med 157:1252, 1983

128. Lopez-Nevot MA, Garcia E, Pareja E, et al: Differential expression of HLA antigens in primary and metastatic melanomas. J Immunogenet 13:219, 1986

129. Whiteside TL, Heo DS, Takagi S, et al: Tumor-infiltrating lymphocytes from human solid tumors: Antigen-specific killer T lymphocytes or activated natural killer lymphocytes. In Stevenson HC (ed): Adoptive Cellular Immunotherapy of Cancer. New York, Marcel Dekker, 1989, pp 139–157

130. Carrel S, Schmidt-Kessen A, Giuffre L: Recombinant interferon gamma can induce the expression of HLA-DR and DQ on DR-negative melanoma cells and enhance the expression of HLA-ABC and tumor-associated antigens. Eur J Neurol 15:118, 1985

131. Van Duinen SG, Ruiter DJ, Broeker EB, et al: Level of HLA antigens in locoregional metastases and clinical course of the disease in patients with melanoma. Cancer Res 48:1019, 1988

132. Brocker EB, Zwadlo G, Holzmann B, et al: Inflammatory cell infiltrates in human melanoma at different stages of tumor progression. Int J Cancer 41:562, 1988

133. Allen CA, Hogg N: Association of colorectal tumor epithelium expression HLA-D/DR with CD8-positive T cells and mononuclear phagocytes. Cancer Res 47:2919, 1987

134. Hata K, Zhang XR, Iwatsuki S, et al: Isolation phenotypic and functional analysis of lymphocytes from human liver. Clin Immunol Immunopathol 56:401, 1990

135. Vitolo D, Zerbe T, Kanbour A, et al: Expression of mRNA for cytokines in tumor-infiltrating mononuclear cells in ovarian adenocarcinoma and invasive breast cancer. Int J Cancer 51:573, 1992

136. Nitta T, Oksenberg JR, Rao NA, et al: Predominant expression of T cell receptor V α 7 in tumor infiltrating lymphocytes of melanoma. Science 249:672, 1990

137. Chomczynski P, Sacchi N: Single-step method of RNA isolation by acid quanidinium thiocyanate-phenol-chloroform extraction. Anal Biochem 162:156, 1987

138. Choi Y, Kotzin B, Herron L, et al: Interaction of Staphylococus aureus toxin 'superantigens' with human T cell. Proc Natl Acad Sci USA 86:8941, 1989

139. Posnett DN: Allelic variations of human TCR V gene products. Immunol Today 11:368, 1990

140. Weidmann E, Whiteside TL, Giorda R, et al: The T-cell receptor VA gene usage in tumor-infiltrating lymphocytes and blood of patients with hepatocellular carcinoma. J Immunol Meth 52:5913, 1992

141. Whiteside TL: Tumor-infiltrating lymphocytes as antitumor effector cells. Biotherapy 5:47, 1992

142. Moy PM, Holmes EC, Golub SH: Depression of natural killer cytotoxic activity in lymphocytes infiltrating human pulmonary tumors. Cancer Res 45:57, 1985

143. Whiteside TL, Heo DS, Sacchi M, et al: Antitumor functions of tumor-infiltrating lymphocytes (TIL) separated from human head and neck tumors and grown in recombinant interleukin 2. In Cortesina G, Krengli M, Pisiani P, Gambaro G (eds): l'Immunotherapia del Tumori della Testa e Collo. Novara, Italy, 1988, pp 45–55

144. Miescher S, Stoeck M, Whiteside TL, et al: Altered activation pathways in T lymphocytes infiltrating human solid tumors. Transplant Proc 20:344, 1988

145. Miescher S, Stoeck M, Quiao L, et al: Preferential clonogenic deficit of CD8-positive T-lymphocytes infiltrating human solid tumors. Cancer Res 48:6992, 1988

146. Whiteside TL, Miescher S, Hurlimann J, et al: Separation phenotyping and limiting dilution analysis of lymphocytes infiltrating human solid tumors. Int J Cancer 37:806, 1986

147. Miescher S, Whiteside TL, Moretta L, et al: Clonal and frequency analysis of tumor-infiltrating T lymphocytes from solid tumors. J Immunol 138:4004, 1987

148. Whiteside TL, Heo DS, Tagaki S, et al: Cytolytic anti-tumor cells in long-term cultures of human liver infiltrating lymphocytes in recombinant interleukin 2. Cancer Immunol Immunother 26:1, 1988

149. Heo DS, Whiteside TL, Kanbour A, et al: Lymphocytes infiltrating human ovarian tumors I. Role of Leu 19 (NKH1)-positive recombinant IL2 activated cultures of lymphocytes infiltrating human ovarian tumors. J Immunol 140:4042, 1988

150. Miescher S, Stoeck M, Qiao L, et al: Proliferative and cytolytic potentials of purified human tumor-infiltrating T lymphocytes: Impaired response to mitogen-driven stimulation despite T-cell receptor expression. Int J Cancer 42:659, 1988

151. Applegate KG, Valch CM, Pellis N: In vitro migration of lymphocytes through collagen matrices: Arrested locomotion in tumor-infiltrating lymphocytes. Cancer Res 50:7153, 1990

152. Shimizu Y, Iwatsuki S, Herberman RB, et al: Effects of cytokines on in vitro outgrowth of tumor-infiltrating lymphocytes obtained from human primary and metastatic liver tumors. Cancer Immunol Immunother 32:280, 1991

153. Cianciolo GJ, Copeland TD, Oroszlan S, et al: Inhibition of lymphocyte proliferation by synthetic peptide homologous to retroviral envelope protein. Science 230:453, 1985

154. Snyderman CH, Klapan I, Heo DS, et al: In vitro production of prostaglandin E2 by squamous cell carcinoma of the head and neck. Arch Otolaryngol Head Neck Surg, in press, 1994

155. Barrett-Lee P, Travers M, Luginani Y, et al: Transcripts for transforming growth factors in human breast cancer. Br J Cancer 61:612, 1990

156. Itoh K, Tilden AB, Balch CM: Interleukin 2 activation of cytotoxic T lymphocytes infiltrating into human metastatic melanomas. Cancer Res 46:3011, 1986

157. Heo DS, Whiteside TL, Johnson JT, et al: Long-term interleukin 2-dependent growth and cytotoxic activity of tumor-infiltrating lymphocytes from human squamous cell carcinomas of the head and neck. Cancer Res 47:6353, 1987

158. Whiteside TL, Heo DS, Takagi S, et al: Characterization of novel antitumor effector cells in long-term cultures of human tumor-infiltrating lymphocytes. Transplant Proc 20:347, 1988

159. Muul LM, Spiess PJ, Director EP, et al: Identification of specific cytolytic immune responses against autologous tumor in humans bearing malignant melanoma. J Immunol 138:989, 1987

160. Itoh K, Platsoucas CD, Balch CM: Autologous tumor-specific cytotoxic lymphocytes in the infiltrate of human metastatic melanomas: Activation by interleukin 2 and autologous tumor cells and involvement of the T cell receptor. J Exp Med 168:1419, 1988

161. Beldegrun A, Muul LM, Rosenberg SA: Interleukin 2 expanded tumor infiltrating lymphocytes in human renal cell cancer: Isolation, characterization and antitumor activity. Cancer Res 48:206, 1988

162. Kurnick JT, Kradin RL, Blumberg R, et al: Functional characterization of T lymphocytes propagated from human lung carcinomas. Clin Immunol Immunopathol 38:367, 1986

163. Morecki S, Topalian SL, Myers WW, et al: Separation and growth of human CD4+ and CD8+ tumor-infiltrating lymphocytes and peripheral blood mononuclear cells by direct positive panning on covalently attached monoclonal antibody-coated flasks. J Biol Response Med 9:463, 1990

164. Itoh K, Shirba K, Shimizu Y, et al: Generation of activated killer (AK) cells by recombinant interleukin-2 (rIL2) in collaboration with interferon-gamma (IFN-gamma). J Immunol 134:3124, 1985

165. Owen-Schaub LB, Gutterman JU, Grimm EA: Synergy of tumor necrosis factor and interleukin 2 in the activation of human cytotoxic lymphocytes: Effect of tumor necrosis factor and

interleukin 2 in the generation of human lymphokine-activated killer cell cytotoxicity. Cancer Res 48:788, 1988

166. Wang YL, Si L, Kanbour A, et al: Lymphocytes infiltrating human ovarian tumors: Synergy between tumor necrosis factor α and interleukin 2 in the generation of CD8⁺ effectors from tumor-infiltrating lymphocytes. Cancer Res 49:5979, 1989

167. Giovarelli M, Santoni A, Jemma C, et al: Obligatory role of IFN gamma in induction of lymphokine-activated and T lymphocyte killer activity but not in boosting of natural cytotoxicity. J Immunol 141:2831, 1988

168. Rosenberg SA, Schwarz SL, Spiess P: Combination immunotherapy for cancer: Synergistic antitumor interactions of interleukin 2 alpha interferon, and tumor-infiltrating lymphocytes. J Natl Cancer Inst 80:1393, 1988

169. Mule JJ, Krosnick JA, Rosenberg SA: IL-4 regulation of murine lymphokine-activated killer activity in vitro. J Immunol 142:726, 1989

170. Rosenberg SA: Immunotherapy of cancer using interleukin 2: Current status and future prospects. Immunol Today 9:58, 1988

171. Kawakami Y, Rosenberg SA, Lotze MT: Interleukin 4 promotes the growth of tumor-infiltrating lymphocytes cytotoxic for human autologous melanoma. J Exp Med 168:2183, 1988

172. Vaccarello L, Wang YL, Whiteside TL: Sustained outgrowth of autotumor-reactive T lymphocytes from human solid tumors in the presence of tumor necrosis factor α and interleukin 2. Hum Immunol 28:216, 1990

173. Ranges GW, Figari IS, Espevik T, et al: Inhibition of cytotoxic T cell development by transforming growth factor-β and reversal by recombinant tumor necrosis factor α. J Exp Med 166:991, 1987

174. Stotter H, Wiebke EA, Tomita S, et al: Cytokines alter target cell susceptibility to lysis. II. Evaluation of tumor infiltrating lymphocytes. J Immunol 142:1767, 1989

175. de Vries JE, Spits H: Cloned human cytotoxic T lymphocyte (CTL) lines reactive with autologous melanoma cells. I. In vitro generation, isolation and, analysis of phenotype and specificity. J Immunol 132:510, 1984

176. Knuth A, Danowski B, Oettgen HF, et al: T cell mediated cytotoxicity against autologous malignant melanoma: Analysis with interleukin 2 dependent T cell cultures. Proc Natl Acad Sci USA 81:3511, 1984

177. Degiovanni G, Lahaye T, Herin M, et al: Antigenic heterogeneity of human melanoma tumor detected by autologous CTL clones. Eur J Immunol 18:671, 1988

178. Ruiter DJ, Bergman W, Welvaart K, et al: Immunohistological analysis of malignant melanomas and novocellular nevi with monoclonal antibodies to distinct monomorphic determinants of HLA antigens. Cancer Res 44:3930, 1984

179. Guerry D, Alexander MA, Herlyn MF, et al: HLA-DR histocompatibility leukocyte antigens permit human melanoma cells from early but not advanced disease to stimulate autologous lymphocytes. J Clin Invest 73:267, 1984

180. Alexander MA, Bennicelli J, Guerry D: Defective antigen presentation by human melanoma cell lines cultured from advanced, but not biologically early, disease. J Immunol 142:4070, 1989

181. Weber JS, Rosenberg SA: Effects of murine tumor class I major histocompatibility complex expression on antitumor activity of tumor-infiltrating lymphocytes. J Natl Cancer Inst 82:755, 1990

182. Parmiani G, Anichini A, Fossati G: Cellular immune response against autologous human malignant melanoma: Are in vitro studies providing a framework for a more effective immunotherapy. J Natl Cancer Inst 82:361, 1990

183. Anichini A, Fossati G, Parmiani G: Clonal analysis of the cytolytic T cell response to human tumors. Immunol Today 8:385, 1987

184. Livingston P: Active specific immunotherapy in the treatment of patients with cancer. In Weber JS, Rosenberg SA (eds): Human Cancer Immunology II. Immunol Allergy Clin N Am 11:401, 1991

185. Chang AE, Shu S, Chou T, et al: Differences in the effects of host suppression on the adoptive immunotherapy of subcutaneous and visceral tumors. Cancer Res 46:3426, 1986

186. Cheever MA, Greenberg PD, Fefer A: Specific adoptive therapy of established leukemia with syngeneic lymphocytes sequentially immunized in vivo and in vitro and nonspecifically expanded by culture with interleukin 2. J Immunol 126:1318, 1981

187. Cheever MA, Greenberg PD, Fefer A, et al: Augmentation of the anti-tumor therapeutic efficacy of long-term cultured T lymphocytes by in vivo administration of purified interleukin 2. J Exp Med 155:968, 1982

188. Kedar E, Weiss DW: The in vitro generation of effector lymphocytes and their employment in tumor immunotherapy. Adv Cancer Res 38:171, 1983

189. Mule JJ, Shu S, Rosenberg SA: The anti-tumor efficacy of lymphokine-activated killer cells and recombinant interleukin 2 in vivo. J Immunol 135:646, 1985

190. Mule JJ, Shu S, Schwarz SL, et al: Adoptive immunotherapy of established pulmonary metastases with LAK cells and recombinant interleukin-2. Science 225:1487, 1984

191. Salup RR, Back TC, Wiltrout RH: Successful treatment of advanced murine renal cell cancer by bicompartmental adoptive chemoimmunotherapy. J Immunol 138:641, 1987

192. Salup RR, Wiltrout RH: Adjuvant immunotherapy of established murine renal cancer by interleukin-2-stimulated cytotoxic lymphocytes. Cancer Res 46:3358, 1986

193. Salup RR, Wiltrout RH: Treatment of adenocarcinoma in the peritoneum of mice: Chemoimmunotherapy with IL-2-stimulated cytotoxic lymphocytes as a model for treatment of minimal residual disease. Cancer Immunol Immunother 22:31, 1986

194. Shu S, Chou T, Rosenberg SA: In vitro sensitization and expansion with viable tumor cells and interleukin 2 in the generation of specific therapeutic effector cells. J Immunol 136:3891, 1986

195. Shu S, Rosenberg SA: Adoptive immunotherapy of a newly induced sarcoma: Immunologic characteristics of effector cells. J Immunol 135:2895, 1985

196. Rosenberg SA, Lotze MT, Muul LM, et al: Observations on the systemic administration of autologous lymphokine-activated killer cells and recombinant interleukin-2 to patients with metastatic cancer. N Engl J Med 313:1485, 1985

197. Rosenberg SA, Packard BS, Aebersold PM, et al: Use of tumor-infiltrating lymphocytes and interleukin-2 in the immunotherapy of patients with metastatic melanoma. N Engl J Med 319:1676, 1988

198. West WH, Taver KW, Yannelli J, et al: Constant-infusion recombinant interleukin-2 in adoptive immunotherapy of advanced cancer. N Engl J Med 316:898, 1987

199. Kedar E, Ikejiri BL, Gorelik E, et al: Natural cell-mediated cytotoxicity in vitro and inhibition of tumor growth in vivo by murine lymphoid cells cultured with T cell growth factor (TCGF). Cancer Immunol Immunother 13:14, 1982

200. Ettinghausen SE, Lipford EH III, Mule JJ, et al: Systemic administration of recombinant interleukin 2 stimulates in vivo lymphoid cell proliferation in tissues. J Immunol 135:1488, 1985

201. Ettinghausen SE, Lipford EH III, Mule JJ, et al: Recombinant interleukin 2 stimulates in vivo proliferation of adoptively transferred lymphokine-activated killer (LAK) cells. J Immunol 135:3623, 1985

202. Rosenberg SA: Observations on the systemic administration of autologous lymphokine-activated killer cells and recombination interleukin-2 patients with metastatic cancer. N Engl J Med 313:1485, 1985

203. Cheever MA: Interleukin 2 (IL2) administered in vivo: Influence of IL2 route and timing on T cell growth. J Immunol 134:3895, 1985

204. Lotze MT: In vivo administration of purified human interleukin 2. II. Half life, immunologic effects and expansion of peripheral lymphoid cells in vivo with recombinant IL2. J Immunol 135:2865, 1985

205. Riccardi C, Giampietri A, Migliorati G, et al: Generation of mouse natural killer (NK) cell activity: Effect of interleukin-2 (IL2) and interferon (IFN) on the in vivo development of natural killer cells from bone marrow (BM) progenitor cells. Int J Cancer 38:553, 1986

206. Talmadge JE, Phillips J, Schindler J, et al: Systematic preclinical study on the therapeutic properties of recombinant human interleukin 2 for the treatment of metastatic disease. Cancer Res 47:5725, 1987

207. Vujanovic NL, Herberman RB, Maghazachi A, et al: Lymphokine-activated killer cells in rats. III. A simple method for the purification of large granular lymphocytes and their rapid expansion and conversion into lymphokine activated killer cells. J Exp Med 167:15, 1988

208. Schwartz RE, Vujanovic NL, Hiserodt JC: Enhanced antimetastatic activity of lymphokine-activated killer cells purified and expanded by their adherence to plastic. Cancer Res 49:1441, 1989

209. Melder RJ, Rosenfeld CS, Herberman RB, et al: Large scale preparation of adherent lymphokine-activated killer (A-LAK) cells for adoptive immunotherapy in man. Cancer Immunol Immunother 29:67, 1989

210. Lafrenier R, Rosenberg SA: Adoptive immunotherapy of murine hepatic metastases with lymphokine activated killer (LAK) cells and recombinant interleukin 2 (rIL2) can mediate the regression of both immunogenic and non-immunogenic sarcomas and adenocarcinomas. J Immunol 135:4273, 1985

211. Papa MZ, Mule JJ, Rosenberg SA: Antitumor efficacy of lymphokine-activated killer cells and recombinant interleukin 2 in vivo: Successful immunotherapy of established pulmonary metastases from weakly immunogenic and non-immunogenic murine tumors of three distinct histological types. Cancer Res 46:3973, 1986

212. Rosenberg SA, Spiess P, Lafrenier R: A new approach to the adoptive immunotherapy of cancer with tumor-infiltrating lymphocytes. Science 223:1318, 1986

213. Greenberg PD: Therapy of murine leukemia with cyclophosphamide and immune LYT2+ cells: Cytolytic T cells can mediate eradication of disseminated leukemia. J Immunol 136:1917, 1986

214. Whiteside TL, Herberman RB: Characteristics of natural killer cells and lymphokine-activated killer cells: Their role in the biology and treatment of human cancer. Immunol Allergy Clin North Am 10:663, 1990

215. Topalian SL, Solomon D, Avis FP, et al: Immunotherapy of patients with advanced cancer using tumor-infiltrating lymphocytes and recombinant interleukin 2: A pilot study. J Clin Oncol 6:839, 1988

216. Sondel PM, Sosman JA, Hank JA, et al: Tumor-infiltrating lymphocytes and interleukin-2 in melanoma [letter]. N Engl J Med 320:1418, 1989

217. Kradin RL, Lazarus DS, Dubinett SM, et al: Tumor-infiltrating lymphocytes and interleukin 2 in treatment of advanced cancer. Lancet 1:577, 1989

218. Rosenberg SA, Aebersold P, Cornetta K, et al: Gene transfer into humans—immunotherapy of patients with advanced melanoma, using tumor-infiltrating lymphocytes modified by retroviral gene transduction. N Engl J Med 323:570, 1990

219. Oldham RK, Dillman RO, Bird R, et al: Treatment of advanced cancer with interleukin-2 (rIL-2) and tumor-derived activated cells (TDAC). Proc Am Assoc Cancer Res 31:261, 1990

220. Aebersold P, Hyatt C, Johnson S, et al: Lysis of autologous melanoma cells by tumor infiltrating lymphocytes: Association with clinical response. J Natl Cancer Inst 83:932, 1991

221. Muul LM, Director EP, Hyatt CL, et al: Large scale production of human lymphokine activated killer cells for use in adoptive immunotherapy. J Immunol Meth 88:265, 1986

222. Topalian SL, Muul LM, Solomon D, et al: Expansion of human tumor infiltrating lymphocytes for use in immunotherapy trials. J Immunol Meth 102:127, 1987

223. Knazek R, Wu YW, Aebersold PM, et al: Culture of human tumor-infiltrating lymphocytes in hollow fiber bioreactors. J Immunol Meth 127:29, 1990

224. Itoh K, Hayakawa K, Salmeron MA, et al: Alteration in tumor-infiltrating lymphocyte tumor cell interactions in human melanomas after chemotherapy or immunotherapy. Cancer Immunol Immunother 33:238, 1991

225. Finke JH, Rayman P, Alexander J, et al: Characterization of the cytolytic activity of CD4+ and CD8+ TIL subsets in human renal cell carcinoma. Cancer Res 50:2363, 1990

226. Uchida A, Kariya Y, Okamato N, et al: Prediction of post-operative clinical course by autologous tumor-killing activity in lung cancer patients. J Natl Cancer Inst 82:1697, 1990

227. Al Maghazachi A, Herberman RB, Vujanovic NL, et al: In vivo distribution and tissue localization of highly purified rat lymphokine activation killer (LAK) cells. Cell Immunol 115:179, 1988

228. Al Maghazachi A: Influence of T cells on the expression of lymphokine-activated killer cell activity and in vivo tissue distribution. J Immunol 141:4039, 1988

229. Basse P, Herberman RB, Hokland M, et al: Confusion about the tissue distribution of lymphokine-activated killer (LAK) cells. Cancer Immunol Immunother 35:428, 1992

230. Basse P, Herberman RB, Nannmark U, et al: Accumulation of adoptively transferred adherent, lymphokine-activated killer cells in murine metastases. J Exp Med 174:479, 1991

231. Lotze MT, Zeh HJ III, Elder EM, et al: Use of T-cell growth factors (interleukins 2, 4, 7, 10, and 12) in the evaluation of T-cell reactivity to melanoma. J Immunother 12:212, 1992

232. Goldfarb RH, Wasserman K, Herberman RB, et al: Non-granular proteolytic enzymes of rat IL2 activated natural killer cells. I. Sub-cellular localization and functional role. J Immunol 149:2061, 1992

233. Sasaki A, Melder RJ, Whiteside TL, et al: Preferential localization of human adherent lymphokine-activated killer (A-LAK) cells in tumor microcirculation: A novel mechanism for adoptive immunotherapy. J Natl Cancer Inst 20:433, 1991

23

GENE THERAPY

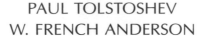

PAUL TOLSTOSHEV
W. FRENCH ANDERSON

Gene therapy as a concept for the amelioration or cure of a genetic disease has been apparent since well before the technical means for isolating and characterizing genes became available in the mid-1970s.[1,2] Modern molecular genetic and biochemical techniques collectively known as recombinant DNA technology allow the isolation, amplification, and characterization of essentially any gene for which a genetic marker, or biologic property, is known. Early techniques of transfection[3,4] or microinjection[5] were developed to introduce DNA, in functioning form, into mammalian cells. Although these techniques were not particularly efficient and often laborious, they constituted the initial technical tools required to contemplate seriously gene therapy manipulations[6–8] of potential clinical utility.

Despite the availability of pure genes and functional delivery systems, the actual clinical implementation of gene transfer and gene therapy in the United States took the best part of another decade. There were a number of reasons for this. First, the ethical, social, and review and oversight considerations needed to be assessed carefully by both the scientific community and the public in general.[7–9] Second, the initial disease focus moved away from the hemoglobinopathies, the first genetic diseases to be characterized at the molecular level. This was a consequence of the realization that not only was there a need in the hemoglobin disorders to replace a defective globin chain gene, but that appropriate regulatory signals were needed to balance the expression of the introduced gene with that of the other nondefective globin genes. Such strict regulation of introduced genes was (and in fact still remains) beyond the capacity of available techniques.

The initial disease target therefore changed[9,10] in the mid-1980s, to one of the severe combined immune deficiency disorders, adenosine deaminase (ADA) deficiency. In this disease, there appeared to be no need to regulate tightly the level of expression of the introduced ADA gene, because, within the normal population, there is an extremely wide range (as much as 500-fold) in the normal levels of the enzyme in lymphocytes. The cell target remained, as it had been for the hemoglobin disorders, the

bone marrow stem cells. Bone marrow is both accessible by biopsy and able to be reintroduced relatively simply via bone marrow transplantation (BMT) techniques. However, it became apparent from early animal and primate studies that introduction into and maintenance of expression of foreign genes in bone marrow stem cells would be difficult to achieve.

When initial clinical testing of gene transfer technology did begin, in May of 1989, it was in fact not directed to any genetic disease, but toward a cell marking technology to study an adoptive immunotherapy procedure for cancer. In the subsequent explosion of clinical studies involving gene therapy, both therapeutic and further marking studies, applications to cancer have been represented strongly.

The major reasons for this early application of gene transfer and therapy to cancer relate initially to the risk-benefit considerations attendant to many of the devastating forms of cancer for which there are few effective therapies. Additionally, they reflect one of the interesting and unanticipated uses of gene therapy techniques, that is, the potential of gene therapy to serve as a sophisticated and effective drug delivery technology for protein drugs. In the past decade, a major focus of new cancer therapies has been in the general field of immunotherapy. This approach uses the properties, cells, and products of the body's own immune defense mechanisms to attempt to augment or strengthen immune responses to cancer. A large number of potent lymphokines, cytokines, and other immune system proteins have been characterized, have had their genes cloned, have been expressed as recombinant proteins, and have been tested as systemic anticancer agents over the last several years. In a number of cases, very short half-lives, toxic side effects at high doses, and difficulties in maintaining therapeutic levels at the desired sites have been observed. These are all classic drug delivery issues, and gene therapy has offered the prospect of an alternative, and possibly more effective, means of delivering these agents.

Clinical studies with cancer patients have been of great significance in the development of gene therapy technologies in humans. Clinical approaches involving gene therapy continue to evolve, with elegant and innovative new approaches to using these extremely powerful techniques. It is the aim of this chapter to describe the current gene therapy applications to cancer treatment, and to describe in detail the clinical studies that currently are being conducted. Additionally, the extraordinary diversity of new and novel approaches to cancer therapies involving gene therapy that are being developed and tested in preclinical studies also is described. First, however, the basic concepts, techniques, and vector systems used in gene therapy are presented, together with the safety issues and studies that are critical to the clinical uses of gene marking and therapy techniques.

BACKGROUND OF TECHNOLOGY

A variety of different ways have been devised to introduce genes into mammalian cells. These are listed in Table 23–1, and span a variety of chemical, physical, and viral methods.[3–5,11–28] The generic term for the agent that constitutes or contains the genes that are to be transferred and expressed in a foreign cell is a vector.

Chemical and Physical Methods of Gene Transfer

The chemical methods[3,4] for gene transfer generally involve generation of some kind of complex with purified DNA, and then application of this complex to cells in culture. A substantial proportion of cells take up the DNA and are able to transport at least some of it to the nucleus of cells, where it is transiently expressed for several days. However, only a very small proportion (generally much less than 1 per cent) of cells permanently retain the DNA, incorporate it into their chromosomes, and continue to express the introduced genes. In these methodologies, the vector is a purified DNA molecule, generally constructed

by gene cloning techniques to contain, in addition to the desired gene, regulatory sequences such as promoters and enhancers to facilitate expression of the gene. However, the DNA vector may be coated with or encapsulated in agents such as lipids or phospholipids,[11,12] or complexed to agents such as binding proteins,[13–15] to facilitate its entry into target cells.

DNA vectors also can be introduced into cells by a variety of physical means. The most straightforward of these, conceptually, is direct injection,[5,17] and sophisticated techniques for injection on the microscopic scale are required to achieve this. This technology, however, is limited by the fact that only a relatively small number of cells can be injected at a given time. There are now attempts to automate microinjection technologies, but the relatively small number of cells that can be injected remains a major limitation. However, it is of interest to speculate that, if a small number of purified bone marrow stem cells[28,29] could be injected, and culture conditions found to expand them substantially, then this method of gene transfer might have significant clinical interest and utility. However, there still remains the issue that only a small proportion of cells injected with vectors are able to sustain long-term, rather than just transient, expression.

Other physical methods of introducing vectors into cells can be applied to larger cell numbers. One of these is electroporation, which can be used to introduce DNA into cells in culture, although viability among recipient cells varies widely with different cell types.[16] A recently developed physical method involves coating very small spheres of a heavy metal[18] (gold, for example), with DNA, and then firing the particles at the cells at high speed so that the particles penetrate the cells. Initial studies with this technique have given encouraging results, and ultimately may provide the opportunity to use such techniques in vivo by directly firing into a selected tissue or organ.

Retroviral Vectors

The most effective vectors that initially have been used clinically have involved viruses that represent naturally evolved gene transfer systems. Viruses, notably the bacterial virus Lambda phage, were the first to be used as vectors to introduce DNA into bacterial cells as part of the development of recombinant DNA techniques. Conceptually, it is therefore not surprising that animal viruses should have been used as vectors for the transfer of genes into mammalian cells. As listed in Table 23–1, several viruses have been exploited in this way. However, for human gene therapy, a mouse retrovirus, Moloney murine leukemia virus (MoMuLV) was the first vector system developed for clinical applications. MoMuLV was developed as a vector system from the pioneering work from a number of laboratories. These studies have been described in a number of reviews[19–20,22] and are not described in detail here.

The general concepts are straightforward. The genes in the viral genome required for reproduction (for MoMuLV, genes called *gag, pol*, and *env*) are removed and replaced

TABLE 23–1. METHODS FOR INTRODUCTION OF GENES INTO MAMMALIAN CELLS

METHOD	REF.
Chemical	
Calcium phosphate (transfection)	3,4
Liposomes	11
Lipofection	12
DNA-protein complexes	13–15
Physical	
Electroporation	16
Microinjection	5, 17
Ballistic particles	18
Viral	
Retroviral vector	19–23
Adenoviral vector	24
Adeno-associated viral vector	25
Herpesvirus vector	26, 27

with a foreign gene. This is accomplished at the DNA level by standard recombinant DNA techniques. What remains from the retrovirus are its regulatory elements, notably the long terminal repeats (LTRs), and a packaging signal, to allow RNA transcripts to be assembled into viral particles. The way in which retroviral vectors are produced is by using a cell line called a packaging cell line.[30] A packaging cell line is a cell line engineered, as described later, to produce the essential components required for generation of a viral vector. The introduction of a vector sequence into a packaging cell line generates what is termed a producer cell line, one that is capable of generating functional vector particles. This concept of packaging, established earlier for avian retroviral vectors,[31] involves engineering a cell line with the genes required to produce the products required for retroviral particle formation (namely *gag, pol,* and *env*). However, the retroviral genes are in such a form that their own RNA transcripts lack a packaging signal and therefore cannot be packaged into a particle. When the retroviral vector genome is introduced into such a packaging cell line, the resultant transcripts are assembled into particles, using the gene products of the *gag, pol,* and *env* genes present in the packaging cell line. The particles that result are what are known as retroviral vectors. They have the ability to enter target cells, to copy their RNA genome into DNA via reverse transcription, and to integrate stably into the target cell chromosomes as a result of the presence of the remaining retroviral regulatory sequences. Once integrated, the inserted gene can be expressed to produce the desired protein product. The retroviral vector, lacking genes for viral reproduction, is not replication competent, and therefore cannot produce more replication-competent viruses from the target cells. Hence the vector acts as a single-hit agent of gene transfer, leaving a copy of the vector sequence in the target cell genome.

Retroviral vectors have a number of desirable features necessary for gene transfer agents for clinical use. These are listed in Table 23–2. The most important of these properties, relative to other methods of gene transfer, is efficiency. In suitable target cells and through the use of selectable markers, essentially all cells of a target population can be modified. This is perhaps the main reason why they were the first vectors used in humans in sanctioned clinical tests.

The first clear indications that retroviral vectors were likely to be the initial vectors for clinical use came around

1984,[10] and spurred a major effort in vector development in many laboratories. From the original retroviral vectors[21,23,32,33] were developed safety-modified backbones such as the LNL and LN[34] series, self-inactivating or SIN vectors in which the LTR enhancer function was eliminated after proviral integration,[35] double copy (DC) vectors in which a foreign gene can be inserted within the 3' LTR,[36] and the MFG vector[37] in which the viral splicing mechanism and region around the start of the viral envelope gene are preserved.

The packaging cell lines used to generate retroviral vectors also have been developed extensively. The major issue has been to reduce the likelihood of generating, through recombination events in the packaging cell line, a replication-competent retrovirus. Under certain circumstances, with particular vector–packaging cell line combinations, this has been observed to occur,[38] but the likelihood of its occurrence has been reduced greatly by safety modifications to the vector backbones, by modifying the viral genes introduced into packaging cell lines such as PA317,[39] or by splitting the packaging functions.[40,41] As a result, there are available today a number of vector–packaging cell line combinations able to generate safe, high-titer (10^6 particles per ml [plaque-forming unit (PFU)] and higher) vectors suitable for clinical studies. The absence of replication-competent virus in vector preparations is one of the major safety issues of retroviral-mediated gene therapy and is discussed in detail later in this chapter.

The size constraint imposed by the need to be able to package the vector RNA genome means that up to about 8 kb are available for introduced genes. This space is sufficient for two average-sized, or three small, genes to be introduced into a single vector. However, there are individual genes, such as that for the clotting protein factor VIII, that are sufficiently large to cause difficulties in introducing them into the Moloney retroviral vector backbone.

A convenient feature of some retroviral vectors has been the presence of selectable marker genes, such as neomycin phosphotransferase, hygromycin phosphotransferase, or several others.[42] Such selection markers both allow a convenient vector titering process and also provide the ability to apply selection to a cell population that has been exposed to the vector to produce a population wherein all cells contain the vector. Hence, the most commonly used vectors contain a selection marker gene as well as a gene of clinical or scientific interest. With such double-gene

TABLE 23–2. PROPERTIES OF RETROVIRAL VECTORS

1.	Well-studied, well-characterized viruses at the molecular level.
2.	Vector and production systems well established, and able to produce good titer vectors, free of replication-competent virus.
3.	Many foreign genes have been expressed with retroviral vectors, in a number of different cell types in vitro.
4.	Functioning genes transferred to cells in vitro can continue to express in vivo when cells are reintroduced into animals.
5.	Efficiency of gene transfer with retroviral vectors can be very high.
6.	Transfer of the proviral sequence into cells is by integration, at random, into chromosomal sites. Transfer is stable and proviral sequences are passed on to progeny when cells divide.
7.	Cells must be replicating to allow retroviral-mediated gene transfer to occur.
8.	Size limit of genes that MoMuLV vectors can accommodate is 7 to 8 kb.

vectors, however, as well as with multiple-gene vectors, the issue of efficiency of expression of the individual genes can be a problem. The viral LTR generally serves as promoter for one of the genes, and internal promoter(s) are used to drive the other gene(s). Genes arranged in vectors in this way are not always expressed at equal efficiency. One solution to the problem is to dispense with the selectable marker and use only a single gene in the vector. This is a feature of the MGF vector,[37] but also has been used in other vector constructs, such as one containing the gene for the human low-density lipoprotein receptor.[43] Such a single-gene vector has been used in a clinical protocol to attempt to correct the low-density lipoprotein receptor defect in the hepatocytes of patients with familial hypercholesterolemia.

Alternative and innovative approaches to size and expression limitations have been of at least two kinds. First, internal ribosome entry sequences of viral origin have been incorporated into retroviral vectors[44–46] and shown to improve markedly the expression of downstream genes in the vector. Second, fusion proteins generated from physically linking together parts of two genes have been generated using retroviral vectors. These include a multiple drug resistance/ADA gene fusion,[47] a neomycin phosphotransferase/β-galactosidase gene fusion,[48] and a neomycin phosphotransferase/hygromycin phosphotransferase gene fusion.[49] This latter construct has been proposed to be used in a clinical protocol to mark cytotoxic T-lymphocyte cell clones that are generated, expanded in vitro, and given back to acquired immunodeficiency syndrome (AIDS) patients with lymphomas after chemotherapy and BMT.[50,51]

The efficiency at which retroviral vectors can be introduced into target cells (a process that is referred to as transduction) can be highly variable. Fibroblasts, epithelial cells, and smooth muscle cells in culture appear to be readily transduced. Additionally, selection procedures often can ensure a fully transduced cell population. However, cells of lymphoid origin often are much more resistant to transduction, and, for peripheral blood lymphocytes (PBLs)[52] and tumor-infiltrating lymphocyte (TIL) cells,[53,54] transduction efficiencies are generally low and rarely exceed 10 per cent. Unfortunately, lymphoid cells grown in suspension culture after transduction are also difficult to select with the neomycin analogue G418. As a potential way to increase the range and efficiency of transduction of cells with retroviral vectors, packaging cell lines using other retroviral envelopes are being developed. One example of this is a packaging cell line that uses the envelope protein of the gibbon ape leukemia virus.[55]

It is a requirement for retroviral vector-mediated gene transfer that the target cells be replicating.[56] This imposes a restriction on the use of retroviral vectors for certain terminally differentiated types that are incapable of being stimulated to divide, and clearly limits the use of these kinds of cells in gene therapy with retroviral vectors.

A final important feature of retroviruses and vectors derived from them is the property of stable integration within the chromosome of the host cell. This property has both its positive and negative aspects. On the positive side, the integration event, which can be limited to one or a few copies within each cell, results in the permanent modification not only of the cell, but all of its progeny. Unlike certain other gene transfer systems, the introduced gene will persist, and, at least in some cases, expression will continue throughout the lifetime of the cell. The maintenance of expression, however, is not obligatory, particularly in vivo where, for example, fibroblasts modified by certain kinds of retroviral vector constructs have been found to shut down expression of the gene over time.[57,58] It has been suspected that this may be related both to the nature of the promoter driving expression of the gene and to the property of the target fibroblast cell. In other situations, such as PBLs modified to express the human ADA gene, expression appears to persist in vivo in human patients with ADA deficiency, although in this case there is almost certainly a strong selection for expressing cells.[50,51]

One of the features of retroviral vector insertion is its random nature. This raises certain questions of safety related to potential activation of oncogenes or inactivation of tumor suppressor genes, and these are discussed in a subsequent section. To be able to extend the applications, and improve the risk-benefit considerations associated with retroviral-mediated gene therapy, two substantial technical advances are required. The first is the development of injectable vectors that have the property of homing to specified target tissues or cells after introduction of the vector in the circulation. The initial approaches to achieving this focus on engineering the retroviral envelope to modify or change its specificity for binding to target cells. A diversity of viral envelopes with different receptor and therefore cell specificities exists.[59] It remains to be established to what extent the specificity and structure of the envelope can be modified and still maintain virus packaging and transduction properties. It also may be necessary to modify the vectors to allow them to survive better the immune system in the recipient. Natural murine retroviruses are highly susceptible to inactivation by the complement system in primate blood.[60,61]

The second feature that likely will be required for vectors will be the ability to integrate in a preselected and "safe" region of the target genome. This could involve the use of a homologous recombination mechanism of a kind that is already known to occur in mammalian cells.[62] Alternatively, it may involve other naturally occurring gene targeting mechanisms, such as that known to exist for the human adeno-associated virus (AAV).[61] Here, the virus has the ability to integrate into a specific site on chromosome 19 in human cells. The generation of these kinds of properties to viral vectors, derived from retroviruses or other viral systems, will extend greatly the already large and growing number of applications of gene therapy techniques, and should increase the safety of the vector systems to the point where they will be able to be used in very large numbers of individuals in non–life-threatening disease situations. The other consequence of such injectable vectors is the prospect of simple and relatively inexpensive treatment regimens that do not depend on expensive, laboratory-intensive, and individual-based therapies that are a feature of many of the initial gene therapy protocols.

Other Vector Systems

There are now rapid advances being made in developing vector systems in addition to retroviral vectors for clinical gene therapy applications. Indeed, the first clinical trial of a cancer therapy that involves a nonviral vector already has commenced. The study, designed to deliver a cell surface antigen to tumor cells to attempt to stimulate the body's immune response, uses a DNA vector encapsulated in a liposome. This protocol, discussed in detail in a following section, is also significant in that it is the first sanctioned in vivo test, because the DNA liposomes are injected directly into the tumor site.

A great deal of attention is being focused on other viral vector systems for gene therapy. The closest to clinical testing is the adenoviral vector system. These vectors[24] are derived from certain strains of human adenoviruses. Replication-impaired vectors have been constructed and these currently have the capacity to accept 7 to 8 kb of foreign DNA. Adenovirus vectors have a number of unique features as gene therapy vectors. Very significant is the fact that they are able to introduce DNA into nondividing cells. These adenovirus vectors have a broad host range in cell types they are able to infect. In addition, unlike retroviruses, they do not integrate into the chromosome of the host, but persist and can express foreign genes in vivo and in vitro for periods of at least several weeks. One study[64] using an adenovirus vector carrying the ornithine transcarbonylase (OTCase) gene to correct a metabolic liver defect in a strain of OTCase-deficient mice (the Spf-ash strain) reports persistence of expression for as long as 1 year. Other features of adenovirus vectors include their stability, which allows them to be concentrated to very high titers, and their tropism for the lung. This enables them to be used in vivo for the delivery of foreign genes to cells of the respiratory tract and makes them well suited as vectors for major genetic diseases that affect the lung, such as cystic fibrosis. The feasibility of this approach in an animal model, the cotton rat, already has been reported, with the delivery and expression of two human proteins, A-1 antitrypsin[65] and the cystic fibrosis transmembrane regulator (CFTR),[66] to the lungs of cotton rats after instillation of the respective adenoviral vectors. Some of the difficulties that may be encountered in the use of adenoviral vectors include potentially short duration of expression, the possibility of immunologic reactions to repeated doses, and questions of safety that are considered separately later in this chapter. It is probable that initial clinical trials in cystic fibrosis patients will have taken place by the time this chapter is published.

Another viral vector system currently the focus of much research is that derived from a human virus, AAV. This virus, which has no known pathogenicity in humans, is still somewhat poorly understood, but vectors and systems for their production have been developed.[67] The vectors can accept approximately 4 kb of foreign DNA and recently have been shown also to be able to correct the chloride channel defect in cultured cells from cystic fibrosis patients by transfer of a functioning CFTR gene.[68] Additionally, much interest surrounds the specific insertion mechanism of the wild-type AAV virus.[63] It is not yet clear which of the elements of the virus are required for this function, but several groups are studying this topic intensively with the objective of developing a vector that retains a specific targeting mechanism.

A variety of other viral systems also are being developed as vectors. Although most of these are still at fairly early stages, they could well be of clinical significance in the longer term because of specific features that they possess. Herpes virus vectors, for example,[26,27,69] have a tropism for cells of the nervous system, and additionally have sophisticated mechanisms of latency and induction. The papillomaviruses, such as bovine papillomavirus[70] and vaccinia virus,[71] for example, have been used extensively as research tools for expression of genes in animal cells, and serious attention now is being focused on them to evaluate any clinical utility they may have for gene therapy.

Finally, an interesting combination of viral and nonviral elements has been developed recently to transfer genes at high efficiency to cells in culture. The approach involves the use of intact adenovirus, and its efficient entry mechanism, to act as a carrier for a complex of DNA and polylysine.[15,72] This system has the capacity to transfer very large pieces of DNA, and the properties of the adenovirus coat are thought to improve the release of DNA from the endosome structures the cell uses to take up such complexes. Because the adenovirus used in this way can be irradiated to render them noninfectious, the method has the potential for eliminating altogether the use of any infectious viral DNA. However, it still remains to be tested how long expression can be maintained with such complexes, and whether they can function efficiently in vivo.

From the large and innovative variety of vector and gene transfer systems that now are being developed, it seems clear that in the future there may be a choice of several different methods for clinical gene therapy applications. Different transfer techniques may have suitability for particular disease applications, and, as a consequence, the opportunities to use gene transfer in the clinical context may be broadened further.

Clinical Concepts

The different kinds of clinical approaches to gene therapy are important to appreciate. The first that was put into effect, and that used in all but one of the subsequent trials, involves the removal of the patient's own cells, effecting the gene transfer in the laboratory and, after testing, returning the gene-modified cells to the patient. This approach is generally termed *ex vivo gene therapy*. It developed from the initial target tissue for gene therapy (i.e., bone marrow), where, with the development of BMT techniques, it is a straightforward approach at least in concept. However, the approach has been extended both experimentally in animals and in the clinic to a variety of other cells and tissues, including different lymphocyte types, hepatocytes obtained by partial hepatectomy and reinfused into the liver, and fibroblasts and smooth muscle cells obtained by biopsy and reintroduced using implantation techniques. Therefore, the approach is generally applicable to several cell types. Ex vivo gene therapy therefore involves an individual patient-specific procedure and to some degree specialized and sophisticated cell culture technique and laboratory expertise, with their attendant costs. However, it clearly also offers the safety features of being able to monitor and test the transduced cells before they are returned to the patient, and the feature that any vector that does not enter the cells can be washed away. As a consequence, the vector itself is not introduced into patients, only cells that have been modified by it.

The second conceptual clinical approach is *in vivo gene therapy*. Here the vector is introduced directly into the body, where the gene transfer takes place. To transduce a particular target cell requires some kind of specific recognition mechanism. Murine retroviral vectors recognize a wide variety of different cell types, and so a specific docking or targeting mechanism generally is required to transduce only a specific cell or tissue. Some of the vector approaches using DNA-ligand complexes have the capacity to achieve this—notably the approach of targeting the asialoglycoprotein receptor on liver cells.[14] Less stringent forms of targeting can be achieved simply by introduction of the vector to the desired organ or target site, and this is the approach that has been taken in a cancer protocol involving direct injection of a liposome-encapsulated DNA vector directly into the tumor site.[73] It is also an approach proposed for retroviral instillation directly into the tumor site in a protocol to treat non–small-cell lung cancer by providing the tumor suppressor gene *p53* (see later in this chapter). In this circumstance, the tumor cells are likely to be the only cells in the local region (apart perhaps from developing vasculature around the tumors) that are replicating and therefore capable of being transduced with the vector.

This latter feature of introducing vector only into cells in a local region that are replicating is an aspect of another delivery modality that may be termed *in situ gene therapy*. The concept, initially proposed and tested in certain animal tumor models,[74,75] involved the implantation at the tumor site of the producer cells that are making a retroviral vector. The vector contains a gene such that any cell acquiring it is rendered susceptible to a certain drug. A clinical protocol to use this approach to treat glioblastoma in the brain has been proposed, and is described in detail in a later section. One of the other early clinical tests of an in vivo approach is likely to involve the use of adenoviral vectors. The natural tropism of adenovirus for the lung makes these vectors ideally suited to approach the treatment of diseases that affect the lung, such as cystic fibrosis, and preclinical studies for this objective are well advanced.

The main issues in in vivo and in situ approaches are those of specificity and to what extent only the desired cell population would be transduced. If other cells in the body are likely to be modified as well, then the safety issues of this event, including the inadvertent modification of germline cells, must be considered very carefully.

SAFETY AND REGULATORY ISSUES

Safety—Retroviral Vectors

Three major issues of safety generally are acknowledged to surround the use of retroviral vectors in humans. The first of these concerns the possible presence in vector preparations of infectious, replication-competent virus generated through a recombination event in the producer cell line. The producer cell line is the engineered packaging cell line, which has had a vector genome introduced into it and therefore generates vector particles. The second concern relates to the potential consequences of the property of random integration into the chromosome of the vector DNA. Finally, the issue of any safety consequences resulting from the nature of the product whose gene is transferred must be considered. This last issue should be considered on a case-by-case basis, and is so done in the discussion of specific protocols.

A number of studies relating to replication-competent virus generation have been conducted. Initial work in primates[60,77,78] has concluded that amphotropically packaged replication-competent murine retrovirus is not an acute pathogen, and in fact confirmed earlier observations of the rapid inactivation of the virus mediated by the complement system. However, a more recent study[79] has reported the development of malignant T-cell lymphomas in three monkeys about 6 months after a BMT/gene transfer protocol. In this study, a replication-competent virus–contaminated vector preparation was used. It was established that the replication-competent virus was associated with the lymphoma generation, because viral inserts were observed in lymphoma cells from all three animals, whereas none of the animals had vector sequences integrated into the lymphoma cell DNA. This observation reaffirms the need, mandated by National Institutes of Health Recombinant DNA Advisory Committee (RAC) and Food and Drug Administration (FDA) review processes for all gene marking and therapy protocols, for the stringent monitoring of vector preparations for the presence of replication-competent virus.

The probability of generation of replication-competent virus from producer cell lines has been studied extensively. The occurrence of the event depends on the degree of homology between the vector backbone and the viral packaging sequences in the producer cell line. The theoretical and practical issues surrounding this safety aspect of vectors of packaging systems have been reviewed extensively.[23,39,80–82] Basically, a minimal overlap exists between the producer cell sequences and the vectors—for example, between the PA317 packaging cell line[39] and the LN and G1 backbones that have been used clinically so far. In such combinations, generation of replication-competent virus is rare.[83] The theoretical probability of occurrence of such recombination events can be reduced further by the use of packaging cell lines[40,41] in which the packaging cell functions are split onto two different DNA constructs that are introduced separately into the packaging cell line. It can be concluded that replication-competent virus generation remains a safety issue for human gene therapy, but that existing vector and production systems do produce virus-free vector, and that sensitive tests are available that will detect a virus breakout should it occur. This seems to be the conclusion being reached on this issue by the regulatory bodies also.[84]

The second safety issue for retroviral vectors is that of a random insertional event causing the activation of an oncogene or the inactivation of a tumor suppressor gene. First, it is important to appreciate that such an event does not obligatorily lead to the formation of a malignancy. Such an event is usually one of a series of required steps that can be as many as ten, as has been demonstrated for certain colon cancers.[85,86] A single random insertion therefore has the potential to constitute one of the required series of steps and to add to already existing environmental or other events. The question then becomes whether the occurrence of such events will statistically affect the frequency of malignancies. Current animal studies (which have involved relatively small numbers) to date have shed little light on this question, because no unequivocal event of association of a retroviral vector insertion with a malignancy has yet been reported. It should be noted that the primate lymphomas mentioned previously were correlated with replication-competent virus, not vector insertion.[79] Replication-competent virus integration occurred at high frequency from virus exposure over a long period of time in immune-suppressed animals. No vector copies were present in the lymphoma DNA of these animals.

The frequency of any such activation or inactivation events will depend on (1) the number of cells transduced, (2) the number of proto-oncogenes or tumor suppressor genes in the human genome that can be affected, and (3) how efficiently the insertion process influences these genes. Only the first of these factors can be measured with any precision at present. A major long-term study in rodents is planned by the National Institute of Environmental Health Sciences, North Carolina, and an initial pilot study has commenced (R. Langenbach, NIEHS, personal communication).

The final point that should be made is that, within conventional and accepted therapies such as radiation, chemotherapy, and immunosuppression, there are significantly elevated risks of subsequent malignancies that are acceptable within normal risk-benefit considerations. It is in this light that this issue should be considered; that is, are the risk-benefit considerations appropriate for the disease and the treatment proposed? The growing numbers of clinical protocols in gene therapy will add rapidly to our safety data base, but it is worth noting that current experience is already more than 100 monkey years and greater than 30 patient years, without any side effects, pathology, or malignancy from retroviral vector-mediated gene transfer. This is not to say the process is without its risks, but only that available information points to the risk as being low.

On the issue of protocol-specific risks, one strategy exists that may have general applicability irrespective of which agent is delivered. This is the concept of a suicide gene within the vector. The prototype of such a system is the herpes simplex virus thymidine kinase (*tk*) gene,[87] but others, such as cytosine deaminase,[88] also have been proposed. The concept is that vector-modified cells will produce the Tk protein and therefore will be sensitive to killing by the agents gancyclovir and acyclovir. Such suicide mechanisms are likely to become standard features of gene therapy vectors. There already exists one protocol related to marking cytotoxic T-cell clones in AIDS patients with lymphomas (see later in this chapter) as well as a brain tumor protocol in which the *tk* gene is used to kill the glioblastoma cells.

Safety—Other Vector Systems

The only nonretroviral vector protocol that has commenced in humans has involved the use of injected liposomes containing DNA. The in vivo efficiency of gene transfer in such systems is rather low, and liposomes in the circulation are cleared rapidly in the reticuloendothelial system. Animal studies with this vector system showed no acute toxicities[73] and no transfer of the gene to other cell types. The review agencies took the view that the risk-benefit equation was appropriate to test this therapy, even though there is a theoretical possibility of transfer of genes to other cell types, including germline cells. The initial patient selection criteria, however, excluded patients who retained reproductive capacity.

The next vector system being tested for gene therapy applications in humans is the adenovirus vector system. Adenovirus of the strains used in vectors are not associated with any serious human disease or malignancy, and attenuated strains have been used as vaccines for many years in over 2 million individuals.[89] Acute safety issues of adenoviral vectors delivered to the lung include the possibilities of inflammation and lung pathology, as well as the generation of a sufficiently strong immune response that would preclude their repetitive administration. Other issues of safety are those of complementation of the vector by other viruses, resulting in continuous production with possible shedding by the patient of infectious virus particles. There is also a theoretical possibility of recombination in vivo with other viruses. These safety issues are being addressed actively in animal studies.

Regulatory Review Process

The evolution of the review process in the United States has been reviewed elsewhere,[50,51,90,91] so only the current status is described here. A protocol initiated in a clinical center is required to receive Institutional Review Board (IRB) and Institutional Biosafety Committee (IBC) approval. If the investigators or institutions are in receipt of federal funding, then approval of the National Institutes of Health (NIH) RAC also is required. Finally, an Investigational New Drug (IND) submission must be approved by the FDA, and a Drug Master File provided for the vector product. Both the RAC and FDA have published Points to Consider for gene therapy protocols.[92,93]

GENE-MARKING PROTOCOLS

Initial Protocol—Tumor-Infiltrating Lymphocyte

The first sanctioned gene transfer experiment was a marking study to introduce a marker gene into a class of white blood cells called tumor-infiltrating lymphocytes. TILs are a cell population of lymphocytes that can be grown out of tumor biopsies from melanoma and renal cell carcinoma patients. They form the basis of an immunotherapy procedure developed at the NIH by Rosenberg and his colleagues.[94,95] The details and applications of this therapeutic approach are not discussed in detail, except as they relate to the gene-marking trial. In summary, the procedure for TIL therapy, which has been studied in patients with metastatic melanoma or renal cell cancer who have failed other conventional forms of therapy and who have a limited life expectancy, is as follows. After biopsy of a tumor, the invading lymphocytic population is grown in tissue culture under the stimulus of recombinant human interleukin 2 (IL-2) for about 1 month until a population of cells in excess of 10^{11} is achieved. The cells are returned intravenously to the patient, who additionally receives several days' IV treatment of high doses of IL-2. Objective response rates of 35 to 40 per cent partial or complete responses have been obtained.[95,96]

A hypothesis for responses observed in this therapy are that the TIL cells contain a subpopulation of cells that have the ability to home back to sites of tumor deposit and mediate killing of tumor cells. The evidence for the hypothesis includes the fact that TIL cell population, although a heterogeneous lymphocyte population, often do have cytotoxic killing properties on autologous tumor in chromium uptake killing assays in vitro.[97] Additionally, labeling of TILs with radioactive ^{111}In as a short-term cell marker (half-life 2.8 days) indicated that a certain fraction of TILs specifically localize to tumor deposits while the majority are found transiently in the lung, liver, and spleen.[98]

Other than these studies, and attempts to correlate production of TIL populations of particular cytokines with the clinical response observed, it has proven difficult to obtain other clinical correlates between the characteristics of the TIL population and a positive clinical response. This difficulty generated the proposal to use a gene marker introduced into TIL cells to track TILs within the body to quantitate their presence in blood and biopsy samples. This, therefore, was the essence of the first sanctioned gene-marking protocol. The protocol had no therapeutic objectives or possible therapeutic benefits for the patient, and was designed only to obtain data about TIL therapy with the hope of improving the therapy in subsequent patients from a better understanding of the TIL procedure.

The protocol was designed to take advantage of some of the features of gene transfer as a cell marking system that are quite unique. These are as follows:

1. Genes inserted into chromosomes of cells are stable markers that can be detected readily by sensitive polymerase chain reaction (PCR) techniques.

2. The gene marker remains in the cell, is not diluted or metabolized to mark other cells on the death of marked cells, and is not diluted but passed on to progeny cells on cell division.

3. Labeling of cells with gene markers is technically not complex and does not expose the cells to toxic or radioactive compounds, which may alter the properties or functions of the cells.

4. Retroviral-mediated gene transfer is the most efficient of gene transfer technologies, and, with TILs, marking is generally around 10 per cent of cells.

5. The marker gene that is used can be a selectable marker—for example, the bacterial gene neomycin phosphotransferase (neo®), which confers on cells the resistance to a neomycin analogue, G418. This can be used to enrich substantially a transduced population by killing with G418 those cells that do not carry the marker.

6. The selection property also, in theory, should allow isolation of labeled cells from biopsy samples.

The TIL marker protocol therefore proposed to take a sample of TIL cells from an early stage of their culture, introduce the marker gene, and then to grow a labeled TIL culture in parallel with the unmarked culture. After carefully testing the marked culture for a variety of parameters, both the marked and unmarked cells would be given to the patient. Then periodic sampling of blood, and of accessible tumor deposits, would allow monitoring for the presence and numbers of the marked TIL cells. A variety of preclinical studies were conducted in support of this protocol, including in vitro studies on transduction and selection of human TIL cultures.[53] Although a mouse model for TIL cell generation is available,[94] it has not proven possible, despite intensive efforts, to introduce genes with the retroviral vector into mouse TIL cells. The reasons for this are still not understood. Nonetheless, a substantial body of preclinical data supported a protocol[99] that was submitted to the NIH internal committees in June 1988 and the NIH RAC in October 1988.

The process of review for this protocol was intense, beginning with approval (conditional) from the NIH Institutional Biosafety Committee, on July 13, 1988, and approval from the NIH director on January 19, 1989. The approval was immediately followed by a lawsuit filed by Jeremy Rifkin on procedural grounds concerning aspects of the review process and was settled on May 15, 1989. The first patient received marked cells on May 22, 1989.

A number of issues were raised during the review process. Among these were the issues of the possibility of replication-competent virus generation during vector production, the potential use of animal model studies, the likelihood of changing the properties of the TIL cell population by the transduction process, issues of informed consent, and technical questions relating to the ability to detect labeled cells once they had been introduced into a patient. A variety of safety tests were mandated by the FDA to test the master seed lot of the producer cells, each batch of retroviral vector supernatant, and also the TIL cells themselves after transduction. These tests represent a mixture of tests already in common use for recombinant DNA products together with tests specifically directed to features of the retroviral vector itself.

It is of interest to note that, although the initial protocol proposed to use the N2 retroviral vector,[32] a safety-modified version of N2, called LNL6, was substituted into the protocol during the course of the review process and was the vector used in the ten patients in this study. The study now has been completed, and the results from the initial five patients have been published.[100] Analysis by PCR of blood samples from patients receiving gene-marked TILs detected marked cells consistently to at least 21 days after infusion. In two patients, gene-marked TILs were detected subsequently at days 51 and 60. One of these patients received a second unmarked TIL infusion on day 94, after which TILs were detected in blood samples out to day 189. The estimates of frequency of marked TILs in the blood ranged from 1 in 300 cells at early times to below 1 in 100,000 cells at later stages (and therefore below the levels of detection). In three of the first five patients, tumor biopsies could be taken, and marked TILs could be detected in all three, the latest being at day 64 after infusion.

In samples from one of the patients (who had a complete response to the TIL therapy), attempts[54] were successful to recover marked TILs by selection with the neomycin analogue G418. Control experiments had established that it was frequently difficult to select G418-resistant TILs from cultures transduced with a vector containing the *neo®* gene. This is presumably because, with low transduction efficiency, G418 selection will kill 90 per cent or more of the cells in the culture that did not receive the selectable marker gene. The remaining resistant cells likely cannot survive the environment of a massive excess of dead and dying cells. The patient studied had TILs that transduced well, and in this case it did prove possible to select transduced cells with G418 and to show that transduced cells in the presence of G418 were able to grow at the same rate as untransduced cells. Nevertheless, in the samples recovered after the infusion of 1.5×10^{11} TILs and 0.6×10^{11} transduced TILs, only samples taken at 1 hour past infusion allowed recovery of G418-selected cells in in vitro cultures. In samples taken at later times, the lower levels of transduced cells were not able to be recovered by selection. Tumor samples also were able to be taken from this patient on days 3, 5, 14, and 19 after TIL infusion. TIL cultures were established and then were subject to G418 selection, initially at low concentration (0.1 mg/mL). In the day 5 and day 14 biopsies, G418-resistant cells grew and could be shown by PCR analysis to contain the *neo®* sequence. For the day 5 culture, a Southern blot signal was observed of equal intensity to that in fully in vitro–selected TIL cells. An analysis of T-cell receptor β chain genes by Southern blotting was conducted on DNA from the infused TIL population and from cells selected and grown from the day 5 tumor biopsy. This study showed that the recovered, selected TILs had several subsets of T-cell receptor in common with the infused cells. Although a possible conclusion is that the TILs selected from tumor were not a random assortment of TILs, it is not possible to exclude the possibility that different subpopulations of TILs grow from tumors during the extended in vitro culture process.

No side effects, or any pathology or other undesirable consequences, were found that could be attributed to the gene transfer protocol. Therefore, the major objectives achieved by this protocol were the demonstration of safe gene transfer in a clinical context, and the technical feasibility of identifying gene-marked cells that had been introduced into patients and then recovered in biopsy samples.

Other TIL Marker Protocols

A second gene-marked TIL protocol, closely based on the first conducted at the NIH, has been initiated at the Centre Leon Bérard in Lyon, France.[101] The study, whose objective was also to study the survival of TILs in the blood stream and their tracking to sites of tumor, began in September 1991. The marked TIL protocol was part of a larger study aimed at examining the efficacy of TIL therapy itself. The vector used, LNL6, was identical to that used in the NIH study. A total of four patients have been studied to date (M. Favrot, personal communication). No toxicity or other side effects were observed that could be related to the gene marking. Analysis of patient samples is currently in progress.

An extension of the NIH gene-marked TIL study has begun at the Pittsburgh Cancer Institute.[102] The clinical objective of this protocol, aside from the gene marking, is to study the potential enhancement of the TIL therapy through the use of recombinant interleukin 4 (IL-4). IL-4, although generally considered as a B-cell–stimulating factor, also is known to be able to mediate expansion of human T cells, and to serve as a major T-cell growth factor in mice.[103] A study involving recombinant yeast-derived IL-4 administered alone or in conjunction with IL-2 to cancer patients has been conducted at the National Cancer Institute, NIH. No responses were found in patients receiving IL-4 alone, but significant responses were found in renal cell carcinoma, malignant melanoma, and one case of breast carcinoma in patients receiving a combination of IL-2 and IL-4. Recombinant IL-4 also has been used, in conjunction with IL-2 in TIL studies at the NIH, to culture TILs in vitro prior to patient infusion. The objectives of the Pittsburgh study were therefore to evaluate TIL therapy in selected melanoma patients in whom TILs are grown in IL-2/IL-4 combinations and in whom combinations of IL-2 and IL-4 also are administered to the patients together with the TILs. A hypothesis that the addition of IL-4 can improve specific localization of TILs to tumor sites is testable most readily by the use of gene-marked TILs. This gene-marking protocol has received RAC and FDA approval, and began in March 1992. A total of two patients have received marked cells in this ongoing study, but no data are yet available.

Finally, a clinical protocol[104] involving gene-marked TILs to be conducted at the University of California at Los Angeles received RAC approval in February 1992. This protocol, designed to study TIL therapy in malignant melanoma and renal cell carcinoma, has two significant features. First, it aims to fractionate TILs into CD4+ and CD8+ components and to derive by in vitro culture separate populations for each of these classes of lymphocytes.

Second, the two cell populations will be marked with one of two retroviral vectors, each of which contains the *neo*® gene but which are sufficiently different so as to be able to be distinguished from each other by PCR techniques. This study, as well as evaluating toxicity and possible efficacy of these kinds of TIL subpopulations, will allow examination of the trafficking patterns and life spans of the administered TIL cells.

Other Marking Protocols

The successful and safe implementation of the TIL marker protocols spurred interest in the use of this marking technology in other clinical contexts. The potential of such marking technology has been realized in other areas, most notably in the area of BMT as a part of therapy in cancers such as the leukemias. Bone marrow marking protocols have begun in several centers over the last 18 months, and preparations for several other studies are in progress. The marking technology also is being proposed clinically in the transplant of liver cells and additionally as an adjunct to the study of putative AIDS therapies.

BONE MARROW MARKING PROTOCOLS

Acute Myeloid Leukemia

In acute myeloid leukemia (AML),[105] most children who respond to chemotherapy (85 to 90 per cent) will relapse subsequently, and the duration of complete continuous remission rarely exceeds 18 months. The currently used cytotoxic drug therapies achieve long-term survival in less than 40 per cent of cases. BMT has begun to be investigated extensively, particularly in patients who relapse. For human lymphocyte antigen (HLA)–matched allogeneic BMT, long-term survival is about 50 per cent for AML patients transplanted at first remission, although there is a significant risk of chronic graft-versus-host disease. Additionally, only 30 per cent of these patients have a suitable matched donor. Consequently, recent focus has been more on the use of autologous BMT (ABMT). The strategy involved here is as follows. Autologous marrow is harvested and frozen during remission. On subsequent relapse, higher doses of chemotherapy and radiation can be used, even to levels that would be lethal were not the stored remission marrow available for rescue. The hope is that the more aggressive treatment will cure a higher proportion of patients than would be possible with conventional regimens, and preliminary data suggest this might be the case. However, even with this approach, a significant number of patients suffer a subsequent relapse. It is the origins of the relapse that a marked bone marrow clinical study was designed to investigate. The central issue is whether the source of the relapse after ABMT has its origins in the marrow transplant or whether it is due to persistence of residual disease in the host. This is a very important clinical question to answer because it will de-

termine which of several significantly different approaches to the treatment of AML should be pursued. Should it prove that the rescue marrow is the source of the relapse, then emphasis must be placed on purging technologies to rid the marrow of residual disease cells. If the origin of relapse is only systemic, then there is little justification to pursue the purging approach with its attendant risks of damage to normal progenitor cells and the slowing of rates of engraftment.

There are several points that serve as the rationale for using gene transfer technology as a method of marking to address this issue in AML.

1. The technology is available and is able to mark not only any leukemic cells, but possibly also normal progenitor cells. Labeling of the latter could shed light on the normal mechanisms of marrow regeneration.
2. The marking technology should be successful in demonstrating relapse origins from the infused marrow, and, moreover, analysis of vector insertion sites could allow a determination of whether the relapse derived from one or multiple cells.
3. The marking protocol also might allow determination in AML as to whether the malignancy derives from a stem cell in the marrow or from a lineage-committed progenitor. In some leukemias, such as chronic granulocytic leukemia,[106] there exists a naturally occurring marker, the Philadelphia chromosome, that confirms the stem cell origin of this disease. No such definitive marker exists in AML, in which gene-marking technology offers the possibility of addressing this issue.
4. The marrow in leukemic patients, particularly in the recovery phase from chemotherapy treatment, may have marrow stem cells that may be cycling, in contrast to stem cells of normal individuals, which are thought to be predominantly quiescent. If this is the case, then there could be the possibility of introducing a marker gene into stem cells that would be reflected by observing marked progeny cells in all cell lineages. There would be benefits from an ability to study the induction of stem cell cycling both in vitro as well as in vivo.

The preclinical data generated in support of this protocol[107,108] were primarily from in vitro transduction studies with normal and leukemic marrow samples. These data included demonstration of the ability of gene-marked colonies grown from transduced marrow to survive in G418, a demonstration that AML blast cells can be transduced with efficiencies of as high as 25 per cent (mean 10 per cent), and demonstration that the transduction process itself had no significant effect on the ability of the marrow to generate in vitro colony growth, particularly after marked and nonmarked marrow are mixed. Finally, PCR techniques were used to confirm the existence of the *neo*® gene in G418-resistant colony DNA.

The protocol received RAC approval in March 1991, and commenced in September 1991. Two patients who suffered a relapse after ABMT have been analyzed, and, in both, the leukemic cells are gene marked, confirming that a marrow origin is responsible, at least in part, for the relapses.

Disseminated Neuroblastoma

This childhood malignancy, the most common extracranial tumor in children under 4 years of age, responds well to current therapies when the disease is localized. Where the disease is disseminated, however, eradication is very difficult even with intensive chemotherapy, and the clinical prognosis for such patients is extremely poor. Again, the ABMT approach with patients in remission has been attempted and the identical question of the origins of subsequent relapse—from rescue marrow or from systemic sites—is at issue. Therefore, a similar gene-marking approach was proposed for this disorder in two different treatment protocols.[108,109] Preclinical studies[110] have shown that freshly isolated malignant neuroblastoma cell lines can be transduced with retroviral vectors with efficiencies ranging from 0.1 to 13 per cent (mean 3.6 per cent). Because of the lower efficiency of transduction values, the statistical considerations of the likelihood of detecting a marked relapse in the clinical study become even more important. It has been calculated[107–109] that, with a 1 per cent transduction efficiency and with 30 per cent of the marrow used for marking, a polyclonal relapse involving only 100 cells would be detected with a greater than 90 per cent likelihood if 12 patients were studied. If greater than 1000 cells are involved in relapse, then the chances are more than 60 per cent of detecting a marked relapse in any one individual. If the relapse stems from 10 progenitors or less, then a very much larger number of patients (more than 50) would be required to have a high likelihood of detecting a marked relapse. These protocols also have received all regulatory approvals and the study began in January 1992.

Chronic Myelogenous Leukemia

Chronic myelogenous leukemia (CML) is most frequent in patients in their 50s and 60s who are frequently not eligible for allograft BMT. In studying therapies for this disease, ABMT has been investigated in conjunction with intensive therapy. However, the majority of such patients still succumb to a second relapse, and the same question arises that is addressed in the AML and neuroblastoma protocols—that is, whether it is the rescue marrow or residual systemic disease that is the source of the relapse. For this reason, gene-marking protocols using *neo*® gene–containing retroviral vectors have been designed and are being conducted.[111,112]

For CML, unlike AML, a genetic marker (the Philadelphia chromosome) and an acute disease-specific transcript (*bcr/abl*) exist, and this facilitates the analysis of cells from relapsed patients who have received retrovirally marked marrow. Additionally, purging methods for removing Philadelphia-positive cells are being developed[111] and these include methods involving DR antigens, late myeloid antigens, and surface cytoadhesion molecules.

The objectives of the marker protocols that have been initiated at M.D. Anderson Cancer Center in Houston and at the University of Indiana are both to study the origins of relapse in AML. Additionally, data also may be obtained from these trials about the introduction of the vector into normal bone marrow progenitor and possibly stem cells. The M.D. Anderson protocol began in July 1991 and currently two patients have received marked marrow. The Indianapolis protocol, which also involves patients with acute lymphoblastic leukemia (ALL), began in May 1992. No data concerning origins of relapse have been reported yet in these studies.

Other Bone Marrow Marker Studies

The continued interest in application of retroviral-mediated gene marking is illustrated by further clinical protocols that are being proposed and that have received recent RAC approval. The first of these, from Dr. Arthur Nienhuis and his colleagues at the NIH, has as its major objective the marking of bone marrow stem cells as part of ABMT in three forms of cancer: multiple myeloma, breast cancer, and CML. In the use of such autologous transplants, it has not been proven formally in humans that it is stem cells from the rescue marrow that reengraft, rather than the rescue marrow simply providing progenitor cells until the endogenous marrow recovers. Gene-marking studies would seem to be the only way to resolve this issue unequivocally in humans. There are several major objectives to this clinical study. First, a fractionated (CD34+ enriched)[113,114] component derived either from the bone marrow or from peripheral blood is proposed to be marked with one of two different, distinguishable marking vectors. Separately marked marrow-derived and peripheral blood–derived stem cells will allow an assessment of the relative contribution of these two sources of stem cells to the reconstruction process (this is the protocol proposed for CML and multiple myeloma; peripheral blood stem cells will not be used in breast cancer patients). The clinical approach also will allow reconstitution kinetics to be studied with these two different cell fractions. This protocol (Dunbar et al., clinical protocol submitted to NIH RAC, June 1992) unlike the earlier marker protocols, proposes the use of specific growth factors, a combination of interleukin 3 (IL-3), interleukin 6 (IL-6), and stem cell factor (SCF), during the transduction process.

In all three disease conditions in these protocols, if residual disease cells remain in the transduction marrow (only a 30 per cent aliquot will be CD34 enriched and used for marking), then relapse cells can be analyzed to see if they contain the marker genes, thereby addressing the same origin-of-relapse question described for the previously mentioned protocols.

Because differing conditioning regimens are used for these ABMTs (e.g., fully ablative for myeloma and CML, not fully ablative for breast cancer), any differences in patterns or efficiencies in reconstitution with these different regimens must be analyzed by the marking patterns of progeny cells. This set of studies, therefore, will be able to address some of the pivotal questions of long-term and short-term reconstitution after BMT in humans. The protocol was approved by the NIH RAC in June 1992.

Another protocol (F.S. Scheuning et al., clinical protocol submitted to NIH RAC, September 1992) that has as its objective the evaluation of repopulating cells isolated from the peripheral circulation also was approved by the NIH RAC in September 1992. The study, to be conducted at the Fred Hutchison Cancer Center in Seattle, proposes to obtain peripheral blood repopulating cells from patients with breast cancer, Hodgkin's disease, or one of several lymphoid malignancies, fractionate them to enrich for CD34+ cells, and introduce a marker gene using a retroviral vector. The cells then would be reintroduced at the time of ABMT, and blood cells followed and tested for the presence of the marker gene. Preclinical studies to support this work have been conducted in dogs.[115] An additional interesting feature of this protocol is that, in one variation, peripheral blood repopulating cells from an identical twin, without a malignancy, would be used.

Finally, two protocols have received NIH RAC approval in September 1992 that aim to pursue and optimize bone marrow purging procedures. The first, from St. Judes in Memphis, aims to purge bone marrow with immunologic procedures in neuroblastoma patients and would replace the existing neuroblastoma marker study. The rationale for pursuing this approach stems from the initial data obtained from the two relapsed patients with marked disease cells in the AML study. The second study, from M.D. Anderson Cancer Center in Houston, aims to study the efficacy of purging in chronic lymphocytic leukemia (CLL). Both these protocols illustrate the continuing clinical applications and significance of gene-marking technology to the development of better clinical strategies for the treatment of a variety of malignancies.

LIVER MARKING PROTOCOLS

A gene-marking strategy is proposed to be used in a clinical protocol that aims to study hepatocellular transplantation as an alternative to whole-liver transplantation. This study was proposed by researchers from Baylor College of Medicine in Houston.[116] The objectives are to isolate hepatocytes from a heterologous donor liver, introduce the *neo®* gene using a retroviral vector, and then reintroduce the hepatocytes into a donor with a diseased liver. In this way, it is hoped that the newly introduced cells will be able to provide essential liver functions, perhaps for a sufficient time until a whole liver is available for transplantation.

GENE THERAPY PROTOCOLS

ADA Deficiency

With the successful initiation of the original TIL marker protocol, it was possible to propose a genuine therapeutic protocol to demonstrate the clinical utility of gene therapy. The ADA protocol began in September 1990 about 15 months after the start of the TIL marker protocol.

ADA deficiency is a rare genetic disorder resulting from a deficiency or total lack of an enzyme of purine metabolism that results in a severe immune deficiency. It is one of the set of severe combined immunodeficiency diseases with a simple single-gene defect as its basis. The disease is manifested in lymphocytes, primarily T but also B lymphocytes, that fail to develop and mature normally as a result of build-up of toxic levels of the metabolite deoxyadenosine. It had become the logical initial gene therapy target[10] since the mid-1980s, with the realization that the other major candidates, the hemoglobinopathies, required a level of control over the expression of the introduced gene that was not possible with existing vector technology. The other feature that made ADA deficiency an attractive candidate was the possibility that corrected cells might have a selective growth advantage over noncorrected cells in the patient. Finally, it was a disorder of the bone marrow and therefore was amenable to an ex vivo gene therapy approach.

ADA deficiency is cured by a matched BMT, and this is the treatment of choice for the approximately 30 per cent of patients for whom a matched donor is available. Untreated patients usually die before the age of 2 from any of a variety of common infections they are unable to combat. A recently developed advance has been enzyme replacement using PEG-ADA[117]—the bovine form of the enzyme modified with polyethylene glycol. This treatment, involving frequent intramuscular injections, usually causes initial clinical improvement, and significantly increases the numbers of circulating lymphocytes from their extremely low values without treatment. However, in the longer term, patients sometimes regress on PEG-ADA therapy, with lymphocyte counts declining and with the patients becoming refractory to increases in PEG-ADA dosage. The reasons for this are not fully understood. Mismatched BMT also has been tried with ADA-deficiency patients, but success rates are not encouraging, although the technology is improving.

The initial gene therapy approach was to attempt to correct the bone marrow stem cells, but introduction and efficient expression of genes in primate bone marrow was technically difficult to achieve in the late 1980s. Two factors were responsible for a change in the clinical objective toward correction of lymphocytes rather than bone marrow. The first was the observation that in matched BMT the patients often retain all of their own cells except the T cells, which are exclusively from the donor.[118] The second was the success of the TIL marker experiment. The lymphocyte correction approach also had the advantage, from a safety perspective, that a terminally differentiated cell population was to be manipulated.

The protocol[119] proposed, therefore, to collect the patient's mononuclear blood cells by leukaphoresis and to culture the isolated cells using the OKT3 antibody and recombinant IL-2 to encourage activation and growth of the T lymphocytes. The T cells would be transduced with the retroviral vector LASN,[34] which carries a normal human ADA gene as well as a *neo®* gene. It was proposed to repeat this procedure once a month, thereby taking account of the temporal changes in the T-cell repertoire with respect to the antigens to which the patients may be exposed. The patients would continue to receive PEG-ADA; treatment with PEG-ADA for at least 9 months prior to gene therapy was an inclusion criterion because this would ensure sufficient T cells in the patient's circulation to make correction possible.

The preclinical data to support the protocol included studies demonstrating the correction of cell lines and primary cells from patients in vitro,[120] as well as the demonstration that corrected lymphocytes survived and continued to express the ADA gene in vivo in immune-deficient mice.[121,122] Studies also were conducted on the survival of corrected lymphocytes in vivo in Rhesus monkeys.[123] The protocol[119,124] received NIH RAC and FDA approval, and began with a 4-year-old girl at the NIH in September 1990.

The patient had been treated for 2 years previously with PEG-ADA and had had an initial good response to the enzyme replacement therapy. However, her T cells subsequently had declined and she was anergic, subject to frequent infections, and restricted to her own home prior to the initiation of gene therapy. Over the initial 15 months, she received eight infusions of cells and showed a significant clinical improvement. Her total T-cell count rose and has been maintained in the normal range, and ADA activity in mononuclear cells has risen steadily to approach 20 to 25 per cent of normal levels. A significant improvement in a number of immune function studies was seen,[51] and she has been able to respond to several vaccinations. The general health status of the patient has improved markedly, and she now leads a relatively normal life and attends a public school. A second patient was commenced on the protocol in January 1991 and is showing similar responses.

Although both patients appear to be showing very encouraging responses, it is still likely that they have not recovered a complete immunologic repertoire, evidenced by the fact that positive skin tests have not been seen for all antigens (M. Blaese, personal communication). For this reason, an addition to the current protocol was proposed. This involves the isolation of a CD34+ enriched peripheral blood cell fraction together with the introduction into these cells (including putative repopulating stem cells) of a human ADA gene via a retroviral vector and the infusion of these gene-corrected cells into the patient. The vector would be slightly different from LASN (and therefore distinguishable by PCR techniques). The lymphocyte correction would continue as before. The monitoring of the patient's circulating blood cells over extended periods of time should allow determination of any contribution of the modified CD34-enriched cells to the mature T-cell component.

No ablative procedures are proposed to make "room" in the bone marrow for any modified repopulating cells. The hypothesis is that any cell that is corrected should have a selective growth advantage. This certainly seems to be the case for corrected lymphocytes; in one of the patients, good evidence for a selective advantage was obtained from the persistence of marked cells during a 6.5-month interval without cell infusions. It is hoped that a similar such advantage may allow corrected stem cells to repopulate the marrow and progressively contribute to the corrected T-cell pool in the circulation. The modification to the ADA protocol has been approved by the NIH RAC and the FDA, and is likely to begin in early 1993.

A second gene therapy protocol for ADA deficiency has begun in Milan, Italy. A 5-year-old patient received a mixture of ADA gene–corrected T cells, and also gene-modified progenitor-enriched bone marrow cells. Two different retroviral vectors, distinguishable at the DNA level, were used in this protocol, which began in March 1992. No reports are yet available with regard to any clinical responses. Based on extensive studies on ADA gene transfer into nonhuman primate bone marrow, it seems likely that a bone marrow clinical study for ADA gene therapy will begin shortly in the Netherlands.

Cancer Protocols

TIL/TUMOR NECROSIS FACTOR

The logical extension of the TIL marking protocol was to attempt to use these cells, modified with genes for therapeutic agents, as delivery vehicles to target substances to the actual tumor sites, provided it could be shown that at least a portion of TILs have the ability to return to the sites of tumor. To attempt to use gene therapy in this way is an excellent illustration of the protein drug delivery potential of the technology.

The basic concept behind this approach is straightforward. A number of lymphokines, cytokines, and antitumor agents have shown promise for cancer therapy, but are clearly agents that are naturally produced only at local sites. When administered by systemic injection, very short serum half-lives (of the order of a few minutes) commonly are seen, and thus very high doses are required to achieve effective local concentrations. With such high doses, unacceptable toxicities frequently are seen. If a cell, particularly a short-lived one, can be modified to produce such a compound by gene transfer, and if that cell can seek out tumor sites, then there is the real prospect of production of effective concentrations locally with consequently much lower systemic levels, toxicities, and side effects.

This approach was taken first with the agent tumor necrosis factor (TNF). TNF, also know as cathexin, is produced by activated macrophages and is known to play a central role in the inflammation process.[125] In addition, a large number of animal modeling studies have demonstrated that injection of recombinant TNF can mediate necrosis and regression of a variety of experimental cancers in mice.[126,127] These observations have led to clinical testing of TNF in patients with advanced cancers.[128,129] No antitumors effects of TNF could be observed, except in circumstances in which high local TNF concentrations could be achieved by intralesional injection.[130] Lack of clinical efficacy by systemic injection of TNF is likely due to an inability to achieve effective concentrations at desired sites. The toxic effects of TNF become clinically limiting in humans at doses of 8 μg/kg, whereas rodents are able to tolerate 50-fold higher levels.[130] This could explain the successes in rodent models compared to lack of clinical efficacy in humans, and points to the need for other ways to deliver TNF in humans to achieve clinical benefit.

For these reasons, the TNF gene was chosen as the first potentially therapeutic agent gene to be introduced into TILs via retroviral vectors. TNF gene–containing retroviral vectors were constructed and demonstrated to be able to transfer the functioning gene into human TILs. For preclinical animal modeling, technical difficulties prevented a direct TIL study. Although a mouse TIL model exists—a fibrosarcoma that can be transplanted and that can yield TILs capable of eliminating these tumors in mice—it has proven extraordinarily difficult to manipulate primary mouse TILs genetically to introduce foreign genes into them. Mouse TILs are very poorly transduced by Mo-MuLV-derived vectors, even when ecotropically packaged. The reasons for this are not understood, because mouse TILs have been shown to contain significant levels of the mRNA for the ecotropic receptor (R. Lyons, personal communication).

Other approaches to preclinical efficacy models therefore were used. The most compelling of these was the introduction, via the TNF gene–containing retroviral vectors, of the TNF gene into the mouse transplantable fibrosarcoma, WP4, in vitro and then its introduction into animals. Whereas tumor cells modified with a control neo® vector grew tumors at the same rate as unmodified tumor cells, the TNF gene–expressing tumor cells developed tumors only to a certain size, after which the tumors regressed completely.[131] The demonstration that this regression could be reversed by the use of anti-TNF antibodies provided further strong evidence that local expression of TNF was responsible for tumor regression.

The protocol received RAC approval in July 1990, but the FDA required an initial phase I toxicity study to be conducted with initially very low doses of TNF/TILs in the absence of recombinant IL-2 and with a gradual dose escalation of the TILs within the same patient. This was requested because of (1) the already established knowledge of toxic effects of TNF in humans and (2) the fact that the bulk of infused TILs are known to be trapped initially, and probably destroyed, in the liver, spleen, and lungs. The phase I study therefore was required to confirm that there would be no side effects from production of large amounts of ectopic TNF at these sites. This study began in January 1991, and four patients received the regimen with no apparent toxicities from the TNF. Five patients have been or currently are being treated with TNF/TILs at therapeutic levels, but no data are yet available to indicate whether the TNF production has improved or augmented the therapeutic benefit of TILs alone.[132] It has proven difficult to obtain good levels of TNF expression in the TILs of many patients,[133] and modifications of the vector to improve expression or even to modify the TNF gene itself to increase the amount secreted[134] still may be required. It is clear that there are a number of other cytokine genes that could be delivered in this way.

TIL/MODIFIED TUMOR CELL PROTOCOLS

One of the objectives of improving TIL immunotherapy is to find ways in which to induce the body to make more effective TILs. An approach to doing this has come from the animal model studies used to support the TNF/TIL protocol. These studies[131] showed dramatic regressions resulting from local TNF production by the introduced tumor cells themselves. This regression was shown to be mediated by the immune system, because it could be abrogated in irradiated mice, and also by depletion in mice of the CD8+ T-cell subpopulation. The tumor cells that produced TNF also could be shown to inhibit the growth of unmodified cells implanted at the same site. Even more significantly, animals that experienced a regression with TNF-modified tumor cells are able to reject a subsequent challenge by unmodified tumor. These data imply that TNF-modified tumor cells are more immunogenic and able to elicit an immunity sufficient to influence unmodified tumor. This same effect has been demonstrated for a variety of other cytokines in similar model systems, and is discussed in more detail later in this chapter. The TNF studies suggested that this may represent a way to generate more effective TILs.

Other studies have suggested that subcutaneous injection of tumor preparations, with or without prior irradiation, sometimes can lead to more cytotoxic TILs (as tested in vitro) or provoke stronger immune responses in human patients. On the basis of these studies, it was proposed[135] to sample a patient's tumor, generate cultures of tumor cells, and introduce via a retroviral vector the TNF gene. The cells then would be injected subcutaneously and intradermally, and 3 weeks later the injection sites and draining lymph nodes would be removed and used to establish cultures of T lymphocytes. These then would be reinfused into patients in a fashion analogous to that used for TIL therapy. This protocol, after additional animal modeling showing that the approach was able to reduce the number of lung metastases in a rodent tumor model, was approved by the regulatory agencies and began at the NIH in October 1991.

A very similar protocol[136] also was proposed by the NIH group, but using a retroviral vector encoding the IL-2 gene in place of TNF. The rationale and preclinical data to support the use of this agent came from a variety of sources. Early studies involving introduction of IL-2 genes by transfection into the CT26 murine tumor[137] was shown to eliminate the ability of these cells to form tumors in animals. CD8+ cell removal restored the ability of these modified cells to cause tumors. Protection against subsequent challenge by the parental tumor also was shown, although this effect was relatively short lived (approximately 4 weeks). The modified cells also were shown to have elicited cytotoxic T-cell activity against the parental line, something that the unmodified tumor was not capable of doing. Further studies[137] with a fibrosarcoma mouse model showed similar effects after introduction of the IL-2 gene, as well as more lasting immunity (several months). Additionally, T-cell–mediated cytolytic activity persisted for more than 2 months.

Rosenberg and his colleagues performed similar studies in support of the clinical protocol.[136] The murine tumor models used were the MCA 205 fibrosarcoma, an immunogenic tumor cell line, and the poorly immunogenic MCA 102 tumor line. This latter tumor cell line has not been observed to generate in vivo immunity, but, after modification with the gene for IL-2, tumor generation was eliminated. Preirradiation of the mice or CD8+ cell depletion restored tumor formation. On this basis, a clinical protocol identical in its approach to the TNF/tumor cell study was submitted and approved. The study began in March 1992, but no clinical response data have yet been reported. It is likely that, because of the lengthy nature of the manipulations involved, clinical data will accumulate slowly.

PROTOCOLS FOR INTRODUCING LYMPHOKINES INTO TUMOR CELLS

HLA-Matched Allogeneic Melanoma Cells Secreting Interleukin 2

An alternative way to deliver IL-2 via its gene, in the context of a tumor vaccine, has been proposed by a group from Memorial Sloan Kettering Cancer Center.[138] The proposal is to make use of a human melanoma cell line, SK-MEL 29, which is an irradiated cell line that already has been tested as a cancer vaccine,[139] or one of two renal cell carcinoma cell lines (B. Gansbacher et al., submission to NIH RAC, June 1992). The human IL-2 gene would be introduced into these cell lines, and, after verification of expression of the IL-2 gene product, the cells would be irradiated and then administered to selected patients with metastatic melanoma or renal cell carcinoma as a subcutaneous injection in the thigh or the arm. This would be followed by a series of booster injections. The patient selection, among other criteria, would be on the basis of matching an HLA antigen, A2.

This protocol is noteworthy in that it makes unnecessary the lengthy and sometimes difficult process of establishing cell lines from a patient's own tumor (i.e., the donor cell is an allogeneic cell line). The irradiation of the cell line eliminates the chance of this cell growing, possibly into a tumor, in the patient. Preclinical studies in mouse models[136,137] provided support for the protocol, which received approval from the NIH RAC in June 1992.

IL-2–Modified Neuroblastoma Protocol

This protocol (M. Brenner et al., NIH RAC clinical protocol submission, June 1992) follows on from the neuroblastoma marker protocol in progress at St. Judes Hospital in Memphis. It proposes to examine as a phase I study the safety of subcutaneous injection of IL-2–modified autologous neuroblastoma cells in relapsed or refractory neuroblastoma patients. Cells are not planned to be irradiated prior to injection, but will represent quantities less than 0.001 per cent of the patient's total tumor burden. The initial study proposes only to look at safety and to determine if it is possible to detect any major histocompatibility complex (MHC)–restricted or -unrestricted antitumor responses that may be induced. It is conceivable, although not likely at the initial early doses, that therapeutic benefits will be seen. No animal models of neuroblastoma exist, although IL-2 introduction into other tumor models (see earlier in this chapter) has resulted in regression of tumors. The preclinical work generated for this protocol therefore has focused on establishment of cell lines from neuroblastoma patients, their transduction with an IL-2/neo® gene retroviral vector, selection with

G418, and demonstration of secretion in vitro of significant levels of IL-2. It also was demonstrated that patient's lymphocytes respond in vitro to levels of IL-2 that stimulate cytotoxic effector cells active against autologous, nontransduced neuroblastoma cells. The protocol was approved by the NIH RAC in June 1992.

IL-4 Gene–Modified Cells for a Tumor Vaccine Protocol

Another lymphokine, and yet another way of delivering its gene and gene product, has been proposed in a protocol from the Pittsburgh Cancer Center (M. Lotze et al., NIH RAC clinical protocol submission, September 1992). The lymphokine is IL-4, which this group currently is using as an injectable recombinant protein to see if it improves the homing of TILs to sites of tumor.[102] The IL-4 gene, introduced by transfection into murine tumors such as the renal tumor cell line Renca, or colorectal carcinoma CT26, was shown to abrogate generation of tumors.[140] In addition, systemic immunity appeared to be generated, and this was tumor specific and mediated via CD8+ cells.[141] Most significantly, introducing IL-4–modified tumor into animals in which unmodified tumor cells had been established 9 days before resulted in a response against the unmodified cells.[141] In the Renca tumor experiments, an infiltration of eosinophytes and macrophages was observed, in contrast to IL-2–modified Renca, in which the infiltrate was predominantly T lymphocytes. A hypothesis for the effects of IL-4 in this context, therefore, is that antigen-presenting cells are recruited to the tumor site and that the local IL-4 generation is responsible.

The other major feature of this protocol is to use autologous skin fibroblasts from the patient as the cell used to express the IL-4. The target patient population proposed is individuals with melanoma, renal cell carcinoma, and breast or colorectal carcinoma who have failed conventional therapies. Fibroblast cultures would be established and transduced with IL-4 vectors. A single cell suspension of tumor also would be obtained, and these two mixed to constitute a vaccine that would be delivered to sites over the left lumbar region after irradiation of the cell mixture. The protocol received RAC approval in September 1992.

Other Lymphokines

This general approach of delivery of cytokines or lymphokines by introduction of their genes into a patient's cells (e.g., tumor cells, fibroblasts) or even allogeneic transplantation is an active area of preclinical and clinical research. Animal model studies have indicated that a wide array of lymphokines and cytokines may have the ability to produce a clinically relevant stimulation of an immune response able to attack tumors. These molecules include IL-2, IL-4, IL-6, IL-7, interferon γ, and granulocyte-macrophage colony-stimulating factor (see ref. 50 for review). It can be argued that the animal models to support this concept are somewhat artificial in that they are transplantable and not spontaneous tumors, as is the case in humans, and that they or their gene-transduced progeny often are selected clonally. Effects on distal, unmodified or preestablished tumors have not been demonstrated. Nevertheless, the potential for this approach is great. Additionally, there is the prospect of delivering combinations of these agents to improve efficacies.

CELL SURFACE MARKER GENE DELIVERY TO TUMORS: IN VIVO PROTOCOL

An illustration of the variety of innovative approaches that are being used to develop cancer therapy involving gene therapy comes from a protocol[73] that already has been initiated at the University of Michigan Medical Center. This protocol, which started in June 1992 with the treatment of a melanoma patient, is of significance also in that the gene delivery system is not a retroviral vector and that the vector (a DNA molecule encapsulated in a liposome) was injected directly into the tumor site of the patient, thereby representing a true in vivo gene therapy approach. A further four patients have received this treatment.

The objective of the protocol is to elicit a strong antitumor immune response by introducing into HLA-B7–negative tumor cells the gene for the human class I MHC HLA-B7, in the hope that an immune reaction to such modified cells also will be effective against other tumor cells. The preclinical studies[142] that supported this protocol have involved a mouse model using an allogeneic class I MHC gene, H-2K^s, into the CT26 mouse tumor cell model. The vector system used consists of a DNA molecule containing the gene for the surface marker driven by a strong viral promoter. This is encapsulated into a liposome preparation by standard procedures and then directly injected into the tumor sites in mice. The development of a cytotoxic T lymphocyte response that was directed to both modified and unmodified tumor cells was observed. Additionally, when vector was injected into preestablished tumors of less than 1 cm diameter, there was regression of tumors in comparison with controls, although preinjection of animals with the H-2K^s gene–modified tumor cells was required to see a definitive response.

The protocol received regulatory approval, but also elicited discussion on the possibility of inadvertent modification of other cells in the patient, including the germline. Although animals studies have failed to show any transfer into other cell types,[142] the patient population has been restricted initially to patients beyond reproductive age. No data are yet available from the study.

TUMOR SUPPRESSOR GENES/ONCOGENE EXPRESSION MODIFICATION PROTOCOL

Lung cancer leads all other cancers as a cause of death among Americans and currently is estimated to be responsible for 140,000 deaths per year.[143] The dominant type of lung cancer is non–small-cell lung cancer (NSCLC), divided into adenocarcinoma and squamous cell types. All current treatment methods for NSCLC have low effectiveness, and about 85 per cent of patients who contract the disease will die of it.

Recently much evidence has accumulated to suggest that genetic events related to mutation or deletion of tumor suppressor genes, or dominant oncogenes, underlie the maintenance of malignancy in NSCLC. For example, the tumor suppressor gene p53 is mutated in greater than 50 per cent of human NSCLC cases,[144] and as many as a third may have mutations in a member of the ras gene family.[145]

A significant proportion of NSCLC patients fail therapy at the primary site of tumor,[146] and these patients, with an unresectable obstructing tumor that is resistant to conventional therapy, have a median survival of months or less. For such cases, a therapeutic approach has been designed that aims, through the use of gene transfer, to reverse a single known genetic event in a proportion of the tumor cells in an attempt to revert the malignant phenotype. Although it is clear that, in most forms of cancer (including NSCLC), multiple genetic events are required to establish a malignant phenotype, in a number of cases it has been demonstrated in vitro and in animal models that reversal of only one of these events[147–150] can lead to a reversal of uncontrolled growth, colony formation in soft agar, or tumor formation in animals.

The clinical approach that has been proposed involves the direct injection of retroviral vector preparations into the local tumor bed. The two retroviral vectors planned to be used clinically are, first, a construct that produces an antisense transcript RNA to the K-ras oncogene, and, second, a construct that produces the normal, wild-type human p53 gene product. The first is designed to block specifically the production of the mutant K-ras protein. The second aims to provide normal p53 protein to replace the function of the mutated protein. Two key features of the protocol are that the vectors should be taken up only by rapidly dividing tumor cells and not the surrounding bronchial epithelium, and that not all tumor cells are required to take up the vector. On the second point, animal modeling studies suggest that it is not necessary to modify all cells in the tumor.

Preclinical studies have been generated to support this approach. A specific anti–K-ras antisense retroviral vector was constructed that was shown to inhibit specifically K-ras mRNA synthesis in human tumor cell lines expressing K-ras.[150] This does not affect the expression of other members of the ras family (e.g., N- and H-ras), which are required for normal cell growth. The antisense-inhibited cells lost their original ability to form subcutaneous tumors in nude mice. Also, a p53 gene transfected into malignant colorectal cells was shown to reduce tumorigenicity.[147] It seems likely that p53 mutations are among the most prevalent mutations in human cancers, and loss of p53 may be the final mutational event required to establish malignancy. This also may be true in the mouse. Recent studies on transgenic mice demonstrated that, when the endogenous p53 gene has been "knocked out," high rates of spontaneous tumors of a variety of types result.[151]

The preclinical p53 studies[150] conducted by the M.D. Anderson Cancer Center group involved the use of human lung cancer cells in which p53 was mutated or deleted. These showed that reintroduction of a normal gene suppressed the transformed phenotype as measured by colony growth in soft agar. The studies also support the notion that the wild-type *p53* is dominant and able to suppress the malignant phenotype in cells with mutant or deleted *p53*.

In vivo studies for both the antisense K-*ras* and *p53* approaches were conducted in an orthotopic lung cancer model, in irradiated nude mice. Endobronchial tumors were established with high efficiency in such animals with the H460a cell line. Prior introduction of the K-*ras* antisense tumors with a retroviral vector prevented tumor development in five of six mice. On the basis of these studies, a clinical protocol (J. Roth et al., clinical protocol submitted to NIH RAC) received approval from NIH RAC in September 1992.

GENE TRANSFER OF THE MULTIDRUG RESISTANCE GENE

A high proportion of human cancers either have intrinsically, or acquire, a resistance to chemotherapeutic agents.[152] This resistance is not to just one agent, but to several different drugs (e.g., doxorubicin, vinblastine, colchicine). The common feature seems to be that all of these are amphipathic hydrophobic substances. The gene product that mediates such resistance in human cells has been shown to be a 170-kDa membrane glycoprotein called P, or the multiple drug resistance (MDR) gene product. The gene for this protein has been cloned[153] and found to be one of a large family of transporter protein genes, including bacterial transporters, the transporters of sex peptides in yeast, the chloroquine pump in malaria, and the CFTR gene. The normal *mdr* gene is expressed in a variety of cells, including the biliary surface of hepatocytes, kidney proximal tubule epithelium, and the large and small intestine.[152] Its general function appears to be to protect the apical surface of a variety of epithelial cells from toxic substances.

The clinical concepts for the use of the *mdr* gene in cancer studies derive first from studies of the introduction of the *mdr* gene, under the control of a β-actin promoter, into transgenic mice.[154] For reasons that are not understood, the *mdr* gene appeared to be expressed almost exclusively in the bone marrow of these mice, and this resulted in resistance of the marrow of these animals to daunorubicin-induced leukopenia. Moreover, this drug resistance phenotype could be transplanted from these transgenic mice by BMT to syngeneic recipient mice. This led to the concept of transferring the *mdr* gene to human bone marrow to induce a higher level of protection during chemotherapy treatment. It also stimulated the construction of retroviral vectors containing the *mdr* gene,[155] which then could be used to transfer the gene to bone marrow stem cells. This was achieved successfully in the mouse model, wherein the gene was shown to be able to be transduced into mouse marrow stem cells, and to give rise to peripheral blood cells containing and expressing the *mdr* gene.[156] Most significantly, on treatment with the cytotoxic drug taxol, a substantial enrichment of bone marrow cells containing the *mdr* gene was observed. Additionally, on rechallenge with taxol, these mice exhibited a smaller reduction in their neutrophil counts than control mice.

These observations provide preclinical support for the concept of the use of *mdr* gene transfer during chemotherapy for such diseases as breast and ovarian cancer. Currently protocols are under review by the NIH RAC.

DELIVERY OF THYMIDINE KINASE GENES TO TUMORS

The viral gene from herpes simplex virus (HSV), thymidine kinase (*tk*), is unusual in that it can be used both as a positive and a negative selection marker. In a background of *tk*$^-$ cells, introduction of this gene can enable selection of cells that possess the gene through use of a specific medium containing hypoxanthine, aminopterin, and thiamine (HAT). The presence of the HSV *tk* gene introduced into a cell also serves to render that cell sensitive to killing by the nucleoside analogues acyclovir and gancyclovir. These selection marker properties have made the HSV *tk* gene a useful research tool in gene transfer studies. However, its properties as a negative selection marker also have led to its use in clinical protocols, including approaches to cancer therapy.

Retroviral vectors containing the *tk* gene first were constructed and used for cancer studies by Moolten and Wells.[87] These studies demonstrated that, when a mouse tumor cell line was modified with this vector, the resulting tumors in animals could be ablated by gancyclovir treatment. Similar studies also were reported[74-76] on a glioma rat tumor cell model. However, even in view of these studies, it seemed unlikely that one could transduce the cells in a tumor to generate gancyclovir sensitivity at efficiencies that might give the potential for clinical benefit in human disease. Therefore, the main interest in *tk* gene vectors was as a safety or "suicide" function. For this concept—a safety feature that could be built into vectors—the presence of the *tk* gene could allow killing of all transduced cells by administration of gancyclovir. This could prove useful to end a gene therapy procedure when an agent was no longer required to be delivered. In addition, it represented another important safety feature. Should a transduced cell, as a consequence of a random insertion event, become a tumor cell, then gancyclovir administration should kill all cells harboring the vector.

Ablation of tumors that contained the *tk* gene in at least a proportion of the tumor cells was demonstrated.[76] These studies were conducted with a variety of animal tumor models and showed a totally unexpected "bystander" effect. This effect means that only as few as 10 or 20 per cent of cells in a tumor needed to contain the *tk* gene to render the entire tumor sensitive to ablation on gancyclovir treatment. The mechanism of the bystander effect is not at all clear; it is possible that some product or metabolite is released by the sensitive cells and enters unmodified cells. Under conditions of sufficiently high cell density, the effect can be demonstrated using cells in culture, and this suggests cell-cell contact may have a role in the process.

Whatever the mechanism involved, the observation led to consideration of appropriate cancer targets where this phenomenon could be put to clinical use. One proposal was for ovarian cancer. The studies,[157] involving an ovarian tumor model in mice, demonstrated that mixing unmodified and modified cells of the tumor could result in tumor ablation after gancyclovir administration. A clinical protocol was proposed (Freeman et al., NIH RAC clinical protocol submission, July 1991) and, after additional studies, was approved in February 1992. The clinical trial has not begun. Another disease target was glioblastoma, specifically the highly malignant primary brain tumor, glioblastoma multiforme (GBM). The prognosis for patients with GBM is poor, and, despite treatment of surgical removal of tumor and postoperative high-dose radiation, median survival is 9 to 10 months. On recurrence, the mortality rate is close to 100 per cent within weeks to a few months.

The approach proposed by an NIH group for a glioblastoma clinical study involves the introduction of retroviral vectors to the site of the tumor, using magnetic resonance imaging–guided stereotaxic intratumoral injections. The concept is that tumor cells are the primary cells undergoing cell division in the brain and therefore will be the primary cells to take up and integrate the proviral sequence. Other cells, not undergoing cell division, should remain unaffected. However, the vector will not be delivered as a vector supernatant. Instead, the protocol is to inject directly into the brain tumor an aliquot of the producer cells that generate the vector. These cells, which are likely to survive for at least a few days even though they are of murine origin, will produce vector particles continuously over an extended period and should increase significantly the proportion of cells that are likely to be transduced. Then, administration of gancyclovir is proposed to kill all vector-transduced tumor cells and, as a result of the bystander effect, perhaps the remainder of the tumor cells as well. Additionally, all producer cells, because they harbor and express the HSV *tk* gene, will be killed, providing an effective way to end the treatment and eliminate the delivery system. The concept of using the producer cell line in situ as a delivery system for retroviral vectors was conceived and tested independently by two groups, both using the rat L-9 glioma cell line in a mouse brain tumor model. One set of studies[74,75] showed that the marker gene β-galactosidase could be introduced efficiently into the tumor. The other study[76] used a *tk* gene vector and was able to show dramatic effects of eliminating the tumor with gancyclovir treatment.

The latter study formed the basis for, and part of the preclinical work in support of, a clinical protocol for glioblastoma (Oldfield et al., NIH RAC clinical protocol submission, June 1992). Studies have been conducted to demonstrate that tumor vascular endothelial cells and tumor cells in the brain of rodents are marked (using a β-galactosidase vector producer cell line), validating the concept that the tumor, because of its rapid proliferation, will be the predominant cell type taking up vectors. This protocol received approval from the NIH RAC in June 1992, and began in December 1992. It is significant that the gene therapy ''product'' that is used for this procedure is not the retroviral vector itself, as is the case for the vast majority of gene therapy protocols conducted so far, but is actually an aliquot of the cells, the producer cells, that generate the vector.

OTHER GENE THERAPY PROTOCOLS

The gene therapy protocols and studies described above have focused primarily on analysis and treatment of cancer. However, in addition to the ADA gene therapy protocol, other clinical studies have begun or are being developed for therapy of several genetic diseases and also for AIDs. A gene therapy approach for the treatment of the genetic disease familial hypercholesterolemia is being tested in a clinical study at the University of Michigan.[158] This disease is characterized by vastly elevated cholesterol levels and early-onset vascular disease, and is due to defective or absent receptor on hepatocytes for low-density lipoprotein. The clinical strategy has been to correct a sample of the patient's own hepatocytes, obtained by a liver resection, using a retroviral vector containing the human low-density lipoprotein receptor gene. The corrected cells then are returned to the patient via an indwelling catheter retained after the initial hepatectomy. Preclinical studies[43] in animals, including in the animal model of this disease, the Watanabe rabbit, have shown that cells corrected in this fashion can survive and function after readministration.

A clinical study to address the blood coagulation disorder hemophilia B has been initiated in Fudan Hospital, China.[159] Low levels or lack of the protein factor IX underlie this genetic disease, and a large body of preclinical work has been conducted to attempt to generate an effective gene therapy approach to this disease. The approach of the group in China has been to use the patient's autologous fibroblasts, modify them with a retroviral vector to make factor IX, and return them to the patient by intraperitoneal and subcutaneous injection. Two patients have been treated.

For approaches to AIDS, two initial clinical studies, both of which have received RAC approval, involve marker protocols. The first[160] seeks to mark amplified clones of autologous cytokine T lymphocytes from AIDS patients undergoing BMT for treatment for leukemia. The marker gene, a fusion between the *neo*® gene and HSV *tk*,[49] will serve both to be able to follow the fate of these cells and as a potential safety feature (through use of gancyclovir) should uncontrolled growth of these cells in the patient be observed. The second, a marker study, (R.E. Walker et al., NIH RAC clinical protocol submission, September 1992) aims to test whether lymphocyte infusion has the potential to benefit late-stage AIDS patients by restoring immune functions, as has been observed for ADA patients. The strategy is to infuse gene-marked PBLs from an uninfected identical twin into the infected sibling.

Gene therapy approaches also are being developed for human immunodeficiency virus (HIV). Most advanced is a vaccination strategy[161] in which the HIV gp160 envelope protein gene is built into a retroviral vector. This is introduced into autologous fibroblasts of a patient, and these cells then are returned to the patient. The concept is that the fibroblasts will produce the HIV gp160 protein and process and present at least parts of the product on their surface. Presentation to the immune system in this way is hoped to generate a stronger cytotoxic T lymphocyte response to the virus than by conventional vaccination ap-

TABLE 23–3. GENE MARKER/THERAPY CLINICAL TRIALS

GENE	VECTOR	TARGET CELL	DISEASE	INSTITUTION	STATUS
Gene Marking Protocols					
1. neo^R	RV	TILs	Malignant melanoma	NIH, Bethesda, MD	Completed
2. neo^R	RV	Leukemic cells in bone marrow	Pediatric acute myeloid leukemia	St. Judes Childrens Research Hospital, Memphis, TN	In progress
3. neo^R	RV	Neuroblastoma blast cells in bone marrow	Neuroblastoma	St. Judes Childrens Research Hospital, Memphis, TN	In progress
4. neo^R	RV	Leukemic cells in bone marrow	Chronic myelogenous leukemia	University of Texas M.D. Anderson Cancer Center, Houston, TX	In progress
5. neo^R	RV	TILs	Malignant melanoma	University of Pittsburgh, Pittsburgh, PA	In progress
6. neo^R	RV	Leukemic cells in bone marrow	Adult acute leukemia	Indiana University, Indianapolis, IN	In progress
7. neo^R	RV	Peripheral stem cell Bone marrow, stem cells, cancer cells	Breast cancer, multiple myeloma, chronic myelogenous leukemia	NIH, Bethesda, MD	In progress
8. neo^R	RV	TILs	Malignant melanoma	Centre Leon Bérard, Lyon, France	In progress
9. neo^R	RV	TILs, CD4 +, CD8 + fractions	Malignant melanoma, renal cell carcinoma	University of California, Los Angeles, CA	RAC, FDA approved
10. neo^R	RV	Peripheral stem cells	Leukemias	University of Washington, Seattle, WA	RAC approved
11. neo^R	RV	Hepatocytes	Liver failure	Baylor College of Medicine, Houston, TX	RAC approved
12. Hygromycin tk fusion	RV	Cytotoxic T lymphocytes	HIV lymphoma	University of Washington, Seattle, WA	RAC, FDA approved
13. neo^R	RV	Lymphocytes (identical sibling)	HIV	NIH, Bethesda, MD	RAC approved
14. neo^R	RV	Leukemic cell purging from bone marrow	Neuroblastoma	St. Judes Childrens Research Hospital, Memphis, TN	RAC approved
15. neo^R	RV	Leukemic cell purging from bone marrow	Chronic myelogeneous leukemia	University of Texas, M.D. Anderson Cancer Center, Houston, TX	RAC approved
Gene Therapy Protocols					
1. ADA	RV	T lymphocyte	ADA-deficient SCID	NIH, Bethesda, MD	In progress
2. ADA	RV	Peripheral stem cells	ADA-deficient SCID	NIH, Bethesda, MD	RAC, FDA approved
3. TNF	RV	TILs	Malignant melanoma	NIH, Bethesda, MD	In progress
4. TNF	RV	Tumor cells	Advanced cancer	NIH, Bethesda, MD	In progress
5. IL-2	RV	Tumor cells	Advanced cancer	NIH, Bethesda, MD	In progress
6. LDL receptor	RV	Hepatocytes	Familial hyper-cholesterolemia	University of Michigan, Ann Arbor, MI	In progress
7. HLA-B7	DNA-liposome	Melanoma cells	Malignant melanoma	University of Michigan, Ann Arbor, MI	In progress
8. HSV tk	RV producer cell	Glioblastoma cells	Brain tumor	NIH, Bethesda, MD/Genetic Therapy, Inc., Gaithersburg, MD	In progress
9. ADA	RV	T lymphocytes, bone marrow stem cells	ADA-deficient SCID	San Raffaele Scientific Institute, Milan, Italy	In progress
10. Factor IX	RV	Autologous skin fibroblasts	Hemophilia B	Fudan University and Shanghai Hospital, Shanghai, China	In progress
11. IL-2	RV	Tumor cell line	Malignant melanoma, renal cell cancer	Memorial Sloan Kettering Cancer Center, New York, NY	RAC approved

Table continued on following page

TABLE 23–3. *Continued*

GENE	VECTOR	TARGET CELL	DISEASE	INSTITUTION	STATUS
12. HSV *tk*	Tumor cell line transduced with RV	Tumor cells	Ovarian cancer	University of Rochester, Rochester, NY	RAC approved
13. IL-2	RV	Neuroblastoma cells	Neuroblastoma	St. Judes Childrens Research Hospital, Memphis, TN	In progress
14. IL-4	RV	Tumor cells	Malignant melanoma	University of Pittsburgh, Pittsburgh, PA	RAC approved
15. Antisense *Ras* or *p53*	RV (in vivo)	Tumor cells	Non–small-cell lung cancer	University of Texas M.D. Anderson Cancer Center, Houston, TX	RAC approved
16. HIV gp160 envelope	RV	Autologous fibroblasts	HIV	Viagene, Inc., San Diego, CA	FDA approved
17. ADA	RV	Bone marrow stem cells	ADA-deficient SCID	Institute for Applied Radiobiology & Immunology TNO with University of Leiden, Leiden, The Netherlands	National review pending
18. CFTR	Adenovirus (in vivo)	Lung epithelial cells	Cystic fibrosis	NIH, Bethesda, MD	RAC approved
19. CFTR	Adenovirus (in vivo)	Lung epithelial cells	Cystic fibrosis	University of Michigan, Ann Arbor, MI	RAC approved
20. CFTR	Adenovirus (in vivo)	Nasal epithelial cells	Cystic fibrosis	University of Iowa	RAC approved

Abbreviations: RV, retroviral vector; SCID, severe combined immune deficiency, LDL, low-density lipoprotein; other abbreviations as in text.

proaches. Extensive animal safety and modeling studies have been done within the limits possible without an animal model that closely resembles human AIDS. This protocol, although not yet having been reviewed by NIH RAC, has received FDA approval.

Finally, therapeutic approaches to the delivery of both extracellular decoys, such as the soluble CD4 receptor or its variants, and intracellular decoys or inhibitory molecules, such as the TAR and RRE target sequences for *tat* and *rev* regulatory proteins of HIV or antisense and ribozyme approaches, have been subjects of intensive preclinical research.[162] An initial protocol to attempt an intracellular decoy approach using autologous lymphocytes and the TAR decoy from a group at Sloan Kettering was submitted to the NIH RAC (C. Smith et al., clinical protocol submission) in June 1992 but was deferred pending more cell culture and animal studies.

SUMMARY AND CONCLUSIONS

The application of gene therapy technologies to clinical research is now expanding rapidly. A complete listing of gene marker/therapy clinical trials that have received RAC or a national approval as of December 1992 is given in Table 23–3. Attempts at cancer therapy have been in the forefront of early gene therapy trials, but there has been no reported demonstration of clinical benefit as yet. Initial proof of the principle for gene therapy has been

obtained in the ADA clinical protocol. Additionally, useful data have been obtained from the initial gene-marker protocols for leukemias. It is a reasonable expectation that efficacious therapies for cancer will be developed through gene therapy.

REFERENCES

1. Friedmann R, Toblin R: Gene therapy for human genetic disease? Science 175:949, 1972
2. Editorial: Repair of genetic defects predicted. Pediatr News 2:1, 1968
3. Graham FL, van der Eb AJ: A new technique for the assay of infectivity of human adenovirus 5 DNA. Virology 52:456, 1973
4. Wigler M, Silverstein LS, Lee A, et al: Transfer of purified herpes virus thymidine kinase gene to cultured mouse cells. Cell 11:223, 1977
5. Anderson WF, Killos L, Sanders-Haigh L, et al: Replication and expression of thymidine kinase and human globin genes microinjected into mouse fibroblasts. Proc Natl Acad Sci USA 77:5399, 1980
6. Friedman T: The future for gene therapy: A re-evaluation. Ann N Y Acad Sci 265:141, 1976
7. Anderson WF, Fletcher JC: Gene therapy in human beings: When is it ethical to begin? N Engl J Med 303:1293, 1980
8. Anderson WF: Gene therapy. JAMA 246:2737, 1981
9. Human Gene Therapy—A Background Paper. OTA BP-BA-32. Washington, DC, U.S. Congress, Office of Technology Assessment, 1984
10. Anderson WF: Prospects for human gene therapy. Science 226:401, 1984
11. Staubinger RM, Papahadjopoulos D: Liposomes as carriers for

intracellular delivery of nucleic acids. Meth Enzymol *101*:512, 1983

12. Felgner PL, Gadek TG, Holm M, et al: Lipofection: A highly efficient lipid-mediated DNA-transfection procedure. Proc Natl Acad Sci USA *84*:7413, 1987

13. Wu GY, Wu CH: Evidence for targeted delivery to Hep G2 hepatoma cells in vitro. Biochemistry *27*:887, 1988

14. Wu C, Wilson JM, Wu GY: Targeting genes: Delivery and persistent expression of a foreign gene driven by mammalian regulatory elements in vivo. J Biol Chem *264*:16985, 1989

15. Curiel DT, Wagner E, Cotten M, et al: High-efficiency gene transfer mediated by adenovirus coupled to DNA-polylysine complexes. Hum Gene Ther *3*:147, 1992

16. Neuman E, Schaefer-Ridder M, Wang Y, et al: Gene transfer into mouse lyoma cells by electroporation in high electric fields. EMBO J *7*:841, 1980

17. Wolff JA, Malone RW, Williams P, et al: Direct gene transfer into mouse muscle in vivo. Science *247*:1465, 1990

18. Yang NS, Burkholder J, Roberts B, et al: In vivo and in vitro gene transfer to mammalian somatic cells by particle bombardment. Proc Natl Acad Sci USA *87*:9568, 1990

19. Gilboa E, Eglitis MA, Kantoff PN, et al: Transfer and expression of cloned genes using retroviral vectors. Biotechniques *4*:504, 1986

20. Eglitis MA, Anderson WF: Retroviral vectors for introduction of genes into mammalian cells. Biotechniques *6*:608, 1988

21. Mann R, Mulligan RC, Buttimore C: Construction of a retroviral packaging mutant and its use to produce helper-free detective retrovirus. Cell *33*:153, 1983

22. Tolstoshev P, Anderson WF: Gene expression using retroviral vectors. Curr Opin Biotechnol *1*:55, 1990

23. Miller AD, Traubner DR, Buttimore C: Factors involved in the production of helper-free retroviral vectors. Somat Cell Genet *12*:175, 1986

24. Berkner KL: Development of adenovirus vectors for the expression of heterologous genes. Biotechniques *6*:616, 1988

25. McLaughlin SK, Collis P, Hermonat P, et al: Adeno-associated virus general transduction vector: Analysis of proviral structures. J Virol *63*:1963, 1988

26. Breakfield XO, DeLuca NA: Herpes simplex virus for gene delivery to neurons. New Biol *3*:203, 1991

27. Anderson JK, Garber DA, Meaney CA, et al: Extended expression of bacterial LacZ in neurons using the neuron specific enolase promoter. Hum Gene Ther *3*:487, 1992

28. Spangrude GJ, Heimfeld S, Weismann IL: Purification and characterization of mouse hematopoietic stem cells. Science *241*:58, 1988

29. Donehower LA, Harvey M, Slagle BL, et al: Mice deficient for p53 are developmentally normal but susceptible to spontaneous tumors. Nature *356*:215, 1992

30. Miller AD: Retrovirus packaging cells. Hum Gene Ther *1*:5, 1990

31. Watanabe S, Temin H: Construction of a helper-free cell line for avian reticuloendotheliosis virus cloning vectors. Mol Cell Biol *3*:2241, 1983

32. Armentano D, Yu SF, Kantoff PW, et al: Effect of internal viral sequences on the utility of retroviral vectors. J Virol *61*:1647, 1987

33. Cepko CL, Roberts BE, Mulligan RC: Construction and application of a highly transmissible murine retrovirus shuttle vector. Cell *37*:1053, 1984

34. Miller DA, Rosman GJ: Improved retroviral vectors for gene transfer and expression. Biotechniques *7*:980, 1989

35. Yu S-F, Rudan T, Kantoff PW, et al: Self-inactivating retroviral vectors designed for transfer of whole genes into mammalian cells. Proc Natl Acad Sci USA *83*:3194, 1986

36. Hantzopoulos PA, Sullenger BA, Ungers G, et al: Improved gene expression upon transfer of the adenosine deaminase minigene outside the transcriptional unit of a retroviral vector. Proc Natl Acad Sci *86*:3159, 1989

37. Ferry N, Dupliessis O, Houssin D, et al: Retroviral mediated gene transfer into hepatocytes in vivo. Proc Natl Acad Sci USA *88*:8377, 1991

38. Muenchau DD, Freeman SM, Cornetta K, et al: Analysis of re-

troviral packaging lines for generation of replication-competent virus. Virology *176*:262, 1990

39. Miller AD, Buttimore C: Redesign of retroviral packaging cell lines to avoid recombination leading to helper virus production. Mol Cell Biol *6*:2895, 1986

40. Danos D, Mulligan RC: Safe and efficient generation of recombinant retroviruses with amphotropic and ecotropic host ranges. Proc Natl Acad Sci USA *85*:6460, 1988

41. Markowitz D, Goff S, Bank A: A safe packaging line for gene transfer: Separating viral genes on two different plasmids. J Virol *62*:1120, 1988

42. Eglitis MA: Positive selectable markers for use with mammalian cells in culture. Hum Gene Ther *2*:195, 1991

43. Wilson JM, Johnston DE, Jefferson DM: Correction of the genetic defect in hepatocytes from the Watanabe heritable hyperlipidemic rabbit. Proc Natl Acad Sci USA *85*:4421, 1988

44. Adam AM, Ramesh N, Miller AD, et al: Internal initiation of translation in retroviral vectors carrying picarnovirus 5' nontranslated regions. J Virol *65*:4985, 1991

45. Morgan RA, Couture L, Elroy-Stein O, et al: IRES vectors: Retroviral vectors containing internal ribosome entry sites. Nucl Acids Res *20*:1293, 1992

46. Jang SK, Krausslich H-G, Nicklin MJH, et al: A segment of the 5' nontranslated region of encephalomyocarditis virus RNA directs internal entry of ribosomes during in vitro translation. J Virol *52*:2636, 1988

47. Germann VA, Chin KV, Pastan I, et al: Retroviral transfer of a chimeric multi-drug resistance adenosine deaminase gene. FASEB J *4*:1501, 1990

48. Fiedrich G, Soriano P: Promoter traps in embryonic stem cells: A genetic screen to identify and mutate developmental genes in mice. Genes Dev *5*:1513, 1991

49. Lupton SD, Brunton LL, Kalberg VA, et al: Dominant positive and negative selection using a hygromycin phosphotransferase-thymidine kinase fusion gene. Mol Cell Biol *11*:3374, 1991

50. Miller AD: Human gene therapy comes of age. Nature *357*:455, 1992

51. Anderson WF: Human gene therapy. Science *256*:808, 1992

52. Culver K, Cornetta K, Morgan R, et al: Lymphocytes as cellular vehicles for gene therapy in mouse and man. Proc Natl Acad Sci USA *88*:3155, 1991

53. Kasid A, Morecki S, Aebersold P, et al: Human gene transfer: Characterization of human tumor infiltrating lymphocytes as vehicles for retroviral-mediated gene transfer in man. Proc Natl Acad Sci USA *87*:473, 1990

54. Aebersold P, Kasid A, Rosenberg SA: Selection of gene-marked tumor infiltrating lymphocytes for post-treatment biopsies: A case study. Hum Gene Ther *1*:373, 1990

55. Miller AD, Garcia JV, Suhr N, et al: Construction and properties of retrovirus packaging cells based on gibbon ape leukemia virus. J Virol *65*:2220, 1991

56. Miller DC, Adam MA, Miller AD: Gene-transfer by retrovirus vectors occurs only in cells that are actively replicating at the time of infection. Mol Cell Biol *10*:4239, 1990

57. Palmer TD, Rosman GJ, Osborne WRA, et al: Genetically modified skin fibroblasts persist long after transplantation but gradually inactivate introduced genes. Proc Natl Acad Sci *88*:1330, 1991

58. St. Louis D, Verma IM: An alternative approach to somatic cell gene therapy. Proc Natl Acad Sci USA *85*:3150, 1988

59. Evans LH, Morrison RP, Malik FG, et al: A neutralized epitope common to the envelope glycoproteins of ecotropic, polytropic, xenotropic, and amphotropic murine leukemia viruses. J Virol *64*:6176, 1990

60. Cornetta K, Wieder R, Anderson WF: Gene transfer into primates and prospects for gene therapy in humans. Prog Nucl Acids Res Mol Biol *36*:311, 1990

61. Bartholomew RM, Esser AF: Mechanism of antibody-independent activation of the first component of complement (C1) on retrovirus membranes. Biochemistry *19*:2847, 1980

62. Smithies O, Gregg RG, Boggs SS, et al: Insertion of DNA sequences into the human chromosomal β globin locus via homologous recombination. Nature *317*:230, 1985

63. Samulski J, Xhu X, Xiao X, et al: Targeted integration of adeno-associated virus (AAV) into human chromosome 19. EMBO J 10:3941, 1991

64. Stratford-Perricaudet LD, Levero M, Chass J-F, et al: Evaluation of the transfer and expression in mice of an enzyme-encoding gene using a human adenovirus vector. Hum Gene Ther 1:241, 1990

65. Rosenfeld MA, Siegfried W, Yoshimuru K, et al: Adenovirus mediated transfer of a recombinant alpha-1 antitrypsin gene to the 1-ng epithelium in vivo. Science 259:431, 1991

66. Rosenfeld MA, Yoshimura K, Trapnell BC, et al: In vivo transfer of the human cystic fibrosis transmembrane conductance regulator gene to the airway epithelium. Cell 68:143, 1992

67. McLaughlin SK, Collis P, Hermonat P, et al: Adeno-associated virus general transduction vector: Analysis of proviral structures. J Virol 63:1963, 1988

68. Egan M, Flotte T, Aflone S, et al: Defective regulation of outwardly rectifying Cl⁻ channels by protein kinase A corrected by insertion of CFTR. Nature 358:581, 1991

69. Palella T, Silverman L, Schroll C, et al: Herpes simplex virus-mediated human hypoxanthine-guanine phosphoribosyltransferase gene transfer into neuronal cells. Mol Cell Biol 8:457, 1988

70. Howley PM, Sarver N, Law M-F: Eukaryotic cloning vectors derived from bovine papillomavirus DNA. Meth Enzymol 101:387, 1983

71. Miner JN, Hruby DE: Vaccinia virus: A versatile tool for molecular biologists. Trends Biotechnol 8:20, 1990

72. Curiel DT, Agarwal S, Wagner E, et al: Adenovirus enhancement of transferrin-polylysine-mediated gene delivery. Proc Natl Acad Sci USA 88:8850, 1991

73. Clinical Protocol—Immunotherapy of malignancy by in vivo gene transfer into tumors. Hum Gene Ther 3:399, 1992

74. Short MP, Choi BC, Lee JK, et al: Gene delivery to glioma cells in rat brain by grafting of a retrovirus packaging cell line. J Neurosci Res 27:427, 1990

75. Ezzeddine ZD, Maruza RL, Platika D, et al: Selective killing of glioma cells in culture and in vivo by retrovirus transfer of the herpes simplex virus thymidine kinase gene. New Biol 3:608, 1991

76. Culver KW, Ishii H, Blaese RM, et al: In vivo gene transfer with retroviral vector producer cells for treatment of experimental brain tumors. Science 256:1550, 1992

77. Cornetta K, Morgan RA, Gillio A, et al: No retroviremia or pathology in long-term follow-up of monkeys exposed to a murine amphotropic retrovirus. Hum Gene Ther 2:215, 1991

78. Cornetta K, Moen RC, Culver K, et al: Amphotropic murine leukemia retrovirus is not an acute pathogen for primates. Hum Gene Ther 1:15, 1990

79. Donahue RE, Kessler SW, Bodine S, et al: Helper virus induced T cell lymphoma in nonhuman primates after retroviral mediated gene transfer. J Exp Med 176:1125, 1992

80. Tolstoshev P: Retroviral-mediated gene therapy—safety considerations and preclinical studies. Bone Marrow Transplant 9(suppl 1):148, 1992

81. Temin HM: Safety consideration in somatic gene therapy of human disease with retroviral vectors. Hum Gene Ther 1:111, 1990

82. Danos O, Heard JM: Recombinant retroviruses as tools for gene transfer to somatic cells. Bone Marrow Transplant 9(suppl 1):131, 1992

83. Lynch CM, Miller AD: Production of high-titer helper virus-free retroviral vectors by cocultivation of packaging cells with different host ranges. J Virol 65:3887, 1991

84. Thompson L: Monkey tests spark safety review. Science 257:1854, 1992

85. Vogelstein B, Fearon ER, Hamilton SR, et al: Genetic alterations during colorectal-tumor development. N Engl J Med 319:525, 1988

86. Goyette MC, Cho K, Fasching CL, et al: Progression of colorectal cancer is associated with multiple tumor suppressor gene defects but inhibition of tumorigenicity is accomplished by correction of any single defect via chromosome transfer. Mol Cell Biol 3:1387, 1992

87. Moolten FL, Wells JM: Curability of tumors bearing herpes thymidine kinase genes transferred by retroviral vectors. J Natl Cancer Inst 82:297, 1988

88. Mullen C, Kilstrup M, Blaese RM: Transfer of the bacterial gene for cytosine deaminase to mammalian cells confers lethal sensitivity to 5-fluorocytosine: A negative selection system. Proc Natl Acad Sci USA 89:33, 1992

89. Chanock RM, Ludwig L, Heubner RJ, et al: Immunization by selective infection with type 4 adenovirus grown in human diploid tissue culture. I. Safety and lack of oncogenicity and tests for potency in volunteers. JAMA 195:445, 1966

90. Carmen IH: Opinion, debates, divisions and decisions: Recombinant DNA Advisory Committee (RAC) authorization of the first human gene transfer experiment. Am J Hum Genet 50:245, 1992

91. Friedmann T: The evolving concept of gene therapy. Hum Gene Ther 1:175, 1990

92. NIH RAC: Revised points to consider. Hum Gene Ther 1:93, 1990

93. FDA draft points to consider on human somatic cell therapy and gene therapy. Hum Gene Ther 2:251, 1991

94. Rosenberg SA, Speiss P, Lafreinere R: A new approach to adoptive immunotherapy of cancer with tumor infiltrating lymphocytes. Science 223:1212, 1986

95. Rosenberg SA, Packard BS, Aebersold PM, et al: Use of tumor infiltrating lymphocytes and interleukin 2 in the immunotherapy of patients with metastatic melanoma. N Engl J Med 319:1676, 1988

96. Rosenberg SA: Immunotherapy and gene therapy of cancer. Cancer Res Suppl 51:5074s, 1991

97. Aebersold P, Hyatt C, Johnson S, et al: Lysis of autologous melanoma cell by tumor-infiltrating lymphocytes: Association with clinical response. J Natl Cancer Inst 83:932, 1991

98. Fisher B, Packard BS, Read EJ, et al: Tumor localization of adoptively transferred indium-111 labeled tumor infiltrating lymphocytes in patients with metastatic melanoma. J Clin Oncol 7:250, 1989

99. The N2-TIL human gene transfer clinical protocol. Hum Gene Ther 1:73, 1990

100. Rosenberg SA, Aebersold P, Cornetta K, et al: Gene transfer into humans—immunotherapy of patients with advanced melanoma, using tumor infiltrating lymphocytes modified by retroviral gene transduction. N Engl J Med 326:370, 1990

101. Clinical Protocol: Treatment of patients with advanced cancer using tumor infiltrating lymphocytes transduced with the gene of resistance to neomycin. Hum Gene Ther 3:533, 1992

102. Clinical Protocol: The treatment of patients with melanoma using interleukin-2, interleukin-4 and tumor infiltrating lymphocytes. Hum Gene Ther 3:167, 1992

103. Renuck D, Roehm N, Smith C, et al: Isolation and characterization of a mouse interleukin cDNA clone that expresses B cell stimulating factor 1 activities and T cell and mast cell stimulating activities. Proc Natl Acad Sci USA 83:2061, 1986

104. Clinical Protocol: The treatment of patients with metastatic melanoma and renal cell cancer using in vitro expanded and genetically-engineered (neomycin phosphotransferase) bulk, CD8(+) and/or CD4(+) tumor infiltrating lymphocytes and bulk, CD8(+) and/or CD4(+) peripheral blood leukocytes in combination with recombinant interleukin-2 alone, or with recombinant interleukin-2 and recombinant alpha interferon. Hum Gene Ther 3:411, 1992

105. Clinical Protocol: Autologous bone marrow for children with AML, use of marker genes. Hum Gene Ther 2:137, 1991

106. Strife A, Clarkson B: Biology of CML. Semin Hematol 25:1, 1988

107. Rill DR, Moen RC, Buschle M, et al: An approach of the analysis of relapse and marrow reconstitution after autologous marrow transplantation using retrovirus-mediated gene transfer. Blood 79:2694, 1992

108. Clinical Protocol: A phase I trial of high dose carboplatin and etoposide with autologous marrow support for treatment of stage D neuroblastoma in first remission: Use of marker genes to investigate the biology of marrow reconstitution and the mechanism of relapse. Hum Gene Ther 2:257, 1991

109. Clinical Protocol: A phase I trial of high dose carboplatin and etoposide with autologous marrow support for treatment of relapse/refractory neuroblastoma without apparent bone marrow involvement: Use of marker genes to investigate the biology of marrow reconstitution and the mechanism of relapse. Hum Gene Ther 2:273, 1991

110. Rill DR, Buschle M, Foreman NK, et al: Analysis of neuroblastoma relapse after autologous bone marrow transplantation using retrovirus mediated gene transfer. Hum Gene Ther 3:129, 1992

111. Clinical Protocol: Autologous bone marrow transplantation for CML in which retroviral markers are used to discriminate between relapse which arises from systemic disease remaining after preoperative therapy versus relapse due to residual leukemia cell in autologous marrow: A pilot trial. Hum Gene Ther 2:359, 1991

112. Clinical Protocol: Retroviral-mediated gene transfer of bone marrow cells during autologous bone marrow transplantation for acute leukemia. Hum Gene Ther 3:301, 1992

113. Berenson RJ, Andrews RG, Bensinger WI: Selection of CD34+ marrow cells for autologous marrow transplantation. In Dicke K, Spitzer G, Jagannith S (eds): Autologous Bone Marrow Transplantation: Proceedings of the Fourth International Symposium. Houston, University of Texas, 1989, p 55

114. Banavali S, Silvestri F, Hulette B, et al: Expression of hematopoietic progenitor cell associated antigen CD34 in chronic myeloid leukemia. Leuk Res 15:603, 1991

115. Schuening FG, Kawahara K, Miller AD, et al: Retrovirus-mediated gene transduction into long-term repopulating marrow cells of dog. Blood 78:2568, 1991

116. Clinical Protocol: Hepatocellular transplantation in acute hepatic failure and targeting genetic markers to hepatic cells. Hum Gene Ther 2:331, 1991

117. Hershfield MS, Buckley RH, Greenburg ML, et al: Treatment of adenosine deaminase deficiency with polyethylene glycol-modified adenosine deaminase. N Engl J Med 316:589, 1987

118. Keever CA, Flomenberg N, Brochsten J, et al: Tolerance of engrafted donor T cells following bone marrow transplantation for severe combined immunodeficiency. Clin Immunol Immunopathol 48:261, 1988

119. Clinical Protocol: The ADA human gene therapy protocol. Hum Gene Ther 1:327, 1990

120. Kantoff PW, Kohn DB, Mitsuya H, et al: Correction of adenosine deaminase deficiency in cultured human T and B cells by retrovirus-mediated gene transfer. Proc Natl Acad Sci USA 83:6563, 1986

121. Culver K, Cornetta K, Morgan R, et al: Lymphocytes as cellular vehicles for gene therapy in mouse and man. Proc Natl Acad Sci USA 88:3155, 1991

122. Ferrari G, Rossini S, Giavazzi R, et al: An in vivo model of somatic cell gene therapy for human severe combined immune deficiency. Science 251:1363, 1991

123. Culver KW, Morgan RA, Osborne WRA, et al: In vivo expression and survival of gene-modified T lymphocytes in rhesus monkeys. Hum Gene Ther 1:399, 1990

124. Culver KW, Anderson WF, Blaese RM: Lymphocyte gene therapy. Hum Gene Ther 2:107, 1991

125. Beutler B, Cerami A: The biology of cathexin/TNF—a primary mediator of the host response. Annu Rev Immunol 7:625, 1989

126. Wang AM, Creasy AA, Ladner MB, et al: Molecular cloning of the complementary DNA for human tumor necrosis factor. Science 228:149, 1985

127. Asher AL, Mule JJ, Reichert CM, et al: Studies of the anti-tumor efficacy of systemically administered recombinant tumor necrosis factor against several murine tumors in vivo. J Immunol 138:963, 1987

128. Feinberg B, Kurzrock R, Talpaz M, et al: A phase I trial of intravenously-administered recombinant tumor necrosis factor-alpha in cancer patients. J Clin Oncol 6:1328, 1988

129. Kahn J, Kaplan L, Ziegler J, et al: Phase II trial of intralesional recombinant tumor necrosis factor alpha (TNF) for AIDS associated Kaposi's sarcoma (KS). Proc Am Soc Clin Oncol 8:4, 1989

130. TNF/TIL human gene therapy clinical protocol. Hum Gene Ther 1:443, 1990

131. Asher AL, Mule JJ, Kasid A, et al: Murine tumor cells transduced with the gene for TNF-α: Evidence for paracrine immune effects of TNF against tumors. J Immunol 146:3227, 1991

132. Rosenberg SA: Gene therapy for cancer. JAMA 268:2416, 1992

133. Hwu P, Yannelli J, Kriegler M, et al: Functional and molecular characterization of TIL transduced with the TNFα cDNA for the gene therapy of cancer in man. J Immunol 150:4104, 1993

134. Kriegler M, Perez C, Defay K, et al: A novel form of TNF/cachetin is a cell surface cytotoxic transmembrane protein: Ramifications for the complex physiology of TNF. Cell 53:45, 1988

135. Initial proposal of clinical research project: Immunization of cancer patients using autologous cancer cells modified by insertion of the gene for tumor necrosis factor. Hum Gene Ther 3:57, 1992

136. Initial proposal of clinical research project: Immunization of cancer patients using autologous cancer cells modified by insertion of the gene for interleukin-2. Hum Gene Ther 3:75, 1992

137. Fearon ER, Pardoll DM, Itaya T, et al: Interleukin 2 production by tumor cells bypasses T helper function in the generation of an anti-tumor response. Cell 60:397, 1990

138. Gansbacher B, Zeir K, Daniels B, et al: Interleukin 2 gene transfer into tumor cells abrogates tumorigenicity and induces protective immunity. J Exp Med 172:1217, 1990

139. Livingston PO, Kactin K, Pinsky CM, et al: Serologic response of patients with stage II melanoma to allogenic melanoma cell vaccines. Cancer 56:2194, 1985

140. Tepper RI, Pattengale PK, Leder P: Murine interleukin-4 displays potent anti-tumor activity in vivo. Cell 57:503, 1989

141. Golumbek PT, Lazenby AJ, Levilsky HI, et al: Treatment of established renal cancer by tumor cells engineered to secrete interleukin 4. Science 254:713, 1991

142. Stewart MJ, Plautz GE, Del Buono L, et al: Gene transfer in vivo with DNA-liposome complexes: Safety and acute toxicity in mice. Hum Gene Ther 3:267, 1992

143. Brown CC, Kessler LG: Projections of lung cancer mortality in the United States 1985–2025. J Natl Cancer Inst 80:43, 1988

144. Hollstein M, Sidransky D, Vogelstein B, et al: p53 mutation in human cancers. Science 253:49, 1991

145. Rodenhuis S, Slebos RJC, Boot AJM, et al: Incidence and possible clinical significance of K-ras oncogene activation in adenocarcinoma of the human lung. Cancer Res 48:5738, 1988

146. Perez CA, Stanley K, Rubin P, et al: Patterns of tumor recurrence after definitive irradiation for inoperable non-oat cell carcinoma of the lung. Int J Radiat Oncol Biol Phys 6:987, 1980

147. Goyette MC, Cho K, Fasching CL, et al: Progression of colorectal cancer is associated with multiple tumor suppressor gene defects but inhibition of tumorigenicity is accomplished by correction of any single defect via chromosome transfer. Mol Cell Biol 3:1387, 1992

148. Mukhopadhyay T, Cavender A, Tainsky M, et al: Expression of antisense K-ras message in a human lung cancer cell line with a spontaneous activated k-ras oncogene alters the transformed phenotype. Proc Am Assoc Cancer Res 31:304, 1990

149. Mukhopadhyay T, Cavender AC, Branch CD, et al: Expression and regulation of wild type p53 gene (wtp53) in human non-small cell lung cancer (NSCLC) cell lines carrying normal or mutated p53 gene. J Cell Biochem 15F:22, 1991

150. Chen P-L, Chen Y, Bookstein R, et al: Genetic mechanisms of tumor suppression by the human p53 gene. Science 250:1576, 1990

151. Harvey M, McArthur MJ, Montgomery CA Jr, et al: Spontaneous and carcinogen-induced tumorigenesis in p53-deficient mice. Nature Genetics 5:225, 1993

152. Pastan I, Gottesman MM: Multidrug resistance. Annu Rev Med 42:277, 1991

153. Veda K, Clark DP, Chen C, et al: The human multidrug resistance (mdr1) gene. J Biol Chem 262:505, 1987

154. Mickisch G, Licht T, Merlino GT, et al: Chemotherapy and chemosensitization of transgenic mice which express the human multidrug resistance gene in bone marrow: Efficacy, potency and toxicity. Cancer Res 51:5417, 1991

155. McLachlin JR, Eglitis MA, Veda K, et al: Expression of a human complementary DNA for the multidrug resistance gene in urine hematopoietic precursor cells with the use of retroviral gene transfer. J Natl Cancer Inst 82:1260, 1990

156. Sorrentino BP, Brandt SJ, Bodine D, et al: Selection of drug-resistant bone marrow cells in vitro after retroviral transfer of human MDR1. Science 257:99, 1992

157. Freeman SM, Whartenby KA, Koeplin DS, et al: Tumor regression when a fraction of the tumor mass contains the HSV-TK gene. J Cell Biochem Suppl 16F:47, 1992

158. Clinical Protocol: Ex vivo gene therapy of familial hypercholesterolemia. Hum Gene Ther 3:179, 1992

159. Clinical Protocol: Clinical protocol for human gene transfer for hemophilia B. Hum Gene Ther 3:543, 1992

160. Phase I study of cellular adoptive immunotherapy using genetically modified CD8+ HIV-specific T cells for HIV seropositive patients undergoing allogeneic bone marrow transplant. Hum Gene Ther 3:319, 1992

161. Jolly DJ: HIV infection and gene transfer therapy. Hum Gene Ther 2:111, 1991

162. Morgan R, Anderson WF: Gene therapy for AIDS. In Kumar A (ed): Advances in Molecular Biology and Targeted Treatment for AIDS. New York, Plenum, 1991, pp 301–308

INDEX

Note: Page numbers in *italics* refer to illustrations; page numbers followed by t refer to tables.

ISBN 0-7216-6483-0